CURRENT PEDIATRIC THERAPY 8

SYDNEY S. GELLIS, M.D.

PROFESSOR AND CHAIRMAN, DEPARTMENT OF PEDIATRICS, TUFTS
UNIVERSITY SCHOOL OF MEDICINE: PEDIATRICIAN-IN-CHIEF, BOSTON
FLOATING HOSPITAL FOR INFANTS AND CHILDREN, TUFTS—NEW ENGLAND
MEDICAL CENTER, BOSTON

AND

BENJAMIN M. KAGAN, M.D.

DIRECTOR, DEPARTMENT OF PEDIATRICS, CEDARS-SINAI MEDICAL CENTER:
PROFESSOR AND VICE-CHAIRMAN, DEPARTMENT OF PEDIATRICS, UCLA SCHOOL
OF MEDICINE, LOS ANGELES, CALIFORNIA

W. B. SAUNDERS COMPANY

Philadelphia · London · Toronto

W. B. Saunders Company: West Washington Square
Philadelphia, PA   19105

1 St. Anne's Road
Eastbourne, East Sussex BN21 3UN, England

1 Goldthorne Avenue
Toronto, Ontario M8Z 5T9, Canada

Current Pediatric Therapy—8   ISBN 0-7216-4089-3

Last digit is the print number: 9   8   7   6   5   4   3   2   1

Preface

As a part of our continuing effort to keep up to date with changing trends in the practice of pediatrics, for the past two editions of *Current Pediatric Therapy* we have been soliciting the comments and suggestions of our readers by means of a postage-paid reply card bound inside the back cover. We are sincerely grateful for the response and have continued the use of the card for this edition. Following are some of the important improvements in the book that have resulted directly from your suggestions:

• The section on disorders of the lungs and pleura has been subdivided into 17 individual articles and considerably expanded with specific therapeutic advice on the problems of bronchitis, bronchiolitis, pulmonary embolism, pulmonary edema and emphysema.

• Many more substances than ever before are covered in the article on acute poisoning.

• Special Problems in the Newborn now includes feeding the premature infant as well as breast feeding, including breast milk jaundice, breast infection and the teaching of proper technique.

• There is a new discussion of the sudden infant death syndrome.

• Recommendations for parents on ways to prevent accidents are discussed in a new article.

• The relation of informed consent to pediatric practice, including a sample consent form, is an entirely new topic that has been much in demand.

• New discussions are provided on the subjects of air travel, infantile colic, neuro-blastoma, viral pneumonia, necrotizing enterocolitis, diabetes insipidus, fractures, the mucocutaneous adenopathy syndrome and acetaminophen intoxication.

In compiling the extensive index, a special effort has been made to provide a ready reference to adverse reactions and other problems encountered in the use of drugs. It is our hope that this edition will prove to be the most helpful so far produced, and we again invite your comments.

For the eighth edition, 294 contributors have prepared 339 articles, over 270 of which are newly written, with virtually all of the rest being carefully revised by their previous authors. Two-thirds of the contributors are new to the book, giving us an opportunity to welcome them and the viewpoints that they represent. When encountering a problem that is new to you, we recommend that you refer not only to this edition but to older editions for a comprehensive review of recognized authorities in pediatrics.

We have a very special obligation to each of our many contributing writers, both new and old, for giving time from their teaching, research and practice to share their therapeutic expertise. We are also in debt to many thousands of readers for a continuing interest in these biennial volumes. Finally, all of us who read and write this book share the most important of all obligations, to pay the best possible attention to the children who are placed in our care.

SYDNEY S. GELLIS

BENJAMIN M. KAGAN

Contributors

PASQUALE J. ACCARDO, M.D.
Assistant Professor of Pediatrics, The Johns Hopkins University School of Medicine; Developmental Pediatrician, The John F. Kennedy Institute for Handicapped Children, Baltimore, Maryland.
Mental Retardation.

MARY M. EICHHORN ADAMS, Ph.D.
Editorial Consultant, Francis A. Countway Library of Medicine, Harvard Medical School; Assistant Editor, *The Journal of Infectious Diseases*, Channing Laboratory, Harvard Medical School, Boston, Massachusetts.
Cholera.

ROBERT M. ADAMS, M.D.
Associate Clinical Professor, Department of Dermatology, Stanford University School of Medicine, Stanford, California.
Topical Therapy: A Formulary for Pediatric Skin Disease.

WILLIAM CURTIS ADAMS, M.D.
Medical Director, Emergency Department, Southeast Alabama Medical Center, Dothan, Alabama.
Aspiration Pneumonia.

JOEL J. ALPERT, M.D.
Chairman and Professor, Department of Pediatrics, Boston University School of Medicine; Pediatrician-in-Chief, Boston City Hospital; Chairman, Executive Committee, Boston Poison Information Center, Boston, Massachusetts.
Acute Poisoning.

BLANCHE P. ALTER, M.D.
Assistant Professor of Pediatrics, Harvard Medical School; Associate in Medicine (Hematology and Oncology), Children's Hospital Medical Center; Senior Clinical Associate, Sidney Farber Cancer Center, Boston, Massachusetts.
Aplastic and Hypoplastic Anemia.

MARY G. AMPOLA, M.D.
Assistant Professor of Pediatrics, Tufts University School of Medicine; Assistant Pediatrician, New England Medical Center, Boston, Massachusetts.
Amino Acid Disorders.

KATHRYN D. ANDERSON, M.D.
Associate Professor of Surgery and Child Health and Development, George Washington University School of Medicine; Senior Attending Surgeon, Children's Hospital National Medical Center, Washington, D. C.
Disorders of the Esophagus. Pyloric Stenosis. Peptic Ulcer. Gastritis.

R. M. APPLEBAUM, M.D.
Instructor, Outpatient Pediatric Clinics, Mount Sinai Hospital; Attending Pediatrician, University of Miami School of Medicine, Miami, Florida.
Breast Feeding.

LEONARD APT, M.D.
Professor of Ophthalmology, Head, Pediatric Ophthalmology, University of California School of Medicine; Staff, Departments of Pediatrics and Ophthalmology, Cedars-Sinai Medical Center, Los Angeles; Consultant in Ophthalmology, St. John's Hospital, Santa Monica; Special Consultant in Pediatric Ophthalmology, Los Angeles City Health Department, and Bureau of Maternal and Child Health, Department of Public Health, State of California, Los Angeles, California.
Spasmus Nutans.

REGINE ARONOW, M.D.
Assistant Professor of Pediatrics, Wayne State University School of Medicine; Director, Poison Control Center; Associate Attending, Department of Pediatrics, Children's Hospital of Michigan, Detroit, Michigan.
Salicylate Poisoning. Acetaminophen Intoxication.

ANDREAS ATHANASIOU, M.D.
Research Fellow in Pediatric Hematology-Oncology, New England Medical Center Hospital, Boston, Massachusetts.
Thalassemia.

FELICIA B. AXELROD, M.D.
Associate Professor of Pediatrics, New York University School of Medicine; Director, Dysautonomia Treatment and Evaluation Center, New York University Medical Center, New York, New York.
Familial Dysautonomia.

GEORGE E. BACON, M.D.
Professor of Pediatrics, University of Michigan School of Medicine; Director, Section of Pediatric Endocrinology, C. S. Mott Children's Hospital, Ann Arbor, Michigan.
Adrenal Disorders.

ANN SULLIVAN BAKER, M.D.
Assistant Professor of Medicine, Harvard Medical School; Assistant Physician, Massachusetts General Hospital, Boston, Massachusetts.
Brain Abscess. Spinal Epidural Abscess.

HENRY H. BANKS, M.D.
Professor and Chairman, Department of Orthopedic Surgery, Tufts University School of Medicine; Orthopedic Surgeon-in-Chief, New England Medical Center Hospital, Boston, Massachusetts.
Fractures of the Extremities.

JAMES W. BASS, M.P.H., M.D.
Professor and Chairman, Department of Pediatrics, School of Medicine, Uniformed Services University of the Health Sciences; Chief, Department of Pediatrics, Walter Reed Army Medical Center, Washington, D. C.
Rhinitis and Sinusitis. Retropharyngeal and Lateral Pharyngeal Wall Abscess. The Tonsil and Adenoid Problem.

STUART B. BAUER, M.D.
Instructor in Urology, Harvard Medical School; Attending in Urology, Children's Hospital Medical Center and Boston Floating Hospital for Infants, Boston, Massachusetts.
Exstrophy of the Bladder.

JULES L. BAUM, M.D.
Professor of Ophthalmology, Tufts University School of Medicine; Senior Ophthalmologist, New England Medical Center Hospital, Boston, Massachusetts.
The Eye.

MARC O. BEEM, M.D.
Professor in Pediatrics, University of Chicago; Wyler Children's Hospital, Chicago, Illinois.
Chlamydial Infections.

A. BARRY BELMAN, M.D.
Chairman, Department of Pediatric Urology, Children's Hospital National Medical Center; Associate Professor of Urology and Child Health and Development, George Washington University Medical Center, Washington, D. C.
Urolithiasis.

GEORGE BENZING, III, M.D.
Professor of Pediatrics, University of Cincinnati College of Medicine; Attending Cardiologist and Pediatrician, Children's Hospital Medical Center; Attending Pediatrician, Cincinnati General Hospital, Cincinnati, Ohio.
Hypotension.

BRUCE O. BERG, M.D.
Associate Professor, Department of Neurology and Pediatrics, Director of Child Neurology, University of California School of Medicine, San Francisco, California.
Disorders of Sleep.

RICHARD S. BERGER, M.D.
Clinical Associate Professor of Medicine, New Jersey College of Medicine and Dentistry, Rutgers Medical School, Piscataway; Attending Staff, Raritan Valley Hospital, Greenbrook; Consulting Staff, Lyons Veterans Administration Hospital, Lyons, New Jersey.
Arthropod Bites and Stings.

ABRAHAM B. BERGMAN, M.D.
Professor of Pediatrics and Health Services, University of Washington School of Medicine; Director of Outpatient Services, Children's Orthopedic Hospital and Medical Center, Seattle, Washington.
Sudden Infant Death Syndrome.

EUGENE M. BERKMAN, M.D.
Assistant Professor of Medicine, Tufts University School of Medicine; Medical Director of Blood Bank, New England Medical Center Hospital, Boston, Massachusetts.
Hemmorhagic Disorders.

BERNARD A. BERMAN, M.D.
Assistant Clinical Professor of Pediatrics, Tufts University School of Medicine; Director of Allergy, St. Elizabeth Hospital; Allergy Consultant, Carney Hospital, Boston, Massachusetts.
Stinging Insect Hypersensitivity.

HELEN K. BERRY, M.A.
Professor of Research Pediatrics, University of Cincinnati College of Medicine; Director, Division of Inborn Errors of Metabolism, Children's Hospital Research Foundation, Cincinnati, Ohio.
Phenylketonuria.

C. WARREN BIERMAN, M.D.
Clinical Professor Pediatrics, University of Washington Medical School; Chief, Division of Allergy, Children's Orthopedic Hospital and Medical Center, Seattle, Washington.
Allergic Gastrointestinal Diseases.

KATHLEEN FOUST BLANE, M.S.
Audiologist, Private Practice, Washington, D. C.
Hearing Loss in Children.

ALFRED M. BONGIOVANNI, M.D.
Dean, School of Medicine, Catholic University of Puerto Rico, Ponce, Puerto Rico; Director of Endocrinology, Children's Hospital of Philadelphia, Philadelphia, Pennsylvania.
Menstrual Disorders.

GORDON BORKAT, M.D.
Assistant Professor of Pediatrics, Case Western Reserve University; Associate Pediatrician, Rainbow Babies and Children's Hospital, Cleveland, Ohio.
Air Travel.

QUELLIN T. BOX, M.D.
Associate Professor of Pediatrics and Microbiology, and Director, Infectious Disease Division, Department of Pediatrics, University of Texas Medical Branch; Director of Bacteriology Laboratory, and Attending Pediatrician, Child Health Center, University of Texas Medical Branch Hospitals, Galveston, Texas.
Diphtheria.

HELEN F. BRICKMAN, M.D., F.R.C.P. (C)
Assistant Professor of Paediatrics, McGill University Faculty of Medicine; Associate Physician, Montreal Children's Hospital; Consultant, Jewish General Hospital, Montreal, Canada.
Familial Mediterranean Fever.

SAUL L. BROWN, M.D.
Clinical Professor of Psychiatry (Child), University of California School of Medicine and Neuropsychiatric Institute; Director, Department of Psychiatry and Family-

Child Section, Cedars-Sinai Medical Center, Los Angeles, California.
Emotional Disorders.

ERIKA BRUCK, M.D.
Professor of Pediatrics, State University of New York at Buffalo School of Medicine; Attending Pediatrician, Children's Hospital of Buffalo, Buffalo, New York.
Shigellosis.

PHILIP A. BRUNELL, M.D.
Professor and Chairman, Department of Pediatrics, University of Texas Health Science Center at San Antonio; Chief of Pediatrics, Bexar County Hospital District, San Antonio, Texas.
Psittacosis.

DAVID P. CAMPBELL, M.D.
Surgeon, Hilo Medical Group; Chief of Surgery, Hilo Hospital, Hilo, Hawaii.
Biliary Atresia. Choledochal Cyst. Diseases of the Gallbladder. Diseases of the Pancreas.

ARNOLD J. CAPUTE, M.D., M.P.H.
Associate Professor of Pediatrics, Johns Hopkins University School of Medicine; Deputy Medical Director, John F. Kennedy Institute for Handicapped Children, Baltimore, Maryland.
Mental Retardation.

IVO J. CARRÉ, M.D., F.R.C.P., D.C.H.
Professor of Child Health, The Queen's University of Belfast; Consulting Paediatrician, The Royal Belfast Hospital for Sick Children and The Royal Maternity Hospital, Belfast, Northern Ireland.
Hiatal Hernia (Partial Thoracic Stomach).

CHARLES A. CARTON, M.D.
Clinical Professor of Surgery (Neurosurgery), University of California School of Medicine; Attending Neurosurgeon, Cedars-Sinai Medical Center, Los Angeles, California.
Brain Tumors.

HUGO F. CARVAJAL, M.D.
Associate Professor, Department of Pediatrics, University of Texas Medical Branch; Chief of Pediatrics, Shriners Burns Institute, Galveston, Texas.
Urinary Tract Infections.

WERNER D. CHASIN, M.D., F.A.C.S.
Professor and Chairman of Otolaryngology, Tufts University School of Medicine, Otolaryngologist-in-Chief, New England Medical Center, Boston, Massachusetts.
Foreign Bodies in the Air Passages. Foreign Bodies in the Ear. Injuries to the Middle Ear.

HARVEY L. CHERNOFF, M.D.
Associate Professor of Pediatrics, Tufts University School of Medicine; Pediatric Cardiologist, New England Medical Center Hospital, Boston, Massachusetts.
Congestive Heart Failure.

JAMES D. CHERRY, M.D.
Professor of Pediatrics, Chief, Division of Infectious Diseases, University of California School of Medicine; Attending Pediatrician, University of California Hospital, Los Angeles, California.
Measles (Rubeola). Rubella (German Measles) and Congenital Rubella.

ROBERT-GRAY CHOTO, M.D.
Fellow in Infectious Disease, Department of Pediatrics, Cedars-Sinai Medical Center and University of California School of Medicine, Los Angeles, California.
Brucellosis. Plague.

DENNIS L. CHRISTIE, M.D.
Assistant Professor of Pediatrics, University of Washington School of Medicine; Chief, Gastroenterology Division, Children's Orthopedic Hospital and Medical Center, Seattle, Washington.
Allergic Gastrointestinal Diseases.

JOHN P. CLOHERTY, M.D.
Instructor in Pediatrics, Harvard Medical School; Senior Pediatrician, Boston Hospital for Women; Associate in Neonatology, Boston Children's Hospital; Assistant in Pediatrics, Massachusetts General Hospital; Member, Joint Program in Neonatology, Boston, Massachusetts.
Infants Born to Diabetic Mothers.

ALAN S. COHEN, M.D.
Conrad Wesselhoeft Professor of Medicine, Boston University School of Medicine; Chief of Medicine, Boston City Hospital, Boston, Massachusetts.
Amyloidosis.

MICHAEL I. COHEN, M.D.
Professor of Pediatrics, Albert Einstein College of Medicine; Director, Division of Adolescent Medicine, Montefiore Hospital and Medical Center, Bronx, New York.
Obesity at Adolescence.

RICHARD A. COHN, M.D.
Research Fellow in Pediatric Nephrology, University of Minnesota Medical School, Minneapolis, Minnesota.
Renal Vein Thrombosis.

HARVEY R. COLTEN, M.D.
Associate Professor of Pediatrics, Harvard Medical School; Chief, Division of Cystic Fibrosis, Children's Hospital Medical Center, Boston, Massachusetts.
Angioneurotic Edema.

FELIX A. CONTE, M.D.
Associate Professor, University of Calfornia School of Medicine; Co-Director, Pediatric Endocrine Unit, University of California, San Francisco, California.
Unusually Tall Stature in Adolescent Girls.

MORTON COOPER, Ph.D.
Private Practice in Vocal Rehabilitation, Speech and Language Therapy, Los Angeles, California.
Management of Voice, Speech, and Language Disorders.

MARVIN CORNBLATH, M.D.
Professor of Pediatrics, University of Maryland School of Medicine; Chairman, Department of Pediatrics, University of Maryland Hospital, Baltimore, Maryland.
Hypoglycemia. Inborn Errors of Carbohydrate Metabolism.

JAMES J. CORRIGAN, JR., M.D.
Professor of Pediatrics, Chief, Section of Pediatric Hematology-Oncology, University of Arizona Health Sciences Center, Tucson, Arizona.
Disseminated Intravascular Coagulation and Purpura Fulminans.

B. PATRICK COX, Ph.D.
Assistant Professor in Pediatrics, Director, Communi-

cation Disorders, Georgetown University School of Medicine, Washington, D. C.
Hearing Loss in Children.

CAROL CROWLEY, M.D.
Instructor in Pediatrics, Tufts University School of Medicine; Assistant Hematologist (Pediatrics), New England Medical Center Hospital, Boston, Massachusetts.
Histiocytosis X.

CHARLES WILLIAM DAESCHNER, M.D.
Professor and Chairman, Department of Pediatrics, University of Texas Medical Branch; Chief of Pediatrics, University of Texas Medical Branch Hospitals, Galveston, Texas.
Perinephritis and Perirenal Abscess.

JANE F. DESFORGES, M.D.
Professor of Medicine, Tufts University School of Medicine; Senior Physician and Hematologist, New England Medical Center Hospital, Boston, Massachusetts.
Sickle Cell Anemia.

LOUIS K. DIAMOND, M.D.
Professor of Pediatrics, University of California School of Medicine; Attending Pediatrician, Moffitt Hospital, San Francisco, California.
Management of the Patient after Splenectomy.

W. EDWIN DODSON, M.D.
Assistant Professor of Pediatrics and Neurology, Washington University School of Medicine, St. Louis Children's Hospital, Barnes Hospital, St. Louis City Hospital, St. Louis, Missouri.
Spinal Diseases.

CARL F. DOERSHUK, M.D.
Professor of Pediatrics, Case Western Reserve University School of Medicine; Associate Pediatrician, University Hospitals of Cleveland, Ohio.
Cystic Fibrosis.

EDOUARD DROUHET, M.D.
Professor of Medical Mycology, Institut Pasteur, Paris, France.
Systemic Mycoses.

BERNARD J. D'SOUZA, M.B.Ch.B.
Assistant Professor of Pediatric Neurology, Milwaukee Children's Hospital, Milwaukee, Wisconsin.
Guillain-Barré Syndrome. Chronic Relapsing Neuropathy. Acute Toxic Encephalopathy and Hypoxic Encephalopathy.

DENNIS P. DURANTE, M.D.
Fellow in Nephrology, University of Colorado Medical Center, Denver, Colorado.
Hemolytic-Uremic Syndrome.

PETER ECHEVERRIA, M.D.
Research Associate, Naval Medical Research Unit 2, Taipei, Taiwan.
Enteroviral Infections.

MILTON T. EDGERTON, M.D.
Professor of Plastic Surgery, University of Virginia Medical School, Charlottesville, Virginia.
Craniostenosis. Crouzon's Disease and Apert's Syndrome. Hypertelorism and Hypotelorism.

THOMAS J. EGAN, M.D., F.R.C.P. (C)
Professor of Pediatrics, University of Toronto School of

Medicine; Director of Ambulatory Services, The Hospital for Sick Children, Toronto, Canada.
Long-Term Total Parenteral Nutrition.

RICHARD M. EHRLICH, M.D., F.A.C.S.
Associate Professor, University of California Center for the Health Sciences, Los Angeles, California.
Malignant Tumors of the Kidney.

MICHAEL F. EPSTEIN, M.D.
Instructor in Pediatrics, Harvard Medical School; Member, Joint Program in Neonatology, Boston, Massachusetts.
Infants Born to Diabetic Mothers.

NANCY B. ESTERLY, M.D.
Associate Professor of Pediatrics, Pritzker School of Medicine, University of Chicago; Director, Division of Dermatology, Department of Pediatrics, Michael Reese Hospital, Chicago, Illinois.
Atopic Dermatitis.

PHILIP R. EXELBY, M.D.
Associate Professor in Surgery, Cornell University Medical College; Attending Surgeon, Chief, Pediatric Surgical Service, Memorial Sloan-Kettering Cancer Center, New York, New York.
Malignant Bone Tumors.

SHIRLEY L. FANNIN, M.D.
Chief, Acute Communicable Disease Control, Department of Health Services, Los Angeles County; Attending Staff, Cedars-Sinai Medical Center; Assistant Clinical Professor, University of California School of Medicine, Los Angeles, California.
Immunization Practice.

RALPH D. FEIGIN, M.D.
Professor of Pediatrics, Washington University School of Medicine; Pediatrician, St. Louis Children's Hospital and Barnes Hospital; Director, Division of Infectious Diseases, St. Louis Children's Hospital, St. Louis, Missouri.
Bacterial Meningitis and Septicemia Beyond the Neonatal Period. Meningococcal Disease.

MURRAY FEINGOLD, M.D.
Professor of Pediatrics, Tufts University School of Medicine; Chief, Genetic and Birth Defect Service, Boston Floating Hospital for Infants and Children, Boston, Massachusetts.
Nevi and Nevoid Tumors.

PATRICIA FERRIERI, M.D.
Associate Professor of Pediatrics, University of Minnesota School of Medicine; Attending Pediatrician, University of Minnesota Hospitals, Minneapolis, Minnesota.
Streptococcal Infections.

LAURENCE FINBERG, M.D.
Professor and Chairman, Department of Pediatrics, Albert Einstein College of Medicine; Chairman, Department of Pediatrics, Montefiore Hospital and Medical Center of the Albert Einstein College of Medicine, New York, New York.
Vitamin Deficiencies and Excesses. Rickets. Tetany. Idiopathic Hypercalcemia. Magnesium Deficiency. Parenteral Fluid and Electrolyte Therapy.

BURTON W. FINK, M.D.
Clinical Professor of Pediatrics (Cardiology), University of California at Los Angeles; Attending Physician and Di-

rector of Pediatric Cardiology, Cedars-Sinai Medical Center, Los Angeles, California.
Pulmonary Edema.

DELBERT A. FISHER, M.D.
Professor of Pediatrics and Medicine, University of California School of Medicine; Research Professor of Developmental and Perinatal Biology, Harbor General Hospital, Torrance, California.
Thyroid Disease.

EUGENE G. FLAUM, M.D.
Assistant Professor of Otolaryngology, University of Southern California; Attending Otolaryngologist, Cedars-Sinai Medical Center, Children's Hospital of Los Angeles, Hollywood Presbyterian Hospital, and Los Angeles County-University of Southern California Medical Center, Los Angeles, California.
Disorders of the Larynx.

LARRY E. FLEISCHMANN, M.D.
Associate Professor of Pediatrics, Wayne State University School of Medicine; Associate Chief of Pediatrics and Director, Renal Service, Children's Hospital of Michigan, Detroit, Michigan.
Renal Hypoplasia and Dysplasia.

M. T. FLIEGELMAN, M.D.
Clinical Professor and Chairman, Section of Dermatology, University of Louisville School of Medicine, Louisville, Kentucky.
Photodermatoses. Diseases of the Hair and Scalp.

ERIC W. FONKALSRUD, M.D.
Professor, Department of Surgery, and Chief of Pediatric Surgery, University of California School of Medicine, Los Angeles, California.
Lymphedema. Lymphangioma.

NORMAN FOST, M.D., M.P.H.
Associate Professor, Pediatrics and History of Medicine, University of Wisconsin School of Medicine; Director, Housestaff Training Program, Department of Pediatrics, Director, Inpatient Service, University of Wisconsin Hospitals; Chairman, Committee for the Protection of Human Subjects, Center for Health Sciences, University of Wisconsin, Madison, Wisconsin.
Informed Consent.

JOHN M. FREEMAN, M.D.
Associate Professor of Neurology and Pediatrics, Johns Hopkins University; Director of Pediatric Neurology, Director, Pediatric Seizure Clinic, Johns Hopkins Hospital and John F. Kennedy Institute, Baltimore, Maryland.
Epilepsy.

STANFORD B. FRIEDMAN, M.D.
Professor of Psychiatry and Human Development, and Pediatrics, University of Maryland School of Medicine, Baltimore, Maryland.
Child Abuse and Neglect.

J. WILLIAM FUTRELL, M.D.
Associate Professor of Plastic Surgery, University of Virginia Medical School, Charlottesville, Virginia.
Craniostenosis. Crouzon's Disease and Apert's Syndrome. Hypertelorism and Hypotelorism.

DONALD C. FYLER, M.D.
Associate Professor of Pediatrics, Harvard Medical

School; Associate Chief of Cardiology, Children's Hospital Medical Center, Boston, Massachusetts.
Pericardial Disease.

STEPHEN L. GANS, M.D.
Associate Clinical Professor of Surgery, University of California School of Medicine; Chief, Pediatric Surgery Service, Cedars-Sinai Medical Center; Attending Surgeon, University of California Hospital and Children's Hospital of Los Angeles, Los Angeles, California.
Preoperative and Postoperative Care of Patients Undergoing Gastrointestinal Surgery. Hernia and Hydrocele.

RICHARD A. GATTI, M.D.
Professor of Pediatrics, University of California School of Medicine; Director, Pediatric Oncology and Immunology, Cedars-Sinai Medical Center, Los Angeles, California.
The Immunodeficiency Disorders.

ANNE A. GERSHON, M.D.
Associate Professor of Pediatrics, New York University Medical Center; Associate Attending, Bellevue Hospital, New York, New York.
Varicella and Herpes Zoster. Herpes Simplex Infections.

SAMUEL T. GIAMMONA, M.D.
Chairman, Department of Pediatrics, Children's Hospital of San Francisco; Adjunct Professor of Pediatrics, University of California, San Diego, and San Francisco, California.
Croup Syndrome (Acute Epiglottitis and Laryngotracheobronchitis). Near-Drowning (Nonfatal Submersion).

BARBARA A. GILCHREST, M.D.
Instructor in Dermatology, Harvard Medical School; Research Fellow, Massachusetts General Hospital, Boston, Massachusetts.
Other Skin Tumors.

BERTIL E. GLADER, M.D.
Associate Professor, Department of Pediatrics, Stanford University School of Medicine; Attending Pediatrician and Associate Director of Hematology, Stanford University Hospital, Stanford, California.
Megaloblastic Anemia.

LOUIS GLUCK, M.D.
Professor of Pediatrics and Reproductive Medicine, University of California School of Medicine; Head, Division of Neonatal-Perinatal Medicine, University Hospital-University of California Medical Center, San Diego, California.
Respiratory Distress Syndrome.

MICHAEL J. GOLDBERG, M.D.
Associate Professor of Orthopedic Surgery, Tufts University School of Medicine; Senior Orthopedic Surgeon, New England Medical Center Hospital, Boston, Massachusetts.
Congenital Muscular Defects. Torticollis.

RICHARD B. GOLDBLOOM, M.D, F.R.C.P. (C)
Professor and Head, Department of Pediatrics, Dalhousie University; Physician-in-Chief, the Izaak Walton Killam Hospital for Children, Halifax, Nova Scotia, Canada.
Nasopharyngitis (The Common Cold). Infantile Cortical Hyperostosis (Caffey's Disease). Acute Infectious Lymphocytosis.

E. S. GOLLADAY, M.D.
Assistant Professor of Pediatric Surgery, University of

Arkansas College of Medicine; Arkansas Children's Hospital, Little Rock, Arkansas
Chest Wall Abnormalities.

EDMOND T. GONZALES, JR., M.D.
Assistant Professor of Urology, Baylor College of Medicine; Director of Pediatric Urology, Texas Children's Hospital, Houston, Texas.
Patent Urachus and Urachal Cysts. Tumors of the Bladder and Prostate. Disorders of the Bladder, Prostate and Urethra. Undescended Testes. Disorders of the Penis and Testis.

DAN M. GRANOFF, M.D.
Assistant Clinical Professor, University of California, San Francisco; Assistant Chief of Pediatrics (Infectious Diseases), Valley Medical Center of Fresno; Adjunct Professor of Biology, California State University, Fresno, California.
Tularemia.

GEORGE A. GREGORY, M.D.
Associate Professor of Anesthesia/Pediatrics, University of California School of Medicine; University of California Hospitals, San Francisco, California.
Resuscitation of the Newborn.

ARTHUR M. GROSSMAN, M.D.
Clinical Professor of Pediatrics, University of Southern California School of Medicine; Associate Clinical Professor of Pediatrics, University of California School of Medicine; Emeritus Attending, Cedars-Sinai Medical Center; Senior Attending, Los Angeles Children's Hospital, Los Angeles, California.
Accident Prevention.

WARREN G. GUNTHEROTH, M.D.
Professor of Pediatrics, University of Washington School of Medicine; Head, Division of Pediatric Cardiology, University of Washington Hospital, Seattle, Washington.
Peripheral Vascular Disease.

ROBERT T. HALL, M.D.
Associate Professor of Pediatrics, University of Missouri School of Medicine; Chief of Neonatal Medicine, Children's Mercy Hospital, Kansas City, Missouri.
Necrotizing Enterocolitis.

J. ALEX HALLER, JR., M.D.
Robert Garrett Professor of Pediatric Surgery, Johns Hopkins University School of Medicine; Children's Surgeon-in-Charge, Johns Hopkins Hospital, Baltimore, Maryland.
Purulent Peritonitis. Chest Wall Abnormalities.

JAMES BARRY HANSHAW, M.D.
Professor and Chairman, Department of Pediatrics, University of Massachusetts Medical School; Lecturer in Pediatrics, Harvard Medical School; Chief of Pediatrics, University of Massachusetts Medical Center, Boston, and St. Vincent Hospital, Worcester, Massachusetts.
Cytomegalovirus Infection.

GORDON HARPER, M.D.
Instructor in Psychiatry, Harvard Medical School; Assistant in Medicine, Psychiatry and Cardiology; Chief, Psychosomatic Unit, Children's Hospital Medical Center, Boston, Massachusetts.
Emotional Problems of Adolescents.

HAROLD E. HARRISON, M.D.
Professor Emeritus of Pediatrics, Johns Hopkins University School of Medicine; Pediatrician, Johns Hopkins

Hospital, Baltimore City Hospitals; Consulting Pediatrician, Sinai Hospital of Baltimore, Baltimore, Maryland.
Parathyroid Disease.

MONTGOMERY C. HART, M.D.
Adjunct Professor of Pediatrics, University of Arizona School of Medicine, Tucson; Co-Director, Arizona State Newborn Transport and Intensive Care Program; Co-Director, Newborn Intensive Care Nurseries, Good Samaritan, St. Joseph's, and Maricopa County General Hospitals, Phoenix; Co-Director, Perinatal Education, Good Samaritan Hospital, Phoenix, Arizona.
Emphysema.

DOUGLAS C. HEINER, M.D., Ph.D.
Professor of Pediatrics, University of California School of Medicine, Harbor General Hospital Campus; Chief, Division of Immunology and Allergy, Department of Pediatrics, Harbor General Hospital, Torrance, California.
Anaphylaxis.

WILLIAM C. HEIRD, M.D.
Assistant Professor of Pediatrics, Columbia University College of Physicians and Surgeons; Assistant Attending Pediatrician, Babies Hospital, Columbia Presbyterian Medical Center, New York, New York.
Total Parenteral Nutrition in Infants.

J. PATRICK HIEBER, M.D.
Assistant Professor of Pediatrics, Southwestern Medical School, University of Texas Health Science Center at Dallas; Consultant in Pediatric Infectious Diseases, Children's Medical Center and Parkland Memorial Hospital, Dallas, Texas.
Listeria Infections.

FRANK HINMAN, JR., M.D.
Clinical Professor of Urology, University of California Medical Center, San Francisco, California.
Hydronephrosis and Ureteral Disorders.

NORBERT HIRSCHHORN, M.D.
Clinical Assistant Professor of Medicine, Harvard Medical School, Boston, Massachusetts.
Cholera.

EDWARD P. HOFFMAN, M.D.
Attending Neurosurgeon, St. Peter Hospital, Olympia, Washington.
Spina Bifida.

JORGE B. HOWARD, M.D.
Instructor in Pediatric Infectious Diseases, Universidad de Chile, Hospital Calvo MacKenna, Santiago, Chile.
Typhoid Fever. Salmonellosis.

JAMES M. HUGHES, M.D.
Fellow, Division of Infectious Diseases, University of Virginia School of Medicine, Charlottesville, Virginia. Career Development Program, Bureau of Epidemiology, Center for Disease Control, Atlanta, Georgia.
Food Poisoning.

WALTER T. HUGHES, M.D.
Eudowood Professor of Pediatric Infectious Diseases, Director of the Eudowood Pediatric Infectious Diseases Unit, Johns Hopkins University School of Medicine, Baltimore, Maryland.
Pneumocystis carinii Pneumonitis. Histoplasmosis.

CAROLE G. H. HURVITZ, M.B. Ch.B.
Assistant Professor of Pediatrics, University of Califor-

nia; Pediatric Hematologist-Oncologist, Department of Pediatrics, Cedars-Sinai Medical Center, Los Angeles, California.
Acute Leukemia.

SIDNEY HURWITZ, M.D.
Associate Clinical Professor of Pediatrics and Dermatology, Yale University School of Medicine; Attending in Pediatrics and Dermatology, Yale-New Haven Medical Center and Hospital of St. Raphael, New Haven, Connecticut.
The Genodermatoses. Diseases of Sweat and Sebaceous Glands.

PETER R. HUTTENLOCHER, M.D.
Professor of Pediatrics and Neurology, University of Chicago; Attending Physician, Wyler Children's Hospital, Chicago, Illinois.
Familial Periodic Paralysis.

YAKUB INATI, M.D.
Fellow in Muscular Dystrophy, University of Pittsburgh, Pittsburgh, Pennsylvania.
Myositis Ossificans.

ALVIN H. JACOBS, M.D.
Professor of Dermatology and Pediatrics, Stanford University School of Medicine; Consultant in Dermatology, Children's Hospital at Stanford, Palo Alto, California.
Papulosquamous Disorders. Melanin Pigmentary Disorders. Miscellaneous Dermatoses.

BURTON F. JAFFE, M.D.
Assistant Clinical Professor of Otolaryngology, Harvard Medical School; Senior Otolaryngologist, Children's Hospital Medical Center; Chief, Division of Otolaryngology, Beth Israel Hospital, Boston, Massachusetts.
Salivary Tumors. Recurrent Parotitis. Thyroglossal Duct Cysts. Branchial Arch Cysts and Sinuses.

JOHN A. JANE, M.D.
Professor of Neurosurgery, University of Virginia Medical School, Charlottesville, Virginia.
Craniostenosis. Crouzon's Disease and Apert's Syndrome. Hypertelorism and Hypotelorism.

NORMAN B. JAVITT, M.D., Ph.D.
Professor of Medicine, and Head, Division of Gastroenterology, New York Hospital-Cornell Medical Center; Attending Physician, New York Hospital; Consultant, Memorial Hospital, New York, New York.
Hepatolenticular Degeneration (Wilson's Disease).

LOIS B. JOHNSON, M.D.
Assistant Professor of Pediatrics, University of Cincinnati; Pediatrician, Health Maintenance Physicians, Inc., Attending Pediatrician, Good Samaritan Hospital and Children's Hospital Medical Center, Cincinnati, Ohio.
Pregnancy. Gynecologic Procedures.

MICHAEL M. KABACK, M.D.
Professor, Departments of Pediatrics and Medicine, University of California School of Medicine; Associate Chief, Division of Medical Genetics, Harbor General Hospital, Torrance, California.
Lipid Storage Diseases.

GUINTER KAHN, M.D.
Director, Pediatric Dermatology Seminar, St. Francis Hospital, Miami Beach, Florida.
Skin Diseases of the Newborn. Eruptions in the Diaper Area. Vesiculobullous Disorders: Dermatitis Herpetiformis, Drug-Induced Toxic Epidermal Necrolysis, Pemphigus Vulgaris and Bullous Pemphigoid.

STEPHEN R. KANDALL, M.D.
Assistant Professor of Pediatrics, Mount Sinai School of Medicine of the City University of New York; Chief, Division of Neonatology, Beth Israel Medical Center, New York, New York.
Hemolytic Diseases of the Newborn.

EDWARD L. KAPLAN, M.D.
Associate Professor, Department of Pediatrics, University of Minnesota School of Medicine; Attending Physician, University Hospitals and Hennepin County Medical Center, Minneapolis. Attending Physician, St. Paul-Ramsey Medical Center, St. Paul, Minnesota.
Rheumatic Fever.

SOLOMON A. KAPLAN, M.D.
Professor of Pediatrics, University of California School of Medicine, Los Angeles, California.
Hypopituitarism.

RIVKA KAULI, M.D.
Lecturer in Pediatrics, Tel Aviv University, Sackler School of Medicine; Senior Physician, Institute of Pediatric and Adolescent Endocrinology, Beilinson Medical Center, Petah Tikva, Israel.
Diabetes Insipidus.

ROBERT KAYE, M.D.
Professor of Pediatrics, Hahnemann Medical College and Hospital; Consultant, Children's Hospital of Philadelphia and St. Agnes Hospital, Philadelphia, Pennsylvania.
Juvenile Diabetes Management.

MARGARET A. KELLER, M.D.
Postdoctoral Fellow, Pediatric Immunology-Infectious Diseases, Department of Pediatrics, University of California Harbor General Hospital Campus, Torrance, California.
Pertussis.

C. HENRY KEMPE, M.D.
Professor of Pediatrics and Microbiology, University of Colorado School of Medicine; Colorado General Hospital, Denver General Hospital, Denver Children's Hospital, Fitzsimons Army Hospital, Denver, Colorado.
Smallpox. Vaccinia.

EDWIN LAWRENCE KENDIG, JR., M.D.
Professor of Pediatrics, Medical College of Virginia, Health Sciences Division, Virginia Commonwealth University; Chairman, Department of Pediatrics, St. Mary's Hospital, Richmond, Virginia.
Infants with Atypical Mycobacteria. Sarcoidosis.

JOSEPH L. KENNEDY, JR., M.D.
Associate Professor of Pediatrics, Assistant Professor of Obstetrics and Gynecology, Tufts University School of Medicine; Director of Nurseries, St. Margaret's Hospital for Women, Boston, Massachusetts.
Birth Injuries.

WAHEED KHAN, Ph.D.
Chief Microbiologist, Research Foundation, Children's Hospital National Medical Center, Washington, D. C.
Hemophilus Influenzae Infections.

SIDNEY KIBRICK, M.D., Ph.D.
Professor of Pediatrics and Microbiology (Virology), Boston University School of Medicine; Visiting Physician for Pediatrics, Boston City Hospital, Boston, Massachusetts.
Warts and Molluscum Contagiosum. Cat-Scratch Disease.

R. A. KLASSEN, M.D.
Instructor of Pediatric Orthopedics, Mayo Medical School, Rochester, Minnesota; St. Mary's Hospital and Methodist Hospital, Rochester; Gillette Children's Hospital, St. Paul, Minnesota.
Disorders of the Spine and Shoulder Girdle.

HOWARD M. KLEIN, M.D.
Fellow in Behavioral Pediatrics and Child Psychiatry, Departments of Pediatrics and Psychiatry, University of Maryland School of Medicine, Baltimore, Maryland.
Child Abuse and Neglect.

JEROME O. KLEIN, M.D.
Professor of Pediatrics, Boston University School of Medicine; Associate Director, Department of Pediatrics, Boston City Hospital, Boston, Massachusetts.
Bacterial Pneumonia.

SAUL KRUGMAN, M.D.
Professor of Pediatrics, New York University Medical Center; Attending Physician, Bellevue Hospital and University Hospital, New York, New York.
Viral Hepatitis.

LOUIS F. KUEHN, M.D.
Active Staff, Northwest Medical Center, Houston; Consultant, Parkway Hospital, Houston, Texas.
Anaphylaxis.

PHILIP LANZKOWSKY, M.D., F.R.C.P., D.C.H.
Professor of Pediatrics, State University of New York at Stonybrook, Health Science Center; Chief of Pediatric Hematology-Oncology and Chairman of Pediatrics, Long Island Jewish-Hillside Medical Center, New Hyde Park, New York.
Hemolytic Anemia.

RAYMOND B. LARAVUSO, M.D.
Assistant Professor of Anesthesiology, Johns Hopkins University School of Medicine; Director of Pediatric Anesthesia, Johns Hopkins Hospital, Baltimore, Maryland.
Anesthesia: Aspects of Significance to the Pediatrician.

ZVI LARON, M.D.
Professor of Pediatric Endocrinology, Sackler School of Medicine, Tel Aviv University; Director of Institute of Pediatric and Adolescent Endocrinology; Director, Israel Counseling Center for Juvenile Diabetics, Beilinson Medical Center, Petah Tikva, Israel.
Diabetes Insipidus.

WILLIAM E. LAUPUS, M.D.
Professor of Pediatrics, East Carolina University School of Medicine; Pitt County Memorial Hospital, Greenville, North Carolina.
Rickettsial Infections.

LUCIAN L. LEAPE, M.D.
Professor of Surgery, Tufts University School of Medicine; Chief of Pediatric Surgery, New England Medical Center Hospital, Boston, Massachusetts.
Malformations of the Intestine. Foreign Bodies of the Gastrointestinal Tract. Intussusception.

JOHN C. LEONIDAS, M.D.
Professor of Radiology, Tufts University School of Medicine; Pediatric Radiologist-in-Chief, New England Medical Center Hospital, Boston, Massachusetts.
Necrotizing Enterocolitis.

WALTER F. LEVER, M.D.
Professor and Acting Chairman, Department of Dermatology, Tufts University School of Medicine; Chief, Dermatology Service, New England Medical Center Hospitals, Boston, Massachusetts.
Discoid Lupus Erythematosus.

RICHARD D. LEVERE, M.D.
Professor and Vice-Chairman, Department of Medicine, State University of New York, Downstate Medical Center; Director, University Hematology-Oncology Division, State University Hospital and Kings County Hospital Center, New York, New York.
Disorders of Porphyrin, Hemoglobin, and Purine Metabolism.

HENRY LEVISON, M.D., F.R.C.P. (C)
Associate Professor of Pediatrics, University of Toronto; Senior Physician, The Hospital for Sick Children, Toronto, Ontario, Canada.
Diseases of the Pleura. Bronchial Asthma.

MICHAEL B. LEWIS, M.D.
Assistant Professor of Surgery, Tufts University School of Medicine; Surgeon, New England Medical Center Hospital, Boston, Massachusetts.
Nevi and Nevoid Tumors.

JOHN E. LEWY, M.D.
Professor of Pediatrics, Cornell University Medical Center; Director, Pediatric Nephrology, New York Hospital, New York, New York.
Glomerulonephritis.

DESPINE LIEBHABER, M.D.
Instructor in Clinical Pediatrics, Washington University School of Medicine; Medical Staff, St. Louis County Hospital; Assistant Pediatrician, St. Louis Children's Hospital, St. Louis, Missouri.
Pica.

JEROME LIEBMAN, M.D.
Professor of Pediatrics, Case Western Reserve University; Director of Pediatric Cardiology, Rainbow Babies and Children's Hospital, Cleveland, Ohio.
Air Travel.

IRWIN J. LIGHT, M.D.
Professor of Pediatrics and Obstetrics and Gynecology, University of Cincinnati College of Medicine; Director, Newborn Clinical Service, University of Cincinnati College of Medicine, Cincinnati, Ohio.
Disorders of the Umbilicus.

HERMAN W. LIPOW, M.D.
Associate Clinical Professor of Pediatrics; Member, Cardiovascular Research Institute, University of California, San Francisco, California.
Bronchiectasis. Atelectasis.

BARBARA M. LIPPE, M.D.
Associate Professor of Pediatrics, University of California School of Medicine, Los Angeles, California.
Disorders of the Vulva and Vagina. Disorders of the Uterus, Tubes and Ovaries. Tumors of the Uterus, Tubes and Ovaries.

IRIS F. LITT, M.D.
Associate Professor of Pediatrics, Stanford University Medical Center, Stanford, California.
Syphilis. Venereal Disease.

JUNE K. LLOYD, M.D., F.R.C.P.
Professor of Child Health, St. George's Hospital Medical School, University of London; Consulting Pediatrician, St. George's Hospital, London, England.
Inborn Errors of Serum Lipoproteins.

LAWRENCE A. LOCKMAN, M.D.
Assistant Professor of Neurology and Pediatrics, Division of Pediatric Neurology, University of Minnesota School of Medicine; Assistant Professor of Pediatric Neurology, University of Minnesota Hospitals; Consulting Pediatric Neurologist, Hennepin County Medical Center, Children's Hospital of St. Paul, Children's Health Center of Minneapolis, Minneapolis, Minnesota.
Headache.

JENNIFER M. H. LOGGIE, M.B., B.Ch.
Professor of Pediatrics and Associate Professor of Pharmacology, University of Cincinnati College of Medicine; Attending Pediatrician, Children's Hospital Medical Center, Cincinnati, Ohio.
Systemic Hypertension.

FREDERICK H. LOVEJOY, JR., M.D.
Assistant Professor of Pediatrics, Harvard Medical School; Associate in Medicine and Clinical Pharmacology, Children's Hospital Medical Center; Executive Director, Boston Poison Information Center, Boston, Massachusetts.
Reye's Syndrome. Vomiting.

JOHN N. LUKENS, M.D.
Professor of Pediatrics, Vanderbilt University School of Medicine; Director of Pediatric Hematology-Oncology, The Children's Hospital, Vanderbilt University Medical Center, Nashville, Tennessee.
Anemias of Iron Deficiency, Blood Loss, Renal Disease and Chronic Infection.

NOEL KEITH MACLAREN, M.D.
Associate Professor of Pediatrics, University of Maryland School of Medicine; Director, Pediatric Endocrinology-Metabolism, University of Maryland Hospital, Baltimore, Maryland.
Hypoglycemia. Inborn Errors of Carbohydrate Metabolism.

LEONARD C. MARCUS, V.M.D., M.D.
Assistant Clinical Professor of Pediatrics and Pathology, Tufts University School of Medicine; Associate Staff, New England Medical Center; Assistant Director of Health Services, State Laboratory Institute, Massachusetts Department of Public Health, Boston, Massachusetts.
Leptospirosis. Rat-Bite Fever. Bites and Bite-Related Infections.

ANDREA MARKS, M.D.
Instructor in Pediatrics, Albert Einstein College of Medicine; Physician-in-Charge, Adolescent Ambulatory Service, Montefiore Hospital and Medical Center, Bronx, New York.
Obesity at Adolescence.

S. MICHAEL MAUER, M.D.
Associate Professor of Pediatrics and Director of Pediatric Dialysis, University of Minnesota Medical School, Minneapolis, Minnesota.
Renal Vein Thrombosis.

GEORGE H. McCRACKEN, JR., M.D.
Professor of Pediatrics, University of Texas Health Science Center, Southwestern Medical School, Dallas; Attending Physician, Parkland Memorial Hospital and Children's Medical Center of Dallas, Texas.
Neonatal Septicemia, Meningitis and Pneumonia.

RAWLE M. McINTOSH, M.D.
Professor of Pediatrics and Medicine, University of Colorado Medical Center, Denver; Member, National Jewish

Hospital and Research Center, Denver, Colorado.
Hemolytic-Uremic Syndrome.

KEVIN M. McINTYRE, M.D.
Assistant Professor of Medicine, Harvard Medical School, Boston; Assistant Chief of Cardiology, Veterans Administration Hospital, West Roxbury, Massachusetts.
Pulmonary Emboli.

GUY M. McKHANN, M.D.
Kennedy Professor of Neurology, Neurologist-in-Chief, Johns Hopkins Hospital, Baltimore, Maryland.
Guillain-Barré Syndrome. Chronic Relapsing Neuropathy. Acute Toxic Encephalopathy and Hypoxic Encephalopathy.

ROBERT L. McLAURIN, M.D.
Professor of Surgery (Neurosurgery), University of Cincinnati Medical Center, Cincinnati, Ohio.
Head Injury. Cerebral Edema. Epidural Hematoma and Subdural Hematoma and Effusion. Intracranial Hemorrhage. Injuries to the Brachial Plexus, Facial Nerve and Sciatic Nerve.

RICHARD H. MEADE, III, M.D.
Professor of Pediatrics, Tufts University School of Medicine, Boston, Massachusetts.
Mycoplasma Infections. Otologic Infections.

HARRY MEDOVY, M.D., D.Sc., F.R.C.P. (C)
Professor Emeritus, University of Manitoba; Consultant Physician, Children's Center, Health Science Center, Winnipeg, Canada.
Pylorospasm.

MARIAN E. MELISH, M.D.
Assistant Professor of Pediatrics, University of California School of Medicine; Attending Pediatrician, University Hospital of San Diego County, Mercy Hospital and Children's Hospital and Health Center, San Diego, California.
Mucocutaneous Lymph Node Syndrome.

WILLIAM M. MICHENER, M.D.
Section of Pediatric Gastroenterology, The Cleveland Clinic Foundation, Cleveland, Ohio.
Constipation. Chronic Nonspecific Diarrhea of Childhood. Intractable Diarrhea of Infancy.

JOHN J. MILLER, III, M.D., Ph.D.
Associate Professor of Clinical Pediatrics, Stanford University School of Medicine; Director, Rheumatic Disease Service, Children's Hospital at Stanford, Palo Alto, California.
The Rheumatic Diseases.

ROBERT A. MILLER, M.D.
Professor of Pediatrics, University of Illinois College of Medicine, Abraham Lincoln School of Medicine; Chairman, Department of Pediatrics, Cook County Hospital, Chicago, Illinois.
Myocardial Disease.

J. GORDON MILLICHAP, M.D., F.R.C.P.
Professor of Neurology and Pediatrics, Northwestern University Medical School; Pediatric Neurologist, Children's Memorial Hospital and Northwestern Medical Center, Chicago, Illinois.
Myasthenia Gravis.

ROBERT R. MONTGOMERY, M.D.
Assistant Professor of Pediatrics, University of Colorado School of Medicine; Pediatric Hematologist, University of Colorado Medical Center, Denver, Colorado.
Hemolytic-Uremic Syndrome.

GRANT MORROW, III, M.D.
Professor of Pediatrics, University of Arizona; Director of Neonatal Biology, Arizona Health Sciences Center, Tucson Medical Center, Tucson, Arizona.
Generalized Undernutrition.

THOMAS S. MORSE, M.D.
Associate Professor of Surgery (Pediatric Surgery), Ohio State University College of Medicine; Attending Surgeon, Children's Hospital, Columbus, Ohio.
The Injured Child: Evaluation and Management.

THOMAS MOSHANG, JR., M.D.
Associate Professor of Pediatrics, Hahnemann Medical College and Hospital; Head, Section of Pediatric Endocrinology and Metabolism, Hahnemann Medical College and Hospital, Philadelphia, Pennsylvania. Consulting Pediatric Endocrinologist, Monmouth Hospital, Monmouth, New Jersey and St. Francis Hospital, Trenton, New Jersey.
Endocrine Disorders of the Testis.

EDWARD GORDON MURPHY, M.D., F.R.C.P. (C)
Associate Professor, University of Toronto; Senior Staff Physician, Hospital for Sick Children; Consultant Neurologist, Ontario Crippled Children's Centre, Toronto, Canada.
Muscular Dystrophy and Related Myopathies.

ALEXANDER S. NADAS, M.D.
Professor of Pediatrics, Children's Hospital, Harvard Medical School; Chief, Department of Cardiology, Children's Hospital Medical Center, Boston, Massachusetts.
Congenital Heart Disease.

J. LAWRENCE NAIMAN, M.D.
Professor of Pediatrics, Temple University School of Medicine; Chief of Hematology, St. Christopher's Hospital for Children, Philadelphia, Pennsylvania.
Idiopathic (Primary) Pulmonary Hemosiderosis.

PRASANNA NAIR, M.B.B.S.
Associate Professor of Pediatrics, University of Maryland School of Medicine; Director, Community Pediatric Center, University of Maryland Hospital, Baltimore, Maryland.
Premarital Counseling for the Adolescent.

ANDREA H. NASH, M.D.
Clinical Instructor in Pediatrics, University of California at Los Angeles; Associate in Pediatrics, Cedars-Sinai Medical Center, Los Angeles, California.
Acute Ataxia.

THOMAS F. NECHELES, M.D., Ph.D.
Professor of Pediatrics, Tufts University School of Medicine; Chief, Pediatric Hematology-Oncology, New England Medical Center Hospital, Boston, Massachusetts.
Thalessemia. Neuroblastoma. Hemorrhagic Disorders. Histiocytosis X.

CATHERINE A. NEILL, M.D., F.R.C.P.
Associate Professor of Pediatrics, and Cardiologist, Johns Hopkins University; Helen B. Taussig Children's Cardiac Center, Johns Hopkins Hospital, Baltimore, Maryland.
Cardiac Arrhythmias. Bacterial Endocarditis.

JOHN D. NELSON, M.D.
Professor of Pediatrics, University of Texas Health Science Center, Southwestern Medical School, Dallas, Texas.
Septic Arthritis and Osteomyelitis.

KARIN B. NELSON, M.D.
Developmental Neurology Branch, National Institute of Neurological and Communicable Disorders and Stroke, Bethesda, Maryland.
Febrile Seizures.

ROSA LEE NEMIR, M.D.
Professor of Pediatrics, New York University School of Medicine; Attending Pediatrician and Director, Children's Chest Clinic, Bellevue Hospital; Attending Pediatrician, University Hospital, New York, New York.
Tuberculosis.

ERWIN NETER, M.D.
Professor of Microbiology and Clinical Microbiology, State University of New York at Buffalo; Director of Bacteriology, Children's Hospital of Buffalo, Buffalo, New York.
Shigellosis.

JAMES CORSON NIEDERMAN, M.D.
Clinical Professor of Epidemiology and Medicine, Yale University School of Medicine, Yale-New Haven Medical Center, New Haven, Connecticut.
Infectious Mononucleosis.

HAROLD M. NITOWSKY, M.D.
Professor of Pediatrics and Genetics, Albert Einstein College of Medicine; Attending Pediatrician, Bronx Municipal Hospital and Hospital of the Albert Einstein College of Medicine, New York, New York.
Genetic Disease: Diagnosis, Counseling and Prevention.

ENRIQUE M. OSTREA, JR., M.D.
Associate Professor of Pediatrics, Wayne State University School of Medicine; Director, University Nursery Service; Chief of Pediatrics, Hutzel Hospital, Detroit, Michigan.
Infants of Drug Addicted Mothers.

L. G. OWEN, M.D.
Associate Clinical Professor of Medicine (Dermatology), Executive Director of Dermatology Section, University of Louisville School of Medicine, Louisville, Kentucky.
Photodermatoses. Diseases of the Hair and Scalp.

ALFRED F. PARISI, M.D.
Associate Professor of Medicine, Harvard Medical School, Boston; Chief of Cardiology, Veterans Administration Hospital, West Roxbury, Massachusetts.
Pulmonary Emboli.

JOHN S. PARKS, M.D., Ph.D.
Assistant Professor of Pediatrics, University of Pennsylvania School of Medicine; Associate Physician and Associate Endocrinologist, Children's Hospital of Philadelphia.
Gynecomastia. Hermaphroditism and Intersex.

ROBERT H. PARROTT, M.D.
Professor, Child Health and Development, George Washington University School of Medicine and Health Care Sciences; Director, Children's Hospital National Medical Center, Washington, D. C.
Bronchiolitis. Viral Pneumonia.

HOWARD A. PEARSON, M.D.
Professor and Chairman, Department of Pediatrics, Yale University School of Medicine; Chief of Pediatrics and Attending Pediatrician, Yale-New Haven Hospital, New Haven, Connecticut.
Disorders of the Spleen.

CHARLES A. PECK, JR., LTC MC
Pediatric Surgeon, Walter Reed Army Medical Center, Washington, D. C.
Burn Therapy.

JAY A. PERMAN, M.D.
Assistant Professor of Pediatrics, University of California, San Francisco, California.
Malabsorption Syndromes and Intestinal Disaccharidase Deficiencies.

JEAN F. PERRAULT, M.D.
Instructor in Medicine, Mayo Medical School; Consultant, Division of Gastroenterology and Internal Medicine, Mayo Clinic and Mayo Foundation, Rochester, Minnesota.
Ulcerative Colitis. Crohn's Disease.

DANIEL A. PIETRO, M.D.
Clinical Fellow in Medicine, Harvard Medical School, Boston; Fellow in Cardiology, Veterans Administration Hospital, West Roxbury, Massachusetts.
Pulmonary Emboli.

SERGIO PIOMELLI, M.D.
Professor of Pediatrics, New York University School of Medicine; Attending Physician and Director of Pediatric Hematology, New York Hospital and Bellevue Hospital, New York, New York.
Lead Poisoning. Iron Poisoning.

ARNOLD C. G. PLATZKER, M.D.
Assistant Professor of Pediatrics, University of Southern California; Director, Neonatal-Respiratory Diseases Division, Children's Hospital of Los Angeles, Los Angeles, California.
Pneumomediastinum and Pneumothorax. Cysts of the Lung. Tumors of the Chest.

STANLEY A. PLOTKIN, M.D.
Professor of Pediatrics, University of Pennsylvania; Director, Infectious Disease Division, Children's Hospital of Philadelphia, Philadelphia, Pennsylvania.
Rabies.

JEFFREY J. POMERANCE, M.D., M.P.H.
Assistant Professor in Pediatrics, University of California School of Medicine; Director of Neonatology, Cedars-Sinai Medical Center, Los Angeles, California.
Intrauterine Growth Retardation and Postmaturity Syndrome.

EDWARD F. RABE, M.D.
Professor of Pediatrics (Neurology), Tufts University School of Medicine; Chief, Department of Pediatric Neurology, Boston Floating Hospital and New England Medical Center Hospital, Boston, Massachusetts.
Infantile Spasms.

AARON R. RAUSEN, M.D.
Professor of Pediatrics, Mount Sinai School of Medicine of the City University of New York; Director of Pediatrics, Beth Israel Medical Center, New York, New York.
Hemolytic Diseases of the Newborn.

HOMER B. C. REED, JR., Ph.D.
Associate Professor of Pediatrics (Psychology), Tufts University School of Medicine; Director, Neuropsychology Service, New England Medical Center Hospital, Boston, Massachusetts.
Reading Disorders.

JACK S. REMINGTON, M.D.
Professor, Department of Medicine, Stanford University School of Medicine, Stanford; Chief, Division of Allergy, Immunology, and Infectious Diseases, Palo Alto Medical Research Foundation, Palo Alto, California.
Toxoplasmosis.

ALAN B. RETIK, M.D.
Associate Professor of Urology, Harvard Medical School; Chief, Division of Urology, Children's Hospital Medical Center; Attending, Boston Floating Hospital for Infants and Children, Boston; Chief of Pediatric Urology, Massachusetts Hospital School for Handicapped Children, Canton, Massachusetts.
Vesicoureteral Reflux. Neurogenic Vesical Dysfunction. Exstrophy of the Bladder.

JULIUS B. RICHMOND, M.D.
Professor, Child Psychiatry and Human Development, Harvard Medical School; Director, Judge Baker Guidance Center; Psychiatrist-in-Chief, Children's Hospital Medical Center, Boston, Massachusetts.
Emotional Problems of Adolescents.

HARRIS D. RILEY, JR., M.D.
Distinguished Professor of Pediatrics, University of Oklahoma College of Medicine; Attending Physician, Children's Memorial Hospital, Oklahoma City, Oklahoma.
Infections Due to Escherichia coli, Proteus, Klebsiella, Pseudomonas and Other Gram-Negative Bacilli.

JEAN E. ROBILLARD, M.D.
Assistant Professor of Pediatrics, University of Iowa Hospitals and Clinics, Iowa City, Iowa.
The Nephrotic Syndrome.

WILLIAM J. RODRIGUEZ, M.D.
Assistant Professor of Child Health and Development, George Washington University Medical School; Adjunct Assistant Professor of Microbiology, Georgetown Medical and Dental Schools; Attending, Children's Hospital National Medical Center, Washington, D. C.
Hemophilus Influenzae Infections.

FRED S. ROSEN, M.D.
James L. Gamble Professor of Pediatrics, Harvard Medical School; Chief, Division of Immunology, Children's Hospital Medical Center, Boston, Massachusetts.
Angioneurotic Edema.

GERALD ROSEN, M.D.
Associate Professor of Pediatrics, Cornell University Medical College; Associate Attending Pediatrician, Memorial Sloan-Kettering Cancer Center, New York, New York.
Malignant Bone Tumors.

AMNON ROSENTHAL, M.D.
Associate Professor of Pediatrics, Harvard Medical School; Senior Associate in Cardiology, Children's Hospital Medical Center, Boston, Massachusetts.
Pericardial Disease.

N. PAUL ROSMAN, M.D.
Professor of Pediatrics and Neurology, Boston University School of Medicine; Director of Pediatric Neurology and Associate Director of Pediatrics, Boston City Hospital, Boston, Massachusetts.
Acute Hemiplegia. Congenital Hypotonia.

SYDNEY ROSS, M.D.
Clinical Professor of Pediatrics, George Washington University School of Medicine; Chief, Microbiology Sec-

tion, Research Foundation, Children's Hospital National Medical Center, Washington, D. C.
Hemophilus Influenzae Infections.

ALAN RUBINOW, M.D.
Instructor in Medicine, Boston University School of Medicine; Assistant Visiting Physician, Boston City Hospital, Boston, Massachusetts.
Amyloidosis.

JOHN F. RYAN, M.D.
Associate Professor of Anaesthesia, Harvard Medical School; Anesthetist, Massachusetts General Hospital, Boston, Massachusetts.
High Fever.

JOSEPH W. ST. GEME, JR., M.D.
Professor of Pediatrics, University of California School of Medicine, Los Angeles; Chairman, Department of Pediatrics, Harbor General Hospital, Torrance, California.
Infections Due to Anaerobic Cocci and Gram-Negative Anaerobic Bacilli. Mumps.

ROBERT B. SALTER, M.D., F.R.C.S. (C), F.A.C.S.
Professor and Head of Orthopaedic Surgery, University of Toronto; Surgeon-in-Chief Emeritus, The Hospital for Sick Children, Toronto, Canada.
Orthopedic Disorders of the Extremities.

FREDERICK J. SAMAHA, M.D.
Professor of Neurology and Pediatrics, University of Pittsburgh; Attending Neurologist, Presbyterian University Hospital and Children's Hospital of Pittsburgh, Pittsburgh, Pennsylvania.
Myositis Ossificans.

JACQUELYN SANDERS, Ph.D.
Lecturer, Department of Education, University of Chicago; Director, Sonia Shankman Orthogenic School, University of Chicago, Chicago, Illinois.
Autism.

RICHARD M. SARLES, M.D.
Associate Professor of Psychiatry and Pediatrics, University of Maryland School of Medicine, Baltimore, Maryland.
Child Abuse and Neglect.

ARTHUR A. SASAHARA, M.D.
Professor of Medicine, Harvard Medical School, Boston; Chief of Medicine, Veterans Administration Hospital, West Roxbury, Massachusetts.
Pulmonary Emboli.

JOHN E. SCHOWALTER, M.D.
Professor of Clinical Pediatrics and Psychiatry, Yale University Child Study Center; Attending in Pediatrics and Psychiatry, Yale-New Haven Hospital, New Haven, Connecticut.
Psychosomatic Illness.

JOHN H. SEASHORE, M.D.
Assistant Professor of Surgery and Pediatrics, Yale University School of Medicine; Attending Physician, Yale-New Haven Hospital, New Haven, Connecticut.
Disorders of the Anus and Rectum.

JAMES S. SEIDEL, M.D., Ph.D.
Assistant Professor of Pediatrics and Lecturer in Microbiology and Immunology, University of California School of Medicine, Los Angeles; Chief of Pediatric Acute Care Clinic, and Acting Chief of Ambulatory Pediatrics, Harbor General Hospital, Torrance, California.
Parasitic Infections.

DAN K. SEILHEIMER, M.D.
Fellow in Pediatric Pulmonary Disease, Cardiovascular Research Institute, University of California, San Francisco, California.
Atelectasis. Bronchiectasis.

DEXTER S. Y. SETO, M.D.
Professor of Pediatrics, University of Hawaii School of Medicine; Director of Research, Kapiolani Children's Medical Center, Honolulu, Hawaii.
Tetanus.

LARRY J. SHAPIRO, M.D.
Assistant Professor of Pediatrics, University of California School of Medicine, Los Angeles; Physician, Division of Medical Genetics, Harbor General Hospital, Torrance, California.
Lipid Storage Diseases.

G. V. R. K. SHARMA, M.D.
Assistant Professor of Medicine, Harvard Medical School, Boston; Director, Coronary Care Unit, Veterans Administration Hospital, West Roxbury, Massachusetts.
Pulmonary Emboli.

EDWARD B. SHAW, M.D.
Professor Emeritus of Pediatrics, University of California School of Medicine; University of California Hospitals, San Francisco, California.
Colic.

SHEILA SHERLOCK, M.D.
Professor of Medicine, Royal Free Hospital School of Medicine (University of London); Consultant Physician, Royal Free Hospital, London, England.
Portal Hypertension. Chronic Active Hepatitis.

HENRY R. SHINEFIELD, M.D.
Clinical Professor of Pediatrics, University of California School of Medicine, San Francisco; Chief, Department of Pediatrics, Kaiser Foundation Hospital, San Francisco, California.
Staphylococcal Infections.

KENNETH SHULMAN, M.D.
Professor and Chairman, Department of Neurological Surgery, Albert Einstein College of Medicine and Montefiore Hospital and Medical Center, New York, New York.
Hydrocephalus.

PAUL A. SHURIN, M.D.
Instructor in Pediatrics, Harvard Medical School and Boston University School of Medicine; Assistant Visiting Physician, Boston City Hospital, Boston, Massachusetts.
Labyrinthitis.

CALVIN C. J. SIA, M.D.
Clinical Professor of Pediatrics, University of Hawaii School of Medicine; Active Staff, Kapiolani Children's Medical Center, Honolulu, Hawaii.
Leprosy.

WILLIAM K. SIEBER, M.D.
Clinical Associate Professor of Surgery, University of Pittsburgh School of Medicine, Pittsburgh, Pennsylvania.
Hirschsprung's Disease.

SHELDON C. SIEGEL, M.D.
Clinical Professor of Pediatrics and Co-director of Pediatric Allergy Clinic, University of California School of Medicine, Los Angeles, California.
Allergic Rhinitis.

WILLIAM D. SINGER, M.D.
Assistant Professor of Pediatrics (Neurology), Tufts University School of Medicine, Boston; Neurologist, New England Medical Center, Boston; Director of Neurological Services, Lakeville Hospital, Lakeville, Massachusetts.
Degenerative Diseases of the Central Nervous System.

RICHARD G. SKINNER, JR., M.D.
Clinical Professor of Pediatrics, University of Florida, Jacksonville Hospitals Educational Program; Active Staff, University Hospital of Jacksonville and Hope Haven Children's Hospital, Jacksonville, Florida.
Specific Learning Disability and Hyperactivity.

FRED G. SMITH, M.D.
Professor and Chairman, Department of Pediatrics, University of Iowa Hospitals and Clinics, Iowa City, Iowa.
The Nephrotic Syndrome.

LAWRENCE M. SOLOMON, M.D.
Professor and Head, Department of Dermatology, University of Illinois College of Medicine, Abraham Lincoln School of Medicine, Chicago, Illinois.
Atopic Dermatitis.

ALEX J. STEIGMAN, M.D.
Professor of Pediatrics, Mount Sinai School of Medicine, New York, New York.
Acute Aseptic Meningitis.

MATTHEW M. STEINER, M.D.
Professor of Pediatrics, Northwestern University School of Medicine; Attending Endocrinologist, Children's Memorial Hospital, Chicago, Illinois.
Obesity.

LEO STERN, M.D.
Professor and Chairman, Department of Pediatrics, Brown University; Pediatrician-in-Chief, Rhode Island Hospital, Providence, Rhode Island.
Bronchopulmonary Dysplasia. Neonatal Atelectasis. Congenital Lobar Emphysema. Meconium Aspiration.

ROBERT C. STERN, M.D.
Assistant Professor of Pediatrics, Case Western Reserve University School of Medicine; Associate Pediatrician, University Hospitals of Cleveland, Ohio.
Cystic Fibrosis.

GUNNAR B. STICKLER, M.D., Ph.D.
Professor of Pediatrics, Mayo Medical School; Chairman, Department of Pediatrics, Mayo Clinic and Mayo Foundation, Rochester, Minnesota.
Ulcerative Colitis. Crohn's Disease.

SYLVAN E. STOOL, M.D.
Professor of Otolaryngology and Pediatrics, University of Pittsburgh School of Medicine; Director of Education, Department of Otolaryngology, Children's Hospital of Pittsburgh, Pittsburgh, Pennsylvania.
Malformations of the Nose. Tumors and Polyps of the Nose. Nasal Injuries. Epistaxis. Foreign Bodies in the Nose and Pharynx.

D. EUGENE STRANDNESS, JR., M.D.
Professor of Surgery, University of Washington School of Medicine; University Hospital, Veterans Administration Hospital, Seattle, Washington.
Peripheral Vascular Disease.

JOSÉ STRAUSS, M.D.
Professor of Pediatrics, University of Miami School of Medicine; Director, Division of Pediatric Nephrology; Attending Pediatrician, Jackson Memorial Hospital and University of Miami Hospital and Clinics, Miami, Florida.
Chronic Renal Insufficiency. Peritoneal Dialysis. Hemodialysis.

RONALD G. STRAUSS, M.D.
Associate Professor of Pediatrics, University of Iowa School of Medicine; Division of Pediatric Hematology-Oncology, University of Iowa Hospitals and Clinics, Iowa City, Iowa.
Transfusion Reactions to Blood Products.

KENNETH F. SWAIMAN, M.D.
Professor and Director of Pediatric Neurology, University of Minnesota Medical School; Pediatric Neurology Staff, University of Minnesota Hospitals, Hennepin County Medical Center, Minneapolis, and St. Paul-Ramsey Hospital and St. Paul Children's Hospital, St. Paul, Minnesota.
Cerebral Palsy.

MELVIN TEFFT, M.D.
Professor of Radiation Medicine, Brown University; Radiotherapist, Rhode Island Hospital, Providence, Rhode Island.
Radiation Exposure in Diagnostic Roentgenology.

J. J. TEPAS, M.D.
Chief Resident in Pediatric Surgery, Johns Hopkins Hospital, Baltimore, Maryland.
Purulent Peritonitis.

THOMAS R. TETZLAFF, M.D.
Fellow in Pediatric Infectious Diseases, University of Texas Southwestern Medical School at Dallas, Texas.
Septic Arthritis and Osteomyelitis.

M. MICHAEL THALER, M.D.
Professor of Pediatrics, University of California; Director of Pediatric Gastroenterology, University of California Medical Center, San Francisco, California.
Idiopathic Unconjugated and Conjugated Hyperbilirubinemias. Cirrhosis and Tumors of the Liver. Galactosemia.

ROBERT F. TILLEY, M.D.
Instructor in Dermatology, Harvard Medical School; Dermatologist, New England Deaconess Hospital and New England Baptist Hospital, Boston, Massachusetts.
Fungous Infections.

JERROLD A. TURNER, M.D.
Associate Professor of Medicine and Microbiology and Immunology, University of California School of Medicine, Los Angeles; Assistant Medical Director, and Chief, Section of Parasitic Disease, Harbor General Hospital, Torrance, California.
Parasitic Infections.

P. JACOB VARGHESE, M.D.
Associate Professor of Pediatrics and Medicine, Johns Hopkins University, Helen B. Taussig Children's Cardiac Center, Johns Hopkins Hospital, Baltimore, Maryland.
Cardiac Arrhythmias.

THOMAS A. VARGO, M.D.
Assistant Professor, Baylor College of Medicine; Associate Cardiologist, Texas Children's Hospital, Houston, Texas.
Visceral Larva Migrans.

VICTOR C. VAUGHAN, III, M.D.
Professor of Pediatrics, Temple University School of Medicine; Attending Physician, St. Christopher's Hospital for Children, Philadelphia, Pennsylvania.
Serum Sickness.

STANLEY L. WALLACE, M.D.
Professor of Medicine, State University of New York, Downstate Medical Center; Associate Director of Medicine and Chief of Rheumatology, Jewish Hospital and Medical Center of Brooklyn, New York, New York.
Disorders of Porphyrin, Hemoglobin, and Purine Metabolism.

LEWIS W. WANNAMAKER, M.D.
Professor of Pediatrics and Microbiology, University of Minnesota; Career Investigator, American Heart Association, Minneapolis, Minnesota.
Rheumatic Fever.

JOHN B. WATKINS, M.D.
Assistant Professor of Pediatrics, Harvard Medical School; Associate in Gastroenterology, Children's Hospital, Boston, Massachusetts.
Malabsorption Syndromes and Intestinal Disaccharidase Deficiencies.

GORDON V. WATTERS, M.D., F.R.C.P. (C)
Associate Professor of Neurology and Pediatrics, McGill University; Director, Department of Neurology, The Montreal Children's Hospital, Montreal, Canada.
Neurocutaneous Syndromes.

PAUL F. WEHRLE, M.D.
Hastings Professor of Pediatrics, University of Southern California School of Medicine; Director of Pediatrics, Los Angeles County-University of Southern California Medical Center, Los Angeles, California.
Influenza.

MARVIN LEE WEIL, M.D.
Associate Professor of Pediatrics and Neurology, University of California School of Medicine, Los Angeles; Chief, Division of Pediatric Neurology, Harbor General Hospital, Torrance, California.
Encephalitis Infections—Postinfectious and Postvaccinal.

MILES WEINBERGER, M.D.
Associate Professor of Pediatrics, University of Iowa School of Medicine; Director, Pediatric Allergy and Pulmonary Division, University of Iowa Hospital, Iowa City, Iowa.
Drug-Induced Disease: Adverse Drug Reactions. Physical Allergy.

KEASLEY WELCH, M.D.
Ingraham Professor of Neurosurgery, Harvard Medical School; Neurosurgeon-in-Chief, Children's Hospital and Peter Bent Brigham Hospital, Boston, Massachusetts.
Cerebral Vascular Disorders. Venous Sinus Thrombosis. Pseudotumor Cerebri (Benign Intracranial Hypertension).

GEORGE F. WILGRAM, M.D., Ph.D.
Professor of Medicine and Dermatology, Tufts University Medical School, Boston, Massachusetts.
Contact Dermatitis. Urticaria. Drug Eruptions.

DANIEL H. WISEMAN, M.D.
Assistant Clinical Professor of Pediatrics, University of California School of Medicine, Los Angeles, California.
Bronchitis.

JAMES A. WOLFF, M.D.
Professor of Pediatrics, Columbia University College of Physicians and Surgeons; Attending Pediatrician, Babies Hospital and Children's Medical and Surgical Center, New York, New York.
Polycythemia. Leukopenia, Neutropenia and Agranulocytosis.

PAUL V. WOOLLEY, JR., M.D.
Professor of Pediatrics, Wayne State University School of Medicine; Director, Growth and Development, Children's Hospital of Michigan, Detroit, Michigan.
Infants of Drug Addicted Mothers.

NORMA WOLLNER, M.D.
Assistant Professor of Pediatrics, Cornell University; Attending Pediatrician, Memorial Hospital, New York, New York.
Non-Hodgkin's Lymphoma.

HARRY T. WRIGHT, JR., M.D., M.P.H.
Professor of Pediatrics, University of Southern California School of Medicine; Head, Division of Infectious Diseases and Virology Research, and Attending Physician, Children's Hospital of Los Angeles, Los Angeles, California.
Coccidioidomycosis.

RICHARD A. WYATT, M.D.
Fellow in Pediatric Allergy and Pulmonary Diseases, University of Iowa School of Medicine, Iowa City, Iowa.
Physical Allergy.

TERRY YAMAUCHI, M.D.
Associate Professor of Pediatrics, University of Arkansas Medical Sciences; Chief of Infectious Diseases, Arkansas Children's Hospital, Little Rock, Arkansas.
Lymphangitis. Lymph Node Infections.

HARVEY A. ZAREM, M.D.
Professor of Surgery, University of California School of Medicine; Chief, Division of Plastic Surgery, University of California Medical Center, Los Angeles, California.
Diseases and Injuries of the Oral Region.

DEBORAH ZEMER, M.D.
Professor, Department of Medicine, Tel-Aviv University Medical School, Tel-Aviv, Israel.
Familial Mediterranean Fever.

EKHARD E. ZIEGLER, M.D.
Associate Professor of Pediatrics, University of Iowa College of Medicine, Iowa City, Iowa.
Feeding of the Premature Infant.

Contents

4

RESPIRATORY TRACT

5
CARDIOVASCULAR SYSTEM

6
DIGESTIVE TRACT

9
ENDOCRINE SYSTEM

10
METABOLIC DISORDERS

11
CONNECTIVE TISSUE

12
GENITOURINARY TRACT

13

BONES AND JOINTS

14

MUSCLES

15
SKIN

16
THE EYE

17
THE EAR

18
INFECTIOUS DISEASES

1

Nutrition

Generalized Undernutrition

GRANT MORROW, III, M.D.

Undernutrition ranks as one of the major health problems throughout the world. Although one usually thinks of undernutrition only when dealing with poverty or underdeveloped countries, as nutrition awareness increases the physician will detect children in affluent societies with varying degrees of protein-calorie malnutrition (PCM). Abnormal intakes due to unusual dietary practices, disrupted maternal-child relationships, as well as a variety of medical problems, may produce PCM. Correction of the underlying social or medical cause has to be achieved before therapy can be effective. The severe syndromes of undernutrition are recognized as edematous and nonedematous PCM. Nonedematous PCM, or marasmus, implies a starved child who has had insufficient caloric intake. Edematous PCM, or kwashiorkor, occurs when protein needs have not been met over a long period of time.

SEVERE PCM

The characteristic physical findings of severe edematous PCM, or kwashiorkor, are edema, irritability or apathy, poor muscle tone, hair changes and skin lesions. Supporting positive laboratory tests include low hemoglobin, depressed albumin, decreased sedimentation rate and a low BUN. Nonedematous PCM, or marasmus, is characterized by skin which is dry, wrinkles easily and has lost its turgor. The cheeks become sunken in severe cases. The child appears weak and is hypotonic. Pulse, blood pressure and temperature may be low.

Initial Treatment

Fluid. In edematous PCM the extracellular fluid space is overexpanded. As a result, fluid *must* be administered cautiously to prevent pulmonary edema and heart failure. Although most children have diarrhea with starvation, the majority can be given liquids orally at the maintenance rate of 1500 ml./m²/day. We prefer to calculate fluid needs on the basis of m² rather than weight since fluid requirements are determined more accurately according to surface area. Also, in the older child, if requirements are calculated on a weight basis, fluid overload can occur if the figures for a smaller child are used. If calculation by weight is desired, then appropriate maintenance values can be determined and used for any particular weight group. By the end of a week of therapy the child should be able to take oral fluids ad lib.

In nonedematous severe PCM, fluid restriction is less critical since these children are more apt to be dehydrated with a contracted vascular space. Daily intake can be 2500 to 3000 ml./m²/day depending upon state of hydration.

Electrolytes. Chronic abnormal potassium losses result in marked hypokalemia. During this phase, oral K^+ can be given at a rate of 8 to 10 mEq./kg./day. If intravenous therapy is required because of diarrhea, a maximal K^+ concentration of 60 mEq./liter can be administered if urine output is adequate. Cardiac monitoring should also be carried out. Supplemental oral K^+ can be given to maintain K^+ intake at 8 mEq./kg./day.

In nonedematous PCM, potassium deficits may be less than in the edematous form. As a result, K^+ replacements of 4 to 6 mEq./kg./day are often adequate. Serum potassium should be monitored until replacement has been completed.

Magnesium losses in severe PCM may occur and may require 2 to 3 mEq./kg./day for replacement. Total body sodium, on the other hand, may be depleted or may actually be in excess in edematous PCM.

In edematous PCM, the physician should be careful not to overload the patient with sodium. Maintenance intakes of 2 to 3 mEq./kg./day are usually adequate. In nonedematous PCM, sodium requirements may be much greater. Monitoring of serum electrolytes during the initial therapy period should be performed. Appropriate adjustments of sodium intake can be made on the basis of serum sodium values.

Protein and Calories. During the first several days of therapy, protein and calories are introduced slowly. On days 1 and 2, 1.5 gm. of protein/kg./day are given. This is increased in a stepwise manner over the next three to four days until the child is taking 3.5 gm./kg./day. The child should then be receiving about 100 cal./kg./day. Whole milk provides the easiest form for administration of protein and calories. However, large volumes may result in excessive protein intake and the lactose can produce diarrhea as the result of a secondary lactase deficiency commonly seen in severe PCM. If lactose intolerance and diarrhea are problems, a nonlactose formula can be used.

As a general rule, the child with edematous PCM, after one week of therapy, should be taking 150 ml./kg./day of fluids orally. The daily (per kilogram) intake should contain 3.5 gm. of protein, 100 calories, 8 mEq. of potassium and less than 4 mEq. of sodium. A convenient mixture is 2 parts of whole cow's milk and 1 part of 15 per cent Dextri-Maltose with 110 mEq. K^+ /liter. Children with nonedematous PCM should be receiving similar intakes except that K^+ requirements may be less and Na^+ may be more.

Infection. Many children with severe PCM have infections, often of the gastrointestinal tract. We do not recommend prophylactic antibiotics but do suggest appropriate treatment of proven infections. The broad spectrum antibiotics tetracycline and chloramphenicol may retard recovery since the former causes a negative nitrogen balance and the latter decreases protein synthesis.

Miscellaneous. Hypoglycemia may complicate severe PCM because of decreased hepatic gluconeogenesis, less adrenal steroid production and lack of glycogen stores. As a result, glucose should always be administered during the initial phase. If the child develops metabolic acidosis or does not respond to the above regimen, the kidneys are evaluated since renal function may be abnormal in severe PCM.

In underdeveloped areas where milk is unavailable or too expensive, fish and vegetable protein supplements may be used instead, e.g., Incaparaina in South and Central America and Pronutro or Superamine in Africa.

Under conditions of hospital crowding, inadequate personnel to feed the children or a high risk of cross infections, outpatient management may be preferable to inpatient care.

Recovery Treatment

After the initial phase of one to two weeks, most children should be gaining weight well with ad lib oral feedings. The physician should expect an initial weight loss due to a decrease in edema. There may also be a transient drop in hemoglobin. Once the child is taking a balanced oral intake, he is probably receiving adequate vitamins and minerals. However, if vitamin preparations are available, they can be given at twice the recommended daily allowance. Daily vitamins D and A intake should be maintained at 800 I.U. and 1500 units during the recovery phase. Children with microcytic anemias should be treated with 6 mg./kg./day of elemental iron as ferrous sulfate.

MILD TO MODERATE PCM

The physical findings of mild to moderate PCM may be quite minimal, i.e., there may only be a decreased weight for age. Treatment of these children consists of supplying adequate protein and calories. During the first year of life approximately 100 calories/kg./day are required. Thereafter, caloric maintenance needs can be approximated according to the formula:

$$\text{Age in years} \times 100 + 1000 = \text{daily calories required.}$$

The distribution of calories should be approximately 10 to 15 per cent protein, 35 to 45 per cent fat and 35 to 45 per cent carbohydrate. If inadequate intake is the primary reason for the child's poor growth, recovery should be rapid once adequate protein and calories are available.

Obesity

MATTHEW M. STEINER, M.D.

Most obese children will not remain in treatment for obesity. Of those who stay in treatment, most will not lose weight; of those who do lose weight, most will regain it if followed long enough. Such sober experience emphasizes the need not only for early prevention of obesity but also for a more enlightened and realistic approach to the management of obesity in childhood.

PREVENTION OF OBESITY

The management of obesity in childhood starts in infancy! The infant at-risk for obesity often has the following background:

Families with one or both parents obese or with a history of obesity and/or diabetes, hyperlipidemia, hypercholesterolemia or vascular degenerative disease.

Disturbed parent-child relationship. Obese children frequently come from disorganized homes where little attention is paid to good family planning and where parents are insecure in their roles as mother and father.

Ethnic and socioeconomic factors play a definite role in the initiative and persistence of obesity. Attitudes concerning quality and quantity of food, even obesity itself, may differ from acceptable norms in our society. Socioeconomic factors can result in a sterile constricted environment with little internal or external stimulation for activities and interests. Food is then likely to become a major source of gratification. Such children often exhibit progressive obesity which is highly resistant to management.

Genetic and other influences. There is divergence of opinion as to whether obesity "runs" in families (genetic) or whether fat hypercellularity differs in families. There is also a good deal of evidence that fatness may be a learned experience for many children.

The physician can set up the following program of preventive measures in high-risk infants:

Education of parents, preferably in prenatal and early postnatal periods, concerning optimal nutrition, the role of calories and composition of food, and the understanding of long-term disadvantages and dangers of progressive obesity.

Instruction of parents in adequate nutrition for optimal weight and growth of the infant without excessive fat accumulation.

Employment of percentile growth charts to plot monthly increments and detect early excessive or accelerated weight gain.

Encourage breast feeding rather than formula feeding so that mothers do not become anxious and persist in having the infant always finish the prescribed amount of formula in the bottle.

Fluids other than extra milk should be offered between feedings. Because of their relatively large surface area infants are often thirsty; mothers mistake this restlessness for hunger rather than a need for more water.

Discouragement of too early solid food feeding. Feeding solids should be delayed beyond the third month since such foods not only add unnecessary calories but also increase the solute load on the kidney. For elimination of extra solutes, infants require extra water. When thirst is mistaken for hunger, and solids rather than water are administered, overfeeding results in a fat child who fails to discriminate between hunger and discomfort. This child later "uses" food as a solace for tensions and boredom.

In general, any program in infancy should be geared to *weight control* rather than *weight reduction*. Otherwise, we will have to deal with distraught parents of fussy babies whose linear growth may be compromised and with reduced chances for effecting a program of long-term weight control.

MANAGEMENT OF CHILDHOOD OBESITY

General Principles. Any medical regimen must be individualized since there is no "typical" fat child. The influence of family, ethnic, socioeconomic, environmental and hereditary factors must be recognized. Hence, we are concerned with the *whole* child, not just the obesity of the child.

Paramount in the management program, and often more important than the diet, is effecting some degree of behavior modification with a built-in system of rewards for weight control and with a mechanism for ensuring regular follow-up sessions over an extended period of time.

Anorexigenic drugs have no place in long-term weight control programs.

An attractive and well balanced dietary program should be used to effect gradual weight reduction (½ to 1 pound per week). Weight control should not compromise linear growth in young children.

Programs of physical and social activity should be adjusted to the socioeconomic and environmental milieu of the family. Many families cannot cooperate with routine prescriptions when there are no available playgrounds or social centers; areas are unsafe for unescorted children; distance to school makes walking dangerous; or opportunities for social contacts are lacking.

Development of responsibility must be fostered within the child for behavior modification, social and physical activities and diet management. Not unlike the approach to the child with diabetes mellitus, the greater the knowledge of nutrition and responsibility for daily activities, the greater the chance for long-term feedback and success.

Practical Management. In the initial interview with the child and parents, the physician should assign enough time to assess the family as to ethnic patterns, socioeconomic and environmental factors. Discussion should include an insight into family conflicts and sibling rivalries, school and peer problems, activities and interests of the child, and possible sources for realistic behavior modification both within the family and in the child's environment. Investigate trends and early conditions which brought about overfeeding and the present obesity. Ascertain attitudes of parents and siblings toward overeating and toward the obese child. What are the chances for family cooperation with a long-term program of changing life styles and dietary management? Discuss the program in general with specific emphasis on gradual behavior modification and long-term weight control.

After a complete physical examination, including neurologic and funduscopic evaluation, the weight should be plotted on a percentile chart (Iowa or Stuart). This should be explained to the parents and child without criticism so that they may understand the optimal weight and height for the age. It may also be appropriate at this time to allay the fears of the obese boy whose prominent breasts are laden with fat and whose diminutive genitalia are sunken within suprapubic fat.

"The How, When, Where, and What Diary." Prior to starting a weight reduction program, ask the child (with the parents' help, if necessary) to submit a three-week diary of food intake, caloric composition, and activity program. Indicate snack periods, day and night, and circumstances associated with urgency to eat between meals. A review of this diary during the second visit serves as the basis for behavior modification and meal planning.

Behavior Modification and Meal Planning. The diet, 1000 to 1200 calories, is adjusted to family and ethnic customs. Printed diets are available from Eli Lilly & Company (Indianapolis) as well as the Carnation Company (Box 610, Dept. 96, Pico Rivera, California 90665). I prefer the American Diabetes Association's Exchange Diet since it offers many choices for the finicky eater or for those who have avoided essential proteins and vegetables. Initially, we use a multivitamin supplement. Stress the use of free foods as snacks after school (e.g., raw vegetables, pickles, celery, lettuce) and avoidance of forbidden foods as bribes for good behavior. A portion of the dessert of the evening meal may be set aside for a snack before bedtime.

Continue the diary and indicate weekly menus with free snack foods and organized activities.

Advocate eating in the same room without television viewing or reading.

Stress the serving of measured single portions of food rather than family style eating in order to avoid the temptation of larger portions and second helpings.

Use smaller plates and include good portions of lettuce, celery and parsley as fillers.

Have the child eat slowly, chew the food well and place utensils down after several swallows. Do not put more food into the mouth until the first mouthful is chewed and swallowed.

The family should avoid table discussions about eating or tension-producing subjects. Attempt to get the parents "off the child's back" and avoid criticism from other members of the family.

Encourage praise for success in some weight loss and make no comment when success is not being achieved immediately.

Forbidden snacks and "goodies" should be eliminated as much as possible. Avoid high caloric condiments—mayonnaise, ketchup, steak sauces and gravies.

Avoid special "miracle" or health fad foods.

Do not skip meals. If the meal is delayed, rely on earlier feeding or free snack foods.

Avoid getting overtired or overhungry with the tendency to overeat or grab high caloric snacks.

In addition, it has been helpful to construct a weight chart on simple graph paper. Using "Weight" as the vertical axis and "Weeks" on the horizontal axis, a straight line depicts the loss at one pound per week. The child should be weighed two or three times weekly and the weight plotted against the declining weight curve.

With the help of the family, the physician can organize a regular program of activity especially after school and during weekends. Stress walking to and from school, enrollment in gym, swimming classes or social activities—any type of program which would substitute for periods of tension or boredom. Positive attitudes at home toward the weight reduction program with overt encouragement from parents and family members are valuable and serve to get the whole family interested in helping the obese child.

Vitamin Deficiencies and Excesses

LAURENCE FINBERG, M.D.

Vitamin deficiency rarely presents in the United States; hence, treatment has become uncommon. Prevention by better dietary advice or in some circumstances by administering vitamins continues to be important for all pediatricians. The easy commercial availability of vitamins makes abuse possible. Clinically significant excess does occur and may warrant corrective measures. Prevention, treating deficiency, and treating or managing the toxicity of overdosage are discussed. For convenience, the fat soluble group, vitamins A, D, E, and K, of special importance in malabsorptive states, is discussed first, followed by the miscellaneous group of water soluble substances.

FAT SOLUBLE VITAMINS

Vitamin A (Retinol). Diets containing butterfat, pigmented vegetables, egg yolks or fortified and skim milk accounting for 15 to 20 per cent of calories will contain sufficient vitamin A to meet the recommended daily requirement of 2000 units for infants or 5000 units for older children. Patients with chronic malabsorption (e.g., cystic fibrosis) should receive 10,000 to 15,000 units daily in a water-miscible vehicle. A similar daily dose for several weeks will correct deficiency.

Overdosage, 200,000 units over a day or two or over 30,000 units daily for an extended time, results in either acute or chronic toxicity. The limiting factor in physiologic protection against toxicity is the capacity of a specific plasma protein to bind retinol. When such capacity is exceeded toxicity occurs; thus, incapacity of the liver, which forms the binding protein, creates susceptibility to poisoning. For either the acute form with increased intracranial pressure and vomiting or the chronic form with generalized periosteal overgrowth, symptomatic measures are all that are available. In almost all instances, recovery is fairly rapid.

Vitamin D (Cholecalciferol and Analogues). The recommended daily allowance of 400 I.U. per day prevents rickets in infants. (A separate section on rickets deals with that disorder in greater depth.) Overdosage with vitamin D occurs at levels of from 10 times the daily dosage in the most vulnerable up to about 40,000 I.U. per day, which probably is universally toxic if absorbed. The complex of steroid hydroxylating enzymes in the liver which both activate (25 OH vitamin D, the precursor of the active hormone, 1,25 dihydroxy D formed in the kidney) and detoxify (by making the molecules more polar and excretable), probably determine the individual vulnerability of patients.

Toxicity is secondary to hypercalcemia which in turn produces vomiting, hypertension and encephalopathy. Management includes immediate withdrawal of all vitamin D intake, furosemide, 2 to 3 mg./kg. several times in 48 hours to promote rapid urinary excretion, and prednisone (or similar corticosteroid), 2 mg./kg./day (up to 80 mg. per day) for up to several weeks. In addition to these measures, symptomatic therapy may also be required on an individual basis.

Vitamin E (α-Tocopherol). This essential nutrient occurs widely in nature and need not be supplemented except in the prematurely born infant, in malabsorptive states and probably in individuals receiving a high proportion of calories from polyunsaturated fat. The recommended dose for infants is 2 to 10 mg. (I.U.) daily. Data concerning toxicity are confusing but certainly no major problem has been described. Megadosage has not proved of value for any of a variety of conditions.

Vitamin K (Menadione and Related Compounds). The newborn infant should be given 1 mg. of vitamin K_1 at birth to obviate failure of production of clotting factors by the liver. Subsequently, the diet and intestinal bacteria provide adequate vitamin K except in those with fat malabsorption who may require daily supplementation of 1 to 2 mg./day.

Toxicity seems limited to the newborn period when overdosage of menadione has resulted in displacement of bilirubin from binding sites and increased likelihood of kernicterus. No specific treatment exists; avoidance of excess dosage is mandatory.

WATER SOLUBLE VITAMINS

Thiamine (B_1). This water soluble compound is found widely in nature so that deficiency is unlikely. However, a polished rice diet or one high in calories from ethanol may reduce the intake below the daily requirement of

0.5 mg. for infants and 1.5 mg. for adults. In that rare event, the result is cardiomyopathy with heart failure and neuropathy, known as beri-beri. Treatment is with thiamine, 5 to 10 mg. daily, parenterally or orally depending on degree of illness.

Riboflavin (B_2). This vitamin is a widely distributed substance and deficiency states are rare. The compound does enhance photosensitivity and will enter into any reactions involving increased light energy absorption by accelerating the biochemical effects. No specific toxic clinical disorders have been described.

Pyridoxine (B_6). Requirements of this vitamin vary from 0.4 mg. for infants to 1.6 mg. daily for adolescents. Deficiency has occurred only when dietary milk formula was subjected to excessive heat. A peculiar result of high dosages in pregnant women (for nausea) may be pyridoxine dependence in the infant. There are also rare inborn errors of metabolism which require high dosage of pyridoxine. For most of these unusual conditions 10 to 20 mg. daily gives maximum benefit. No serious toxicity is known.

Niacin. This vitamin, for which tryptophan may be substituted, prevents pellagra. The recommended dosage, assuming low tryptophan intake, is 8 mg./day for infants, up to 20 mg. for adolescents. In treating pellagra, 100 mg./day of niacinamide provides rapid recovery. No serious toxicity is known.

Folacin. The recommended daily dosage is small, ranging from 0.05 mg./day in infants to 0.4 mg./day in adolescents. Patients who have rapid bone marrow turnover (chronic hemolytic anemias) may have a greater need in order to prevent megaloblastic anemia. Certain anticonvulsive drugs, such as phenytoin or primidone, may increase requirement also. Deficiency states are adequately corrected with dosages of 5 mg./day.

Cyanocobalamin (B_{12}). The requirement of B_{12} is normally less than 1 μg./day. However, if there is congenital (rare) or acquired lack of gastric intrinsic factor or an intestinal disorder blocking absorption of the B_{12} intrinsic factor complex, deficiency results. When this occurs, intramuscular injection of 25 to 50 μg. per month is corrective.

Vitamin C (Ascorbic Acid). The recommended daily dose is 30 mg./day for infants and 60 mg. for adolescents; even less will effectively prevent scurvy. Ascorbic acid is not found in sufficient amounts in cow's milk and should be supplemented daily if neither fortified feedings nor natural fruits are given. Once the infant has progressed to a liberal in-take of fruits and vegetables, no further supplement is required. Large (1500 mg./day) doses have been tried for prevention of infection and for other reasons without notable success. Toxicity is not common but may occur in the form of oxalate renal stones or, when renal impairment is present, as acidemia. The homeostatic protection from ascorbic acid overdosage is excretion of the ascorbate in the urine. When large amounts are given the compound is simply excreted, since the total body pool of ascorbic acid will not exceed 2.5 to 3.0 gm., and any additional given becomes overflow in the urine. Impaired renal function prevents this protective mechanism.

Total Parenteral Nutrition in Infants

WILLIAM C. HEIRD, M.D.

Total parenteral nutrition, first described approximately 10 years ago, has been used widely in many areas of medicine. In pediatrics the technique has been used largely in patients requiring multiple operative procedures for correction of congenital anomalies of the gastrointestinal tract and in patients with intractable diarrhea. It has also been used in the nutritional management of low birth weight infants, but its efficacy in this particular group of patients is not as well established.

Although the technique has been responsible for a marked reduction in mortality of patients with surgically corrected anomalies of the gastrointestinal tract (such as gastroschisis) as well as patients with intractable diarrhea, the presence of an indwelling catheter increases the likelihood of infection, while the complex nutritional mixture results in a large number of metabolic complications. An unacceptable incidence of both groups of complications results largely from the usual tendency to "hang" the nutrient infusate once the catheter is in place and "wait for the infant to start growing." In addition to possible deleterious effects upon the patient, this approach leads inevitably to total disenchantment with the technique. On the other hand, with realization that the technique requires careful and rigid control, both groups of complications can be controlled sufficiently to allow patients requiring this therapy to benefit maximally from it. Only with such understanding can the technique assume its proper role as an adjunct in nutritional management of pediatric patients with deranged gastrointestinal function.

The concentrated nutrient mixture must

be infused continuously and at a constant rate. While many reliable and relatively simple pumps are available to assure constant infusion, none is completely foolproof. Thus the patient receiving total parenteral nutrition requires close observation by personnel who are aware of the technique's complexities. Such observation is rarely available outside of an intensive care unit. The optimal environment is a small unit in which only patients receiving total parenteral nutrition are housed. However, the small number of patients who require total parenteral nutrition at any one time makes such an arrangement infeasible for most hospitals. Nonetheless, if the technique is to be used successfully, areas that provide at least semi-acute nursing care must be made available.

Once the complexities of total parenteral nutrition are realized, the technique can be used to produce weight gain and positive nitrogen balance until gastrointestinal function is recovered. Weight gains of 7 to 20 gm./kg./day and nitrogen balances of 100 to 250 mg./kg./day can be expected with this form of nutrient management, provided the regimen delivers 110 to 125 cal./kg./day and approximately 2.5 gm. of amino acids/kg./day. In general, the higher values are observed in patients who experience little or no stress during the technique (such as patients with intractable diarrhea), whereas the lower values are observed in patients requiring multiple operative procedures or experiencing episodes of sepsis or other stress during total parenteral nutrition.

The Nutrient Infusate. The requirements for any infusate serving as the sole nutrient source include amino acids, calories, electrolytes, minerals and vitamins. A suitable infusate is depicted in Table 1.

Two general sources of amino acids are available—hydrolysates of either fibrin or casein or crystalline amino acid mixtures. Both provide essential as well as nonessential amino acids, although none of the currently available preparations contains an ideal mixture of amino acids. While there is no evidence for increased efficacy of one type of preparation over the other, the crystalline amino acid mixtures allow administration of a more rigidly controlled amino acid intake. Whichever is used, the amino acid intake should approximate 2.5 gm./kg./day. Doses of 4 gm./kg./day were used initially; however, neither nitrogen balance nor weight gain is significantly better with this intake than with an intake of 2.5 gm./kg./day. Further, the fact that azotemia is observed frequently with the higher intake suggests that it is excessive. While use of any of the available preparations results in positive

TABLE 1. Composition of a Suitable Parenteral Nutrient Infusate

COMPONENT	AMOUNT (PER KG. DAILY)
Nitrogen source (hydrolysate or crystalline amino acid mixture)	2.5 gm.
Glucose*	25–30 gm.
Sodium (NaCl)	3 to 4 mEq.
Potassium†	2 to 3 mEq.
Calcium (Ca gluconate)	0.5 to 1.0 mEq.
Magnesium (MgSO₄)	0.25 mEq.
Chloride	3 to 4 mEq.
Phosphorus*	2 mM.
M.V.I.‡	1 ml.
TOTAL VOLUME	120 to 130 ml.

*Glucose can be reduced depending on amount of intravenous fat emulsion used. Amount provided on initial day should not exceed 15 gm./kg./day (see text).

†Hyperphosphatemia often develops when more than 2 mM./kg./day is used; thus, if potassium intake of more than 2 mEq./kg./day is required, a mixture of KCl and KH₂PO₄ should be used.

‡Multi-Vitamin Infusion, U.S. Pharmaceutical, Tuckahoe, New York. This preparation (1 ml.) contains adequate amounts of all required vitamins except folic acid and vitamins B₁₂ and K. These can be added to the daily infusate (5 μg. of vitamin B₁₂, 50 μg. of folic acid and 500 μg. of vitamin K); alternatively vitamins B₁₂ and K can be given by intramuscular injections.

nitrogen balance, none results in an absolutely normal plasma aminogram.

Fructose, or a mixture of glucose and fructose, is sometimes used as a caloric source; however, the most commonly used agent is glucose alone. Intravenous fat preparations have been used for a number of years outside the United States and have recently become available for use in this country. While use of a sufficient amount of these preparations to supply essential fatty acid requirements (such as 2 to 5 per cent of the total caloric intake) appears warranted, use of larger amounts cannot be unequivocally recommended at the present time. Although lipid doses of up to 4 gm./kg./day have been used without apparent complications, the tolerance of intravenous lipid from infant to infant is unpredictable and quite variable; thus, while some infants may tolerate up to 4 gm./kg./day, or even more, others may tolerate only a fraction of this amount.

Failure to metabolize the intravenous fat emulsion results in accumulation of the emulsion in the blood stream. Such accumulation, in both human volunteers and animals, results in decreased pulmonary diffusion capacity. On the other hand, complete metabolism of the infused emulsion results in increased plasma levels of free fatty acids, which can displace albumin-bound bilirubin. In vitro studies suggest that the plasma levels of free fatty acids necessary to displace bilirubin from albumin are unlikely to occur, even with infusion of large amounts of these agents; nonetheless, this possibility remains a serious consideration, particularly in icteric infants.

Another reason preventing unequivocal recommendation for use of intravenous fat emulsions is the possibility that a fat calorie, although equivalent to a carbohydrate calorie with respect to energy, is not equivalent to a carbohydrate calorie with respect to nitrogen sparing. Thus, even though intravenous fat emulsions could be safely used to increase total caloric intake, such use may not result in better nitrogen retention unless "adequate" carbohydrate (which cannot be defined) is provided as well.

Another concern with respect to use of intravenous fat emulsions concerns the effect of these agents on plasma lipid levels—for example, the plasma concentration of both triglyceride and cholesterol increase at least transiently with infusion of fat emulsions. In addition, pigment granules are routinely observed in the reticuloendothelial system of both patients and animals that receive these preparations.

Electrolyte, mineral and vitamin content of the infusate can be provided in the form of various additives. Electrolytes are usually added in amounts approximating established oral or intravenous maintenance requirements. Since most minerals are incompletely absorbed from the gastrointestinal tract, the parenteral needs for these are significantly less than oral needs. Thus the amounts supplied rarely exceed half of the usual oral recommendations. Adequate information concerning the parenteral requirements (or need) for trace minerals is lacking; thus, these nutrients are usually not provided, a potentially serious omission. While parenteral vitamin requirements are likely to be different from oral requirements, the usually recommended daily oral allowances for most vitamins are provided.

The nutrient infusate should be prepared frequently (daily or every other day) under laminar flow by a pharmacist or similar individual trained in aseptic additive techniques. Rather than use a standard mixture for all patients, the content of each patient's daily infusate should be determined by a physician after careful assessment of the patient's clinical and biochemical status. Most infants can tolerate the suggested amino acid intake on the first day of parenteral feeding, but few if any can tolerate the full caloric intake initially, especially if the total caloric requirement is provided as glucose.

The initial daily infusate should deliver 2.5 gm./kg./day of amino acids but only 10 to 15 gm./kg./day of glucose. The glucose content can then be increased gradually to a level of 25 to 30 gm./kg./day in accordance with the patient's tolerance of glucose and the amount of intravenous lipid being used. Rarely can full caloric maintenance from glucose alone be achieved in less than 4 or 5 days. In low birth weight infants the time required is closer to 10 to 14 days. Intravenous fat emulsions may help somewhat in this regard, but the variable tolerance for lipid makes the extent of this help unpredictable. Small doses of insulin (0.25 to 0.5 μ/kg.) have been used to increase glucose tolerance, but there is no evidence that such therapy is of particular benefit.

Catheter Insertion and Care. See also p. 10. Specific steps for catheter insertion by the jugular vein are as follows:

1. The child is appropriately restrained, the hair is shaved from the scalp and both the scalp and neck are prepared with a standard surgical preparation.

2. A skin incision is made in the neck and the external or internal jugular vein is exposed.

3. A silicone rubber (Silastic) catheter of appropriate size is inserted into the vein, directed into the mid to lower portion of the superior vena cava and fixed in place with ligatures. The length of catheter that should be inserted is approximately equal to the distance from the neck incision to the second intercostal space.

4. Before proceeding further, the position of the catheter tip should be verified radiographically. If a radiopaque catheter is not available, contrast material (approx. 0.5 ml.) must be injected aseptically into the catheter.

5. After the catheter is in proper position and secured, the proximal portion is directed subcutaneously to exit through the parietal scalp, just behind and above the ear. The subcutaneous tunneling is accomplished by threading the catheter onto a modified Kirschner wire or by directing it through the lumen of a large bore Vim-Silverman needle. When the wire or needle is removed, the catheter remains enclosed in a long subcutaneous tunnel.

6. The catheter is secured to the scalp with a ligature and the neck wound is closed, usually with fine nylon sutures.

7. An antimicrobial ointment (such as Betadine) is applied to both the catheter exit site and the neck wound. A sterile occlusive dressing is applied to the catheter exit site, and a regular dressing is applied to the neck wound.

8. After inserting a 0.22μ membrane filter between the catheter and the administration tubing, the nutrient infusate is delivered continuously and at a constant rate using a constant infusion pump.

Regular meticulous care of the central venous catheter is mandatory for prolonged, safe, and complication-free use. The catheter must never be used for purposes other than delivery of the nutrient infusate (such as blood transfusions or blood sampling). The catheter exit site should be dressed at least three times per week. On each such occasion, the occlusive dressing is removed and the skin area is cleaned with defatting and antiseptic agents. The antiseptic ointment should then be reapplied, followed by a fresh occlusive dressing. With meticulous care, a single catheter can be used safely for up to 90 days. The average life of a catheter, however, is closer to 30 days.

Complications. See p. 11. Most metabolic complications can be prevented or detected early if an adequate biochemical monitoring schedule is rigidly followed (Table 2).

Team Approach. The approach to total parenteral nutrition that has been described is a team approach. Most institutions at which the technique has been used successfully have established a team approach. The team consists of a physician, who is primarily responsible for overseeing the entire program. Other key members of the team include a nurse, who assists the physician in all aspects of the program, a pharmacist or technician trained in aseptic additive techniques and responsive microbiological and microbiochemical laboratories. Such laboratories are necessary for detection and diagnosis of infections and metabolic complications. The exact makeup of the team will differ from institution to institution. Such

minor details are unimportant; the important fact is that a team is mandatory if successful total parenteral nutrition is to be achieved.

Despite the efficacy of total parenteral nutrition in some groups of pediatric patients, the long-term effects have not been assessed nor can they be assessed until the experience with the technique increases. Until more experience is available, careful attention must be directed toward patient selection to assure that patients in whom nutritional management can be achieved by other methods are not subjected unnecessarily to a technique that might have deleterious long-term effects. However, in patients with markedly deranged or absent gastrointestinal function, the immediate positive results of total parenteral nutrition when applied correctly seem to outweigh consideration of potentially harmful long-term effects.

Long-Term Total Parenteral Nutrition

THOMAS J. EGAN, M.D.

Malnutrition for a prolonged period increases mortality in infants and children with disease in the gastrointestinal tract. Some of these lesions can be approached surgically, but the general physical deterioration secondary to inanition at the time of diagnosis makes surgical procedures very hazardous. Similarly, some patients with chronic diarrhea develop a state of malnutrition which can reach a point where normal body repair processes cannot take place. Eight years ago, Dudrick and coworkers first showed that normal growth and weight gain could be achieved through the intravenous infusion of an amino acid-glucose solution. Since that time, use of this technique has become more widespread with sufficient success to warrant its continued use in selected patients. Initially, the technique required insertion of a central venous catheter and infusion of the very hypertonic feeding solution into a large central vein. In recent years, two new approaches to total parenteral nutrition have been described. One technique involves the infusion of fat solutions along with glucose and amino acids into peripheral veins, thus avoiding the need for a central venous catheter. Because the intravenous fat solution was not commercially available in the United States until 1976, a technique of total parenteral nutrition through a peripheral vein without using lipids has been tried with success. Development of these techniques utilizing peripheral veins

TABLE 2. Suggested Monitoring Schedule During Total Parenteral Nutrition

VARIABLES TO BE MONITORED	SUGGESTED FREQUENCY (TIMES PER WEEK)*	
	Initial Period	*Later Period*
Plasma electrolyte	3 or 4	2 or 3
Blood urea nitrogen	3	2
Plasma calcium, magnesium, phosphorus	3	2
Blood glucose†		
Blood acid-base status	3 or 4	2 or 3
Blood ammonia	2	1
Serum protein (electrophoresis or albumin/globulin)	1	1
Liver function studies	1	1
Hemoglobin	2	2
Urine glucose	7 (daily)	14 (twice daily)
Clinical observations (activity, temperature, etc.)	7 (daily)	7 (daily)
WBC count and differential	As indicated	As indicated
Cultures	As indicated	As indicated

*Initial period is the period before full glucose intake is achieved or any period of metabolic instability. Later period is the period during which the patient is in a metabolic steady state.

†Blood glucose should be monitored closely during periods of glucosuria (to determine the degree of hyperglycemia) and for 2 or 3 days following cessation of parenteral nutrition (to detect hypoglycemia). In the latter instance, frequent Dextrostix determination constitutes adequate screening.

has decreased the rate of complications and allowed use of the technique in a much wider variety of pediatric feeding problems.

INDICATIONS

Total parenteral nutrition should be reserved for infants and children whose lives are endangered because feeding by the gastrointestinal tract is not possible, is inadequate or inadvisable. Criteria for selection of suitable patients include reasonable expectation for eventual return or development of enough gastrointestinal function to support life and the absence of associated incurable disease states in which heroic efforts to maintain life may be contraindicated.

Total parenteral nutrition found its earliest use in the management of surgical problems including chronic intestinal obstruction, peritoneal sepsis, bowel fistulas, intestinal resections with residual inadequate intestinal length, and omphalocele repairs. Prior to total parenteral nutrition, many patients with these conditions succumbed during the postoperative period as a direct or indirect consequence of malnutrition. From this beginning, the treatment was extended to other patients with chronic nutritional problems including severe chronic diarrhea, extensive body burns, and chronic inflammatory bowel disease. Total parenteral nutrition has been used to treat uremia and hyperkalemia of acute renal failure with a consequent reduction of need for dialysis.

With increasing experience and knowledge and the advent of new intravenous feeding preparations and techniques, total and supplementary parenteral nutrition has been used in very small premature infants when oral feedings cannot meet nutritional needs for satisfactory growth and weight gain.

There remain enough known and unknown hazards to make it imperative that good clinical judgment be used in choosing candidates for such therapy. Total parenteral nutrition should not be used when nutrients can be absorbed from the gastrointestinal tract. The introduction of elemental diets, when tolerated, has reduced the number of patients who might require total parenteral nutrition. However, the ability to use this technique by peripheral vein has reduced morbidity considerably and permits its increasing application to clinical nutritional problems.

Total parenteral nutrition should not be attempted in any setting lacking skilled medical, nursing, and pharmacist supervision. Laboratory facilities must be constantly available to monitor treatment.

METHODS

Preparation of the formulas for total parenteral nutrition is dealt with elsewhere in this text. Formulations should be selected to suit the individual requirements of each patient depending on size, stage of maturity, and clinical conditions which may modify the metabolic turnover of various nutritional components. Infusion rates are calculated to provide approximately 100 to 150 ml. water/kg./24 hours, 2 to 5 gm. of protein/kg./24 hours, and about 100 cal./kg./24 hours. Intakes in this range have been shown to result in reasonable weight gain and positive nitrogen balance. While the base solution contains some minerals, additional amounts of sodium and potassium salts may be required. Required amounts of these electrolytes are similar to oral requirements, but other minerals such as calcium, phosphorus and magnesium are much less than oral requirements because only a fraction of the oral intake would be absorbed. Vitamins are usually added to the daily solution. Data are lacking concerning parenteral vitamin requirements and care should be taken to guard against overdosage of vitamins A and D in particular. Iron requirements can be met by either blood transfusion or intramuscular injections of iron dextran. There are three basic techniques of total parenteral nutrition—central feeding, and peripheral feeding with and without fat.

Central Feeding. Prior to the introduction of intravenous fat feedings, adequate caloric content could be achieved only by the addition of large quantities of glucose in the solution. The resulting solution is very hypertonic and must be given by a constant infusion pump through a central venous catheter placed in a large vein. The usual procedure consists of passage of a silicone rubber catheter through the internal or external jugular vein to the superior vena cava. To minimize the danger of blood stream infection, the catheter is placed in a skin tunnel at the point of entry and exits through a scalp wound several centimeters away. The location of the catheter tip must be established roentgenographically. The procedure is best performed in an operating room under local or general anesthesia, and strict aseptic technique is mandatory. Silicone rubber catheters were selected to minimize irritation to vessel walls, but they are soft and easily occluded by malpositioning or improper suture placement around the vein. A well inserted catheter can remain in place for several weeks without replacement. (See also p. 8.)

Antibiotics should not be given prophylactically but may be required in treatment of the infant's or child's primary disease. A millipore filter is placed in the intravenous line to remove any particulate matter or microorganisms in the solution itself. The feeding solution is an excellent culture medium and, in spite of the best precautions, can easily become contaminated. It is good practice to change solution bottles and intravenous tubing every 24 hours and to restrict wound care and blood sampling by the catheter to a minimum number of well trained personnel. Part of the tubing which cannot be exchanged and the wound area itself are frequently cleansed with povidone-iodine solution or ointment because of its effectiveness against both bacteria and fungi.

Peripheral Feeding with Fat. The recent availability of a commercial intravenous fat feeding (Intralipid) has allowed total parenteral nutrition to be administered without a central venous catheter. Fat has a high caloric density (9 cal./gm.) and exerts no osmotic effect; therefore, the amount of glucose required in the infusate can be reduced considerably. Two parallel infusion systems are required; one bottle contains the fat emulsion and the other contains the amino acids, glucose, minerals and vitamins. Individual infusion pumps are required since each solution must be infused at an independent rate. The parallel systems should join in a Y connection as close as possible to the entry point since prolonged mixing of the two solutions can lead to deterioration of the fat emulsion. The resultant solution is isotonic and can be infused through a peripheral vein by needle rather than by an indwelling catheter. Even a scalp vein needle can be used in small infants. The millipore filter must be omitted from the final intravenous line since the fat emulsion cannot pass.

Peripheral Feeding without Fat. This technique, developed prior to the general availability of intravenous fat emulsion, came into use in an effort to avoid the significant complications of using a central venous catheter. The use of a peripheral vein required marked reduction of total osmolarity of the infusate by reduction of amino acid, and glucose concentration. The final solution contains approximately 0.56 cal./ml. compared with about 0.9 cal./ml. in the hypertonic central catheter infusion fluid. Thus a larger volume of fluid must be infused by peripheral vein to provide a similar caloric intake to that provided by central catheter infusions.

OBSERVATIONS OF RESPONSE

It is important to monitor the adequacy of treatment during total parenteral nutrition by recording daily body weight, accurate intake and output of fluids, and weekly estimations of serum electrolytes and blood cell counts. More frequent monitoring will be required if the patient has impaired liver or renal function. Patients should show a steady weight gain after an initial plateau period of about two weeks in debilitated infants or small children. Weight gains vary but may range between 20 and 30 gm./day in the neonate, which is almost comparable to rates of gain expected from oral feedings.

During the first day or two of feeding, the large glucose load can lead to glucosuria and an osmotic diuresis. Sometimes it is necessary to use a half-strength solution to initiate therapy. The body quickly adapts to the increased glucose load, and full-strength solution will be well tolerated in 48 to 72 hours.

COMPLICATIONS

Complications can be divided broadly into three categories—septic, metabolic, and technical.

Septic Complications. The major drawback of the earliest techniques of total parenteral nutrition through a central venous catheter has been the high rate of blood stream infection. Organisms can gain access by the catheter or by contaminated solutions. As a foreign body in the vascular channels, the catheter becomes a prime target for bacterial growth. Unexplained fever, leukocytosis, or the appearance of glycosuria after the first two or three days of treatment may herald the onset of sepsis. While in various patient series the incidence of sepsis has ranged from 16 to 27 per cent, the mortality rate is much lower. Candida infections are most common and a variety of gram-positive and gram-negative organisms have been implicated in various reports. The infection is often low-grade, and withdrawing the catheter often clears the blood stream infection without antibiotic treatment, particularly in the case of Candida infections. The lowest rates of sepsis have occurred in centers in which stringent precautions have been taken to minimize external contamination.

While septic complications have been reduced by techniques which eliminate the need for a central venous catheter, there remains an appreciable risk in patients receiving total parenteral nutrition by a peripheral vein and continued meticulous aseptic techniques must be employed.

Metabolic Complications. Hyperglycemia has been observed during the first 2 or 3 days of infusion of hypertonic glucose, and infusion rates and/or concentration must be adjusted to avoid osmotic dehydration. Such intolerance can persist in low birth weight premature infants, and may occasionally make it necessary to discontinue total parenteral nutrition. The advent of fat infusions has almost eliminated this hazard but, as usual, brings new problems to the fore.

Hyperlipidemia can occur with infusions of Intralipid if plasma clearance rates are exceeded. The clearance rate is dependent on lipoprotein lipase activity. Premature infants demonstrate a slower clearance rate and plasma Intralipid levels may rise producing visible lactescence and hyperlipidemia. While adults, children, and term infants can usually assimilate 3 to 5 gm./kg./day, lower rates of infusion may be required in the small premature infant. It is good procedure to monitor serum by nephelometry to keep Intralipid levels below 100 mg. per 100 ml. The use of heparin to promote Intralipid clearance by activation and release of lipoprotein lipase is not recommended as there may be deleterious effects on the myocardium.

Intralipid should be avoided in jaundiced infants as the free fatty acids released by hydrolysis can displace unconjugated bilirubin from albumin-binding sites increasing the risk of kernicterus. Anaphylactic reactions experienced with earlier fat emulsions have not been described. Most patients develop an eosinophilia but it does not appear to be harmful. Since Intralipid is rich in polyunsaturated fatty acids, essential fatty acid deficiency seen with fat-free central venous catheter feedings is no longer a problem. If Intralipid cannot be used, it has been shown that the daily application of sunflower seed oil to the chest of infants can prevent or treat essential fatty acid deficiency.

Other reported metabolic complications have included abnormal serum concentrations of sodium, potassium, magnesium, chloride, phosphate, and calcium, and at least weekly monitoring of serum levels is a necessity. Some earlier amino acid formulations caused metabolic acidosis, hyperammonemia, or worrisome elevations of specific serum amino acids. Adjustment of the amino acid formulations has solved most of these problems. Hypocupremia and zinc deficiency has been noted on occasion and addition of trace metals to basic solutions has been advocated. It is important to point out that there are undoubtedly new metabolic hazards yet to be discovered and clinical vigilance is mandatory.

Technical Complications. The central venous catheter technique has many hazards such as venous perforation, transitory cardiac arrhythmias, kinking producing obstruction, thrombophlebitis and thrombosis. Phlebitis is minimal when silicone rubber catheters are used. Hypertonic fluids given in peripheral veins do cause phlebitis but the almost isotonic Intralipid solution has been well tolerated. More problems occur when calcium ions are deposited interstitially when the peripheral vein needle is accidentally dislodged. Frequent monitoring of flow can minimize the occurrence of tissue slough.

2

Mental and Emotional Disturbances

Mental Retardation

ARNOLD J. CAPUTE, M.D., M.P.H.,
and PASQUALE J. ACCARDO, M.D.

Mental retardation occupies a prominent place in the spectrum of chronic handicapping conditions of childhood, both as a primary disorder and as a complication of numerous other neuropathologic syndromes. The early diagnosis and long-term management of this disability is perhaps the most challenging task for the pediatrician as developmentalist. Those who undertake to accept this challenge must be prepared to work in cooperation with numerous medical and paramedical disciplines, to interpret to the parents the complex shades of difference inherent in these various approaches, and ultimately, as the primary advocate for the child and his family, to resolve the various cross purposes frequently evident in bureaucratically organized services. The pediatrician's willingness to involve himself in what at first appears to be a totally nonmedical and time-consuming field of endeavor receives one of its strongest supports from a long historical legacy in which all the great innovators in the realm of retardation were themselves physicians of the first order—Itard, Seguin, Howe, Ireland, Langdon Down and Montessori. But what most fits the pediatrician for his preeminent role in mental retardation is his long training in the phenomena of both normal and abnormal development, an experience unique in its comprehensiveness compared with the more limited scope of the other professions involved in the management of retardation.

If the concept of treatment were taken in its most limited sense as a cure of disease, a total eradication of underlying pathology, then this chapter would be at an end. Except for a few metabolic disorders (e.g., phenylketonuria, galactosemia, cretinism, maple syrup urine disease, and certain abnormalities of ammonia metabolism), "treatment" of retardation is virtually nonexistent; prevention of other selected disorders through genetic counseling, amniocentesis, and therapeutic abortion presents an ever lengthening list of "treatable" diseases which, unfortunately, account for only a minute fraction (less than 10 per cent) of the retarded population. It would reflect an unrealistic optimism to expect this rough statistic to change appreciably in the next generation. An admirable goal, prevention nevertheless remains distinct from treatment.

If, however, a broader and somewhat older concept of treatment is employed, the physician assumes the responsibility of caring for the whole patient and of educating family and community as to the nature of the disorder and the method of its habilitation. It is within the context of this latter concept of treatment as caring rather than curing that the following pages will depict the pediatrician in the role of an educator entering into a chronic therapeutic dialogue with the family of the retarded

Supported in part through Project 917, Maternal and Child Health Service, Department of Health, Education and Welfare.

Page 13

child. In so doing, some of the wiser developmental insights of psychiatry, psychology and education will be seen to return to the medical source of their original impetus. With upwards of 30 trained personnel for each handicapped child and perhaps twice as many involved professions, the skilled pediatrician emerges as the only individual with a background of sufficient breadth to qualify in the role of primary manager.

DEFINITIONS

Mental retardation refers to a significantly subaverage general intellectual functioning existing concurrently with deficits in adaptive behavior, and manifested during the developmental period (AAMD 1973). Although mental retardation is a symptom rather than a disease, the infrequency with which an underlying etiology is identified justifies its usage as a primary diagnostic label.

In the absence of an independently valid measure of adaptive behavior (the Vineland Social Maturity Scale yields social quotients consistently 10 to 20 points higher than simultaneously administered intelligence quotients), retardation is reduced to an individual's performance on a standard intelligence test, properly administered by a professional experienced in the evaluation of deviant children. This last qualification cannot be overstressed; many dramatic variations in IQ scores can be attributed to improperly performed tests. A mislabeled psychometric category can at times be more damaging to a child than an erroneous medical diagnosis.

The grades of mental retardation are defined by the number of standard deviations ($\sigma = 15$ points on the Wechsler scales) from the mean IQ of 100. Although almost all current intelligence tests are based on this refined statistical concept of a standard deviation for each age level tested, the older developmental quotient (DQ = mental age ÷ chronologic age × 100) offers a rule of thumb quite useful. Borderline individuals (IQ range 84 to 70) are educationally slow learners, children whose retardation is obvious only in an academic setting; as adults in a technological society they may experience significant difficulty blending into the normal population unless adequate support services (educational and later vocational) are available. Mildly retarded individuals (IQ range 69 to 55) are referred to etiologically as sociocultural or familial (polygenic) retardates; educationally they are classified as educably mentally retarded (EMR). The goals for the EMR still include both social competence and economic independence.

The IQ of 55 represents a significant demarcation point: 5/6 of the retarded population are above this level, only 1/6 fall below it. Those patients with an IQ greater than 55 are unlikely to have an identifiable organic etiology, whereas with an IQ below 55 a chromosomal, genetic, metabolic or encephalopathic etiology is much more probable. Retardation less than IQ 55 associated with either short stature or some other major organ system malformation is an indication for chromosome studies; the

advisability of banding needs to be discussed with local laboratory facilities.

Moderate mental retardation (IQ range 54 to 40) comprises the group referred to educationally as trainable mental retardates (TMR); the severe (IQ range 39 to 25) and profound (IQ range below 25) retardates are classed educationally as subtrainables (SMR, PMR). The ordinate on the right of the accompanying figure gives approximate levels of academic achievement to be expected for each age and level of mental retardation. Since it is apparent from this graph that the high trainable child will not achieve functional literacy (i.e., 4th grade reading comprehension level), it is a tragic waste to spend more than a decade of schooling attempting to instill basic academic skills to the exclusion of the needed self-help, vocational and social skills.

Psychological theories in vogue are understandably hostile to the narrowness of a purely psychometric concept of cognition, but unfortunately they extend this critical attitude to the point of considering intellectual and adaptive function as completely environmentally determined. The truth in this latter position remains to be demonstrated; however, the highly political philosophy which espouses the total plasticity of an organically defective human organism is simply not verified in clinical reality. Thus, with rare exception, the various grades of mental retardation can be used as predictive categories when counseling the parents of handicapped children. Whereas the great majority (greater than 75 per cent) of retardates are globally retarded (uniformly delayed in all major functional areas of behavior), a smaller percentage demonstrates a significant scatter of abilities that makes accurate long-term prediction difficult. While it is hoped that a child with discrepant abilities will ultimately function at the level of his highest abilities, his poorer skills often severely limit the use of his higher ones.

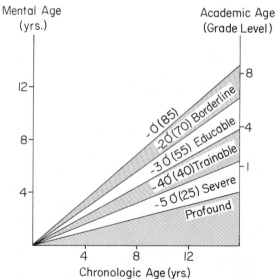

Level of academic achievement to be expected with different degrees of mental retardation at successive ages.

PEDIATRIC EVALUATION

Screening tools for developmental assessment breed quickly, each one briefer than the one preceding. These "quickie" tests for use by health paraprofessionals in no way relieve the pediatrician of his fundamental responsibility to assess neurodevelopmental status in earliest childhood. While recognizing the poor predictive validity of infant IQ tests for the normal range (especially IQ greater than 85), it is nevertheless true that as the developmental quotient drops the predictive validity increases, so that even below a year of age a DQ less than 55 (especially when it is duplicated by sequential assessments) achieves a high predictive validity. The old myth of the pediatrician's "built-in Gesell scale" has been questioned by several studies; however, numerous pediatric residency programs are beginning to realize how important training in developmental assessment is to the general pediatric practitioner. Ultimately the pediatrician must know how to evaluate the normality of children who fail (and even of those who pass) currently available screening tools. Alterations in the developmental course are certainly among the most sensitive indicators of the well being of the whole patient.

In infancy and early childhood developmental assessment focuses on language, problem-solving ability, perceptual and fine motor integration, self-help and personal-social skills; in middle childhood the attention shifts to academic performance with formal psychometric evaluation being indicated only when school failure becomes apparent. In adolescence and adulthood the accent is on vocational and job skills. Whereas those on the borderline of mild retardation may not be noticed until school age, moderately to profoundly retarded children should be recognized within the first year of life. (Indeed, except where careful developmental assessment is being routinely carried out, a child suspected of developmental delay within the first year of life is most probably moderately to profoundly retarded.)

The physician is careful to rule out a significant visual or auditory problem as a cause for pseudo-retardation; however, it must not be forgotten that once a diagnosis of primary retardation is made, children so identified are still at a high risk for associated submaximal impairments of vision and hearing. The difficulties inherent in adequate testing of these sensory modalities in retarded children are multiple and, in addition to close cooperation with an ophthalmologist and audiologist, the pediatrician needs to be familiar with Sheridan's STYCAR tests for both vision and hearing. (For information on Sheridan's tests, write NFER Publishing Company, Ltd., 2 Jennings Building, Thames Avenue, Windsor, Berks, England.)

When a suspicion of mental deficiency has been confirmed by serial pediatric developmental evaluations (and verified by the appropriate psychometric tests), the pediatrician uses clinical judgment to determine the extent of the biomedical evaluation. At this point he will keep in mind, on the one hand, the low diagnostic yield for organic etiology in children with an IQ greater than 55 and, on the other hand, the high priority parents place on establishing an etiology for purposes of prognosis, possible treatment and recurrence risks. While careful medical evaluation reveals a specific etiology in only a small percentage of patients, if mental retardation is considered to be the result of a major organ system malformation, it will be seen that in as many as two thirds of patients, major problems in another organ system will be uncovered, with about one third of the children actually demonstrating more than two involved systems; i.e., these are often *multiply handicapped children*. Frequently the management of these handicaps will involve the close cooperation of several different medical and paramedical specialists. The service model has been successively referred to as the multi-, inter-, and trans-disciplinary team; unfortunately, the degree of cooperation is often less than perfect. The child, who in one sense nobody wanted, becomes ironically the object of interprofessional rivalry.

Note that the recommended schedule of immunizations for normal children is to be followed in retarded children. The myth that active immunizations need to be deferred with some retarded children reflects the prevalent concept of "separate but equal" medical care for the handicapped.

COUNSELING

As complex as it may appear, the diagnostic evaluation presents the easier task compared with the long-term goals of parent counseling. Much has been written of the difficulty of getting parents of retarded children to accept their child's diagnosis—as if the diagnostic label were some kind of magic pill that when swallowed would suddenly make all things well. It is often overlooked that parental resistance to poorly presented and inadequately documented findings may reflect an attitude that is both appropriate and healthy. There is rarely any need to ram the word "retarded" down the parents' throats. They have already begun to accept the fact of the child's slowness by bringing him in for diagnostic evaluation. Nevertheless, the word "retarded" ought to be used during the counseling; no number of cautious euphemisms will protect the parents from hearing this word in the community.

Rather than open the session with a diagnostic label or a psychometric number, let the parents review *their perception* of the child's development. It is amazing how accurate parents (even of only children and often with little or no familiarity with popular child-rearing literature) can be in assessing their child's mental age when queried, "How old a child would you say he acts like?" (Indeed, they are even adept in noting discrepancies between different areas of development.) When they have successfully depicted the child's actual behavior with its implicit level of functioning, this picture can be interpreted to them utilizing the results of the pediatric and psychological evaluations. (A mental age range is often much more intelligible than an IQ score.) The parents thus play an *active* role in the diagnostic process itself, a mode to be fostered in all future interactive processes.

It is extremely important that both parents be present so as to relieve the one parent of the overwhelming burden of explaining the results of such an evaluation to the absent spouse (or, as is not infrequent, from either deliberately or subconsciously distorting the findings to protect the other parent). Watches, clocks and other timepieces need to be outlawed from the room in which the counseling is held; interruptions must be placed under absolute prohibition. The parents must in no way feel the usual rush and pressure that is part of the doctor's daily routine. Technical language is avoided as much as possible; diagrams of the brain localizing potential lesions often impress the speaker with his own status and hinder free communication by reducing the parents to silent bewilderment. Questions are to be not only allowed but encouraged; they should in no wise be considered as delaying the progress of the session, but rather their absence signals a breakdown in communication.

Regardless of the certitude of the diagnostic evaluation, the results should be qualified so as to allow the parents to hope—even in the face of imminent death, hope is fostered. One of the most effective means to avoid "doctor shopping" is to offer, at the beginning, a referral to (other) competent specialists for confirmation; if openly volunteered, this gesture will often solidify parental confidence in the pediatrician, and if the parents do seek elsewhere, the physician will have helped to guarantee that their search will be directed toward a reputable resource.

In the initial counseling session it is unwise to plot predictions for the child's entire life cycle; no matter how accurate these may be, they will probably overload the parents' information processing abilities. (The greatest difficulty in sketching the life history of a retarded child rests in the marked potential variation in future social attitudes determining the role to be imposed on deviant individuals.) One should attempt to answer specific questions concerning behaviors such as reading, toileting, speech, and ambulation. The positive—the humanness of the handicapped child—must be stressed throughout. The most frequent misunderstanding caused by a diagnosis of mental retardation is that the child will remain static and never develop; therefore, one of the points that needs repetition is that retardation refers to a slower than normal *rate* of development. All children demonstrate change with time—even the most profoundly handicapped children (some exhibiting a slight depression in an already low IQ score) will show some progression along the various substages of Piagetian sensorimotor schemas. Compared to normal children with their seemingly rapid rates of development, retarded children may appear to plateau, but compared to themselves they demonstrate a steady, if predictably slow, progress.

When etiology is discussed, extreme caution in phraseology must be exercised if any possible diagnoses can be interpreted as assigning responsibility to either parent. Feelings of guilt and inadequacy are to a certain extent inevitable and should not be fueled by careless reference to the possible contribution of, for example, a suspected history of mental defect in a distant relative on the maternal or paternal side of the family. Marriages burdened with retarded children show a significantly higher rate of disintegration, and any means of shoring up the family's strengths need to be utilized. The extent to which medicine has forgotten its ethical dimension is reflected in the physician's frequent failure to explore the possibly positive contribution of the family's religious faith.

The conclusion of a counseling session focuses on the present situation—how the child is currently functioning and what are the most appropriate means available to attain immediate short-term habilitation goals. Finally, the pediatrician involved in this therapeutic process needs to maintain an open-door policy—ready availability to answer questions, to review the patient's status and to assess the appropriateness of major changes in placement.

The pediatrician must demonstrate sensitivity to the successive emotional stages through which the family evolves: denial, anger, bargaining, depression and acceptance. The reaction to the initial diagnosis of retardation has been compared to grief upon the death of a child, the death of the hoped-for normal child who has inexplicably been replaced by this changeling. Perhaps the stage of "acceptance" is never really reached, but rather a continuing process of "chronic sorrow," an intelligible, healthy response to a tragic and irreversible fact. Complicating the doctor-patient relationship is the emotional reaction (frequently hostility) toward the physician who first imparts the diagnosis.

At first glance, an intensive psychiatric experience would appear necessary to respond to the subtle cues presented by these different emotional stages; however, only one basic skill is essential—the art of listening. When mentally reviewing the long list of points to be covered during a counseling session, it is best to discard all but the most significant, leaving the remainder for later sessions. The better part of the time should be spent in listening, for this is as significant a part of the practice of medicine as is imparting technical information. It is important to remember that even with the commonest problems of pediatric practice, the most frequent parental complaint is that the physician never heard *their* concerns.

Parents and siblings of retarded children can derive a great deal of emotional support from specially structured group sessions. Participation in group dynamics also can be educational for the interested physician.

INTERVENTION

When a diagnosis of mental retardation is made in the pre-school period a concern is frequently expressed over the efficacy of various programs to stimulate the child to achieve his maximal potential. The pediatrician needs to be thoroughly familiar with facilities in his community for the exceptional child. When the syllabus suggests the potential to cure mental retardation, it is promising more than is reasonable to expect. Infant stimulation programs have not produced scientifically verifiable permanent results. This is not to say that children will not make progress in such programs, for the simple reason that retarded children are not children who do not make progress. Keeping this last observation in mind, it is easy to see why all such programs achieve some striking "successes." And, of course, when failure occurs, it is the parents' fault (as if their guilt were not great enough already) for not religiously following a rigid "25 hour day" schedule of exhausting perceptual-motor exercises designed (and documented in rat experiments) to stimulate the regeneration of damaged cortical structures. Failure of the pediatrician to volunteer prophylactic advice in this area will only complicate later counseling. In the face of absent documentation on the efficacy of such programs, other relevant variables such as time, expense, travel, waiting lists, respite care, etc. need to receive priority.

Many parents with a school-age retarded child wage long battles with the school system to get their special child placed in classes for children with emotional disorders or learning disabilities rather than in a class for retarded children. There is currently a movement among educators to avoid this problem through several administrative tactics: (1) change the labels of the special education classes to some neutral term that parents will not find objectionable; (2) lump all categories of deviant children into one of these classes with a nondescript label; and/or (3) mainstream deviant children into regular classes.

The movements toward mainstreaming and away from labeling are in many cases quite justifiable. However, when the social scientist's attack on incorrect labeling exceeds reasonable bounds by suggesting that accurate diagnosis and prognosis are impossible (again the myth of the infinite plasticity of human nature in the hands of the social engineer), then his idealistic hope is not in the best interests of the child. While a few of the higher functioning children at each level of retardation may perform well (especially in the learning of social competence) in a class geared to the next higher level, one cannot ultimately hope to educationally mix children needing basic instruction in self-help skills with those who have already achieved competence at this level and have advanced to early academic skills. In this regard, some educational programs demonstrate little contact with developmental reality.

Finally, although many state teachers' lobbies place legal restrictions in the way, the most appropriate teacher for the severely and profoundly retarded child is often not a "teacher" at all, but rather an occupational or physical therapist. These latter persons have the requisite expertise to facilitate in mentally and physically handicapped individuals the basic fine and gross motor skills in the relevant areas of upper and lower extremity functioning, respectively (feeding, dressing, toileting, and gait training).

BEHAVIOR DISORDERS

In some older and a few younger retarded children behavior becomes the major obstacle to the child's acceptance by society, school and family. At the root of such behavior problems is frequently a failure to adjust expectations to the child's level of maturation. With children whose functional profile demonstrates a significant scatter of abilities, it is an easy trap for school and parents to expect the child to behave consistently at the level of his highest abilities; this then leads to a vicious cycle characterized by increasing frustration and deteriorating behavior. The necessary help often resembles common sense advice—not because the parents lack common sense, but because they have become so entangled in the infighting, like front line combatants, that they are unable to place issues in proper perspective. In such a situation, a skilled neutral observer can be effective.

Successful methods for handling such problems have been delineated by the school of behavioral psychology. The most important single fact for the practitioner to keep in mind is that the successful application of behavior modification techniques is completely independent of an extreme behaviorist viewpoint. Centuries before Watson and Skinner, Rousseau advocated the behavioral treatment for temper tantrums still utilized by most pediatricians. In short, the use of operant conditioning techniques—analytically focusing on the simpler components of complex behaviors with careful observation of the frequency of these components as well as the nature of the reward inherent in the situation in which the behavior occurs in order to extinguish undesired and shape desired outcomes—in no way implies an acceptance of the underlying nondevelopmental philosophy.

Child psychiatrists claim that up to 50 per cent of retardates have psychotic manifestations characterized by poor eye contact and self-stimulatory, repetitive mannerisms such as head banging, rocking and body rolling, with occasional hallucinations. The developmental pediatrician, on the other hand, frequently interprets this behavioral complex as reflecting what may be called the "expanded Strauss syndrome," amenable to behavior modification and psychotropic drug therapy. The Strauss syndrome, manifested by attentional peculiarities such as short attention span, perseveration, emotional instability, distractibility, hyperactivity and fidgetiness, is found in the child with minimal cerebral dysfunction and usually associated with a learning disability. Since this behavioral pattern becomes more pronounced as the degree of brain damage increases, an "expanded Strauss syndrome" occurs most often in those retardates who are trainable or below and have organicity as a major component. (Unless they also have acquired brain damage, children with Down's syndrome do not demonstrate this syndrome.)

Particularly in brain-damaged retardates, behavior modification, although helpful, may not be sufficient to control organically driven hyperactivity, short attention span, and other stimulus-bound behavior. Psychotropic drugs then provide an excellent adjunct, with the caution that these never be employed in the absence of a careful overview of the whole patient and in association with ongoing behavioral counseling. Dextroamphetamine* and methylphenidate,† both of which produce excellent results in controlling the hyperactivity syndrome in children of normal or near-normal intelligence, rarely have this positive effect in more retarded individuals. Among the phenothiazines, thioridazine (Mellaril)‡ is effective in treating behavior disorders in significantly retarded children. Its dosage is between 1 and 3 mg./kg., divided in three to four daily doses; in addition to tablet form, it is conveniently available in a 30 mg./ml. elixir. Thioridazine is started at a dose of 10 to 25 mg. three times a day, and increased according to its effect on behavior; the commonest side effects include weight gain and constipation. Dystonic reactions are treatable with diphenhydramine. An initially positive response may wear off after a few weeks, necessitating one or more dosage increments. It is also not infrequent to see a retarded child whose behavior is nicely responsive to a dosage somewhat higher than the range recommended here; obviously treatment needs to be individualized, and this decision has considerable ethical content. Chlorpromazine (Thorazine), prochlorperazine (Compazine), and other members of this group have also been used with success. The list of side effects for these drugs is extensive, and the physician will need to monitor these patients closely. Diphenhydramine (Benadryl) for sleep problems frequently results in marked tachyphylaxis, but is useful brief therapy. Medication should never be employed as a short cut to

---

*Manufacturer's precaution: Dextroamphetamine is not recommended for use in minimal brain dysfunction in children under 3 years of age.

†Manufacturer's precaution: Methylphenidate is not recommended for children under 6 years of age since the safety and efficacy in this age group have not been determined.

‡Manufacturer's precaution: Thioridazine is not intended for children under 2 years of age.

replace rather than supplement behavioral counseling. Finally, remember that older retardates are not dissimilar to very young children who cannot tell the pediatrician what is wrong. Not infrequently sudden inexplicable changes in behavior are secondary to occult physical illness that must be diligently sought.

With the adolescent retardate, sexual acting out is a frequent parental concern. Oral contraception is relatively ineffective in the female owing to poor compliance; however, irreversible surgical procedures pose serious legal and ethical questions. With various movements to foster the sexual rights of the retarded, multiple cross purposes are pursued which have the effect of clouding certain basic concepts. Sex can be viewed as a predominantly cerebral activity: as intelligence decreases, so does sexual drive. The myth of the hypersexuality of the retarded was based on the frequency with which masturbation and indecent exposure were observed in institutionalized retardates. In reality these attention-getting behaviors were quite appropriate both to these patients' mental age and to their state of enforced boredom. Contraception of any sort cannot be considered a substitute for adequate supervised activity, appropriate sex education, and protection from sexual abuse by the more intelligent deviates in the community. Not infrequently hysterectomy will be recommended for "hygienic" reasons despite the fact that with minimal nursing supervision the care of menstrual flow is less complicated than toileting. Surgery should not replace social and behavioral services.

(A problem-solving age of approximately 18 months suffices for toileting in older retardates, although the age for this skill in normal children is closer to 3 years. In these latter children toilet training appears to be reflective of a higher and more complex level of ego functioning than in the retarded.)

CONCLUSION

Mental retardation presents a financial and social problem of immense magnitude. Various solutions—institutional and bureaucratic, de-institutional and humane—have been tried. Ultimately society's definition of humanity is a cognitive one with purely intellectual criteria; those who do not meet the standards are placed in a deviance role. The integration of the most advanced contributions of scientific medicine, psychiatry, psychology, education and related disciplines for the purpose of relieving the burden of the family with a retarded child, for the purpose of working through an understanding of this most incomprehensible problem of childhood suffering, is the singular contribution of the developmental pediatrician. In a society that has committed itself to the large task of de-institutionalization, but has not appropriated funds for the adequate support services necessary for normalization to work, the pediatrician as gadfly must continue to be a most vocal advocate for the rights of all children.

Emotional Disorders

SAUL L. BROWN, M.D.

Therapy in all branches of medicine succeeds best when the patient is receptive to what we offer. A child with emotional disturbance is usually mistrustful of adults. He is often, therefore, less than receptive to the initial offers of help that a physician makes to him. He needs to be won over. This is a delicate process.

Very often it is time consuming. Not all physicians have the inclination for this kind of activity. Moreover, a child's receptivity to psychological help is very much dependent upon the attitudes of his parents. A child who is not functioning successfully in a psychological or emotional sense has a powerful impact upon his parents and also upon his siblings. Conversely, emotional problems in the parents may very well have preceded or precipitated problems in the child. Thus helping a child with emotional disturbance may turn into a complex project involving parents and siblings as well. Time and patience are needed.

My clinical experience with the emotional disturbances of children has led me to be concerned less about ultimate etiology and more with defining those factors that appear to be perpetuating a disturbance: (1) attitudes of the parents toward the child; (2) how the child's behavior affects the parents; (3) how the siblings react and also how their attitudes may be reinforcing the disturbed child's behavior; (4) environmental forces that may be playing into and perpetuating the child's disturbance, such as the quality of life in the neighborhood, family economic stresses and, most important, the nature of the child's school experience; and finally (5) chronic illness in one of the parents or siblings, a recent death, marital strife, an aging grandparent living in the home, and the child's own physical status and recent medical or surgical procedures that he may have undergone.

Usually, emotional disturbance in children is evidenced through behavioral patterns or syndromes. Disturbance may also be evidenced through physiological reactions. There are differences of opinion about the latter, but my own experience suggests that this is frequent.

Underlying a child's disturbed behavior or psychogenic physiologic reactions are certain feeling states that may be responses to one or more of the factors listed in the preceding section. Psychotherapists usually look first for underlying *anxiety*, then for underlying *hostility*, and finally for underlying *guilt*. If we can discern any of these at work, we have some first notion of how to talk with a child and also of how to talk with his parents. If we can see some connection between any of these feelings and any of the factors that I referred to, we can then talk about this with the child and the parents.

Underlying Anxiety.   If we discover that a child's behavior reflects anxiety about violent arguments between his parents, or about his mother's recent illness, or about a recent earthquake, or about his father's job loss, it becomes possible to talk with the child about how that particular situation has made him feel. A child derives enormous relief from hearing a warm, friendly adult put those fears into words and thereby help make his irrational feelings understandable.

Underlying Anger.   When we sense that a child is very angry (remember that he can be *both* anxious *and* angry!) we need to tell him so. Again, if we have gained some intuition or evidence about what factors in his family or school life are making him angry, we can try to tell him what we think. Clearly, we will get nowhere if we sound judgmental or pedantic. If the factors are on the surface, such as being severely teased and "put down" by an older, or even a younger, sibling, we may find the child able to ventilate his feelings to us. This is especially productive if his parents are receptive and understanding and can be present and a part of the talk.

Often, however, the sources of a child's hostility are complex. When, for example, they are a result of punitive or rejecting parental attitudes, or of actual deprivation and neglect, offering psychological help may turn out to be frustrating and difficult. The skills of a full-time psychotherapist may be needed, since such children tend to be distrustful while at the same time demanding and controlling.

There are some neglected children who are able to experience profound reassurance if a physician just talks sympathetically with them. The child's feeling of relief comes out of the sharing and understanding he receives. Actual change in his situation may not be possible. Once the physician realizes this and settles for small gains, he may feel gratification even in the small help he provides such a child.

Underlying Guilt.   Guilt in a child is an elusive phenomenon. Often children are provocative or troublesome precisely because they feel badly about themselves or about their ideas or aggressive impulses. In effect, they bring about their own punishment for their imagined misdeeds. Children from closely knit middle class homes are particularly subject to this subtle kind of underlying guilt. Because their parents are reasonable and nice, the children feel guilty or ashamed of their normally primitive impulses to be occasionally disorderly or rebellious or hard on their siblings. This sometimes extends into the sexual sphere. Such children may feel guilty because of their impulses to look at the genitals of adults or children or because they have touched others or their own, or because they have talked about "forbidden" subjects. It often requires a long time and a trusting relationship with the physician before a child will share the "inner world" of thoughts and fantasies that may be producing underlying guilt.

Situational or family factors may be more immediate reasons for a child's "guilt." For example, a child may be angry at an aging grandma who lives with the family and is always scolding him, but he feels guilty for having such "bad" feelings. Where the factors are on the surface, a physician may be more easily effective in helping the parents and child ventilate his feelings and thereby reduce his sense of guilt.

When, however, guilt relates to more subtle "inner world" ideas and feelings, it is often deeply entrenched and is the essence of what we usually refer to as a "neurosis." In the case of neurotic states, the efforts of a psychodynamically trained psychotherapist are usually needed if true relief for the child is to be achieved. Reassurance or sympathetic support just is not enough.

BASIC TECHNIQUES OF THERAPY

Emotions are least troublesome if they can be expressed openly but in such a way that they do not lead to a destructive result. Certain physicians have a natural ability to make patients feel safe in ventilating their emotions. Others need to learn techniques for this. The primary action in any humanistic psychotherapy is to "hear a patient out." This applies to both children and adults. A nonjudgmental listener is worth his weight in gold!

If a pediatrician elects to work on an emotional disturbance, he needs to be explicit in a friendly way.

Jim, I get the idea you have some troubles. I don't know if I can help you get over them or not. First I'd like to know if you think you have troubles. Your parents seem to think so, but I don't know if you do. Would you like to talk a little?

Children rarely respond with expanded commentary. We need to observe their nonverbal reactions in order to judge whether they are "with us."

I find that beginning with parents present is often valuable, although this can backfire if the parents are so angry that the session turns into an inquisition. A good way to begin is to clarify that you as physician can only help with words, that if the family wants a chance to "just talk" you would like to listen. The attitudes of the family will determine whether to carry out the discussion with everyone present or whether to suggest that you talk with the child alone and with the parents separately.

Usually when the latter avenue is chosen, it is important to tell all of them that you are not going to report to the parents about everything the child tells you. Hopefully the child can discern the difference between a general report to his parents and a detailed quoting of him. He needs reassurance that your purpose in reporting to his parents is for them to better understand what might be troubling all of them and to make things better in the family.

The usual sequence is to meet first with parents on one day in order to hear their concern. On another occasion meet with the family for a while and possibly with the child alone for a while. On a third occasion, a report to the parents is indicated. A few more sessions with all of them or with the child alone may follow.

It is very important to give clear messages about your own intentions. If you intend to meet only two or three times, say so in the beginning so that there will not be a feeling of rejection or letdown when the sessions are at an end. Early clarification of the extent of your involvement helps the family to monitor their own expectation of you.

ENURESIS

A first step is to ask the child how he (or she) feels about his symptom. Is he troubled about it? Would he like to overcome it? Does he believe he can? What kind of help would he like? Coincidentally, a similar exploration of the parents' expectation should occur. My preference is to do both together, in a family interview, but family interviewing requires skills which a pediatrician may not have learned.

A second step is to discuss with the child and his parents those factors that seem to be contributing to the enuresis. If those factors are "situational" or environmental, discussion and clarification can help the child and parents be more objective and reduce the secondary guilt and shame in both. Also the ventilation of feelings that occurs with this kind of frank and uncritical discussion helps provide the child with the feeling that he can develop mastery of his own bodily functions.

If the factors contributing to the enuresis are more subtle than situational stresses—undercurrent hostility or anxiety in the family—referral to a skilled psychotherapist is usually indicated.

Behavior reinforcement methods, such as a "conditioning device" which awakens the child when the bed becomes wet, may be worth trying, but only if the child commits himself to wanting such help. If a child is not enthusiastic about such an approach, he can only feel assaulted and deprecated if it is imposed upon him. The long-term effectiveness of such devices is still open to considerable doubt, even though they sometimes produce immediate "cures."

Medication has been recommended by some. The complications inherent in relying upon drugs to overcome psychological disturbances are easily apparent. The greatest complication is that drug therapy provokes a dependency upon outside resources and distracts from an effort to understand and master the sources of emotional distress. If a psychiatrist or psychotherapist is not available, the pediatrician's openly verbalized sympathy for the distress the child experiences from his symptom is nevertheless of extreme value to him. Reassurance ought to be reserved, however, until the child's distress has been talked about and some of his emotions ventilated.

ENCOPRESIS

Fecal soiling can be a most stubborn symptom. It usually reflects a subtle mixture of anxiety and anger in a child, neither of which has become clearly evident to the parents. The symptom, because of its noxious nature, tends to block reasonable thought about it. More often it evokes irritation, anger, disparagement of the child and despair in the parents and in the siblings as well. Usually the mother becomes locked into a futile struggle with the child who has, through his symptom, discovered a most powerful mechanism for reducing his mother (and father) to relative helplessness.

The physician's first efforts need to be in the direction of eliciting the child's interest in overcoming his symptom. Often the child seems remarkably oblivious of the noxious effect of the symptom upon others, but this is usually a cover-up. Given an opportunity to reveal his feelings in a nonjudgmental and supportive interview, such a child will often acknowledge his wish to overcome the symptom.

The next step is for the physician to share with the child his belief that he (the child) must be angry about some things but is perhaps afraid to say what these things are. Often this may be anger at siblings; other times at father's unavailability or at his authoritarian attitudes; other times at mother's overdominance.

A third step is to try to talk with the child about being the boss of his own body functions. The physician may share with a child the notion that he and he alone can control his own bowel movements. Surprisingly, this statement may awaken in the child a sense of his own voluntary power over the symptom.

Familial factors may be so subtle as to require a psychotherapist's skill. But the physician may do well to make some initial efforts to reach the undercurrent feelings in child and family. Even if he fails, his uncritical and supportive exploration reduces the negative emotional pressure upon the child and may begin to disrupt the cycle of mutually defeating feelings in the family.

Exhorting the child has no place in this situation, even though one may be tempted. A child who soils usually cannot stop the tendency in a short time. Even if successful discussion of his anger and his anxiety occurs, the symptom may not stop for several months. Recurrences need to be expected and parents and child both need reassurance.

STEALING AND LYING

A judgmental attitude toward children who steal or lie is difficult to avoid. Nevertheless, that is just what we must do if we are to be of help to such children and to their parents. The challenge to us is to get through to the "inner person" in the child who lies or cheats or steals. Viewing such behavior as symptomatic makes it possible for us to be helpful. Rarely, however, is success rapidly achieved, because such behaviors often reflect serious underlying problems in the child and in the family system. Diagnostic assessment of motivating factors is therefore crucial.

Moving from the simple to the complex, consideration of the following causes may help.

Attention Seeking. If, having talked with the parents and the child, we conclude that the child's antisocial behavior is a reaction to feeling "left out" or to being devalued or underrated in the family, we may be able to arouse the parents' awareness of this. We can encour-

age them to think of some remedies. Even the most responsible of parents become preoccupied or distracted and fail to realize that their child is feeling neglected. The sources for this can be myriad—arrival of a new baby, illness in a parent or sibling, family financial problems or marital tensions. Searching out what may be going on in the family life that could be provoking a child to act in disruptive or negative ways may require time.

Hostility Toward Authority. Some children are extremely angry at adults and are determined to "get even." A sympathetic physician can sometimes talk with such a child about those feelings. Great care is needed not to betray the child's trust, especially if his parents tend to be punitive or insensitive. If, however, the parents seem open to self observation and change, they can be confronted with the idea that their child's antisocial and disruptive behavior seems to be a rebellion against overcontrol.

It seems he feels he can't win against so much authority and control. Could you reconsider some of your rules and punishments? Maybe some talk with him and some negotiation and compromise is in order, with the idea that you would let up on some rules if he'll show you he can be trusted.

If parents are obtuse or opinionated it may not be fruitful to attempt this. In such instances, a pediatrician may need to work in two directions at once. On the one hand, he may need to show the parents that he understands how it feels to put up with a child who is so difficult. With the child, however, the pediatrician may need to appeal on another level.

Your parents are really angry at your fibbing (or "taking things"). I guess you're pretty mad at them too. I can see they are very strict. But when you keep doing some of those things it only makes them get stricter. What if we try to think of ways you could go along with their rules even if you don't always want to.

Of course a child who has reached such a level of anger at rigid parents is not likely to take kindly to the advice of an authority figure such as a physician. Additionally, there are many rigid parents who seem determined to have a scapegoat for their own angry feelings. So asking the child to make compromises may be futile. Nevertheless there are some families in which initial rigidity can melt, especially if it arises from parental insecurity.

I have learned that if I can be supportive and sympathetic to such parents, even when I feel they are being overly punitive, they can bit by bit let go and take on a more flexible attitude with their child.

Deprivation. Absence of emotional warmth from parents may lead to antisocial behavior and especially a compulsion to steal objects. Again, the life circumstances of the family needs to be evaluated. Possibly the parents can do no better because of their own deprivation. Once again, discussion with the child of these feelings can be helpful, even though the facts of his life may change little. A physician needs to tread a narrow line in these situations—sympathizing with the child's feeling "gypped" but nevertheless avoiding positive sanction of the antisocial behavior.

MASTURBATION

It appears that most children masturbate from time to time. Indeed, there is evidence that periodic masturbation is an essential component of body image development and of basic acceptance of genital sensation and function. For some children, however, masturbation becomes compulsive and therefore must be viewed as a symptom.

A crucial first step is to find out from the parents just what they have said about masturbation, about genitals and about sex. Their own emotional attitudes are thereby revealed. Are they embarrassed? Ashamed? Fearful? If so, what do they fear will happen? Are they "morally offended?" What do they think is causing the problem? What have they heard from others about masturbation?

Exploration is in itself therapeutic. It frees up the parents to be more objective and the child may benefit.

Secondarily, the child needs to be talked with, possibly in the presence of the parents. What is talked about depends on the child's age and intelligence as well as upon what factors are apparently operating (see earlier sections of this article).

If it appears that the masturbation reflects a deep personality disorder, comments from the pediatrician can be of value if they relate to the child's feelings of anxiety: "It looks like you have a lot of scary thoughts. You touch yourself a lot and maybe that's because you feel troubled." This kind of comment helps a disturbed child feel understood and relieves some of his shame and guilt.

The pediatrician may invite the child to talk about what's troubling him. In such instances, a little bit of talk can be relieving to the child and reduce his compulsivity. Rarely does it dissolve the symptom all at once. It usually helps to reassure the child that his worries are understandable and that touching himself is not necessarily bad.

If the diagnostic evaluation suggests that the child's personality is intact but that his masturbation is reflective of ordinary childhood anxieties, fairly direct verbal discussion with the child may be of value.

Your parents tell me you touch your penis (or your vagina) a lot. I guess it may feel good to you. But maybe you could learn not to do it in front of other kids so much. It's kind of a private thing. Maybe you could just remember if you touch yourself there too much it will make your skin sore.

By way of light commentary the child is guided toward moderation.

Usually a supportive and reassuring attitude to parents reduces pressure in all directions. If exaggerated parental fears can be talked over, the parents themselves may avoid becoming locked into an excessive preoccupation with their child's masturbation.

When there is a major feeling of anxiety in the child because of family circumstances such as parental discord or a new sibling's arrival or illness in the family, the pediatrician needs to find a way to help the child talk about these concerns.

TICS

Often a tic syndrome is transient. Once established, however, it tends to be stubborn. Usually tics occur as localized bodily expressions of aggressive feelings. Not uncommonly they occur in children of very loving parents. The child feels guilty if he shows aggression openly. Tics can become reduced when a child feels freer to express anger but that freedom may be only slowly achieved. Children with tics are often rather compulsive and well ordered. They have carefully trained themselves not to let emotions spill over. Not infrequently their parents are quite similar. Careful and sensitive encouragement to the family members that they "let out" their angry feelings to each other may help. Medications have been tried but are rarely practical.

CRUELTY

Persistence of this kind of behavior usually reflects a fairly deep kind of hostility in a child. Superficial factors of the kind defined earlier as "environmental" or "situational" may be at work and if so, the cruelty can usually stop when those factors are discussed. First step is to try to gain the child's trust and explore whether he understands his actions. Next, his motivation for change needs to be explored. If the child wants to stop his cruelty, family discussions about the origins of the behavior and candid talk about what might be provoking the child's hostility can be helpful. More often, the help of a skilled psychotherapist will be needed.

SETTING FIRES

Fire setting usually reflects a combination of angry feelings in a child and a tendency to master anxiety through creating an exciting distraction. Searching out the sources of anxiety and hostility requires careful family study. Often such a child is angry because he feels siblings are receiving favored treatment. He may also be anxious about parental attitudes toward him.

Logical talk about the dangers of fire rarely helps, unless it is combined with discussion of the feelings that he is experiencing. Parental participation is essential, particularly if they can allow their child to verbalize his angry feelings toward them. What makes this symptom particularly difficult is the fact that usually such a child fears retaliation for revealing his angry feelings to one or both of his parents openly. Often his fear is justified if in fact his parents tend (or one of them tends) to respond with hostility or in a punitive fashion when they are offended.

Sometimes children who set fires are reacting to excessive sexual arousal resulting from seeing their parents in the nude or from being exposed to adult sexuality. It may be useful to obtain a close history from the parents about what the child is being exposed to.

BREATH HOLDING ATTACKS

Breath holding episodes are more typical of very young children and are manifestly efforts to control parents or adults. Usually such children have been cued to "get their way." They then experience overwhelming rage when their parents change the rules of the game and do not comply with each demand. They succeed in frightening their parents into compliance once the breath holding symptom evolves.

Parents usually need considerable guidance in these situations. They need support to wait out the episodes of breath holding while at the same time they must be encouraged to help their child to feel secure without overindulging him. Such parents often are confused about how to draw limits and they tend to view limit setting as hurtful. They need to learn to differentiate permissiveness from benign warmth.

Specific advice should be offered to the parents about how to hold the child firmly and protectively when he has a tantrum or holds his breath. Often such parents are at a loss about how to physically contain their child in a firm and definitive, non-hurtful fashion. Also one often finds they are in conflict with each other about how firm to be. When that is the case, no advice will work until they have been guided to standing together on whatever rules are set up.

PSYCHOTIC REACTIONS

A diagnosis of a psychotic state in a child is difficult to establish. Usually psychological studies are important. Once established, a program of therapy requires a full scale study of the family's resources, community clinical resources, and clarity about the school's capacity to work along with such a child. Medication may be indicated but it must be made very clear to parents that medicine will not "cure." Its purpose is to help the child settle down and get along better.

Usually the parents of a psychotic child are committed to the idea that an "organic" problem underlies the behavior. Even when this is the case, educational and psychotherapeutic approaches are at the center of clinical effort. Parents will need to be led to appropriate community resources such as special schools and to psychiatrists or child therapists who can help them manage their problem and make realistic plans.

Medications such as chlorpromazine or thioridazine are useful if the child's behavior is excited or overly aggressive. Trifluoperazine HCl (Stelazine) is useful if the child's thinking is suffused with fragmented or very frightening content. Methylphenidate can be helpful if the child's psychosis is accompanied by hyperkinetic behavior.

Use of medication requires careful observation through trial and error. There is great variation in the reactions children have to medications.

HYPERACTIVITY

Assuming that a substantial effort has been made to clarify the origins of a child's hyperactivity, pediatric efforts will need to be aimed at several targets more or less simultaneously. If such potential sources of hyperactivity as plumbism or hypoglycemia occurring with poverty or nutritional deficits, or reading and learning deficits, have all been ruled out, the next focus of effort will need to be on interpersonal factors. These include those listed earlier in this chapter including environmental and situational ones as well as intrafamilial ones. Generally, the approach is similar to what has been described in relation to anxiety and for behavior disorders.

Because a hyperactive child is almost always in trouble at school, a successful interpersonal effort will need to include some contact with his teacher. The latter will usually be the best barometer for reflecting changes, both positive and negative. Also a teacher's cooperation in planning is crucial. Possibly this can be accomplished by enlisting the help of a school nurse. Teachers and parents need to talk matters over together with the pediatrician, specifically:

1. Ways to calm the child by making appropriate comments to him when he gets excited, and through introducing quieting distractions.

2. Mutually agree upon methods for removing the child from exciting group activities, but in a fashion that is not punitive nor shaming.

3. Ways to enhance the child's self-esteem even while talking candidly with him about the fact that he has "a problem" with "nervousness." This includes being openly complimentary every time he manages to "cool it" and to contain his overactivity.

When medications are used, careful cooperation is needed from both of the parents, the child himself, and the school. There should be no mystique about the purpose of the medication. It should be described as a "nerve calmer." It is crucial that the child be asked to talk about his own concept of why he needs medicine. If he reveals that he thinks it's because he's "crazy" or "something is wrong" with his "brain," opportunity presents to help him understand that his trouble is only that his "nerves work too fast" and he needs help to slow them down.

Medication appears to be useful in up to one third of hyperactive children. The choices are usually (1) dextroamphetamine given two or three times a day or (2) methylphenidate given two or three times a day. Usually the last dose of either should be given no later than midafternoon. A trial of one medication over a 2 week period is usually needed in order to establish dosage and validity. The teacher's observations are the most reliable measure of success or failure, since parents tend to have unrealistic expectations of a medication.

When neither of the above two medications succeeds, a trial of chlorpromazine or of thioridazine, 25 mg. four times a day (maximum dosage not to exceed 3 mg./kg./day), may be indicated, with some reduction if drowsiness becomes a problem. Neither of these medications is desirable unless a child's behavior is extreme, since they are major tranquilizers and they may affect levels of central nervous system function which are important for basic learning.

Autism

JACQUELYN SANDERS, PH.D.

The autistic child is one who, convinced that he cannot influence the external world, has retreated from it. It is as though he dwells in what Bettelheim called an "empty fortress." He appears not to even notice the events around him, much less make any effort to relate to them, but seeks gratification from inner directed, isolated and repetitive self-stimulation. While a child can suffer from various degrees of autism, and exhibit any of a variety of rather typical symptoms, this quality of extreme unrelatedness is that which sets the autistic child apart. At five years or older it makes the child obviously different from "normal" and fairly easy to identify. However, the onset of autism is considered to be in the first two years of life. Though early diagnosis is difficult, since some autistic-like symptomatology is developmental, the earlier treatment is instituted the better.

The treatment is psychological and must be as pervasive as possible. The autistic child is isolated and has stopped growing emotionally because he has given up all efforts to interact with and influence those around him. In order to enable him to resume such interaction, he must be convinced that his efforts *will* influence those around him and will thereby affect what happens to him. This is the first part of treatment. The child has to be carefully attended so that his initiative is detected, understood, and responded to.

The typical autistic child seems to express no desire for meaningful communication. However, it has been our experience upon careful observation of any autistic child that this is not so. He is expressing something meaningful and reacting to what happens around him. His expressions are not ordinary and so are hard for us to understand, but he does express himself through his unique system of communication. When the small signs of this initiative are responded to, the child communicates more fully and is often then able to work through some of the reasons for the initial retreat from the world.

For example, since we recognized that his repeated pouring of water down the bathroom drains was a meaningful activity for one autistic boy, rather than simply a repetitious isolated occupation, we did what we could to try to understand it by watching him and playing with him. It gradually became clear that his pervasive fascination with drains was related to his anxiety about people disappearing. He then revealed both in play and verbally more and more of his ideas about disappearance. His interaction with us around the drains over a long period of time was an important part of his overcoming a great anxiety about people disappearing.

When the child begins to believe that what he does will be responded to, will make a difference in his life, he begins to make more and more efforts in the world, and toward other people. In other words, he begins to change his autistic position.

A second aspect of treatment is helping the child to feel that neither his nor others' emotions are overwhelming. Though the etiology of autism is the subject of debate, it is generally agreed that autistic children are unusually sensitive and, therefore, events that would be relatively easy for a normal child to cope with, are experienced as unmanageably painful by the autistic child. We speculate that from the start the autistic child has experienced life as more painful and emotions as more devastating than normal children.

It is fairly typical that there is a history of behavior that the parents found themselves unable to cope with, such as seemingly incessant crying, removal of clothes and self mutilation. It is also not unusual that the mother had been under intense stress during the child's infancy, that she coped by staying away from the child, often so as to protect him from her negative emotions. Thus, frequently, the child's own inability to cope with his painful emotions in any way other than by retreating has been intensified by the parents' inability to cope with the child's and their own painful emotions.

To overcome this requires, again, pervasive attentiveness so that the child does not feel deserted or feared when feeling or expressing painful emotions. That is, it is of utmost importance that the child not be left alone either when expressing great distress by difficult behavior, or when isolating himself because of inner distress. The person who is with the child must, of course, be able to deal with his own emotions, including those that are aroused by the difficult behavior of the autistic child.

When the child begins to feel that it is safe to experience emotions, great care must be taken because he has not learned to express them in a modulated way and therefore they can be primitive and potentially destructive. To deal with this so that expression is neither harmful nor again repressed requires a good deal of skill. This is often a necessary step on the way to humanity for the autistic child.

The third facet of treatment is providing stimulation to and structure for growth. Since the autistic child has early in life given up trying to do things vis-à-vis his environment, he misses the tremendous amount of learning that takes place in the normal child almost naturally as he grows. It is important to provide for this learning in the course of treatment. However, the manner in which this is done is crucial. Since the critical issue in the disturbance is the child's feeling of not being in control of what happens to him, to impose learning that has nothing to do with his own efforts or desires reaffirms his lack of influence and reinforces the autistic position.

In the course of such treatment, learning is likely to take a long time. The lack of learning in the case of the autistic child is not due to a particular block, as in some other kinds of emotional disturbance, but to a lack of the developmental learning that accompanies ego growth. Therefore, once the learning begins, it is certainly no quicker than normal and might even take longer. An added problem is that in dealing with such children as they begin to learn, it is harder for us to do naturally the things that make such learning easier for the small child.

For example, the acquisition of speech in the normal child is a slow process. The child who says his first words at age 1 does not actually have speech for months or years after. When the autistic child begins to talk the acquisition of complete speech is likely to take even longer. Thus, on the one hand, the child coming out of an autistic position still does not have the normal freedom to learn and, on the other hand, the adult does not so naturally engage in such developmentally helpful activities as endless repetition. These difficulties must be recognized and dealt with so that the child, once he has become able to grow and is free to feel, may be able to learn the many skills and tools that are necessary to live successfully.

Since to effect the above requires a pervasive environment, the treatment of choice is milieu therapy. It is, of course, long-term treatment. The convictions of the autistic child are not reversed without a total effort of years' duration, requiring special skills. Our direct experience has been with children 4 years and older. For these children residential treatment is indicated. In all of the children who have come to us, the onset of autism has been described as no later than 18 to 24 months. Most often this description is from parental report, though there are some reports of clear diagnosis by a professional at that early age. There is not enough evidence regarding children who have been similarly described at 18 months and subsequently developed "normally," though there are certainly many reports of children with autistic symptoms who "outgrow" them, such as lack of speech development until four or so. When autism is suspected at an early age, it is best for the parents to be guided in their relationship with the child by a professional. There are some analysts, social workers, psychologists and workers at child guidance clinics who will do such counseling, providing assistance in the three areas described above. It is possible that when the parents get help early enough in dealing with the child and in dealing with their own emotions regarding the child, retreat can be reversed and the self can begin to grow.

Pica

DESPINE LIEBHABER, M.D.

Pica is the persistent search for and ingestion of nonfood substances beyond the age of 18 months, the age at which a child normally ceases mouthing and even occasionally swallowing inedibles as a primary means of exploring his environment. About this time, ongoing developmental gains, including ambulation and the coordination of visual, auditory, and tactile senses, enable the child to learn about surroundings in a manner more sophisticated than hand-mouth behavior. The child finds ways of achieving comfort and pleasure by means other than oral gratification, and coincident with this, finger and thumb sucking also diminish. Simultaneously, repeated and consistent admonition from the child's caretaker teaches discrimination between the acceptable ingestion of foods and the unacceptable mouthing, biting, chewing and ingestion of nonfoods.

The incidence of pica varies according to age groups of children studied and to the definition of pica applied with respect to the intensity and frequency of the habit. In some children, pica is an activity which simply persists beyond the age at which it normally disappears; in other children, pica gradually emerges after an interim of normal oral behavior. Pica may involve the ingestion of many kinds of available objects, or may be selective and limited to one specific substance; it may be random and sporadic, or persistent and highly motivated. Consequences of pica include parasitic infestation, accidental poisoning, trichobezoars, gastrointestinal obstruction, perforation or hemorrhage, and most commonly, lead intoxication.

Careful questioning for pica should be a part of every child's health assessment. Mothers often exhibit more concern for other types of hand-mouth behavior, such as thumb sucking or prolonged attachment to the pacifier, and rarely spontaneously mention the existence of pica in a child. In some cultures, certain forms of oral behavior including pica are condoned, and pica itself in the form of clay or starch eating may be practiced by the child's mother or caretaker. Most cases of pica in the 18 to 30 month age group can be stopped if the child's caretaker is educated concerning the potential dangers of pica.

The causes of severe pica are complex and have been variously attributed to inadequate parenting, deprivation of early normal sucking or other oral activities, perverted appetite associated with various feeding problems, and inappropriately learned behavioral patterns.

Autistic and mentally retarded children are known to have a high incidence of pica, including pica for lead. The retarded child with additional physical handicaps or serious behavioral problems is even more prone to pica.

Nutritional deficiencies have not been clearly established as a cause of pica in children, except in anecdotal case reports. Since children with pica or with elevated lead levels often come from lower economic backgrounds, and since children with pica may have poor appetites or unusual food preferences, the nutritional anemias or other nutritional deficiencies seen in these children cannot be considered to be predisposing factors in pica.

Inadequate mothering has been implicated most consistently as a cause of pica. Some mothers have been found to be emotionally passive or depressed. They may fail to communicate adequately with the child or to satisfy the child's emotional needs. They may fail to assist the child in developing adequate patterns of control over the persistent mouthing or ingestion of nonfoods. They may even covertly sanction pica in the same way that pacifiers and bottles are condoned long after they should have been removed, because the child's gratification from these oral pleasures, including pica, may allay maternal anxieties.

A recent longitudinal study of a small group of British children with highly motivated pica identified several additional causative factors, which include adverse environmental conditions, distorted developmental patterns, and psychodynamic stresses. In some instances, housing was old with inadequate play space. Several parents had mental or chronic physical illness, and there were instances of an emotionally disturbed, retarded, or ill sibling. Some children suffered from inadequate parental supervision, or were lonely and isolated. Several were retarded or had additional behavioral disorders, and some had speech difficulty which frustrated efforts to communicate satisfactorily.

Since the causes of pica are multifactorial, and since the threat it poses depends on its severity and on the kinds of substances consumed, each case must be dealt with individually and will benefit from the intervention of various disciplines working in concerted effort with the child and family.

Children living in old and dilapidated housing have easy accessibility to leaded paint chips, chunks of old window putty and crumbling lead-containing plaster. Under these conditions, pica is almost always implicated in the development of lead toxicity.

Dust on floors and window sills of homes such as these has been found to contain lead, presumably from pulverized paint and plaster. Lead has also been identified in soil surrounding these homes. It is therefore possible that even normal hand-mouth activity in a child can result in some lead absorption.

With the exception of children with lead toxicity requiring chelation treatment, a successful therapeutic approach to elevated lead levels may be directed toward eliminating the child's pica; so long as the pica is random rather than highly motivated, it represents little more than a slight excess of oral activity, and the child is otherwise developmentally normal. In addition, the child's caretakers must have the motivation and capacity to respond appropriately to education by health personnel, direct the child's energies and interest to other activities, keep house floors swept and surfaces dusted, and make some simple home repairs.

Under these conditions, by eliminating the child's pica, it may be possible to avoid the large expenditures of money which would be necessary to completely eliminate lead from the child's home environment.

Thus the treatment of lead pica requires the services of an interdisciplinary staff to first identify the child whose pica can be eliminated before lead toxicity occurs, to vigorously educate the child's caretakers, to help families cope with the child's environmental hazards and to maintain close surveillance of the child who continues to remain at risk.

For the child with highly motivated pica not specific for lead, major changes may need to be made in the physical environment, in the child's activity schedule, or in parental attitude toward the pica. Where indicated, admission to a day-care center, nursery school, or change of secondary school can offer a child who has been lonely or unstimulated opportunities for meaningful play and for new exciting experiences. The mother who works or whose absence from home appears to be a motivating factor in the emergence or continuation of pica might be encouraged to remain at home. The inadequate mother must be helped to develop nurture and affection for the child, to respond to his needs, and to give the child consistent direction. Parents must be helped to change attitudes toward the child which are depriving, punitive, or uncaring. At the same time, assistance must be offered to improve those financial, social, or environmental circumstances which overwhelm families and reduce parental effectiveness. The child must be helped to develop positive relationships with adults or peers, loneliness must be avoided, and speech and language therapy might be offered to the child who is isolated or frustrated by an inability to communicate adequately. Nutritional deficiencies and abnormal dietary patterns have been found to occur with pica and should be corrected.

Psychosomatic Illness

JOHN E. SCHOWALTER, M.D.

Over the past decade it has become less fashionable to define certain illnesses as "psychosomatic." There are a number of reasons for this trend. First, since psychologic stress can cause the organism to be less resistant to whatever pathologic forces are present, "psychosomatic" becomes such a general term that it means both more and less than is usually intended. Second, it is clear that "psychosomatic" and "somatopsychic" effects are so intertwined that they seldom can be extricated for any practical purpose in a given patient. Third, since controlled studies failed to support them, enthusiasm has disappeared for various theories which purported a particular symbolic meaning, conflict, or personality type to be etiologic for a specific disorder.

There are certain illnesses, such as asthma, ulcerative colitis, and neurodermatitis, for which psychosocial stresses play a specially important role in triggering exacerbations. Headaches and bellyaches are even more common problems in the practice of the pediatrician. For example, only about 5 per cent of children with recurrent abdominal pain ever reveal an organic cause.

It is generally assumed that illness is the result of constitutional givens in conjunction with physiologic and/or psychosocial stimuli. Any one stimulus might be necessary but not sufficient to cause symptoms. For example, some children are so inclined constitutionally toward asthma that almost any stimulus, be it infectious, allergic or psychologic, triggers an attack. Other children wheeze mainly or only as a result of a certain stimulus or a certain combination of stimuli.

While few pediatricians intellectually would deny that psychologic factors play a role in altering personal susceptibility to illness, it is also true that we all tend to ignore the relevance of variables not within the scope of our own familiarity. The reason that the mind-body problem has plagued physicians since earliest recorded time is that those interested in each have their own approaches and their own language. It is this fact which still makes the treatment of the so-called "psychosomatic" disorders so difficult and frustrating.

What might a pediatrician do to alleviate the psychosocial factors which aggravate a patient's condition? In most cases the pediatrician can be more helpful here than a child psychiatrist or psychologist. The reason for this is that the pediatrician usually already has longitudinal knowledge of the family and has their trust. By recognizing and inquiring about concerns which parents and child have about "fault" in the cause of the illness and about its prognosis, by helping the family and patient reduce the seeming but actually only illusory "gains" from the environment which accrue secondarily in response to the patient's disabilities, and by offering suggestions about child rearing practices which at the time may be poorly handled, the pediatrician can do much to lessen the psychologic reasons contributing to the disorder. Especially helpful will be anything the pediatrician can do to decrease feelings of helplessness and hopelessness.

Although bowel surgery for ulcerative colitis is often the most striking cause of psychologic improvement with that disorder, in general it is best to keep medication and procedures to a minimum in patients with "psychosomatic" illness. Iatrogenic problems secondary to steroids are distressingly common, and procedures strongly reinforce a self-concept of invalidism. It has been suggested correctly that for these patients the laying on of hands is not as important as the laying back of ears. Whatever the pediatrician can do to aid the patient and family either to understand the problem or to feel understood is likely to foster symptomatic relief.

At times the pediatrician may believe it best to separate the child from the family. Before such drastic action is taken, however, it is best to consult with a child psychiatrist. Practically speaking, probably the most important step in treating the more major "psychosomatic" illnesses is to enlist the help of a good child psychiatrist. This may prove as difficult as it is important. Of all the subspecialists, many pediatricians feel least comfortable conferring with child psychiatrists. Pediatricians often believe child psychiatrists are unavailable when needed, overly passive, and more interested in theory than results. Child psychiatrists frequently feel ignored and undervalued by pediatricians. Both groups are oftentimes right. Keeping a professional relationship cordial between pediatrician and child psychiatrist may require the patience of Job. In my experience, when it works, the two collaborators have previously gotten to trust one another either through social contact or in group activities such as professional societies or jointly attended seminars. In any case, it is well worth the pediatrician's time to find a child psychiatrist (or child psychologist or social worker) with whom he or she is comfortable. Conversely, it is well worth the child psychiatrist's time to find a pediatrician with whom he or she can collaborate effectively.

Individual psychotherapy has been the traditional approach to "psychosomatic" patients referred by the pediatrician. A number of other approaches are growing in popularity. These include family therapy, so parents can take a more active and enlightened role in their child's treatment, and group therapy, so patients can share their concerns with other patients who are at various stages of coping with the same illness. If family therapy is to be used, it is important that the therapist be knowledgeable about children as well as adults. Behavior modification is being used more, and with the present intense study of feedback effects on the brain from the viscera, it is hoped that autonomic conditioning will prove increasingly useful.

Disorders of Sleep

BRUCE O. BERG, M.D.

Sleep disturbances of children often go unrecognized for a considerable period of time before medical advice is sought because of the uncertainty about what is "normal" sleep for a child. Disorders of nocturnal sleep are usually more readily observed because the sleep of the parents is interrupted, but excessive daytime sleep, unless extreme, may persist unnoticed because the child is quiet without attracting parental attention. Much has been learned about normal and abnormal sleep physiology during the last few decades, and some methods of management of sleep disturbances have been introduced.

The most common sleep disturbances are secondary to some *environmental discomfort* or *illness.* A child may be too cold, too warm or be wearing uncomfortable night clothes. Febrile illnesses, endocrine disorders and convulsive phenomena may also disturb a child's sleep. These conditions are usually readily apparent and treated by appropriate measures.

Insomnia. There are a wide variety of lifestyles in the United States and whether a child goes to bed at seven or nine o'clock depends upon the family's sleep habits. Settling refers to the adjustment of the infant to sleeping from night to the next morning, and commonly by the end of the first year most infants have established a "settling pattern." Those infants with organic brain dysfunction may "settle" at a later age. Transient periods of awakening during the night are common and are often secondary to minor environmental changes. Usually, however, a child will adapt to the family's sleep pattern from the age of 2 years through 4 years. This period of adaptation is often one of great anxiety for the parents and the family as a whole.

True insomnia is relatively uncommon in the child, and one should only attach such a diagnostic label with care. Usually, the inability to fall asleep or the lack of sleep is indicative of some intrafamilial problem or other personal upset. A careful history regarding sleep habits and the circumstances related to sleep must be obtained. It is of particular importance to know whether or not the child takes any medication and the dosage of the medication throughout the 24 hour period. Central nervous system stimulants, particularly amphetamines and methylphenidate hydrochloride, distributed so often to our child population, may be given late in the afternoon or early evening and this may be the cause of the child's inability to fall asleep at the usual bedtime. It is generally inadvisable to give such medication after late afternoon.

Drug dependency may also be a cause of insomnia in childhood. Most, if not all, hypnotic medications lead to the development of drug tolerance and dependency. Transient sleep disturbances of children should, therefore, not be too readily treated by hypnotics, for drug dependence insomnia may develop within one or two weeks. The physician should always carefully explore the possibility of intrafamilial psychopathology before recommending any such medication. Hypnotics should be used most judiciously in the presence of a true disorder of sleep.

Episodic disturbances of sleep occur during stage III or IV of the nonrapid eye movement (non-REM) phase, and include somnambulism (sleep walking), pavor nocturnus (night terrors) and nocturnal enuresis. One person may have any or all of these episodic disturbances of sleep and there is often a history of other family members having had similar sleep disturbances.

Somnambulism (sleep walking). Persistent sleep walking is usually seen in the school age child, occurring in 1 to 6 per cent of the population and affecting males more than females. Occasional episodes are thought to occur in 10 to 15 per cent of all children, and may be associated with enuresis.

The child usually sits upright in bed and appears dazed, as if in a trance. Although his movements are somewhat clumsy, the child may carry out rather complex maneuvers, meandering throughout the room or house. The child's response to commands or conversation during the episode is somewhat garbled and not clearly related to what was asked. They are not "acting out," contrary to some psychiatric viewpoints. Purposeful movements or walking, however, and meaningful speech in monologue or in response to questions are suggestive of a psychological disturbance. The duration of the sleepwalking episode may be from a few minutes to about one-half hour. Children with true somnambulism are amnesic for this nocturnal event.

In the case of occasional sleepwalking no treatment is indicated, although obvious dangers to the child during this event should be removed, for the child may hurt himself while walking in his sleep. Potentially dangerous doorways and stairways should be obstructed. If sleep walking is a persistent problem, diazepam, 5 to 20 mg. orally, given at bedtime, will usually suppress stage III or IV of non-REM sleep and effectively reduce sleepwalking.* The matter of somnambulism should be carefully discussed with the parents, emphasizing that there is usually no serious psychological disturbance in the child who walks in his sleep and, further, these nocturnal episodes become less frequent as the child grows older.

Pavor nocturnus (night terrors). Night terrors most commonly occur in the preschool child and are often confused with nightmares

---

*This use of diazepam is not mentioned in the manufacturer's instructions.

or convulsive phenomena. They usually begin anywhere from 15 to 90 minutes after the child goes to sleep, when the child abruptly sits up, often screams or groans and appears terrified. There is an increase in respiratory rate and pulse rate and the face may appear flushed. Consoling parents find little response to their efforts and the child may only mumble. After 5 to 10 minutes, occasionally somewhat longer, the child will calm down and return to sleep. There is no recollection of this nocturnal event the next morning.

Nightmares, on the other hand, are characterized by unpleasant, frightening recall and usually occur during rapid eye movement (REM) sleep. Nightmares occurring in children are often related to daytime activities and indicate no psychological disturbance. When nightmares are frequent and persistent, they are more commonly accompanied by other symptoms of psychopathology.

Night terrors usually occur rather infrequently, do not indicate psychopathology and require no treatment. However, should the night terrors occur frequently, diazepam, given in doses of 5 to 20 mg. orally at bedtime, will effectively eliminate their recurrence.

Nocturnal enuresis has been reported in 5 to 15 per cent of children between the ages of 3 and 15 years. It is essential to rule out structural, metabolic and inflammatory processes of the genitourinary system that could be responsible for the bedwetting. Gastaut and Broughton have described an "enuretic episode" that usually occurs one to three hours after the child falls asleep, when progressing from stage III or IV of sleep to the first rapid eye movement (REM) episode. At that time, body movements have been noted with increased muscle tone, followed by increased pulse and respiratory rate, and sometimes erection in the male. Urination occurs a few minutes after the start of the episode during a moment of relative quiet. The child is difficult to arouse and is amnesic for the episode.

Imipramine is generally the drug of choice for this episodic disturbance of sleep in doses ranging from 25 to 75 mg. daily, given one hour before bedtime. There may be a tendency for recurrence of enuretic episodes when the drug is withdrawn. Imipramine is recommended for children 6 years and older.

Narcolepsy is characterized by sudden short attacks of sleep throughout the day, often occurring in situations not particularly conducive to sleep. In addition to the attacks of episodic sleep, there may be additional symptoms of cataplexy, hypnagogic hallucinations and sleep paralysis. It is uncommon for one patient to manifest all of the symptoms, and about 80 per cent present with recurring sleep attacks and cataplexy. The peak age of onset is between 15 and 25 years, but 20 per cent of one representative group of narcoleptics complained of excessive daytime drowsiness and sleep before the age of 11 years.

Cataplexy refers to recurring episodes of abrupt loss or inhibition of muscle tone resulting in momentary weakness, either generalized or localized, to particular muscle groups. The patient may slump to the ground. Cataplectic attacks are typically initiated by laughter, a surprise or sudden anger and are believed to be characteristic of the narcoleptic syndrome.

Hypnagogic hallucinations are usually terrifying visual or auditory experiences that occur while falling asleep or waking up. They may occur with sleep paralysis upon awakening, or may occur during the sleep attack. Sleep paralysis lasts for only a matter of seconds, and there is usually awareness of the environment; the patient is unable to move. Sometimes the patient will scream but then fall asleep, remembering this frightening experience as an event at the beginning of sleep.

Once the diagnosis of narcolepsy is clearly established, it is worth the time and effort to discuss the disorder with the parents and child. Such an explanation will often clarify some questions of behavioral disturbance and poor school performance, and provide the child and his family with much needed reassurance.

Methylphenidate hydrochloride,* in doses of 5 to 10 mg. three times daily, seems to provide effective control of the sleep attacks, but does not control the other symptoms as well. Imipramine is more effective for treating sleep paralysis, cataplexy, and hypnagogic hallucinations, but it is not recommended for children under the age of 6 years.†

Management of Voice, Speech, and Language Disorders

MORTON COOPER, PH.D.

Children of all ages may experience voice, speech, and language disorders. Some of these children, depending upon the severity of the problem, the age of the child, and other relevant considerations, may need the assistance of a voice therapist, a speech therapist, an au-

---

*Manufacturer's precaution: Methylphenidate hydrochloride should not be used in children under six years, since safety and efficacy in this age group have not been established.

†Manufacturer's warning: Administration of imipramine in pediatric conditions other than enuresis or in children under 6 years of age is not recommended.

diologist or other specialists as recommended by the pediatrician.

A child's speech and language development proceeds through stages which may overlap or run concomitantly. These stages include crying, babbling, lallation, echolalia and jargon. By the end of the first year of age, the child usually is beginning to use words. From this point, the child's vocabulary increases rapidly, and gradually speech becomes more intelligible as more sounds are correctly articulated.

If speech and language are not developing normally, that is, if the child is not speaking by 2 to 2½ years or is not basically intelligible by 3½ to 4 years, speech and language evaluations are advisable. The child may be diagnosed as having delayed language or an articulation disorder (sound substitution, distortion, omission or addition). Other tests (hearing, psychological, physical, etc.) may also be appropriate.

Speech.   Table 1 may be used as a guide for speech sound development, although speech sounds may appear earlier or later than the chart indicates. Speech sounds correctly produced in isolation or in single words do not constitute correct speech; the pediatrician must listen to the child's spontaneous, connected speech. The chart also indicates language development as depicted by sentence length.

TABLE 1.   **Speech and Language Development**

Ages	Speech (Sound development)*	Language (Sentence length in words)†
1		1
1½		1.2
2		1.8
2½		3.1
3	All vowels and diphthongs: *m, n, ng, p, f, h, w*	4.1
3½	*y*	4.7
4	*b, d, k, g, r*	5.4
4½	*sh, ch, s*	5.4
5		5.7
6	*t, th* (unvoiced), *v, l*	6.6
7	*th* (voiced), *z, zh, j*	7.3
8		7.6

*Sounds listed by age at which 75% of children tested produced sounds correctly in all positions in words, except in consonant blends (Templin).

†McCarthy (1 to 2½), Templin (ages 3-8).

In referring the child for speech therapy for articulation disorders, the pediatrician must take into account factors other than the sound development. These include the child's reaction to his speech, the parents' reaction to the child's speech, and the importance the parents (and the family) place upon correct speech.

Speech or language disorders may be either functional or organic in origin. Functional causes may include lack of speech stimulation, acceptance of gesture language by parents, inadequate speech models, bilingual influence, an environment which penalizes speech, an older sibling speaking for the child, an accident or illness, and any incident or continuing situation which creates psychological trauma. Organic causation may be neurologic, such as a hearing loss (slight or severe), mental retardation, brain damage, aphasia, and cerebral palsy, or it may involve structural deviations, such as cleft palate, submucus cleft, and "tongue-tie." ("Tongue-tie," although infrequently encountered, from a speech standpoint basically should be treated surgically as early as possible, before the child is one or two years of age, to avoid any interference with normal speech development.)

The length of speech and language therapy depends upon the severity of the disorder, the age of the child, parental support, motivation, and the child's emotional and psychological reactions to the speech or language problem, among other factors. Children with organic involvement require early diagnosis and may need long-term speech and language therapy, special school programs and extensive parent counseling.

Methods of Therapy.   In speech and language therapy with a child who has delayed language (functional or organic causation), the child must learn that using language is enjoyable and is the only realistic means of controlling his environment. The therapist may begin with an initial babbling of bilabial sounds, such as *b, p, w,* combined with physical movement (jumping, clapping, etc.) which encourages the child to participate and to imitate. Any attempt at speech imitation by the child is rewarded by appreciative verbal approval. Language used in the therapy session must be direct and simple, with constant repetition.

The therapist may initiate a structured framework to develop such concepts as colors, animals, family, and community helpers. As therapy progresses, concepts may be combined, such as talking about environmental objects and colors, i.e., "blue car," "brown shoes." When the child's language begins to develop, introduction of familiar words with initial bilabial sounds may be instituted with auditory, visual and tactile stimulation. Throughout the therapy program, the parents are guided by the therapist to reinforce the same type of program into the home environment.

Various approaches can be utilized by the therapist in the treatment of articulation disorders. After determining which sounds are incorrectly produced, the therapist may choose that sound which the child can most easily produce correctly. Success is essential at the initial stage of therapy so that the child develops a positive attitude toward therapy and its goals.

Personalizing the speech sounds for the younger child within a construct of speech activities geared to correct production of the sound helps the child remember the sound. The reward of a move on a speech game board, a picture he can paste in a book or a bell he can ring further reinforces the child's use of the correct sound in words, phrases and sentences. Carry-over of the speech sound into spontaneous speech can be accomplished by structuring situations that approximate those in the child's world. Doll families, manipulative toys, story telling, and puppets are some of the ways in which to move the child toward his final goal of carry-over of correct speech production into his everyday life. For the older child, speech activities emphasize the positive aspects of acceptable sound production and stress a more direct approach to therapy with the use of tape recordings, advanced speech materials, reading, and acting in plays.

Tongue Thrust. Children may experience a condition referred to as "tongue thrust." Tongue thrust occurs when the child places his tongue against the front teeth and pushes the tongue forward during swallowing or speaking. Speech therapy is often recommended by orthodontists in conjunction with orthodontic treatment. Speech therapy consists of alerting the child to the thrust of the tongue against the teeth and providing simple, direct exercises to retrain the position of the tongue during swallowing and speaking.

Stuttering. Some children may have the problem of stuttering. Stuttering is an interference with the normal flow of speech, actual (physical) or anticipated (psychological), and a reaction to the interference (or stuttering) which involves an attempt to avoid the interference (or stuttering). Stuttering usually involves noticeable and excessive dysfluencies, such as repeating, hesitating, prolonging, or blocking on speech sounds. Stuttering may be due to psychological tension which has been created by an attempt to avoid the normal dysfluencies that are present in normal speech.

Stuttering usually develops in two stages, primary and secondary. In the primary stage, the child appears to be without self-awareness or self-concern for the noticeable dysfluencies in his speech. In the secondary stage, the child either becomes aware or is made aware of the dysfluencies, seeks to minimize, prevent or avoid them, and attempts to produce perfect speech. Complicating factors of the secondary stage may include facial grimaces and other contorted body movement by which the child tries to prevent stuttering.

For a child in the primary stage of stuttering, play therapy encourages positive speech experiences and affords the child an opportunity to directly express his feeling state and to structure a more relevant self-image. The use of direct speech therapy depends upon the therapist's discretion. For a secondary stutterer, the therapist needs to develop a close relationship with the child, to meet the child's specific needs, and to work with the child on his own individual manner of stuttering. This approach allows the child to understand how he stutters, why he stutters, and how to cope with the stuttering.

An essential part of the therapy program is parent counseling. The parent(s) should be given information regarding the problem and suggestions to attenuate the emotional and psychological tensions which may contribute to or which may be activated by stuttering.

The following suggestions are for parents of primary stutterers: (1) As the child speaks, listen attentively and help the child to enjoy talking. (2) Provide experiences which the child can describe, such as visits to the park, museum, zoo and library. (3) Plan times to play, read and talk to the child. (4) Guide the child toward self-discipline, but avoid strict discipline. (5) Accept the child and his efforts, praising him whenever possible. (6) Do not refer to the child as a stutterer or discuss the stuttering in his presence. (7) Do not interrupt or correct the child when he is speaking. (8) Do not provide the child with words to complete his thoughts when he hesitates. (9) Do not pressure the child unrealistically in speech, in school work or in other activities. (10) Do not force the child to perform or participate in events which are threatening to him. (11) Do not criticize, ridicule or reject the child by words or actions.

In addition to these suggestions, parents of secondary stutterers should accept the child, his behavior and his speech; they need to provide reassurance, understanding, support and love, which in turn helps the child accept himself. The child needs to be encouraged to develop himself and his talents and to become a self-sufficient individual according to his age and his capabilities.

Dysphonias. Voice disorders in children may be either functional or organic. Functional dysphonias seen most frequently include nasality, falsetto, and functional misphonia (tired or weak voice with hoarseness present), which is the most prevalent type. Organic dysphonias which are encountered most often are nodules, polyps and papillomas on the vocal folds.

Voice problems are evidenced by negative vocal symptoms, visual, auditory, or sensory. Visual symptoms may be inflammation, edema or growths on the vocal folds. Auditory symptoms may include hoarseness, nasality, breathiness, limited vocal range, voice breaks and reduced volume. Sensory symptoms may include throat clearing, a sore, tight or strained throat, a feeling of a foreign substance in the throat, effortful voice and progressive vocal fatigue.

Childhood dysphonias are most frequently caused by vocal misuse and abuse, such as use of incorrect pitch, tone focus, volume or breath support, imitation of inadequate or inappropriate vocal models (vocal image), group singing in an incorrect pitch range, voice change at puberty, or poor vocal hygiene (shouting, screaming or talking frequently above noise). Contributing factors or causes may be a cold or upper respiratory infection if pitch and tone focus are affected; medical conditions, such as allergy, postnasal drip, hay fever, sinusitis, or infected tonsils; emotional or psychological problems; and organic involvements, such as a hearing loss, cleft palate or mental retardation.

Most childhood dysphonias may be alleviated or eliminated through vocal rehabilitation, which essentially eliminates vocal misuse by retraining the individual's voice in the use of pitch, tone focus, quality, breath support, volume or rate. The practice of good vocal hygiene is instituted to minimize or eliminate vocal abuse. Good vocal hygiene is a vital aspect of vocal rehabilitation.

The habitual pitch level may be above or below the optimal or natural pitch level. With the exception of falsetto, most children with dysphonias are using too low a pitch level. The child is taught to use the natural or optimal pitch level (Cooper and Cooper, 1977).

Tone focus (sound resonance) may incorrectly emphasize nasal resonance (from nasopharynx), oral resonance (from oropharynx), or laryngeal resonance (from laryngopharynx); the last is the most frequently heard resonance in dysphonias, except in nasality. Proper tone focus involves a balanced oro-naso-laryngo-pharyngeal resonance, which the child must develop.

Voice quality is determined by the vocal folds which produce the sound and by the resonating areas which modify the sound. Im-paired vocal folds may create a hoarse or a breathy voice; excessive nasal resonance may cause nasality. Correct pitch level and proper tone focus usually result in the resolution of a deviant voice quality.

Breath support may incorrectly stress clavicular breathing or upper chest breathing. Midsection breath support has been found to be the most effectual for speech.

Incorrect volume may be too loud or too soft; inappropriate rate may be too fast or too slow. Vocal rehabilitation involves appropriate volume and rate.

As the voice is being retrained, the child usually requires brief or extended *vocal psychotherapy* to help him adjust to the new voice and the new vocal image. The vocal image involves the positive or negative feelings and reactions toward a voice and determines the type of voice a child likes (and will use) or dislikes (and will not use). Children usually have a positive vocal image toward the old voice and a negative vocal image toward the new voice. Vocal psychotherapy allows a vocal catharsis, an expression of feelings and reactions toward the old and new voices. The extent of vocal psychotherapy, which varies from one child to another, is dependent upon the strength of the old vocal image. If the child does not become adjusted to and accepting of the new voice and the new vocal image, he will not use the new voice, and vocal rehabilitation will not be successful. In a few selected cases, psychotherapy may be necessary alone or in conjunction with vocal rehabilitation (Cooper, 1973).

The pediatrician's role in the management of voice, speech and language disorders is that of (1) recognizing disorders of speech, language and voice, (2) counseling the parents regarding the child's problem, (3) referring the child to appropriate specialists, (4) serving as a coordinator of the various specialists assisting the child, in some cases and (5) providing continual support for the rehabilitative programs.

References

Cooper, M.: Modern Techniques of Vocal Rehabilitation. Springfield, Illinois, Charles C Thomas, 1973.

Cooper, M., and Cooper, M. H. (eds.): Approaches to Vocal Rehabilitation. Springfield, Illinois, Charles C Thomas, 1977.

McCarthy, D.: Language development in children. *In* Carmichael, L., ed.: Manual of Child Psychology 2nd ed. New York, John Wiley & Sons, 1964.

Templin, M. C.: Certain Language Skills in Children: Their Development and Interrelationships. Minneapolis, University of Minnesota Press, 1957.

Specific Learning Disability and Hyperactivity

RICHARD G. SKINNER, JR., M.D.

Specific learning disability and hyperactivity are considered in one article because they probably represent a spectrum of disease or normal variation. At one end of the spectrum is the child with hyperactivity and at the other end is the child with specific learning disabilities. Each exists in a relatively pure form with a much larger group of patients manifesting a mixture of the two problems with symptoms of each, but with varying expression of symptoms.

To be considered in the above category it is assumed that the patients have intact organ systems, and thus their difficulty is not due to visual or hearing impairment; nor are children with mental retardation in this category. The latter problems can be identified by visual and auditory testing and by administration of a standard intelligence test.

Hyperactivity caused by emotional problems is more difficult to evaluate, because a number of children with primary emotional difficulties have a secondary hyperactivity. It is also common to see children with hyperactivity and specific learning disabilities have secondary emotional disorders.

The importance of obtaining a detailed assessment of the family background and culture cannot be over-emphasized; frequently a sibling or parent (usually male) may have had similar difficulties.

The symptoms associated with specific learning disability and hyperactivity can be lumped into four broad categories: (1) increased motor activity; (2) difficulty in learning, usually in the language area; (3) inattention; and (4) personality disorder.

Treatment should be a broad-based and consider the personality of the individual. In children who are outgoing, aggressive, and extremely active, management is directed at reducing the activity and allowing the person to function at a more normal level. Assuming this child has no major learning disability, he can function effectively in a regular classroom. At the other end of the spectrum is the shy, somewhat withdrawn child who has a negative self-image and may have significant learning problems. Since learning requires participation, the primary goal of treatment is to find ways to encourage the child to participate and make an appropriate attempt to learn.

Patients who manifest primary inattention usually respond quite dramatically to medication, provided the inattention is not due to some emotional disturbance. Some patients with hyperactivity and/or learning disabilities have significant personality disorders which make them objectionable companions. They may be grouchy, prone to argue, and generally present a rigid, noncompliant personality. These children are sometimes more compatible when taking medication.

The basis of all treatment regimens is to get the family to be supportive of the patient, rather than destructive. Frequently in order to help the child to overcome learning disabilities, the family spends hours and hours working with him in the areas of his educational deficits; thus the child sees himself as a nonproducer not only all day in the classroom, but in the eyes of his family as well. Generally it is difficult for the parents to serve in the dual role of parent and educator. Parents can assist the child in the educational process by providing appropriate space free of distractions and a regular time for the child to carry out his homework. It may be necessary for one parent to sit in the room and read while the child does his homework to ensure that he persists at the task. Far better, however, is a system that rewards the child for accomplishing homework in a reasonable period of time and with a reasonable degree of accuracy. It is the role of the teacher to ensure that the child understands what he is supposed to do and to review with him the completed homework, making necessary corrections and explanations. Frequently the doctor can act as a catalyst to get the teacher and the parent to work together as a team.

The child with hyperactivity will generally not function well in the classroom due to an inability to sit in his seat and pay attention to the task at hand. If the activity and attention can be improved with behavioral management techniques and/or medication, the child may be able to learn in a normal fashion.

The child with learning disabilities has problems with the thought process system and may require special teaching techniques. He will learn best in situations approaching one-to-one instruction; however because of the cost, this type of instruction is generally not financially feasible. Alternatives are classes for children with specific learning disabilities or the use of resource room teachers. Most schools now have exceptional education departments, and the physician can be a tremendous help to families with his knowledge of community resources, both public and private. In addition, some communities have tutoring programs outside of school hours.

The child with moderate or severe learning disabilities will have great difficulty learning to read, and may never be a competent reader. The physician can serve as a resource to the family to guide them to those capable of making adequate diagnosis and treatment, but should continue to monitor the problem to be sure that the emphasis on education is not out of proportion to the child's ultimate capabilities. The child may be sacrificed to the idol of education without due regard for the overall personality growth of the individual, and the recognition that there are other alternatives open to the child commensurate with his abilities.

Several general principles regarding medication should be rigidly adhered to. (1) The physician should become familiar with the basic medications usually involved in the management of these problems, and use first those drugs that have stood the test of time. (2) He should begin with the smallest possible dose to achieve the desired result. (3) He should obtain an objective evaluation of the effectiveness of the drug.

One method of obtaining an objective evaluation of a drug's effectiveness is by employing the double blind system. This can be done through arrangements with a local pharmacist to dispense the drug in a capsule. The family is given four vials of medicine with two containing the active drug and two placebo. The pharmacist randomly picks which weeks will contain the active ingredient and fills the capsules accordingly. This information is returned to the physician in an envelope to be opened at the completion of the study. The family reports on the effectiveness of the capsule each week for four weeks. If the child is in school it is extremely helpful for the teacher to be included in the reporting system. Not infrequently, medication seems to improve a child's organizational abilities in regard to schoolwork, and this benefit may be discernible only by the teacher. Although this is a somewhat complex system, it is well worth the effort.

Another method of evaluation is to have the mother begin the child on medication without telling the teacher. The parent should then have a conference with the teacher after about one week, giving the teacher an opportunity to volunteer whether the child's behavior and learning capabilities in school were better.

A third method of assessing the effectiveness of the drug is to have the family discontinue the medication for 24 to 48 hours, after the child has been taking it for three to four weeks, to see if they can tell the difference. Generally speaking, the family should be able to give fairly precise ideas as to the time that it takes for the medicine to take effect, and the approximate length of time they feel that it works.

Another method for monitoring the effectiveness and side reactions of the medication is to provide the parents with a reporting form with the prescription and require that they return the form prior to the issuance of another prescription. This provides a permanent record for the chart, and a system for the orderly renewal of the prescription.

Since some children who require the medication frequently have difficulty getting along with their peers without medication, they should be given the medication seven days a week and throughout the summer. For increased motor activity and inattention medication may be required only during the school day.

The specific drugs that may be used are amphetamine, methylphenidate, thioridazine, chlorpromazine, and pemoline. The amphetamines (Dexedrine) have been used the longest. It appears that the dextrorotatory form is considerably more effective than the levorotatory form. It is available in tablet form in 5 mg. size, in elixir with a concentration of 5 mg./5 ml. and in sustained release form in 5 mg., 10 mg., and 15 mg. capsules. Amphetamine should be avoided in patients with cardiac disease, hypertension, and hyperthyroidism and should not be used with monamine oxidase inhibitors. Tablets usually take effect in 30 to 45 minutes, and will last from three to five hours. The sustained release capsules take effect in 30 minutes to an hour, and last up to 8 to 12 hours. Amphetamines tend to interfere with appetite more so than does methylphenidate, and also are more likely to cause sleeplessness. They should be prescribed only with the greatest caution in teenagers or in those children in whom the possibility of drug abuse is likely because of the euphoria that is produced. On a fixed dose the euphoria quickly disappears, and if the administration of the medication is rigidly controlled, this is no great problem. If the child himself has access to the medicine, he may take increasing doses to overcome the tolerance that he has developed. Amphetamine also has the disadvantage that a higher percentage of patients seem to develop a tolerance to its effectiveness in the control of hyperactivity. If this occurs the medication can be stopped for a period of time and then restarted, apparently with full resumption of effectiveness. The amphetamines are not recommended for use in children under age three and it is highly desirable not to use this medication in children under six years. For those between the ages of three and six, amphetamine, 2.5 to 5 mg. per dose in the nonspansule form, is given no more than three to four times a day. This dose may have to be increased slightly as the child becomes older. The usual dose of the sustained release capsules for children six years of age and older is 10 to 15 mg. per day.

Methylphenidate (Ritalin) is an excellent and reasonably safe drug. It does not produce euphoria, but excessively high doses may cause tolerance and drug dependence. It is available in 5, 10, and 20 mg. tablets and is not recommended for use in children under six years. A child six years of age may be started on 5 mg. two to three times a day, increased if necessary to 10 mg., but rarely beyond that. If the dose is kept below 1 mg. per pound, the side reactions of headaches, abdominal cramps, dizziness, appetite impairment, or growth disturbance are rare. Other side reactions are drug sensitivity with rashes, tachycardia, and arrhythmias. Methylphenidate usually takes effect in 20 to 30 minutes, lasts from three to five hours, and is given before meals. Occasionally a hyperactive child will have trouble settling down to sleep, in which case a trial of a small dose of methylphenidate may be given after supper to determine its effectiveness in calming him and allowing sleep. However, the drug may also cause sleeplessness. Methylphenidate may inhibit the metabolism of phenobarbital, phenytoin, and primidone, and their doses may need to be adjusted if given with methylphenidate.

Thioridazine (Mellaril) is another drug sometimes used. Classified as being "possibly effective" in treating hyperactivity, it is approved for use in children over two years of age. Again the dose should be the smallest possible within the range of 0.5 to 3.0 mg./kg./day in divided doses. It is available in 10, 15, 25, and 50 mg. tablets. Side reactions are unusual, but may include drowsiness, pseudoparkinsonism and other extrapyramidal symptoms plus other reactions associated with phenothiazine drugs.

Chlorpromazine (Thorazine) is another drug that should be used infrequently. Occasionally though, it is valuable in calming the extremely wild child who seems not to benefit at all from his previous experiences, and is in constant danger of hurting himself because of his wild activities and extreme personality difficulties. Chlorpromazine should be used with caution in children with chronic or severe respiratory problems. It decreases the cough reflex and intensifies the action of central nervous system depressants. It should be started in low dose in children receiving phenobarbital for seizures. A dose of 0.25 mg./lb. every four to six hours should not be exceeded. In children six years old, 10 mg. three times a day can be given. The drug occasionally causes jaundice, allergic reactions, skin pigmentation, phototoxicity, and symptoms of phenothiazine toxicity. It is sold in 10, 25, and 50 mg. tablets, and syrup containing 10 mg./ 5 ml.

Pemoline (Cylert) is a relatively new drug that is supposed to be effective for hyperactivity and has the advantage of its action lasting 8 to 12 hours. Although peak blood levels occur in two to four hours, it may take three days for the blood levels to plateau. Clinical improvement is gradual and may take three to four weeks, making it difficult to assess the effectiveness of the drug. Many parents can tell the exact time that the medication begins and ends, even on a daily basis; if so, this drug can be a useful alternative to the drugs mentioned above. Many 11 and 12 year old children object to taking medications in school since it makes them feel "different." Pemoline may be useful because of its long action and because it has not yet shown any serious side reactions. It is begun in a dose of one 37.5 mg. tablet in the morning. This may be increased up to two or three tablets at one week intervals but should not exceed 112.5 mg. It is supplied in 18.75, 37.5, and 75 mg. tablets. Pemoline is not recommended in children under six years of age since safety and efficacy in this age group have not been established.

Imipramine (Tofranil) is occasionally used in children who have a combination of enuresis with hyperactivity and learning disorders; but it has been approved for use in enuresis only and should not be used for other reasons.

In most instances the above mentioned drugs will enable the physician to manage the great majority of patients with learning disability and hyperactivity. He should become familiar with a few drugs and use them appropriately and avoid the random use of large varieties of drugs of questionable value. Periodically the drug being used should be discontinued to see if it is still needed; if not, the medication should be stopped.

Recently Dr. Feingold has brought up the concept of the possible toxic effects of natural salicylates in foods as well as effects of food additives and coloring agents. Although it is difficult to keep any child on a diet, the diet he proposes seems to be safe and provides dramatic results in some children. This diet will have to pass the test of time and needs to be researched.

Megavitamin therapy does not seem to be have been as effective as some originally thought. It has the disadvantage of requiring very large doses of vitamins, the long-term effects of which are unknown.

Food allergies can also be incriminated as causative agents in hyperactivity and specific learning disorders and should be managed by traditional elimination diet methods.

Drugs are only a part of management. The physician should use his medical skills and knowledge of the family and community to monitor and coordinate this complicated and often exasperating problem. His genuine support of all concerned can sometimes be the difference between success and failure on the part of the child.

Reading Disorders

HOMER B. C. REED, Jr., PH.D.

Reading disorders exemplify one major aspect of school problems, a field in which pediatricians are becoming increasingly involved. The failure of a child to progress satisfactorily in school has potentially momentous significance for the future welfare of that child. Pediatricians represent a logical line of defense for many parents when they first become aware of their child's school problems. Although effective treatment of school problems is rarely the province of the pediatrician, he must nevertheless possess sufficient skill in diagnosis to give appropriate advice and to make appropriate referrals.

The significance of school problems for the overall health and welfare of the child can hardly be overstated. The problems may be symptomatic of some covert condition of which the pediatrician needs to be aware. Such is the case, for example, when the school problems are related to seizure activity or to metabolic disease, or represent one aspect of the residual effects of an earlier illness or handicapping condition. The percentage of school problems in which there is an easily identified medical component is not large. In the majority of cases, the school problem does not signify any identifiable previous or current illness, but its significance for the child's future is not thereby diminished. The future psychological well-being of the child may be jeopardized, parental

peace of mind is threatened, and on both counts the pediatrician must be prepared to respond.

Reading disorders are said to exist when the child reads much less well than would be expected on the basis of his previous educational experience and general intelligence. Reading problems may also be said to exist when the child reads much less well than his peer group. In the latter instance, reading difficulties may be part of a pervasive disorder in mental and educational development. Although it is misleading to describe such a child as having a reading problem, this is nevertheless frequently done.

There are no clinical procedures or laboratory examinations specifically useful in revealing medical problems associated with reading and learning disorders. Rather, what is required is a thorough general examination, a procedure that will, admittedly, yield negative findings more often than not. Most reading problems are attributable to factors not revealed by physical and laboratory examination. These factors include inadequate teaching, poor home environment, impaired general intelligence, emotional disturbance, and subtle neurologic deficit.

It is debatable just how much direct responsibility the pediatrician should assume for the diagnosis and management of reading problems not associated with an identifiable organic disturbance. What is not debatable is the pediatrician's responsibility for helping the parents to find adequate diagnostic and treatment services for their child. In urban communities, psychologists can be located who specialize in the diagnosis and management of school problems, including reading disorders. In small and large communities alike, school systems employ reading specialists and learning disability specialists who can frequently provide the necessary services. In certain instances, it may not be wise to utilize school personnel on an initial basis because of negative feelings that may have developed between the parents and the school.

Pediatricians who desire to develop some degree of personal skill in the diagnosis and management of reading problems may be frustrated by the lack of formal training opportunities. Probably as sound a way as any to proceed is to develop a collegial relationship with a child psychologist or reading specialist. For pediatricians interested in office examination routines, there is an abundance of formal reading tests that can be used to identify problems. Both the Gray Oral Reading Test and the Gilmore Reading Test are examples of tests that are well recommended and that can be used in a routine office examination. There are also many diagnostic reading tests to explore the importance of different components of the reading process, but such instruments are too specialized and too time-consuming for routine use by pediatricians.

The management of reading disorders and other school problems must always include helping parents to understand the issues, and in this area pediatricians can be quite active. Serious reading disorders are notoriously difficult to treat, and it is frequently true that everyone involved—teachers, parents, and child—becomes frustrated with the limited success of remedial programs. Pediatricians can help ensure appropriate parental expectations and can also be alert to the need to provide the child with special psychological support services. Finally, pediatricians can frequently help both child and parents by acting in the role of child advocate with local school personnel. The right of a child to appropriate special educational services is now guaranteed by federal law. By being aware of both federal and state laws pertaining to the education of handicapped children, pediatricians can help ensure local availability of appropriate educational services.

3

Nervous System

Head Injury

ROBERT L. McLAURIN, M.D.

Head injuries occur frequently in the pediatric age group but fortunately only few are of sufficient seriousness to leave permanent residuals. In general, the pediatrician's responsibility is in making a decision about which injury requires hospitalization and possible neurosurgical care.

There are three basic mechanisms responsible for most head injuries: the head may be struck by a relatively small rapidly moving object; the stationary head may be suddenly accelerated; or the moving head may be suddenly decelerated. The first mechanism results in tearing of the penetrated tissues. The others, acceleration and deceleration, cause damage to intracranial contents by movement of the brain against bony prominences and by tearing of vascular channels. Some knowledge of the mechanism of injury, therefore, can be of assistance in evaluating the possible damage.

Injuries to the head may cause damage to the coverings of the brain, to the brain itself or to blood vessels which in turn may lead to hematomas and secondary brain compression. The present section deals only with injuries to the coverings (scalp, skull and meninges) and direct injury to the brain. It is apparent that in most cases these occur simultaneously, but for purposes of evaluation and treatment they should be considered as separate aspects of the same injury.

LACERATIONS

Most injuries of the scalp result in laceration or in bleeding into the subgaleal space causing a cephalohematoma. Laceration should not be dealt with lightly but should be surgically cleansed and closed at the earliest possible time. Fortunately, the high degree of vascularity of the scalp helps prevent infection and the occurrence of a vascular necrosis of the skin. Nevertheless, meticulous surgical technique is of value, and suturing should be done without burying foreign material. Adequate preparation of the skin adjacent to the laceration includes shaving an area extending at least 1 inch from the laceration. Antibiotics are not used unless the laceration has remained unclosed for more than 4 hours or unless there is extensive soft tissue damage and wound contamination.

There is no specific treatment needed for subgaleal hematomas not compounded by adjacent lacerations. Such hematomas may persist for several days but invariably subside spontaneously. Tapping of hematomas is not only unnecessary but probably risks introduction of organisms. The presence of a hematoma may obscure an underlying depressed fracture, and therefore x-ray evaluation is usually indicated. Moreover, a subgaleal hematoma may resemble a depressed fracture to palpation. Subgaleal hematomas probably do not ever become calcified, but occasionally hematomas occurring beneath the periosteum in association with skull fracture may calcify. The latter can usually be distinguished in infancy and childhood because they do not cross the cranial sutures where the periosteum is attached.

FRACTURES

Fractures of the skull may be classified as linear, diastatic, basal and depressed; each has its own significance. In general, any infant or child who has received a sufficient impact to cause skull fracture should be hospitalized for observation of his intracranial status if seen initially within a few hours after injury. The commonest fracture is the simple linear fracture in one or more of the bones of the cranial vault. Those occurring to the frontal and parietal bones are usually of no significance clinically. Commonly, such fractures are not recognized for several days; since the impact is not witnessed, there are no signs of intracranial damage, and the parent only later becomes aware of a subgaleal hematoma. Under these circumstances, hospitalization is usually not necessary since the danger period has already passed.

The linear fractures which require careful observation are those occurring in the temporal area and crossing the middle meningeal artery, those crossing the sagittal plane with potential injury to the underlying sagittal sinus and its tributaries, and those in the occipital bone extending to the foramen magnum. This last fracture usually results from falls on the back of the head and may be accompanied by injury to the brain stem. Persistent vomiting is quite common following fractures in the occipital area. Thus, undisplaced linear fractures in these three locations must be treated with respect, and a period of hospital observation is usually indicated.

Another type of linear fracture which should be recognized for its potential hazard is the one in which the fracture line is greater than 3 mm. in width. Such a fracture implies a rather severe impact to the skull and also suggests that the underlying dura mater is also torn, since there is firm fixation of the dura to the suture lines, especially in infancy. This type of fracture may require surgical repair of the meningeal defect if there is evidence of underlying brain damage. It is also imperative that such a fracture be followed by a radiograph 3 months later to be certain that the fracture line is not becoming progressively wider as occurs with the development of a leptomeningeal cyst. This has been termed a "growing fracture" and when encountered it should be explored surgically so that dural and cranial repair can be done.

The term diastatic fracture is usually applied to separation of cranial bones along a suture line as a result of mechanical force. This is more likely to occur in infants and toddlers and the fracture itself is simply an index of the severity of the impact. The most frequent sutures involved are the sagittal and lambdoid, and since both of these sutures happen to be closely related to subjacent major venous channels, the possibility of intracranial bleeding must be suspected. No specific treatment of the fracture is necessary unless there is significant inward or outward displacement of a bony plate. Over a period of several weeks the bones become reapproximated and the suture line resumes a normal appearance.

The third type of fracture with clinical significance is the basal fracture. Since this fracture is usually accompanied by tear of the dura which is closely adherent to the skull base and since the fracture usually communicates with an air-filled space—the mastoid, middle ear, paranasal sinus or nasal cavity—the fracture is, by definition, compound. Most fractures involving the temporal bone, and characterized by cerebrospinal fluid otorrhea, heal sufficiently in 24 to 72 hours to stop the fluid leakage. Therefore, in this clinic for the past 10 years antibiotics have not been routinely employed and no increase in intracranial sepsis has occurred. If, however, the child has a purulent upper respiratory infection at the time of injury or if the drainage persists longer than 48 hours antibiotics are used. Pencillin G, 300,000 to 600,000 units/24 hours, is employed since the contaminating organism is usually pneumococcus. Basal fractures involving the anterior fossa and paranasal sinuses are more likely to result in persistent CSF drainage lasting from several days to indefinitely. For this reason, antibiotic treatment is to be given as soon as the drainage is recognized or suspected and continued until it ceases. Repeated spinal taps, previously advocated to diminish leakage, should not be done as there is no evidence that CSF rhinorrhea is diminished and there is a theoretical hazard of organisms being drawn into the cranial cavity from the air-containing cavities. In older children, maintaining the head in an elevated position may reduce CSF drainage by decreasing intracranial pressure. If cerebrospinal fluid drainage from the nose persists for 7 to 10 days after the injury, surgery is recommended to close the dural defect.

The final type of fracture requiring special management is the depressed fracture. Such a fracture usually results from impact of a relatively small object against the head and there may be an associated scalp laceration. There is no convincing evidence that all depressed fractures need to be corrected surgically but the following criteria are used to determine whether elevation is necessary: (1) if the wound is compounded and the fragments are severely comminuted, removal of the fragments is part of adequate debridement; (2) if the depressed fracture is accompanied by a local neurologic deficit corresponding to the fracture site, elevation of the depressed fragment should be done urgently; and (3) if the inner table depression is greater than 3 mm. over the sensorimotor strip or greater than 5 mm. over other portions of the cerebral surface, as measured on tangential views, elevation of the depressed element, repair of the dural tear, and restoration of normal cranial contour are indicated. Thus, with the exception of compound injuries, emergency treatment of depressed fractures is not necessary.

BRAIN INJURIES

The usual classification of brain injuries includes concussion (mild closed head injury) and contusion (severe closed head injury). The criterion for concussion is generally considered to be loss of consciousness, but in the pediatric age group there are many injuries which are not accompanied by definite loss of contact but which are followed by lethargy, pallor, confusion and vomiting which may last for several hours. A common symptom of concussion in children not rendered unconscious is transient loss of vision.

The principles of management of concussion include close observation for possible intracranial bleeding and control of vomiting. Thus, hospitalization is recommended for any child who has had a definite period of unconsciousness, visual loss, confusion lasting longer than a few minutes or vomiting persisting more than 2 hours. Observation is concerned mainly with level of consciousness and the patient should be watched from this standpoint at hourly intervals for the first 6 hours after injury and then the frequency of observation decreased if the patient appears stable.

In addition to observation of consciousness the observer should also note pupillary symmetry and response to light and symmetry of movement of the extremities. Changes in vital signs (pulse, blood pressure, respiration) are of little importance in the management of the child with simple concussion. They are late manifestations of intracranial complications and are usually not required for evaluation of associated bodily injuries in patients with concussion only. It is therefore unwise to use nurses' time taking and recording vital signs at frequent intervals; that can be used to greater advantage in observation of conscious level.

If vomiting persists more than 2 to 3 hours it should be treated with promethazine (Phenergan), 12.5 to 25 mg. suppository, or prochlorperazine (Compazine), 2.5 to 5 mg. suppository. The patient should take nothing by mouth until approximately 4 hours have elapsed after the injury or the most recent episode of vomiting. He may be started on clear liquids in small amounts with progression to regular diet over 8 to 12 hours if tolerated. The total period of hospitalization for a simple concussion may be overnight or, at most, 2 days if vomiting is controlled and the patient remains alert and responsive. There is no evidence that limitation of subsequent activity has any beneficial effect.

Any child who has a convulsion following a head injury, however minor, should be hospitalized. Trauma may initiate the first seizure in a child with idiopathic epilepsy. Moreover, focal seizures after injury suggest cerebral contusion regardless of the conscious level of the patient. Therefore, electroencephalography should be performed if seizures are part of the post-traumatic course.

Contusion of the brain is a much more serious injury, is apt to be associated with other bodily trauma, and may be followed by prolonged or permanent neurological deficits. It is usually accompanied by unconsciousness lasting from one half hour to an indefinite period. As with concussion, however, the most important aspects of neurologic observations concern consciousness, pupillary function, and motor responses. The presence of decerebrate extensor posture is an indication of brain-stem injury and therefore suggests a more serious prognosis. Vital signs are of less importance except as they may be used to evaluate other aspects of bodily injury.

In addition to neurologic observation certain specific therapeutic measures are indicated. If the child remains comatose following hospitalization, care of the respiratory function is of paramount importance, since pulmonary complications account for the greatest mortality in comatose patients. Endotracheal intubation is usually indicated in deeply comatose patients because of the lack of cough reflex. The endotracheal tube should be attached to a device for assisted or controlled respiration until a period of observation has established that adequate exchange would be maintained otherwise. Close observation of blood gases should be done and an effort made to keep the patient mildly hypocarbic ($Paco_2 \pm 30$ mm.) since elevation of Pco_2 leads to vascular dilatation and aggravation of intracranial hypertension which may already be present from cerebral bruising. Meticulous care of the respiratory system should be maintained by frequent suctioning and constant humidification. Antibiotics are not routinely used unless pulmonary complications occur.

Nasogastric suction should also be a routine part of the management of a child comatose from cerebral contusion. Aspiration of gastric contents may easily occur otherwise, leading to chemical pneumonitis. The gastric suction should be measured carefully and volume replaced as normal saline in addition to other fluid requirements. Fluids and electrolytes are administered entirely parenterally during the first week of post-traumatic coma. Since hypotonicity of body fluids accentuates cerebral swelling, the serum osmolality or sodium should be monitored at least daily for the first 3 days. The total osmolality should not be allowed to drop below 280 mOsm./liter or the serum sodium below 140 mEq./liter. If there are no fluid losses other than gastric suction and insensible loss the daily volume should not exceed 1200 ml./m². Administration of nitrogen substances is not a necessary part of nutritional replacement during the first few days after injury.

After severe cerebral contusion prophylactic anticonvulsant medication should be used. Since a minimum sedative effect is advisable, phenytoin is used in daily divided dosages totaling 3 to 8 mg./kg. Hyperthermia is treated most effectively by means of a cooling blanket. For lesser degrees of temperature elevation, aspirin by rectum may be employed. For control of intracranial pressure glucocorticoids have been recommended, but there is not good evidence of their effectiveness against traumatic cerebral edema. Hypertonic agents (urea, mannitol, glycerol) may be used for short-term control of pressure only. Lumbar puncture has no role in the diagnostic or therapeutic management of acute head injury and may indeed be hazardous.

Cerebral Edema

ROBERT L. McLAURIN, M.D.

DEHYDRATION

True cerebral edema implies an increase of water within either the intracellular or intercellular (extracellular) compartments. Two basic types of edema are recognized: cytotoxic and vasogenic. In the former there is increase of intracellular water, in the gray or white matter, without enlargement of extracellular spaces and without breakdown of the blood-brain barrier. Examples of this type of edema are seen in lead encephalopathy and water intoxication. In vasogenic edema there is damage to the blood-brain barrier and extravasation of protein-rich fluid into the extracellular space, especially of the white matter. Examples occur

in the vicinity of brain tumors, following head trauma and with inflammatory lesions.

Management of both forms of edema include measures to reduce water content: (1) restriction of water intake, (2) administration of sufficient NaCl to ensure normotonicity of body fluids and (3) use of osmotically hypertonic agents to withdraw water from the brain tissue.

1. While overhydration per se does not *cause* cerebral edema, the edema resulting from some other disease state may be reduced by moderate water restriction. The total volume administered should be a normal daily maintenance to ensure adequate renal function. In infants this does not exceed 1200 ml./m² unless there are other extrarenal sources of water loss. Adequacy of water intake for renal function should be monitored by blood urea and creatinine levels as long as water restriction is being employed.

2. A greater threat than overhydration to the patient with potential or actual cerebral edema is hypotonicity of body fluids. This results from the fact that since water crosses the cell membrane more easily than electrolytes there is a consequent passage of water into the cells and resulting cellular swelling when systemic hypotonicity is present. The ultimate of cellular overhydration is seen in water intoxication in which cellular functions are altered by the intracellular hypotonicity. Sodium chloride intake should be 50 mEq./m² for patients over 5 kg. and 2 mEq./kg. for those less than 5 kg. The tonicity should be monitored daily during periods of active therapy. Serum osmolality should be maintained above 280 mOsm./liter and the serum sodium should be held between 140 and 145 mEq./liter.

3. The most rapid method of reducing cerebral edema and lowering intracranial pressure is by use of hypertonic agents. Such agents create an osmotic gradient between the intravascular and extravascular compartments and thereby reduce the extravascular water content. These substances are probably most effective in the presence of a stable blood-brain barrier and are relatively less effective in areas of vasogenic edema. The substances most frequently employed for this purpose are urea and mannitol.

Although diuresis is not a necessary occurrence in the effectiveness of osmotic agents, it does routinely occur. For this reason an indwelling catheter should always be inserted to prevent bladder distention and so that output can be accurately assessed.

Urea is administered as a 30 per cent solution intravenously and is given in dosages of

0.5 to 1.5 gm./kg. It should be given rapidly, over a period of 15 to 30 minutes. Lowering of intracranial pressure usually occurs within about 30 minutes and the effect is maintained for 4 to 6 hours. This dosage can be repeated as often as every 6 to 8 hours for several times, but repeated use may lead to systemic dehydration and hypertonicity. Thus, serum osmolality should be determined at least every 12 hours and should not be allowed to exceed 320 mOsm./liter. Urea should not be used if renal insufficiency is suspected. In general, the osmotic agents should be considered as effective short-term treatment and should rarely be relied on for intervals longer than 48 hours. There is not general agreement as to whether there is a "rebound" after the effect of urea ceases. While rebound is less likely to occur in cytotoxic edema, it may occur in vasogenic edema due to the accumulation of the substance in the extravascular space. Nevertheless, this rebound effect is seldom troublesome.

Mannitol* has increased in popularity as an osmotic agent during the past few years because it is less expensive than urea and possesses other favorable characteristics. Mannitol is a hexahydric alcohol which is rapidly excreted by the kidney and produces a diuresis. The molecular weight is larger than that of urea and therefore a greater weight must be administered to achieve a similar osmotic effect. It is given intravenously in a 20 per cent solution and in amounts of 1.0 to 2.0 gm./kg. over 30 to 45 minutes. The effect on intracranial pressure lasts 5 to 8 hours, and equilibrium between brain and serum mannitol does not occur until 6 hours after administration. As with urea mannitol can be used repeatedly for limited times but the same hazards are present with repeated administration—systemic dehydration, hemoconcentration, hypotension and tachycardia. These effects, however, can be rapidly counteracted by infusion of isotonic glucose solution. Mannitol, like urea, is contraindicated in the presence of impaired renal function.

Glycerol, a trivalent alcohol which is not metabolized completely when given in large doses, may also be used as an osmotic agent. It acts promptly, can be given repeatedly over a prolonged period of time and is not toxic. The dosage is 0.5 to 2.0 gm./kg. given through a nasogastric tube. While the substance is of advantage in dealing with chronic types of cerebral edema, it is not as effective as urea or mannitol in treating acute edema.

*Manufacturer's precaution: The use of mannitol in pediatric patients has not been studied comprehensively.

STABILIZATION OF BLOOD-BRAIN BARRIER

The osmotically active agents described above are used principally for short-term management of acutely elevated intracranial pressure. The corticosteroids, which probably act by restoration or stabilization of the blood-brain barrier, have become extremely useful in treating certain types of edema over a protracted period of time. Since the principal effect is on the blood-brain barrier, steroids would be thought to be most effective against vasogenic edema, but in fact there is no good evidence that this therapy prevents or decreases edema resulting from mechanical trauma. There is definite evidence, however, that it is effective against edema due to inflammatory reaction or adjacent to a mass lesion.

The most commonly used drug is dexamethasone. Lowering of intracranial pressure may be recorded within 1 to 2 hours after administration, but the clinical effect is usually noted within 6 to 8 hours and reaches a maximum at 18 to 24 hours. The effect of a single loading dose lasts for 10 to 12 hours and it is customary to follow such a dose with maintenance doses at 6 to 8 hour intervals. In the child whose weight exceeds 50 kg. an initial intravenous dose of 10 mg. is followed by maintenance intramuscular doses of 4 mg. If the body weight is between 20 and 50 kg. the doses are halved, and when the body weight is less than 20 kg. doses of 2 mg. initially and 1 mg. thereafter are used.

Because of the increased likelihood of gastric ulceration during steroid therapy, antacids are used routinely through a nasogastric tube in any comatose patient. Preparations containing aluminum hydroxide are administered every 4 hours. There seem to be no other significant complications of dexamethasone therapy, as the salt-retaining effect of this steroid is not marked. If the acute stage of cerebral edema is followed by the need for more prolonged treatment, it is frequently possible to decrease the maintenance dose admininstration to 12 hour intervals. If corticosteroids are used for periods less than 7 days it is not necessary to taper the dose but rather it may be discontinued abruptly. If administration has been longer than 7 days, dosages should be tapered over a period of a week to allow resumption of normal adrenocortical function, which has been suppressed during therapy.

As previously indicated, corticosteroids are of doubtful value in the treatment of post-traumatic edema despite their popularity in such situations. They are of unquestionable help in treating edema which surrounds a tumor or is adjacent to an abscess or hematoma, as these are clear examples of vasogenic edema. They are also effective as an adjunct in the treatment of swelling due to heavy metal intoxication, as in lead encephalopathy, and should be part of the standard treatment of that condition. Steroids are also effective against the edema which leads to pseudotumor cerebri, an entity which is poorly understood pathophysiologically but which is characterized by generalized swelling of the cerebral tissue and consequent intracranial hypertension. Finally, the cerebral edema which follows withdrawal or decrease of steroids after prolonged use responds appropriately to increase of dosage.

VASOCONSTRICTION

"Cerebral edema" is often synonymously used with "cerebral swelling" which may be due to enlargement of the vascular compartment rather than to an excess of extravascular water. Moreover, in the presence of true cerebral edema intracranial pressure can be partially controlled by reduction of the vascular compartment. Thus, treatment of cerebral edema should include efforts to reduce the vascular bed by vasoconstriction.

The most potent agent affecting cerebral vasomotor tone is carbon dioxide. Lowering arterial Pco_2 leads to vasoconstriction and consequent reduction of the vascular compartment. In any condition, therefore, in which there is intracranial hypertension (such as cerebral edema) it is imperative that the $Paco_2$ be maintained at normal or hypocarbic levels. Since this is dependent on ventilatory function, particular attention must be directed toward adequate ventilation. Respiratory function may be depressed by elevated intracranial pressure and a vicious circle thereby created. Thus, if there is depression of conscious level accompanying the cerebral swelling, attention must be directed toward maintaining a clear airway and sufficient pulmonary exchange to prevent accumulation of CO_2. If cerebral swelling has occurred to the point of causing progressive neurologic deterioration it may often be reversed by mechanical hyperventilation.

Hyperventilation is achieved by a 25 to 50 per cent increase over the patient's normal minute volume. Initially the hyperventilation should be done with 100 per cent O_2 and this can then be reduced to maintain the arterial oxygen tension between 100 and 200 mm. Hg. The $Paco_2$ may be maintained in the 20 to 25 mm. range with a corresponding vasoconstriction of the cerebral vessels and reduction of the

total intracranial mass. Respiratory alkalosis will occur during hyperventilation but is usually of no consequence in the presence of normally functioning kidneys. In addition to causing vasoconstriction artificial hyperventilation prevents the compounding of cerebral swelling with edema which can result from a combination of hypoxia and hypercapnia.

HYPOTHERMIA

This method of edema control has been advocated in the past, but recent experience has led to the conclusion that it simply retards and does not prevent the occurrence of edema. For this reason, and because of complications, hypothermia is seldom used. However, it is important to maintain normothermia in the patient with cerebral edema or swelling, as the intracranial dysfunction seems to be aggravated during hyperthermia.

MECHANICAL DECOMPRESSION

The therapeutic measures described above have depended on biological effects to prevent or reduce cerebral edema. When these measures fail, mechanical decompression of the swollen brain may be used. Since one of the lethal effects of cerebral edema is herniation of the brain through the tentorial incisura and resulting brain stem damage, decompression of the supratentorial compartment may prevent this herniation. Modified decompressions may be done in the subtemporal areas. The squamous portion of the temporal bone is removed and the dura is incised, allowing outward herniation of that part of the cerebrum. If more extensive decompression is needed bilateral frontotemporoparietal craniectomies can be done. This has been effective in the past in the treatment of cerebral swelling due to trauma, lead intoxication and encephalitis. After subsidence of cerebral edema the bone flaps, if preserved, may be replaced or some other type of cranioplasty performed.

Epidural Hematoma and Subdural Hematoma and Effusion

ROBERT L. McLAURIN, M.D.

Accumulation of blood or fluid in a localized area over the surface of the brain leads to several pathophysiologic events. An understanding of these events is helpful in planning management. A surface hematoma or effusion is an added mass within the limited intracranial space and in certain instances progressively enlarges. By virtue of its mass it raises intracranial pressure and if unilateral displaces the brain toward the opposite side and downward through the tentorial incisura. If bilateral, the lateralward displacement does not occur. Intracranial pressure is further increased by edema which occurs beneath the surface lesion, and progression of the edema may be responsible for neurologic deterioration despite a static size of the surface mass. In addition there may be obstruction to the surface circulation and reabsorption of cerebrospinal fluid leading to hydrocephalus. In the case of effusions associated with meningitis there may be further interference with CSF circulation by the basic inflammatory process.

EPIDURAL HEMATOMA

Epidural hematoma, usually the result of traumatic laceration of the middle meningeal artery, is a true surgical emergency. Arterial laceration most often occurs in the temporal fossa and the hematoma expands rapidly in that area which is adjacent to the uncal gyrus and brain stem. When the diagnosis is made, therefore, the patient is usually losing consciousness and showing signs of uncal herniation with pupillary asymmetry and respiratory irregularity leading to decerebrate rigidity and respiratory failure. The objective of management at that stage is to maintain respiration, attempt to minimize intracranial pressure and herniation, and proceed as quickly as possible to surgical decompression.

If the diagnosis is suspected from the classical history of a minor injury with unconsciousness followed by a lucid interval followed by neurologic deterioration, all within a few hours, time should not be wasted in obtaining x-rays of the skull. While the operating room is being made ready measures should be taken to retard the intracranial pathophysiology. The most important measure to accomplish this is the rapid intravenous administration of urea (1 gm./kg.) or mannitol* (1.5 gm./kg.). While these are being given a catheter should be inserted into the bladder.

If the conscious level has deteriorated sufficiently and respiratory function is being affected, the child should be intubated and hyperventilated. This maneuver assures adequate oxygenation and also produces hypocarbia which further reduces intracranial pressure by vasoconstriction. If seizures have occurred during the stage of neurologic dete-

rioration, diazepam (Valium) should be administered. There is no indication for steroids under these conditions. Definitive treatment, of course, consists of craniotomy to release the rapidly expanding arterial hematoma and location and coagulation of clipping of the bleeding meningeal vessel. Providing irreversible brain stem damage has not occurred, the prognosis is excellent for survival and recovery. Epidural bleeding is rare in infancy because of the attachment of the dura to the skull at the suture lines. It is more likely to occur after 5 years of age.

SUBDURAL HEMATOMA

Whereas extradural hematomas are usually acute lesions, subdural hematomas, because they are most often of venous origin, are usually chronic. In the occasional instance of an acute subdural hemorrhage the treatment is the same as that for extradural hematomas. One significant difference is that in infancy, subdural bleeding may be of sufficient volume to render the patient hypovolemic. Therefore, hypotension may occur in the early phase or anemia later; in the former blood replacement should be done by transfusion, while in the latter situation the use of whole blood or iron depends on the severity of the anemia.

The clinical picture of chronic subdural hematoma varies according to the age of the patient. The condition is most common in infancy, where it presents as intracranial hypertension with macrocrania and frequently with seizures. Management, therefore, includes control and prevention of seizures, followed by investigation of the cause of increased intracranial pressure. Seizure control in this age group is best done by phenobarbital in doses of 5 mg./kg./day. If the intracranial hypertension has led to vomiting prior to diagnosis, dehydration may be present and should be corrected by appropriate fluid replacement.

The objective of definitive treatment is, of course, removal of the subdural hematoma or control of intracranial pressure regardless of the persistence of some fluid and blood in the subdural space. Diagnosis is usually confirmed by insertion of a 21-gauge needle through the lateral border of the anterior fontanelle or through the coronal suture (at least 1.5 cm. from the midline) and treatment begins as the fluid is removed for diagnosis.

Subdural hematomas in infancy are usually bilateral and therefore bilateral subdural taps are always necessary. Fluid should not be aspirated from the subdural space. Generally, fluid containing blood and with xanthochromic supernatant fluid is allowed to run through the

---

*Manufacturer's precaution: The use of mannitol in pediatric patients has not been studied comprehensively.

needle until it stops. It must be remembered that when this occurs the subdural fluid is equilibrated with atmospheric pressure, but the subdural accumulation has not been completely eliminated; indeed, if significant macrocrania is present, some craniocerebral disproportion is bound to be present and the subdural space cannot be completely collapsed. There is no limit to the amount of fluid which may be drained at one sitting, but rarely does it exceed 50 ml.

Following the initial tap, subsequent taps are performed only when there is evidence of build-up of pressure as judged by fontanelle tension or clinical signs such as vomiting, lethargy or irritability. The intracranial pressure may become elevated again within 24 hours, may require several days or occasionally does not recur. If hypertension does not recur, no further taps are necessary. This method of treatment is based on the principle that fluid in the subdural space is itself not harmful but only if accompanied by intracranial hypertension. Moreover, membrane removal is not done, as it is untenable that subdural membranes are capable of restricting cerebral growth which normally is not restricted by the scalp, skull and dura mater.

Rarely intracranial pressure cannot be controlled by tapping alone. If after 8 to 10 taps fluid accumulation and pressure continue to recur, shunting of the subdural space may be necessary. Shunting may be done into the pleural or peritoneal spaces or into the vascular system. Shunting of ventricular fluid to other body compartments is the method of treatment necessary in those rare cases of hydrocephalus.

Chronic subdural hematomas occurring in older children are similar in management to those occurring in adults. They are the result of injury and present within several weeks as expanding surface lesions which cause symptoms and signs of intracranial hypertension and focal neurologic impairment or irritation. They are more often unilateral than those of infancy. If the sutures and fontanelle have functionally closed, diagnosis can be made most easily by angiography, best performed via the femoral route. Brain scanning is also of assistance by demonstrating increased uptake of nuclide over the brain surface. Definitive treatment is done by two or more cranial burr holes, incision of dura, and drainage of fluid from the subdural space. Reaccumulation is rare and complete recovery is the rule unless there was serious cerebral contusion at the time of initial injury.

Subdural effusion occurs in some cases of meningitis and occasionally may be responsible for the increased intracranial pressure. Treatment is similar to that described above: subdural tapping only in response to intracranial hypertension. Since effusion is not chronic, craniocerebral disproportion does not occur and reaccumulation is therefore uncommon.

Intracranial Hemorrhage

ROBERT L. McLAURIN, M.D.

Intracranial hemorrhage includes bleeding into the substance of the brain or into one or more of the meningeal compartments—epidural, subdural or subarachnoid. The bleeding may be a direct result of trauma or it may occur spontaneously from a vascular abnormality (aneurysm, angioma, arteriovenous malformation) or as a result of a coagulation defect. While there is no constant relationship between the location of hemorrhage and its etiology, there are certain relationships which occur with sufficient frequency to be of diagnostic value. Thus, trauma most frequently leads to surface bleeding, aneurysms commonly rupture into the subarachnoid space, and ateriovenous malformations and angiomas usually bleed into the brain substance.

The first goal of management is to define the cause and primary location of hemorrhage. In rare instances immediate treatment of intracranial hypertension is needed, either by administration of osmotically active agents, by needling of the hematoma or ventricles, or by craniotomy. More often, however, emergency treatment is not necessary and diagnostic investigation can be pursued in a more orderly way. History is especially important in relation to injury and to prior history of bleeding tendencies. When vascular deformity is responsible there is usually no historical assistance in the pediatric age group as the hemorrhage is likely to be the first that has occurred.

Examination is of limited help with the etiology but may provide evidence of head trauma or of other areas of spontaneous bleeding. On the other hand, examination may provide considerable help as to location of hemorrhage. Subarachnoid blood leads to signs of meningeal irritation without localizing neurologic signs, since blood diffuses rapidly and evenly throughout the CSF compartment. An acute or progressive focal neurologic deficit may occur with localized hematomas (which are primarily unilateral) either within or compressing the brain. Infantile subdural hematomas, being chronic and usually bilateral, may cause signs of intracranial hypertension only, manifested by macrocrania (see p. 46). Seizures are more apt to be present with localized surface hematomas. Transillumination of the skull may be possible in infants of less than 6 months of age who harbor subdural hematomas. Cranial bruit may accompany arteriovenous malformation but does not occur with aneurysm.

More definitive diagnostic studies are usually necessary. Lumbar puncture is of limited value, but it differentiates meningeal signs due to blood from those due to infection. The presence of blood in the CSF does not mean that the primary source of bleeding was in that compartment; bleeding may have occurred within the brain substance with rupture into the ventricular or subarachnoid space. Spinal tap has no therapeutic value and may contribute to brain herniation through the incisura if a supratentorial hematoma is present. If the diagnosis has otherwise been confirmed, therefore, or if hemorrhages are present on funduscopic examination, lumbar puncture is not recommended.

Subdural taps are used to detect the presence of blood in that space and can be done with ease up to about 2 years of age. The needle is introduced at least 1.5 cm. from the midline and just through the dura mater. Aspiration should not be done since liquified hematoma, if present, will spontaneously flow from the needle. Thus, when the diagnosis is made, therapy is automatically begun by release of the hematoma contents. If the infant is in extremis and subdural fluid is not obtained, the needle may be inserted through the cortex and brain substance to the lateral ventricle. This may allow life-saving intracranial decompression for a brief period of time as well as detect evidence of blood within the ventricular system.

Angiography is the most definitive diagnostic study in those patients whose hematomas have not been detected by subdural tapping. In children over 3 years of age angiography should always be done if there is clinical evidence of a post-traumatic progressive neurologic deficit suggesting hemorrhage. In this situation the exact location, intra or extracerebral, and the size of the hematoma can be determined. In addition, it should be done in all cases, regardless of age, of spontaneous hemorrhage with neurologic localization and in cases of subarachnoid bleeding unexplained by trauma or blood dyscrasia. In the latter circumstance the presence of a vascular anomaly may be determined.

After diagnostic determination of the loca-

tion of intracranial hematoma, therapy is directed toward its removal as expeditiously as possible. If neurologic deterioration is progressing rapidly it may be arrested temporarily by relief of intracranial pressure. As stated previously ventricular tapping may cause transient relief of pressure, but this can be done by needle in only the first few years of life because of subsequent fusion of cranial sutures. Moreover, it provides relief for only 30 to 60 minutes in most instances. A more prolonged reduction of pressure can usually be achieved by dehydrating agents such as hypertonic mannitol or urea solutions. Mannitol is given intravenously in a 20 per cent solution in amounts of 1 to 2 gm./kg. over a period of 20 to 30 minutes.* The pressure reduction occurs within 30 minutes and may be maintained for 4 to 6 hours. Urea is administered in a 30 per cent solution in dosages of 0.5 to 1.5 gm./kg. with the same duration of effectiveness. Both of these agents can be repeated after 6 to 8 hours but should not be used in lieu of hematoma evacuation. After hematoma removal it is seldom necessary to repeat them.

Maintenance of an adequate airway during neurologic deterioration is of utmost importance since any increase of P_{CO_2} is immediately reflected in the intracranial pressure due to its vasodilatory effect. Ideally, the P_{CO_2} should be maintained at 25 to 30 mm. Hg., and this may require use of tracheal intubation or tracheostomy with mechanical respiratory assistance or control.

Removal of the hematoma is accomplished by whatever is appropriate in relation to the patient's age and the location and age of the blood clot. Hematomas become liquified after 10 to 12 days and can then be removed by needle. The chronic subdural hematoma of infancy is illustrative of this lesion. It is noteworthy that sufficient bleeding may occur into the infant's subdural space to cause hypovolemia, and blood replacement may be necessary. Acute meningeal hematomas usually require burr holes or craniotomy for removal, and intracerebral hematomas should be removed only through a craniotomy approach.

Subarachnoid hemorrhage does not require specific treatment unless it leads to hydrocephalus. Blood within the subarachnoid compartment disperses rapidly throughout the cerebrospinal fluid and does not act as a localized mass lesion. However, due to blockage of CSF absorptive pathways, it may lead to acute hydrocephalus with accompanying signs

---

*Manufacturer's precaution: The use of mannitol in pediatric patients has not been studied comprehensively.

of acutely raised pressure or herniation. Ventricular tapping or drainage may be necessary to control intracranial pressure.

Definitive treatment of hematomas due to vascular anomalies includes, in addition to hematoma removal, consideration of measures to prevent future bleeds. If an aneurysm is present (rare in the pediatric age group), craniotomy for clipping or trapping of the lesion may be done. If an arteriovenous malformation is found, the decision will be between surgical excision, embolization with plastic spheres, or no definitive treatment on the basis of size and location of the malformation combined with the clinical residuals of hemorrhage.

Anticonvulsant therapy should be part of the treatment of any intracranial hemorrhage other than subarachnoid. Phenobarbital, 5 mg./kg./day, should be started immediately and continued or replaced with phenytoin, 3 to 8 mg./kg./day, until there is no clinical or electroencephalographic evidence of seizure tendency.

Hydrocephalus

KENNETH SHULMAN, M.D.

Hydrocephalus is a disease state associated with an abnormal increase in the amount of cerebrospinal fluid (CSF) under increased pressure within the cranial vault. In infancy and childhood this volume increase is accommodated by head expansion leading to an enlarged head, a full tense anterior fontanelle and prominent scalp veins. The child becomes irritable, with lethargy and vomiting. The time of onset and the severity of the signs and symptoms of hydrocephalus depend upon the degree of cerebrospinal fluid abnormality, specifically the absorption deficit. Available physiologic data indicate that most instances of clinical hydrocephalus are due to an absorption deficit resulting from a blockage within the CSF transport system, that is, the cerebral ventricles, or at the site of CSF-venous absorption in the subarachnoid space. Infantile hydrocephalus is largely congenital. Acquired hydrocephalus does occur in infants and children after head injury or meningitis due to particulate matter (red and white blood cells) clogging the CSF absorption mechanism. Rare instances of hydrocephalus are associated with tumors strategically located so as to obstruct CSF flow. Vascular malformations of the vein of Galen and large hemispheric arteriovenous malformations can also result in hydrocephalus.

The pediatrician presented with an infant whose head circumference exceeds the normal rate of growth, either by exceeding the absolute head circumference for age or by moving rapidly from the third to the 97th percentile over time, should seek neurosurgical consultation. Differential diagnosis includes familial megalocephaly and chronic subdural hematoma. The latter condition, for reasons unclear, seems to be less frequent at the present time than in the past decade. The current availability of computerized transaxial tomography (CTT) permits imaging of the head and the ventricular system in a noninvasive fashion, with easy ascertainment of hydrocephalus, chronic subdural hematoma, or no cause of the enlarged head. Accepting the need for short-term hospitalization for this test because of the need for anesthesia to immobilize the child, CTT permits earlier diagnosis of hydrocephalus and will probably yield better surgical results. It is currently my policy to utilize CTT without subsequent air study to diagnose and follow children with hydrocephalus unless some particular information is needed about the pathophysiology of the CSF system or there is serious question of infection.

Therapy. Having ruled out a specific cause of CSF obstruction, i.e., tumor, vascular malformation or arachnoid cyst, the surgical treatment of hydrocephalus is largely based upon diversion of CSF from the head into various other extracranial sites by means of shunt systems. Each of the variety of CSF shunt systems comprises a proximal ventricular cannula, a valve and a distal catheter which can be placed into a number of places. I presently favor peritoneal placement of the distal catheter.

The timing of therapy is related in a general way to effectiveness so that intervention should be deliberate once the diagnosis is made. On clinical grounds there are some children whose heads go through rapid growth phases and then seem to stop growing rapidly. Observation has been useful in such children but should be accompanied at the present time with CTT scanning to distinguish those with progressive hydrocephalus. CTT scanning can be done without contrast agent (iodinated organic compounds) unless a tumor or vascular malformation is suspected on other grounds, such as focal neurological deficit, seizures or cranial neural findings.

The ventriculoperitoneal shunt is placed with the ventricular catheter in the right lateral ventricle via a posterior parietal burr hole. I am accustomed to use a valve in series at the site of the burr hole (Holter valve manufactured by Extracorporeal Devices). The valve, which really is composed of two fish-mouth plastic slit valves in series with a chamber between, becomes a pump so that the compressibility of the chamber tests CSF flow. Easy compressibility means that the distal peritoneal catheter is patent; rapid refilling of the chamber indicates an open ventricular catheter. The distal catheter is passed subcutaneously and via a subxyphoid incision into the peritoneal cavity, where approximately 20 to 30 cm. of tubing is placed in no specific location. This relatively simple operation can be done on any size infant or child and requires about 40 minutes. Prophylactic antibiotics are not used. The effect of the shunt is seen soon afterward with a depressed anterior fontanelle and a less irritable child. If venous engorgement or pupillary sunsetting is present, it will clear within 12 hours. Subsequent head circumference should not increase further until the child's body growth curve catches up with the head curve, and then both somatic and head growth should become parallel and appropriate.

Follow-up and Complications of Treatment. The mechanical concept of hydrocephalus and its treatment by CSF diversion suggest that careful follow-up for shunt malfunction is mandatory if satisfactory long-term results are to be obtained. This must be done by neurosurgeon and pediatrician working in concert in such a fashion that the parents do not become either anxious or discouraged about frequent follow-up visits. Each month after shunt placement the head circumference is measured and the pump can be tested. By six months of age developmental assessment of the child's neurological function can be estimated. Subsequent to this, x-rays should be obtained at yearly intervals to look for any disconnection of the shunt tubing, which is radiopaque, or displacement of the distal catheter from the peritoneum with somatic growth. Signs of shunt obstruction, such as irritability and vomiting, should be assessed as early as possible, and a decision made promptly as to whether or not shunt revision is necessary. Urgent shunt revisions can be somewhat limited if such routine follow-up is performed. However, multiple revisions will be necessary in most shunts, and if done well should not prejudice the ultimate outcome of treatment.

Ordinarily elective shunt revisions will be required for growth. However, some children will outgrow the need for a shunt. With brain growth the CSF absorption deficit will diminish, decreasing the need for the shunt. The best estimate is that approximately 30 per cent

of children, particularly those with communicating or extraventricular obstructive hydrocephalus, will not need subsequent shunts and will become shunt independent. With a shunt dependent child the first revision of the shunt is ordinarily at 2 years of age, again at 5, and perhaps again at 10 years. It is unsafe to remove a shunt which may or may not be working without a prior period of shunt ligation to ascertain absolute need of a shunt. It is also not my practice to remove shunts assuming shunt dependency without now obtaining a CTT scan. On CTT scan, the child who tends to be shunt independent has ventricles two to three times normal size, whereas the shunt dependent child has normal or small ventricles.

Over the past years many neurosurgeons have adopted peritoneal shunting instead of shunting into the vascular system. However, there remains a large group of somewhat older children with ventriculojugular shunts placed between 1960 and 1970, and the pediatrician should be aware of the specific technical problems with regard to these shunts, particularly late infection and septicemia. Between 5 and 8 per cent of children with jugular shunts will develop a low grade staphylococcal infection characterized by fever, anemia, lassitude and easy tiredness. Blood cultures and cultures of the cerebrospinal fluid obtained during febrile illness will generally show modest growth of gram-positive cocci sensitive to ordinary antibiotics. In rare instances a shunt nephritis due to antigen-antibody reaction in the kidney to the capsular polysaccharide of *Staphylococcus* will ensue, generally demanding shunt removal. The shunt infection without glomerulonephritis should be treated with intraventricular and intravenous antibiotics for 10 to 14 days in the attempt to eradicate the infection without shunt removal. If this is unsuccessful the shunt should be removed under appropriate antibiotic coverage and placed in the peritoneal cavity. Methicillin, 50 mg.; gentamicin, 2 mg.; or chloramphenicol, 50 mg. can be used in the ventricle, instilled through the shunt tubing.*

Finally, specific complications of peritoneal shunts related to bowel perforation and catheter extrusion have been reported and should be recognized early.

Prognosis. The prognosis in the various forms of congenital and acquired hydrocephalus is generally good. Some 70 per cent of children are educable in normal schools and are quite functional. Less than 10 per cent are

---

*Intraventricular use of methicillin, gentamicin, and chloramphenicol is not mentioned in the manufacturers' instructions.

grossly retarded. It is still not possible at the inception of treatment to distinguish children who will be grossly retarded. The number of shunt revisions is not directly related to prognosis, nor is infection or other treatable complications of shunting. Therefore, a generally hopeful attitude should be maintained with vigorous surveillance of the shunt system and a ready willingness to revise shunts as these revisions become necessary.

Brain Tumors

CHARLES A. CARTON, M.D.

Several generalizations are helpful in the recognition and treatment of brain tumors in children: (1) Symptoms and signs are produced by the local signature of the lesion and by its relationship to the ventricular system (and consequent obstructive hydrocephalus). (2) Although adult types of tumors occur in children, the incidence of certain of these is quite low (such as meningioma). (3) There is a high incidence of so-called "congenital" tumors in children.

GLIOMA

Supratentorial tumors, such as astrocytoma, oligodendroglioma, glioblastoma, ependymoma, are best handled by aggressive surgical removal via craniotomy. Frontal, occipital, and temporal lobectomies are possible, with care not to leave the patient aphasic or hemiplegic; a homonymous hemianopsia as a residual defect may be an acceptable trade-off for adequate decompression. In other areas, such as motor or speech, biopsy or judicious decompression or cyst evacuation, followed by radiation, is all that can be done without severe neurological deficit. Radiation should be started approximately one week after surgery. Chemotherapy can be used concomitantly with radiation.

Infratentorial tumors are approached by suboccipital craniectomy, usually in the sitting position, using a midline incision and a right occipital burr hole with ventricular drainage during surgery. Central venous pressure catheter in right atrium (for control of possible air embolism) and an arterial line are standard during surgery. The face-down position is used sometimes as well.

ASTROCYTOMA. These may be cystic with a mural nodule which, if removed, is curative. In the hemisphere, much of a solid tumor can be removed. The solid tumors are of low-grade malignancy, but radiotherapy is still given. Vermis location may make total excision difficult and again radiotherapy follows.

MEDULLOBLASTOMA. A vermis-splitting incision will allow the tumor to be lifted from the floor of the fourth ventricle (it usually arises from the vermis) and for aqueduct decompression. Radiotherapy follows; the tumor is unusually sensitive and cures have been reported (80 per cent); the entire neuraxis must be irradiated.

EPENDYMOMA. Separating the cerebellar tonsils and splitting the vermis will reveal the ependymoma rising from the floor of the fourth ventricle. Much of the tumor can be removed, leaving a thin layer. The aqueduct is decompressed by tumor removal; radiation follows.

HEMANGIOBLASTOMA. A cystic lesion and vascular mural nodule (delineated angiographically) can be removed completely. A highly vascular lesion involving hemisphere and brain stem may make extirpation impossible; radiation follows.

Pontine Glioma. Radiation without exploration has been the procedure of choice, unless other studies (particularly CAT scan) suggest abscess, cyst or localized hemorrhage. In these latter situations, exploration within the fourth ventricle may reveal elevation of the floor of the ventricle and the lesion may be removed completely or partially, or the cyst decompressed. Shunting also may be required if there is significant ventricular obstruction.

Thalamic Glioma. If there is no ventricular obstruction (at the foramen of Monro or occasionally of the third ventricle), radiation has been the procedure of choice. With hydrocephalus, however, air study has been helpful in indicating intraventricular protrusion, which can be biopsied by a transcortical or transcallosal approach. The ventricles are intercommunicated at that time by making an opening in the septum pellucidum; shunting from one ventricle only then follows; or shunting from both ventricles without biopsy, followed by radiation, is frequently done.

Optic Nerve Glioma. Biopsy is carried out via frontal craniotomy. The posterior extent of the lesion can be determined and the optic foramen opened and the optic nerve decompressed, both as a prelude to radiation. If the lesion appears to be limited to the optic nerve alone, the roof of the orbit is removed and an attempt is made to excise completely the optic nerve with tumor.

PINEALOMA

The proximity of this tumor to the aqueduct and posterior third ventricle requires shunting of the resulting hydrocephalus. Direct attack on the lesion can best be carried out via the infratentorial supracerebellar approach. Many of these lesions cannot be removed totally, but will respond to radiation. On occasion, radiation without exploration is indicated.

CRANIOPHARYNGIOMA

Small tumors can be totally excised as can an occasional larger tumor. However, the morbidity of total excision is high and must be weighed in the context of relatively short-term, good quality survival, and the increased morbidity with repetitive surgery for recurrences. Decompression of the visual apparatus and relief of ventricular obstruction and hypothalamic involvement are the goals of surgery. Shunting is required frequently.

PITUITARY TUMORS

A surgical approach is required via frontal craniotomy for biopsy and relief of optic nerve, chiasm, and optic tract compression. Total removal of chromophobe adenomata has not been advocated; rather radiation has been employed in these cases after appropriate decompression.

INTRAVENTRICULAR TUMORS

Colloid cyst or epidermoid of third ventricle. These tumors are most easily approached via a transcortical frontal incision when the lateral ventricles are enlarged, and via a transcallosal approach when the ventricles are small. Total removal and cure can be expected.

Choroid papilloma of lateral ventricle. Usually there is hydrocephalus (communicating) and the tumor can be approached by a transcortical parieto-occipital incision. The tumor can be removed, either piecemeal or in toto, along with the choroid plexus. Care should be taken that blood does not get into the ventricular system, since it may obstruct the aqueduct. Occasionally a choroid plexus papilloma may occur in the fourth ventricle (see above).

MISCELLANEOUS TUMORS

Epidermoid. Skull. If confined to the skull, total excision of bone (after x-ray localization, if necessary) will effect a cure. Occasionally, these lesions may be huge, usually epidural in localization. The epidural component can be removed, although small pieces of capsule can lead occasionally to recurrence. The tumor does not usually go transdurally.

Intracranial. Occasionally these lesions are located within the fourth ventricle or cerebellopontine angle. Removal of the "cottage cheese"–like tumor is relatively easy, but again, portions of capsule may be left.

Dermoid. These tumors may be associated with congenital dermal sinuses in the mid-line, usually in the suboccipital area. The dermal sinus is excised and the intradural dermoid removed as well as possible; radiation follows.

PREOPERATIVE MANAGEMENT

Decadron, 4 mg. by intravenous push or orally, every six hours, will be helpful in combating cerebral edema and buying time for appropriate diagnostic studies. The clotting mechanism should be checked. Note should be made of aspirin derivatives (such as for headache) used by the patient, which may adversely influence clotting during surgery despite normal parameters of clotting mechanism. Prophylactic anticonvulsants are initiated prior to surgery, if time permits (see below). Fluids are limited to bare maintenance (using surface area formula); isotonic fluids are used such as 5 per cent dextrose in one-half normal saline rather than 5 per cent dextrose in water. Occasionally, when there is associated hydrocephalus, external ventricular drainage is used to relieve pressure and to improve the patient's condition preoperatively.

OPERATIVE MANAGEMENT

Monitoring vital functions is essential. An arterial line, introduced either percutaneously or by cutdown, affords continuous pressure levels and intraoperative and postoperative blood gases and electrolytes. Monitoring central venous pressure in the sitting position is mandatory to control possible air embolism. It is also useful in determining the adequacy of fluid replacement. Temperature is controlled with cooling or heating blankets and is monitored by a rectal or esophageal thermometer. Wrapping the limbs with webril can help reduce heat loss. Drapes and solutions should be warmed for infants. Warming and cooling blankets and external heat sources (lights) are used for infants.

Antibiotics are used prophylactically. Methicillin is given by intravenous push, and gentamicin is given intramuscularly. Ventricular drainage is used when associated hydrocephalus is present. Hyperventilation also helps to reduce increased intracranial pressure. Mannitol, 1.5 gm./kg., is used to reduce increased intracranial pressure (also used postoperatively).*

POSTOPERATIVE MANAGEMENT

The patient is kept relatively dehydrated at a serum osmolality of 300 to 305 mOsm.

---

*Manufacturer's precaution: Dosage requirements of mannitol for patients 12 years and under have not been established.

Careful intake and output measurement of fluid balance is made. Anticonvulsants and antibiotics are continued. Phenobarbital, 3 to 5 mg./kg. 2 or 3 times daily, and phenytoin, 5 to 8 mg./kg. 2 or 3 times daily, are given.

Radiotherapy. Radiation dosage depends upon factors such as type of tumor, daily dosage, and age of patient. For example, in malignant glioma of the hemisphere (glioblastoma), 6000 rads are given to the entire brain. Another plan might be to use 5000 rads to the entire brain with a boost of 1500 rads to the local tumor area. In medulloblastoma or malignant ependymoma, 4500 rads are delivered to the entire brain with 5500 rads total to the posterior fossa; the spinal cord would receive 4000 rads. In general, in patients under 2 years of age, the dosage is reduced 10 per cent. The rate of radiation is usually 800 to 1000 rads per week. Additional local treatment to a cumulative dose of 5000 rads is given to spinal metastases, should they occur.

Brain Abscess

ANN SULLIVAN BAKER, M.D.

Early diagnosis followed by antibiotic and surgical therapy is crucial for the successful treatment of brain abscess. The abscess usually arises from one of four mechanisms: direct extension of infection from a contiguous focus such as a sinus or middle ear infection; in relation to congenital heart disease with right to left or pulmonary arteriovenous shunting; by hematogenous dissemination from distant sites of infection; or by direct introduction of bacteria into the brain such as following trauma.

The cardinal symptom of a brain abscess is headache, relentless and progressive, which is usually followed by focal neurological manifestations. Fever is present in only two-thirds of the patients. Papilledema and other manifestations of increased intracranial pressure are common later in the course.

Antibiotic Treatment. Because of the great variety of aerobic and anaerobic microorganisms isolated from cerebral abscesses, broad-spectrum antimicrobial therapy is used initially. Three categories of microorganisms are predominant in brain abscess: streptococci, Enterobacteriaceae, and staphylococci. Anaerobic microorganisms are present in one-third of abscesses and multiple organisms in one-quarter of abscesses. Most of the bacteria isolated from cerebral abscesses are susceptible to either penicillin or chloramphenicol. Initial therapy with this combination is suggested, started prior to surgery (see below).

When a brain abscess follows penetrating skull trauma or a neurosurgical procedure, staphylococci are likely bacteria, requiring a penicillinase-resistant penicillin (oxacillin, methicillin, or nafcillin, 200 mg./kg./day intravenously). If there is a history of a severe allergy to penicillin, erythromycin, 40 mg./kg./day intravenously, is substituted for penicillin. The final antimicrobial regimen should be devised based on results of Gram-stained smears and cultures of material obtained at surgery. Brain abscess requires treatment for 3 to 4 weeks following aspiration of pus. Actinomycotic abscesses require 2 to 3 months, therapy with penicillin.

Surgery. The lesion is initially localized by scan. When the abscess is deep or does not have a well formed capsule, the abscess is aspirated. Subsequent treatment by drainage or repeat aspiration is guided by results of the scan. When the abscess is in an accessible region, a craniotomy is carried out. If there is a well formed capsule, the lesion is totally excised and the incision closed. The abscess material should be immediately Gram-stained and cultured aerobically and anaerobically.

The clinical course of the patient should be carefully monitored daily, with computer tomography evaluations at needed intervals. If the abscess resolves, there is no need for exci-

TABLE 1.   Intravenous Antibiotic Dosages

	CHILDREN	ADULTS
Penicillin	300,000 units/kg./day divided in 6 doses	24 million units/day
Chloramphenicol	100 mg./kg./day div. in 4 doses (max. 4 gm./day)	3 to 4 gm./day
Semisynthetic penicillin		
Oxacillin	⎫	10 to 12 gm./day
Nafcillin	⎬ 200 mg./kg./day divided in 6 doses	6 to 10 gm./day
Methicillin	⎭	16 to 24 gm./day
Erythromycin	40 mg./kg./day divided in 3 doses	3 to 4 gm./day
Gentamicin*	Under age 2: 7.5 mg./kg./day; over age 2: 5 mg./kg./day; divided in 3 doses	3 to 5 mg./kg./day

*Brain penetration of intravenous gentamicin is poor; local instillation may be required. Local instillation of gentamicin is not mentioned in the manufacturer's instructions.

sion. If the abscess remains unchanged or increases in size, repeat aspirations or excision may be needed. The presence of a foreign body or a nonresolving abscess is indication for excision. A cerebellar abscess is harder to tap repeatedly and may also require excision.

The patient with an acute brain abscess will usually have associated brain edema. If the pressure is elevated, agents such as dexamethasone, 1 mg./kg. followed by 0.3 mg./kg. every six hours, or glycerol, 1 to 2 gm./kg./24 hours divided into 6 to 8 doses, may be necessary. Patients with brain abscesses are prone to seizures and these should be prevented by prophylactic anticonvulsant medication such as phenytoin, 10 to 30 mg./kg./day, to a maximum dose of 300 mg.

Definitive therapy of a cerebral abscess must also include effective treatment of the predisposing extracranial lesion. Anticonvulsant therapy is maintained for several years after eradication of the brain abscess.

Spinal Epidural Abscess

ANN SULLIVAN BAKER, M.D.

Spinal epidural abscesses may be classified as acute and chronic. The acute abscess is associated with a rapid clinical course of less than two weeks and a purulent collection of epidural material. Chronic abscesses are associated with an interval of more than two weeks between back symptoms and surgical intervention and the presence of granulation tissue in the epidural space.

The primary source of infection is usually hematogenous, secondary to skin infection or, less commonly, to dental infection, upper respiratory infection, urinary tract infection, osteomyelitis or direct spread from a contiguous source, such as a dermal sinus, or an operative wound.

The clinical picture of an acute epidural abscess was classically described by Heusner as a progression from spinal ache, root pain and weakness to paralysis. Time from onset of back pain to appearance of root symptoms averages three days. Weakness follows within four days in the patient with acute abscess. Symptoms in the patient with a chronic abscess may progress over weeks to months.

S. aureus is the organism most commonly isolated. Streptococci, gram-negative bacilli such as *E. coli* secondary to urinary tract infections and, rarely, anaerobes or mixed organisms often secondary to upper respiratory infections, are also involved.

The patient with back pain, fever and localized spinal "tenderness" requires immediate evaluation to prevent progression to root pain, weakness and paralysis. The first step should be radiography of the spine. If spine films are negative, a bone scan should be obtained. Tomography is helpful in detecting defects not seen on the plain film. This information is especially valuable for planning the surgical approach (anterolateral versus posterior). If there are signs or evidence of cord compression, a myelogram is imperative for localization prior to surgical decompression. Spinal puncture for myelography should be performed distal to the involved area to prevent introduction of infection into the subarachnoid space during performance of the lumbar puncture.

Surgery. With the finding of a block or epidural mass on myelogram, decompression should be performed without delay, exposing the entire longitudinal extent of the abscess. For acute abscesses, the area is drained. If the abscess is chronic and consists primarily of granulation tissue, the spinal cord is fully decompressed and the wound closed.

It is crucial to evaluate the presence or absence of accompanying osteomyelitis, usually associated with an anterior spinal epidural abscess. The surgical approach for posterior abscess differs from that for an anterior abscess associated with osteomyelitis. When the primary abnormality is anterior, the extradural exposure should be done by removal of a pedicle or by a lateral or anterior approach. Careful follow-up is imperative for years following the laminectomy to detect the occurrence of scoliosis.

Antibiotic Therapy. Blood cultures should be obtained prior to surgery. Material obtained at operation should be immediately examined by Gram stain and cultured. Antibiotic therapy should be started just before opening the abscess, or earlier if the process is acute, because of concomitant bacteremia or complicating meningitis.

A semisynthetic penicillin (oxacillin or nafcillin) should be employed in high dosage by the intravenous route when a staphylococcal or streptococcal etiology is suspected (such as following a skin infection). The combination of semisynthetic penicillin and gentamicin is recommended in the setting of a known urinary tract focus. If penicillin allergy is present, a cephalosporin might be used in place of penicillin or semisynthetic penicillin. If severe allergy is associated with urticaria or anaphylaxis, erythromycin or vancomycin (40 mg./kg./day every eight hours) might be substituted for B-lactam type antibiotics. If there are no predisposing foci and no clues to the bacterial cause on examination of the Gram stain, a penicillinase-resistant penicillin in combination with gentamicin or chloramphenicol should be started initially until cultures are reported (see below). The intravenous dosages of antibiotics are the same as for brain abscess on p. 53.

An epidural abscess merits treatment with parenteral antibiotics for three to four weeks; concomitant vertebral osteomyelitis should be treated with parenteral antibiotics for six to eight weeks.

Cerebral Vascular Disorders

KEASLEY WELCH, M.D.

A number of processes may lead to infarction of the brain or bleeding into its substance or beneath its membranes. Spontaneous intracranial hemorrhage during childhood is most commonly due to rupture of an arteriovenous malformation, which may be extremely small. Arterial aneurysms figure less prominently, while blood dyscrasias, rupture of collateral channels, tumors and hypertension each may play a role. Predisposing to ischemia are dehydration, congenital and valvular heart disease, polycythemia, sickle cell anemia, trauma to the vessels of the neck, inflammation of the blood vessels due to continuous infection (meningitis, tonsillitis) or noninfective vasculitis and homocystinuria. The goals of treatment include preservation of life and function, prevention of complications, the assurance, when possible, that the condition will not recur and the rehabilitation of the patient.

In general the clinical features will allow tentative classification into three groups: ischemic infarction, subarachnoid hemorrhage and parenchymal hematoma; but overlaps and uncertainties will occur. More precise diagnosis requires special studies which include computed tomography and angiography, but a number of problems of therapy are shared.

For the critically ill patient, constant care is required. Blood pressure, pulse and respiratory rates, the level of consciousness, the size of the pupils and patterns of posture and movement are observed and recorded, initially at 15 minute intervals and later, when the situation is more stable, hourly. Blood gases are monitored. Position in bed is changed frequently and the skin is kept clean and dry. In unconscious patients, the eyes may be taped shut to avoid corneal drying. Excessive tracheal secretions are aspirated and postural drainage may be necessary. Hyperthermia is treated by using temperature control blankets. Overhydration is avoided by adjusting the volume of fluid administered according to urine volume.

For swelling of the brain, dexamethasone, 1 to 4 mg. every 6 hours, may give relief after 12 to 24 hours. Osmotic therapy with mannitol,* 0.5 to 1.5 gm./kg., administered slowly intravenously is more rapidly effective as is glycerol, 0.5 to 2 gm./kg., as an initial dose and 0.5 to 0.7 gm./kg. every 3 hours, administered orally or by stomach tube.

If there are signs of parenchymal insult, it is wise to use anticonvulsants in anticipation of seizures. Phenytoin, 6 mg./kg./day, and phenobarbital at half that level are begun and final dosage is adjusted according to blood levels. A similar schedule may be used if a seizure occurs. If seizures are incessant or continuous, more vigorous methods (see page 77) are necessary for their control.

Passive movement of paralyzed parts is begun early. Deformities due to rigidity or spasticity may require splinting. During convalescence active exercises are encouraged and the patient is taught to cope with residual disability.

Infarction of the Brain.   Ischemic softening may result from vascular occlusion on the arterial or venous side and in the former case may be thrombotic or embolic. Arterial embolism and cortical venous thrombosis may lead to multiple foci of softening which are hemorrhagic. Seizures which may be intractable are especially characteristic of venous occlusions.

If infarction is not accompanied by severe swelling, treatment is supportive and directed at underlying processes. Rarely, especially in cerebellar infarction, life may be threatened and decompression is indicated.

Subarachnoid Hemorrhage.   The patient is nursed and closely observed in a quiet environment. Sedatives may be required for restlessness or excitement and analgesics for pain. Lumbar puncture for the relief of pressure often helps both. Vasospasm, which may accompany subarachnoid hemorrhage, is manifested by obnubilation and lateralizing, often changing neurological signs. No specific treatment is known. Failure of the patient to improve or later deterioration may also signal that communicating hydrocephalus has set in and that a shunting procedure is necessary.

When the condition of the patient is stable, consideration needs to be given to surgical treatment of the offending lesion.

Intracerebral Hemorrhage.   Massive parenchymal hemorrhage, whatever its origin, may threaten life by causing herniation of the brain before there is any opportunity for inves-

---

*Manufacturer's precaution: The use of mannitol in pediatric patients has not been studied comprehensively.

tigating the situation. Endotracheal intubation, hyperventilation and osmotic therapy may buy time to get the patient to the operating room or even to obtain a computed tomogram on the way.

In less severe instances decision about evacuation of a hematoma will need to be made in the individual case. Subcortical clots and those in the cerebellum lend themselves to removal; deep hemispheral hematoma is best treated expectantly unless deterioration occurs.

See also p. 47.

Venous Sinus Thrombosis

KEASLEY WELCH, M.D.

Septic dural venous sinus thrombosis arising from infection of the face, ear, scalp or upper respiratory apparatus is now a rarity. Treatment with antibiotics should not await the result of cultures. When appropriate, as in mastoiditis or other loculated collections of pus, surgical treatment is indicated. The thrombus may extend into cortical veins and the process may be accompanied by meningitis, subdural empyema or brain abscess.

Bland thrombosis complicating severe dehydration due to gastrointestinal disturbances in infancy is also rare. Its onset is usually signaled by focal seizures due to cortical venous obstruction; however, cerebellar infarction with acute hydrocephalus has been seen.

The most common clinical presentation is benign intracranial hypertension with lateral sinus thrombosis, and in this setting parenchymal damage due to spread into veins does not occur. Aural infection is predisposing but in the majority of cases no causative factors are discovered. Treatment is the same as it is for pseudotumor.

Pseudotumor Cerebri

(Benign Intracranial Hypertension)

KEASLEY WELCH, M.D.

Headaches and papilledema, sometimes with visual loss but without demonstrable hydrocephalus or space-taking process, constitute the syndrome of pseudotumor cerebri. Patients seem remarkably well and do not exhibit signs of involvement of the parenchyma of the brain, but the sixth nerve may be affected.

The objective of therapy is to preserve vision until the process subsides. Treatment depends upon the setting in which the disorder appears. In children the most common cause is bland dural venous sinus thrombosis, usually of a lateral sinus (when associated with otitis media the condition is called otitic hydrocephalus), but the thrombus may extend into the internal jugular vein or the latter may be compressed. Endocrine disturbances such as Cushing's disease, the administration or discontinuance of adrenal steroids, hypoparathyroidism and pregnancy have been implicated. Obese young women with menstrual disorders are at risk as are women taking contraceptive steroids. Tetracycline therapy in infants and vitamin A overdosage are also predisposing factors.

Discontinuation of offending drugs or correction, when possible, of the metabolic effect of endocrine disturbance is effective when appropriate. Repeated lumbar puncture with release of fluid for reduction of pressure is effective and often only one or a few taps are required before the pressure returns to normal. Chlorothiazide, 5 mg./kg./day, has been advocated as has acetazolamide, 25 to 50 mg./kg./day. When manifestation of the syndrome is concurrent with the discontinuation of adrenal steroids, these ought to be reinstituted and the dosage reduced gradually. Dexamethasone is frequently prescribed and may be useful.

The course of therapy needs to be followed by frequent measurement of visual acuity, when possible, and examination of the optic discs; in older children who can cooperate, mapping of the blind spot gives graphic evidence of recovery. In the occasional intractable case the question of surgical treatment will be raised. Subtemporal decompression, formerly commonplace, rarely is considered now and then only as a last resort.

Neurocutaneous Syndromes

GORDON V. WATTERS, M.D.

Included in this group of disorders are those in which the skin and nervous system are the principal organ systems involved by an inheritable and/or embryological defect. Aita lists 42 such disorders but many would argue that inclusion of some of the entities is stretching a point.

The two commonest entities in the group are neurofibromatosis (von Recklinghausen's disease) and tuberous sclerosis (Bourneville's disease). Less common entities included in the group are cerebelloretinal angiomatosis (von Hippel-Lindau's disease), multiple mucosal neuroma syndrome and nevoid basal cell carcinoma syndrome. These five disorders are inherited as autosomal dominants. Ataxia-telangiectasia (Louis-Bar syndrome) is usually included in the group also, but is an autosomal recessive. Some sporadic disorders also included under this rubric are encephalotrigeminal angiomatosis (Sturge-Weber syndrome), linear nevus sebaceus, and nevus unis lateris. These disorders are discussed below.

NEUROFIBROMATOSIS (VON RECKLINGHAUSEN'S DISEASE)

This disorder may be diagnosed in the newborn period if café-au-lait spots are present. Its multiple protean manifestations must be anticipated to ensure early recognition and hence early treatment. A balance must be struck between conscientious follow-up and avoidance of undue anxiety on the part of the parents and child over potential future problems.

Although neurofibromatosis is inherited as an autosomal dominant disorder, about 50 per cent of the children who present with the disorder appear to be new mutations. A central form with few or no skin lesions and a peripheral form with multiple café-au-lait spots are said to occur. The majority of children with the disease have five or more café-au-lait spots which are greater than 1.5 cm. in diameter; this remains the hallmark of the disease. Involvement of the nervous system in neurofibromatosis may include lesions of the eye, brain, meninges, spinal cord, cranial, peripheral, and autonomic nerves as well as skin, bone, soft tissue, endocrine, vascular, gastrointestinal and pulmonary lesions.

An annual assessment of a child with neurofibromatosis should include the interval history, physical examination, and ophthalmological examination including visual acuity, fields, optic nerve head appearance (optic nerve or chiasmal glioma) and perhaps intraocular pressure (glaucoma). A biannual radiologic survey at least should include the skull, optic foramina, and spine, plus other sites if lesions are suspected there. Blood pressure recordings are essential to detect systemic hypertension which may be due to renal artery lesions or a pheochromocytoma. Both lesions are of increased incidence in neurofibromatosis. An audiogram may detect an acoustic neuroma early, although this complication usually manifests at the earliest in the second decade.

Some degree of intellectual deficit occurs in about 25 percent of children with neurofibromatosis. This may be accounted for by the demonstrated defect in cerebral architectonics. It is essential however to be sure the poor mental performance is not due to a progressive lesion of the central nervous system such as increased intracranial pressure due to aqueductal stenosis, or direct brain involvement by a glioma of brain stem, optic chiasma, or cerebral hemisphere. Poor academic performance may also be due to failing vision caused by an optic glioma, or a hearing deficit secondary to an acoustic neuroma. The degree of mental deficiency is usually mild to moderate. Assessment of the child's capabilities and the design of special school programs to accommodate them are important. It is essential that the school and family understand the child's disorder, his abilities and disabilities.

Convulsive disorders occur with a slightly increased frequency in children with neurofibromatosis. They are managed in the usual way after appropriate studies to exclude a progressive intracranial lesion have been performed. Macrocrania is a feature in neurofibromatosis and may be due to the complications mentioned or to megalencephaly. Computerized tomography should help in differentiating these disorders. If aqueductal stenosis is present or a tumor is suspected, neurosurgical consultation is indicated. Management of optic nerve or chiasmal gliomas is controversial in regard to conservative management, surgical management and/or radiation therapy. A combined consultation with the neurosurgeon, ophthalmologist, and radiation therapist is essential. The optic chiasmal glioma may encroach on the third ventricle and the hypothalamic-pituitary axis. In obstructions of circulation of the cerebrospinal fluid, conservative therapy such as a shunt may be appropriate in view of the difficulties which may ensue with attempts at resection of the tumor and its slow growth. Endocrinologic consultation is indicated for assessment of endocrinologic deficits and replacement therapy. Acoustic nerve tumors are surgically removed but are complicated surgical problems requiring special expertise in this area.

Scoliosis and kyphoses which occur more frequently in neurofibromatosis may be due to neuromuscular imbalance (idiopathic), a neurofibroma in the region of the scoliosis, spinal dural meningioma, spinal cord glioma, angioma, or syringomyelia, or a bony anomaly of the spine and/or dural sac. Scoliosis in a patient with neurofibromatosis always requires spine films and usually requires myelography to ensure that there is no tumor present. Orthopedic and neurosurgical consultation is necessary.

Bony lesions in neurofibromatosis include pseudoarthrosis, subperiosteal and bony cysts in the region of the epiphysis, pathologic fractures but rarely malignancies of bone. Orthopedic consultation is mandatory.

Plexiform neuromas may occur at any site and may produce effects due to location such as in the orbit, but usually do not require removal. Subcutaneous neurofibromas where recurrent abrasion occurs, such as on the under surface of the forearm, may be removed if necessary. Encroachment on adjacent nerve trunks by neurofibromas may occur in the brachial and lumbar plexuses and poses a difficult therapeutic problem. Excision has been necessary in some, but postoperative fibrotic reactions and recurrences are common; generally surgery should be avoided. Sarcomatous change has occurred in these tumors but is rare.

Local gigantism of one limb or one digit may be so unsightly as to require excision, but careful weighing of all the factors is essential. No treatment for neurofibromatosis-associated hemihypertrophy syndromes has been found. Association of hemihypertrophy with visceral tumor and especially Wilms' tumor has been documented, and a careful assessment of the patient with this in mind is required.

Pharyngeal and gastrointestinal neurofibromas may occur and if symptomatic require surgery. Pheochromocytomas occur with increased frequency in neurofibromatosis and treatment is as for this disorder. Another cause for arterial hypertension in neurofibromatosis is renal artery stenosis which requires renal arteriography for diagnosis. Surgical therapy is indicated.

TUBEROUS SCLEROSIS (BOURNEVILLE'S DISEASE)

Tuberous sclerosis is an autosomal dominant with a mutation rate as high as 80 per cent in some series. In the patient originally described by Bourneville and in many patients with tuberous sclerosis there is a convulsive disorder, mental retardation, hemiplegia, and hard nodules in the cerebral hemispheres (tubers).

Characteristic, almost pathognomonic skin abnormalities include areas of hypopigmentation (white macules often with an ash leaf configuration), adenoma sebaceum of the face, a shagreen patch on the trunk, and periungual (and periodontal) fibromas. Retinal gliomas, cerebral tumors, cerebral tubers, and subependymal nodules, rhabdomyomas of the heart, angiomyolipomas of the kidney, cysts of bone and lung, and hamartomatous tumors of pancreas, thyroid and adrenal glands occur.

The adenoma sebaceum of the face primarily affects the cheeks, the perinasal region and midline chin, and may be present at birth, but more usually appears at about age five. Proliferation of this angiofibroma may occur resulting in severe disfigurement. Dermabrasion and treatment with liquid nitrogen may be helpful in some cases but such decisions require consultation with a dermatologist. Repetition of treatment courses may lead to complications and less good results. If severe, the periungual fibromas of fingers and toes may require surgery with recurrence also common. Periodontal fibromas and the shagreen patch usually do not require treamtent.

The fundal lesions, whether they be the opalescent gliomas of the nerve head or the more subtle mound of the peripheral retinal gliomas, are not deleterious to vision and do not require therapy. The intracranial tumors of tuberous sclerosis, usually benign by cell type, require treatment as for any tumor of that region. Commonly the region of the foramen magnum is involved producing obstructive hydrocephalus. Treatment will depend on the extent of the lesion, its involvement of adjacent structures, and the clinical state of the patient. Palliative shunting may be appropriate.

The seizure disorders associated with tuberous sclerosis are probably due to the disturbances in cerebral architectonics, tumors, tubers, or subependymal nodules. In the first two years of life, infantile spasms with or without an hypsarrhythmic electroencephalogram require treatment. Adrenocorticotrophic hormone (ACTH) or corticosteroid therapy (prednisone) is advocated as for infantile spasms in general. Clonazepam is one of the more effective anticonvulsants, but response to medications is often poor to fair. The typical infantile spasms usually subside over the period of a year or two, and are replaced by complex, generalized or myoclonic seizures, or a combination of both. Phenytoin is as effective an anticonvulsant as any, but the gingival hyperplasia and "Dilantin facies" may worsen an already grievous cosmetic problem. Phenobarbital or primidone may be used, but behavioral disorder may prove a problem. Carbamazepine may be a preferable agent controlling seizures equally well and ameliorating behavioral difficulties in some. If myoclonic attacks and major seizures occur, the combination of carbamazepine and clonazepam may be used. If absences occur, ethosuximide remains the drug of choice.

Although a child with tuberous sclerosis may have normal intelligence, moderate to severe intellectual deficits occur in about 50 to 60 per cent. The child with tuberous sclerosis who has moderate to severe mental deficits, a seizure disorder, some degree of motor handicap, and often either an endogenous or exogenous behavior disorder poses a major problem in management, even in the presence of excellent school facilities and understanding parents and educators. The behavioral disorder may be improved by behavior modification programs, and on occasion hyperactivity is ameliorated by methylphenidate and less often by thioridazine. Parents require support and regular, periodic review of the educational and pharmacological treatment program.

Hemiplegia, a motor defect seen in some patients with tuberous sclerosis, requires orthopedic consultation for appropriate operative and bracing procedures.

Rhabdomyomas of the heart may be present at birth or present later. They may lead to cardiac failure, cyanosis and sudden death. The tumor is usually multiple in tuberous sclerosis and no specific treatment is known.

About 50 per cent of all renal angiomyolipomas occur in patients with tuberous sclerosis and in these patients they are almost always bilateral. About 50 per cent of patients with tuberous sclerosis at autopsy have angiomyolipomas. In life these tumors are frequently mistaken for polycystic kidney disease. Biopsy for diagnosis should be avoided since serious hemorrhage may result. Where complications result from the tumor itself, nephrectomy is necessary. Most of these tumors do not present until the third decade with flank pain and hematuria.

Lung cysts are an uncommon feature of tuberous sclerosis. Bony changes are common in tuberous sclerosis but in childhood rarely cause symptoms requiring treatment.

Tumors in the region of the hypothalamus may produce precocious puberty, and endocrinologic and neurosurgical consultation is indicated.

MULTIPLE MUCOSAL NEUROMA SYNDROME

The multiple mucosal neuroma syndrome shares features with neurofibromatosis. However, café-au-lait spots are not a major or even minor feature. It appears to be an autosomal dominant disorder, but most cases are sporadic. There is a characteristic facies due to neuromas of the subcutaneous tissue. These are most prominent deep to mucous membranes of the tongue and lips, while the eyelids are affected to a much lesser degree. The incidence of pheochromocytoma is increased in these patients, but of even greater importance is the high incidence of medullary thyroid carcinoma. The presence of malignancy may be confirmed by an assay showing an increase in serum calcitonin. Early excision of the thyroid tumor can achieve a cure for this otherwise often fatal malignancy.

CEREBELLORETINAL ANGIOMATOSIS (VON HIPPEL-LINDAU'S DISEASE)

This is an autosomal disorder usually presenting in early adult life but sometimes in childhood with visual symptoms due to a retinal hemangioblastoma or signs of increased intracranial pressure due to a posterior fossa hemangioblastoma. Polycythemia occurs in 50 per cent of patients with cerebellar hemangioblastomas.

Other associated abnormalities include renal carcinoma, pheochromocytoma, and cysts of pancreas, kidney, and epididymis. There are no characteristic skin lesions. Treatment of the cerebellar lesion is surgical removal. A variety of therapies have been advocated for retinal lesions and a decision requires ophthalmologic consultation. Treatment of pheochromocytoma is as indicated elsewhere as is treatment for renal carcinoma.

NEVOID BASAL CELL CARCINOMA SYNDROME (BASAL CELL NEVUS SYNDROME)

The nevoid basal cell carcinoma syndrome is an autosomal dominant disorder characterized by multiple basal cell carcinomas of the skin, usually appearing after puberty, benign jaw cysts, "pits" of the palms and soles, calcification of the falx cerebri, and endocrinologic and bony abnormalities. Anteceding the skin changes in these patients, there is an increased incidence of early onset medulloblastoma. Other types of brain tumor and congenital developmental abnormalities of the nervous system also occur. The medulloblastomas present in the first five years of life and require surgical treatment. The skin lesions which develop later are treated by electrodesiccation, and if small by curettage. Radiation therapy is not recommended. Dermatologic consultation and follow-up are necessary.

ATAXIA-TELANGIECTASIA

Ataxia-telangiectasia, a complex disorder inherited as an autosomal recessive, is characterized by neurologic, dermatologic, immunologic, and neoplastic abnormalities. Progressive cerebellar ataxia begins as early as one year of age followed by oculomotor apraxia, choreoathetosis, and a neuromyopathy. About a third of patients have some degree of mental deficiency. Telangiectasia of bulbar conjunctiva occurs at about age four, and telangiectasia of cheeks, ears and other sites then evolves with eczema and seborrheic dermatitis occurring in some.

Immunologic deficits in humoral and cell-mediated immunity of varying degrees are present in all and correlate with the severity and complications of recurrent viral and bacterial infections, which occur so often in these patients. The infections primarily affect the respiratory tract and to a lesser extent the skin.

There is a strikingly increased incidence of lymphoreticular neoplasms, lymphomas and leukemia in patients with ataxia-telangiectasia. Other organ systems are also affected and include an unusual type of diabetes mellitus, gonadal abnormalities, hepatic dysfunction and growth failure.

The cerebellar ataxia of ataxia-telangiectasia is unresponsive to any treatment at present, although intention tremor may be improved by propranolol,* 10 to 30 mg. three times daily. The choreoathetosis has been unresponsive to a multitude of drugs, but recently some improvement was noted using dantrolene sodium. The neuromyopathy may be a result of the primary nervous system disorder or a form of diabetic neuropathy. The latter seems unlikely. The oculomotor apraxia which occurs in most is progressive. Surgical therapy of any strabismus must take this into account.

Recurrent respiratory infections due to bacteria require prompt treatment with appropriate antibiotics. Viral infections with pulmonary involvement may require supportive physiotherapy.

In those patients in whom the severity of the neurologic disease renders them deficient in respiratory toilet, or those with chronic sinusitis or bronchiectasis, more vigorous antibiotic and physiotherapy programs are required. The deficiency of IgA in the secretions of many patients with ataxia-telangiectasia may contribute to these recurrent respiratory and skin infections, but administration of IgA by plasma infusions has not been helpful, nor have plasma infusions been successful in correcting their IgE deficiency.

Treatment with recurrent administration of intramuscular gamma globulin, fresh or frozen plasma intravenously, or isologous white cells has not been widely used and has not been shown to be beneficial. Transfer factor has had some recent trials as have thymus and/or bone marrow transplants with long-term results to be reported. Most patients with ataxia-telangiectasia die in the second or third decade of life as a result of severe respiratory infection or the effects of a malignancy.

The treatment of the malignancies of the lymphoreticular system which occur in 10 per cent of patients with ataxia-telangiectasia requires special caution since patients show increased sensitivity both to radiation therapy and the immunosuppressants used in chemotherapy. Further, the presence of neurologic and pulmonary disabilities renders these patients less able than others to tolerate the stresses of neoplasia. Consultation with the oncologist and radiation therapist is required.

In the special diabetes mellitus of ataxia-telangiectasia there is a markedly elevated renal threshold for glucose, a resistance to the development of ketosis, and hypersecretion of insulin with apparent reduced insulin sensitivity of peripheral tissues. The hepatic disease of ataxia-telangiectasia may accompany or be related to this diabetes. Treatment of the diabetes or the hepatic disease is usually not necessary. An elevation of alpha fetoprotein has been documented in the serum of patients with ataxia-telangiectasia and may prove to be a reliable marker of the disease. Gonadal abnormalities are not present in all and do not seem to require treatment. Growth failure has not been severe and has been shown not to be due to deficient growth hormone.

ENCEPHALOTRIGEMINAL ANGIOMATOSIS (STURGE-WEBER SYNDROME)

This sporadic disorder is characterized by: (1) venous angiomatosis of the leptomeninges overlying the cerebral cortex usually in the parieto-occipital region; (2) gyriform calcifications in the cortex underlying the angiomatosis; (3) ipsilateral nevus flammeus (port wine stain) of the face; (4) focal or generalized seizure disorder and hemiplegia appropriate for the cerebral lesion; (5) involvement of the eye with the nevus flammeus adjacent, by buphthalmos, choroid angioma, or glaucoma; (6) mental retardation in some.

If the ophthalmic and maxillary division is involved by the nevus flammeus, in about 50 per cent of cases the eye on that side will develop glaucoma. Anticipatory assessment by an ophthalmologist is necessary to provide early treatment.

Nevus flammeus of the face may or may

---

*This use of propranolol is not listed in the manufacturer's instructions. Data on the use of propranolol in the pediatric age group are too limited to permit adequate directions for its use.

not be associated with intracranial involvement. If the port wine stain does involve the ophthalmic division, it is much more likely the patient will also have intracranial involvement. The presence at birth of a nevus flammeus involving the first division or more of the face had been considered by some to be an indication of neurosurgical exploration and an excision of the suspected angiomatous lesion of the meninges. Almost all would regard this as inappropriately aggressive. Seizure disorder in these patients is treated with anticonvulsants, including phenytoin, phenobarbital, primidone or carbamazepine. Indications for surgical interference are intractable seizures, worsening school and mental performance, and increasing neurologic deficit. In such cases consultation with neurosurgery is indicated. Treatment of the nevus is usually accomplished by a covering cosmetic cream.

LINEAR NEVUS SEBACEUS (NEVUS SEBACEUS OF JADASSOHN)

Linear nevus sebaceus is a sporadic disorder characterized by a linear nevus present at birth most often in the midline of the face and scalp. The nevus evolves from a smooth to a verrucous plaque. In most of the patients there are neurologic deficits including convulsions, mental retardation, and hemiplegias or quadriplegias. Other congenital anomalies especially involving the eye may also occur. In adolescence and adulthood basal cell carcinomas and some benign tumors may develop in the skin lesions; thus excision of the lesion through full thickness of the skin is advocated where feasible. Dermatologic and plastic surgery consultation is indicated.

NEVUS UNIS LATERIS

Nevus unis lateris is a linear configuration of light to dark brown papules histologically different from linear nevus sebaceus and located on any part of the body. It is a sporadic disorder present at birth and associated with mental deficiency, convulsions, and bony abnormalities. Malignant change in the nevus may occur later and excision may be appropriate. Dermatologic consultation is indicated.

Acute Ataxia

ANDREA H. NASH, M.D.

Ataxia is incoordination resulting from dysfunction of the cerebellum or its connections with other parts of the nervous system. It may be so subtle that the patient is unaware of it, or so severe that it is incapacitating. Ataxia may be manifested by nystagmus, dysarthria, intention tremor, dysmetria, dysdiadochokinesia, exaggerated rebound, damaged check mechanisms, unsteady broad-based gait, difficulty with tandem gait, titubation, and primary truncal ataxia, occurring singly or in various combinations, sometimes with associated hypotonia. To make matters more complicated, sensory deficits, weakness, myoclonus, chorea, athetosis, tremor, vertigo and diffuse, undefinable incoordination or clumsiness may all be confused with ataxia even by well trained, experienced observers. This discussion is concerned with a number of disorders in which acute, usually generalized, ataxia is the first or major symptom. When therapy is available, it will be described, or the reader will be referred to other sections of this volume.

Acute Cerebellar Ataxia of Childhood. The term "acute cerebellar ataxia of childhood" is usually used to refer to a syndrome with abrupt onset of ataxia, which worsens over a period of one to several days. The cerebellar signs are often accompanied by irritability, vomiting, mild meningeal signs, headache, and variable alterations in deep tendon reflexes. The disorder occurs equally in both sexes and is most common in children between 1 and 5 years of age. At least half of the reported cases have been associated with a nonspecific, mild, probably viral illness occurring a week or so prior to the onset of neurologic symptoms, whereas others have been associated with such definable infections as mononucleosis, varicella, or other exanthems. Lumbar puncture may reveal a mild lymphocytic pleocytosis (usually no more than 25 cells) and perhaps slight increase in protein, but normal pressure. Most patients recover completely without therapy within days to months. However, about a third of children who are hospitalized with severe symptoms are left with a permanent, although usually mild, neurologic deficit. This residuum is usually in the form of ataxia, but alterations in behavior and learning ability may occur. Since no medications are known to be effective, and most patients improve rapidly without treatment, no therapy is recommended.

Ataxia and Opsoclonus. A syndrome of ataxia and opsoclonus (wildly chaotic, dancing eye movements, with jerking of the eyes in all directions) may occur in three forms in childhood. In its most benign form, it resembles acute cerebellar ataxia of childhood except that the ataxia is more severe and opsoclonus is present. In this situation, no therapy is usually necessary, since improvement occurs without treatment in most cases. However, in severely affected patients, ACTH gel, 40 units intramuscularly 3 times a week, may result in more rapid improvement of the movement disorder. After 1 to 2 weeks of therapy, tapering should be performed over weeks to months, depending on the clinical response. Prednisone, 1 mg./lb./day, may also be used, with a similar schedule of full daily dosage for 1 to 2 weeks, followed by gradual tapering. Although the use of ACTH or prednisone may improve the ataxia and opsoclonus initially, it does not alter the long-term prognosis. At least one third of these patients have persistent and significant alterations of behavior, intellectual ability, or cerebellar function. A second, probably congenital, form of the syndrome occurs in young infants and has an even worse prognosis. It is almost invariably associated with at least mild mental retardation and persistent ataxia and abnormal eye movements. It is not known whether ACTH or steroids are of value in this variant. Most importantly, the syndrome of ataxia and opsoclonus at any age in childhood may be the first sign of an occult neuroblastoma. All children with this syndrome should have a thorough evaluation to rule out this neoplasm. If such an evaluation is negative, it should be repeated every 6 months for at least 2 years. The movement disorder may improve or even disappear after an underlying tumor has been effectively treated, and it may reappear if the tumor recurs. If the ataxia does not respond to therapy for neuroblastoma (see p. 278), then a search for metastases is indicated, and a trial of ACTH or steroids for symptomatic relief may be worthwhile. Success in treating ataxia and opsoclonus with ACTH or prednisone does not imply that neuroblastoma is absent, and does not prevent neurologic sequelae whether or not tumor is present.

Drug Intoxication. Acute ataxia in childhood is frequently caused by drug intoxication, usually by accidental ingestion, but occasionally as the result of iatrogenic overdosage. A multitude of sedatives, tranquilizers, and antipsychotic medications may produce ataxia, as can alcohol and other drugs affecting the central nervous system. Treatment of such poisonings is discussed elsewhere. Iatrogenic ataxia occurs most commonly with anticonvulsants. Intolerance to phenytoin because of a defect in parahydroxylation may cause intoxication and ataxia within 48 to 72 hours, even at low doses. Parents should be warned about this possibility whenever phenytoin is prescribed. Phenobarbital frequently causes ataxia, since many physicians are unaware that the commonly quoted dosage schedule for phenobar-

bital (5 to 6 mg./kg./day) is too high for many children over the age of 5 years. Intoxication can be prevented by using lower doses (2 to 3 mg./kg./day) of phenobarbital in older children, and obtaining a blood level after 2 weeks of oral therapy before altering the patient's drug regimen. Treatment of drug intoxication is discussed elsewhere in this volume. An important point to make here, however, is that if a patient has taken an anticonvulsant for over 1 week, the drug should be discontinued slowly. Once the blood levels have fallen within the therapeutic range, dosage should be tapered over at least 3 to 4 days and preferably a week. Abrupt discontinuation of anticonvulsants is the most frequent cause of status epilepticus.

Trauma, Tumor and Hydrocephalus. Acute ataxia can be caused by trauma even when no intracranial hematoma is present. It may present a diagnostic problem when the trauma has been unrecognized or unreported. Posterior fossa or bilateral supratentorial subdural hematomas may cause ataxia acutely, but other signs and symptoms of these lesions are usually present as well. Patients with chronic hydrocephalus that is incompletely or only intermittently arrested may suddenly develop ataxia, with or without signs and symptoms of increased intracranial pressure or long tract signs. In particular, aqueductal stenosis and mild variations of the Arnold-Chiari malformation may present in this way, since they may be unrecognized in early childhood, especially if only mild megalencephaly has been produced. Patients with posterior fossa or midline supratentorial tumors frequently develop chronic ataxia, usually with other evidence of neurologic dysfunction. In these children, ataxia may be perceived as arising acutely even if it has not actually done so. In addition, ataxia may in fact develop acutely, especially after hemorrhage into a tumor or cyst. When subdural hematoma, hydrocephalus, or tumor is suspected, lumbar puncture should be deferred if possible. These diagnoses can be made most safely with computerized axial tomography. The treatment of these disorders is neurosurgical.

Guillain-Barré and Fisher Syndromes. Patients with the Guillain-Barré syndrome or tick paralysis may have apparent ataxia because of weakness. In some of these children, however, ataxia occurs without sufficient weakness or sensory loss to account for it. In at least one such patient, damage to spinocerebellar pathways has been demonstrated at autopsy. Patients with the Fisher syndrome present with ataxia, areflexia, and ophthalmoplegia of abrupt onset. This syndrome appears to lie within a spectrum including both the Guillain-Barré syndrome and acute cerebellar ataxia of childhood. The associated signs and symptoms make the differential diagnosis less difficult. The use of steroid therapy in Guillain-Barré syndrome is controversial. It is not recommended here because its benefits are not well documented and its potential side effects are undesirable. (For a discussion of this and other forms of therapy, see p. 91.) The Fisher syndrome is benign and requires no therapy.

Ataxia Following Sleep or Associated with Fever. Acute ataxia of mild degree may occur in some neurologically intact children in association with fever or following sleep. In these circumstances, parents are usually aware of the recurrent, benign, and frequently familial nature of the problem; nevertheless, the first episode may be frightening. In many cases, tremulousness rather than true ataxia is present. Treatment is not indicated for patients whose ataxia follows sleep; reassurance is sufficient. In patients with ataxia precipitated by fever, as in patients with febrile convulsions, aspirin and acetaminophen may be alternated in full dosage every 2 hours, so that neither drug is given more often than every 4 hours, but 1 antipyretic is given every 2 hours (e.g., aspirin at 4 p.m., acetaminophen at 6 p.m., aspirin at 8 p.m., etc.). In evaluating the febrile child with ataxia, however, it is well to keep in mind that rarely acute ataxia may be the presenting sign of bacterial meningitis.

Rare Disorders. Acute ataxia may be the first sign of metachromatic leukodystrophy, infantile neuroaxonal dystrophy, lipofuscinosis, ataxia telangiectasia, or multiple sclerosis. Recurrent ataxia may occur in several rare disorders, including familial intermittent cerebellar ataxia, Hartnup disease, pyruvate decarboxylase deficiency, the intermittent form of maple syrup disease, hyperalaninemia, and diseases which eventually resemble spinocerebellar degenerations. In all of these disorders, other signs and symptoms eventually make the diagnosis clear; treatment is discussed elsewhere.

Degenerative Diseases of the Central Nervous System

WILLIAM D. SINGER, M.D.

Deterioration of motor and/or intellectual function occurs in the course of many diseases affecting children. Recent advances, such as lysosomal enzyme analysis in storage diseases (Niemann-Pick or Tay-Sachs disease), and biochemical analysis (Leigh's subacute necrotiz-

ing encephalitis), have afforded us a greater understanding of some of the degenerative diseases of the central nervous system, enabling us to provide improved diagnostic services and improved genetic counseling through carrier detection. However, whether the etiology is known or not, the degenerative diseases share a course of progressive deterioration of neurologic function lasting several months to many years, do not exhibit significant periods of spontaneous remission and, in general, their treatment is aimed at symptomatic relief, not at arresting the underlying disease process.

While these degenerative disorders are categorized by the predominant element of the nervous system involved—such as disorders of gray matter, disorders of white matter, those affecting interrelated areas of the CNS or system disorders such as those involving extrapyramidal or corticospinal system—as the diseases progress, many common features and in turn common problems develop. There are basic principles of care applicable to all these disorders. Where available, specific therapeutic modes will be briefly discussed for individual disorders.

Therapeutic Plan. The therapeutic plan must be comprehensive and flexible enough to accommodate patients and their families whose needs change month to month and year to year. When the diagnosis is confirmed, the physician must provide the family with a frank and comprehensive discussion of the nature of the disease, its genetic implications (if known) and the expected course. The family should be assured of the willing involvement of the primary care physician and all those who will be caring for the child, and an acceptance by the physician of a role in providing emotional support to the family. Families benefit greatly when they feel that they may turn to the physician and allied health personnel for assistance in all aspects of the disease. The availability of community services and the role of visiting nurses, physiatrists, physiotherapists, occupational therapists, home health aides, and other social service agencies should be discussed, as well as the supervisory role of the physician in coordinating these services.

The family should be helped to understand that in all but a limited number of cases treatment is geared to the relief of symptoms and that these symptoms change periodically, progressing in spite of treatment. Encouraging active family participation often makes it easier for them to accept that all available therapeutic modes are being used and provides them with a sense of personal involvement in relieving symptoms.

Neuromuscular Function. Characteristic of these diseases is a loss of motor function through weakness, atrophy, spasticity or movement disorder individually or in combination. The aim of supportive care is to maintain useful function as long as possible and to remove those factors which make motor activity inefficient.

Physical therapy, including passive range of motion exercises for paretic or paralyzed limbs, is used to prevent contractures and maintain a full range of motion. This is provided initially by physiotherapists and nursing personnel in a hospital, clinic or home setting, and then is taught to family members to be carried out on a daily basis at home with periodic evaluation and supervision. Exercises may be supplemented by splints to passively stabilize joints when exercises are not being done, braces to stabilize weight bearing joints, wrist splints to maintain the wrist and hand in the most efficient position for grasping, and spring braces to correct foot drop. In addition crutches, and tripod canes, pickup or rolling walkers are available to assist ambulation.

Orthopedic procedures such as tendon lengthening and immobilizing casting should be considered only in light of the patient's condition, rapidity of progression and expected course. Rapid ambulation following surgery is necessary because of the frequent finding that patients with marginal neuromuscular function may no longer be able to ambulate independently following prolonged bed rest.

Spasticity can be reduced with diazepam (Valium), 0.25 to 0.5 mg./kg./day in 3 or 4 divided doses. The daily dose may be increased in children less than 3 years of age by 1 to 2 mg. and in older children by 2 to 4 mg. at 4 or 5 day intervals until the effectiveness of the drug plateaus or sedation is encountered; the dosage is then decreased to the lowest amount giving maximum effect without sedation. By increasing the dosage slowly, patients are able to tolerate surprisingly high daily dosages before sedation (the major limiting factor in using diazepam) is encountered.

An alternative medication is dantrolene sodium (Dantrium),* introduced at a dose of 1 mg./kg./day and increased at weekly intervals to a maximum of 3 mg./kg. two to four times per day, with total dosage not to exceed 100 mg. four times daily. Before using dantrolene sodium, a therapeutic goal should be established, such as utilization of braces or transfer maneuvers, and dosage should be increased

until maximum performance consistent with the dysfunction due to the underlying disease is reached. No further increase in dosage is then indicated.

Dystonia, accompanying spasticity or presenting alone, may be treated with dantrolene sodium or levodopa * at an initial dose of 15 to 25 mg./kg./day, with increases in dosages of 5 to 10 mg./kg. at weekly intervals to a total of 100 mg./kg./day, not to exceed 8 gm./day. Sinemet,† a preparation containing levodopa and carbidopa (an inhibitor of aromatic amino acid decarboxylation in peripheral blood), permits a reduction in dosages of levodopa administered, while it increases the percentage of drug entering the central nervous system, thus decreasing gastrointestinal discomfort frequently encountered with levodopa. Increased dystonia, the development of choreoathetosis and tardive dyskinesias may be seen with levodopa preparations and are an indication for withdrawal of the medication.

Respiratory Function. As their overall condition deteriorates, these patients are at increased risk for atelectasis and aspiration with subsequent pneumonia as a result of decreased activity level with large amounts of time spent in bed, weakness of intercostal musculature, decreased total lung volume, poor cough reflex and in some cases a diminished or absent gag reflex. Frequent change in position with as little time spent at bed rest as can be tolerated, encouragement to breathe deeply and maintenance of adequate hydration at all times, combined with an active program of postural drainage, initiated at the first indication of respiratory tract infection and subsequently as a routine daily activity, will help to minimize respiratory tract difficulties. These measures may be supplemented by the use of oral mucolytic agents and expectorants.

Intermittent positive pressure breathing via home-based respiratory therapy equipment may help to expand lungs and deliver mycolytics. As the patient's cough reflex and respiratory reserve diminish, the use of tracheal and hypopharyngeal suctioning should be introduced. Tracheostomy, to facilitate respiratory care by providing easy access to trachea and bronchi for suctioning of secretions and prevention of aspiration, may be carried out pre-terminally.

---

*Manufacturer's precaution: The safety of dantrolene sodium (Dantrium) in children under the age of 5 years has not been established.

---

*Manufacturer's precaution: The safety of levodopa in children under the age of 12 years has not been established.

†Manufacturer's precaution: The safety of Sinemet in patients under 18 years of age has not been established.

The use of respirators for ventilatory support should be limited to the early stages of the disease when episodes of respiratory failure such as aspiration, atelectasis and pneumonia represent transient problems.

Nutrition. Adequate caloric and fluid intake may be complicated in those disorders affecting the buccopharyngeal musculature and gag reflex. When solid foods are no longer tolerated, blenderized diets prepared at home containing appropriate caloric, protein and fluid proportions or commercially prepared liquid diets (Sustacal, Ensore, Complete B, and so on) can be administered by large syringes fitted with rubber or plastic feeding tips or by nasogastric feeding tubes. Adjustments in intake should take into consideration the level of activity currently undertaken. If this route is not adequate, a feeding gastrostomy will facilitate feeding and decrease the possibility of aspiration. The patient may be unable to handle three feedings per day as a result of slow transit time producing gastric distention, excessive vasovagal responses to the dilatation, and diarrhea which occasionally accompanies these diets.

Bowel Function. The regulation of bowel function may become a significant problem, with constipation and fecal impaction being sources of discomfort and much concern. Foods with natural laxative effects, oral stool softeners such as dioctyl sodium sulfosuccinate in dosages of 40 to 120 mg./day, and lubricants such as mineral oil (where the danger of aspiration is not great) may aid in regulating bowel function. Oral laxatives may be of value in patients able to communicate their needs and able to use the toilet, commode or bedpan. If these modes fail, regularly scheduled enemas may be necessary. Attention should be paid to gastric and intestinal dilatation as a source of respiratory embarrassment.

Genitourinary Tract. Incontinence frequently occurs due to either spastic or atonic bladders. When overflow incontinence is present, Credé's method of expressing urine is preferred. Recent studies have shown intermittent catheterization to be preferable to chronic indwelling catheters. When a spastic bladder is present, a spasmolytic agent such as propantheline bromide (Pro-Banthine) may be helpful.

When chronic indwelling catheters are used, infection is a frequent sequela. Initial management calls for acidification with ascorbic acid, and prophylactic use of drugs such as methenamine mandelate. Urine must be acidic in order for the methenamine mandelate to dissociate into formaldehyde, its active form

(maximal efficiency at urine pH of 5.5). When infection occurs, antibiotic therapy should be determined on the basis of urine culture and sensitivity.

Prolonged immobilization results in mobilization and excretion of large amounts of calcium. Large volume of dilute urine is preferred in an effort to prevent calculus formation. Urine calcium should be determined periodically in an effort to predict calculus formation.

Skin Care. Immobilization encourages pressure injury to skin, especially in patients with sensory loss. Bony prominences and areas receiving pressure as a result of braces or other appliances should receive protective padding. In bedridden or otherwise immobilized patients, repositioning should be done at 2 to 3 hour intervals. Water or air flotation mattresses or alternating pressure mattresses may allow longer intervals between repositioning. Adequate protein intake, bland oils to maintain appropriate moisture over dry areas, drying powders to absorb perspiration, and protective creams and salves to prevent maceration in skin creases as a result of urine and feces are essential. When skin breakdown occurs, relief of pressure, drying and early treatment of superficial infection should be undertaken.

Seizures. Seizures are a frequent accompaniment of degenerative disorders, especially those of gray matter. Treatment should be with usual anticonvulsant modes as outlined elsewhere.

Behavior. Behavioral changes frequently accompany degenerative disorders of the central nervous system. Irritability, aggressive behavior and agitation often become major difficulties. Therapy should begin with medications producing mild tranquilizing effects such as diphenhydramine (Benadryl), 5 mg./kg./day in 4 divided doses (to a maximum of 150 mg./day); promethazine (Phenergan), 50 to 75 mg./day; or hydroxyzine (Vistaril or Atarax), up to 10 mg. 3 or 4 times per day. If necessary, haloperidol (Haldol)* beginning at 0.25 mg./day, thioridazine (Mellaril)† beginning at 10 mg. 2 or 3 times per day, or chlorpromazine (Thorazine), 0.5 mg./kg. every 4 to 6 hours, can be used. Their individual doses should be raised slowly to controlling levels.

Education. Where the progression of the disease is slow, and the stage of the disease

---

*Manufacturer's precaution: The safety and effectiveness of haloperidol in children have not been established; therefore, this drug is not recommended for use in the pediatric age group.

†Manufacturer's precaution: Thioridazine is not intended for children under 2 years of age.

permits, adapted educational programs for the handicapped or retarded should be encouraged. In many schools physiotherapy and occupational therapy are available and may serve as an adjunct to home-based programs.

Death.   In spite of all efforts, progression of the disease process may continue, requiring frequent or prolonged hospitalization. The physician must be alert to signs of preterminal state as an indication for possible hospitalization, and the need for increased emotional support. The family should be informed that death is inevitable, and that all measures to promote the patient's comfort are being taken.

SPECIFIC PROBLEMS

Ataxia-Telangiectasia.   The neurologic deterioration in this condition is not treatable. Recurrent infections, especially sinopulmonary, resulting from a defect in T-cell function and decreased IgA and IgE are common and should be managed according to their bacterial flora.

Ceroid Lipofuscinosis.   These disorders have been treated with doses of 800 to 1000 units per day of vitamin E; however, the efficacy of treatment is not established.

Charcot-Marie-Tooth Disease (Perineal Muscular Atrophy). This disorder is characterized by a slowly progressive myopathy and peripheral neuropathy. Regular mild exercise of weak muscles should be encouraged, since disuse of a partially atrophic muscle may accelerate disability. Spring braces to minimize foot drop may extend the period of independent ambulation. Where sensory loss is significant, the patient must learn to protect partially anesthetic extremities from inadvertent injury.

Dystonia Musculorum Deformans.   As there is intellectual sparing while the movement disorder and dystonic posturing progress, surgical intervention and medication may produce significant improvement. The production of stereotactically placed lytic lesions in the posterior half of the ventral lateral nucleus of the thalamus may reverse involuntary movements and dystonia. However, bilateral lesions may be necessary and recurrence of symptoms may necessitate repeating surgery. Levodopa has produced improvement in some cases and should be tried prior to surgical intervention. If symptoms persist, adjustments in the educational setting may be necessary, such as the use of tape recorders and the use of oral examinations when written work is impaired.

Familial Spastic Paraparesis.   This slowly progressive disorder lends itself to an active physiotherapy program. Spasticity may be relieved by diazepam or dantrolene sodium. Surgical procedures, unless essential to release contractures, should be discouraged. When surgery is required, early ambulation should be encouraged.

Friedreich's Ataxia.   Specific treatment is not available. To accommodate the loss of proprioceptive sense, emphasis should be placed on the development of visual cues to aid coordination. Coordination exercises should be encouraged as tolerated. Bracing and casting may be used to treat scoliosis. Surgical correction of foot deformities and scoliosis should only be undertaken when the disease is in a slowly progressive phase. Cardiomyopathy may accompany this disorder, requiring treatment of heart failure with diuretics and digitalis preparations.

Hepatolenticular Degeneration (Wilson's Disease).   This rare disease is characterized by excessive accumulation of copper in body tissues, producing extensive damage to liver and brain, if not treated. The drug of choice is D-penicillamine (0.3 to 2.0 gm./day orally taken on an empty stomach), which forms soluble complexes with tissue-stored copper, facilitating its excretion. A strict low copper content diet to limit exposure is necessary. Other chelating agents such as BAL and EDTA have been used but show no significant advantage over D-penicillamine.

Huntington's Chorea.   Choreiform movements may be controlled using phenobarbital (6 mg./kg./day), reserpine (0.02 mg./kg./day), phenothiazines and haloperidol. Dipropylacetate, gamma aminobutyric acid, clonazepam, tetrabenazine and levodopa are now undergoing evaluation in the treatment of the chorea. Treatment is symptomatic and does not alter the course of the disease.

Hypertrophic Interstitial Neuritis.   Treatment is similar to that of Charcot-Marie-Tooth disease. Steroids have been administered but fail to alter the course of the disease.

Juvenile Paralysis Agitans.   Levodopa or levodopa-carbidopa combinations and amantadine hydrochloride may relieve the bradykinesia and rigidity. Benztropin (Cogentin) may also reduce rigidity.

Laurence-Moon-Biedl Syndrome.   No specific treatment is available. Obesity, if not controlled, may limit the activity of these children. The progressive decrease of vision and mental subnormality should be considered in educational planning.

Leigh's Disease (Subacute Necrotizing Encephalopathy).   This disorder is characterized by the presence of a thiamine pyrophosphate-adenosine triphosphate phorphoryl transfer inhibitor. Large doses of thiamine hydrochloride (0.6 to 4.0 gm./day) have produced transient remission. Substituted thiamine derivatives, thiamine propyldisulfide (0.15 to 0.8 gm./day) and thiamine tetrafurfuryl disulfide (0.5 to 1.0 gm./day) are more efficacious in raising cerebrospinal fluid and blood thiamine levels. Intravenous administration of any of the thiamine derivatives produces the highest levels of cerebrospinal fluid and blood and is the preferred route in acute exacerbations. Thiamine tetrafurfuryl disulfide has the advantage of imparting little odor to patients.

Lesch-Nyhan Syndrome. This disorder is characterized by an error in purine metabolism, hyperuricemia, mental retardation and an irresistible urge for self-mutilation. Treatment with allopurinol is successful in reducing serum urine acid levels; however, the self-mutilation has been refractory. Mechanical aids and restraints have been individually designed to limit self-mutilation but allow participation in social situations.

Progressive Myoclonic Epilepsy of Unverricht-Lundborg. The seizures accompanying this disorder have been refractory to most commonly used anticonvulsants. Recently L-5 hydroxytryptophan in conjunction with the peripheral decarboxylase inhibitor carbidopa, and clonazepam have been shown to be effective.

Trichopoliodystrophy (Kinky Hair Disease). Recent reports indicate that if diagnosed early, some patients may have neurologic and biochemical dysfunctions altered by the intravenous administration of cupric salts. Subcutaneous or intramuscular administration of cupric salts has not been effective.

Cerebral Palsy

KENNETH F. SWAIMAN, M.D.

Many forms of therapy are available for patients with the varied perinatal motor disabilities subsumed under the rubric of cerebral palsy. Many patients improve with or without therapy; therefore the results of therapy must be compared with the natural improvement of function and coordination that accompanies maturation. There are several aspects of therapy that can be considered individually.

Patient and Family Knowledge. The physician must explain carefully the symptoms and signs of the form of cerebral palsy which affects the patient. An attempt should be made to discuss the known pathophysiologic features that result in cerebral palsy. The expected course should be explained to the parents. Cerebral palsy should be contrasted with other conditions with which it is frequently confused. The expected lack of progression and if appropriate the possibility that the patient suffers from mental retardation are discussed candidly. The usual lack of hereditary pattern is stressed unless there is some doubt concerning diagnosis.

General Therapeutic Measures. It is important that children with suspected or confirmed cerebral palsy have ophthalmologic and audiologic examinations. Both visual and auditory impairment are common in children with cerebral palsy. Every attempt should be made to reduce their communication handicap.

Seizures occur in approximately one-third of children with cerebral palsy although the incidence varies with the type of motor impairment. Patients with hemiplegia experience seizures more commonly than those with choreoathetosis. Electroencephalography and other necessary studies are performed. Anticonvulsant medication appropriate to the seizure disorder is administered.

If limitation of intelligence is suspected, adequate and appropriate psychometric evaluation is necessary. The patient with speech delay and articulation errors should be evaluated by an experienced speech pathologist.

Medication. A number of medications have been used to reduce spasticity. Regardless of medication used, the child should be given a small dose initially and the dosage increased gradually over 4 to 8 weeks.

Diazepam,* .03 to .05 mg./kg./day in 3 to 4 divided doses, is often effective in severe spasticity and may benefit patients with athetosis; on occasion, drowsiness or incoordination is induced.

In recent years dantrolene,† 2 to 10 mg./kg./day in 2 to 4 divided doses, has also been of value in treating both spasticity and athetosis. The drug has a more long-acting effect than diazepam and is of benefit in one-third to one-half of my patients. Dantrolene may cause marked loss of tone and weakness to the point that it must be discontinued even though the dose is reduced greatly. Leukopenia and hepatotoxicity may occur; initial laboratory monitoring at monthly intervals and then quarterly is recommended.

---

*Manufacturer's precaution: The safety and efficacy of diazepam have not been established in the neonate.

†Manufacturer's precaution: The safety of dantrolene in children under 5 is not established. Long-term safety and efficacy in humans are not established.

I have had no experience with fonazine, a phenothiazine thought to reduce decerebrate rigidity and produce relatively little sedation.

Levodopa,* 0.5 to 4.0 gm./day in 4 divided doses, has been of value to a few patients with athetosis and spasticity.

Bracing, Injections, and Surgery. The use of surgery to overcome secondary contracture formation associated with spasticity is often necessary. Attempts should be made to modify the contracture with casts and exercise before surgery is recommended.

Spasticity has also been treated with motor point block (intramuscular neurolysis). A motor point is located within the muscle by stimulation and a 5 per cent phenol solution is injected. The effects of the injection last approximately 4 to 12 months. Attempts to repeat therapy in the same location may be unsuccessful or less successful because of arborization of nerve fibers after regrowth. This therapy must be used selectively, but has proved valuable in some patients.

Leg bracing is helpful for some patients. Long leg braces with a knee spring lock and adjustable ankle stop are used. Braces should not be used for children who can ambulate reasonably well without them; however, bracing should not be postponed if a patient is having progressive difficulty with ambulation.

Subcutaneous tenotomies of the Achilles tendons are of particular value in children with severe equinovarus deformities. The foot and leg must then be casted to maintain the position until the operative site has healed. Flexion contractures of the hip may be surgically released. Application of a long leg brace immediately afterward is necessary.

If surgery is contemplated in which tendon transplants are indicated, infiltration of the peripheral nerve with local anesthetic to induce weakness and decrease spasticity may make possible evaluation of the expected effects of surgery.

Before surgery on the arm and hand, the extent and type of involvement must be assessed. Limitation of active and passive motion must be recorded. Impairment of sensory function must be sought carefully. The patient should have some degree of voluntary control of grasp and release mechanisms if surgical therapy is to be successful. It is important in planning to know the patient's overall intelligence and the likelihood that patient and parents will cooperate in a therapy program after surgery. Surgery is most often performed on

patients with spasticity and limited wrist extension and supination. Most often surgery for the wrist flexion and forearm pronation deformity consists of tenotomy of the pronator teres and a transfer of the tendon of the flexor carpi ulnaris with insertion into the tendon of the extensor carpi radialis longus. There are approaches to other problems which are less common.

I have had no personal experience with chronic cerebellar stimulation in cerebral palsy. Proponents proclaim significant short-term and long-term improvement in spasticity and in athetosis, speech and functional status. As with any new invasive therapy, meticulous evaluation should be performed before the technique is accorded a place in routine therapy.

Physical Therapy. Physical therapy improves leg function more than hand function in patients with spastic quadriplegia. Usefulness of the hand despite therapy and operation often depends on the integrity of deep and superficial sensation pathways. Patients with mild spastic hemiparesis usually develop a serviceable gait pattern whether or not they receive physical therapy. On the other hand, therapy may improve patients with more severe hemiparesis. Dyskinesias such as choreoathetosis and dystonia are affected little by physical therapy. The initial severity of the symptomatology appears to be the most important factor in eventual serviceable function.

Occupational Therapy. Occupational therapy may be most important in the development of self-help skills, particularly those involving the arms. The child may be helped to develop head control and trunk stability such that the use of the arms will be optimal. Occupational therapists may also recommend the use of special dressing techniques. Specifically designed spoons and dishes may be a great help.

Educational-Social Program. Every effort should be made to provide the child with cerebral palsy with as near-normal a social and educational environment as possible. Day-care centers, nursery schools, and regular grade schools should be used when feasible. Unfortunately a number of patients with cerebral palsy are in need of individualized educational programs and individualized concomitant physical therapy. Coordination is important. Problems with educational planning are complicated further because children may have associated difficulties with intellectual ability, hyperactivity, distraction and dependency. The child with severe physical difficulty and normal intellect provides an intricate educa-

---

*Manufacturer's precaution: The safety of levodopa in children under 12 has not been established.

tional and vocational planning problem, and school placement must be carefully individualized.

Spinal Diseases

W. EDWIN DODSON, M.D.

TRAUMA

Avoidance of additional neurological injury and facilitation of rehabilitation are key in the management of patients with spinal cord damage. For the purposes of this discussion, the management of spinal trauma is divided somewhat arbitrarily into three phases: acute (1 to 3 days), convalescent (1 to 6 weeks), and rehabilitative (after 6 weeks).

Acute spinal injuries are medical emergencies and require expert care by experienced specialists. Patients should be immobilized and transported without manipulation of the spine to minimize the risk of iatrogenic injury to the spinal cord. Careful reduction and immobilization of the spine are essential and in most instances require neurosurgical assistance. Patients with spinal cord lesions which are partial and progressing or patients with bony fragments in the spinal canal are candidates for surgical exploration. Dexamethasone should be administered to minimize the development of edema of the spinal cord. The usual dosage is 0.1 mg./kg. every six hours. Patients with immediate, complete spinal cord lesions after trauma usually are not helped by surgical exploration. Spinal mobility, when persistent, may be treated electively by spinal fusion. Patients developing signs and symptoms of spinal cord injury after trivial spinal trauma should be suspected of harboring vertebral or craniocervical anomalies which permit abnormal mobility of the spine. After these anomalies are defined radiographically, they should be treated by reduction and immobilization and then surgically by fusion to prevent further spinal cord damage.

Spinal shock accompanies acute trauma to the spinal cord and results in autonomic disturbances including urinary retention. The bladder should be catheterized to prevent overdistention. When there is impaired thermoregulation it may be necessary to use heating or cooling blankets to maintain a normal body temperature. Hypotension due to interruption of sympathetic pathways may be treated by the judicious use of vasopressors if attempts to restore blood pressure by wrapping the extremities with elastic bandages or by expanding plasma volume by fluid replacement are unsuccessful.

Gradual recovery from spinal shock usually occurs within six weeks after spinal trauma. Bowel and bladder function gradually become autonomous. Sterile technique in handling urinary catheters is required throughout the patient's management. A culture of the urine should be obtained several days before changing an indwelling catheter so that specific antibiotic therapy can be administered in the preceding 18 hours. The purpose of this treatment is to sterilize the urine during the period of catheter manipulation to minimize the chance of sepsis. Whereas bacteriuria is often present when indwelling catheters are used, treatment with antibiotics should be guided by the occurrence of symptoms, evidence of upper tract inflammation on urinalysis, and bacteriological culture and sensitivity data.

Some urologists recommend administering methenamine mandelate (Mandelamine) and ascorbic acid to patients with indwelling catheters. The former suppresses bacteriological growth in the urine collection system and the latter acidifies the urine. An adequate fluid intake should be maintained to keep urine flow high. When adequate bladder tone and spontaneous emptying are recovered, indwelling catheter can be discontinued. Training the patient to perform Crede maneuvers can be undertaken to help empty the bladder. Decreased bowel motility can result in constipation and the development of fecal impactions. Thus varying combinations of stool softeners, stimulant laxatives and occasional enemas may be indicated.

Care of the patient's skin requires careful attention to avoid the development of decubitus ulcers. This is best accomplished by maintaining the patient on a soft dry surface with frequent changes of position. The use of Stryker frame beds, alternating air pressure mattresses, and sheep skins aid in providing the conscientious nursing care required to maintain good skin condition. Physical therapy should be initiated during the convalescent phase to minimize the development of contractures. During the convalescent phase plans for rehabilitation should be initiated.

The rehabilitation of patients with permanent neurological deficits due to spinal injuries is a challenging and important problem. An attitude of realistic optimism on the part of the medical staff can provide valuable support for the patient and his family. Academic programs for children of school age should be initiated as soon as the patient's condition permits. Among adolescents, preinjury career plans should be assessed and reevaluated sensitively but realistically. During this phase of the illness, the social worker can help identify resources within the community for continued education and/or specific vocational training.

The medical problems of the convalescent phase of the injury may persist and periodic follow-up is required. Good habits developed during early periods of care regarding bowel and bladder training, skin care and the use of physical therapy to reduce contractures facilitate the patient's rehabilitation. Patients having neurogenic bladders after spinal trauma remain vulnerable to the development of urinary tract infections, and periodic urinalysis and culture are indicated. Recurrent infections, intractable ureterovesical reflux or deterioration of the upper urinary tracts are indications for consulting the urologist regarding a ureteral reimplantation or urinary diversion before renal function deteriorates irreversibly. Incomplete emptying of the bladder producing a large residual volume may be treated by intermittent catheterization. Lifelong attention to skin care is required for patients having permanent anesthesia. The education of these patients to deal with their special disabilities is an important responsibility shared by the entire health care team.

A variety of methods are available to improve the motor function of patients with spinal cord damage. The aggressive use of physical therapy, assistive devices, and braces permits the development of independent ambulation among most patients with spinal cord levels at or below L3. Similarly, the use of splints and other devices may improve function of the upper extremities in patients sustaining lower cervical cord damage. Obviously, the treatment program must be individualized. Patients developing excessive spasticity or flexion spasms after spinal cord injury may be benefited by medications. Among these patients a trial of diazepam (Valium) or dantrolene sodium (Dantrium) may be indicated. Appropriate dosage varies considerably. Treatment is initiated at low dosage and gradually increased until spasticity is reduced or toxicity supervenes.

MASS LESIONS

Mass lesions involving the spinal cord can also present as medical emergencies. In acute situations neurosurgical consultation is indicated prior to myelography because this procedure may precipitate worsening of a neurological deficit requiring an immediate decompressive laminectomy. Steroids should

be administered to minimize edema of the spinal cord.

Spinal mass lesions have been classified as extradural, intradural or intramedullary depending on the site of occurrence. Extradural and intradural lesions are most often neoplastic or infectious in origin. Metastatic tumors such as lymphomas or neuroblastomas are often intradural. Surgical exploration for decompression and diagnosis is usually indicated. Intramedullary mass lesions of the spinal cord in children are usually neoplastic, most often astrocytomas or ependymomas. These intramedullary lesions may be approached by the neurosurgeon's dividing the posterior columns to visualize the areas of concern. In certain cases of spinal ependymoma a complete removal may be possible. Other nonresectable spinal cord tumors may have cystic components which can be evacuated to alleviate symptoms. Postoperatively, radiotherapy is usually indicated and referral should be made to the radiotherapist. The appropriate role of chemotherapy of spinal tumors is undefined. Guidelines for chemotherapy of intrinsic spinal tumors will be forthcoming only after a significant number of patients have been referred to centers for controlled clinical trials.

MISCELLANEOUS SPINAL LESIONS

Diastematomyelia, tethered cord, and vascular disorders of the spinal cord are rare. *Diastematomyelia* producing progressive neurological dysfunction should be treated by surgical removal of the bony or fibrous band which transects the spinal cord. A *tethered cord*, often associated with other spinal abnormalities such as lipomas or lipomeningoceles, should also be considered for surgical treatment. *Arteriovenous malformations* of the spinal cord producing symptoms in childhood usually are large and located posteriorly. They can produce sudden severe neurological impairment because of a tendency to bleed. These lesions are thus best treated surgically by an experienced neurosurgeon skilled in operating with the use of a microscope. Careful preoperative evaluation of vascular malformations with the use of selective spinal angiography is indicated. In all these conditions, the goal of surgery is to prevent worsening of the disability. Recovery of function after surgery is generally unpredictable.

Vascular occlusion producing *spinal cord infarctions* may be associated with abdominal or craniocervical trauma, vasculitis, or can occur iatrogenically in association with clamping of the aorta. Usually the result is an anterior spinal artery syndrome. Steroids should be administered initially to reduce edema, and spinal shock, if present, should be treated as outlined above. Sensory and autonomic dysfunction in patients with spinal cord infarction usually improves. The use of braces and physical therapy can significantly help rehabilitate patients with residual motor handicaps.

Degeneration of the intervertebral discs in childhood is rare and is most often due to infection in younger children. In such cases a specific bacterial etiology should be sought by percutaneous aspiration of the disc space followed by culture of the aspirate. The optimal duration and route of antibiotic administration are not firmly established. However, it seems prudent to initiate therapy intravenously with a penicillinase-resistant penicillin until a specific bacterial etiology and antibiotic sensitivity are known. Whereas immobilization of the spine by use of a spica case or traction may produce relief of pain, similar results may sometimes by produced by bed rest. Children with infections restricted to the disc space enjoy a good prognosis for recovery without residual neurological disability. Herniated discs occurring in older children as a result of physical trauma should be treated initially with immobilization and bed rest. Surgery may be considered if there is persistent pain, radiculopathy or a complicating vertebral anomaly such as a narrow spinal canal.

Spina Bifida

EDWARD P. HOFFMAN, M.D.

The infant born with myelomeningocele presents a difficult problem of medical management. The dilemma has not been solved by the recent advances of surgical technology. Fortunately, the management of spina bifida occulta is not a serious problem in most cases.

TREATMENT OF OCCULT MYELODYSPLASIA

Generally no treatment is necessary for spina bifida occulta, the malformation being limited to the spine. However, occult spinal dysraphic lesions may be present including the following: thickened and shortened filum terminale; aberrant nerve roots or adherent bands with tethering effect, restricting ascent of the spinal cord; diastomatomyelia; congenital dermal sinus, with or without epidermoid or dermoid tumors; lipoma or lipomyelomeningocele. Any cutaneous anomaly along the spinal axis should lead one to suspect an associated intraspinal lesion and the possibility of a congenital dermal sinus. The spine should be investigated if there are malformations of the lower extremities. The presence of sensory impairment or weakness of the lower extremities, urinary incontinence or perianal numbness, fecal incontinence or back pain warrants investigation. Certainly, any progressive deficit demands evaluation. Changes may be subtle in infancy and are easily overlooked. Delayed onset of symptoms and progression are common.

X-rays of the spine are taken. In most cases structural changes of the spine will be present but roentgenograms may be normal or show only minor variations. Myelography is usually done, the exception being an infected dermal sinus. Myelography should include studies in the prone position.

The presence of any neurologic deficit, and particularly any progressive deficit, may dictate surgical intervention. The primary aim of surgery is prevention of further neurologic impairment; only in 25 per cent of cases will actual improvement occur. This fact should be made clear to the relatives of the patient before surgery.

Surgery is done to remove intraspinal lesions so that there is elimination of direct pressure on the spinal cord or cauda equina and pressure on the vascular supply of the spinal cord. Multiple lesions should be sought. Total excision should be attempted if possible, but with lipomatous lesions this may be dangerous. In such case, it may be safest to leave behind some of the fatty tissue. Adhesive fibrous bands and hypertrophied filum terminale are sectioned to prevent the detrimental tethering effect of the spinal cord associated with elongation of the spinal canal as the child grows. Use of the microscope, bipolar forceps and nerve stimulator reduces surgical morbidity. The stimulator is used before sectioning any fibrous bands or filum terminale and is frequently applied during resection of lipomatous tissue.

It is mandatory that a dermal sinus be explored since intraspinal extension predisposes to the devastating consequences of meningitis. The sinus tract must be traced and excised to the end of its innermost terminus. In the lumbosacral area it will course cephalad. Total excision of the sinus should be carried out if it can be done safely.

SELECTION FOR TREATMENT OF SPINA BIFIDA CYSTICA

Perhaps the most difficult problem of management is selecting those patients who should be treated actively. Recommendations in the recent literature are contradictory. A number of workers have recommended that no active treatment be given if the infant has one or more of the following conditions: (1) a large thoracolumbar or thoracolumbosacral lesion; (2) severe paraplegia with no innervation below the L3 segmental level, with at most function of hip flexors, adductors and quadriceps; (3) kyphosis or scoliosis clinically evident at birth; (4) gross hydrocephalus with head circumference exceeding the 90th percentile by at least 2 cm., related to birth weight; (5) severe cerebral birth injury or intracranial hemorrhage; and (6) other congenital defects such as cyanotic heart disease, mongolism or serious malformations of the genitourinary tract.

Active treatment should be withheld in those infants who already have hydrocephalus and significant neurologic impairment and who, after closure of the spinal defect, develop meningitis and ventriculitis. Also, no treatment should be considered in the severely handicapped child who later develops a life-threatening episode. Another factor to be considered is the social situation of the family. Even if the physical condition is a little better than the severe handicaps listed above, the fate of such a child is grave if he is unwanted or abandoned. Finally, x-ray demonstration of Lückenschädel (lacunar skull deformity) in the infant with multiple adverse physical findings or gross congenital anomalies is a contraindication to aggressive treatment. If any question arises, a second opinion can always be obtained.

Once the decision not to operate has been made, nothing should be done that might prolong the child's survival. However, all patients should receive normal nursing care and they should be protected against any suffering. The defect should be dressed accordingly. Analgesic and anticonvulsant medications are administered if indicated, but the use of tube feeding, resuscitation, and antibiotics for infection should be withheld. Once the decision not to actively treat the patient is made, one should not be tempted to shunt hydrocephalus because progressive hydrocephalus is an important cause of early mortality.

Elective early treatment is now widely accepted, and there has been improvement in the quality of survival with this approach. The results of early operation without selection have been disheartening. In spite of some increase in survival rate, a large percentage of survivors are mentally retarded and have serious medical problems and physical handicap. These patients will require many surgeries. In addition, the social life of the involved family is adversely affected. Contrary to the concern that a fair number of untreated infants may survive with handicaps greater than they would have had if they were not treated from the beginning, nearly all of the untreated have died within six months, usually from hydrocephalus or meningitis. If such an individual survives to the age of six months, the decision could then be made to carry out operation if it appears likely that the child will continue to live. Once such treatment is started, further therapy should not be withheld. Therefore, the initial decision not to actively treat is not necessarily a final one.

The method of selective treatment is far from ideal, but is the best that can be offered today. The most promising possibility is that of in utero selection for therapeutic abortion. Investigation is being carried out for detection by amniocentesis of elevated alpha fetoprotein of the amniotic fluid of a high risk fetus in the early months of pregnancy, occurring in a woman who has already given birth to an infant with myelomeningocele or in whom there is a strong family history of the condition. In addition, research is being directed to the detection of alpha fetoprotein in the maternal serum. If this is fruitful, the risk of amniocentesis would be avoided.

WHEN TO OPERATE

If the decision is made for surgery, the meningocele or myelomeningocele should be repaired as soon as possible in order to lessen the risk of meningitis and to prevent the possibility of drying of the sac and damage to neural structures. It is generally agreed that rupture or imminence of rupture of the sac is indication for immediate surgery. Prophylactic antibiotics will not prevent meningitis. The existence of progressive hydrocephalus is *not* a contraindication to myelomeningocele repair. Lesions already infected or ulcerated should not be repaired until the infection is controlled and the ulcer is healed. When surgery is delayed, the sac should be covered with sterile gauze soaked in saline; daily soap baths are performed.

In those patients selected for active treatment, shunting procedures for control of hydrocephalus are mandatory to prevent irreversible brain damage with subsequent mental retardation. Unless there is rapidly progressive hydrocephalus, generally it is best to defer shunt operations until 4 to 6 weeks of age because there is a high incidence of complications from a procedure done before one month. Obstruction of the ventricular end of the shunt and shunt dependence are particularly apt to occur. There has been no significant increase in the proportion of retarded children by such a judicious delay. The presence of infection of a myelomeningocele sac has *not* yet been a contraindication to shunt procedure, and in some cases primary treatment of hydrocephalus has led to the clearing of infection and healing of myelomeningocele defect. At that time, repair of the sac could be carried out.

SURGERY

Prior to surgery the sac is protected with sterile moist dressings. X-rays are taken in the region of the defect to delineate the bony abnormalities at the site of the myelomeningocele and to demonstrate the presence of other associated congenital abnormalities. The following antibiotic combination has been recommended for preoperative administration: gentamicin, 4 mg./kg. intramuscularly, and oxacillin, 100 mg./kg. intravenously, daily for five days. General anesthesia is used and the infant must be properly positioned on padding so that pressure necrosis is avoided. A warming blanket is usually used. The extremities are wrapped to lessen heat loss. There should be an intravenous line with a needle caliber large enough to administer blood. Blood must be available for surgery.

A circumferential elliptical incision is made along the line of demarcation between the normal skin and the atrophic covering of the myelomeningocele sac. Strict attention to hemostasis should be maintained. Dissection is carried down through the subcutaneous tissue and the dural neck of the sac is defined. The dura is opened at cranial end of the sac to lessen the chance of damage to the nerve roots. As much dura as possible is left intact to allow later closure. The scarred sac is carefully dissected free from the neural tissue, great care being taken to identify and preserve neural structures. This is facilitated by the use of the nerve stimulator, microscope and bipolar forceps. If damage to the nervous tissue can be avoided, all adherent epithelial tissue should be removed to prevent subsequent development of an intraspinal dermoid cyst. Nerve roots and meninges are separated from surrounding tissues to avoid the development of traction on them with the later growth of the vertebral column. Neural tissue should be repetitively irrigated with saline solution to prevent damage from drying.

Dural closure should be water-tight and there should be no tension on the enclosed nerve roots. If there is not enough dura available, duroplasty may be necessary. A small piece of fascia would be suitable for this. Rotation of fascial flaps may be necessary to reinforce the thin dura or the suture line. No attempt is made to close the vertebral defect with bone. However, the displaced spinous processes and adjacent paraspinal muscles can be rotated up and over the dural closure in the upper lumbar region. In the lower lumbar area muscle-fascia mass alone is mobilized and approximated by absorbable suture.

Skin closure must be water-tight without undue tension. This usually requires undermining the skin from multiple directions. Rotation flaps may be

necessary. Skin grafting over the muscle may be preferable to extensive undermining.

Postoperative fecal contamination of the wound site is prevented by sealing the lower part of the dressing with waterproof plastic adhesive tape. Daily inspection of the wound is necessary. If any spinal fluid accumulates beneath the skin, it is aspirated. If there is recurrent accumulation, ventricular shunting is usually necessary.

Daily measurements of head circumference are taken. If there is excessive growth of the head size above the normal curve or if a rapid persistent increase in size develops, shunting will be necessary. Ventriculoperitoneal shunts have several advantages over the ventriculoatrial procedures: avoiding direct infection of the blood stream if there has been any threat of contamination of the spinal fluid; and deferring the time of revision due to growth of the child since positioning of the peritoneal end of the shunt is less critical than placement of the distal end of an atrial shunt.

OVERALL MANAGEMENT

Total care of the patient requires coordinated effort, and the pediatrician is probably best suited to oversee this. Counseling the family should begin immediately with explanation of the problem and potential difficulties to be encountered. Social workers may be helpful in guiding the family and dealing with problems as they arise. Educational requirements are best altered to fit the particular handicap or potential of the individual; most ambulatory children may be able to attend public schools. Vocational training may be indicated at the appropriate time.

Periodic follow-up is necessary for orthopedic, neurosurgical and urological evaluation. Deformities should be discovered and corrected at an early age, before the stage of significant deterioration of function occurs. One should also look for associated abnormalities. Failure of the ventriculoatrial or ventriculoperitoneal shunting apparatus must be detected early to prevent fatality or brain damage.

MANAGING DEFORMITIES IN PATIENTS SURVIVING WITH MYELOMENINGOCELE

Orthopedic management is necessary for correction of deformity and maintenance of that correction as well as for obtaining the greatest possible degree of mobility and self-sufficiency. In order to determine the appropriate management, one must evaluate the pattern of remaining neurologic function and the presence of spastic and flaccid muscle groups as well as the status of their antagonists. Assessment should be done as soon as possible after birth and at regular intervals throughout the growth period of the child and adolescent.

By this means developing deformity and contracture may be prevented.

Conservative means to correct deformity, such as casting and bracing, are usually contraindicated because of the risk of causing skin breakdown in the presence of sensory deficit or existing deformity. Even if there is initial success with such methods, recurrence is likely if muscle imbalance exists. If immobilization or fixation with bracing or plaster casts is carried out, it should rarely be done longer than one month.

Muscle balance is achieved by tendon transfer or lengthening and by denervation or excision of overactive muscles. It may be necessary to correct the remaining deformity by osteotomy or excision of bone and cartilage. The ideal time of corrective surgery on the limbs is between 6 months and 2 years of age, and additional procedures are often done between 2 and 5 years. Deformities of the spine are most often corrected in adolescence.

About one third of the patients develop severe lumbar lordosis and scoliosis in adolescence. Recommended treatment has been multiple wedge osteotomy and fusion using Dwyer staples and cable fixation. The main indication for surgery in this case is rapidly increasing spinal deformity with loss of mobility. Kyphosis tends to be progressive and difficult to treat. Gibbus formation may lead to an overlying skin ulceration. Closing-wedge spinal osteotomies or ostectomy have been used. The latter procedure is hazardous and there is a tendency for gradual recurrence of gibbus with the former procedure.

Hip flexion contractures have been treated by anterior hip release. Iliopsoas transfer, with or without osteotomy, has been used to correct hip dislocation with limited success. Whatever procedure is done, hip mobility must be maintained. Dislocated mobile hips are preferable to immobile ones. In some cases surgery may be obviated by abduction–internal rotation splinting from an early age.

Hyperextension deformity is the most frequent associated knee problem. It has been corrected by serial plaster casting in the position of flexion to prevent elongation of the quadriceps. Knee flexion deformity is treated by transfer of hamstring tendons. The two most common foot deformities with myelodysplasia are equinovarus and equinocavovarus. These are best treated by tissue-releasing and tendon transfers. Arthrodesis of the feet may be necessary in more severe cases.

Orthotic devices may facilitate ambulation and should be tailored to the specific needs of the individual.

TREATMENT OF GENITOURINARY SYSTEM COMPLICATIONS

Until the age of 2 years the majority of deaths from spina bifida cystica occurs from effects on the brain or spinal cord; after this age the principal cause of fatality is chronic renal failure. Surgical repair of myelomeningocele has little bearing on the incidence of urinary complications. Most patients with spina bifida cystica who survive the first two years of life have urinary incontinence, and the majority of these have recurrent or persistent pyuria. There is often urinary retention and vesicoureteral reflux. Complications predisposing to death are hydronephrosis with infection, bilateral chronic pyelonephritis and hydronephrosis with contralateral renal agenesis.

Avoiding renal complications requires the diagnosis of urinary anomalies in infants with myelodysplasia and active preventive therapy. Intravenous pyelography and micturition cystography should be performed within the first few weeks of life. The following principles have been recommended for the treatment of renal disorders associated with myelomeningocele: (1) long-term suppressive doses of antibacterial drugs to reduce the incidence of urinary tract infection; (2) reduction of residual vesical urine by scheduled frequent voiding, aided by the Credé maneuver; (3) prolonged indwelling catheter drainage to decrease vesicoureteral reflux and hydronephrosis; and (4) urinary diversion procedure (uretero-ileostomy) in those patients with intractable severe hydronephrosis or urinary incontinence that persists to school age.

MANAGEMENT OF ASSOCIATED PROBLEMS

Constant vigilance is necessary to prevent skin breakdown from the combination of immobilization, lack of sensation and deformity leading to local skin pressure. Ulcers over the feet are usually treated by padding or alteration of shoes. Occasionally sympathectomy or even amputation is necessary. Local inflammation may develop near the vulva or anus from urinary or fecal incontinence. Sometimes urinary tract diversion procedures may be necessary to eliminate this problem.

Prolapse of the rectum is not uncommon and usually requires only conservative management. It generally disappears within one year. Bowel control is usually achieved by training, diet manipulation and stool softeners. Sometimes constipating agents are necessary. Parents should be advised to restrict diet since the relative inactivity of the patient predisposes to weight gain.

It is apparent that the treatment of spina bifida entails the coordinated effort of multiple medical specialties. Only by this means can the prognosis of the patient be improved and the possibility of prevention be attained.

Acute Hemiplegia

N. PAUL ROSMAN, M.D.

Acute hemiplegia of childhood is a rapidly evolving postnatally acquired unilateral paralysis that occurs in the absence of detectable antecedent neurological disability. Although the etiology of this syndrome is frequently unknown, many disorders have been reported as causative. These include a variety of cerebral diseases, arterial occlusions, venous occlusions, vascular malformations and intracranial hemorrhages.

Cerebral diseases that can be complicated by acute hemiplegia include hypoxic encephalopathy induced by seizures associated with fever, meningoencephalitis, post-infectious and post-vaccinal demyelinative encephalopathies, brain tumor, brain abscess and lead encephalopathy. *Arterial occlusions* can be caused by trauma to the neck, resulting in thrombosis of the extracranial carotid artery, or by paratonsillar trauma, causing thrombosis of the internal carotid artery. Other causes include arteritis from neighboring infection, collagen disease, amphetamine abuse, or dissecting aneurysm and emboli (septic or bland) that originate in the heart, lungs, or long bones (fat emboli). Arterial occlusions can also complicate metabolic disorders, such as homocystinuria and diabetes mellitus, and hematologic disorders such as sickle cell disease. In certain cases of acute hemiplegia, angiography will demonstrate multiple intracranial arterial occlusions that usually are of obscure etiology.

Venous occlusions are predisposed to by dehydration, cerebral thrombophlebitis from bacterial meningitis, head trauma, and hematologic disorders such as polycythemia. *Vascular malformations,* such as arteriovenous malformations and saccular aneurysms, may rupture into the brain parenchyma and cause acute paralysis; arteriovenous malformations may also cause motor deficits by siphoning blood away from vital regions of brain. *Extracerebral hemorrhages* in the extradural or subdural spaces are an additional cause of acute hemiplegia in childhood. Such hemorrhages are usually of traumatic origin, but also may complicate blood dyscrasias such as leukemia or hemophilia.

CLINICAL FINDINGS

Acute childhood hemiplegias usually occur in the first 5 years of life and are most frequent in children less than 3 years. The paralysis is typically of rapid onset, and the deficit almost always is maximal immediately or very early in the course of the illness. Characteristically, the arm and face are more severely affected than the leg. Consciousness is usually depressed. There may be an associated hemianopia, hemisensory deficit or dysphasia, the last particularly in older children. Two rather distinct clinical syndromes can be seen. In the more common, hemiplegia develops in a child less than 3 years as an immediate sequel to recurrent seizures (status epilepticus) triggered by an antecedent infection. Fever is often associated. Patients frequently show clinical and laboratory evidence of increased intracranial pressure, and vascular thromboses are characteristically absent. It is important to distinguish these hemiplegias from the transient ones that may persist for hours or days as a sequel to focal seizures in childhood (Todd's paralyses). The less common acute hemiplegic syndrome in childhood is more frequently seen after 3 years, and in such children the hemiplegia usually develops in the absence of seizures. In this second group, intracranial angiography will frequently demonstrate a vascular occlusion. This latter variety may be mimicked by an episode of hemiplegic migraine, a diagnosis that should be considered, particularly in children with a history of more than one hemiplegic attack.

LABORATORY STUDIES

A complete blood count and examination of a blood smear may disclose evidence of an underlying hematologic disorder. Urinalysis may show lipid globules in cases of fat embolism and a positive cyanide nitroprusside test in homocystinuria. The erythrocyte sedimentation rate is frequently elevated in patients with systemic infection or collagen disease. Skull films may demonstrate a fracture, as in acute epidural hematoma. An electroencephalogram may show diffuse slowing caused by increased intracranial pressure, or localized slowing owing to an intracranial mass lesion. A radioisotope (technetium) brain scan may demonstrate a tumor, abscess, vascular malformation, hematoma, infarction, contusion, or subdural fluid collection. Results of cerebrospinal fluid examination are frequently normal, but may disclose increased intracranial pressure, subarachnoid hemorrhage or meningoencephalitis. Echoencephalography may show a shift of midline intracranial structures, as with an acute subdural hematoma. Intracranial angiography can demonstrate vascular occlusions and mass lesions, and will provide an assessment of ventricular size. Computerized axial tomography (CT scan), a recently developed, noninvasive neuroradiologic technique, can be of enormous diagnostic assistance, for it can delineate a diverse array of intracranial disease processes.

TREATMENT

The effective treatment of acute hemiplegia includes general supportive measures, specific measures to correct any treatable underlying disorder, and management of complicating seizures and intracranial hypertension.

General Supportive Measures. An adequate airway should be maintained and, if necessary, ventilatory assistance provided. Secretions should be removed by suctioning. The stomach should be emptied by aspiration through a nasogastric tube and a urinary catheter should be placed. Vital signs, state of responsiveness, pupillary size and reactivity should be monitored carefully. Complicating shock should be treated. Fluid intake should be restricted to about 1000 ml./m.²/day. Temperature elevation should be treated with vigorous sponging and, if necessary, antipyretics. Controlled hypothermia, to 34° C. (93.2° F.), may provide some added benefit.

Specific Measures. If possible, the condition that gave rise to acute hemiplegia should be treated directly. Bacterial meningitis should be treated with antibiotics. Certain intracranial hematomas (parenchymal, epidural, subdural) require surgical evacuation, although many subdural fluid collections in infancy can be managed by repeated aspirations. Brain tumors or abscesses should be removed surgically. Lead encephalopathy should be treated with chelating agents. Anticoagulants should be used in cases of recurrent emboli caused by cardiac arrhythmias, and may be of benefit in certain cases of cerebral thrombophlebitis and venous thrombosis. Corticosteroids may be of value in the treatment of cerebral arteritis. In certain cases of extracranial carotid occlusion, the obstruction can be treated surgically, providing a restoration of circulation and benefit to the patient.

Management of Complicating Seizures. Seizures that accompany acute hemiplegia should be treated with parenteral anticonvulsants. If the child presents with status epilepticus, diazepam* (Valium) is a drug of choice. It should be given intravenously, undiluted, in a dose of 0.3 mg./kg., at a rate not exceeding 1 mg./minute. If necessary, the dosage can be repeated in 15 to 30 minutes, to a maximum of 2 to 4 mg. in the infant and 5 to 10 mg. in the older child. Alternatively, phenobarbital can be given intravenously in a dose of 6 to 10 mg./kg. If the seizures do not subside within 20 to 30 minutes, the same dosage of phenobarbital can be repeated. If phenobarbital and diazepam are given within minutes of one another, they may act synergistically and cause hypotension and/or respiratory depression. Paraldehyde is a useful therapeutic adjunct in the acute management of seizures. A dosage of 1.0 to 1.5 ml. per year of age to a maximum of 7 ml. can be given rectally (with an equal volume of mineral oil), by intravenous drip or by deep intramuscular injection. Once seizure control has been achieved, anticonvulsant therapy should be maintained. Either phenobarbital or phenytoin, in a dose of 5 to 8 mg./kg./day, are the most useful drugs for long-term management of seizures.

Management of Complicating Intracranial Hypertension. When acute hemiplegia is complicated by signs of increased intracranial pressure, the intracranial hypertension should be treated promptly. Passive hyperventilation, by which means the pco_2 should be lowered from 40 to 25 mm. Hg, is an effective means of treating elevated intracranial pressure, regardless of cause. Mannitol,* given intravenously in a dose of 1.5 to 3.0 gm./kg., will rapidly reduce intracranial hypertension, but its repeated administration causes a secondary rise in intracranial pressure ("rebound") and fluid and electrolyte imbalance. Also, it promotes or worsens intracranial bleeding, and thus is potentially hazardous in acute hemiplegia caused by head trauma or by hemorrhagic diathesis. Corticosteroids, such as dexamethasone, given intravenously in a dosage of 0.1 to 0.2 mg./kg., act more slowly than do the hyperosmolar agents such as mannitol, but can be used for prolonged periods (days to months) and do not cause secondary "rebound" or promote intracranial bleeding. Corticosteroids are particularly effective in the treatment of intracranial hypertension associated with brain tumor.

Intracranial hypertension associated with acute hemiplegia occasionally requires surgical treatment such as subdural aspirations, ventricular drainage and, on rare occasions, decompressive craniectomy.

---

*Manufacturer's precaution: The safety and efficacy of injectable diazepam have not been established in the neonate.

*Manufacturer's precaution: The use of mannitol in pediatric patients has not been studied comprehensively.

PROGNOSIS

The outlook in acute hemiplegia is related most directly to the underlying cause. The neurological morbidity in young children, in whom hemiplegia evolves in association with seizures, is usually much greater than in older children, in whom hemiplegia is unaccompanied by seizures. The most frequent sequelae are motor deficits, recurrent seizures, mental retardation, specific learning disabilities and behavioral abnormalities. A number of children die during the early stages of illness, either as a complication of status epilepticus or from the underlying disease process. Fortunately, many of the deficits in the survivors are relatively short-lived and others are benefited by a variety of long-term therapies.

Epilepsy

JOHN M. FREEMAN, M.D.

A seizure is an alteration in either motor function or behavior due to electrical disturbance within the central nervous system. Epilepsy is recurrent seizures. Since seizures are a symptom and not a disease, therapy should first be directed at discovering and correcting the primary cause, i.e., hypoglycemia, hypocalcemia, renal disease, infection, vascular disease, or tumor.

Only when the underlying cause is not discernible or not treatable are anticonvulsants utilized in the management of seizures. The choice of anticonvulsant is dictated to a large extent by seizure type; therefore, classification of the seizures is important.

Drugs, however, are only one part of the management of the patient with seizures. Psychological factors in the patient, in his or her family and in the environment, at school or work, may play a significant role in the seizures and in the patient's general well-being. Therapy and management of these psychosocial factors are as important as the control of the seizures themselves.

Diagnosis of a seizure disorder is based *solely* on the interpretation of the history of the paroxysmal event and the circumstances in which it occurred. The electroencephalogram does *not* establish the diagnosis nor does it rule out epilepsy. Seizures occurring within 48 hours of head trauma or in conjunction with intracranial infection may require acute man-

Supported in part by grant 03-11-000143-06 HEW, PHS, Philadelphia, Region III, for Pediatric Supervision of the Epilepsy Clinic, John F. Kennedy Institute.

agement, but do not necessarily require long-term therapy. Seizures associated with fever in young children are also a special case and are discussed below.

CLASSIFICATION

Proper interpretation of the events during a seizure is the key to diagnosing that this was an electrical event (a seizure) as well as to proper classification of seizure type. This classification has implications for the etiology of the seizures, the prognosis, and the choice of drug therapy.

Focal Seizures. Focal seizures are sensory or motor events which begin locally and usually suggest a focal brain abnormality, such as scars, focal infection, vascular abnormalities, or tumors. Since focal seizures in older children and adolescents may be caused by progressive processes, they deserve particular evaluation.

Psychomotor seizures, also called temporal lobe seizures, or partial seizures with complex symptomatology, are a special form of focal seizures and often respond to particular medications. Their pleomorphic manifestations include staring with automatism, abdominal discomfort, fear, or disorders of perception. These symptoms may progress to a generalized seizure.

Absence seizures (staring spells with automatism) are commonly confused with petit mal (Table 1) and are classified as one form of psychomotor seizure.

Generalized Seizures. Generalized seizures may start locally, but spread so rapidly to involve the whole cortex that no focal signs are apparent. They include:

GENERALIZED TONIC-CLONIC—GRAND MAL. These are the most frequently recognized, but from a diagnostic and therapeutic

TABLE 1. Differentiation of Petit Mal from Absence Seizures

PETIT MAL	ABSENCE (PSYCHOMOTOR)
No automatisms	Lip smacking, fumbling, automatisms
Brief, less than 15 seconds in duration	Often longer than 15 seconds in duration; postictal confusion may occur
Many seizures per day	Less than one or two seizures per day
Rare in children under 4 years and usually end at puberty	Any age
3 per second spike and wave	2½ to 4 per second spike and wave, often temporal lobe activity
Ethosuximide	Carbamazepine, primidone, phenytoin, etc.

standpoint they are no different from seizures which are just tonic or clonic.

PETIT MAL. This form is rare, often confused with the absence spell of psychomotor epilepsy (see Table 1), and has a benign prognosis. Despite common usage by physicians and laymen alike, everything which is not grand mal does not become petit mal. True petit mal and some absence spells respond dramatically to ethosuximide.

MINOR MOTOR. Akinetic, kinetic and myoclonic seizures are a special form of generalized seizure. They are often age-dependent, are associated with mental retardation and have a poor prognosis. They rarely respond to the usual anticonvulsants and therefore require special therapeutic approaches (see below). These seizures include those of the child who suddenly slumps or falls to the ground with only momentary loss of consciousness, as well as those with head nodding and sudden muscular jerks or massive spasms.

DRUG THERAPY

The drug therapy of epilepsy is an art, not a science. Risks of side reactions and effects of toxicity must be weighed against benefits in every case. The benefits to be derived depend on seizure type, frequency and time of occurrence. The goal of therapy—total seizure control—is attainable in 70 to 80 per cent of patients without undue side effects.

Initiation of Therapy. Drug therapy is begun *after* an adequate history has established that the patient has a seizure disorder and its type, and after an adequate neurological examination to establish a baseline and to rule out acquired or progressive neurological deficit. While an electroencephalogram and routing blood chemistries (calcium, PO$_4$, BUN, and *fasting* blood sugar) usually should be performed, therapy need not be delayed.

There is no unanimity of opinion about initiating therapy after a single seizure. This must be left to the judgment of the physician and the desires of the patient and the family, and will depend on the circumstances, character and duration of the seizure. Single seizures related to trauma or acute intercurrent illness may require either no anticonvulsant therapy or only short-term therapy.

The initial evaluation and initiation of therapy can be carried out by the primary physician. Referral to a child neurologist or specialist in epilepsy should be carried out if: (1) there are signs or symptoms suggesting a progressive neurological disease, such as acquired focal neurological deficit, increased intracranial pressure, or slow wave (delta) forms on the EEG; or (2) the patient continues to have seizures despite adequate trials of the primary medication (see below).

The guiding principle in therapy is not to give a fixed dosage, but to give enough of the drug to control seizures completely without toxicity. When toxicity occurs and seizures persist, the dosage should be reduced and another drug added.

The pediatrician should be thoroughly familiar with a few drugs used in the initial therapy of varying types of seizures. When he has given these an adequate trial, and the child is continuing to have seizure problems, he should consider getting consultative help. Drugs commonly utilized in the pediatric seizure clinic at Johns Hopkins are shown in Table 2.

Use and Abuse of Blood Levels. The major recent advance in the management of patients with epilepsy is the availability of techniques to measure blood levels of anticonvulsants and the consequent knowledge of their pharmacokinetics. The level of drug in the blood is roughly correlated with its anticonvulsant effect and with its toxicity. The amount of medication in the blood is determined by the amount of drug prescribed, the amount ingested, the amount absorbed and the rate of degradation and excretion. The commonest causes of continuing seizures are inadequate

TABLE 2.   **Drugs Commonly Used in Epilepsy**

FOCAL OR GENERALIZED SEIZURES	PETIT MAL OR ABSENCE	PSYCHOMOTOR	MINOR MOTOR, AKINETIC, MYOCLONIC, OR INFANTILE SPASMS
Phenobarbital	Ethosuximide	Carbamazepine	Clonazepam (Clonopin)
Methyl phenobarbital (Mebaral)		Primidone	Diazepam (Valium)
Phenytoin (Dilantin)		Phenobarbital	Ketogenic diet
Carbamazepine (Tegretol)		Phenytoin	ACTH
Primidone (Mysoline)			Diamox

dose prescribed, inadequate amounts ingested (noncompliance) and, on occasion, inadequate absorption. The determination of the level of medication in the blood is the *only* method of assuring adequacy of therapy in the patient who is continuing to have seizures. In addition, blood levels are the *only* method of ascertaining the agent causing toxicity in the patient who is on multiple medications.

Blood levels of anticonvulsants are readily available in hospital or commercial laboratories; however, a recently conducted study showed that many laboratories were unreliable. Unreliable results may be worse than no results at all. Be certain that the laboratory you are using is participating in an outside quality control study.

Anticonvulsant blood levels should be determined:

1. Ideally 2 to 3 weeks after starting a new drug in order to assure compliance, absorption, and lack of effect on blood levels of other anticonvulsants.

2. If the patient is continuing to have seizures; in order to assure compliance, absorption, and adequacy of levels. (In the absence of the availability of accurate levels, increasing the dose up to toxicity and discussing compliance may suffice).

3. In the presence of signs of toxicity, such as lethargy or ataxia, in order to establish which drug of multiple drugs is producing the toxicity. Since one drug may influence the metabolism of another, the physician cannot assume that the drug he increased is the one producing toxicity.

4. Once a year in the patient who is well controlled or taking drugs prophylactically (i.e., for febrile seizures) to assure compliance and adequacy of the dose.

INTERPRETATION OF ANTICONVULSANT BLOOD LEVELS. The "therapeutic" ranges of some commonly utilized anticonvulsants are shown in Table 3. This range indicates the *usual* serum levels which control seizures and do not produce toxicity. An individual patient's seizures may be controlled at "subtherapeutic" levels, or the patient may require levels above those listed. Toxicity is unusual within the therapeutic range, but a patient requiring higher than "therapeutic" blood levels to control seizures, who does not show signs of toxicity, may continue to have his dosage increased.

Just as there is no set dosage of anticonvulsant for an individual person, there is no set blood level which will either control that person's seizures or produce toxicity.

Concepts of Drug Half-Life and Loading.

For most anticonvulsant drugs, the rate of elimination of the drug determines the amount of time required for a constant dosage to reach a steady state in the serum. The rate of elimination is expressed as the time required for the drug to fall to one-half of its original value, the metabolic half-life (T-½). It should be noted that the T-½ of an individual drug varies with the age of the child, varies between individuals, and may be modified by other drugs.

It takes five half-lives for a drug to reach 97 per cent of its steady state value. Thus if a patient is given a daily dosage of a drug with a T-½ of 24 hours, it will take five days for that drug (or new dose) to reach steady state.

If a patient is given phenytoin (formerly called diphenylhydantoin) in the usual daily amounts (5 to 7 mg./kg.), therapeutic blood levels are likely to be achieved in 4 or 5 days. (For phenobarbital the time required is considerably longer).

To achieve therapeutic levels more rapidly, a loading dose must be given. This loading dose, however administered, is roughly three times the usual maintenance dose. Such a dose should produce approximately 85 per cent of the therapeutic blood level within the first 6 to 12 hours, depending on the route of administration.

Drug half-lives also enable us to know how frequently to administer the drug. For drugs such as phenobarbital or phenytoin, which in older children have long half-lives, there is *no* pharmacological reason for giving the drug more than once a day. There may be psychological reasons for splitting the dose into twice daily aliquots.

The half-lives, "therapeutic" blood level, usual daily dosage, and frequency of administration of commonly used drugs are shown in Table 3.

Selection of Drug. The seizure type determines the group of drugs to be used (see Table 2). The choice of drugs within each category is arbitrary and open, based not on demonstrated differences in effectiveness, but rather on cost and side effects.

Termination of Therapy. There is no data on how long therapy should be continued. One study (Holdwach) discontinued medication after the patient was free of seizures for four years, and found that 80 per cent of patients had no recurrence of seizures. Pending further studies we recommend that a patient who has had few, mild, easily controlled seizures, and a "mildly abnormal EEG" be continued on medication until seizure free *at least* 2 to 3 years. With a more severe seizure disorder, a very abnormal EEG, or definite evidence of cortical damage, therapy is continued until the patient is seizure free for at least four years. If the seizures have occurred only during one brief period of time, associated with a specific illness or trauma, long-term therapy may not be necessary.

When therapy is terminated, the drug should be gradually withdrawn over 3 to 4 months or longer. For the patient on multiple drugs, only one drug should be withdrawn at a time. There is little evidence to support the concept that puberty is a poor time to withdraw medications.

EEG in Epilepsy Therapy. There is *no* reason to repeat the initial EEG in a patient whose seizures are well controlled. The EEG *should* be repeated if seizures are breaking through medication, if they are changing in pattern, or if there is progressive deficit in intellectual or motor function. The EEG is a poor predictor of the likelihood of recurrence of seizures when anticonvulsants are discontinued.

Management of Toxicity. Any patient on anticonvulsant medication who shows evidence of progressive intellectual or physical deterioration should be assumed to be drug-intoxicated until proved otherwise. In such situations, blood levels should be obtained. A rare patient may manifest intellectual impairment with normal blood levels.

With intoxication, the drug may be completely discontinued for one or two days to foster a more rapid decrease in blood levels, and reinstituted at a lower dose when signs of toxicity have cleared.

MAJOR ANTIEPILEPTIC DRUGS

Therapy for Focal or Generalized Seizures

Phenobarbital. Phenobarbital is, in general, a safe, effective and cheap anticonvulsant. The usual starting dose is 4 to 6 mg./kg. Since phenobarbital has a long half-life, it need only be given once a day. The long half-life also means that therapeutic levels will not be achieved for 10 to 14 days. Loading the patient with triple doses the first day and double doses the second day will speed this process, but also result in marked sedation. Drowsiness is common during the first days of therapy, but subsides without alteration of the dose. Dosage is increased as necessary to achieve seizure control or until sedation becomes a problem. Hyperactivity is common, particularly in younger children or in those with evidence of "minimal cerebral dysfunction." If hyperactivity persists, the patient should be switched to another anticonvulsant. Methyl phenobarbital and primidone (Mysoline) are both metabolized to phenobarbital, but appear to be less likely to produce hyperactivity—even when the child was hyperactive on phenobarbital.

Phenobarbital appears to be equally well absorbed orally, intramuscularly or intravenously, and while time of absorption may differ, the patient may be switched from one route to the other with equivalent doses.

In the newborn, the half-life of phenobarbital is in excess of 100 hours. A single intravenous dose of 15 to 20 mg./kg. produces therapeutic blood levels without excess sedation. These levels are maintained for at least five days without additional medications. Higher doses may be given if blood levels are monitored and the child observed for excess sedation or respiratory depression. Drug reactions to phenobarbital are rare.

Phenytoin. Phenytoin is a relatively safe and effective medication for focal, generalized or psychomotor seizures. With a half-life of about 24 hours, it may usually be given once a day, but requires five to seven days to achieve steady state levels. The usual dose is 5 to 7 mg./kg. in children, 300 to 400 mg./day in adults, but as with all anticonvulsants requires individual titration. Comparable doses may be given orally or intravenously, but when administered by the latter route phenytoin should be given slowly (not more than 50 mg./min.) while monitoring the blood pressure and EKG. Arrhythmias and hypotension are common with too rapid injection. Loading requires three times the maintenance dose to achieve "therapeutic" levels and may be done intravenously or orally depending on the speed desired.

Special Cautions. The use of phenytoin by the intramuscular route is *not* advised since absorption is slow, irregular and unpredictable. There is suggestive evidence that oral phenytoin may be poorly absorbed by the intestinal tract of the newborn and young infant. Therefore if it is given orally in this age group, blood levels must be monitored.

The use of phenytoin suspension is to be avoided. It is rarely possible to maintain the same concentration of drug at the top and bottom of the bottle; therefore the child tends to be undermedicated at the start of the bottle and overmedicated at the bottom. In addition, it is difficult to give accurate dosage of liquid medication. Chewable Infatabs provide more reliable therapy.

When plasma levels of phenytoin are already in the therapeutic range, small increments in dose may cause large increases in plasma levels. Therefore, at higher dosages, increases should be made in small increments.

One further caution: phenytoin absorption for the gastrointestinal tract is particularly susceptible to particle size, formulation and the filler in the capsule. Since each individual patient will be titrated for control and blood levels, it makes little difference which brand of phenytoin is given, *as long as the same brand continues to be prescribed.* If this cannot be assured, brand name prescriptions should be used instead of generic prescriptions.

SIDE EFFECTS. *Hypertrichosis* is a common and irreversible side effect of phenytoin. Some feel that this is one reason to utilize other anticonvulsants first, particularly in young girls.

Gingival hyperplasia is a second common, distressing side effect of phenytoin. It appears to be idiosyncratic, but related to therapeutic levels in susceptible individuals. Meticulous dental hygiene with vigorous gum massage may decrease the extent of the hyperplasia. Gingivectomy may be necessary in severe cases.

Allergic reactions to phenytoin occur and may progress from rashes to the Stevens-Johnson syndrome, hepatitis and even death. The occurrence of a rash, usually within the first three weeks of institution of phenytoin, requires immediate inspection by the attending physician. While most rashes are unrelated to the drug, only the doctor's inspection can differentiate erythema multiforme from flea bites, viral rashes, and so forth. When in doubt, discontinue the drug. The drug rash should fade over a number of days. If such an individual needs phenytoin again, he may be rechallenged with a single dose of phenytoin to see if allergic symptoms recur. Lymphoid hyperplasia and pseudolymphoma syndrome have also been reported.

Hypocalcemia and *osteomalacia* have been reported in patients receiving phenytoin. Their significance is, in general, unclear. Osteomalacia is preventable with vitamin D. We do not routinely supplement all patients with vitamin D, but in institutionalized patients or those with inadequate diet or little exposure to sunlight, such supplementation should be considered.

DOSE-RELATED SIDE EFFECTS. Nystagmus occurs at a serum phenytoin level of 20 μg./ml., ataxia at serum levels above 30 μg./ml., and lethargy at levels above 40 μg./ml. The latter two side effects are indications for checking the blood level and decreasing the dose.

Primidone (Mysoline). Primidone is effective for preventing grand mal, focal and psychomotor seizures. Some feel that it is more effective than phenobarbital in psychomotor seizures, although evidence to support this is lacking. Primidone is metabolized to phenylethylmalonamide (PEMA) and phenobarbital,

both of which have anticonvulsant action. It is administered orally.

Since primidone has an initial tendency to produce sedation and personality changes, we usually begin with 50 to 100 mg. twice daily and increase every 3 to 4 days to the usual dose of 10 to 15 mg./kg. (750 to 1500 mg./day). Since primidone and PEMA have short half-lives, it has been traditional to give this drug in 2 or 3 divided doses. The pharmacology and pharmacokinetics of primidone are not well established and while levels of primidone, PEMA and phenobarbital can be measured, the first two are rarely useful. Phenobarbital levels give an index of compliance, but levels higher than 40 μg./ml. may be well tolerated. There would seem little reason to give both phenobarbital and primidone to the same patient.

SIDE EFFECTS. Primidone, like phenobarbital, may produce hyperactivity, but some children who had been hyperactive on phenobarbital may tolerate primidone. In other patients, negativism and personality changes may require discontinuing the drug or altering the dosage. Rash, megaloblastic anemia and a lupus-like syndrome have been reported rarely.

Carbamazepine (Tegretol). While only recently introduced as an anticonvulsant in this country, Tegretol has achieved widespread popularity in Europe for focal and generalized tonic-clonic seizures as well as psychomotor seizures. It may be the treatment of choice for the latter group. Its reported toxic side effects in adults have limited its use in this country, but appear to be far less common in children. The recommended dosage is 200 to 400 mg. given three or four times per day (10 to 20 mg./kg./day). Although the half-life is approximately 48 hours, its rapid absorption may produce nausea or diplopia if given in large single or twice daily dosages.

The therapeutic serum level is not well established, but appears to be 6 to 8 μg./ml. Large doses of the drug (800 to 1200 mg. or more per day) are required to achieve this range.

SIDE EFFECTS. Dose-related side effects include sedation, nystagmus, nausea and diplopia. In many cases these effects may be avoided by giving the drug in 3 or 4 divided doses.

IDIOSYNCRATIC REACTIONS. Granulocytopenia occurs in up to 10 per cent of adults, but is less common in children. In many the lowered white count returns to normal despite continuation of carbamazepine. However, if the white count drops below 2500, the drug should be discontinued. Agranulocytosis, aplastic anemia, hepatic dysfunction or allergic skin rashes may occur. The literature recommends that blood counts and liver function tests be performed monthly for the first year and every three months thereafter. At Hopkins, however, we have seen no such reactions and blood work is done less frequently. In general, carbamazepine would appear to be a safe and effective drug in children and should achieve growing popularity.

Therapy of Petit Mal and Absence Seizures

All little spells have been called "petit mal." We feel that the distinction between petit mal and absence spells has both therapeutic and prognostic importance. That distinction, shown in Table 1, is not universally accepted and accounts for the varied approach to patients with these seizure types.

We feel that pure petit mal is a rare seizure type and is benign. We find that it readily responds to ethosuximide alone and is not associated with grand mal spells. When the spells occur only a few times per day, when they last longer than 15 seconds, or are associated with lip smacking, automatism, or an EEG which is other than classical 3 per second spike and wave, we believe that the spells derive from the temporal lobe with "secondary bilateral synchrony." We usually initiate therapy with phenobarbital, phenytoin, primidone, or carbamazepine, and only add ethosuximide if the staring spells persist.

Livingston does not draw this distinction between petit mal and absence seizures, and because of the association of absence with grand mal spells, he initiates therapy with barbiturates and subsequently adds ethosuximide. Penry and Dreifus start therapy with just ethosuximide unless the absence spells have a period of postictal confusion or last longer than 45 seconds.

Ethosuximide (Zarontin). Ethosuximide is effective in petit mal or absence spells, but seems to have no effect on cortical seizures. It is rapidly absorbed from the gastrointestinal tract and has a half-life of 30 to 60 hours. The usual dose is 10 to 15 mg./kg. per day, and 750 to 1250 mg. per day is usually required to achieve therapeutic blood levels of 40 to 80 μg./ml. We usually give the drug in 2 or 3 divided doses. Ethosuximide may be given as the 250 mg. capsule or as a suspension (250 mg./5 ml.), which should be well shaken before use. As with all liquid medication, calibrated syringes or measuring devices should be utilized.

SIDE EFFECTS. Ethusoximide may cause gastric irritation which can be avoided if the drug is administered with or after meals. Dose-related side effects include tiredness, headache, and unsteadiness. Idiosyncratic side effects include skin rashes and exfoliative dermatitis, rare agranulocytosis or leukopenia, and lupus-like syndrome. These side effects are uncommon.

Clonazepam (Clonopin). Clonazepam is discussed below. One double blind controlled study suggests that this drug is more effective than ethosuximide in the control of absence seizures. However, about one-third of children in the study could not tolerate clonazepam because of drowsiness or other side effects. We have not utilized it for absence seizures.

Trimethadione (Tridione). Trimethadione is also an effective agent for petit mal, but because of its frequent and serious side effects, it should be employed only when ethosuximide has failed, and then with great caution.

A number of other drugs (Atabrine, Diamox, amphetamines and Tofranil) have been used in the treatment of "refractory petit mal." However, utilizing the distinction between petit mal and absence seizures and the approach indicated above, we have not found it necessary to use any of them.

Therapy of Minor Motor Seizures

Minor motor seizures include head nods and head drops, akinetic, kinetic and myoclonic spells. They are often associated with slow spike and wave discharges or a "Lennox-Gastaut" pattern on the EEG. They are the most difficult types of seizures to control and are often associated with retardation. Indeed, in some previously normal children, the onset of these seizure types is associated with progressive loss of motor and intellectual function. Despite (and because of) the poor prognosis, this form of seizure should be treated particularly vigorously.

Minor motor seizures rarely respond to the usual anticonvulsant drugs discussed above. Therefore when they occur in the absence of generalized or focal seizures, it is our practice to initiate treatment with the therapies indicated in Table 3.

Benzodiazepines. The benzodiazepine group of anticonvulsants has only recently been introduced. Diazepam has achieved wide use as a tranquilizer and for the management of status epilepticus. Clonazepam is the newest and perhaps the most useful of the group in minor motor seizures and absence spells (see above).

Pharmacokinetic data are incomplete for clonazepam, and biotransformations to other

TABLE 3.   Half-Life, Usual "Therapeutic" Range, Usual Dosage and Frequency of Administration

DRUG	HALF-LIFE (hr.)	THERAPEUTIC RANGE (μg./ml.)	USUAL DOSAGE* (mg./kg./day)	FREQUENCY OF ADMINISTRATION (times/day)
Phenobarbital				
Newborn	ca 100		see text	see text
Child	37 to 73	10 to 20	4 to 6	1 to 2
Adult	96		2 to 3	1 to 2
Phenytoin				
Newborn and infant	ca 100	10 to 20	see text	see text
Child	24		5 to 7	1 to 2
Adult			3 to 5	1 to 2
Carbamazepine	16 to 40	5 to 15	10 to 20	1 to 2
Primidone	5 to 7 Primidone 30 PEMA	9	10 to 15	2 to 3
Ethosuximide	30 to 60	40 to 80	15 to 25	2 to 3

*See text under individual drugs.

potentially active compounds make clinical correlations difficult. While it is said that the therapeutic range is 15 to 30 ng./ml., serum determinations are difficult and not readily available. The half-life of the drug and many of its metabolites appears to be 20 to 40 hours, but pharmacologic effectiveness seems much shorter, so that drug is usually utilized 3 or 4 times per day.

Drug interactions with other anticonvulsants occur. Clonazepam may depress or elevate serum phenytoin levels, and phenobarbital may decrease diazepam levels. Therefore, blood levels of the standard anticonvulsants should be remeasured 2 to 3 weeks after the addition of diazepam or clonazepam to a stable therapeutic regimen, and if toxicity occurs after such an addition.

DIAZEPAM (VALIUM).   While diazepam has achieved widespread use as an intravenous drug for status epilepticus, the tendency for patients to break through with further seizure after weeks to months of administration has limited its usefulness as an oral chronic anticonvulsant. Nevertheless, an occasional patient may have marked benefit in seizure control. The dose of the drug is limited only by the sedation produced, and even large doses (20 to 30 mg./day) may be tolerated by small children if the drug is increased in small amounts every 3 or 4 days.

CLONAZEPAM (CLONOPIN).   Clonazepam was released for general use in the United States in 1975, therefore its limitations and effectiveness are not widely known. It produces few serious side effects other than hypotonia or the dose-related sedation. The sedative side effect is reduced by increasing the drug in small increments 0.5 to 1 mg. every 3 or 4 days until seizures are controlled or sedation becomes a constant problem. The initial sedation with each increment usually wears off

in 1 or 2 days. Behavioral disorders and aggressive personality changes are not uncommon and may require discontinuation of the drug.

Hypersalivation and bronchial hypersecretion may cause problems in young children. Seizure control may be established with exceedingly small doses (1 to 3 mg./day) but breakthrough is common. Control may be reestablished with increased dosage, but may require 20 to 30 mg./day. However, in these refractory forms of epilepsy, perseverance is indicated.

THE KETOGENIC DIET

The ketogenic diet represents a time-honored and effective therapy for refractory seizures, particularly the minor motor seizures, which are least likely to respond to medication. The diet has several advantages over medication in this group of patients. When effective, it completely controls seizures and allows discontinuation of most or all medications. In the child with progressive intellectual deterioration and a Lennox-Gastaut pattern on EEG, the ketogenic diet may be the only way of sorting out whether deterioration is due to drugs, electrical status, or underlying cerebral deterioration.

The major disadvantage of the diet is in the eye of the prescriber. A diet of high fat, low protein and low carbohydrate would seem to be aesthetically unpleasing and difficult for families. However, a good dietitian, who can accurately calculate menus to the prescribed ratios, is the key to the diet, and can readily help the family to prepare the diet. Rigidity on the part of the physician in demanding prolonged fasting to initiate the diet is also important. When the diet is helpful, it is a rare family or child who does not tolerate it. When it is ineffective, it becomes a major burden and should be discontinued.

The medium chain triglyceride (MCT) diet, while ideally allowing a greater variety of foods, has been less successful in our hands. Several children with Lennox-Gastaut syndrome whose seizures did not respond to the MCT diet responded well to the ketogenic diet.

Since we do not know the mechanism of the anticonvulsive effect of either diet, we cannot necessarily assume that they are identical.

STATUS EPILEPTICUS

Status epilepticus is a medical emergency. Continued prolonged seizures may cause damage to the brain and even death. There are myriad definitions of status epilepticus, and myriad forms, depending on whether the seizure is focal, hemi, or has no motor component. We are particularly concerned with the individual with generalized tonic-clonic activity.

A generalized tonic-clonic seizure of more than 30 minutes may begin to damage the brain. The damage is due to local brain edema, acidosis, alterations in local circulation as well as hypoglycemia. With longer seizures, the local changes may lead to lowered seizure threshold, and the seizures may become increasingly difficult to control.

Therefore, whenever a generalized tonic-clonic seizure lasts more than 20 minutes, it should be treated as a medical emergency with oxygen, glucose and intravenous medication. The same may also be true for a hemiconvulsion (involving only one side of the body).

It is not the choice of drug, but rather the timing, route of administration and vigor of therapy which are the major determinants of the duration of status epilepticus, and its subsequent morbidity. Vigorous intravenous therapy within the first half-hour of a generalized seizure may prevent status. Early therapy is far more effective than later therapy.

The therapy and dosage for status are shown in Table 4. While each drug has its proponents, there is at present no demonstrable superiority of one drug over another.

Three major errors are made in the management of status: (1) Drugs are given intramuscularly or rectally rather than intravenously. The intravenous route is the only route which provides rapid and reliable absorption in this emergency. (2) Not enough drug is given. Status is an emergency because the continuous electrical activity compromises brain function as well as respiration and circulation. Physicians are afraid of giving "too much" drug and causing respiratory depression and arrest. Status should only be treated intravenously where a respiratory arrest can be managed with an artifical respirator. It is better to have a patient with respiratory arrest due to overdosage of medication than to continue to have impaired cardiorespiratory function with continued seizures. The former can be managed medically, the latter cannot. (3) Once seizures have been stopped, the patient should be loaded with an anticonvulsant which will provide continued seizure control. Too often a patient is treated in the emergency room, then sent to the ward, only to awaken in status again. This is particularly true with the use of intravenous diazepam, which has an effective duration of 15 to 20 minutes. It is better to have a patient oversedated for 2 or 3 days after an episode of status than for him to have a second episode of status.

I prefer to begin with phenobarbital, 20 mg./kg., giving half as an immediate dose. If the seizures continue, I administer in the following order, until the seizures are controlled: (1) the third quarter in 5 to 10 minutes; (2) the last quarter after another 5 to 10 minutes; (3) phenytoin, 20 mg./kg. at a rate not to exceed 1 mg./kg. min., monitoring EKG and blood pressure; and (4) (this is rarely necessary) paraldehyde as a 4 per cent solution in 10 per cent glucose as rapidly as necessary to control the seizures. Paraldehyde should be used with caution in individuals with pulmonary problems.

We have had virtually no patients whose

TABLE 4.   Intravenous Drug Therapy of Major Motor Status Epilepticus

DRUG	DOSE	COMMENTS AND CAUTIONS
Diazepam	1 mg./kg., max. 10 mg.	Repeat every 10 min. three times. May cause respiratory depression or arrest. Do not dilute. Short acting.
Phenobarbital	15 to 25 mg./kg.	Give ½ stat, then ¼ every 5 minutes if seizures persist. May cause respiratory depression or arrest.
Phenytoin	15 to 20 mg./kg.	Give slowly, not more than 1 mg./kg./min. Monitor EKG and blood pressure.
Paraldehyde	Enough (up to 1 gm. for single dose)	May give undiluted in glass syringe or as a one or two per cent solution.

status could not be controlled on this regimen whose seizures could ultimately be controlled at all.

For prolonged status (greater than one hour), the use of drugs such as dexamethasone, mannitol, or furosemide should be considered.

Oxygen and a continuous intravenous administration of 10 per cent glucose are utilized from the start of therapy. Close attention is paid to the amount of fluid given, so as not to foster cerebral edema. In addition, patients are observed for signs of infection or hyperthermia which may exacerbate the cerebral damage. While the status epilepticus is being managed, an adequate history and physical examination are carried out to elucidate the cause.

In young children without a previous history of epilepsy who present with status, the ingestion of drugs, particularly cholinergic agents, should be suspected and, where possible, serum and urine are screened. These children may require specific treatment with atropine rather than the anticonvulsants listed.

PSYCHOSOCIAL MANAGEMENT OF EPILEPSY

Drug therapy is only one part of the management of epilepsy. While it has taken a disproportionate share of this section, the psychosocial management is equally important.

Seizures are frightening experiences both to those who have them and to those who witness them. For the former, the loss of control and the uncertainity of when a seizure will recur represent a significant burden. For the observer, fright and inability to help make seizures an unpleasant and frustrating experience.

Superimposed on these feelings are the still present myths and prejudices about epilepsy and the epileptic. These represent a significant handicap to the individual with epilepsy as he or she goes about the activities of daily living.

Parents tend to be overprotective: What if the child had a seizure on the playground? While crossing the street? While riding a bike? This overprotection is natural, but for many children with seizures, it creates dependency and immaturity which ultimately become the major handicaps at the time of adolescence.

Frank and open discussion of the issues with parents is as important as the medication. Discussion with the child of his fears and concerns about what seizures are may alleviate or prevent some of the psychological disability. Parent groups and teenage groups have been exceedingly useful in our experience. Nothing is sadder than to see a young adult whose seizures are under control, but who is unable to obtain or hold a job because of avoidable psychological problems.

Febrile Seizures

KARIN B. NELSON, M.D.

At the onset of a feverish illness that is not of itself likely to injure the brain, an otherwise normal young child may have a seizure. This tendency to seizures with fever is common, is most often expressed between the ages of six months and three years, and appears to cluster in families. Previously abnormal children may also have seizures with fever; the prognosis in such children is related to the nature and degree of their preexisting abnormality.

Most workers exclude from the definition of febrile seizures those seizures with fever which are associated with recognizable acute neurological illnesses, such as meningitis or lead encephalopathy. In the following discussion, it is assumed that such conditions have been excluded or will be ruled out during the course of treatment.

Management of the Acute Attack. Tight clothing should be loosened, especially about the neck, and the child protected against physical injury. A clear airway must be established and maintained, and suctioning may be required. If the convulsion has ended, the child should be placed in a semiprone position to minimize the risk of aspiration. Fever should be reduced by uncovering, sponging with tepid water, and aspirin by mouth or suppository.

If the convulsion is in progress and has lasted less than 10 minutes, it is likely to stop spontaneously. Intramuscular phenobarbital, 4 mg./kg., may be administered, its chief purpose being to reduce the chance of recurrence in the next hours.

If a continuing convulsion of longer duration is in progress, it should be terminated as rapidly as consistent with safety, and the agent used should be the one with which the clinician is most experienced. Diazepam (Valium) may be administered, 0.3 mg./kg., slowly intravenously* or by intramuscular injection. If necessary this dose may be repeated in 10 minutes. Careful attention should be given to cardiac and respiratory rate and blood pressure, especially if barbiturates have previously been administered.

---

*Manufacturer's precaution: The safety and efficacy of injectable diazepam have not been established in the neonate.

Alternatively, paraldehyde may be given rectally (1 ml. per one year of age, not to exceed 5 ml. regardless of age). If not already in a hospital, the child with a lengthy seizure should be transferred to such a facility. Where respiratory support is available, a lengthy seizure can be treated with intravenous phenobarbital or with paraldehyde by intravenous drip (10 mg. in 100 ml. of solution, slowly over 10 to 20 minutes). In rare instances, short-acting barbiturates or volatile anesthetics may be required and are best administered by an anesthesiologist.

Once the seizure has been controlled, a diagnosis of the illness associated with the fever should be sought, and treatment instituted if possible. The clinician must be alert for any indication, from history or physical or laboratory findings, of an underlying illness requiring prompt and specific action. Even for a child with a family or personal history of past febrile seizures, confident determination that the current attack is a febrile seizure requires exclusion of graver possibilities. It is of primary importance to rule out meningitis; therefore, lumbar puncture should be performed in all infants under the age of six or eight months who have a seizure, in those of any age whose history or physical signs are suggestive of meningitis, and in any child who cannot be carefully observed by a reliable adult for some hours after an acute attack and returned rapidly for medical care if clinical change should warrant.

If signs suggestive of increased intracranial pressure are observed there should be caution in the performance of lumbar puncture, and consultation with a neurologist or neurosurgeon if possible. The child should, in the absence of heavy sedation, return to a normal state of consciousness and neurological functioning within half an hour or so after the acute attack; failure to do so should lead to reconsideration of the diagnosis and immediate further clinical evaluation.

Prevention of Recurrences. Approximately one-third of children who have one febrile seizure experience a recurrence, and about half of those who have a second later experience at least one further recurrence. There is no general agreement as to the need for, or efficacy of, medical efforts to prevent recurrences. Administration of phenobarbital at the time of febrile illnesses is not an effective means of seizure prevention, both because the seizure may be the first sign of illness and because of the length of time required to establish stable therapeutic levels of barbiturate in the blood.

Committing a child to long-term treatment with anticonvulsant medication is justified only if the risk of preventable sequelae is judged to be clearly greater than the risk of treatment. Because the data available for estimation of these risks are still incomplete, no dogmatic statement is warranted, and the following suggestions are subject to alteration as further information becomes available.

Chronic prophylaxis is recommended only in the presence of two or more of the following characteristics:

1. The initial febrile seizure was focal, or lasted longer than 15 minutes, or more than one seizure occurred on the day of onset.

2. The neurological or developmental status of the child was abnormal prior to the occurrence of the first febrile seizure.

3. There is a history of nonfebrile seizures in a parent or sibling.

4. The first febrile seizure occurred before the child's first birthday.

5. Two febrile seizures or more have occurred in separate episodes.

6. The parents express such anxiety about the possibility of recurrence that the physician judges there may be a harmful effect upon the relationship between parent and child if prophylaxis is not provided.

If treatment is undertaken, it is suggested that phenobarbital, 4 mg./kg., or a dose sufficient to provide a serum barbiturate level of 15 to 20 μg./ml., be given in a single dose shortly before bedtime. Initiation of therapy with half the anticipated dose, with an increase over a two week period, may minimize side effects. Parents must be strongly urged to administer medication regularly, as abrupt interruption of anticonvulsant medication can precipitate withdrawal seizures. Serum drug level determinations at intervals of four months or so will allow adjustment of dosage for growth and provide a check on compliance.

If a rash appears, medication should be withdrawn. If changes in behavior, sleep pattern or activity level are troublesome at doses required to maintain a therapeutic blood level of barbiturate, a trial of lowering the dose with gradual resumption, or substitution of mephobarbital may be made. If intolerance is still apparent, it is probably wise in most instances to reduce and then eliminate medication, advising the use of antipyretics and sponging at the onset of feverish illness. Only if the first seizure lasted longer than 20 minutes would efforts to continue barbiturate medication in the presence of changes in behavior appear warranted; in such instances, the addition of small doses of dextroamphetamine may sometimes be helpful in the control of side effects.

Approximately 90 per cent of recurrent febrile seizures take place within two years of the first attack, and of the small proportion who have a subsequent nonfebrile seizure, a majority begin within two years after the first febrile seizure. Prophylactic treatment, if elected, might therefore reasonably be continued for two years, at the end of which medication should be withdrawn gradually, over a period of two months. If any nonfebrile seizure occurs, prolonged treatment with anticonvulsant medication is indicated.

General Considerations. Certain therapeutic measures may contribute to a lowering of seizure threshold in susceptible individuals. Overhydration is such a factor. Large doses of penicillin administered parenterally are epileptogenic. Diphenhydramine (Benadryl) may activate subclinical seizures as monitored by electroencephalography, and has been shown to potentiate induced seizures with fever in immature mice; many decongestant medications are potential central excitants. Whether these medications contribute to the likelihood of seizures with fever in young children has not been established, but some caution would appear warranted.

The child who has had one febrile seizure has one chance in three of having another febrile seizure, and one chance in thirty to forty of having a later nonfebrile seizure. Although subsequent seizures are usually brief and self-limited, an occasional attack is not. Therefore, whatever course is elected with regard to chronic prophylaxis, it is important to discuss with the parents of each child who has had a febrile seizure what they would do if a seizure occurred which did not stop within 10 minutes or so. The distance of the home from the nearest medical facility, and availability of transportation and of possible caretakers for other young children of the family should be thought out and telephone numbers of emergency vehicles posted. Such contingency plans will help to ensure that if a subsequent seizure should occur, it need not continue long uncontrolled.

A final consideration is the need for, and appropriateness of, reassurance. During the seizure or the postictal period, parents unfamiliar with febrile seizures sometimes think that their child is dying. Once the youngster has roused, they may worry about sequelae. It is possible to provide realistic reassurance in most cases, because most children who were normal before a febrile seizure, and who experience only occasional and brief attacks, are not known to suffer any lasting damage from febrile seizures.

Infantile Spasms

EDWARD F. RABE, M.D.

This syndrome includes an electroencephalographic (EEG) abnormality (hypsarrhythmia) and an unusual type of seizure. The EEG abnormality consists of three parts: (1) multiple, independent, usually asynchronous, high voltage spikes occurring at some time in every lead; (2) recurrent, often asynchronous, high voltage slow waves (1.5 to 3 Hz., 250 to 300 microvolts); and (3) irregularly occurring periodic decreases in voltage to near isoelectric levels, a state which lasts several seconds. The EEG abnormality is most fully developed in sleep. As a result, sleep tracings must be obtained for diagnosis or for comparison of serial tracings when evidence for change is being sought.

The characteristic seizures are massive myoclonic jerks which often occur with lightning speed. They involve the trunk and extremities simultaneously. They may be flexor, extensor or mixed (flexor and extensor), and can occur singly or in "trains" of variable duration. They appear most often in the "twilight state" between waking and sleeping and are often felt by the parent holding the infant while feeding. Other types of seizures occur concomitantly in one-third of these patients and are most frequently generalized tonic and clonic seizures.

The syndrome responds most consistently to ACTH, perhaps less consistently to corticosteroids, unpredictably to benzodiazepines and not at all to the usual anticonvulsants such as phenobarbital or phenytoin or to the ketogenic diet.

When a diagnosis is established, aqueous ACTH is given intramuscularly in a dose of 20 units every 12 hours. Because up to 55 per cent of affected infants have or develop other seizure types concurrently, phenobarbital is given in two or three divided daily doses in an amount which maintains a serum level between 20 to 30 μg./ml. (6 mg./kg./day is often adequate to do this but the serum levels should be monitored). The aims of therapy are (1) to obliterate the peculiar irritability consistent with the early stages of the syndrome; (2) to stop the massive myoclonic jerks; (3) to hasten the return of the EEG to normal; and (4) to obtain a normal rate of global development.

Disappearance of the initial irritability occurs within 48 hours of onset of treatment. Decrease in the daily number of seizures may be noted within 1 to 10 days after starting treatment, and seizures (massive myoclonic jerks) stop within days up to six months of therapy in 81 per cent of patients. Seizure control can occur in 86 per cent but relapses of massive myoclonic jerks may be seen in as few as 8 per cent or as many as 53 per cent of therapeutic responders. EEG change toward normal can be seen by the end of the first week, whereas maximal improvement usually occurs after 3 to 17 weeks of treatment. Up to 13 per cent may show complete resolution of any EEG abnormality, 43 per cent may show improvement and 44 per cent may show little or no change with treatment.

As soon as seizures decrease, the EEG changes toward normal and the irritability disappears. When these changes begin, intramuscular aqueous ACTH is changed to gel form and is given every two days intramuscularly in a dose of 80 units. The infant is now observed at 2 to 4 week intervals.

When serial changes in EEG's, frequency of seizures, and rate of change in the developmental performance reach a plateau which persists for three months, the ACTH dose is gradually decreased by 20 units per dose at two month intervals. The change at 20 units every two days is to 10 units every two days, three times per week for one month, then five units every two days three times a week for one month, and then to discontinuation of the ACTH. During this time, phenobarbital is continued. If another seizure type intervenes and is not controlled by adjusting the serum phenobarbital level, an appropriate anticonvulsant is added or substituted for phenobarbital.

If, during the period of decremental ACTH dosage, clinical exacerbation occurs in any form—that is, if massive myoclonic jerks recur or increase in number, or the EEG pattern of modified hypsarrhythmia regresses, or the rate of developmental change clearly slows—the ACTH dose is immediately increased to 80 units of gel intramuscularly every other day. The dosage is continued at this level until repeated evaluations substantiate the return of a three-month plateau in all three parameters. Again, the ACTH dose is systematically lowered.

Expectations for therapeutic results are modified by several factors. The syndrome appears to be the response of the brain of an infant to many known and to some unknown insults. Thus the cases are divided into two large groups: symptomatic and idiopathic. Patients who can be classified as idiopathic, who show little or no evidence of developmental lag or focal neurologic deficit at the time of diagnosis, and who are treated immediately with ACTH as described, have a 50 per cent chance of surviving with a normal developmental quotient (DQ). Although treatment within one month or less of the onset of symptoms is thought to favor a good therapeutic result, this impression lacks statistical proof. Nonetheless, early treatment should be a therapeutic goal until this is proved to be unnecessary.

Infants with the syndrome who are classified as symptomatic, who are moderately to severely retarded developmentally when diagnosed and who are treated with ACTH can be expected to have an obliteration of massive myoclonic jerks within three to six months in 81 per cent of cases, to have a rapid change in EEG toward normal in 56 per cent of cases and to evidence disappearance of the initial irritability in all. However, one-half of symptomatic patients with low initial developmental quotients who are treated have a lower DQ on follow-up one or more years later than initially and the remainder have the same or insignificantly higher DQ's.

From 14 to 32 per cent of patients will not respond to ACTH as defined by significant reduction in massive myoclonic jerks. When they do respond, 71 per cent have done so within three months of the onset of treatment and 81 per cent within six months. It is therefore recommended that every infant who meets the diagnostic criteria should be treated with ACTH for a minimum period of three months.

Unwanted side effects of ACTH treatment with this regimen are seen unpredictably and not in all patients. The most frequent symptoms and signs include cushingoid obesity, seborrheic dermatitis, hirsutism, and skin pigmentation. None of these has necessitated stopping therapy and all of the signs and symptoms have disappeared when treatment stopped. Side effects reported by others include electrolyte imbalance, congestive heart failure, and increased susceptibility to infection.

Any neonatal infant suspected of having massive myoclonic jerks should have an EEG, especially during sleep. ACTH therapy should follow the discovery of hypsarrhythmia. Although therapy does not favorably affect the developmental lag in infants severely retarded at the onset of treatment, and although therapy has not increased the number of normal survivors in idiopathic cases with normal DQ's when patients are alternately treated or not treated, since no such series has been reported, the therapeutic regimen described does cause cessation of seizures and a lower number of clinical relapses than any other reported series.

There are variations of this syndrome which should be mentioned. Hypsarrhythmia occurs without infantile spasms and when it does, the prognosis for survival and for normal development is worse than when the two occur simultaneously. Until evidence accrues to the contrary, hypsarrhythmia without infantile spasms, or with other seizure types only, should be treated with ACTH for a minimum of three months. Infantile spasms without hypsarrhythmia also occur. If two successive EEG's in such a patient are normal, if there are no neurologic abnormalities clinically and if the DQ is normal, the prognosis is excellent without treatment.

Spasmus Nutans

LEONARD APT, M.D.

Spasmus nutans is an uncommon disorder characterized by head nodding, nystagmus, and an abnormal head tilt. The disorder is self-limited. Manifestations usually appear between 4 and 12 months of age, and generally subside spontaneously in 4 to 36 months.

Poor illumination, malnutrition, viral infection, and genetic factors have been implicated in the etiology of spasmus nutans, but the actual cause is unknown.

Various methods of treatment, including vitamins, diet, sunlight, and so forth, have not altered the course of the disease. No treatment is necessary.

On occasion, manifestations suggestive of spasmus nutans may be seen in patients who primarily have an ophthalmologic disorder or a neurologic disease (e.g., brain tumor, brain stem dysfunction). A complete eye examination or, if other neurologic signs or symptoms are present, a neurologic evaluation is recommended.

Headache

LAWRENCE A. LOCKMAN, M.D.

ACUTE HEADACHES

Trauma. Severe headache may result from head trauma even in the absence of skull fracture or superficial hematoma. Appropriate attention to the potential serious intracranial complications of trauma diverts concern from the pain which is more often present.

Analgesics such as morphine, meperidine, codeine, and other agents which depress the level of consciousness or elevate intracranial pressure are contraindicated. Aspirin is also to be avoided because of possible adverse effects on clotting. Acetaminophen used in doses appropriate for the patient's age and size does offer some measure of relief. Local application of cold packs over the area of maximal tenderness, with some pressure if a hematoma is developing, may reduce pain. Many children over the age of two whose consciousness is preserved will participate in the management of an effective cold pack.

Post Lumbar Puncture Headache. The headache following lumbar puncture is thought to be due to a shift in intracranial structures with traction on pain-sensitive dura and blood vessels. While not as common in children as in adults, these headaches sometimes occur and may persist if there is continuing leak of spinal fluid through the dural tear. Vomiting may be prominent. Immediate relief is almost always obtained by placing the patient in the recumbent position without a pillow. Analgesics are not usually effective in the absence of postural adjustment. These headaches usually clear within 24 hours but occasionally last for several days. Since resolution of the headache is dependent upon sealing the meningeal leak and reconstitution of the normal volume of cerebrospinal fluid, adequate fluid intake must be maintained. If vomiting is a problem intravenous fluids may be necessary. The child remains recumbent, except to use the bathroom, for 24 hour blocks of time. Then upright posture is attempted. If headache recurs, lying down is then advised for another 24 hours. This very conservative therapy has been sufficient to alleviate severe postspinal tap and postpneumoencephalogram headaches within three to four days in almost all instances. Surgical repair of the dural leak or blood patching, advocated in the literature, has never been required in the author's experience.

Inflammation. Headache is one of the cardinal signs of inflammatory disease of the meninges, due not only to increased intracranial pressure but also to direct inflammatory involvement of pain-sensitive structures within the cranial cavity and spinal canal. Although complete relief of this headache is not usually possible during the acute course of the disease, therapeutic removal of spinal fluid during lumbar puncture may help. Use of a mild nonsedative analgesic (acetaminophen) should be routinely employed; its influence, if any, on the course of fever over the first few days of therapy does not alter the mode or duration of antibiotic therapy.

RECURRENT HEADACHES

Recurrent headaches are a common human affliction; unfortunately, children do not escape. Headache is always a symptom; therapy therefore begins with a conspicuous, rational diagnostic approach to the underlying process. Fascination with medical topics nurtured by television, radio, and the printed word has made parents and older children aware of many serious diseases which may present as headache. Although the overwhelming majority of recurrent headaches in childhood are due to non-life-threatening causes, therapy will rarely succeed if the patient is not given reasonable assurance that a careful medical history and physical examination have excluded such commonly promoted causes of headache as sinusitis, brain tumor, aneurysm, meningitis, encephalitis, and "simple nervous tension."

Concern with these serious causes of headache is implicit when the patient seeks medical help and may impel consultation more than the desire to achieve relief from a disabling symptom. Much of the anxiety surrounding the headache may be alleviated at the time of the physical examination by specific mention of those signs which exclude, for practical purposes, such diseases as acute sinusitis, hypertension, increased intracranial pressure from brain tumor, arteriovenous malformation, otitis, brain abscess, tooth abscess, and "pinched nerves." Occasionally parents will have concern for a specific unusual etiology. Directed inquiry may allow specific reassurance.

Muscle Contraction or Tension Headaches. Muscle contraction or tension headaches are the most common recurrent headaches at any age. These headaches are a psychophysiologic response to emotional stress. Although usually radiating from the neck to the frontal region bilaterally, sometimes they are frontally predominant, vise-like, or pressure-like. Generally they do not begin suddenly, but build over several minutes to an hour; they may throb. Occasionally the pain is severe enough for the child to seek a dark, quiet place for repose; vomiting may occur. Treatment should be directed toward removing the underlying cause as well as removal of the symptom itself. The psychological cause is rarely immediately obvious ("I always get headaches during math"), but often is more subtle and complex. Depression, a mechanism for muscle contraction headache, is common in

children, often has a strong family history, and may be exacerbated by environmental demands. The cardinal symptoms of depression in childhood—significant mood change, failure to seek or maintain friends, decreasing school performance, appetite loss, enervation, sleep disturbance, and a family history of affective disorder—should lead one to consider this as the most likely diagnosis.

Therapy begins with parental education and informal counseling. A trial of amitriptyline, 30 to 75 mg./day in divided doses, may be used in children over 12 years of age for symptomatic relief of the depression. (Amitriptyline is not recommended for children under 12.) Generally several weeks are needed for response and a definite trial period of three to six months is arbitrarily picked at the outset of therapy. There is some risk in families with a history of chemical dependency. In children between 6 and 12 years of age, imipramine hydrochloride, 10 mg. three times a day, increasing to 25 mg. three times a day, may be used.* Simple analgesics such as aspirin or acetaminophen in adequate age-related and size-related doses may offer additional help during the headaches. Local measures such as warm packs to the cervical musculature and warm or cool packs to the forehead can be tried.

Headaches as a Form of Epilepsy. The differentiation between headaches due to epilepsy and migraine headaches is difficult. Both forms of headache are recurrent, stereotyped, and may be preceded by feeling of malaise, or aura. Severe throbbing hemicrania may occur with either, accompanied by an apparent alteration in consciousness, and leading to post attack sleep. Vomiting is common in both. The decision that a headache is a seizure manifestation is made using ancillary information such as a past history of other seizures, positive family history, consistent bilaterality of the headache, peculiar experiential aura, or extremely deep post-headache sleep. Some patients with seizure disorders of other types develop apparent migraine as their anticonvulsant dose is being adjusted. Appropriate increase in medication will alleviate these headaches.

A waking, drowsy, and spontaneous sleep electroencephalogram is needed to decide whether to treat the headaches as migraine or as epilepsy. The presence of paroxysmal activity, that is, spikes or paroxysmal bursts of slow-

---

*Manufacturer's warning: Use of imipramine (Tofranil) in pediatric conditions other than enuresis or in children younger than 6 years is not recommended.

ing, on the electroencephalogram influences one to begin therapy with anticonvulsant medication. The electroencephalographic abnormalities seen in many patients with migraine are usually not paroxysmal. Anticonvulsants used are phenobarbital, primidone, phenytoin, or carbamazepine, in that order. A single drug is used; its dose is· adjusted on the basis of clinical response and blood concentrations as in the treatment of other seizure disorders. Greatest success has been obtained with primidone, although carbamazepine has been useful in resistant cases.

Migraine Headaches. The diagnosis of migraine is suggested by hemicrania, typical visual aura, photophobia, vomiting, relief by sleep, and a normal electroencephalogram. A family history is very common, but specific clinical details of affected relatives should be elicited, as it is popular to label all severe headaches as migraine. The majority of attacks should involve only half the head. Failure of migraine to shift sides at least on occasion raises suspicion of intracranial arteriovenous malformation.

Some patients have attacks precipitated by eating specific foods; of note are chocolate, nuts, dairy products and cheeses, citrus fruits, certain fried foods, onions, tea, pork, frankfurters, and seafood. Historical inquiry may alert the patient to this association. If the migraine attacks are frequent and intractable, a diet which will eliminate all of these foods may be given a one month therapeutic trial. Individual foods are then re-introduced if the elimination diet is successful.

Therapy is selected on the basis of severity and frequency of attacks, and the response to previous modalities of therapy. Some children with migraine achieve sufficient relief from their very infrequent attacks with salicylates and a one hour nap. Other patients have very frequent attacks occurring weekly or more often, accompanied by intractable vomiting and excruciating photophobia.

INTERMITTENT THERAPY. Cafergot is used in patients whose attacks occur once per month or less frequently.* In children under 12 years of age one tablet is given at the onset of the attack and an additional tablet every half hour, for a maximum of four tablets per attack. Children over 12 years old start with two tablets. This agent has its maximal efficacy in the early phases of the attack before vasodilatation has occurred. The patient therefore must be allowed to carry the medication so that de-

pendence on other people being available at the onset of the attack is eliminated. Suppositories may be used if oral medication cannot be retained. Therapy is not always successful, by any means, and caution against overdosage must be specific as ergotism may occur. Generally no more than 10 tablets are dispensed at a time so that the physician is aware if attacks increase in frequency or if this medication with significant toxic effects is being overused.

CONTINUOUS THERAPY. In patients with migraine attacks several times monthly, maintenance ergotamine and phenobarbital therapy has been found effective. Bellergal in a dose of 3 to 4 tablets daily is given for a three month trial.* Cafergot may still be required although the frequency of attacks generally diminishes. Because migraine tends to improve over a period of time, medication should be cautiously discontinued at least every six months.

Methysergide (Sansert)† has been widely used in adults and in some children for the prophylaxis of severe recurrent migraine. We are no longer using this agent because of the serious side effect of retroperitoneal fibrosis.

Recently, in patients with frequent and intractable migraine headaches, propranolol orally has demonstrated a degree of efficacy not previously described with any prophylactic agent. Dosage is begun at 10 mg. three times a day and increased as needed to 25 mg. three to four times a day. Propranolol is a potent beta-adrenergic blocking agent and familiarity with its effects is essential. Particularly cardiovascular and central nervous system effects may be a problem. Propranolol has not been approved for use in children nor for use in migraine, but it is widely used for both at the present time.

Guillain-Barré Syndrome

BERNARD J. D'SOUZA, M.B.Ch.B., *and*
GUY M. McKHANN, M.D.

This syndrome is characterized by a progressive, flaccid paralysis. The early symptoms are often aching muscles and distal paresthesias. The motor weakness is often symmetrical and ascending. Facial and bulbar musculature may be involved. The course is not relentlessly progressive, and the patients may plateau and then progress again, often

---

*Cafergot tablets contain ergotamine tartrate 1.0 mg., and caffeine 100 mg.

*Bellergal tablets contain ergotamine tartrate 0.3 mg., phenobarbital 20 mg., belladonna alkaloids 0.1 mg.

†Manufacturer's precaution: The use of methysergide in children is not recommended.

skipping areas of the nervous system. Thus the combination of weakness of the face and legs is not uncommon. Objective sensory findings are minimal.

The majority of patients have a history of a previous gastrointestinal or respiratory illness, progression of symptoms over several days, and signs of improvement after 2 or 3 weeks. Complete recovery occurs in most patients, but some have residual weakness, contractures, and areflexia. Other features which aid in the diagnosis are an afebrile course and the characteristic findings in cerebrospinal fluid of elevation of protein, primarily albumin, and a normal cell count. Nerve conduction velocities are usually normal during the acute phase but may be delayed when recorded 5 to 6 weeks after onset.

Support of Respiration. Impaired respiratory function may result from involvement of the intercostal muscles and the diaphragm. In addition, the patient may have depressed swallowing, with pooling of secretions and aspiration. Postural drainage and mechanical suction should be used as needed. Sweating, persistent tachycardia and restlessness are early warnings of hypoxia. Significant respiratory dysfunction is accompanied by stupor, coma and seizures.

It is mandatory to monitor vital capacity, blood gases, and such clinical criteria as respiratory rate, strength of voice and depth of respiration. A useful clinical test is to ask the patient to take a deep breath and count as many numbers as possible. In a younger child, the ability to blow out a match gives similar information.

If there are signs of deterioration in respiratory function, oxygen by mask or by endotracheal intubation with intermittent positive pressure may be indicated. Tracheostomy should be performed if an endotracheal tube must be left in place for more than 4 or 5 days. Periodic cultures of pulmonary secretions and chest x-rays should be obtained in order to assure appropriate antibiotic therapy should pneumonia develop.

Cardiovascular Function. Acute pulmonary edema and arrhythmias may occur as a consequence of myocarditis, hypoxia, or fluid and electrolyte imbalance. Cardiac monitoring and frequent observation of vital signs are advised for all patients. In addition, there may be the inappropriate secretion of antidiuretic hormone. Thus daily input and output charts and periodic checks on serum electrolytes and urine specific gravities should be recorded.

Autonomic Dysfunction. Despite the improvements in respiratory care, a few patients with the Guillain-Barré syndrome die during the acute phase of the disease. It is now apparent that autonomic dysfunction can be life-threatening. Hypertension, orthostatic hypotension, cardiac arrhythmias, ileus and urinary retention are all manifestations of autonomic dysfunction.

Blood pressure measurements may show wide fluctuations. It is advisable to treat hypertension with short acting preparations, such as diazoxide.

Postural hypotension can be corrected with intravenous fluids, vasopressors, leg stockings and avoidance of rapid changes in posture. Bowel and bladder dysfunction may occur as a result of involvement of either the abdominal musculature or the autonomic nervous system. The Credé maneuver is helpful in emptying the bladder. Catheterization is rarely necessary.

Supportive Measures. Fever is not usually part of the syndrome and indicates infection, dehydration or a disturbance in temperature regulation. In patients with prolonged disease a nasogastric tube or feeding gastrostomy may be necessary to maintain adequate nutrition. Close attention must be paid to serum osmolality, volume of intake and possible aspiration.

Acute glomerulonephritis has been reported in association with this syndrome. The clinical presentation of nephritis may go undetected, therefore serial chemical and microscopic urine examinations are advisable.

Skin care and frequent changes in position are needed to avoid decubitus ulcers. Psychological support is also necessary, as patients often demonstrate changes in mood and behavior. Fatigue and irritability may persist after recovery of motor function. Diazepam (Valium) used cautiously may be employed to treat the anxiety. During convalescence—that is, when the neurological status is stable—a graduated physical therapy program including active and passive exercises should be instituted to prevent contractures.

There is no convincing evidence that any specific drug therapy, including steroids, will alter the course of the Guillain-Barré syndrome.

Chronic Relapsing Neuropathy

BERNARD J. D'SOUZA, M.B.Ch.B., *and*
GUY M. McKHANN, M.D.

Chronic relapsing neuropathy is a rare disorder which predominantly presents with motor problems and relatively minor sensory complaints. Cranial nerves, particularly the seventh nerve, are frequently involved. Weakness and atrophy in the distal musculature and thickening of the nerves may be observed on clinical examination. The evolution of the clinical picture varies from days to weeks with a similar pattern of recovery. A correlation between relapses and immediately preceding infection, particularly upper respiratory infection, is not uncommon.

The cerebrospinal fluid protein may increase during exacerbations. This rare condition may be a variant of the Guillain-Barré syndrome, but some cases are distinguished by their relapsing course and the therapeutic effect of steroids. Nerve conduction velocities are delayed and some patients show electromyographic evidence of denervation.

Suppression of the clinical and laboratory manifestation of this form of neuropathy may be achieved with the use of steroids. Prednisone in a dose of 60 mg./m²/day is recommended. An alternate day regimen may be considered when the disease process has stabilized. The dosage of steroids is slowly decreased to avoid exacerbations.

Claims of therapeutic success have been reported with the use of immunosuppressive agents such as azathioprine, methotrexate and 6-mercaptopurine.

Familial Dysautonomia

FELICIA B. AXELROD, M.D.

Many of the clinical manifestations of familial dysautonomia are caused by a deficit in autonomic homeostatic function and sensory appreciation of peripheral pain and temperature. Both deficiencies can be accounted for by the decreased number of unmyelinated neurons noted in sural nerve biopsies and autopsies. Prominent manifestations include feeding difficulties, delayed developmental milestones, labile body temperature and blood pressure, absence of overflowing tears and corneal anesthesia, recurrent aspiration pneumonia, breathholding episodes, ataxia, spinal curvature and intractable vomiting.

There is no specific treatment for this condition; thus therapy is directed to specific symptoms and complications. Feeding and swallowing difficulties are mitigated by avoiding liquids and thickening feedings. The infant may be completely incapable of sucking, necessitating the use of gavage feedings or gastrostomy to maintain nutrition and prevent aspiration.

Fevers. Hyperpyrexia should herald an intensive search for a source, but the fever may remain unexplained. Fever is often accompanied by shaking chills, cold extremities, and lack of sweating. Antipyretics may not be sufficient therapy. Massaging the cool extremities, and cooling the trunk by sponging or even a hypothermic mattress may be necessary. Chlorpromazine is often helpful in reducing anxiety and muscular spasms during hyperpyrexia.

Vomiting. Vomiting crises are often associated with hypertension, personality changes and occasionally hyperpyrexia. Occasionally they are precipitated by infection or emotional anxiety, but there may be no obvious cause. Some patients even exhibit a cyclical pattern with vomiting occurring once a month or even once a week. The crises can last from 3 to 72 hours and can lead to severe dehydration and the requirement of parenteral fluids. Chlorpromazine continues to be the most effective antiemetic for the dysautonomic vomiting crisis. The initial dose is usually 0.5 to 1 mg./kg. given intramuscularly. The dose should be effective in producing sleep, which seems to be necessary for resolution of the crisis. Seconal or Valium may aid inducement of sleep rather than giving additional chlorpromazine. Subsequent doses of chlorpromazine should be repeated at approximately 6 hour intervals and tapered until the crisis resolves.

Pneumonia. Recurrent pneumonias are frequent. Repeated aspiration is probably the major factor in causing pulmonary disease, with most of the damage to the lung occurring during infancy and early childhood. The signs of pneumonia may be subtle. Cough is not consistently present and is rarely productive. The child is more likely to vomit increased pulmonary secretions. Tachypnea is generally not evident and auscultation may be unrewarding because of decreased chest excursion. Radiographic examination is often necessary for diagnosis. Pathogens cultured from tracheal aspirations are often uncommon agents, such as *E. coli*, *S. proteus* or *Serratia*. Broad spectrum antibiotics should be used until bacteriological study permits more specific therapy. In the seriously ill child, blood gases must be monitored to detect CO_2 accumulation, which may be severe enough to cause coma and require assisted ventilation.

Bronchiectasis is a common sequela of the repeated pneumonias. Pulmonary hygiene, consisting of postural drainage and intermittent positive pressure, is helpful not only in the acute situation but as a daily routine for those children with chronic lung disease. Suctioning is often required because of ineffective cough. Chest therapy should be administered at home by the parents on a regular basis. Chest surgery is rarely indicated, as the disease is usually diffuse.

Spinal Curvature. Spinal curvature (kyphosis or scoliosis or both) will develop in 95 per cent of dysautonomic patients by adolescence. Spinal curvature may start as early as 3½ years or as late as 14 years. There may be rapid progression at any time. The completion of puberty generally halts the progression of scoliosis, as it does in the idiopathic adolescent form, but puberty is commonly delayed in dysautonomia. Spinal curvature further compromises respiratory function, adding the component of restrictive lung disease to bronchiectatic disease.

Annual radiographic examination of the spine is recommended after the child starts to walk. Splinting with a Milwaukee brace is the only effective conservative treatment. The brace must be carefully fitted and the skin inspected daily at pressure points because of the risk of ulceration as a result of decreased sensitivity to pain. The brace may also impair pulmonary ventilation. It is important to continue the program of pulmonary hygiene, including intermittent positive pressure breathing, during the period of bracing. If the brace is not successful in halting progression, or if the patient presents with a severe curve, spinal fusion is recommended.

Corneal Abrasions. Corneal complications have been decreasing with the regular use of artificial tear solutions containing methylcellulose. Artificial tears are instilled three to six times daily depending on the child's own baseline of eye moisture, environmental conditions and whether or not the child is febrile or dehydrated. Moisture chamber spectacle attachments help to maintain eye moisture and protect the eye from wind and foreign bodies. If an ulcer occurs, the eye can be patched. Tarsorrhaphy of the medial or lateral part of the palpebral fissure has been reserved for the unresponsive and chronic situations. The newest development is soft contact lenses, which are effective in promoting corneal healing.

Breathholding (Seizures). The phenomenon of prolonged breathholding with crying in the early years can result in actual cyanosis, syncope and seizure activity. This is due to lack of awareness that it is necessary for the next inspiration to be initiated, i.e., the patients are manifesting insensitivity to hypoxia and hypercapnia. This may become a manipulative maneuver with some children. This type of episode is frightening but self-limited and, in our experience, has never been fatal. The cyanosis which occurs as a result of breathholding must be differentiated from that which occurs with mucous plugs and must be treated by suctioning. Both types of cyanotic spells can go on to produce seizure-like movements and decerebrate posturing. Electroencephalograms are usually normal or nonspecific, and the frequency of either type of spell is unaffected by anticonvulsant therapy.

Due to the lack of appropriate response to hypoxia and hypercapnia, diving, underwater swimming and air travel at high altitudes are potential hazards. If the plane's altitude exceeds 37,000 feet, then supplemental oxygen will probably be necessary.

Azotemia. A large proportion of patients have a moderate degree of azotemia (20 to 30 mg./100 ml.) and variable values for creatinine clearance. These patients do not exhibit clinical signs of dehydration, and the urea nitrogen may often be reduced by simple hydration. In two patients whose urea nitrogen was greater than 40 mg./100 ml. and unalterable by intravenous hydration, renal biopsies were performed which showed greater than 40 per cent glomerulosclerosis. Further work is needed in this area prior to recommendations for specific therapy.

Anesthesia. Anesthesia for surgical procedures is associated with an increased risk because of extreme lability of blood pressure and diminished responsiveness to variations in blood gases. Local anesthesia with chlorpromazine as preoperative sedation is preferred whenever possible. Large amounts of epinephrine should not be infiltrated because of the exaggerated response to sympathomimetic drugs. If general anesthesia is indicated the gas anesthetics are preferred because of the rapid reversibility of their effects. An intravenous drip is maintained to assure adequate hydration and to permit the rapid administration of norepinephrine to combat profound hypotension. The amount and duration of norepinephrine administration are determined by the blood pressure response. In prolonged surgical procedures, an arterial line should be inserted for frequent monitoring of blood gases and blood pressure. If the patient is going to have a prolonged postoperative course, as in spinal fusions, elective tracheostomy performed one week prior to major surgery can facilitate postoperative recovery. It is during this inactive period when the patient is most likely to develop pneumonia, mucous plugs and aspiration.

Therapy. The administration of bethanechol (Urecholine) to a group of children with familial dysautonomia has been reported to have a favorable effect on some of the manifestations of this syndrome. Increased lacrimation, as measured by the Schirmer test, is consistent and dose-related when pharmacologically adequate amounts of bethanechol are administered. The effective dose has been 0.2 to 0.4 mg./kg./day subcutaneously in four divided doses, with about 4 hours between doses.* It is preferable to give bethanechol one half hour prior to meals and with an antacid. There is usually a 3 to 4 day lag period before the patient demonstrates the optimal effect. After two weeks of four subcutaneous injections a day, oral medication may be instituted. A 5 mg. tablet by mouth appears to be equivalent to 1 mg. subcutaneously, but absorption may not be reliable. However, an oral dose at mid-day allows greater flexibility, especially if the child is of school age.

Bethanechol improves esophageal motility as demonstrated by cine-esophagogram (five of six patients), but it does not always relieve the vexing problem of vomiting. In 12 of 17 patients, the number and severity of vomiting crises were reduced, with success more frequent among the younger patients. The eventual appearance of side reactions has prevented the long-term use of bethanechol in all but a very few patients. If vomiting is caused by accumulation of secretion, frequent nasopharyngeal aspiration and postural drainage are indicated. Chlorpromazine remains the most effective agent at our disposal for the usual vomiting problem.

Although the therapy of dysautonomia is nonspecific, the physician can render the family a great deal of support and comfort by thoroughly familiarizing himself with the varied manifestations of this condition. Living with the dysautonomic child imposes a great burden on the parents, who are aware of the serious prognosis and are faced with the care of a chronically handicapped child with repeated life-threatening crises. A sympathetic, artful physician can provide needed reassurance.

Injuries to the Brachial Plexus, Facial Nerve and Sciatic Nerve

ROBERT L. McLAURIN, M.D.

BRACHIAL PLEXUS

Brachial plexus injuries may occur at any age due to either penetrating injury or to sudden stretch of the plexus, but the most frequent cause is the stretch which may occur

at birth. If the head and shoulder are forcibly separated, as may occur when traction is applied to the shoulder during breech extraction or to the head during cephalic presentation, the resulting damage is to the upper portion of the plexus. Maneuvers that apply traction to the hyperabducted arm may lead to lower brachial plexus damage. In either case the basis of the injury may be simply stretching of the nerves distal to their emergence from the spine or true avulsion of the nerve roots from the cord. Neural function is usually recovered in a stretch injury, whereas there is no chance of recovery of neural function in avulsion of the nerve roots. It is apparent that any given traumatic event may result in a combination of these processes.

Upper brachial plexus injury (Erb) leads to paralysis of the shoulder and upper arm muscles. The result is loss of abduction of the shoulder, weakness of external rotation of the humerus, and weakness of the biceps muscle. The triceps and forearm and hand muscles are preserved. The biceps reflex is usually absent. Trauma to the lower plexus (Klumpke) leads to paralysis of the intrinsic hand muscles and flexor group of muscles in the forearm, whereas movements of the proximal portion of the extremity are preserved. In the newborn the grasp reflex is absent. If avulsion of the lower plexus has occurred, Horner's syndrome (miosis, drooping lid, and decreased facial sweating on the side of the nerve damage) may be present and has an ominous prognosis regarding recovery.

Management of brachial plexus injury includes proper diagnostic evaluation, surgical exploration in a few instances, and intensive physical therapy. Proper evaluation in turn includes clinical as well as electrical examination. If a penetrating wound has occurred in the supraclavicular region, surgical exploration for nerve repair is necessary. If, on the other hand, there is no evidence of trauma to the extraspinal plexus, surgery is not indicated since either stretch or avulsion has occurred. Electrical studies are helpful to establish the extent of denervation as well as to detect evidence of regeneration long before it may be detectable clinically.

In older children who sustain a severe impact to the shoulder with consequent brachial paralysis, myelography may be useful to help delineate the pathology. During the acute post-traumatic phase myelography may demonstrate passage of contrast medium into the chest or soft tissues; this results from avulsion of the root and surgery is valueless. After the acute stage myelography will demonstrate diverticulae which occur at the site of avulsion.

---

*This use of bethanechol is not mentioned in the manufacturer's instructions.

These findings automatically exclude surgery.

The only definite indication for surgical intervention is the penetrating injury from knife or gun. The remaining injuries are not assisted by surgery, although the presence of hematoma or swelling has been used as a basis for deciding to explore the plexus.

Regardless of the decision as to nerve exploration, it is apparent that the extremity requires vigorous physical therapy. This should include range-of-motion manipulation of the shoulder and joints of the arm. An abduction ("airplane") splint is frequently helpful, although it is more difficult to apply to a newborn infant. Muscle and tendon transplants may be considered at a later age if the extremity has useful sensation but limited motor function. Spontaneous recovery of nerve function is much greater in upper than in lower plexus injury.

FACIAL NERVE

There are three causes of facial nerve paralysis in the pediatric age group. The first is external trauma to the nerve at the time of birth, usually associated with the use of obstetrical forceps. The nerve is injured as it emerges from the parotid gland. The resulting paresis is frequently incomplete and affects only the lower part of the face. There is noted asymmetry of movement of the face on crying, especially the lower corner of the mouth. Less often there may be inability to close the eye due to weakness of the orbicularis muscles. The prognosis is quite good since the nerve is not severed and the injury is outside the facial canal.

The second type of facial nerve injury accompanies fracture of the temporal bone. The paralysis may be partial or complete, immediate or delayed. Complete paralysis is accompanied by the hazard of exposure keratitis since the child is unable to close the affected eye. This complication may be avoided by use of methylcellulose drops in the eye several times daily and by taping the eye closed at night. If there has been simultaneous injury to the trigeminal nerve, so that corneal insensitivity has resulted, partial or complete tarsorrhaphy should be considered. If the nerve injury is partial, these measures are usually unnecessary since the eye can be closed weakly.

Immediate facial paralysis occurs with a significant impact to the nerve or with transection of the nerve at the site of bone fracture. While these cannot be distinguished clinically initially, there may be evidence from electrical testing during the ensuing few days. Nerve excitability to external stimulation is tested daily.

If there is progressive evidence of denervation as demonstrated by an elevation of threshold, nerve exploration should be undertaken since the nerve frequently can be anastomosed and successful recovery ensured. This should be done within 10 days of the injury to achieve maximum recovery. If the facial paralysis is delayed after head injury it may be assumed that the nerve has not been divided but swelling and/or hemorrhage have occurred within the facial canal. Steroids have been used in these circumstances, although it is not possible to prove their efficacy. Electrical testing is again used to determine whether a reaction of degeneration is occurring and, if so, surgical decompression of the nerve should be considered. Meanwhile, protection of the eye and massage of the face to prevent loss of tissue tone are indicated.

The third type of facial paralysis occasionally seen in childhood is Bell's palsy. The etiology is unknown but is thought to be due to swelling of the nerve within the temporal bone. Clinically it is characterized by rather rapid onset of partial or complete facial paralysis accompanied by pain referred to the ear. The role of steroids in the treatment of Bell's palsy is still uncertain but is advisable. Recovery occurs in approximately 90 per cent of patients but may require 2 or 3 months. Electrical testing should be done frequently after the onset, and if there is evidence of nerve degeneration decompression should be considered.

SCIATIC NERVE

The most frequent cause of sciatic nerve injury in the pediatric age group is faulty intramuscular injection. Factors which may contribute to this are the small size of an infant, cachexia due to illness with loss of subcutaneous tissue, uncontrolled squirming during injection, and the normal variant of the nerve emerging above the pyriformis muscle (18 per cent) which leads to fixation and a more superficial position of the nerve. For all these reasons injection injury to the sciatic nerve is more common in pediatric than in adult practice.

Numerous types of medication have been implicated. The most frequent offenders are antibiotics, none of which appear to be innocuous if injected directly into the nerve. The antibiotic and the vehicle have been shown to be neurotoxic. While antibiotics are probably not responsible for nerve damage if injected outside the nerve, certain substances, such as paraldehyde, may cause significant perineural scarring.

The offending injection is probably accompanied by immediate pain, although in older children there is occasionally no good history of such an immediate onset of discomfort. Later the pain may assume a burning, hyperesthetic quality characteristic of causalgia. The physical findings are dependent on the portion of nerve involved and the completeness of paralysis. Since the sciatic nerve may be divided into its two principal components even up to the sciatic notch, one component part may be separately injected. The peroneal portion is laterally placed and more susceptible to injury; therefore, foot-drop with loss of eversion of the foot is the most frequent finding on examination. This is easily detected in infants by lack of dorsiflexion on withdrawal from a pinprick on the sole of the foot and in older children by a slapping gait. If the entire nerve is injured, the plantar flexors, innervated by the posterior tibial nerve, are also paralyzed. Under these circumstances there may be no voluntary movement below the knee, the ankle reflex is absent, and the sole and a part of the dorsum of the foot are anesthetic.

Management of injection sciatic injury depends on the severity of pain and the extent of neurologic deficit. Immediate surgical exploration of the nerve is never justified. There is no evidence that steroids are of benefit in minimizing the damage caused by nerve injection. The discomfort may respond to analgesics but narcotics should be avoided since the pain may persist for weeks or months. The causalgic type of pain may require sympathetic blocks or even sympathectomy in extreme cases. The nerve deficit should be observed only for a period of several months. Caution should be exercised to ensure that the anesthetic sole of the foot or the toes do not become ulcerated and infected. The child will be able to walk more comfortably with less chance of tripping if a foot-drop brace is provided.

The role of surgery is still uncertain but it should not be considered until at least 3 to 6 months have elapsed and there is no clinical or electrical evidence of nerve recovery. When these criteria have been met, nerve exploration and internal or external neurolysis may be undertaken.

Prevention of sciatic nerve injury requires education in proper intramuscular injection technique. Injections may be safely given in the anterior and lateral portions of the thigh or in the deltoid region above the midpoint of the upper arm. If the gluteal area must be used, the upper-outer quadrant is safe provided the needle is not angled caudally and medially.

While nerve injection is by far the commonest means of injury, the sciatic nerve can be damaged by posterior hip dislocation. A rare cause of bilateral sciatic paralysis in the newborn has been attributed to injection of therapeutic agents into the umbilical artery with resulting thrombosis of the inferior gluteal arteries. There is no specific treatment for the nerve injury in this condition.

Acute Toxic Encephalopathy and Hypoxic Encephalopathy

BERNARD J. D'SOUZA, M.B.Ch.B., *and* GUY M. McKHANN, M.D.

Acute toxic encephalopathy is characterized by the abrupt onset of alteration of consciousness, increased intracranial pressure and seizures. Initially, patients are febrile without signs of meningeal irritation and signs of systemic illness. The process occurs in patients between the ages of 6 weeks and 12 to 14 years. There is often a preceding history of vomiting, possible upper respiratory infection, and the use of antiemetic or antipyretic drugs. Despite the name, there is no evidence of any specific toxin being the causative agent.

The clinical picture can resemble that of acute bacterial meningitis, viral encephalitis, subarachnoid hemorrhage, poisoning with known agents, such as lead or organic phosphates, or Reye's syndrome. Acute toxic encephalopathy is distinguished from Reye's syndrome by having normal or only moderate abnormalities in liver function, normal blood ammonia levels, and normal levels of blood glucose. However, the distinction is difficult and there are some cases which could be classified as either entity.

The brain has a high, continuous demand for oxygen. *Hypoxic encephalopathy* can be produced by interruption of delivery of oxygen (as in cardiac arrest), drop in oxygen concentration (high altitude or carbon monoxide poisoning) or, in unusual circumstances, increased oxygen demand (seizures occurring when perfusion is already impaired).

The duration of symptoms and the rate of recovery are variable and difficult to predict. The length of the period of hypoxia, the age of the patient, and the adequacy of brain perfusion are all factors in the prognosis. Rarely patients have a biphasic course with the first phase being acute coma, and the second being some degree of recovery, followed by a progressive decline in function.

The management of acute toxic encephalopathy and hypoxic encephalopathy is similar, and they will be considered together.

Supportive Measures. POSITIONING. Patients in a stuporous or comatose state should be kept on their sides or stomach, in a slightly head-down position. They should be turned every one-half to one hour to avoid aspiration pneumonia and pressure sores.

TEMPERATURE REGULATION. Hyperthermia increases oxygen demand by the brain; thus patients who have decreased perfusion of the brain should be kept normothermic or hypothermic if possible. A body temperature of 32 to 33°C. reduces brain metabolism by approximately one-half. Temperature can be regulated by rectal antipyretic agents, acetaminophen, and a cooling blanket.

AIRWAY AND RESPIRATION. An adequate airway should be established and maintained by mechanical suctioning, endotracheal intubation and artificial respiration. An endotracheal tube can be left in place up to 4 or 5 days. After that, tracheostomy is required.

BLOOD PRESSURE. The patient with impaired brain perfusion must not be allowed to become hypotensive. Blood pressure can be maintained by plasma volume expanders and careful attention to fluid volume and central venous pressure. Special care must be exercised to maintain blood pressure when hyperosmotic agents such as mannitol or arteriographic dye are being used. Supportive drug therapy includes the use of isoproterenol (0.2 μg./min.) or levarterenol bitartrate (Levophed) (0.5 ml./min.). Constant blood pressure and central venous pressure monitoring is required when these pharmacologic agents are being used.

Cerebral Edema. Cerebral edema can be counteracted by hyperosmotic agents, steroids, hyperventilation and, rarely, surgical decompression.

Hypertonic solutions provide an osmotic gradient across the blood-brain barrier. They are the most rapidly active in decreasing brain volume, but their effects are of short duration. In addition, with some agents, particularly urea, there is a "rebound phenomenon" as urea gradually enters the brain. With hypertonic solutions, diuresis should be monitored by urine output and serum osmolality.

A 20 per cent solution of *mannitol,* given intravenously at a rate of 1.5 gm./kg. over 20 minutes, is most commonly used.* The dose can be repeated every 6 to 8 hours. *Urea* is given intravenously as a 30 per cent solution in a dose of 1 gm./kg. over 30 minutes, repeated every 6 hours.

Glycerol may be given by nasogastric tube in a dose of 0.5 to 1.0 gm./kg. and repeated every 6 hours. This agent can be given over a long period of time. However, in an unconscious patient, aspiration of glycerol is a potential problem which must be recognized. A 10 per cent intravenous glycerol solution can also be used, but hemolysis has been reported as a complication.

Steroids, particularly dexamethasone, appear to affect cerebral edema by altering vascular permeability. There is a lag period of 12 to 24 hours before they become effective. Dexamethasone is given either intravenously or intramuscularly in a dose of 0.25 to 0.5 mg./kg./day in four divided doses. An additional loading dose of one-third the daily dose is used to

---

*Manufacturer's precaution: The use of mannitol in pediatric patients has not been studied comprehensively.

TABLE 1. Use of Anticonvulsants in Patients with Central Nervous System Depression

ANTICONVULSANTS	DOSAGE AND ROUTE OF ADMINISTRATION	COMMENTS
Diazepam*	Intravenous diluted in sterile water, 0.5 to 0.75 mg./kg. given slowly over minutes. Repeat × 2 every 15 minutes. Single dose not to exceed 10 mg.	Hypotension and respiratory depression, particularly following barbiturates or paraldehyde.
Paraldehyde	Rectal 0.3 ml./kg., repeat every 4 to 6 hours.	Action delayed one-half hour.
	Intramuscular 0.15 ml./kg., repeated every 4 to 6 hours.	Sterile abscesses.
	Intravenous perfusion 10 ml. in 90 ml. normal saline, titrated according to patient's needs (5 to 40 ml./hr.).	Solution should not be allowed to stand in plastic bags.
Phenytoin	Loading dose: intravenous perfusion 15 mg./kg. in normal saline at the rate of 50 mg./min. Then 5 to 8 mg./kg. once daily. Should not be given intramuscularly.	Monitor blood pressure and cardiac rate.

*Manufacturer's precaution: Safety and efficacy of injectable diazepam have not been established in the neonate.

initiate therapy. The duration of therapy is dictated by the clinical state of the patient.

Hyperventilation will decrease brain volume acutely. It can be a helpful adjunct to therapy when a marked increase in intracranial pressure is encountered, and hypertonic solutions are being prepared.

Surgical decompression, consisting of removal of the bones overlying the temporal, frontal and parietal regions of brain, has occasionally been done as a last resort. In the authors' opinion, this type of heroic surgery is rarely, if ever, justified.

Fluid therapy should be directed toward maintaining normal serum osmolality. In the presence of cerebral edema, intravenous therapy should be limited to 75 per cent of the average daily requirements.

Control of Seizures. Like hyperthermia, seizures increase cerebral metabolism, and should be controlled. The problem is to obtain an anticonvulsant effect without further suppressing consciousness and respiratory function. Thus, barbiturates are not used acutely, but only as the patient stabilizes or starts to improve. The preferred drugs and the details of their use are given in Table 1.

Rehabilitation. Early advice and treatment by a therapist can avoid the threat of contractures. Attention to the socio-psychiatric aspects are helpful in restoring the patient to his environment at home.

Reye's Syndrome

FREDERICK H. LOVEJOY, Jr., M.D.

Reye's syndrome was first described from Australia in 1963 in 21 children who manifested severe encephalopathy and fatty degeneration of the liver. Although its clinical manifestations, course and prognosis as well as biochemical, physiologic and pathologic aberrations have been clarified and broadened since that time, its etiology remains unclear. Initially it appeared to be a new or at least rare phenomenon. Increased awareness of the syndrome and occurrence of the disease in epidemic form have made Reye's syndrome one of the most common causes of acute encephalopathy in childhood.

Reye's syndrome occurs in all pediatric ages from six months through adolescence. One to seven days following a mild respiratory infection, gastroenteritis, or occasionally varicella, the patient becomes lethargic and drowsy and begins to vomit. The parent's concern is heightened shortly thereafter by the child's restlessness, irritability, delirium and combativeness. It is at this point that the patient often presents to the physician.

STAGING

A system of staging has been adapted to describe the progression of the disease: Stage I—lethargy, drowsiness, vomiting, elevation in serum liver enzymes, grade I electroencephalogram; Stage II—disorientation, combativeness, hyperventilation, tachycardia, pupillary dilation, hyperactive reflexes, purposeful response to painful stimuli, bilateral Babinski reflex, elevation in blood ammonia and serum liver enzymes, grades II, III, or IV electroencephalogram; Stage III—coma, persistent tachycardia and hyperventilation, upper midbrain involvement (loss of ciliospinal reflex, pupillary dilation, decorticate posturing in response to painful stimuli, bilateral Babinski reflex), persistent elevation in blood ammonia and serum liver enzymes, grades II, III, or IV electroencephalogram; Stage IV—deepening coma, further rostral-caudal progression of midbrain involvement (loss of doll's head maneuver and response to ice water calorics, sluggish pupillary response to light, decerebrate rigidity and decerebrate posturing to painful stimuli, bilateral Babinski reflex), decrease in blood ammonia and serum liver enzyme activity, grade III or IV electroencephalogram; Stage V—coma, loss of response to painful stimuli, to light, to doll's head maneuver and to ice water calorics, cessation of spontaneous respiration, continued improvement in blood ammonia and serum liver enzyme activity, grade V electroencephalogram.

Other important laboratory findings include normal protein and sugar with absent pleocytosis and negative bacterial cultures on lumbar puncture, normal serum bilirubin, elevated serum creatine phosphokinase activity reflecting skeletal muscle involvement and respiratory alkalosis with a superimposed metabolic acidosis. Common complications seen during the illness include gastrointestinal and urinary tract bleeding, inappropriate secretion of antidiuretic hormone, severe electrolyte derangements and disseminated intravascular coagulation.

Management is influenced by clinical and laboratory factors suggesting a severe course and poor prognosis such as: (1) rapid progression through clinical stages; (2) a blood ammonia concentration at any time during the illness greater than 300 μg./100 ml.; (3) serum enzyme alteration (serum creatine phosphokinase, serum glutamic-oxalo transaminase, serum glutamic-pyruvic transaminase) indicative of both hepatic and skeletal muscle involvement; (4) severe metabolic acidosis on admission (HCO$_3$<10 μg./liter); and (5) grade III or IV electroencephalogram indicating a severe course and a grade V or worse associated with a fatal outcome.

MANAGEMENT

Logical management must take into consideration the wide variability in the disease process, which ranges from mild illness and full recovery with supportive therapy alone to highly fulminant disease with a rapid fatal outcome. Reversal of a downhill clinical course is attainable in Stages I through IV, and only in Stage V does this not appear possible. Thus therapy must be adjusted to the severity of the illness. Further, as outcome is related to prompt institution of treatment, early diagnosis is of critical importance. Because of the need for greater study and understanding of the disease, all but the mildest cases should be referred to centers with intensive care capabilities familiar with the care of Reye's syndrome. Present mortality rates range from 20 to 40 per cent, contrasting to the previous figure of 80 per cent.

Therapies have included intensive anticerebral edema measures for control of increased intracranial pressure, peritoneal dialysis, exchange transfusion, hypertonic glucose to prevent excess mobilization of fat with subsequent fatty acidemia, and therapy with various amino acids (ornithine, citrulline, arginine) for lowering blood ammonia. Evidence to date would indicate that no one method of therapy is clearly superior to another and that supportive care with attention to prompt correction of biochemical or physiologic alterations is a logical approach. In hospitals in which intensive care facilities are not available, the following basic principles of support can be initiated while awaiting transfer of the patient:

1. Restrict fluids to 40 to 70 ml./kg./day with hourly adjustment of input and output (one third normal saline with 10 per cent glucose). Central venous pressure should be maintained between 2 and 4 cm. of water while maintaining optimal tissue perfusion as determined by urinary output and systemic blood pressure. Serum sodium concentrations should be maintained between 140 and 155 mEq./liter. Serum osmolarity should be monitored frequently to prevent rapid lowering that would exacerbate cerebral edema (osmolarities in Stage II maintained between 290 and 310 mOsm./liter, Stage III between 310 and 320, Stage IV between 320 and 330).

2. Fluid restriction alone should be used in clinical Stages I and II with anticerebral edema therapy upon entrance into Stage III (mannitol,* 0.5 to 1.5 gm./kg. intravenously

*Manufacturer's precaution: The use of mannitol in pediatric patients has not been studied comprehensively.

per dose, glycerol by nasogastric tube, 3 to 6 gm./kg./day, and dexamethasone, 0.5 mg./kg./day intravenously).

3. Nasogastric and endotracheal intubation is initiated upon entrance into Stage III.

4. Vitamin K, 5 mg. intravenously, is given every other day.

5. Fresh blood transfusion is carried out for correction of clotting factors and maintenance of venous hematocrit greater than 35 per cent.

6. When blood ammonia concentrations exceed 300 μg./100 ml., neomycin, 50 mg./kg./day by nasogastric tube, and neomycin enemas are given.

7. Maalox, 5 to 10 ml. every two hours by nasogastric tube, is given upon patient's entrance into Stage III.

8. Avoid drugs predisposing to respiratory depression (sedative and anticonvulsant drugs), gastrointestinal bleeding (salicylates) and drugs with hepatotoxic potential (salicylates and acetaminophen).

9. Seizures are treated with low doses of phenobarbital, phenytoin or paraldehyde.

10. Treat excessive temperature elevation with a cooling blanket.

11. Monitor arterial blood gases with maintenance of P_{CO_2} greater than 20 mm. Hg and P_{O_2} greater than 80 mm. Hg.

12. A new approach to therapy involves the use of intraventricular or subdural monitoring and prompt treatment of elevated pressure waves with anticerebral edema measures. Though seemingly a logical approach to therapy, greater experience is needed to assess its effect on outcome.

13. Once the patient is fully stabilized, transfer may be more safely accomplished.

The health care team needed to care for the acutely ill patient with Reye's syndrome includes the pediatrician, neurologist, gastroenterologist, physical and respiratory therapist, intensive care nurse and social worker. On recovery, long-term follow-up by the pediatrician is important in coordinating care of the neurological and psychological sequelae of the illness. At present this spectrum includes severe motor deficits with mental retardation, expressive and receptive language deficits, behavioral disorders and severe family stress.

4

Respiratory Tract

Malformations of the Nose

SYLVAN E. STOOL, M.D.

There are two major considerations in malformations of the nose: the physiological effect of airway obstruction and the cosmetic defect. The abnormalities of the nose which are present at birth and produce signs of respiratory obstruction usually involve absence of normal structures, persistence of embryonic membranes or anomalous anatomic development. Although external deformities may cause much concern to the parent and physician, they frequently are not of as much physiological significance as are internal abnormalities of the nose.

Most of the abnormalities in the newborn are congenital and involve various facial clefts and abnormalities such as Crouzon's and Apert's syndromes. The external deformity is obvious and surgical intervention is usually not warranted in the newborn. A minor-appearing congenital malformation is the presence of a small, dermal sinus usually presenting at the junction of the bony and cartilaginous nose in the midline. These sinuses may be extensive and even extend intracranially. Therapy is usually surgical. The time of operation will depend upon the patient's age, general condition, and whether there is evidence of infection in the sinus tract. Some of the other abnormalities associated with this are discussed in the following section on "Tumors and Polyps of the Nose." It is important to emphasize early that any midline defect may be extensive.

One of the most important malformations for the physician to be aware of is atresia of the posterior choanae. The symptoms usually occur immediately after birth. When the child makes respiratory efforts, he is unable to breathe through the nose and will close his mouth while making strong, inspiratory effort. Unless the mouth is opened so the child is able to breathe, he will suffocate. This fact is usually appreciated when the child opens his mouth and starts to cry. He is able to breathe, but with the mouth closed there is marked respiratory obstruction. The diagnosis should be suspected whenever this clinical picture presents.

Diagnosis may be confirmed in a number of ways. A small probe may be passed into the nose and will usually strike a firm ridge about 1¼ inches from the anterior nares. A catheter may be passed into the nose, the nasopharynx and pharynx, where it may be visualized or palpated. Dye studies using colored dyes or contrast media are of value in establishing the patency of the nose and in ascertaining the site of obstruction. When the nose is aspirated, very thick mucoid nasal discharge is usually present.

Treatment is accomplished by inserting either a catheter or an airway into the mouth, so that the baby will be able to breathe through the mouth. I usually prefer to pass a large catheter through the mouth into the stomach. This maneuver opens the mouth and breaks the glossal palatine seal and also provides a means for nutrition. Small, metal oral airways may also be taped into the mouth. Once an oral airway has been established, the patient can then be evaluated and a decision made as to the method and time of repair. If the child's general physical condition is satisfactory, repair by either transnasal or transpalatal surgery can be accomplished in the first few days of life.

There is a lack of agreement among various surgeons as to the preferred method of therapy, but under any circumstances, the patient will have to be followed for several months to make sure he maintains an adequate airway. It usually takes about four months for the child to learn to breathe through his mouth or to be able to breathe through the mouth when eating.

Tumors and Polyps of the Nose

SYLVAN E. STOOL, M.D.

Although tumors of the nose are relatively rare, a great variety of them may be seen. Any tumor that occurs in the midline is usually related to abnormality of development. These include nasal gliomas, encephaloceles, dermal sinuses and dermoids. These tumors are invariably benign; however, because of either size, location or intracranial connections, they may be very difficult to remove. It is usually necessary to differentiate the solid tumors from those that are extensions of the intracranial contents and may be of a cystic nature. In general, the solid tumors do not have intracranial connections. Evaluation of these patients should include radiographic examination. Usually, tomography is difficult to obtain in small children unless anesthesia is used, and in recent years, computerized axial tomography has been helpful in evaluating these lesions. When an intracranial extension is shown to be present, a team approach, with the neurosurgeon and otorhinolaryngologist working together, is necessitated.

Among the benign tumors, nasal papillomas—wartlike projections—may occur in the vestibule or on the anterior portion of the inferior turbinate. They usually have a high incidence of recurrence after removal. Intranasal tumors most commonly encountered are polyps and cysts. Nasal polyps have been found frequently in patients with cystic fibrosis and in spite of adequate surgical removal are prone to recur. They may also be found in other allergic children. These patients are difficult to treat satisfactorily, as the etiology remains obscure. Occasionally, a polyp may originate in the maxillary sinus and be large enough to present in the oropharynx; this is referred to as an antral choanal polyp. These polyps are usually single and may be attached to a long pedicle; therapy consists of surgical removal and usually there is no recurrence. A variety of malignant tumors occur in the nose, but fortunately these are rare. Not infrequently, by the time the diagnosis is made the child has an extensive tumor, and surgical removal along with radiation and chemotherapy is necessary. In general, it is best to avoid mutilating surgery in tumors of the nose and nasopharynx in children.

One of the most frequently encountered tumors of the nose in young male children is the angiofibroma which frequently presents because of nasal obstruction and epistaxis. The epistaxis may be life-threatening. Diagnosis of these tumors is usually made because of a high index of suspicion. Radiographic examination using angiography is frequently diagnostic and biopsy may not be necessary; however, if there is any doubt, a biopsy should be performed. Prior to surgical removal, in some instances estrogen therapy is used to decrease the tumor size; however, the side effects of this therapy may not be desirable. Prior to the actual surgical procedure, embolization of the blood supply to the tumor has been used with an encouraging degree of success to decrease blood loss during the operative procedure. Although this is a benign tumor, it may be extensive and extend intracranially.

Nasal Injuries

SYLVAN E. STOOL, M.D.

Nasal injuries are common in children and because of this, there is a tendency to treat them lightly. The nose is the most frequently injured part of the face. This is especially true in the young child because of his instability when walking, and in the newborn because of birth trauma. When older children engage in contact sports, nasal injury is not uncommon. Severe nasal injuries are increasingly common in adolescents because of automobile and motorcycle accidents.

An injury frequently seen in the newborn is dislocation of the nasal septum, usually manifest by some external nasal deviation and easily diagnosed by inspection. In the newborn, it is relatively easy to replace this deviation of the septum if the abnormality is recognized. This may be accomplished by grasping the nose firmly between the thumb and index finger and pushing it to the midline. If this maneuver is not successful, it is necessary to elevate the nose and manipulate it with a special infant nasal elevator or, if such an instrument is not available, a hemostat whose blades are covered with a segment of rubber tubing may be used to elevate the nose, and then the external nose and septum may be manipulated. If the pediatrician is unable to accomplish this, consultation with an otorhinolaryngologist may be indicated. Reduction of these fractures in the newborn may prevent subsequent marked deformities.

Injuries in infants and young children usually occur secondary to falls and are usually accompanied by hematoma formations. Occasionally there is a marked hematoma of the nasal septum and it is necessary to provide drainage, accomplished using general or local anesthesia, and a segment of nasal mucosa is usually excised to provide adequate drainage. If a septal hematoma becomes infected, complications may ensue and occasionally meningitis develops. Many young children who suffer from this type of trauma develop discoloration from extravasated blood beneath the eyes. This is frequently of marked concern to the family and it is well to advise them that discoloration beneath the eyes will probably persist for several weeks. If there is marked nasal swelling and the child is cooperative, a dressing may be applied using adhesive tape to support the nasal tip.

Nasal injuries in older children are usually more extensive and frequently include fractures of the nasal bones as well as hematoma, abrasions and lacerations. The most important aspect of diagnosis is palpation of the nasal bone. Palpation should be used to ascertain the mobility of the nasal bones, the presence of crepitation, and the relationship of the nasal bones to the cartilages. Radiographic examination may be of value; however, any extensive injury is probably accompanied by fracture of the nasal bones. The important decision is whether there is displacement. After any extensive injury, swelling is usually rapid and it may not be possible to do an adequate evaluation. When the swelling decreases in 7 to 10 days the position of the nasal bones can be ascertained. The reflection of light on the nasal dorsum is a good clue as to the symmetry of the nose. If displacement is noted, the fracture should be elevated. In the past, it was felt that the nasal bones were firmly fixed within 10 days; however, it is frequently possible to mobilize the fragments for three or four weeks. It is advisable to have a child who has obvious deformity of the nose evaluated by a rhinologist to consider realignment of the nasal bones.

Extensive nasal injuries are frequently accompanied by fractures involving the frontoethmoid complex or the maxilla. In these instances, accurate evaluation by physical examination and radiographic examination including tomography may be necessary to delineate the extent of the injury. These fractures may be accompanied by cerebrospinal fluid rhinorrhea. Fortunately, in many instances this will heal spontaneously and may not require extensive surgical repair. Injuries of the maxilla may be accompanied by blow-out fractures of the sinus. These fractures may require open reduction to prevent marked deformities.

Epistaxis

SYLVAN E. STOOL, M.D.

Nosebleed is one of the most common disorders seen in infancy and childhood. The majority of nosebleeds are not serious and indeed are more of a nuisance rather than a life-threatening condition. In many instances, the initial condition is made worse by attempts at therapy.

The majority of nosebleeds are related to trauma. Excessive drying of the mucous membranes because of inadequate humidification is common in childhood. Inflammation because of allergy, bacteria, and viruses may also result in nosebleeds. Abnormalities of the clotting mechanism are an infrequent cause of nosebleeds. In general, any child who does not bleed from other sites, and who does not have a family history of bleeding, probably does not have a nosebleed secondary to a coagulation disorder. Foreign bodies and tumors, however, may have their initial presentation with severe epistaxis.

In the management of nosebleed, the first thing the physician should do is remain calm and do all he can to urge the patient, parent, friends and relatives to do the same. A nosebleed sufficiently severe to cause a serious illness and death is extremely rare in childhood. The first and simplest method of therapy is to apply pressure to the external nose by pinching the nares closed with the child sitting on the mother's lap. It is advisable to do this for from 5 to 10 minutes, since it takes this long for the blood to clot. If this is not effective, the next step is to apply pressure by using a small piece of cotton that has been coated with a lubricant or a pledget of absorbable, oxidized cellulose. This is inserted into the anterior nares and pressure is applied. The child should sit upright with the head tilted slightly forward so blood will not enter the oropharynx.

If these simple methods do not control the situation, it is advisable to ascertain the site of the bleeding. In order to do this, illumination is necessary and suction is mandatory. It is desirable to sedate the child adequately; in many instances this stops the nosebleed. Occasionally, it is necessary to use general anesthesia. If excessive force is used to conduct this examination, the nose may bleed more excessively. After the child has been properly prepared and adequate illumination is available, the nasal speculum is inserted into the nose and the nasal space is aspirated of all blood clots. Frequently, just removing the blood clot is sufficient to control epistaxis.

Topical vasoconstrictors may be used and are applied by moistening a pledget of cotton with quarter per cent Neo-Synephrine. One or two per cent cocaine may be used. This is an excellent vasoconstrictor and provides topical anesthesia. Two per cent lidocaine (Xylocaine) with 1:1000 epinephrine will provide vasoconstriction and anesthesia. It is important to use discretion with topical anesthetics as they are rapidly absorbed from the mucous membrane.

A search is made for a local bleeding point. If this is found, there are a number of ways it may be treated. In general, local pressure is preferable and may be accomplished by using oxidized cellulose or nasal packing. When the nose is packed, it is important that it be done properly, so other areas of the mucosa are not unduly traumatized. I prefer to use an absorbable packing such as oxidized cellulose in the treatment of young children, as it is not necessary to remove this type of packing. The pack is inserted gently through the anterior nares using a bayonet forceps, and the anterior nasal space is firmly packed. The nares may then be packed with a firm, cotton pledget and tincture of benzoin applied to the external nose so that adhesive tape may be used over the cotton in the nares to hold it in place. Usually, if the cotton is removed after 24 hours, the pack will spontaneously come out. If gauze packing is used, the pack is placed in a continuous grip by applying it in layers using a bayonet forceps and packing from the floor of the nose upward.

The majority of nosebleeds in children come from the area just inside the vestibule and on the nasal septum. This is an area that is subject to trauma from nose picking, rubbing and dry air. This may be treated by using a variety of lubricants, such as petrolatum, skin creams and in recent years, steroid creams have been available. These are especially effective in decreasing the inflammatory reaction. The child who has nosebleeds from this area can be treated by advising the parent to apply one of these ointments or creams to the nose in the morning and evening. This is especially important in the evening as the child frequently will rub his nose on the pillow during sleep. Have the parent apply the ointment liberally for about five days, both morning and evening, and following this, use the ointment in the evening. This will effectively protect the area.

In rare instances when anterior packing and other measures are not successful, it may be necessary to provide a posterior pack. Patients requiring posterior packing should be hospitalized. The insertion of a posterior pack may be very traumatic, and it is advisable to sedate the child. For some patients, general anesthesia may also be necessary. The pack is inserted by passing a catheter through the nose into the oropharynx, and there the tip of a catheter may be picked up with a hemostat. The pack is then attached to the catheter with a string, and the catheter withdrawn from the nose so that the pack may be heated in the posterior choanae. It is important that the pack not be too large, as it will cause pressure in the nasopharynx and this may result in marked respiratory obstruction. After the posterior pack is inserted, anterior packing is usually performed.

Prevention of epistaxis is most important. This can best be accomplished by providing adequate humidification, especially during the winter time, improving nasal hygiene and encouraging the child to refrain from nose picking. Children who have allergies should be treated with control of specific allergens. If the bleeding site is in the anterior portion of the nasal septum, drying and crusting should be prevented. It is important to show the parents where the bleeding area is, and encourage them to treat the child properly. I prefer to show the parent the affected region using an otoscope with a nasal speculum, thus permitting the parent to see the inflamed region with the numerous small blood vessels. With this knowledge, the parent will be less frightened and will be able to accept the fact that the child may have recurrent nosebleeds and can initiate treatment that is simple and effective.

Foreign Bodies in the Nose and Pharynx

SYLVAN E. STOOL, M.D.

An amazing number and variety of foreign bodies may be found in the nose and pharynx during childhood. The symptoms and signs will depend upon the size of the object, as well as its composition. In general, organic substances produce a more violent inflammatory reaction than does inorganic material. This has been especially true in recent years since a

Sympathomimetic-antihistamine mixtures are even available in oral drop dosage form. These may carry particular risks for young infants in whom we have observed hypercapnia attributable to respiratory depression following their use, especially if the infant happened to be mildly dehydrated. Too often these mixtures are prescribed principally as a result of advertising pressure or as the easiest way to deal with parental pressure to "do something." This sort of parental anxiety is normal and should be dealt with more directly through reassurance and explanation of what can be expected in the normal course of the illness. The emotional tolerance of different families for the normal frequency of respiratory illness in their children is variable. Many parents are unaware of the fact that the average North American preschooler and young school-age child have 5 or 6 minor respiratory infections per year.

Removal of the tonsils and adenoids is without effect on the frequency of viral upper respiratory infections, and the empirical administration of gamma globulin under such circumstances is completely without logical foundation or demonstrated value. Kleenex and "tincture of time" remain the bulwarks of treatment of the common cold.

Rhinitis and Sinusitis

JAMES W. BASS, M.D.

A runny nose, though seemingly trivial, is one of the most common single symptoms the pediatrician manages. This specialist can ill afford to ignore the subtleties of the modest subject. Infants and young children with nasal congestion require careful evaluation and treatment based on accurate diagnosis.

Acute Viral Rhinitis with clear mucinous nasal discharge and mucosal congestion is caused by numerous respiratory tract viral pathogens. It usually runs a benign course lasting only a few days and requires little treatment. Probably the most important aspect of treatment is the education of the young parent. The causation, course, and symptomatic management should be discussed as well as the common complications and criteria for intervention by the physician. Children older than six months are traditionally treated with any of a number of vasoconstrictive and/or antihistamine combination drugs which are of questionable benefit but fortunately are of low toxicity. The list of over-the-counter and prescription drugs of this nature is legion, and so long as the recommended dosage is not exceeded their use is guided only by the art of medicine.

Vasoconstrictive nose drops should be used conservatively for no longer than four to seven days as excessive use may result in paradoxical "rebound" congestion. Commonly used nose drops are Neo-Synephrine 0.25 per cent (0.125 per cent for small infants), Afrin 0.05 per cent, or Otrivin 0.05 per cent—all at a dose of 2 to 4 drops in each nostril every four to six hours (with the exception of Afrin which is given every 12 hours). Pediatric tetrahydrozoline hydrochloride (0.05 per cent) even at the recommended dose has produced lethargy and depression in young infants and should probably be avoided. Oral fluids, room humidification, and aspirin or acetaminophen for low grade fever and myalgia are time-honored.

Infants under three to four months old are obligate nose breathers and often present a special problem when they develop rhinitis; choking episodes may occur and feeding is difficult. Nasal irrigation with 0.9 per cent saline nose drops followed by suction of each naris with a rubber bulb aspirator may be especially helpful before feeding (this procedure should be demonstrated to the parent). Neo-Synephrine nose drops may also be used but sparingly. Stronger local or systemic medications are best avoided in this age group. Due to a realistic increased concern and expense in following infants in this age group with respiratory illness, it is wise to avoid exposure to older children with respiratory tract infections as may occur in day care centers, nurseries, and crowded pediatric waiting rooms.

Bacterial Rhinitis should be suspected when nasal congestion is accompanied by a thick yellow or green purulent discharge. Fever, toxicity, and leukocytosis are often present. Though numerous bacterial pathogens may be implicated, at least two fairly distinct clinical pictures exist. In some infants and children with these findings culture of the discharge often yields a heavy growth of pneumococci. Surprisingly, blood cultures taken on many such children have also been positive for pneumococci, and this combination of findings has become known as "pneumococcal fever." Sick young infants with this entity should be hospitalized and have a septic work-up including a blood culture and studies of cerebrospinal fluid, with parenteral penicillin therapy initiated pending culture results. Older children with purulent rhinitis usually are not as sick and can be managed as outpatients. Treatment with oral penicillin (Pen-Vee K, 50 mg./kg./day in four divided doses with maximum dose of 2 gm./day) or erythromycin (35 to 50 mg./kg./day in four doses with maximum dose of 1 gm./day) frequently results in remarkable improvement within 24 to 48 hours, although antibiotic administration should be continued for at least 7 to 10 days.

A second well described cause of bacterial rhinitis is group A beta hemolytic streptococci. It usually presents in children under six months of age as a persistent (sometimes for weeks) "cold" with a low grade fever. Nasal discharge is watery to slightly serosanguinous; the nares are often cracked and fissured. A culture of the nasal discharge grows an almost pure culture of group A beta hemolytic streptococci and penicillin therapy produces a dramatic cure.

Other causes of bacterial rhinitis include foreign bodies. Sponge rubber from torn furniture cushions is now probably most often encountered; others include paper, small pieces of toys, fruit seeds, small nuts, etc. There is usually a secondary foul-smelling purulent unilateral nasal discharge which upon culture most often grows gram-negative enteric organisms, primarily *Pseudomonas, Proteus, Klebsiella,* or *Escherichia coli*. Removal of the foreign body and drainage usually effects a cure unless there is an associated cellulitis and fever. Appropriate systemic antimicrobial therapy is then indicated. A less common cause of unilateral nasal discharge is nasal diphtheria. If speculum examination of the nares reveals a membranous growth on the mucosa, nasal diphtheria should be considered especially in the individual not immunized. Though less serious than tonsillopharyngeal diphtheria, diphtheria antitoxin (some would withhold this for nasal diphtheria) and penicillin or erythromycin therapy should be initiated immediately pending culture confirmation of the diagnosis.

Allergic Rhinitis may be seasonal or perennial. Seasonal allergic rhinitis is more responsive to therapy as specific allergens are more easily identified. In most cases they may then be eliminated from the child's environment or exposure can be minimized. Air conditioning with high efficiency filtration is often beneficial. Oral antihistamines and nasal decongestants usually help control symptoms. Nasal aerosol dexamethasone (Decadron Turbinaire) frequently produces dramatic results but should be used with caution for only a short period of time and in a highly controlled dosage, since systemic absorption of this drug by this route is significant. If seasonal allergic rhinitis cannot be controlled with these measures, skin testing and hyposensitization against demonstrated offending inhalant allergens should be undertaken. Hyposensitization against food allergens is of no proven benefit; identified food allergens simply are eliminated from the diet.

Perennial allergic rhinitis is less responsive to treatment. The child with watery nasal discharge and puffy eyelids, often wiping his nose upward with his hand (the allergic salute) can be an exasperating problem to manage. When no inhalant allergen can be identified, a broad based approach is recommended. In addition to air conditioning, all possible inhalant irritants should be removed. The child should have a Dacron pillow and his mattress should be enclosed in an air-tight plastic casing. Lint, dust, mold, or mildew from soiled fabric toys, rugs, carpets, and draperies should be eliminated; house plants and pet animal danders should be ruled out. Rarely (in some young infants with apparent persistent perennial rhinitis) a change from cow's milk to a soy bean milk formula has produced dramatic relief. The child with perennial allergic rhinitis without demonstrated specific inhalant allergens by skin testing rarely, if at all, responds to nonspecific hyposensitization with allergens such as mold or house dust. Long-term antihistamine therapy may be helpful in the management of these children but treatment with either nasal aerosol or systemic corticosteroids is definitely to be avoided.

Sinusitis. A simple outpatient regimen is all that is needed to provide significant relief of symptoms and promote resolution. Humidity during sleeping hours is achieved by a mist vaporizer in a closed bedroom. Warm mist or steam inhalation several times a day may produce beneficial drainage. Nose drops administered within the limits described above may relieve acute pressure symptoms; oral antihistamine-decongestant regimens may be helpful for allergic disorders complicated by sinusitis. Associated fever and/or purulent discharge are indications for appropriate antimicrobial therapy.

Staphylococcus aureus, Hemophilus influenzae, the pneumococcus, and less frequently group A beta hemolytic streptococci are the most common bacterial invaders of an obstructed sinus. Ampicillin, 100 mg./kg./day in four divided doses, provides rationale therapy in the uncomplicated case pending culture reports and/or clinical response. If a penicillin-resistant staphylococcus proves to be the primary pathogen, oral cloxacillin or nafcillin in the same dose and interval is substituted. Treatment is continued for at least 7 to 10 days. Surgical drainage is seldom required in uncomplicated sinusitis in children.

Complicated Sinusitis. Sinusitis occurring with bacterial invasion of other tissues is a serious complication. This includes all local extensions such as orbital cellulitis and frontal cellulitis associated with frontal sinusitis (Potts' puffy tumor). Ethmoidal sinusitis with developing orbital cellulitis is particularly difficult to diagnose early in the young child where it may follow an explosive course worthy of the utmost respect. Prompt hospitalization with otolaryngology consultation is indicated with techniques directed toward obtaining culture material, and adequate drainage should follow. High dose intravenous antimicrobial therapy is indicated. It should be directed at the same organisms listed above as the most common agents causing uncomplicated sinusitis. The gravity and rapid progression of these complications warrant the use of a penicillinase-resistant penicillin from the outset such as either nafcillin,* 100 mg./kg./day, or methicillin,* 200 mg./day given intravenously in divided doses at four hour intervals. Since *H. influenzae* organisms are frequently implicated in these serious complications, ampicillin should be given along with nafcillin or methicillin from the outset at a dose of 200 mg./kg./day intravenously in divided doses at four hour intervals. Should cultures of purulent material from the nasopharynx grow ampicillin-resistant *H. influenzae,* intravenous chloramphenical sodium succinate, 100 mg./kg./day in four divided doses, should be substituted for ampicillin.

Retropharyngeal and Lateral Pharyngeal Wall Abscess

JAMES W. BASS, M.D.

Retropharyngeal Abscess occurs primarily in infants and young children of preschool age. In this age group the prevertebral space contains lymphatics and several lymph nodes which drain the nasopharynx. Purulent infection with abscess formation of this space occurs as extension of primary nasopharyngeal infection. On occasion, purulent infection of this space occurs after traumatic perforation of the posterior pharyngeal wall, as may occur when children fall with sticks or other objects in their mouths. The classic presentation is abrupt onset of high fever and signs of upper airway obstruction as well as difficulty in swallowing. Most retropharyngeal abscesses are visible through the oral pharynx as a bulging of the posterior pharyngeal wall. Lateral roentgenograms of the head and neck will substantiate the diagnosis even when the abscess is confined to the posterior nasopharynx or hypopharynx and cannot be seen directly by inspection.

Lateral Pharyngeal Wall Abscess occurs more commonly in school age children frequently as an extension of peritonsillar infection though it may occur in tonsillectomized individuals. Similar symptoms of airway obstruction with pain and difficulty on swallowing occur. Since the abscess is in the lateral wall, the lateral head and neck roentgenogram is not as helpful a diagnostic aid as it is for retropharyngeal abscess.

The major cause of both of these types of abscesses is group A beta hemolytic streptococci followed closely by *Staphylococcus aureus.* Other organisms are less commonly implicated. With either type of infection there is a stage of development when only fullness of the area without frank fluctuant bulging or "pointing" is observed. Signs of airway obstruction or swallowing difficulties are not present. If the disease can be recognized in this "prefluctuant" period, aggressive appropriate antimicrobial therapy alone may resolve the process without the need for surgical drainage. Since nafcillin* is effective against penicillin G-resistant staphylococci and it is almost as effective as penicillin G against group A beta hemolytic streptococci, it would seem prudent to initiate antimicrobial therapy with this drug, 100 mg./kg./day intravenously in divided doses at four hour intervals. This approach has additional support from the observation that presently even non-nosocomial staphylococci are mostly penicillin-resistant. If laboratory reports substantiate the causative organism to be group A beta hemolytic streptococci or penicillin-sensitive staphylococci, treatment should then be changed to intravenous aqueous penicillin G, 100,000 units/kg./day in divided doses at four hour intervals.

In patients presenting with symptoms of overt airway obstruction and difficulties in swallowing, life-threatening abscess formation has probably already developed and provisions for surgical incision and drainage of the abscess should be made immediately. In addition to antimicrobial therapy outlined, team

---

*Manufacturer's precaution: Clinical experience with intravenous use of nafcillin and methicillin in infants and children is too limited to permit specific intravenous dosage recommendations.

---

*Manufacturer's precaution: No clinical experience exists with intravenous use of nafcillin in infants.

management of this patient is best accomplished by the pediatrician, otolaryngologist, and anesthesiologist. Surgical drainage is performed with the patient in the Trendelenberg position with care to provide immediate suctioning should spontaneous rupture occur before surgical drainage is achieved. Should purulent material be aspirated, bronchoscopy with removal by lavage should be performed immediately. In the early postoperative period parenteral analgesics may be needed for pain; in the older more cooperative patient intermittent oral irrigation with warm saline may hasten resolution of the infection. Warm broths or soups are then offered as first feedings as tolerated.

The Tonsil and Adenoid Problem

JAMES W. BASS, M.D.

Tonsillectomy usually with adenoidectomy (T and A) is the most common operation performed upon children in the United States today. It is most likely that many of these are not indicated but it is difficult to establish simple, clear-cut indications for this procedure based upon scientific evidence. A number of retrospective, and several prospective, studies have attempted to better define these indications but none to date have been adequately controlled. More recently there has been a tendency by many physicians to individualize and perform only a tonsillectomy or adenoidectomy when the child's problem appears clearly related to one or the other.

There are only a few criteria for tonsillectomy on which there is general agreement: (1) a peritonsillar abscess, (2) tonsilloadenoidal hypertrophy producing significant obstruction to the pulmonary outflow with developing cor pulmonale, (3) persistent diphtheria carrier state, and (4) suspected tonsillar malignancy. The most debated criteria is chronic (or frequently recurrent) tonsillitis. There is no proof that the child with frequently recurring tonsillitis, who clears completely between bouts, is benefited by tonsillectomy. Nor is the child benefited who has only chronic cryptic exudates on his tonsils. The diagnosis of chronic tonsillitis seems appropriate when the child is sickly, has otherwise unexplained bouts of low grade fever, and has longstanding anterior cervical lymphadenopathy with pus repeatedly expressible from the tonsillar crypts. Removal of the tonsils in such children has on many occasions produced dramatic improvement. It

is this gray area that requires the most objective clinical judgment.

Adenoidectomy without tonsillectomy has become a generally accepted procedure when enlarged adenoids can be shown to obstruct the eustachian tube, playing a role in causation of recurrent or chronic otitis media. Unfortunately, this is most common in young children (one to four years of age) where the operative risk is high. Limitation of the performance of this procedure to a qualified specialist would seem indicated. In all children with recurrent or chronic otitis media without enlarged adenoids, adenoidectomy has been largely replaced by placement of a polyethylene tube or other device in the eardrum promoting pneumatization and drainage of the middle ear. Results with this procedure have been generally satisfactory. The tubes are often spontaneously extruded after several months to a year or more. Many of these patients have no further chronic problems and the drum heals without incident. However, it should be noted that this approach is not without potential complications. Permanent perforation of the drum, cholesteatoma, and foreign body granuloma have been observed in some patients.

Adenoidectomy is generally agreed to be indicated in children who have enlarged adenoidal tissue (not due to treatable causes such as allergy or infection) and normal nasal breathing is impaired. Mouth breathing is an almost constant feature. If allowed to persist, the child develops a typical "adenoidal facies" with the mouth open, eyes drooping, a nasal quality to the voice, and noisy breathing during sleep. Secondary facial bone developmental abnormalities may result. The profile and frontal facial features may be changed producing a completely avoidable permanent cosmetic injury. The resulting dental malocclusion may require orthodontic treatment. A recently reported condition titled "sleep apnea" may become a recognized criteria for adenoidectomy.

Numerous criteria for tonsillectomy and/or adenoidectomy have been advanced for which there is little or no supporting evidence of benefit. These are compounded by pressure from misinformed parents and account for most unwarranted procedures. There is no evidence that frequent sore throats or recurrent viral respiratory infections are reduced. Although often performed in children who have had three or more attacks of streptococcal pharyngitis in the previous year, there is no evidence that the subsequent incidence of streptococcal pharyngitis in operated individuals is less than in nonoperated comparable controls. Allergic rhinitis is not benefited by removal of the adenoids. Frequent bouts of acute or chronic sinusitis are not benefited except where hypertrophied adenoids block the posterior choana causing nasal secretions to pool and become infected with extension into the sinuses. Children who have had rheumatic fever do not have fewer subsequent episodes after tonsillectomy so long as adequate penicillin prophylaxis is maintained. There is no proven benefit or rationale for tonsillectomy in children who have had acute glomerulonephritis. Exceptionally large tonsils alone are not an indication for removal except in the uncommon specific situation mentioned previously.

A conservative approach is best taken in any discussion on the tonsil and adenoid problem. Tonsillectomy and/or adenoidectomy is still a major surgical procedure with a significant operative morality even today. The parents should have knowledge of these risks before committing their child to surgery. A number of deaths are still reported annually, primarily due to anesthesia or hemorrhage as complications during the procedure. In general, pediatricians are becoming increasingly cautious and more resistant toward recommending a T and A for their patients.

Disorders of the Larynx

EUGENE G. FLAUM, M.D.

The severity of the symptoms in a child with laryngeal obstruction usually dictates the appropriate therapy. A patient with obvious acute epiglottitis should not be sent for x-rays when establishment of an airway (endotracheal tube or bronchoscope) is the reasonable course of action. Medical treatment with drugs such as racemic epinephrine and/or dexamethasone is warranted in many cases of severe laryngotracheobronchitis, but if there is no change in the clinical picture, a change in action must be quickly considered. Endoscopic evaluation may reveal the expected narrowed subglottic airway, but occasionally an unexpected foreign body is found. In short, be aware that the unexpected problem may be the cause of the symptoms.

Neonatal stridor or an abnormal or absent cry is usually the result of a congenital malformation or neurological defect, although tetany due to hypocalcemia may also present in this manner.

Hemangiomata of the glottic or subglottic airway become symptomatic at approximately 2 months of age. Stenoses of the subglottic area may not be noted before 2 to 4 months of age because of the greater need for an increased airway in the growing child, and are usually seen at the time of an upper airway infection with croup-like symptoms. As the infant grows and becomes more active, foreign body aspiration is possible. Acute laryngotracheobronchitis is not usually seen prior to 9 months of age and is more common in the 18 month and older age group. Acute epiglottitis is not commonly seen under 2 years of age and is more common in the 3 to 5 year old age group.

Treatment depends on the severity of the disease. The use of a home vaporizor or bathroom steam and a mucolytic agent such as a glycerol guaiacolate-containing compound (50 to 100 mg. 3 or 4 times a day) is recommended. Never use antihistamines or atropine-like drugs, as they will cause dry, tenacious secretions and increased respiratory distress. Probably over 90 per cent of patients respond to this conservative approach. The child whose symptoms are severe enough to require an emergency room visit may be febrile or mildly dehydrated. Encouragement of oral fluids and the use of antibiotics (ampicillin, 100 to 150 mg./kg./day) should be added to the regimen.

A child in moderate to severe respiratory distress requires further medical treatment. The pulse rate often is 160 beats/minute or more and the respiratory rate in the range of 60 respirations/minute. Racemic epinephrine may be effective if administered by a capable therapist. A mixture of 2.5 per cent racemic epinephrine is diluted 1:8 with water and delivered nebulized by compressor through a face mask. An inexperienced therapist may use an excessive amount of the drug or administer it at unusually high levels in an IPPB machine nebulizer, thus causing catastrophic changes in the cardiovascular system.

Many children exhibit a rebound phenomenon, with increased stridor following a period of so-called improvement. I advise a period of post-treatment observation of at least one hour prior to considering discharge from the emergency facility. The sicker child should be admitted to the hospital for continued therapy and observation. In such a sick child I frequently use dexamethasone. The amounts given do not follow a set pattern. Because of its quick breakdown following intravenous or intramuscular administration, up to 4 mg. (average dose between 2 and 3 mg.) has been given as an initial dose in children under 1 year of age. Repeated doses and amounts (1 to 2 mg./6 hr.) are dictated by the severity of the signs and symptoms. Sedatives must not be used.

If the child continues to tire and becomes more stridulous, an artificial airway is established following endoscopic evaluation of the larynx. Because of the narrowed subglottic airway, I believe that a tracheostomy is the better choice, as an endotracheal tube may cause increased local tissue reaction. Continued application of mist with oxygen concentrations up to 40 per cent is recommended. Intravenous antibiotics and fluids should be used until oral intake is sufficient. The period of hospitalization following tracheostomy is usually 6 to 7 days, with the patient being extubated on about the fourth or fifth day.

As soon as the diagnosis of acute epiglottitis is made, consultation with an otolaryngologist and an anesthesiologist should be quickly carried out. An individual not trained as an endoscopist should not traumatize the child while attempting to examine the epiglottis, as laryngospasm may ensue and possibly worsen the respiratory distress. An injection of dexamethasone may stabilize the patient long enough to get to the operating room safely. A child who is more comfortable sitting up, in moderate stridor, drooling, and febrile must be considered to have epiglottitis, and time wasted (such as in x-ray department) may lead to an untoward result.

Various centers throughout the country differ regarding tracheostomy versus intubation as the treatment of choice. The child who is intubated has to be sedated for the three days or so that the tube is in place; the tracheostomized child is awake and active during the 4 or 5 days in which the tube is in place. If excellent 24-hour in-house coverage by a pediatric anesthesiologist is readily available, intubation may be considered. The antibiotic of choice is ampicillin, 150 mg./kg./24 hrs. The cephalosporins are recommended if the patient is sensitive to penicillin. Once again, there is no place for decongestants in treatment, and since the trachea is usually normal, the use of mucolytic agents or mist is less important.

Acute epiglottitis and severe laryngotracheobronchitis are the only laryngeal infections which necessitate emergency therapy. Acute laryngitis may be either of allergic or of viral etiology. Mist, voice rest, and a mild cough mixture is probably sufficient for less severe cases. Antihistamines should be avoided in children under 8 years of age because respiratory obstruction may occur with an increase in thickened secretions.

Hemangiomata of the glottic or subglottic airway are treated differently in various parts of the world. Low dosage irradiation, sclerosing agents, and cryotherapy have been used. The wait-and-see attitude with a tracheostomy

tube in place is frequently recommended. I believe a safe method to be use of corticosteroids in the acute period when respiratory distress is the greatest (at about 2 to 3 months of age). Prednisone, 60 mg./m²/24 hrs. in divided doses, is recommended until stridor decreases, and then the dosage is gradually increased to a maintenance dose of about 5 mg. of prednisone every other day. These low doses can be given up to 6 months or more without causing changes in growth pattern. If there is exacerbation of stridor with associated upper respiratory infection, the dose may be increased until recovery occurs; it may then be lowered to maintenance levels.

With myasthenia gravis there may be generalized weakness as well as stridor and aspiration. The treatment is that of myasthenia gravis (see p. 459).

Other laryngeal disorders (such as clefts, webs, paresis, cysts, laryngomalacia, stenoses) are diagnosed by endoscopy, and management is at the discretion of the endoscopist.

Croup Syndrome

(Acute Epiglottitis and Laryngotracheobronchitis)

SAMUEL T. GIAMMONA, M.D.

Croup or croup-like syndrome is a clinical term used by physicians to describe obstruction, inflammation or infection of the structures of the upper respiratory tract affecting the laryngeal area. This includes clinical problems that may extend from the pharynx to the larger bronchial divisions. Each of the disorders producing croup should be more precisely defined to denote site of the disorder and causative agent if known, in order to plan definitive rational therapy.

The most important life-threatening type of acute upper airway obstruction is epiglottitis, most often due to *Hemophilus influenzae* type B infection, which if not properly diagnosed and treated may result in death in a short period of time. The onset of supraglottic croupiness and stridor due to epiglottitis is usually abrupt with rapid progression over a few hours with fever, sore throat, dysphonia, dysphasia, drooling and progressive signs of air hunger (dyspnea), with marked irritability and apprehensiveness. Immediate differentiation from subglottic or glottic inflammation is essential and yet procedures which involve directly observing these structures are fraught with the danger of producing acute total obstruction.

Anterior, posterior, and lateral x-ray projections of the neck during inspiration have proved to be the most reliable alternate method of examination by demonstrating swelling of the epiglottis and aryepiglottic folds and/or ballooning of hypopharynx with normal appearing larynx and subglottic trachea. Direct visualization by cautious depression of tongue or indirect laryngoscopy of a greatly enlarged fiery, cherry-red epiglottis is confirmatory, but should only be attempted by personnel capable of providing immediate intubation and respiratory resuscitation if this should prove necessary. All children with supraglottic obstruction must be hospitalized.

The most important therapeutic measure in supraglottic obstruction, once properly diagnosed, is determination of whether an airway is needed immediately. Because of many deaths and increased morbidity in many centers with only observation, many physicians recommend immediate establishment of an airway in all children with epiglottitis as soon as the diagnosis is confirmed. If so, either a nasotracheal intubation or tracheostomy can be used for 3 or 4 days until symptoms and signs abate. There are now many documented reports of excellent results using nasotracheal intubation and, currently, if expert staff is available, nasotracheal intubation with a properly sized, noncuffed, plastic tube would be recommended as the preferred method of maintaining airway patency. Alternatively, direct endotracheal intubation by the oral route has been found effective. The institution of a tracheostomy, after direct intubation, is felt by others to be the choice procedure. The risks (which appear to be equivalent) that these procedures may produce long-term complications, such as subglottic stenosis, are extremely small. In certain hospital environments with highly skilled pediatricians, nurses, surgeons, anesthesiologists and respiratory therapists, some children may be prudently followed without airway intervention, but the risk of sudden fulminating complete obstruction is always present, especially in the first 12 hours after admission.

Other supportive therapy includes meticulous handling of airway secretion by periodic use of sterile tracheal suction, frequent changes in position with postural drainage and the use of cold water nebulization (aerosol) to maintain airway humidity and to liquefy secretions. Intravenous fluid therapy will often be required to keep the child hydrated and free of acidosis. Maintenance fluids can be given at a rate of 120 to 140 cc./100 cal. metabolized with maintenance sodium (3 mEq./100 cal.) and potassium (3 mEq./100 cal.). Antibiotic therapy should be started immediately with ampicillin, 300 to 400 mg./kg./day,* and chloramphenicol sodium succinate, 100 mg./kg./day, given by the intravenous route to treat the probable *H. influenzae* B organism. When *H. influenzae* B is cultured from blood or directly from supraglottic secretions, sensitivity studies are needed to determine if beta-lactamase production is present, which indicates that the organism is ampicillin-resistant.

There is no proven therapeutic value to adding steroids, adrenergic, antihistaminic or sedative drugs to the regimen. Relief of obstruction always results in cessation of anxiety and irritability, which are indications of hypoxia and/or hypercapnia and not indications for sedative drugs.

Subglottic obstruction or acute laryngotracheobronchitis is most commonly a viral infection (chiefly the para-influenza-myxoviruses group) resulting in edema of subglottic folds, vocal cord attachment, upper trachea and/or lower bronchial tree. This edema leads to inspiratory stridor and barking, raspy cough, most often occurring suddenly in the young child with mild coryza symptoms, in the evening after going to sleep. Suprasternal and supraclavicular inspiratory retraction without tachypnea may be noted. This may be associated with signs or symptoms of hypoxemia and hypercapnia, depending on degree of obstruction and extent of disease; but in general, there is slow progression of the disease without increasing respiratory rate or signs of bronchial inflammation, parenchymal consolidation or lung collapse.

In the mildly affected child, a change of environment to one with increased humidity and hot or cold air may be beneficial. At home, sitting the child on the lap of a parent in the bathroom with a hot shower running may provide relief. In the hospital treatment room setting, the use of nebulized racemic epinephrine has been found to provide temporary, acute relief in some but not all children. This is administered as 2.5 per cent racemic epinephrine (Vaponefrin) diluted 1:8 with water by a face mask aerosol. It may be repeated in 30 minutes if significant improvement was shown by first administration. In evaluating its usefulness it is

---

*This dosage of ampicillin is higher than that recommended by the manufacturer but has been found to be safe and effective.

clear that it in no way shortens the duration of the disease or reduces the number of children whose disease may progress to a degree of airway obstruction requiring intubation or tracheostomy.

If the clinical status dictates that inpatient status is indicated, the child should be kept in high humidity (usually a mist tent with cold water nebulizer), and diagnostic procedures should be minimized with gentle handling of child by parent and by all personnel. Close careful observation with adequate oral hydration may be all that is required.

Antibiotic therapy is almost never indicated unless the clinical status suggests a rare bacterial origin of the disorder, or secondary infection is confirmed by blood or tracheal cultures. There is no documented evidence of the usefulness of steroid therapy or any other drugs in this disorder, except that subemetic doses of syrup of ipecac (1 ml. per year of age) may reduce mild laryngospasm in a home situation. It should never be used in severe cases. One must never forget that these children may progress to respiratory failure, and in most children the use of arterial blood gas analysis will enable the physician to decide more appropriately that hypercapnia or hypoxemia has developed, requiring airway intervention or supplemental oxygen. Judgment of the degree of hypoventilation on a clinical basis often is not only inaccurate but is a hazardous assumption, so that close monitoring of arterial blood gas analysis is needed. Absolute signs for establishment of an artificial airway are cyanosis and/or apneic episodes, increasing fatigue with pallor, restlessness and increasing or decreasing pulse rate, and an arterial blood gas with a pH less than 7.2 P_{CO_2} greater than 50 to 60 mm. Hg and/or P_{O_2} below 70 mm. Hg with supplemental inspired oxygen greater than 80 per cent.

In all children presenting with signs of upper airway disease, the possibility of foreign body aspiration must never be forgotten. If clinical progression is atypical or unsatisfactory, diagnostic examinations for foreign body aspiration (fluoroscopy, laryngoscopy or bronchoscopy) should be carried out immediately.

In children with measles, a form of severe croup has occasionally been encountered that may require therapeutic intervention as outlined above. Rarely, diphtheritic laryngitis has been encountered in a susceptible population. Tumors or congenital lesions, such as hemangioendothelioma or laryngeal polyps, intrinsically or by external compression may narrow the upper airway as they grow in size, but these are exceedingly rare causes of croup.

Foreign Bodies in the Air Passages

WERNER CHASIN, M.D.

Foreign bodies in the respiratory passages are seen most commonly in children between the ages of 14 months to 6 years. They may lodge in the hypopharynx, larynx, trachea, or bronchi. The severity of the obstructive symptoms depends on four factors: the size of the foreign body relative to the size of the lumen in which it is impacted; the shape of the object which determines whether the obstruction is partial or total; the site at which the foreign body is lodged, since an object located in the distal portion of one of the major bronchi causes relatively few obstructive symptoms; and the degree of inflammatory swelling which the foreign substance incites in the mucosa. For example, the oil in a peanut is particularly irritating.

All foreign bodies of the air passages require endoscopic removal. The presence of a foreign body should be suspected in any child with respiratory signs and symptoms which are unusually persistent or recurrent.

The assessment of a child with a known or suspected foreign body should include the following radiographic studies: a lateral x-ray of the neck taken during inspiration if possible; an anteroposterior chest x-ray taken during both inspiration and expiration; and a lateral film of the chest. Fluoroscopic study of the chest may also be useful to study air-trapping and mediastinal shifting during respiration in very young children and in instances wherein the foreign body is not radiopaque.

The plans for removal of foreign objects include the following considerations. If the child is not in severe distress due to a high impaction of the foreign body, the urgency to remove the substance is not great and the procedure can be safely delayed for hours or more. A maximum attempt should be made to obtain an exact replica of the foreign body so that the optimal foreign-body removal forceps can be chosen. There exists a broad array of such forceps and each instrument is designed for an object of a specific shape and size. The endoscopic procedure is best performed in the operating room at a center which has the personnel, equipment, and experience required for the removal of such foreign bodies.

The endoscopic removal is performed either with or without general anesthesia depending upon the location of the foreign body. In either case an experienced pediatric anesthesiologist should be in attendance. Objects which are lodged in the hypopharynx or larynx are removed without anesthesia so that the object is not accidentally dislodged or inhaled and so that the child retains an active cough reflex. Foreign objects which are located in the trachea or bronchi are usually best removed with the child under general anesthesia. Endotracheal intubation is not employed, both because this maneuver may dislocate the foreign body and because the laryngeal lumen of a child is too small to accommodate both a tube and a bronchoscope. Anesthesia is first administered by mask and consists of nitrous oxide, halothane, and oxygen. The subsequent anesthesia and ventilation are carried out either by means of the Sanders venturi apparatus which is attached to the bronchoscope or by means of intermittent bag-compression via the ventilating arm of the bronchoscope.

The foreign body is extracted by one of a variety of endoscopic maneuvers depending on the type and size of foreign body. Some objects may be grasped with the appropriate forceps and removed through the bronchoscope. Others, which are too large, may have to be grasped and pulled up to the distal opening of the scope and then removed as a trailing object by removing the endoscope and forceps holding onto the object as a unit.

If the foreign substance in a bronchus cannot be visualized or safely grasped because of edema of the mucosa proximal to the object, it may be best to discontinue the procedure. The child is treated for 24 to 48 hours with a systemic corticosteroid and antibiotic to reduce the mucosal edema and facilitate the subsequent procedure to remove the object. An occasional foreign object which has migrated or has been pushed into a peripheral bronchus will have to be removed in the x-ray department under the guidance of the biplane fluoroscope.

Bronchopulmonary Dysplasia

LEO STERN, M.D.

This condition, which is also known as chronic respirator lung disease, was initially described as a separate entity in infants with hyaline membrane disease who were subjected to respirator therapy on positive pressure respirators with the use of endotracheal tubes and who were in high oxygen concentrations at the same time. Although its original namegivers attributed the disease to the toxic effects of oxygen, there has been considerable controversy regarding not only the etiology of the disease but the role of oxygen in its produc-

tion. Thus a similar picture can be seen in adults on positive pressure respirators, but neither newborn infants nor adults have ever been clearly described with the syndrome when negative pressure ventilation (which does not require an endotracheal tube) is utilized.

The currently accepted views can probably be best synthesized in ascribing the major component of the production of the condition to both the endotracheal tube and the time over which positive pressure ventilation takes place. If oxygen is indeed responsible for some of the changes, then it is not oxygen alone but the oxygen superimposed on an already damaged lung which appears to be involved. In this connection it is interesting to note that the newer techniques of assisted ventilation in hyaline membrane disease, whereby low pressures and low rates are being substituted for the previous high pressure, high rate methods, have yielded a much lesser incidence of this complication.

Clinically the disease supervenes on respirator management with chronic respiratory insufficiency and is supported by radiographic findings which reveal areas of fibrosis, compensatory emphysema with evidence of scarring and diffuse septal thickening on pathologic examination. The picture is often complicated by suppurative changes resulting from additional superimposed bacterial infections, and in the end stages changes not unlike bronchiectasis in adults have been noted. It is generally assumed that all of these changes are secondary to both the initial disease and the ventilation process, although the possibility has been raised that some patients may have a hereditary or genetic predisposition to their development. In this connection there have been several studies of alpha-1-antitrypsin activity in both patients and their parents, but the results as yet do not warrant any such assumptions.

Treatment is primarily the avoidance or minimization of those factors which lead to its occurrence. Thus since the disease seems to be related to the use of intratracheal tubes, the proponents of negative pressure ventilation have used this as an argument for substitution of negative as opposed to positive pressure methods when feasible. Earlier use of continuous distending pressure (either positively or negatively applied) appears to reduce the need for more drastic ventilator therapy and may also reduce the inspired oxygen concentration in initial management of the infant with hyaline membrane disease. In this connection there have been some recent experimental reports of the preventive effect of vitamin E on the development of oxygen toxicity in the lung, but such therapy remains experimental.

Antibiotics should be given where suppurative complications have occurred, and graded use of oxygen with frequent blood gas monitoring is indicated to control difficulties with oxygenation. Corticosteroids are of no use in the disease and are clearly contraindicated where suppurative complications (such as pneumonia or abscess formation) have already occurred. Cor pulmonale with right heart failure, which supervenes in the extreme cases, may need to be managed with digitalis and diuretics.

The outcome for infants with this disease appears to be changing rather rapidly, as the incidence and severity of the complications become less with improved methods and techniques of assisted ventilation. In the initial reports, there was a high mortality incidence from chronic pulmonary infection and respiratory failure within the first year of life. Happily, such cases are now becoming fewer, but still occur. Together with respiratory failure, the cause of death in several instances has been at least in part cardiac owing to the occurrence of cor pulmonale and right heart failure. In many children who ultimately recover functionally, there is evidence of residual fibrosis and cyst formation in the lungs. Although functionally these appear to be of little importance in childhood, the question as to the long-term prognosis for the possibility of chronic pulmonary disease in the survivors cannot be answered. It would seem advisable to maintain a cautious outlook for these children in this regard.

Neonatal Atelectasis

LEO STERN, M.D.

Atelectasis, or collapse of one or more lobes or portions thereof, is not an uncommon finding in the newborn. Its most characteristic diffuse form is idiopathic respiratory distress syndrome (hyaline membrane disease). In this condition atelectasis is diffuse and is the direct result of an inactivation or lack of surfactant preventing stability of the smaller alveoli in expiration. Although major areas of collapse of contiguous alveoli are unusual, in hyaline membrane disease when the alveoli begin to collapse in expiration, the smaller ones which collapse quicker tend to empty into the larger ones rapidly because of the reduced resistance to air flow in the larger still-open alveoli. Under such circumstances, it is possible to arrive finally at the complete "white-out" lung, which has not only the radiographic appearance but the functional physiologic findings of more or less total intrinsic atelectasis of both lungs.

Atelectasis, which is due to a failure to initially expand the lungs, secondary either to birth asphyxia or central nervous system trauma as well as to peripheral nerve injuries (phrenic or diaphragmatic paralysis), can be present from birth on, since the initial opening pressure to expand the lungs with the first breath is much higher than the pressure required to sustain the expansion with subsequent breaths. Unless hyaline membrane disease is present, lungs once expanded do not collapse totally from such neurologic causes, although individual lobes may do so with prolonged immobility in the supine position.

Extrinsic compression on bronchi will lead to collapse of the alveolar segment distal to the pressure. These include neurenteric cysts and dermoids, diaphragmatic hernias, and the pressure collapse from a pneumothorax. The latter two are readily apparent on characteristic x-ray appearance, but smaller extrinsic lesions may not be visible radiographically, as the collapsed area obscures them and the true cause becomes apparent only on surgical exploration.

Intrinsic obstruction of a bronchus, which would lead to collapse of its distal alveolar segment with resorption of the air in it, needs to be either total, or partial and moveable. Total obstruction, such as from an atretic segment or webs, can also be mimicked by the aspiration of pus, blood, mucus, or meconium, thus allowing for atelectatic episodes in pneumonias, aspiration of blood or pulmonary hemorrhage, excessive mucus production in tracheoesophageal fistulas, and meconium aspiration. The latter, however, tends to give partially fixed rather than partially moveable obstruction because of the stickiness of the meconium with the resultant physiologic production of segmental emphysema and pneumothorax rather than alveolar collapse.

This difference is critically important to appreciate in the etiologic production of collapse from partial obstructions, which, if they are moveable, ultimately act as a ball-value arrangement, with collapse of the distal alveoli as the descending material is inhaled further down the bronchial tree. In contrast, the partially fixed obstruction tends to permit progressive emphysematous overfilling of the distal alveoli as the bronchi constrict in expiration around the unmoveable obstruction and will ultimately yield interstitial emphysema, pneumomediastinum and pneumothorax (see below under Meconium Aspiration).

Pathophysiologically, what is produced is both restriction of alveolar surface with subsequent respiratory exchange difficulty and disturbances in blood gases. The continued perfusion of collapsed areas of a lung is, however, the primary contributor to the oxygenation defect. Therefore, mere attempts at ventilation will not restore the low Pao_2 unless either the circulation to the collapsed area can be altered or that portion of the lung which has collapsed can be re-expanded.

Treatment consists of removal of the obstructing agent by needle aspiration, or drainage via a chest tube in the case of a pneumothorax. In the latter, it should be emphasized that since the infant is lying on his back the tube should be placed anteriorly, as the free air will rise to the anterior portion of the chest. Treatment of the underlying pneumonia with appropriate antibiotics, and supportive therapy with intravenous fluids and electrolytes, should be undertaken where this is the identifiable cause. Aspiration of maternal blood requires relatively little therapy, but pulmonary hemorrhage of the intrinsic variety may require blood replacement to substitute for the losses which occur from the circulating hemoglobin pool.

Bronchoscopy in the newborn infant is an extremely difficult procedure and unlikely to be productive, in that the agents one is trying to reach tend to be much more distal than the bronchoscope can reach. Moreover, with meconium, the fixity to the bronchial wall is sufficiently difficult to make anything other than aspiration of the meconium from the upper air passages highly unlikely.

Since newborn infants do not cough very well, physiotherapy gently but expertly applied to the chest wall with frequent positioning may be helpful in relieving obstruction. The use of high humidity is contraindicated, particularly in incubators, since there is no evidence that any further lysis of secretions occurs, and the propensity for multiplication of bacterial organisms in the humidified atmosphere is exceedingly high.

Disturbances in blood gases can be corrected by either increasing the inspired oxygen concentration to raise a low Pao_2 or increasing ventilation to reduce a high $Paco_2$. The disturbances are often due to the diffuse underlying disease, but even where no disease exists, it is extremely unlikely that a low Po_2 is the result of the collapse itself as opposed to the continued perfusion of the collapsed area. While increasing the inspired oxygen concentration may be helpful, complete correction will occur only once the lobe or that part of it responsible is re-expanded.

The long-term prognosis for any or all of these causes is good, depending upon correction of the underlying cause. All of the intrinsically aspirated agents which can cause collapse tend to resorb and leave no residua in the lungs. In diaphragmatic hernia, the lung on the side on which the hernia occurs (usually the left) tends to be hypoplastic from prolonged in utero compression, but the long-term prognosis is nonetheless good since there is progressive postnatal growth and multiplication of alveoli, so that adequate pulmonary function and appearance on the affected side is usually apparent by the first or second year of life.

Congenital Lobar Emphysema

LEO STERN, M.D.

Although the major manifestations are those of progressive and emphysematous enlargement of the lobe of the lung with progressive collapse of noninvolved areas due to compression and ultimate shifting of the mediastinum, the basic underlying cause of this condition resides not in the alveolar tissue itself but in the bronchus leading to it. Congenital lobar emphysema is effectively the result of a weakening of the cartilaginous support of the bronchus (bronchomalacia), such that there is inability to evacuate air during expiration and progressive emphysematous enlargement of the lobe distal to the abnormality. The resultant disturbances in blood gases are due to reduction of available gas exchange alveolar surface as well as to the continued perfusion of nongas-exchanging areas with the resultant production of a large physiologic right-to-left shunt.

Treatment is surgical removal of the involved lobe, since it is rarely possible to correct the underlying bronchial defect in any meaningful way. The long-term prognosis for overall pulmonary function under such circumstances is excellent.

Meconium Aspiration

LEO STERN, M.D.

Although the aspiration of meconium may present primarily as a pulmonary problem, it is inseparable from the birth asphyxia which is now generally agreed to be invariably associated with its occurrence. The majority of perinatal mortality classifications have shifted away from permitting meconium aspiration to be classified with the other pulmonary causes of perinatal mortality and morbidity, and have requested that they be classified together with the other causes of birth asphyxia. Such a change in the positioning of the disease is likely to become universal by 1980 with the adoption of the new World Health Organization classification by sufficient member states.

The asphyxia may be either intrapartum or occur just at the time of birth. Forewarning can often be obtained through the appearance of meconium (especially in a vertex presentation) in the amniotic fluid either on amnioscopy or at rupture of the membranes just prior to delivery. It is assumed that under asphyxiating conditions, increased gastrointestinal movements result in the expulsion of meconium into the amniotic fluid. It is not known for certain whether the breathing movements which the fetus makes can actually inhale meconium into the lungs prior to birth, but there is clear evidence that the swallowing movements permit presence of large amounts of meconium in the upper pharynx and airways, which can subsequently be inhaled with the initial respiratory efforts of the newborn.

The aspiration of the meconium into the smaller bronchi and alveoli results in both alveolar and bronchiolar obstruction, although the major brunt of such obstruction mechanically is probably at the level of the smaller bronchioles, resulting in an obstructive bronchitis which may give enormous elevations of $Paco_2$. In addition, the tendency of the meconium to stick to the bronchial walls yields a partially fixed type of obstruction with alveolar overdistention as the alveoli tend to overexpand in expiration. Pathophysiologically there is both a loss of effective ventilating surface and continued perfusion of underventilated areas of the lung, resulting in the reduction in arterial oxygen tension and in the extreme elevation of Pco_2 in the blood.

Treatment consists primarily of the avoidance of peripartum asphyxia and its minimization where it can be detected either clinically or through intrapartum fetal monitoring. An infant born with meconium in the amniotic fluid or suspected of being asphyxiated should be removed from the delivery table immediately, since there may be further expulsion of meconium directly onto the infant's face and mouth if he is left lying in the vicinity. Attempts at aspiration of the meconium from the upper pharynx and airways seem profitable, although it is not possible to reach areas lower down. Bronchoscopy is contraindicated because of the difficulty in its performance in the newborn and the sticky nature of the meconium, which makes it extremely difficult to remove from the bronchial passages by such means.

Although meconium has been reported experimentally as favoring the growth of bacteria, there is no evidence that the meconium itself is unsterile, and antibiotics are probably not indicated for the meconium alone. However, many of these cases occur after prolonged rupture of the membranes, and under those circumstances antibiotic coverage has been advocated in view of the high incidence of infection, which increases as the time of membrane rupture begins to exceed 24 to 48 hours.

The use of corticosteroids is highly controversial, but there is no real evidence that it is helpful. If corticosteroids are being used, they will not "break up" the meconium or hasten its disappearance. They are used solely for their anti-inflammatory propensity, since meconium is highly irritating and results in secondary edema and swelling of the bronchial walls around it. The dosage used should be high, 100 to 200 mg. of hydrocortisone initially, given preferably within the first three hours and certainly no later than 6 hours after birth, and sharply tapered and discontinued by 48 to 72 hours of age.

Severe respiratory failure has been known to occur and may require management with oxygen and a ventilator. If assisted ventilation is necessary, continuous distending pressure either in the form of continuous positive airway pressure or continuous negative pressure is *contraindicated* since the alveoli are already overdistended and any further pressure will tend to increase an already high $Paco_2$. The underlying central nervous system injury may often predominate either as clinical respiratory difficulty or as convulsions and cerebral edema. The seizures should be managed with anticonvulsant therapy, and the cerebral edema may require mannitol for its treatment and control.

Complications include alveolar collapse and pneumothorax. Pneumothorax is by far more common, and a variety of extrapulmonary air complications ranging from interstitial emphysema to pneumomediastinum with or without pneumothorax commonly occur. On occasion, subcutaneous emphysema, pneumopericardium, and pneumoperitoneum have been reported as well.

The major reason for the occurrence of extrapulmonary air collections stems from the partially fixed obstructive nature of meconium in the smaller bronchi with resultant overdistention in expiration as the bronchi narrow in the expiratory phase of the respiratory cycle. Unlike hyaline membrane disease, however, where the reduced compliance of the lung makes it relatively resistant to large shifts when collapse occurs, no protective mechanism exists in the meconium aspiration syndrome, and there is a greater tendency toward large tension pneumothoraces, which need to be treated rapidly and aggressively by either needle aspiration or tube drainage of the air. If continued air collection occurs in the form of a bronchopleural fistula, the constant application of a small amount of negative pressure to the drainage tube may help.

In the long term, no residua are to be expected from meconium aspiration. Because the disease is associated with birth asphyxia, the prognosis for intellectual and developmental outcome represents the major problem. Thus the outcome can be predicted easily for the lung irrespective of how bad the situation may look radiographically, since the meconium will invariably be removed from the lung without any apparent permanent damage. It is the central nervous system, which has sustained a greater or lesser degree of injury at the same time, for which the prognosis must for obvious reasons be more guarded.

Pneumomediastinum and Pneumothorax

ARNOLD C. G. PLATZKER, M.D.

Pneumomediastinum. Pneumomediastinum per se rarely if ever causes symptoms, but it should alert the physician that there is sufficient pulmonary disease and air trapping to cause alveolar rupture. Any attempt to "drain" the mediastinum is bound to fail since it is not a discrete well-bounded space like the pleural cavity. Rather, it is filled with areolar tissue that assumes the appearance of an air-filled sponge when air is present. No single drainage tract or tube can begin to drain these multiple loculations. The mediastinal space is unbounded at its upper and lower ends so that no pressure will build up within it. Rather, the air will dissect freely into the neck or less commonly through the esophageal or caval hiatus into the retroperitoneum or leaves of the mesentery.

Pneumomediastinum in the infant with hyaline membrane disease or aspiration pneumonitis needs no specific therapy but warns the clinician that the infant is at risk to develop pneumothorax. It may occasionally be difficult to differentiate pneumomediastinum from pneumopericardium, a much less common but potentially lethal complication. When the air is within the pericardial sac in any quantity, the chest roentgenogram will have a sharp radiolucent line between the diaphragmatic portion of the pericardium and the inferior border of the heart.

In the older child, bronchiolitis, acute asthma, pertussis, cystic fibrosis, and bronchial rupture from cough or trauma may cause pneumomediastinum. If the history is suggestive, an esophageal perforation by penetration, blunt trauma or ingested foreign body must also be considered. Esophageal perforations are usually accompanied by mediastinal widening or air-fluid levels within the mediastinum and can be further studied by a contrast roentgenographic examination of the esophagus using dilute Gastrografin. Esophageal perforations may require both surgical (such as mediastinal drainage and closure of esophageal perforation) and medical intervention (such as antibiotic treatment); thus immediate surgical consultation is necessary.

Pneumothorax. Any infant who has pneumomediastinum should be followed closely for development of pneumothorax since the same air-trapping conditions predispose to both problems. Any sudden deterioration of an infant with lung disease should be considered as resulting from a tension pneumothorax until this has been ruled out. When present, the distended "pigeon-breasted" chest, shifted cardiac apical beat, tympanitic percussion note, tracheal shift and absent breath sounds can lead to swift and accurate diagnosis. When these findings are associated with a sudden drop in the systolic blood pressure and a narrowing of the pulse pressure, the clinical suspicion of a tension pneumothorax is further supported. If the patient has continuous electrocardiographic monitoring, with the onset of the pneumothorax, there may be a sudden decrease in QRS voltage when air enters the pleural space. Recently, transillumination of the chest with a very bright fiberoptic light (Medgeneral, 10800 Lyndale Avenue, Minneapolis, Minnesota) has been shown to be helpful in confirming the presence and location of a pneumothorax. The presence of air in the pleural space will cause a large area of transillumination around the site of the pneumothorax. Frequently, however, pneumothorax defies clinical diagnosis in a tiny infant receiving positive pressure ventilation. Often the most rewarding radiographic examination is the cross-table lateral with the patient in supine position. As air accumulates in the chest, the lung settles posteriorly, and its anterior border forms a sharp line behind and roughly parallel to the sternum.

When a pneumothorax is suspected clinically, the chest can be safely aspirated with a needle to confirm the presence of free air in the pleural space. If air is found, a chest tube should be placed as soon as possible, especially if the infant is receiving positive pressure ventilation. While preparing for the tube thoracostomy, the pneumothorax can be evacuated with a 23-gauge scalp vein needle (connected to a three-way stopcock and a 20 ml. syringe). The needle is placed in the pleural space at a point adjacent to the site of the tube thoracostomy. The thoracocentesis can be continued until the thoracostomy tube is placed.

For the tube thoracostomy in infants we prefer a No. 12 French Argyle catheter with a self-contained stylet. These tubes have an end hole and three side holes, so that they are unlikely to plug with clot or fibrin. The outermost hole is at the radiopaque stripe, so that the position of the last hole in relationship to the chest wall can be determined by routine chest roentgenogram.

We prefer to place the tube in either the second intercostal space slightly lateral to the midclavicular line or in the third or fourth intercostal space in the anterior axillary line. With more medial placement there is risk of injuring the large infant thymus or of the tube's ending up in the mediastinum. Placement of the tube requires aseptic technique to reduce the risk of infection. After the skin has been prepared with povidone-iodine solution, we infiltrate the skin and the chest wall over the pectoral fold with 0.5 per cent lidocaine, we make a 5 mm. skin incision and place a purse-string suture encircling the incision.

The intercostal space is defined and spread with the tips of a small hemostat. We insert the chest tube, controlling the depth of the initial penetration through the chest wall by grasping the tube and trocar firmly between the thumb and forefinger about 1.5 cm. from the tip and pressing the tip firmly into the intercostal space. When the pleural space is entered, the trocar is then pulled back slightly so that the sharp tip is protected by the tube, and then the entire unit is directed superiorly and introduced until the last hole is well within the chest. In penetrating the chest wall it is essential to direct the trocar toward the center of the pleural space. Failure to do so may result in the tube's being placed subcutaneously or coiled up in the axilla without entering the pleural space.

Once the thoracostomy tube is placed, the purse-string suture should be pulled firmly around the thoracostomy tube and tied; the tube is sutured securely and supported by tape applied to the tube and the skin, after it has been coated with tincture of benzoin. Vaseline gauze is applied to further seal the thoracostomy tube site and a small sterile dressing is applied. Immediately after placement of the thoracostomy tube, a chest roentgenogram is essential to check the position of the chest tube and completeness of lung expansion.

Water seal drainage is usually adequate to re-expand the lung completely, but if there still is residual pneumothorax or a large air leak, negative pressure up to -15 cm. H_2O may be required. The visceral pleura must be held tightly against the parietal pleura to seal an air leak.

An alternate method of tube placement is that of making a 5 mm. skin incision, placing a purse-string suture, and plunging the tip of a hemostat into the pleural space. When there is an audible escape of air, the tip of the chest tube is forced through the same hole while grasped in a hemostat. The chest tube is connected to water seal drainage and the purse-string suture is tightened and tied. The chest tube is left in place until the lung is completely expanded and no air has leaked for 12 or more hours. The chest is then clamped for several hours, and a chest roentgenogram is obtained. The chest tube is removed if the roentgenogram does not reveal free pleural air.

An otherwise healthy infant occasionally will develop a small pneumothorax. He may have mild tachypnea, but no significant respiratory distress, even though a chest roentgenogram reveals a small pneumothorax. Chernick and Avery have shown that this pneumothorax will absorb rapidly if the infant is placed in an oxygen-enriched atmosphere. A small pneumothorax in the premature infant must not be treated with high oxygen exposure since there is a risk of producing retrolental fibroplasia in premature infants if arterial Po_2 remains elevated for even a short period of time.

In the older child, pneumothorax may occur spontaneously or can complicate asthmatic attacks, bronchiolitis, cystic fibrosis, staphylococcal pneumonia, and lung tumors. Most of these conditions require insertion of a chest tube to re-expand the lung until the leak is sealed. Spontaneous pneumothorax can occur in adolescent females associated with menses. Idiopathic spontaneous pneumothorax is uncommon in small children but occurs frequently in teenagers. A significant number of these teenagers have recurrent pneumothorax because of congenital subpleural blebs occurring usually in the apical segments of the upper lobes. After several episodes these patients should be considered for resection or oversewing of apical pulmonary blebs which are invariably present.

Pleurodesis obtained by injecting quinacrine through a chest tube has been tried with success in some patients. In teenagers 100 mg. of quinacrine in 15 ml. of normal saline is instilled into the pleural space through the thoracostomy tube using sterile technique on four successive days. Following each instillation of quinacrine into the pleural space, the patient should be repositioned to allow for uniform distribution of the quinacrine in the pleural space.

Traumatic pneumothorax in children may occur without broken ribs since the child's ribs are so flexible. In general, all chest injuries sufficiently severe to produce pneumothorax require drainage with a chest tube.

Cysts of the Lung

ARNOLD C. G. PLATZKER, M.D.

Lung cysts are rare. They may arise from major airways or from dysplasia, hypoplasia, or infection of small airways or parenchyma (such as staphylococcal pneumonia). When these disorders present in the newborn period, they often provoke a surgical emergency.

Lung cysts may arise following severe respiratory distress syndrome as a part of the post-respiratory distress syndrome, lung disease, or bronchopulmonary dysplasia. In this instance, the treatment is usually medical. On rare occasions, one of the multiple cystic lesions may expand to cause compression atelectasis of adjacent lung tissue and a shift to the mediastinum to the contralateral side of the chest. Oxygen therapy is indicated to relieve the hypoxia which might result, though the inspired oxygen concentration should be limited to provide the infant with an arterial oxygen tension of 50 to 60 torr. Supportive therapy should include aerosolized bronchodilators (for bronchospasm), chest percussion and postural drainage, maintenance of an adequate oxygen-carrying capacity by packed red blood cell transfusion, and provision of adequate calories (by gastric or parenteral nutrition) to allow for growth.

Occasionally diuretic therapy is required when this disease is severe and complicated by interstitial pulmonary edema. Although furosemide, 1 mg./kg./dose, is the drug of choice initially, we prefer to use chlorothiazide, 20 mg./kg./day, given as one-half the daily dose every 12 hours, when chronic diuretic therapy is required. Frequent determinations of electrolytes and often supplemental potassium and/or Aldactone therapy are required to reduce and replace salt losses when infants are receiving long-term diuretic therapy. In infants with the most severe manifestations of bronchopulmonary dysplasia, digitalis therapy is indicated when cardiac failure complicates the chronic respiratory failure. On rare occasions, massive enlargement of a single lung cyst will produce deepening respiratory distress, and then surgical resection of the single cyst should be considered.

Pneumatoceles resulting from pulmonary infection may rupture during the acute stages of the infection, causing a pneumothorax or pyopneumothorax, requiring tube thoracostomy for drainage and re-expansion of the lung. If the cysts do not rupture during the acute phase of the pneumonitis, they usually regress completely as the pulmonary infection responds to medical management.

Cystic lesions originating from the trachea or major bronchi require surgical resection. Cystic adenomatous malformation of the lung in the neonate and small infant is a rapidly progressive disease and should be treated as a surgical emergency by resection of the affected lobe. Lobar emphysema, on the other hand, most often produces only mild to moderate respiratory distress and may be treated conservatively by medical management as described above, unless the respiratory symptoms become markedly severe. If surgical resection of the emphysematous lung is not required, the emphysematous changes resolve over a period of years, and often by the teens or early adulthood the chest roentgenogram no longer reveals any localized hyperinflation of the lung.

Hyperlucency of a single lung or entire lobe may result from absence or dysplasia of one or more tracheal or bronchial cartilaginous rings. Therefore, before considering surgery to resect a hyperlucent lung, it may be advisable to perform an air or high contrast cineroentgenographic study of the airway to determine whether the overinflation is due to collapse of a major bronchus from congenital absence or dysplasia of one or more cartilaginous rings. This form of airway abnormality leads to ball valve airway obstruction and hyperinflation of the affected lung. Although there are reports of successful resection of the abnormal cartilaginous rings and reanastomosis of the bronchus, we prefer to manage these infants medically, as already described. We reserve surgery for infants not responding to the medical management.

Tumors of the Chest

ARNOLD C. G. PLATZKER, M.D.

Primary tumors of the lung are exceedingly rare. By far the most common malignancy affecting the lung is the metastatic spread of a primary malignancy from another organ. However, tumors affecting the lung, even when histologically benign, can cause severe respiratory distress by compression of airways or lung parenchyma. Thus they must receive prompt diagnosis and treatment.

In addition to the initial anterior-posterior and lateral chest roentgenogram to determine the localization of the tumor, diagnostic studies may include tomograms of the area of the lung in which the tumor is located to determine the size and relation of the tumor to the airway and major blood vessels. When a highly vascular tumor of the lung is suspected, a radioisotopic perfusion study of the lung may confirm this suspicion. Ventilation lung scanning identifies whether the tumor is causing airway obstruction. When a nonvascular tumor is situated in or impinges on the lumen of a large airway, bronchoscopy allows visualization and biopsy of the tumor, and resection when it is polypoid. Tomography of the lung or bronchography may, in some instances, help outline a tumor impinging on or located in airways too small to be seen with bronchoscopy.

Current treatment of lung tumors frequently includes utilization of surgical, chemotherapeutic, and radiotherapeutic modalities together. Except in the instance of solitary or superficial metastatic tumors of the lung, which may be treated surgically, most metastatic tumors of the lung are treated either by chemotherapy or radiotherapy or both.

Benign tumors of the lung, such as a bronchial adenoma or a papilloma of the bronchus, are treated by surgical resection of the tumor. Vascular tumors of the lung are occasionally treated surgically, but may also be treated with radiotherapy or corticosteroids.

Mediastinal tumors are rare, but of great clinical importance due to their proximity in the mediastinum to the major airways. Untreated, these tumors frequently lead to severe major airway compression and life-threatening respiratory distress.

Therapeutically and prognostically, the mediastinal tumors can be divided into two major groups. Anterior and middle mediastinal lesions consist mainly of cystic and vascular lesions, such as thymoma or thymic cysts, teratoma, retrosternal thyroid or thyroglossal duct cyst, vascular ring lesions encircling the trachea and esophagus, blood vessel tumors, neurofibromatosis, and esophageal diverticula, duplication, and benign tumors. Tumors also invade the anterior mediastinum by metastatic spread. The most common of these tumors are non-Hodgkin's lymphomas, Hodgkin's disease, and T-cell leukemias. Frequently these tumors have been diagnosed prior to their spread to the anterior mediastinum. The therapy for these lesions may include corticosteroids, chemotherapeutic agents and radiotherapy.

Posterior mediastinal lesions are frequently malignant neurogenic tumors with a serious prognosis, and rarely lateral meningoceles, neurenteric cysts, and bone or cartilaginous tumors. The diagnostic studies required to define the masses are similar to those employed in diagnosing primary and secondary lung tumors. Therapy of the anterior mediastinal tumors is usually surgical as most are discrete and resectable, whereas posterior mediastinal tumors, frequently malignant, often require combined surgical, chemotherapeutic or radiotherapeutic management. In the small infant, when the anterior mediastinal mass is suspected of being a large thymus, one to two days treatment with prednisone, 1 mg./kg., will cause temporary involution if the mass is thymus, differentiating the mass from nonthymic tissue, often making it possible to avoid surgical intervention.

Bronchitis

DANIEL H. WISEMAN, M.D.

Bronchitis is a common disorder characterized by the combination of cough and excessive bronchial secretions which usually lasts from 1 to 4 weeks. This diagnosis is not tenable when the findings are only those of a brief cold with cough. Many episodes of bronchitis occur following a viral respiratory infection which has produced bronchial mucosal damage and needs time to heal. Of greater concern are those cases in which bronchitis is the initial event in a serious or chronic pulmonary disease. Over the years this concern apparently has been communicated to parents because many parents become extraordinarily distressed when their child has a severe or persistent cough. Their concern only increases when their child receives less therapy than they expected. It is particularly difficult to convince such people that cough is a defense mechanism and not a disease.

Therapeutic Evaluation. Management of bronchitis begins during the examination of the child as the physician discovers and discloses the major features of the illness. Most cases occur in otherwise healthy children and the parents are usually relieved to know this. Useful clues that help predict a prolonged, recurrent or complicated course may present with the initial episode. Infants with a past history of prematurity, respiratory distress syndrome, bronchiolitis or pneumonia have more frequent respiratory illnesses during their first two to three years of life. One fourth to one third of infants who have bronchiolitis or pneumonia in their first year of life will have another severe lower respiratory infection in the subsequent 24 months. Whether these recurrences are due to some injury occurring during the "initial" illness or due to a primary predilection is not always clear.

A history of more than the expected 6 to 8 respiratory illnesses per year should prompt a search for underlying allergies or high levels of exposure to respiratory pathogens (large families, day care centers, new enrollment in school, and so on). Chronic and recurrent bronchitis is often seen in mentally retarded children (especially Down's syndrome) and in children with pharyngeal incoordination and other causes of recurrent aspiration. A sudden onset of cough and choking should make the physician suspect a foreign body aspiration. Recurrent or persistent cough in an older child or adolescent should prompt questions regarding the use of tobacco and, when found, be followed by a full and frank discussion of the effects of tobacco.

On examination, sneezing, nasal rubbing (itching), wheezy cough, and pale, edematous nasal mucous membranes suggest respiratory allergy. The nasal sinuses should be palpated (for tenderness) and sometimes transilluminated or x-rayed because of the frequent association of sinusitis and postnasal drip with bronchitis. Often the only evidence of excessive bronchial secretions is the presence of a few pulmonary rhonchi or scattered wheezes, as infants and children rarely raise their sputum. The chest usually sounds "clear." If there are more impressive findings or any other doubts, chest x-rays are obtained to rule out pneumonia, atelectasis, foreign body or cardiac enlargement.

Once it is clear that the child has uncomplicated bronchitis, the physician should take the time to explain the importance of cough in clearing the airways, to discuss the dangers in suppressing cough, and to justify withholding antibiotics when there is no evidence of bacterial infection. Parents are more likely to accept this approach when they observe that the physician is knowledgable of the nature of their child's condition, sincerely concerned for his well being, and available to them to follow the patient to a satisfactory resolution of the illness.

Antihistamines, Decongestants and Antitussives. These medicines are widely used for cough and bronchitis despite the lack of evidence of their value and their potentials for counterproductive side effects. All possible single and multiple drug combinations are available either over-the-counter or by prescription. In the early phases of an episode of allergic bronchitis, antihistamines may decrease the symptoms but they should not be used if the cough persists because they may cause drying of secretions (an anticholinergic effect) and interfere with the ciliary escalator.

The decongestants contained in most "cough medicines" are either alpha-adrenergic stimulants or beta-adrenergic stimulants. Alpha-adrenergic stimulants (such as phenylephrine) cause vasoconstriction and thereby decrease respiratory mucous membrane edema, when present. Beta-adrenergic stimulants (ephedrine, pseudoephedrine, propanolamine, isoproterenol, and so on) are bronchodilators. In high doses they may cause tachycardia, tremulousness, irritability or sleep disturbances.

Narcotic antitussives (codeine, hydrocodone) suppress cough by a direct effect on the medulla and do so at about one-third the dose required to achieve analgesia. However, they can depress respiratory drive (decrease alveolar ventilation) and increase airway resistance (by increasing bronchial muscle tone, a cholinergic effect). Therefore, they should not be prescribed in patients with small airways (infants and small children) or in patients with preexisting chronic airway disease (asthma, chronic bronchitis, crystic fibrosis, etc.). The non-narcotic antitussive dextromethorphan is also effective and much less likely to produce toxic side effects. Antitussives may be useful in the child with a dry (nonproductive), irritating or exhausting cough, but they should be avoided if there is evidence of much mucus because the cough is needed to clear the secretions.

"Mucolytics" and "Expectorants." The only mucolytic or expectorant to receive wide and permanent acceptance is water. The universal recommendation to "take fluids" has several potential benefits. The sick child often refuses to eat solids but will continue to take liquid foods. The increased volume intake ensures that there will be sufficient water to form new secretions, humidify the incoming air and possibly prevent dehydration. Any liquid the child will accept may be given. I do not believe that "milk makes more mucus," rather it coats the mucus already in the pharynx and makes it more obvious. Greater volumes will be ingested if the parents are advised to give relatively small amounts frequently rather than trying to "force fluids." Fluids may also be administered by inhalation; the simplest method is a shower before bedtime. Cold mist nebulizers are widely available for home use but are more helpful for croupy, laryngeal coughs than for the deeper cough of bronchitis.

In children with copious and recurrent accumulations of secretions, it is useful to teach the parents how to do postural drainage, chest percussion and expiratory vibration to assist in mobilizing secretions and augmenting the natural cough.

Antibiotics.   When bronchitis is due to allergic or viral causes, antibiotics are neither useful nor necessary. When associated with streptococcal upper respiratory infection, bacterial otitis media or pneumonia, antibiotics are given for the associated infection. In the absence of these recognized specific bacterial infections, proof that the episode is related to bacterial infection is difficult to obtain. All currently available culture methods (throat culture, expectorated sputum, and tracheal aspiration) require that the specimen be drawn through the oropharynx and, in the process, be mixed with oropharyngeal flora. In spite of these problems, it is best to guide antibiotic therapy by using respiratory tract cultures and to suspect underlying major pulmonary disease when antibiotics seem to be necessary.

Bronchiolitis

ROBERT H. PARROTT, M.D.

Most cases of bronchiolitis are due to viral infection, particularly respiratory syncytial virus (RSV). In the absence of rapid virus diagnostic techniques, a good indication that RSV is likely to be the cause of a case at hand is the occurrence of an excess of bronchiolitis and pneumonia in the community. Especially at such times antibiotics can be avoided, as they have been shown to be of no value in epidemic bronchiolitis.

Management depends upon the severity of bronchiolitis, which can vary from mild tachypnea and wheezing to severe lack of oxygen and death. The infant with mild signs can be observed at home with advice to watch for increase in respiratory rate or distress. In bronchiolitis of increasing severity, hospitalization is indicated. Evidence of excess air in peripheral lung fields on percussion of the chest or chest x-ray confirms the diagnosis. Attention must be given to the potential need for ventilatory assistance; there may be increased functional residual capacity and hypoxemia. Forty per cent humidified oxygen should be administered by tent or by mask and/or nasotracheal tube if necessary to maintain arterial saturation at 80 to 90 per cent. Frequent blood gas measurements are indicated.

Downes' criteria for acute respiratory failure include: decreased to absent inspiratory breath sounds; severe thoracic retraction on inspiration; maximal hyperinflation of the thorax; cyanosis of lips and mucous membranes in 40 per cent oxygen; and decreased to absent response to painful stimuli. Three of these criteria sustained for more than one hour with a Pco_2 of 65 torr or higher indicates respiratory failure and warrants ventilatory assistance. Nasotracheal intubation, neuromuscular blockage with d-tubocurarine and positive pressure ventilation may be necessary for 2 to 9 days.

After initial hydration, maintenance hydration and electrolytes are given intravenously; dehydration is also assessed and corrected. Avoid overhydration. Because of difficulty with breathing and excess respiratory secretions, oral feeding is avoided or limited for the first day or two. Careful suctioning to remove secretions is helpful. Although provision of a highly humidified atmosphere has been popular in recent years, we now feel that this is indicated only if there is evidence of dry upper respiratory secretions which adequate systemic hydration should prevent. There is a danger of bacterial infection with the prolonged use of mist tents. Also, ultrasonic or jet nebulizers must be used with caution because small particles may actually increase airway resistance. Under any condition the child should never be lost from sight because of dense mist.

Occasionally an older infant or child with bronchiolitis may get symptomatic relief from bronchodilators possibly because certain such children are in fact undergoing an initial episode of asthma. If epinephrine (0.01 ml./kg./dose of 1:1000 aqueous solution) seems to give relief and the child does not respond to oxygen and hydration in 18 to 24 hours, we sometimes use intravenous theophylline (12 mg./kg./24 hours in 3 doses over 4 to 5 minutes).

Steroids have not proved helpful in controlled trials.

Many infants with bronchiolitis progress to clinical and roentgenographic signs of pneumonia within a few days as the respiratory distress is alleviated. If fever is protracted and respiratory distress returns, and especially if much airway manipulation, extensive mist therapy or intubation has been necessary, consider the possibility of bacterial superinfection with "hospital" strains of bacteria such as Pseudomonas or *Staphyloccus aureus* or a foreign body.

About 25 per cent of infants who have bronchiolitis requiring hospitalization irrespective of the specific etiology will have at least one episode of asthma subsequently. Presently there is no practical way to distinguish which children will be affected. However, the primary physician should keep this observation in mind in following the infant who has had severe bronchiolitis.

Aspiration Pneumonia

WILLIAM CURTIS ADAMS, M.D.

Treatment of aspiration pneumonia varies, since proper therapy is dictated by the amount and composition of the material aspirated. Prevention is paramount and may be accomplished by educating the public as to the potential hazards of inhaling dangerous substances. An excellent example of prophylaxis is lessening the inhalation of zinc stearate powder by reduced usage and more effective containerization.

The susceptibility for aspiration pneumonia is created by a large number of debilitating conditions, such as prematurity, Guillain-Barré syndrome, poliomyelitis, collagen disease, and congenital abnormalities. Therapy of the traumatized patient resulting in immobilization makes such a patient a prime candidate for developing aspiration pneumonia. No debilitated patient should be fed too rapidly or overfed, and it is imperative that ingestion of oily substances by oral or nasal route be avoided totally. If any compromise of respiratory exchange occurs, respiratory support techniques will reduce the potential danger of aspiration. All infants should be placed on the stomach or right side after every feeding to lessen the chance or regurgitation and aspiration.

Once aspiration occurs, the symptomatology varies with the components and amount of substances inhaled. Symptoms will range from a minor cough to complete respiratory failure. If respirations are severely compromised by excessive foreign bodies lodged in the major airways, bronchoscopy is indicated and may be followed by tracheostomy to permit repeated therapeutic aspiration. If minor symptoms occur, therapy may be as simple as inhalation of air moisturized by a 20 per cent solution of alcohol-water. When administration of intermittent positive pressure breathing is needed, it should be provided with a 20 per cent alcohol-water solution with a 3 to 5 second amnestic pause. This mixture will provide a pH of 6.8 to 7.0, which is within normal range, and will not alter the normal surface tension of the mucous membranes within the air passages. The addition of racemic epinephrine to the mixture will stimulate the escalator activity of the ciliary mucous membrane and will promote production of thin watery secretions.

Careful monitoring of the arterial blood gas provides an excellent guide to the mode of therapy needed to maintain normal pH, CO_2, Po_2, and so on. Postural drainage and enhancement of cough are also important adjuncts to adequate therapy.

Antibiotic therapy is generally reserved for instances of known superimposed infections, especially with petroleum distillate and lipoid aspirations. However, if severe gastric juice aspiration occurs, carbenicillin therapy is indicated for the aerobic and anaerobic gram-negative infection which will follow.

Following hydrocarbon ingestion, both olive oil and saline cathartic should be introduced into the gastrointestinal tract to minimize absorption of the harmful substances and to enhance the excretion of the petroleum distillates.

Children with recurrent esophageal regurgitation are always prime candidates for aspiration. A significant percentage of adults who have developed intrinsic asthma in later years have been shown to have symptomatic hiatal hernias with reflux which probably originated in childhood.

Children with esophageal reflux should be considered for antacid and antireflux (foam) therapy to prevent the various complications of aspiration and reflux. This need is even more evident and apparent in the debilitated and immobilized traumatized patient. The use of pulverized alginic acid–antacid combinations after meals and on retiring may prevent many complications of regurgitations and aspirations. The administration of a pulverized tablet of Gaviscon followed by or mixed with a glass of water may provide this protection.

In summary, the basic principles of therapy remain the same in all types of aspiration pneumonia: respiratory support, removal of foreign material (bronchoscopy) if practical, correction of pH and electrolyte changes, general supportive measures, special measures as applicable to each individual case, that is, correct identification of character and components of ingested material.

Bronchiectasis

HERMAN W. LIPOW, M.D., *and*
DAN K. SEILHEIMER, M.D.

The clinical diagnosis of bronchiectasis implies a child with chronic pulmonary illness whose symptoms include a chronic productive cough. Bronchiectasis literally means widening of the bronchi, but it varies in form, extent, distribution and reversibility. Radiologists divide bronchiectasis into three types based on their bronchographic appearance: cylindrical (tubular), varicose and saccular (cystic).

Cylindrical (tubular) bronchiectasis is characterized by mild uniform dilation of the bronchi and the absence of a normal peripheral tapering pattern. Cylindrical bronchiectasis is extremely common with any bronchial inflammation and is almost always reversible unless the child suffers from a systemic disease that causes bronchial dysfunction. This bronchial change would be better labeled cylindrical *dilatation,* rather than bronchiectasis, and the term bronchiectasis reserved for the two other types, varicose and saccular. Using the term dilatation would alert the clinician to the fact that the patient may have a reversible lesion.

The best example is cylindrical dilatation of the right middle lobe bronchus in the asthmatic child. Because of the geometry of the airway and unfavorable position for gravity drainage, the right middle lobe drains less well than the other lobes. The coupling of difficult bronchial drainage with the increased volume of airway secretions in the asthmatic child results in mucus impaction in the right middle lobe bronchus, distal atelectasis and some dilatation of the bronchus. This happens frequently in asthmatic children, and if a bronchogram is performed at that stage (and we do *not* recommend it), cylindrical dilatation will always be present. Careful follow-up studies reveal almost no evidence that cylindrical dilatation of this origin progresses to varicose or saccular bronchiectasis. There is a great tendency for the right middle lobe bronchus to return to normal diameter with time. Management should be directed toward improving treatment of the asthma, including removal of allergens, regular use of bronchodilators (orally and by aerosol inhalation) and respiratory physiotherapy. Classifying an increased radiodensity in the right middle lobe as a separate syndrome, right middle lobe syndrome, tends to divert attention from the known etiologies and too frequently results in unnecessary surgical removal of the right middle lobe. This usually leaves the basic asthmatic condition unchanged and unimproved. Cylindrical dilatation (bronchiectasis) is never an indication for surgical extirpation in our opinion.

Varicose and saccular (cystic) bronchiectasis refer to grossly dilated bronchi associated with a decreased number of bronchial subdivisions on bronchogram. These patients are usually symptomatic with chronic productive cough. Bronchial changes of this magnitude are only rarely reversible and, depending upon the underlying etiology, remain static or progress to widespread bronchiectasis.

Children with varicose or saccular bronchiectasis usually acquire the disease secondary to a severe bronchial infection that causes a localized destruction of the bronchial segment. This infection may occur fortuitously or may follow an inhaled foreign body or toxic substance. A congenital bronchial anomaly may predispose the area to dilatation and infection. Bronchiectasis after a localized insult tends to remain static and, contrary to some opinions, does not spread to involve other areas of the lung. The occurrence of this localized type of varicose or saccular bronchiectasis as a sequela to pertussis, rubeola or tuberculosis has dropped precipitously over the past 30 years as the incidence of these diseases has declined. Also, the early use of antibiotics in treating bacterial pneumonia may prevent destructive changes in the bronchi.

There are a group of children who have a systemic disease associated with bronchial dysfunction that predisposes them to develop bronchiectasis. The treatment programs for these children require special modifications. The three generalized disease states associated with bronchial dysfunction that are currently recognized as being prone to develop widespread bronchiectasis are cystic fibrosis, Kartagener's syndrome and some of the immunodeficiency diseases. Bronchiectasis in these disorders tends to be progressive, gradually involves both lungs and makes these children, with rare exceptions, unsuitable candidates for a surgical approach to their disease.

Medical treatment of all types of bronchiectasis can be divided into two general categories: respiratory physiotherapy to help remove secretions from the airway and antibiotic treatment to *reduce* the amount of infection in the airway.

Respiratory Physiotherapy. A good program of respiratory physiotherapy is remarkably effective in helping patients clear their lungs of retained secretions. The physical principles of bronchial drainage are simple and have been aptly described as analogous to trying to get "ketchup out of a bottle." By placing the lobe to be drained in the superior position and the corresponding draining bronchus in a gravity dependent position, the patient utilizes gravity to help carry the mucus into a major bronchus. The chest is percussed (clapped with a cupped hand) to loosen the sputum, then vibrated in the same fashion as one shakes the ketchup bottle and at the same time compressed to help with exhalation. Once the mucus approaches a larger airway, cough is spontaneously or volitionally induced, and the mass of sputum is coughed up without difficulty.

For teenagers and young adults living on their own, electrical percussors made by modifying saber saws with rubber padded applicators are available. Although electrical percussors are not as effective as good manual percussion and vibration, they seem a reasonable compromise. Inhaling an aerosol bronchodilator just before starting bronchial drainage may increase the volume of sputum removed, as bronchospasm is present in many patients with bronchiectasis.

Antibiotics. Children with localized bronchiectasis (but without systemic disease associated with bronchial dysfunction) will need periodic treatment with antibiotics for 1 to 2 weeks when they develop respiratory infections. These patients are apt to be infected with *Hemophilus influenzae,* pneumococcus and other common respiratory pathogens, and they will usually respond to ampicillin, penicillin, or cephalexin. There is no need for continuous antibiotic therapy.

This contrasts sharply to patients with systemic disease associated with bronchial dysfunction (cystic fibrosis, immunodeficiency disease and Kartagener's syndrome), who have developed *widespread bronchiectasis* and may need continuous *suppressive* antibiotic therapy. Labeling this prophylactic treatment is incorrect and a contradiction in terms, as these patients usually have a continuous infection of their bronchi. Sputum culture and sensitivity testing should be obtained before selecting an antibiotic. Patients frequently require intensive antibiotic therapy with penicillinase-resistant penicillins, co-trimoxazole, chloramphenicol, tetracycline (if over eight years of age) or intravenous aminoglycosides (gentamicin, tobramycin or amikacin). If their bronchi become colonized with Pseudomonas, these patients probably continue to harbor Pseudomonas in their bronchi for the rest of their lives, despite intensive antibiotic treatment. Even with a continuing program of daily respiratory physiotherapy, many of these patients will have exacerbation of bronchial infection whenever suppressive antibiotic therapy is discontinued.

Acceptance of the need for continuous suppressive antibiotic therapy is difficult for physicians who have had limited experience in treating patients suffering from systemic diseases associated with bronchial dysfunction. Discontinuing long-term suppressive anti-

biotics in patients with far advanced bronchiectasis is frequently associated with an increase in bronchial suppuration within a period of one to two weeks. The need for continuous suppressive antibiotics is greatest during the winter months when viral respiratory infections are frequent and trigger exacerbations of the chronic bacterial infection. Often antibiotics can be stopped during the summertime, if a vigorous respiratory physiotherapy program is continued.

The most common error in patient management is caused by the failure of physicians to separate bronchiectatic patients into one of the two groups described above. One group, with localized destruction of a bronchus, has static well localized bronchiectasis, whereas the other group, with a systemic disease process associated with bronchial dysfunction, tends to develop progressive bronchial involvement. Surgical extirpation of an area of localized bronchiectasis (usually in a lower lobe), causing repeated pulmonary infection in spite of medical therapy, should be curative for the patient with focal bronchiectasis and no systemic disease. The indications for surgical removal of an infected lobe in patients with cystic fibrosis, immunodeficiency disease or Kartagener's syndrome are life-threatening gross hemoptysis, definitely localized to a specific lobe, or a child with persistent fever and toxicity who has far advanced bronchiectasis localized to one lobe, while the remaining lung is still relatively uninvolved.

Atelectasis

DAN K. SEILHEIMER, M.D., *and* HERMAN W. LIPOW, M.D.

Atelectasis refers to collapse of part of a lung following loss of air from previously aerated alveoli. Atelectasis is common and may be due to one or more of many factors. Since successful therapy may depend upon correction of each contributing factor, a thorough search to identify all possible causes should be made.

Complete obstruction of an airway from any cause may lead to resorption of the gas distal to the occlusion. Therapy depends upon removing the obstruction. The most common cause of airway obstruction in children is the accumulation of mucus which has not been cleared from a bronchus by the normal mucociliary "escalator" and coughing. This mucus accumulation causes lung collapse in cystic fibrosis, asthma and bronchial infections. Therapy is directed both at the underlying disorder (bronchodilators for asthma, antibiotics for infections) and at the abnormal mucus transport by instituting respiratory physiotherapy (postural drainage, percussion and vibration of the chest).

Airway secretions accumulate and atelectasis may develop whenever the normal cough reflex is severely diminished. The cough reflex is suppressed by narcotics, anesthetics and many diffuse central nervous system diseases. Weakness or paralysis of the trunk muscles, particularly the abdominal muscles necessary for the forced expiration of coughing, may cause mucus retention. Ineffective coughing may also occur after extensive thoracic or abdominal surgery. The patient avoids increasing incisional pain by shallow respirations and suppressing his normal cough reflex.

Whenever retained secretions cause atelectasis, it is important to maintain an optimal state of hydration to prevent the patient's bronchial mucus from becoming dry and inspissated. Postural drainage and percussion help remove accumulated secretions. The patient's position should be changed (side to back to side) every two hours to prevent pooling of mucus in a dependent segment of lung. When atelectasis occurs in an upper lobe, the patient should be placed in a sitting position for several hours a day to aid in draining mucus from the affected airway. Children with dysfunction of their central nervous system often have pharyngeal dysfunction and tend to aspirate secretions and food. When atelectasis occurs, aspiration should be suspected and, if present, the airway protected.

Patients who have an ineffective cough can be aided by a parent, nurse or therapist to expel their airway secretions by a maneuver known as "assisted coughing." The assistant spreads his hands over the supine patient's abdomen. After the patient inspires maximally, he closes his glottis and performs a vigorous Valsalva maneuver. Simultaneously the assistant pushes firmly, but gently, on the abdomen to further increase the intra-abdominal pressure. When the child opens his glottis a more forceful cough is produced than could have been achieved without assistance. This may be repeated several times until secretions are cleared. It can be done after postural drainage or any time the patient feels the need to cough.

Extrinsic compression of airways by enlarged mediastinal structures may also lead to atelectasis. Radiographs of the hilar area may reveal enlarged lymph nodes compressing the contiguous bronchus. Appropriate antibiotics for infection (tuberculosis) or chemotherapy for malignant lymphadenopathy (lymphoma,

leukemia) should relieve the compression. Mediastinal tumors (bronchogenic cyst, teratoma) or aberrant vessels which compress airways usually require surgical correction. The lung parenchyma may become atelectatic when it is compressed by pleural effusion, hyperinflated adjacent lung or ascites. Removing the compressing mass allows the lung to reexpand.

The physiologic derangement produced by atelectasis is hypoxemia. Blood passing through the atelectatic area is exposed to airless alveoli and fails to become fully saturated with oxygen. If the atelectatic area is large, serious hypoxemia and cyanosis will develop from the large intrapulmonary shunt. Reexpansion of the collapsed lung is necessary for normal gas exchange. Supplemental humidified oxygen will not correct hypoxemia due to shunting, but it will improve oxygenation in areas of the lung where partially obstructed airways cause ventilation-perfusion inequality.

Occasionally, massive atelectasis with severe hypoxemia and respiratory insufficiency makes mechanical ventilation necessary. Since the intubated patient cannot cough, aggressive respiratory physiotherapy and endotracheal suctioning (after instilling a small amount of normal saline) are necessary to ensure continued removal of bronchial secretions.

Since medical management has become successful in removing airway secretions, the need for bronchoscopy has decreased. However, occasionally a patient does not improve with medical management and requires bronchoscopy. The acutely ill child with hypoxemia who fails to improve after a few days of receiving vigorous respiratory physiotherapy is a bronchoscopy candidate. If such a child is deteriorating clinically, the need for bronchoscopy is urgent.

When a carefully obtained history does not suggest the possibility of foreign body aspiration (which would argue for early bronchoscopy), we do not recommend immediate bronchoscopy for patients without acute respiratory symptoms. We continue a hospital or home respiratory program (two to three times daily) for several weeks. If the atelectasis persists in spite of aggressive medical care, elective bronchoscopy is performed to lavage mucus plugs. Rarely this will uncover an unsuspected foreign body, bronchial adenoma or airway stenosis.

A persistently atelectatic area along the medial basal area of a lung suggests a sequestered segment. Sequestered lobes are congenitally anomalous portions of lung that often have no connection with the tracheobronchial tree and are therefore airless. Absence of an airway predisposes these segments to infection. Their arterial supply usually comes from the aorta; venous drainage is to the pulmonary or azygous veins. The systemic arterial to pulmonary venous connection may be large. Consequently, blood shunting through a pulmonary sequestration may place an additional load on the left ventricle.

Pulmonary sequestrations are classified anatomically, and certain types have been associated with particular complications. However, these associations are not absolute, and we base our therapy upon the presence of complications rather than upon anatomical classifications. Definitive therapy is surgical excision. This is indicated for sequestered lobes which are chronically or recurrently infected or when the volume of blood shunted through the sequestration gives rise to evidence of cardiac strain. The surgeon removing the sequestered lung must be aware that its systemic arteries may arise in the abdomen, penetrate the diaphragm and enter the under surface of the sequestration. When these arteries are divided, they retract through the diaphragm into the abdomen. If they are not ligated before division, exsanguination is likely.

Emphysema

MONTGOMERY C. HART, M.D.

Idiopathic Pulmonary Emphysema. A common problem in adults, idiopathic pulmonary emphysema is virtually never observed in childhood. Irreversible emphysema of any type is seldom seen in the pediatric age group except rarely as a complication of cystic fibrosis, severe intractable asthma or severe bronchiectasis. When pulmonary emphysema does occur in children, it may be a localized finding secondary to localized obstruction, either intraluminal (foreign body, mucous plug, secretions, infections, granuloma) or extraluminal (such as hilar or mediastinal lymphadenopathy) or as a generalized finding resulting from widespread inflammatory disease (such as tuberculosis). Therapy is aimed at the cause, utilizing bronchoscopy, bronchography, angiography, antibiotic chemotherapy and possibly surgery.

Congenital Lobar Emphysema. Congenital lobar emphysema, once considered rare, is recognized more frequently at present. In one-half of the cases, symptoms occur in the first few days of life, in the other half before four months of age. The condition almost always occurs in the upper or middle lobes and is usually associated with bronchial cartilage defects. Definition, morphologic aspects and pathogenesis are controversial and incompletely defined. The entity is here defined to exclude lobar enlargement secondary to such phenomena as secretions, plugs, foreign bodies and the like, all successfully reversible by removal of the cause.

Treatment of congenital lobar emphysema depends on the severity of the condition. When symptoms are moderately severe to life-threatening, surgical removal of the affected lobe(s) is indicated. Operative mortality is low (7 per cent). Conservative therapy has been associated with a mortality rate of 50 per cent and persisting emphysema in 75 per cent of the remaining survivors. When symptoms are mild or absent, conservative therapy may be safely undertaken, though some persisting hyperinflation of the affected lobe(s) occurs.

Pulmonary Interstitial Emphysema. This condition represents a form of pulmonary air leak that is being increasingly recognized clinically, especially in newborn infants, though it has been reported in older children and even in adults. It occurs more commonly in preterm than in term infants and is especially frequent in infants with hyaline membrane disease, particularly those requiring ventilatory support. Pathogenesis begins with alveolar rupture usually near the hilum. Following this alveolar leak, interstitial air tracks along the peribronchial and perivascular spaces, usually leading to pneumothorax, pneumomediastinum or more rarely to pneumoperitoneum or pneumopericardium. Less frequently, air embolism into the vascular system and even into the cerebral ventricular system has been reported.

Increasingly, persistence of interstitial emphysema, usually unilateral, is being recognized. This condition interferes both with pulmonary blood flow and ventilation in the affected lung. Death usually ensues when the emphysema is severe and bilateral, and frequently occurs even when the disease is unilateral. Treatment is controversial. Surgical management (lobectomy or pneumonectomy) is subject to considerable risk, yet severity and mortality are so high, that aggressive management is appropriate. Conservative medical management has been recommended and includes: vigorous physical therapy including instillation of saline, suctioning, vibration, percussion and positioning to favor secretion drainage from the affected side; recurrent intermittent usage of 100 per cent oxygen in an attempt to favor reabsorption of the interstitial gas; and selective intubation of the mainstem bronchus of the unaffected lung for periods of one to several days with careful ventilation of only that lung, anticipating reabsorption of the interstitial gas from the affected lung. It is reasonable to consider any or all of the above modalities given the high morbidity and mortality of the disorder. Should conservative measures fail, lobectomy or pneumonectomy of the affected tissue may then need to be undertaken. Recently, when the disorder is unilateral, incising or stripping the visceral pleura of the affected lung has been shown to be successful. Again, when emphysema is generalized and bilateral, no therapeutic mode has been successful.

Bullous Emphysema (Pneumatoceles). These cyst-like air pockets are usually noted following infectious processes (such as staphylococcal pneumonia, Klebsiella, tuberculosis). No symptoms are generally present and no therapy is required. Resolution is usually spontaneous in weeks. Treatment is necessary only if rupture leads to pulmonary air leak.

Subcutaneous Emphysema. This disorder, associated with tracking of gas into the subcutaneous area of the chest, neck and head usually follows disease, injury, or surgery involving the respiratory tract. It may also occur secondary to hyaline membrane disease in infants, in association with other pulmonary air leaks, with injury or surgery to the esophagus or trachea, including tracheostomy, or as a complication of cystic fibrosis, pertussis, asthma, bronchiolitis, foreign bodies, and so on. Treatment is aimed first at the primary disease including evacuation of any large pulmonary air leaks. Symptoms occur with surprising rarity, and the gas usually resolves quickly. When symptoms do occur, it is often in a patient on a ventilator, and may be associated with compression of the structures in the neck. Treatment with a supraclavicular surgical window leads to dramatic relief in these patients.

Pulmonary Edema

BURTON W. FINK, M.D.

Treatment of pulmonary edema should be directed at both immediate relief of the acute symptoms and correction of the basic cause.

If the cause is increased capillary pressure, as seen in acute heart failure or obstructed pulmonary venous return, efforts are required to reduce that pressure. Digitalis will increase cardiac output and re-direct fluid into the systemic circulation and is administered according to the dosage schedule in the chapter on congestive heart failure (p. 137), but there will be a time delay prior to reaching effective drug levels. Lasix, 1.0 mg./kg., will draw fluid from the lungs by raising colloid osmotic pressure. This fluid then will be eliminated through the kidneys. Tourniquets in the form of blood pressure cuffs, with pressures raised between arterial and venous levels, placed on three extremities and rotated every 15 minutes, will immediately decrease venous return. Positioning the patient with the head elevated will tend to pool blood in the lower half of the body and decrease venous return. Venisection will immediately decrease blood volume. Morphine sulfate, 0.1 to 0.2 mg./kg. intramuscularly, has been found to be effective but the mechanism of action remains obscure. Aminophylline, 3 to 4 mg./kg. intravenously slowly over 30 minutes, can be useful. Although ganglionic blocking agents such as hexamethonium or phenoxybenzamine have been used in adults to dilate peripheral arterioles, there is no experience with their use in pediatrics. If all medical modalities fail to alleviate the acute symptoms, positive pressure respiration will reduce venous return by increasing intrathoracic pressure, will improve blood gas exchange by distending collapsed alveoli and will counteract forces favoring filtration into the lungs.

If the edema is due to an acute decrease in intrathoracic pressure as seen in massive atelectasis, the treatment is directed to raising the intrathoracic pressure by guaranteeing a clear airway and the use of positive pressure respiration.

If the edema is secondary to increased capillary permeability which may result from trauma, pneumonia, inhalation of gaseous or chemical poisons, following central nervous system damage, or after near-drowning, the therapeutic challenges are increased. One can only utilize the treatments already discussed combined with overall supportive care until the capillaries heal.

Pulmonary Emboli

DANIEL A. PIETRO, M.D.,
G. V. R. K. SHARMA, M.D.,
ARTHUR A. SASAHARA, M.D.,
ALFRED F. PARISI, M.D.,
and KEVIN M. McINTYRE, M.D.

Although pulmonary embolism in adults is a common and extensively investigated condition, it is considered rare in children, the pediatric literature containing only a few small series and case reports. Several investigators, however, consider it to be significantly more prevalent than most clinicians realize. As in the adult population, a high index of suspicion is clearly needed for early diagnosis and prompt treatment.

Predisposing risk factors in the pediatric age group include local infection (especially of lower extremity), sepsis, trauma, immobilization, surgery, intravenous and umbilical catheterization, and hypercoagulable states (such as sickle cell disease, marked dehydration, and malignancy). The most common sources for pulmonary emboli in adults remain the lower extremity and pelvis; although these appear to be the most frequent areas of concern in children, other sources for venous thrombosis have been identified. These include nasopharyngeal, cerebral and umbilical veins, ventriculoatrial shunts, congenital heart disease, and congestive cardiomyopathy.

Deep venous thrombosis of the lower extremity (DVT) in children is considered infrequent. In a retrospective study, lower extremity venous thrombosis was reported in 28 patients over 20 years (1.2 per 10,000 hospital admissions). Three of these had evidence of pulmonary emboli. Another retrospective study in England documented 36 cases of venous thrombosis, 10 of which were DVT, the remainder including renal, cerebral, axillary, jugular, and umbilical vein thrombosis. Pulmonary embolism from these other sources has also been described.

Diagnosis of DVT in children is rarely entertained except when the evidence is striking. The typical signs and symptoms include increased diameter of one extremity, local tenderness and warmth, a positive Homan's sign (calf tenderness with dorsiflexion of foot) and a palpable venous cord. This set of findings represents only the most dramatic presentation. In contrast, cases have been reported which demonstrated venous thrombosis two days after operation in children who had no signs or symptoms. These patients had thrombosis of the femoral and popliteal veins, which has been shown to be far more likely to result in pulmonary embolism in the adult population than thrombosis of smaller distal veins. Clinical manifestations can be found in less than 50 per cent of adult cases; while such data are not yet available in the pediatric age group, it must be remembered that DVT can occur without symptoms and the initial presentation may be insidious or even a pulmonary embolus.

The clinical presentation of pulmonary embolus may be highly suggestive or may be nonspecific. The diagnosis is easily entertained if pleuritic pain, pleural friction rub, and hemoptysis occur acutely. Many of the nonspecific manifestations of pulmonary embolism, including dyspnea, tachycardia, tachypnea, fever, and pulmonary infiltrate, however, are common to a number of cardiopulmonary disorders, viz., pneumonia, atelectasis, and congestive heart failure. When these latter are considered in this clinical setting, pulmonary embolus should be included in the differential diagnosis. A poorly resolving pneumonia, in retrospect, may have been an unsuspected pulmonary embolus.

TREATMENT

Experience with therapeutic interventions in pulmonary embolic disease in the pediatric population is almost nonexistent. As in the adult, prevention is the most profitable treatment. This requires careful attention to the risk factors considered above. Early diagnosis and treatment are required when prevention has failed. Anticoagulation is the mainstay of treatment and should be instituted immediately after the diagnosis is made. Bed rest, sedation, and oxygen also play important roles in therapy.

Anticoagulation, by the very nature of the patient population, carries certain risks. Careful monitoring of coagulation parameters may help reduce the incidence of bleeding complications. The following is the currently accepted technique of anticoagulation employed in the pediatric population for thromboembolic disease.

Heparin sodium is the anticoagulant of choice and should be administered intravenously in a bolus or continuous infusion. Continuous intravenous infusion is preferred because the marked fluctuations in clotting parameters seen with the bolus administration technique are avoided. The partial thromboplastin time (PTT) immediately after administration of a bolus of heparin approaches infinity and gradually returns toward normal. Adequate heparinization is achieved when the PTT at 4 hours after the last dose is 2 to 2.5 times control. Heparin is administered every 4 hours and regulated on the basis of the partial thromboplastin time.

The usual dosage of heparin in the intermittent technique is 50 units/kg. of intravenous bolus followed by 100 units/kg. every 4 hours. The continuous infusion technique requires an accurate delivery system with an infusion pump. The initial dose is 50 units/kg. of intravenous bolus followed by a maintenance infusion of 20,000 units/m²/24 hours. The PTT can be evaluated after 2 to 3 hours of infusion and any time thereafter. The infusion rate should be adjusted to maintain a PTT or 2 to

2.5 times control. Clinical response dictates the duration of heparin therapy. A minimum of 5 to 7 days is considered the time required for fresh thrombus to adhere to vessel walls and, accordingly, the minimum duration of heparin therapy. Fixation of thrombus is felt to reduce the incidence of further embolic episodes during this stage of therapy.

Long-term oral anticoagulation in the adult population reduces the incidence of recurrent deep venous thrombosis and pulmonary embolic disease. Whether similar practice in children is useful in reducing recurrent venous thromboembolism is purely conjectural. Based on our experience in adults, however, anticoagulation for a period of 3 to 6 months may reduce the incidence of recurrence. This must be balanced against the risk of anticoagulation in a young, active, and often accident prone patient population. Another important factor to be considered is whether or not the predisposing factor is self-limited or chronic. In the latter case, continuing anticoagulation may be advisable. Effective oral anticoagulation can be readily achieved with warfarin sodium.

Warfarin is a vitamin K antagonist and depresses the production of clotting factors by the liver. These include factors VII, II, IX, and X. Depression of these factors takes 36 to 48 hours and, therefore, the anticoagulant effect will not be reflected until this time has elapsed. Warfarin treatment should be initiated while the patient is maintained on heparin, 2 to 3 days before discontinuation of heparin, so that a hiatus in anticoagulation is avoided. Warfarin should be administered in 10 to 20 mg. doses for 2 days followed by a maintenance dose of 2.5 to 10 mg. each day. The maintenance dose should be adjusted 1 to 2 mg. every other day based on the results of the Quick one-stage prothrombin time, which should be maintained at 2 to 2.5 times control. It is important to note that heparin also affects the prothrombin time; a final adjustment of warfarin dosage is therefore needed when heparin is discontinued. After stabilization, prothrombin times should be performed every 2 to 3 weeks and dosage adjusted accordingly. Overdosage of warfarin may be reversed with vitamin K and/or fresh frozen plasma.

Drug interactions are common with warfarin, and the level of anticoagulation can be altered as a result. The more commonly used drugs which increase anticoagulation includes salicylates, quinidine, and sulfonamides. Reduction in the effectiveness of warfarin is caused by vitamin K, barbiturates, and meprobamate, among others. Surgical therapy for pulmonary emboli in adults includes ligation of the inferior vena cava or umbrella filter placement. In massive pulmonary embolism with hemodynamic decompensation, embolectomy has been performed occasionally. At present, the use of these procedures in the pediatric age group can only be considered investigational.

Venous thromboembolic disease in pediatric patients has not been well studied. Early recognition and treatment are most important. Further investigation is clearly indicated and will undoubtedly improve diagnosis and management.

Diseases of the Pleura

HENRY LEVISON, M.D.

The commonest disease of the pleura is due to a pleural effusion which is usually secondary to underlying pulmonary disease. In the investigation of pleural effusion, a diagnostic thoracocentesis is almost always indicated. Occasional exceptions may be made such as in the presence of minimal effusions occurring in typical pneumococcal pneumonia or viral pneumonitis. When aspiration yields air, frank pus, blood or chyle the type of pleural disease is readily diagnosed and appropriate therapy can be instituted.

Purulent Pleurisy (Empyema). This is a collection of purulent material in the pleural cavity or occasionally in both pleural cavities. In most instances empyema is secondary to bacterial pneumonia, especially staphylococcal pneumonia, although more recently cases due to pneumococci, beta-hemolytic streptococci, or *Hemophilus influenzae* have been reported. When a diagnosis of empyema is made, the pleural fluid should be examined and a blood culture taken; specific therapy can then be instituted.

PLEURAL DRAINAGE. The pleural cavity should be drained using a large-bore, siliconized intercostal catheter, which can readily be inserted under local anesthesia. The catheter should be connected to a closed under-water sealed drainage system with suction. Rib resection is usually not necessary, although one must be prepared to do this at short notice if needed. Closed pleural drainage should be continued until the empyema cavity has been evacuated and the lungs reexpanded.

ANTIBIOTIC THERAPY. A good combination to begin with is penicillin-G, 200,000 to 400,000 units/kg./day in six divided doses, and methicillin,* 400 mg./kg./day in four divided doses, both given intravenously. The latter preparation may cause methicillin-mediated nephritis, so that the urine should be checked weekly. An alternative to methicillin is nafcillin, used in similar dosage. It is usually recommended that antibiotic therapy be continued for at least three weeks after the patient has become afebrile and the white cell count has returned to normal.

An alternative approach to prolonged intravenous therapy is to use intravenous antibiotics for one to two weeks and, with clinical improvement, to change to an oral antistaphylococcal preparation such as cloxacillin or dicloxacillin in a dose of 300 to 400 mg./kg./day in four divided doses.† Oral dicloxacillin or cloxacillin should be continued for at least four to six weeks after the patient has become afebrile and the white cell count has returned to normal.

The clinical status cannot be judged by the appearance of the chest x-ray alone, as this may remain abnormal for many months after the patient is well. Antibiotic treatment should not be discontinued too early; it is better to err in the direction of too long rather than too short a period of antimicrobial therapy.

Patients not responding to the above treatment should be examined for a secondary focus of infection such as cerebral abscess, septic arthritis, osteomyelitis, perinephric abscess or pericarditis. When an organism is isolated from blood or pleural fluid, its antibiotic sensitivity should be determined so that the appropriate antibiotic can be used parenterally. Chemotherapy should be under continual review, and should be modified if the clinical response is not satisfactory or if the sensitivity pattern of the isolated organism indicates the use of alternative drugs.

Hemothorax. The usual cause of hemothorax in the pediatric age group is thoracic trauma, which is most commonly seen in multiple system injuries including multiple rib fractures with pneumothorax or hemothorax. The diagnosis of hemothorax requires thoracocentesis. Sometimes a single evacuation of blood will suffice, however, a number of thoracocenteses may be required and, in a few instances, continuous chest drainage is indicated. The associated injuries will require im-

mediate attention, so that as well as evacuation of blood from the pleural cavity, frequent evaluation of respiratory function, which includes measurements of arterial carbon dioxide and oxygen tensions, will be required. These patients are best managed in a pediatric intensive care unit.

In some instances, hemothorax may be associated with hemorrhagic disease or hemorrhage from an aneurysm that may occur in conditions such as Marfans' syndrome.

The treatment of hemothorax, as in many pleural diseases, is treatment of the underlying cause. Small amounts of blood in the pleural cavity require no treatment since the blood will be absorbed spontaneously. A large hemothorax should be aspirated as completely as possible. Closed continuous drainage may be required. If active bleeding continues into the thoracic cavity, surgical exploration may be necessary to locate and ligate the bleeding areas. Attention should also be given to appropriate correction of any associated clotting defects.

Chylothorax. Chylothorax usually occurs in the neonatal period and generally no cause is found. In the older child it may occur following thoracic surgery, especially cardiovascular surgery.

Treatment is by thoracocentesis; clearing usually occurs after a single tap, although in a few patients several taps may be required to give permanent relief. Occasionally, continuous drainage using a large-bore tube with gentle suction is necessary. After thoracocentesis a chest x-ray should always be taken because of the possibility of pneumothorax.

Growth may become a problem when nutritional loss owing to repeated thoracocenteses is excessive. Most reports advocate a fat-free, high-carbohydrate, high-protein diet. Recently a diet containing medium-chain triglycerides as the sole source of fat has been suggested. Some physicians prefer to keep the patient on nasogastric suction with nothing by mouth and to rely completely on parenteral alimentation. New techniques of intravenous alimentation now in use will undoubtedly augment this approach.

Idiopathic (Primary) Pulmonary Hemosiderosis

J. LAWRENCE NAIMAN, M.D.

Idiopathic or primary pulmonary hemosiderosis is rare; its course usually chronic and occasionally fatal, and its management controversial. It is wise, therefore, for the pediatri-

---

*Manufacturer's note: The number of instances in which methicillin was administered intravenously to infants and children is not large enough to permit specific dosage recommendations.

†Manufacturer's note: Experience with dicloxacillin in the neonatal period is limited; therefore a dose for the newborn is not recommended at this time.

cian who suspects the diagnosis to refer the affected child (for initial consultation at least) to a specialist who has had considerable experience in treatment of the disorder. Before any therapeutic regimen is adopted it is important to exclude those causes of secondary pulmonary hemosiderosis which may respond to specific medical or surgical measures, such as chronic left-sided cardiac failure and collagen-vascular diseases. Moreover, since pulmonary hemorrhage may on occasion be the first manifestation of Goodpasture syndrome, renal function tests should be obtained initially and at intervals throughout the course of any illness carrying the diagnosis of idiopathic pulmonary hemosiderosis.

Current evidence suggests that this disorder results from immunologic injury to the alveolary capillaries. For control of acute pulmonary hemorrhage, therefore, we have relied upon large doses of corticosteroids, upon transfusion of packed red cells for severe anemia, and upon administration of oxygen, depending on the degree of hypoxemia. Prednisone, in a total dose of 2 mg./kg./day, is given orally in three or four divided doses. In the rare circumstance in which severe dyspnea precludes oral medication, we give an equivalent intravenous dose of hydrocortisone (e.g., Solu-Cortef, 2.5 mg./kg. every 6 hours, or a similar preparation). Antibiotics are reserved for patients in whom bronchopneumonia is suggested by the presence of high fever and inspiratory rales, an interstitial or lobar pattern on chest roentgenogram, or recovery of pathogens in cultures of sputum or tracheal aspirate.

In the child who presents mainly with chronic anemia from repeated relatively minor pulmonary hemorrhages, corticosteroids alone may suffice to arrest the bleeding. Once active bleeding has subsided, the anemia will usually respond to adequate doses of oral iron in the form of ferrous sulfate (sufficient to supply 6 mg. of elemental iron/kg./day in 3 divided doses). In a child such as this who often appears well but pale, transfusions usually are not required unless the hemoglobin level is below 5 to 6 gm./dl. or there is significant tachycardia. Because the child who is only moderately anemic may suffer an acute pulmonary hemorrhage at any time, such children must be observed carefully, with blood in readiness for transfusion at the first sign of bleeding.

A favorable response to the above therapy can usually be anticipated within three to five days, with diminished respiratory rate, a reduction in abnormal densities on the chest roentgenogram, a rise in hemoglobin level,

and a fall in reticulocyte count toward normal. Since complete normalization of the above measures of active disease often takes one to two months, we usually continue the same dose of oral prednisone and iron during this period. If the patient is comfortable and showing progressive improvement, he or she may be followed as an outpatient, while we obtain hemoglobin levels and reticulocyte counts weekly (or more or less often, depending on the severity of the anemia), and chest roentgenograms about every two weeks. Oral iron is continued until the child has been free of pulmonary bleeding for at least two months. After the hemoglobin level reaches 12 gm./dl. and the peripheral blood smear shows no hypochromic red cells, iron is given for another two months to replenish tissue stores.

After signs of activity of the disease subside, we reduce the daily dose of prednisone in 10 mg. decrements, observing for at least one month following each reduction of dosage before proceeding to the next dosage level. When the dose has reached about 20 mg./day, we adopt decrements of 5 mg./day. If at any time the child's condition worsens (as reflected in increasing cough, dyspnea, abnormal chest roentgenogram, fall in hemoglobin or rise in reticulocyte count), we return the dosage of corticosteroids to the initial dose level, which is maintained until the situation is under control. In our experience most children can be eventually weaned from steroids, but the duration of therapy required for control of the disease may vary from a few months to a few years.

In those children who seem to require maintenance dosages of prednisone of 10 to 15 mg. daily for longer than 4 months, we have recently attempted to circumvent some of the side effects of steroid through a gradual replacement of steroid therapy by immunosuppressant therapy using azathioprine.* While the patient is still on the minimal prednisone maintenance dose, we add azathioprine in an initial dose of 2 to 3 mg./kg./day, given as a single dose. Side effects of this drug are minimal and infrequent, but with larger doses or more prolonged therapy one must watch for evidence of bone marrow suppression or disturbed liver function. In patients receiving azathioprine, additional monitoring studies should include monthly white cell counts and differentials, and liver function tests (SGOT and SGPT) every three months. After the patient has been on azathioprine for approxi-

---

*This use of azathioprine is not listed in the manufacturer's instructions for azathioprine.

mately two to three months without any recurrence of symptoms, we attempt to reduce the daily dose of prednisone in 5 mg. decrements. If there is no worsening of the child's condition, we stop the prednisone completely and keep the child on azathioprine alone. If at any point the child becomes worse, the daily dose of prednisone is increased by 10 to 20 mg. (depending upon the severity of the situation) and the dosage of azathioprine is also increased by 25 mg./day (to a maximum of 5 mg./kg./day). The goal of such therapy is to eventually achieve a complete transfer to azathioprine. If this can be achieved and if the child remains free of symptoms or signs of recurrent pulmonary bleeding for at least 6 months, we try to stop this drug completely. Any recurrences that develop after this time are managed by short-term prednisone therapy and reinstitution of azathioprine at the previous dose level.

In children on long-term immunosuppressive therapy with corticosteroids or azathioprine, the risk of severe infection with varicella must be kept in mind, and the parents appropriately alerted. If in spite of reasonable precautions the child is exposed, zoster immune globulin should be administered within 72 hours. Zoster immune globulin is not available commercially but may be obtained from the Center for Disease Control in Atlanta, Georgia: day—(404) 633-1311; night—(404) 633-2176. Also if at any time the child develops pneumonia, one must consider the possibility that this might represent infection with *Pneumocystis carinii* (or a similar opportunistic organism). Where the clinical and roentgenographic picture suggests this, a lung biopsy should be carried out and appropriate therapy begun without delay.

Diets free of cow's milk have been recommended by a number of authors. We have not had much success with such regimens but would consider them in any child who seems to have persistent evidence of disease activity beyond three to four months, and prior to giving a trial of azathioprine.

Splenectomy has been recommended also by others, but we have not had to resort to this in any of our patients. Because pulmonary hemosiderosis so often affects children in the first few years of life in whom the risk is great of overwhelming infection following splenectomy, we have been discouraged from trying this measure.

In patients with uncontrolled recurrent pulmonary hemorrhage, accumulation of iron in the lung parenchyma may contribute to progressive pulmonary fibrosis. In a situation such as this, efforts to remove iron by one of the iron-chelating agents such as deferoxamine might be considered. We believe, however, that aggressive efforts to control and prevent bleeding are a more rational way of dealing with this problem. If in spite of such efforts recurrent bleeding and pulmonary fibrosis develop, a trial of deferoxamine should be made (see p. 259). Also, in the child older than 5 or 6 years, the degree of lung damage should be assessed periodically by pulmonary function studies. Progressive deterioration would be an indication for more aggressive therapy.

Discussions of prognosis with the parents should stress the fact that the course of this disease tends to be chronic, and of unpredictable duration and outcome. Some encouragement can be derived from current survival statistics which show that approximately 60 to 80 per cent of children are eventually well and free of signs of pulmonary disease.

5

Cardiovascular System

Congestive Heart Failure

HARVEY L. CHERNOFF, M.D.

The goal of treatment in congestive heart failure is to enable the failing ventricles to pump more efficiently. The major therapeutic approaches involve reduction of the cardiac work load and enhancement of myocardial contractility. Determination of the cause for congestive heart failure is a necessity since the cause influences the therapy.

Although digitalis is the mainstay of long-term treatment, reduction of the cardiac work load by decreasing the expanded circulatory volume present in cardiac failure offers the patient more immediate relief. The latter involves the use of rapid acting diuretics and, rarely, in severe situations, phlebotomy.

Diuretics. In overt congestive heart failure rapid acting diuretics are administered, almost always parenterally (Table 1). This is done even prior to obtaining chest films or the electrocardiogram if clinical findings suggest distressing pulmonary congestion.

Diuretics are also used as an adjunct to digoxin in the longer term treatment of congestive heart failure when digoxin alone does not result in the desired level of compensation. Not infrequently diuretics are employed because of the difficulty in maintaining children on more than only minimally salt-restricted diets. Rapid acting agents used long term are given only several days a week since they are likely to cause electrolyte imbalance if given daily. This is especially true in infants, who are prone to develop hypochloremic alkalosis. The less rapid acting diuretics can be given daily. Electrolytes should be monitored several times over the initial 4 to 6 weeks in all patients who

are receiving diuretics regularly to determine if potassium supplementation is necessary. Spironolactone is usually reserved for those in whom potassium depletion cannot be compensated with potassium supplements (Table 1).

Digitalis. Digoxin is the digitalis preparation used almost universally in pediatrics. It has a rapid onset, is rapidly excreted and is available in parenteral and oral preparations in convenient dosage:

Parenteral: ampules	Pediatric 0.1 mg./cc.
	Adult 0.25 mg./cc.
Oral: Elixer	0.05 mg./cc.
Tablets (unscored)	0.125 mg.
(scored)	0.25 mg.
(scored)	0.5 mg.

The dose of digoxin varies according to age and weight (Table 2). To achieve a rapid therapeutic effect requires that the patient be given a loading ("digitalizing") dose. This is administered in stages since there can be considerable variation in patient response. Prior to administration of each aliquot the rhythm is evaluated and the P-R interval is measured in the electrocardiographic limb leads to be certain that there is no evidence of toxicity. An increase of 0.02 second over the predigoxin administration P-R interval is acceptable. Any further increase is considered toxicity.

The maintenance dose is one tenth of the actual amount of digoxin required to obtain clinical evidence of compensation, or the accumulated dose resulting in an 0.02 second increase in the P-R interval, and is given every 12 hours. Each dose can be given an hour earlier or later to arrive at a convenient time schedule.

Children in mild congestive heart failure or who are compensated at rest and in failure

TABLE 1. Diuretic Agents

PREPARATION	DOSAGE	ROUTE
Potent natriuretics		
Ethacrynic acid*	1 mg./kg./dose	Intravenously only
	2 to 3 mg./kg./day	Orally
Furosemide	1 mg./kg./dose	Intravenously or intramuscularly
	2 to 3 mg./kg./day	Orally
Thiazides		
Chlorothiazide	20 to 40 mg./kg./day	Orally
Hydrochlorothiazide	2 to 5 mg./kg./day	Orally
Aldosterone antagonists		
Spironolactone	1 to 2 mg./kg./day	Orally

*Manufacturer's note: Until further experience in infants is accumulated, therapy with oral or parenteral ethacrynic acid is contraindicated.

only during exertion (active play in older children, sucking and crying in infants) may be digitalized by mouth. All others should receive parenteral digoxin.

Although determination of digoxin levels is a readily available procedure, there is poor correlation between the serum level and the clinical status. The level in children with good clinical response to digoxin may be below 0.5 ng./ml. or as high as 5 ng./ml. Individuals manifesting signs and symptoms of digoxin toxicity may have serum measurements lower than the expected toxic levels of 2 ng./ml. in older children and 5 ng./ml. in infants. Despite this, digoxin levels are helpful when they support a clinical suspicion of toxicity.

Digoxin Toxicity. Manifestations of digoxin toxicity are listed below:

I. Bradycardia for age
   A. In infants, pulse below 100 per min.
   B. In older patients, bradycardia must be determined according to age but ranges below 60 to 80.
II. Arrhythmia
   A. Any arrhythmia having its onset during digoxin therapy must be considered a result of digoxin toxicity until proved otherwise.
   B. Usually different from initial arrhythmia in those with congestive heart failure secondary to arrhythmia (e.g., supraventricular tachycardia).
   C. Great variation in different individuals; combinations are seen often.
   D. Approximate sequence of electrocardiographic changes:
      1. First degree atrioventricular block
      2. Wenckebach periods
      3. Intermittent dropped ventricular beats without Wenckebach periods
      4. Bigeminy or trigeminy
      5. Second degree atrioventricular block
      6. Complete atrioventricular block
      7. Premature ventricular beats
      8. Ventricular tachycardia
      9. Atrial fibrillation
      10. Atrial arrest
      11. Ventricular fibrillation
      12. Ventricular arrest
III. Anorexia and vomiting
IV. Lethargy and confusion
V. Intractable failure

If the patient does not have a significant arrhythmia (second or third degree atrioventricular block, atrial arrest, premature ventricular contractions, ventricular arrhythmia) and it has been four hours since the last administration of digoxin, close monitoring and discontinuation of digoxin are usually adequate. If treatment is needed potassium chloride is the first agent employed. It is given by slow intravenous infusion and titrated against the patient's response on the continuously monitored electrocardiogram (Table 3). Atropine may be helpful if bradycardia is a problem.

Digitalis-induced arrhythmias not responding to potassium chloride may require administration of propranolol. This drug is usually effective by mouth. If the arrhythmia is life-endangering, intravenous propranolol, 0.1 mg/kg, is used. A pediatric dose for propranolol has not been established by the manufacturer. Lidocaine may be useful in suppressing

TABLE 2. Dosage Schedules for Digoxin

ROUTE	ONSET OF EFFECT (MIN.)	INTERVAL BEFORE MAXIMUM EFFECT (HR.)	PREMATURE INFANTS UNDER 2.5 KG. (MG./KG.)	PATIENTS UNDER 1 MONTH, OVER 2.5 KG. (MG./KG.)	PATIENTS FROM 1 MONTH TO 2 YEARS, OVER 2.5 KG. (MG./KG.)	PATIENTS UNDER 2 YEARS, UNDER 30 KG. (MG./KG.)	PATIENTS OVER 2 YEARS, OVER 30 KG. (MG./KG.)
Intravenous	5 to 10	2 to 4	0.03‡	0.05‡	0.075‡	0.04‡	0.03‡
Intramuscular	15 to 60	4 to 6	0.03‡	0.05‡	0.075‡	0.04‡	0.03‡
Subcutaneous	15 to 60	4 to 6	0.03‡	0.05‡	0.075‡	0.04‡	0.03‡
Oral	120	4 to 6	1.5 times parenteral‡	1.5 times parenteral‡	1.5 times parenteral‡	1.5 times parenteral‡	1.5 times parenteral‡

Maintenance dosage in all cases is $^1/_{10}$ to $^1/_8$ of actual digitalizing dose every 12 hours.
Mature adolescents may require up to 3.0 mg. as a total digitalizing dose.
‡Half is given immediately and ¼ is given 4 to 8 and 8 to 16 hours later.

**TABLE 3.   Agents Used in the Treatment of
Spontaneous or Induced Arrhythmias**

Potassium chloride	Slow intravenous infusion of 1 mEq./10 ml. of 5 percent glucose in water, titrated against electrocardiographic response. Total dose not to exceed 0.5 mEq./kg./24 hours.
Propranolol	1 mg./kg./24 hours orally in 4 divided doses; 0.1 mg./kg. intravenously as single dose
Lidocaine	1 mg./kg. slow intravenous push; 20 to 50 μg./kg./min. intravenously, titrated against electrocardiographic response
Phenylephrine	0.1 to 0.2 mg. diluted to 5 or 10 ml. and given intravenously to produce an acute transient blood pressure elevation
Quinidine	3 to 6 mg./kg./dose orally every 2 hours for five doses until desired effect or toxicity (QRS prolongation, fall in blood pressure). Maintenance: effective total dose divided 4 times daily or with long-acting tablets, twice daily
Atropine	Infants, 0.02 mg./kg. intravenously or intramuscularly Children, 0.015 mg./kg. intravenously or intramuscularly Adolescents, 0.01 mg./kg. intravenously or intramuscularly

ventricular arrhythmias. Rarely, exchange transfusion or dialysis is required if the above measures do not maintain an acceptable rhythm.

Arrhythmia. Congestive heart failure caused by arrhythmias requires restoration to a more normal rhythm. The majority of arrhythmias are paroxysmal supraventricular tachycardias. Vagal stimulation by carotid massage or anal dilation is rarely helpful. Eyeball compression should not be used because of the danger of retinal detachment.

Digoxin is usually effective in converting supraventricular tachycardia to a normal rhythm. It often achieves this with administration of only the first half of the calculated digitalizing dose (Table 2). For patients not responding to digoxin, phenylephrine (Table 3) is given intravenously to produce a sudden increase in arterial pressure. A second dose may be tried when the blood pressure returns to the predrug level if the tachycardia has not been converted. If digoxin and phenylephrine fail or if the patient is in severe congestive heart failure, defibrillation is used. The direct current defibrillator settings in watt seconds are 20 to 50 in newborns, 50 to 100 in children and 100 to 300 in adolescents. The conscious patient should be sedated. Diazepam, 0.1 mg./kg. intravenously, usually suffices.* (In neonates

an agent not containing sodium benzoate should be used.)

All patients should be maintained on an antiarrhythmic medication for at least one year to prevent recurrence. Digoxin is the agent of choice even if it has not resulted in the restoration of the normal rhythm. The maintenance dose should be based on the calculated digitalizing dose. If digoxin does not prevent recurrence quinidine or propranolol may be helpful. Occasionally digoxin in combination with one of these agents will be needed.

Pulmonary Edema. Pulmonary edema may accompany congestive heart failure. If the pulmonary edema is not so severe that it is producing asphyxia, the treatment of the heart failure with diuretics and digoxin will likely cause a sufficiently rapid reduction in vascular volume to bring about relief. If, however, the degree of pulmonary edema is producing respiratory embarrassment, morphine sulfate can be used in a dose of 0.05 to 0.1 mg./kg. intravenously or subcutaneously. This agent will reduce the bronchospasm present with pulmonary edema and aid in reducing apprehension. Aminophylline, 3 to 6 mg./kg. given intravenously over a 10 to 15 minute period, is effective in relieving more severe degrees of bronchospasm.

Severe symptoms due to pulmonary edema can be temporarily but quickly reversed by administration of a continuous positive airway pressure of 6 to 8 cm. water. This can be accomplished depending on the age and condition of the patient with nasal prongs, face mask, head bag or hood or tracheal intubation. Measures to reverse the cause of the problem must go forward in parallel or an equilibrium will be reached between the vascular space and pulmonary interstitial tissue and alveoli, and edema fluid will begin to reaccumulate at the higher airway pressure.

Special Considerations. Infants not responding to medical management of congestive heart failure require early definitive diagnostic procedures (echocardiography, cardiac catheterization, angiography) since they may require surgery on an urgent basis to restore them to a compensated state.

Preterm infants in congestive heart failure due to a patent ductus arteriosus who are not improved by conventional medical therapy may be helped by nonsurgical closure of the patent ductus arteriosus with indomethacin. This agent is instilled into the stomach by gastric tube. The rectal route has also been used. The dose is 0.1 to 0.2 mg./kg. It should not be given if the infant has any evidence of renal dysfunction or necrotizing enterocolitis. Clo-

---

*Manufacturer's precaution: The safety and efficacy of injectable diazepam in the neonate have not been established.

sure of a patent ductus arteriosus with indomethacin may take 12 to 24 hours; the drug may require readministration once or twice more. If at any time during the attempt at medical closure the infant's condition seems to be deteriorating, surgical closure should be done. Indomethacin is not approved for this use and an informed consent protocol should be followed.

When to Refer.   All children suspected of having cyanotic heart disease or developing heart failure in the first month of life should be transferred to a center in which facilities are available to perform cardiac catheterization, angiography and echocardiography. This is important since those infants responding unsatisfactorily to medical management will require such studies to determine if surgical intervention is indicated.

Beyond the first month of life if the degree of congestive heart failure is mild and a diagnosis apparent, digitalization may be done on an outpatient basis if the patient is seen at 4 or 5 day intervals and if the parents are good observers. Rather than using the usual method of giving a loading dose of digoxin over several hours, the patient is started on the calculated oral maintenance dose. Four or five days later the patient is seen and evaluated for clinical response, rhythm and P-R interval. Once compensated, the children with suspected anatomic lesions should undergo procedures to establish a definitive diagnosis.

The group of patients with congestive heart failure secondary to arrhythmias should be treated in a hospital. The availability of personnel able to institute emergency measures such as defibrillation is essential.

All infants with congestive heart failure due to an anatomic defect should undergo cardiac catheterization or other definitive diagnostic procedure soon after satisfactory cardiac compensation is achieved. Those responding poorly to medical management will require such studies when the lack of progress in the direction of improved function becomes evident.

Patients in severe congestive heart failure at any age require hospital care. Here, too, the 24 hour presence of qualified personnel is a paramount consideration. Also important is the availability of the necessary supportive equipment and services. Those patients who are to be transferred to a center should have treatment started prior to transfer. This includes both a rapid acting diuretic and the first aliquot of the calculated digitalizing dose. In the case of infants, transfer should be in an incubator in the company of personnel able to institute emergency measures such as tracheal intubation.

At some point after treatment of congestive heart failure, those not already seen by the pediatric cardiologist should be given the benefit of a consultation.

Future Considerations.   The increasing sophistication of noninvasive techniques for measurement of cardiac function may enable determination of the degree of cardiac improvement being achieved by treatment. This "quantification," when evaluated and available clinically, will likely alter the present clinical techniques for restoring cardiac function and may result in greater dependence on large centers for treatment of children with congestive heart failure.

Congenital Heart Disease

ALEXANDER S. NADAS, M.D.

GENERAL PRINCIPLES

Major changes have occurred in the management of children with congenital heart disease since the first report of successful surgical treatment of a congenital cardiac lesion by Robert E. Gross from Boston in 1938. Surgery then was limited to one lesion, patent ductus arteriosus, making up no more than 10 per cent of the total congenital cardiac population; today close to 90 per cent of such patients may be offered surgical treatment. Operative intervention in the late 1930's and early 1940's was proposed principally to eliminate an anatomic and physiologic abnormality in asymptomatic children and thus avoid its putative consequences; the majority, though surely not all, of the patients with congenital heart disease undergoing surgery today are severely symptomatic and often face immediately life-threatening situations. Finally, at least in our institution, and in most large congenital cardiac centers in the United States, the age of patients at operation is progressively younger and the procedures of choice are curative rather than palliative.

DIAGNOSTIC TECHNIQUES

Cardiac Catheterization remains the "deluxe" method of evaluating patients with congenital heart disease. Detailed physiologic studies relating to blood flow and pressure in all chambers of the heart and all the great vessels, coupled with contrast visualization performed by skillful operators with large experience in infants and children, in a well equipped laboratory, will yield maximal information not only as to diagnosis but also, and often more importantly, in regard to severity. Overall catheter mortality in the proper hands is minimal (0.1 per cent) and restricted almost exclusively to babies under three months of age (1 per cent) with critical disease. Morbidity is equally negligible, but the psychological trauma should not be underestimated, particularly if the procedure is performed, as it probably should be, without general anesthesia.

No patient is too sick or too young to undergo cardiac catheterization with proper indications. Major indications are: (1) evidences of hypoxia or congestive heart failure in a patient with heart disease; (2) estimation of severity in patients with firm clinical diagnosis; (3) follow-up studies of patients with previously established moderate or even mild disease in whom progression may be suspected; (4) postoperative evaluation of patients with complex heart disease; and (5) diagnostic study in late adolescence of youngsters with clinical diagnosis of mild or even trivial disease, in order to assist them with conclusive evidence in their life planning.

Echocardiography. Other opinions notwithstanding, echocardiography is seldom a substitute for cardiac catheterization today. Future technology may change this opinion. Presently, ultrasonic examination is a substitute for cardiac catheterization only in cases of hypoplastic left heart syndrome, in establishing the inoperative nature of the malformation and, possibly, in the rare situation where the differential diagnosis between primary heart disease and lung disease is not possible on clinical grounds. Even in the latter situation one should be leery in excluding the diagnosis of total anomalous venous return, an occasionally difficult feat.

Although, in this author's opinion, echocardiography is seldom a substitute for catheterization and contrast studies, it indeed is a useful complementary tool in helping to determine the urgency of the study, guiding the course of the catheterization procedure and, most importantly, as a post catheterization and postoperative follow-up measure.

Radionuclide Angiocardiography is a more complex technological feat than ultrasonic examination. It shares with the former the noninvasive characteristic, no hospitalization is required for either, and the tests may be performed repeatedly so that the patient's course may be monitored over a short or long time period. While to the best of our present information echocardiography is without any hazard whatsoever, radionuclide angiography exposes the patient to some radiation, probably less than a tenth of that involved in catheterization and angiography and about the same as an intravenous pyelogram. Of course the information obtained cannot be compared, in terms of details, with that obtained from a complete catheter study, but it can serve as a useful screening tool excluding sizeable left to right and right to left shunts, in the clinic or in the postoperative state. The instrumentation is complex, expensive and demands close cooperation between radiology and cardiology; a saving in dollars is not a good reason to rely on radionuclide studies.

MANAGEMENT OF SPECIFIC DEFECTS

Ventricular Septal Defect. CATHE-TERIZATION. Patients of any age with clinically suspected large ventricular defect and congestive failure should be subjected to cardiac catheterization as soon as practical. It is important to stress that at least moderate cardiac enlargement, with or without failure to thrive, may be the only manifestation of a failing heart. Asymptomatic children and adolescents with signs suggesting a small ventricular defect (normal x-ray and cardiogram) may be catheterized (electively) to confirm the diagnosis in the late teens. All patients beyond infancy with suspected ventricular defect and right ventricular hypertrophy in the cardiogram deserve immediate catheterization to clarify the diagnosis and to measure the pulmonary arterial pressure.

SURGERY. Only patients with elevated pulmonary arterial pressure (mean pressure >20 mm. Hg) should be considered for surgery. Exceptions to this rule are certainly toddlers with large hearts and persistent failure to thrive, and possibly older children with a left to right shunt resulting in a pulmonary systemic flow ratio of 2:1 or more. Among those with elevated pulmonary arterial pressure, only those with a pulmonary systemic flow ratio of 2:1 or more can be operated upon safely with reasonable expectations of success. The older the patient at surgery, the less likely is the pulmonary arterial pressure and resistance to return to normal range. We prefer to operate on our patients with ventricular defect and severe pulmonary hypertension electively between six months and two years. Since at least 25 per cent of the defects diminish in size within the first year, judicious procrastination combined with recatheterization six months after the initial study is acceptable in patients doing reasonably well clinically. Pulmonary artery banding is probably outmoded. Primary closure is the approach of choice at the risk of between 5 and 10 per cent in infancy and around 1 per cent for older children.

FOLLOW-UP. Recatheterization one year postoperatively is indicated. If the postoperative study reveals that the defect was completely closed and the pulmonary arterial pressure is normal, the patient can live an entirely normal life. Clinical reevaluation at 2 to 5 year intervals is recommended. Whether these patients with proven ventricular defect closures should continue to receive bacterial endocarditis prophylaxis is debatable.

Transposition of the Great Arteries.
CATHETERIZATION. All patients for whom there is a clinical suspicion of this diagnosis are catheterized as soon as possible. If during the study the diagnosis is confirmed, balloon septostomy is attempted on all those two months old or younger.

SURGERY. *Transposition of the great arteries with an intact ventricular septum.* After balloon septostomy, the infant's pH and oxygen saturations should be monitored carefully at least daily. In the absence of acidemia and with satisfactory clinical progress, arterial saturations of over 55 per cent may be acceptable for discharge 10 days after ballooning. If under frequent and careful clinical follow-up the baby progresses satisfactorily, repeat catheterization is performed electively between six and eight months, to be followed by elective Mustard procedure before the first birthday. Early recatheterization is indicated by an unsatisfactory clinical course (cyanosis, failure to thrive, congestive failure). Mustard's baffle procedure may be performed after ballooning if indicated by the physiologic and clinical picture. The earliest successful Mustard operation in our institution was performed within the first 36 hours of life on a baby weighing 2.2 kg. Hospital mortality is estimated to be 10 per cent or less.

FOLLOW-UP. Elective recatheterization one year postoperatively is mandatory. Clinic visits, at least yearly, are strongly recommended even in the face of good physiologic results, in view of the relative newness of the corrective operation. Antibiotics for bacterial endocarditis are indicated. Activity is to be limited only by the patient's fatigue. Long-term course is unknown, but one should be mindful of the dangers of arrhythmias, of baffle obstruction, and competence of the right ventricle and the tricuspid valves in terms of several decades.

Transposition of the great arteries with large ventricular septal defect. After balloon septostomy one may proceed right away to pulmonary artery banding, with debanding, ventricular defect closure and a Mustard operation to follow two years or later. Alternatively, since primary operation in the neonatal period is dif-

ficult, one might attempt medical management of heart failure for the first three months and then attempt closure of the ventricular defect with Mustard operation without palliative procedure. Whichever way one chooses to proceed, some type of surgery, aimed at reducing the pulmonary arterial pressure, is mandatory before three months of age and certainly by six months of age. For follow-up, see the preceding section.

Transposition of the great arteries with ventricular defect and pulmonary stenosis. Some of these patients with optimal degrees of pulmonary stenosis may be relatively asymptomatic throughout infancy and early childhood, as though they had undergone pulmonary artery banding. For these children, primary repair, electively, is recommended at two years of age, or if asymptomatic, even later.

Those with marked hypoxia due to severe pulmonary stenosis probably should have an arterial (Blalock-Taussig, Waterston) shunt operation in early infancy to be followed by secondary repair in early childhood. Follow-up is the same as for those with intact ventricular septum.

Hypoplastic Left Heart Syndrome.
CATHETERIZATION. Whether patients with this firm diagnosis should undergo cardiac catheterization is debatable. Excellent pediatric cardiologists recommend that if ultrasonic diagnosis of hypoplastic left heart syndrome is definitely established by a competent echocardiographer, cumbersome and life-threatening physiologic and contrast studies do not alter the almost mandatory conservative management of these babies during their short existence. Other equally competent but more adventurous pediatric cardiologists and cardiovascular surgeons require physiologic and morphologic details before deciding on a plan of management. On the whole this author's prejudice lies with trusting a total clinical picture rather than relying exclusively on the echocardiogram.

SURGERY. No curative operation is available for any of these lesions. Palliative procedures attempted with various degrees of uncertainty include atrial defect creation, pulmonary artery banding, by-pass procedures or relief of coarctation and systemic pulmonary artery shunts for those with severe hypoxia.

FOLLOW-UP. This is not a group of curable patients. As a consequence, if they survive with, without or in spite of surgery, close follow-up with skillful management of anticongestives, careful attention to infections and wise counsel recommending a life style as nearly normal as tolerated are recommended.

Tetralogy of Fallot. CATHETERIZA-

TION. All patients with the clinical diagnosis of tetralogy of Fallot should be catheterized and first rate angiograms should be obtained, immediately if the patients are symptomatic and around the first birthday even if they are doing well clinically.

SURGERY. Palliative shunt procedures, with rare exceptions, are outmoded today in the treatment of tetralogy of Fallot. Corrective surgery in skillful hands carries a mortality not much higher than 5 per cent in early infancy and below this number in children. Severe cyanosis or hypoxic spells are indications for surgery in infancy. Exercise intolerance sufficient to limit full participation in peer activities is sufficient operative indication for toddlers and older children. Probably all patients, irrespective of symptomatology, should be treated surgically before they enter school.

FOLLOW-UP. Careful, at least yearly, follow-up is recommended for all postoperative patients, indefinitely. A life centered around competitive athletics is discouraged, but recreational sports are highly desirable. Bacterial endocarditis prophylaxis is adhered to.

Patent Ductus Arteriosus. CATHE-TERIZATION. Infants and particularly children with classic clinical signs of patent ductus arteriosus need not be catheterized. Those with less than typical murmurs, or with right ventricular hypertrophy demonstrated on the cardiogram, or other unusual features should have detailed physiologic studies preoperatively.

SURGERY. All infants and children with a net left-to-right shunt through a patent ductus arteriosus should be operated upon, with the possible exception of medically manageable premature infants in whom the ductus might be expected to close spontaneously within the first three months of life. Mortality, except in the sickest patients with pulmonary artery hypertension, is less than 1 per cent.

FOLLOW-UP. This is one of the few congenital cardiac lesions that does not require routine postoperative follow-up unless pulmonary artery hypertension was noted preoperatively. Even antibiotic prophylaxis may be omitted.

Simple Coarctation of the Aorta Without Congestive Heart Failure. CATHETERIZA-TION. The diagnosis is easily suspected at routine physical examination by absent or delayed femoral pulses, and is confirmed by a right arm blood pressure that is 20 mm. Hg or more above that of the leg pressure. Under ordinary circumstances, without additional cardiac anomaly suspected, catheterization is not necessary for diagnosis preoperatively. Children with simple coarctation of the aorta seldom have left ventricular hypertrophy and strain in the cardiogram. If this is noted, catheterization should be performed to exclude coexisting aortic stenosis.

SURGERY. Elective relief of the aortic obstruction is recommended any time after two years of age with an expected mortality of 1 per cent of less. Earlier operation in symptomatic patients or those with excessive hypertension may be performed at any age, although restenosis is said to be more frequent in those operated upon in infancy at a somewhat higher risk.

Coarctation of the Aorta with Congestive Heart Failure. CATHETERIZATION. In contrast to patients with asymptomatic coarctation of the aorta, these infants, usually neonates, should undergo detailed physiologic and angiographic studies as soon as possible. An outline of the coarctation and knowledge of the presence and nature of associated cardiac anomalies are essential for intelligent management.

SURGERY. *Patients with simple coarctation and no associated anomalies* with congestive failure may respond promptly to vigorous anticongestive measures. If clinical improvement persists, and the baby gains weight, medical management is continued and surgery may be postponed to two years of age. If the immediate response to digitalis and diuretics is less than completely satisfactory, or if after a satisfactory response the baby suffers a relapse, immediate resection of the coarctation is recommended. Mortality is less than 10 per cent even in the sickest babies.

Patients with coarctation and a hypoplastic aortic arch, or even interrupted arch, usually associated with ventricular defect and other anomalies, present within the first few days of life in severe failure. If cardiac catheterization studies confirm this diagnosis, immediate surgery is recommended. Whether the operation should be palliative or an attempt at complete correction is a matter of controversy. Either way a mortality of 25 to 50 per cent has to be expected. High as this figure is, it is still preferable to the almost 100 per cent mortality associated with conservative management.

FOLLOW-UP. Patients with coarctation surgery of any kind (for simple or complex lesions) should be followed at least yearly as outpatients. X-rays and cardiograms are recommended routinely every two or three years. Exercise studies are helpful in determining the level of activities allowed to patients. Restrictions are difficult to enforce in these usually athletically inclined youngsters. Bacterial endocarditis prophylaxis is strongly recommended. Repeat catheterization five years postoperatively is advisable for those with complex lesions or residual relative hypertension.

Atrial Septal Defect Primum (Incomplete A-V Canal). CATHETERIZATION. Physiologic and contrast studies to assess the size and location of the septal defects and the degree of mitral regurgitation are recommended as soon as the patient is symptomatic or by five years of age at the latest. No patient should be operated upon without catheter studies.

SURGERY. A pulmonary to systemic flow ratio of at least 2:1 with or without pulmonary hypertension is the primary indication for surgery. The degree of mitral incompetence should be carefully assessed preoperatively and the nature of surgical intervention tailored accordingly. Atrial defect closure with significant residual mitral regurgitation leads to pulmonary edema and disaster. Symptomatic patients may be operated upon at any time. Elective surgery is recommended between 5 and 10 years with a risk of less than 5 per cent.

FOLLOW-UP. Careful yearly checkups and routine catheterization five years postoperatively are recommended. Bacterial endocarditis prophylaxis is in order. Normal activities are permitted including, with proven excellent repair, competitive sports.

Atrial Septal Defect Secundum. CATHETERIZATION. The clinical profile may be classic enough, with typical echocardiograms and a radionuclide angiocardiogram showing a pulmonary to systemic flow ratio of 2:1 or more preoperatively, so that catheterization may be omitted. In less typical cases physiologic studies are recommended.

SURGERY. All secundum atrial defects should be closed electively; mortality is around 1 per cent in children five years old or older. Slightly higher risks should be quoted for young children and infants on account of heart failure. Atrial defects with pulmonary artery hypertension represent unusual, relatively high-risk situations, without guarantee of normal pulmonary artery pressure postoperatively.

FOLLOW-UP. Infrequent outpatient visits are recommended on account of the tendency to arrhythmias and the association of prolapsed mitral valve. Bacterial endocarditis prophylaxis may not be necessary in patients without mitral valve disease. Postoperative catheterization may be omitted if clinical evidence suggests excellent repair.

Pulmonary Stenosis with Intact Ventricular Septum. CATHETERIZATION. Children with classic auscultatory, cardiographic and radiological evidence of severe valvar pulmonary stenosis may be operated upon without preoperative physiologic studies. All infants with this diagnosis should be catheterized.

SURGERY. Patients with valvar pulmonary stenosis and right ventricular pressure, documented or inferred from clinical evidence, at 75 mm. Hg or more should have valvotomy on cardiopulmonary bypass. Inflow occlusion may be used only in patients with catheter-proven uncomplicated valvar obstruction. Mortality beyond early infancy is less than 1 per cent.

FOLLOW-UP. Recatheterization is not necessary except for specific indications, such as residual right ventricular hypertrophy in the cardiogram or other unusual features. Bacterial endocarditis prophylaxis may be omitted and even competitive sports may be allowed in those with proven good surgical results. Return visits may be kept at a minimum.

Valvar Aortic Stenosis. CATHETERIZATION. All infants with the clinical diagnosis and congestive failure need immediate catheter studies. Children with angina, exercise intolerance, syncope or left ventricular strain pattern should also be urgently studied. Asymptomatic children without ST-T wave changes, but with loud murmurs of aortic stenosis should undergo physiologic studies electively at 5 to 10 years. Repeat studies, even in consistently asymptomatic individuals, are recommended at 5 to 10 year intervals. The cardiogram and the vectorcardiogram are presently the best noninvasive tools for follow-up.

SURGERY. Valvotomy on cardiopulmonary bypass is recommended for all infants in congestive failure and for all children with symptoms, strain patterns or a gradient of over 75 mm. Hg.

FOLLOW-UP. Checkups have to be particularly careful and frequent, every 6 to 12 months, as restenosis and bacterial endocarditis are relatively common. Irrespective of operative success, competitive sports should not be allowed.

CLOSING REMARKS

The summary statements on the nine common lesions should be viewed only as guidelines. They should serve the pediatrician as a yardstick by which to measure the opinions of the "experts."

Choose a pediatric cardiologist whom you can trust and who is independent of the cardiac surgeon. There is nothing mystical about all this. Indications for catheterization and cardiac surgery can be discussed rationally with one's colleagues.

Do not procrastinate with infants in congestive heart failure or severe cyanosis. If possible get them operated upon at an early age. You can pick your time in asymptomatic patients, with the possible exception of aortic stenosis.

Do not lose contact with postoperative patients; they may be a lot better but rarely do they have a "perfect" heart.

Cardiac Arrhythmias

CATHERINE A. NEILL, M.D., F.R.C.P., and
P. JACOB VARGHESE, M.D., M.R.C.P.

GENERAL PRINCIPLES

The management of arrhythmias has changed significantly in the past 10 years. Their importance as a cause of morbidity and occasional mortality in the young is more widely recognized, evaluation is more precise, and therapeutic options are greater due to a combination of improved monitoring methods, new and more effective drugs, and to the use of serum levels of the drug.

Because in the past pediatric training in arrhythmias has been highly empiric, the pediatrician often approaches these disorders with little confidence and sometimes less logic. It is helpful to recognize that pediatric arrhythmias fall into five basic groups: (1) sinus arrhythmia; (2) premature contractions, which may be atrial, junctional ("nodal"), or ventricular in origin; (3) tachyarrhythmias, which may be supraventricular or ventricular in origin: supraventricular tachycardias include atrial flutter and fibrillation and also paroxysmal supraventricular tachycardia, which is divided into two types, the more common type due to a reentry mechanism and the second due to an ectopic focus; (4) bradyarrhythmias, including sinus bradycardia and heart block; the latter may be either congenital or acquired in origin and partial or complete; (5) others include sinus bradycardia-tachycardia syndromes and other complex arrhythmias which may require detailed electrophysiologic study for recognition. In any patient with recurrent tachycardias, the possibility of Wolff-Parkinson-White syndrome should be considered and repeated electrocardiograms taken, since the characteristic electrocardiographic pattern may be intermittent.

Management of any arrhythmia should be based on several basic principles. First, the presence of an arrhythmia should be confirmed and its nature defined, both as to site of origin and basic mechanism. Second, knowledge of the natural course of the arrhythmia, once identified, may help in deciding if any intervention is needed; for example, sinus arrhythmia and many of the premature atrial and ventricular contractions seen in children with normal hearts require no therapy. Third, there should be reason to believe that the therapy selected is likely to modify or abolish the arrhythmia without unacceptable side effects or toxicity, and that control of the arrhythmia will indeed make a difference to the patient's course.

The latter criterion is easy to fulfill in, for example, supraventricular tachycardia in infancy which is life-threatening if not controlled, but associated with normal life expectancy if adequately treated. However, in complex arrhythmias in individuals with already malformed hearts, limited understanding of the underlying mechanism and the precise mode of action of various drugs may make the risk-benefit ratio of therapy much less clear.

Finally, once therapy is decided on, the choice of a particular drug depends on knowledge of its site and mode of action. In general, it is advisable to use only one antiarrhythmic drug at a time and attention should be given to possible differences in the appropriate dose and side effects between children and adults. Serum blood levels are often valuable, since in most cases therapeutic activity is closely related to plasma concentration. The pharmacokinetics of antiarrhythmic drugs may vary considerably between individuals and an arrhythmia should only be defined as resistant to a specific medication if it is not controlled even with an adequate blood level.

Resistant arrhythmias may require the use of more than one drug. Such patients should always be followed carefully by a cardiac group, including a cardiologist with special interest and expertise in arrhythmia management.

Electrical methods of arrhythmia control include cardioversion, intracardiac "overdrive" pacing, and pacemaker therapy. DC cardioversion is the treatment of choice for ventricular fibrillation or ventricular tachycardia and in rare episodes of supraventricular tachycardia when the rate is very rapid and the clinical condition deteriorating. In selected patients with supraventricular tachycardia, electrical pacing of the atrium at a rate faster than the tachycardia ("overdrive") pacing followed by switching off the pacemaker may result in sinus rhythm. This technique also has the advantage of recording an intracardiac electrocardiogram and allowing a precise diagnosis of the site and mechanism of the arrhythmia.

Pacemaker therapy is used for patients with bradycardia resulting in cardiac symptoms. Many types of pacemakers are available, and although all have some inherent disadvantages, a rechargeable pacemaker may at the present time be optimal in childhood so that frequent changes of wires and batteries are avoided.

Surgery has a very limited role in management of arrhythmia, but surgical division of the accessory pathway has proved useful in a few children and young adults with Wolff-Parkinson-White syndrome and with severe recurrent tachyarrhythmias resistant to all medical therapy.

EVALUATION OF ARRHYTHMIA

Exact definition of the problem is usually easier if the arrhythmia is present on the electrocardiogram when the patient is first seen. In infancy most arrhythmias present as tachycardia for a period of time may lead to congestive cardiac failure. Older children may present with symptoms of palpitations or rarely episodes of syncope. The majority of arrhythmias during childhood are detected only on routine examination.

The pediatrician usually has little difficulty in recognizing sinus arrhythmia because of the marked variation of the cardiac rate with respiration. However, evaluation of tachyarrhythmias may prove more difficult. The aim should be to localize the site of origin and basic mechanism. For example, in supraventricular tachycardia the electrocardiogram usually shows a QRS complex of the same duration as in sinus rhythm; occasionally, however, the QRS complex is widened due to aberrant conduction, thus leading to confusion with ventricular tachycardia. In aberrancy the initial vector of the QRS is the same as that of the sinus beat and a right bundle branch block pattern is frequent because of the inherent increase in the refractoriness of the right bundle. Despite these differentiating points it is occasionally difficult to differentiate ventricular from supraventricular tachycardia with an aberrancy and specialized physiologic studies may be necessary.

The *mechanism* of a tachyarrhythmia may often be understood by analyzing an electrocardiogram taken at its onset or termination. For example, a reentry tachycardia involving the atrioventricular node, the mechanism of most of the supraventricular tachycardias of infancy, often starts with a premature beat with a prolonged PR interval. This conduction delay is a prerequisite for a reentry tachycardia. Continuous electrocardiographic recording for a 12 to 24 hour period using a Holter monitor is often useful in planning treatment, since this type of reentry tachycardia will usually respond well to digitalis alone, whereas if an ectopic focus is present, another drug such as quinidine may be necessary for suppression of the focus before the arrhythmia may be completely controlled (Table 1).

Children or adolescents with symptoms such as palpitations or syncope possibly due to an arrhythmia, but with a normal resting electrocardiogram, present a special problem. Again, a 24 hour Holter tape recording accompanied by a careful diary kept by the patient of his activities and symptoms during this period will aid in determining whether episodes of palpitation or syncope can be correlated with an arrhythmia. Monitoring can also be useful after therapy has started to document reduction in episodes of arrhythmia.

In some patients, particularly those who have undergone prior open heart surgery, careful history taking shows the onset of arrhythmia is related to exercise. Again, the resting electrocardiogram may be completely normal; however, exercise electrocardiography not only can identify the arrhythmia, but is a clue to correct management. For example, in one child with an operated tetralogy of Fallot the resting electrocardiogram was normal except for right bundle branch block, but short bursts of ventricular tachycardia occurred once the heart rate rose to 110 with exercise. The use of propranolol in a dose adequate to prevent such a rise with exercise has controlled this potentially life-threatening problem. Some bradyarrhythmias, both in premature infants and adolescents, may be due to altered autonomic tone rather than to any structural abnormality of the heart. When sinus bradycardia of adolescence is due to increased vagal tone, intravenous atropine will abolish the bradycardia, whereas in bradycardia due to structural disease at the sinus node "sick sinus" syndrome, atropine will have little or no effect.

Evaluation of cardiac arrhythmias resistant to conventional therapy or of complex nature may require more invasive techniques including intracardiac electrography and stimulation studies. Occasionally such studies may also be useful in the rapid evaluation of an antiarrhythmic agent.

SPECIFIC ARRHYTHMIAS

Once the presence of an arrhythmia has been documented and its nature defined, the decision needs to be made if treatment is warranted. If it is, it should be undertaken with the maximal understanding of the therapeutic principles involved and with regard for

TABLE 1.   Drugs Used in Cardiac Arrhythmias in Children and Adolescents

NAME AND FORM OF DRUG	MAJOR ACTIONS	USES	DOSE
Digoxin (Lanoxin) Ampule, 0.1 mg./ml. Tablets, 0.125, 0.25, 0.5 mg.	Inotropic effect on myocardial contractility. Increases refractory period of atrioventricular node.	Supraventricular tachycardia; atrial fibrillation	*Digitalization:* Infants: 40 μg./kg./day in 3 divided doses (½, ¼, ¼) Children: 20 μg./kg./day in 3 divided doses (½, ¼, ¼) *Maintenance:* 10 μg./kg./day Maximum adult dosage of 2 mg./day digitalizing and 0.25 mg./day maintenance.
Quinidine sulfate Tablets, 200 mg.	Depresses myocardial excitability; suppresses ectopic foci; prolongs refractory period (prolongs QT interval); slows conduction velocity; enhances atrioventricular conduction	Suppresses ectopic foci, especially premature auricular contraction; atrial fibrillation, especially prior to cardioversion; prophylactic in supraventricular tachycardias, attacks in Wolff-Parkinson-White syndrome or ectopic foci	Test dose: 2 mg./kg., then 20 mg./kg./day (5 mg./kg./6 hrs.). Maximum adult dosage of 2 gm./ day.
Procainamide (Pronestyl) Ampule, 100 mg./ml. (10 ml.) Capsule, 200 mg.	Similar to quinidine	Suppresses ectopic foci, especially premature ventricular contractions due to digitalis toxicity	3 mg./kg. IV over 5 min., then IV drip 5 mg./kg. at 0.5 to 1.0 mg./ kg./hr. PO 30 mg./kg./day in 4 divided doses every 6 hrs. Maximum adult dosage of 1.0 gm. IV and 2.0 gm. PO daily.
Lidocaine (Xylocaine)* Ampule, 0.5% (2.5 or 50 ml.)	Depresses myocardial excitability; suppresses premature ventricular contractions	Ventricular arrhythmia, especially intraoperative or digitalis-induced	1 mg./kg. IV over 2 to 5 min., then 4 mg./ml at 0.5 to 1.0 mg./min. Maximum adult dosage of 1 mg./ kg. every 20 min., and 750 mg./ day.
Propranolol (Inderal)† Ampule, 1 mg./ml. Tablets, 10 mg.	Inhibits myocardial response to catecholamines; decreases automaticity; increases refractory period; suppresses ectopic foci	Supraventricular tachycardia; supraventricular tachycardia with block due to digitalis; multiple premature ventricular contractions; recurrent ventricular tachycardias	0.01 to 0.05 mg./kg. IV in 2 divided doses 5 min. apart (maximum of 1 mg. per dose). PO 1 mg./ kg./day in 4 divided doses every 6 hrs. Maximum adult dosage of 160 mg./day.
Phenytoin (Dilantin) Capsule, 30 mg. or 100 mg.	Suppresses ectopic foci; affects ionic movement through cell membrane	Transient or recurrent ventricular arrhythmia, including digitalis-induced*	2 to 4 mg./kg. by slow IV injection (can repeat after 15 min.); maximum dose not to exceed 600 mg./day. PO 3 to 8 mg./kg./day in 3 divided doses every 8 hrs. Maximum adult dosage of 1 gm./day.
Atropine sulfate Ampule, 0.4 mg./ml.	Vagolytic effect; increases rate of sinoatrial nodal contractions.	Sinus bradycardia due to sick sinus syndrome or vagal stimulation, especially during cardiac procedures	0.01 mg./kg. IV. May be repeated in two hours.

*This use of phenytoin is not mentioned in the manufacturer's instructions.

minimizing the risks of toxicity, side effects and the undesirable sequelae of prolonged medication.

Sinus arrhythmia is in almost all instances benign and does not require therapy. Exceptions include children on digitalis in whom increasing sinus arrhythmia may indicate early toxicity and the rare child with sinus tachycardia-bradycardia syndrome associated with syncope who will usually require Holter monitoring and electrophysiologic studies for complete elucidation and may need pacemaker therapy. Sinus tachycardia may be due to many causes, but the use of cardiac medications to reduce the sinus rate is virtually never indicated.

In general, when confronted with any arrhythmia, it is valuable to consider whether medications or toxins may be the underlying cause.

Tachyarrhythmias are the largest group of concern to the pediatrician. The most frequent is *supraventricular tachycardia*, usually of the reentry type, but occasionally due to an ectopic focus. Most infants do not respond to vagal maneuvers, but do well with digitalization. In typical reentry tachycardia of infancy the return to sinus rhythm is abrupt, usually after about three-quarters of the total digitalizing dose has been given (Table 1). Because of the risk of recurrence, maintenance digitalis is usually given for six months to one year after the onset. In a few infants ectopic beats or brief runs of tachycardia persist, indicating an ectopic focus which may require suppression with quinidine or propranolol (Table 1). Often

TABLE 1. Drugs Used in Cardiac Arrhythmias in Children and Adolescents (continued)

NAME AND FORM OF DRUG	THERAPEUTIC BLOOD LEVELS	CONTRAINDICATIONS	TOXIC SIDE EFFECTS	COMMENTS
Digoxin (Lanoxin) Ampule, 0.1 mg./ml. Tablets, 0.125, 0.25, 0.5 mg.	1 to 2 ng./100 ml. (more than 3 ng./100 ml. in children and 3.5 ng./100 ml. in infants is probably toxic. Check levels 6 hrs. after last dose.)	Digitalis toxicity	Vomiting, premature atrial and ventricular contractions; atrial tachycardia with block; late toxicity; atrio-ventricular dissociation; cerebral irritation	Toxicity: discontinue digitalis (for other measures see text)
Quinidine sulfate Tablets, 200 mg.	5.8 mg./liter. Check levels 4 hrs. after last dose.	Quinidine sensitivity; adverse reaction to test dose (hypotension); atrioventricular block	Diarrhea; nausea; tinnitus; premature ventricular contractions, prolonged QRS interval; syncope, thrombocytopenia	
Procainamide (Pronestyl) Ampule, 100 mg./ml. (10 ml.) Capsule, 200 mg.	4 to 8 mg./liter	Hypotension	Prolonged QRS interval; hypotension; lupus-like syndrome	Discontinue if QRS prolongation is greater than 50% or if multiple premature ventricular contractions present. Long-term use in children rarely warranted
Lidocaine (Xylocaine)* Ampule, 0.5% (2.5 or 50 ml.)	1 to 6 μg./liter	Atrioventricular dissociation; slow nodal or ventricular pace maker; liver failure	Drowsiness; diplopia; sweating; medullary depression; seizures	
Propranolol (Inderal)† Ampule, 1 mg./ml. Tablets, 10 mg.	20 to 50 μg./liter	Hypotension; asthma; bradycardia; atrioventricular block; cardiac failure	Bradycardia; hypotension; nausea; dizziness; hypoglycemia	Not yet approved by FDA for use in children. Antidotes are atropine or isoproterenol. Major use in arrhythmia precipitated by catecholamine release (following exercise or excitement)
Phenytoin (Dilantin) Capsule, 30 mg. or 100 mg.	10 to 20 μg./liter	Usually ineffective in supraventricular tachycardias; avoid in hypoxia or acidosis	Ataxia; nystagmus; tremor; confusion	
Atropine sulfate Ampule, 0.4 mg./ml.			Hypothermia; urinary retention	

*Manufacturer's warning: Evidence for proper usage of lidocaine in children is limited.
†Manufacturer's note: At this time the data on the use of this drug in the pediatric age group are too limited to permit adequate directions for use.

both digitalis and quinidine may be discontinued after some months when the ectopic focus is no longer active.

In older children treatment of supraventricular tachycardia includes not only management of the attack, but prevention and management of recurrences. If the acute attack responds to vagal stimulation, the child may learn to abort later attacks himself by use of the Valsalva maneuver, induced vomiting, sipping of ice water, and so on. Digitalization is usually effective, and it is well known that vagal stimulation may be more successful once the child is partially digitalized. In recurrent attacks every effort should be made to avoid frequent hospitalization. Management in the home or by a brief outpatient visit requires maximal cooperation between the pediatrician and cardiologist.

If the acute episode does not respond to digitalis and vagal maneuvers, a single intravenous injection of methoxamine hydrochloride (Vasoxyl), 1 to 5 mg., may result in an abrupt ending of the tachycardia, particularly if it is associated with a mild degree of hypotension. Medications most frequently used in the prevention and therapy of recurrent attacks in children are digoxin with or without propranolol (Table 1).

Atrial tachycardia with block is the characteristic rhythm of digitalis toxicity. It should be treated by discontinuing digitalis, potassium chloride, 0.3 mEq./kg./hr. up to a maximum of 2 to 3 mEq./kg./24 hrs., and treatment with phenytoin. A new serum containing digitalis antibodies is currently under development. It is not yet available for general use, but promises to prove most valuable in this extremely difficult problem.

Atrial flutter responds well to electroconversion; however, in most instances the optimal procedure is digitalization to slow conduction through the atrioventricular node, followed by quinidine in gradually increasing doses (Table 1). If sinus rhythm does not return after 48 to 72 hours of therapy or if the child is deteriorating, electroconversion may be undertaken. In children with anatomically normal hearts (including postoperative atrial septal defects), quinidine may be continued for a few days after conversion and then all medication discontinued. However, when flutter supervenes in a child with a prior Mustard procedure or other complex intracardiac anatomy, maintenance quinidine for many years may be indicated.

Atrial fibrillation is rare in children and usually responds well to a course of management similar to that outlined for atrial flutter.

Ventricular tachycardia may respond rapidly to lidocaine (Table 1). Electroconversion should be undertaken if there is not an immediate response to lidocaine or if hypotension is present.

Ventricular fibrillation is an immediate life-threatening emergency associated with cardiopulmonary arrest; adequate airway should be obtained, ventilation started and external cardiac compression undertaken while arrangements are being made for electrical defibrillation. An electrocardiographic monitor should be available and an intravenous cutdown put in place so that hypotension and acidosis can be treated.

Bradyarrhythmias are relatively frequent in the premature nursery and then are rarely seen during the childhood years, but may again become a problem during adolescence.

Sinus bradycardia (a resting heart rate of under 60 per minute in children and under 90 per minute in infancy) may be noted during sleep or in athletic individuals and does not normally require therapy. It is not infrequently seen following head injury and, under such circumstances or if due to the increased vagal tone of adolescence, will show a good response to atropine, as will the bradycardia seen in vasovagal attacks.

Sick sinus syndrome may occur in individuals with otherwise normal hearts, but more frequently occurs in those who have undergone surgery such as repair of sinus venous defects, Mustard procedures, and so on, impairing the vascular supply to the sinoatrial node. Episodes of severe bradycardia and sinus arrest may be associated with syncope and sometimes with sudden death. All such patients require a very detailed study including Holter monitoring and electrophysiologic studies before a decision is made as to the need for permanent pacemaker therapy.

Atrioventricular block, whether partial or complete, may be due to a congenital defect of the conduction system or may be acquired postoperatively. The latter is now becoming rare. In general terms, it is usually well tolerated in children as long as the ventricular rate at rest is at least 40, and the rate rises to 60 or more with exercise. If these conditions are not met, or if there is evidence of ventricular irritability, permanent pacemaker therapy may be required.

Premature contractions rarely require therapy during childhood. However, if they are associated with recurrent episodes of tachycardia, or if they become more frequent with exercise, suppression of the ectopic focus may be warranted. It is our present practice to undertake Holter monitoring of such patients to document the frequency of the premature contractions during the average day, and also to perform exercise electrocardiography before making a decision regarding suppressive medications. In most children (approximately 90 per cent of those seen in our institution), premature contractions are not associated with symptoms or episodes of tachycardia, and tend to decrease or disappear with exercise. We believe no therapy is warranted, though we have been obtaining follow-up electrocardiograms at one to two year intervals and have not restricted activity. Suppression of the ectopic focus with quinidine is useful in many instances, whereas propranolol has proved valuable if premature contractions appear as the ventricular rate increases with exercise.

ADDITIONAL COMMENTS

The drugs mentioned in Table 1 have all been in use for a number of years, though newer work on electrophysiology and pharmacokinetics allows now for their more rational use than in the past. New medications available in some centers for use in children include aprindine and verapamil. Aprindine is valuable in suppressing ectopic foci and has been used in some intractable tachycardias due to Wolff-Parkinson-White syndrome and in some recurrent ventricular arrhythmias refractory to all other medications. Verapamil has also been shown useful in some intractable supraventricular tachycardias associated with Wolff-Parkinson-White syndrome. Both these drugs are still considered experimental and require special prescription by a group skilled in cardiac pharmacology.

In summary, we would encourage the pediatrician to approach an arrhythmia in the logical sequence we have outlined above. First, determine whether an arrhythmia is present, recognizing that if it is not present on the resting electrocardiogram, we now have techniques for documenting it with a Holter monitor. Second, define the exact nature of the arrhythmia, since this influences therapy decisions. Third, decide if therapy is indicated, recognizing that many arrhythmias in the pediatric age group are entirely benign and not associated with symptoms or cardiac difficulty. Fourth, undertake therapy if indicated with the maximal understanding of the pharmacokinetics of the drugs involved.

Myocardial Disease

ROBERT A. MILLER, M.D.

The myocardial diseases of infancy and childhood cause many deaths in otherwise healthy children. So little is known about the cause and the pathogenesis of these diseases that even their names vary from year to year. One example is idiopathic hypertrophic subaortic stenosis, also called obstructive cardiomyopathy or asymmetric septal hypertrophy of the obstructive type.

Myocardial Disease Associated with Infective Agents. *Acute or chronic disease of the myocardium associated with a significant change in titer of specific viral antibodies, or positive culture for specific viruses.* So-called viral myocarditis is usually, but not exclusively, a disease of infancy. The therapy for these patients is directed against the two most common manifestations, congestive heart failure and disturbances of cardiac rhythm. Although the management of heart failure and dysrhythmias has been discussed on pp. 137–149, it should be emphasized that the treatment of both conditions must be continued long after the clinical manifestations have ended—in my experience, at least one to two years from the onset even though the heart size and the electrocardiogram have returned to normal sooner than that. A recurrence of congestive heart failure following an untimely termination of digitalization may be impossible to control.

Infection of the myocardium with bacteria or other infectious agents. Specific antibiotic therapy will usually control myocardial infections with two notable exceptions. (1) Diphtheritic myocarditis. In addition to penicillin or erythromycin, the intramuscular or intravenous use of the specific antitoxin, 20,000 to 40,000 units, shortens morbidity and lowers mortality. (2) The development of myocardial abscesses secondary to infective endocarditis, especially when they occur in the region of the aortic valve, may create a surgical emergency.

Myocardial disease associated with acute or chronic immunological (collagen) diseases. Myocardial involvement in acute rheumatic fever is less important than the destructive lesions of the aortic and mitral valves. Rapid cardiac dilatation and congestive heart failure of acute rheumatic carditis are indications for steroid therapy. Used with or without digitalis and diuretics, prednisone therapy (1.5 mg./kg./day) often results in increased cardiac output, slowing of heart rate, and improvement in the symptoms and signs of heart failure. The use of steroids has diminished the mortality rate and shortened morbidity in acute rheumatic carditis.

Inflammatory myocardial disease associated with rheumatoid arthritis and lupus erythematosus is rarely extensive enough to cause heart failure in childhood. Pulmonary edema or other signs of congestive heart failure in patients with acute glomerulonephritis are associated with an increased volume load and systemic hypertension rather than with extensive involvement of the myocardium.

Noninflammatory Diseases of the Myocardium. *Inherited neurological or muscular diseases.* Muscular dystrophy and Friedreich's ataxia are examples of autosomal dominant genetic diseases associated with myocardial degenerative changes and diffuse interstitial fibrosis. There is no specific therapy. Although rarely a serious problem in Friedreich's ataxia, the myocardial disease of muscular dystrophy is not infrequently associated with congestive heart failure that may be the terminal event in these children and young adults. Pompe's disease, a type of generalized glycogenosis resulting from a genetically determined deficiency of acid maltase, results in extensive infiltration of the myocardium with glycogen and severe congestive heart failure.

Obstructive cardiomyopathy; idiopathic hypertrophic subaortic stenosis; asymmetric septal hypertrophy of the obstructive type. This poorly understood myocardial disease causes sudden death in about 30 per cent of individuals with it who are referred to cardiologists. It is usually familial and is recognizable in the first year of life. Characteristic of this disease is the marked increase in left ventricular outflow tract obstruction produced by infusion of the beta-adrenergic agent isoproterenol. The "medical therapy" of this disease usually means the use of a beta-adrenergic blocking agent (propranolol). The use of this agent is associated with a lessening or disappearance of the pressure difference across the left ventricular outflow tract recorded during cardiac catheterization. In adult patients, the efficacy of propranolol can be judged by its relief of symptoms, such as angina or syncopal episodes. It is much more difficult to evaluate the drug in children in whom this disease may produce little disability. In an adequate dose, propranolol can abolish the resting pressure difference between the body of the left ventricle and the outflow tract and can block the characteristic response to infused isoproterenol. Therefore it is possible to maintain these patients for years without a significant left ventricular outflow tract obstruction. Sudden death, however, has occurred occasionally in patients without a pressure gradient maintained on therapeutic doses of propranolol.

Surgical therapy consists of left ventricular myotomy and myectomy, which can also result in elimination of the pressure gradient, both at rest and after isoproterenol infusion. Surgery has been, in most cases, limited to those patients with a significant obstruction at rest who also have symptoms, most often angina or syncope. There is little question that adequate surgery prolongs the life of individuals properly selected for the procedure. The risk of the operation and the knowledge that sudden death may occur years after adequate surgical correction of the obstruction make it difficult to recommend surgery in asymptomatic children with significant obstruction. The following therapeutic recommendations, however, are based on the high incidence of sudden unexpected deaths in apparently healthy teenagers with this obstructive cardiomyopathy.

1. Patients with no demonstrable obstruction at rest who develop a significant pressure difference in response to isoproterenol infusion are treated with propranolol. We start with a dose of 1 mg./kg./day in divided dosage, increasing over the first month of therapy to a final dose of 2 mg./kg./day.*

2. Patients with a significant (40 mm. Hg or greater) pressure gradient recorded at cardiac catheterization but with electrocardiogram showing upright T waves over the left-sided chest leads are also treated with propranolol as above. They should be re-studied after six months to determine the effect of the beta-adrenergic blockade on the outflow tract obstruction.

3. Patients with a significant pressure gradient at rest (40 mm. Hg or more) whose electrocardiogram shows inverted T waves (left

ventricular strain pattern) over the left-sided chest leads are initially treated with propranolol as above. If the patient is asymptomatic and if the T waves become upright on propranolol therapy, surgery is not recommended.

4. Patients with a significant pressure gradient at rest whose electrocardiogram shows the left ventricular strain pattern with inverted T waves and whose echocardiogram and electrocardiogram do not change despite propranolol therapy at 2 mg./kg./24 hours over a period of six months are now considered surgical candidates by the author, despite a lack of symptoms and ability to take part in sports and games.

Not all patients tolerate propranolol in this dosage for reasons that are not entirely clear. The three most common complaints in such individuals are fatigue, angina and depression. Since these symptoms are more likely to occur with the use of propranolol in patients with cardiac enlargement, it is tempting to attribute them to the depressant effect of propranolol on ventricular function. Propranolol is contraindicated in patients with congestive heart failure and should be used with great caution in individuals with cardiac enlargement. The beta-adrenergic blocking effect should be evaluated every six months by echocardiography, or by cardiac catheterization if the attending physicians do not consider the former as dependable as the latter.

Pericardial Disease

DONALD C. FYLER, M.D., *and* AMNON ROSENTHAL, M.D.

Pericarditis and Pericardial Effusion. The management problems of patients with suspected pericarditis center around the questions: Is pericarditis present or not? and, if it is, Is tamponade present or likely to develop? Often the answers to these questions are not certain.

Pericardial disease is present if a pericardial friction rub is audible. Other helpful signs are suddenly enlarging heart, chest pain (precordial and left shoulder), pericardial ST and T changes on the electrocardiogram and a clinical course suggesting a disease which is known to involve the pericardium. Often repeated observations are required to become confident of the diagnosis. Treatment for pericarditis without tamponade is directed toward the underlying cause. Otherwise no specific intervention is required.

It is necessary to know whether tamponade may be developing. Marked right

*Manufacturer's precaution: Data on use of propranolol in children are too limited to permit adequate directions for use.

sided congestive heart failure with little or no dyspnea should be interpreted as tamponade until proved otherwise. The classic findings of cough, anxiety, distended neck veins, enlarged liver, "paradoxical" pulse, "paradoxical" blood pressure, narrowed pulse pressure, tachycardia and an enlarged heart which is not palpably pulsatile are well known. Unfortunately, few physicians see more than a rare child with pericardial effusion of sufficient magnitude to cause tamponade and, consequently, rigid ideas based on limited experience are common.

None of the clinical features of tamponade is a sine qua non. In any patient some of the classic findings will be present and others will not. For example, "paradoxical" pulse or blood pressure theoretically should be present in all but is not always readily observed in every patient. In practice, this sign is also observed under other circumstances (hydrothorax). When a child has or may have pericardial inflammation and the heart size is large or, even more ominous, is enlarging, close clinical observation is mandatory.

With the conviction that tamponade is developing, pericardial drainage becomes inescapable. Reticence to do a pericardial tap because of inexperience or fear of doing an unnecessary tap is common. Often the differential diagnosis comes down to either pericardial effusion and tamponade or gross myocardial failure due to myocarditis. Since myocarditis is more common, some unproductive pericardial taps are inescapable. Still, pericardial tapping has little risk compared to the danger of missed tamponade.

Inexperienced physicians should consult a cardiologist or surgeon. If no help is available, puncture of the pericardium is best accomplished by inserting the needle beneath the sternum at the xiphoid and directing it posterior, leftward and upward. Care should be taken not to puncture the liver; fluoroscopic control may be helpful. If aspiration produces blood, removal of a small amount (10 to 20 ml. in an infant, 50 ml. in an adolescent) should produce notable improvement if the blood is removed from the pericardium. If doubt exists as to the source of blood, comparative hematocrits of the supposed pericardial blood and venous blood may be helpful. Blood that has been in the pericardium for more than a few hours will have a lower hematocrit. If serious fluid is obtained, samples should be taken for culture, protein content, cell counts and pathological examination for tumor cells. The total amount of fluid to be removed is a subject of too much debate. Enough fluid to clarify the diagnosis and remove the threat of tamponade is all that is required; all additional fluid which can be aspirated easily is usually removed. The introduction of air into the pericardium may be helpful for later radiographic diagnosis, but it is necessary to be certain that the needle is in the pericardium. Close observation following pericardial tapping is required to recognize recurrent tamponade.

Bacterial Pericarditis. Having recognized this disease because of signs of pericardial effusion and a septic course, it is necessary to drain the pericardium while using appropriate antibiotics for the organisms present. Whether the pericardium is drained through repeated pericardial taps, through a tube placed in the pericardium or by opening the pericardium into the pleural cavity and drainage of the pleural space does not seem to matter. Without drainage recurrent tamponade is a life-threatening danger until antibiotics have brought the infection under control. Late constrictive pericarditis has not been a problem where drainage has been adequate and the infection eliminated.

Viral Pericarditis. Pericardial inflammation and effusion is commonly encountered in the course of viral illnesses, Coxsackie viruses being a common cause. Treatment is rarely more than expectant and pericardial taps are uncommonly required.

Tuberculous Pericarditis. This disease is now rare. Treatment with antituberculous drugs attacks the primary cause. Pericardial tapping is avoided unless tamponade is a threat. Thickening and constriction of the pericardium may occur, often having a prolonged course; the treatment is then pericardiectomy.

Collagen Disease Pericarditis. Pericarditis is sometimes the presenting feature of rheumatoid arthritis, rheumatic fever or lupus erythematosus. Pericardial tapping may be needed either for diagnostic or therapeutic reasons, but rarely because of large collections of fluid. Treatment for the underlying cause will usually result in a satisfactory regression of the pericardial inflammation.

Pericardial Effusion with Other Diseases. Neoplastic invasion of the pericardium, radiation damage to the pericardium, pericardial effusion as a manifestation of leukemia. Cooley's anemia, congenital hypoplastic anemia, or uremia may require drainage of the pericardium if tamponade is threatened while efforts to control the underlying problems are underway.

Chronic Constrictive Pericarditis. This condition is rare in childhood and consequently is difficult to recognize. The cause is sometimes easily recognized, as in the case of prior x-radiation, but the disorder may be idiopathic. With evidence of chronic tamponade and a thickened pericardium, an attempt should be made to remove the constricting pericardium. This may be dramatically beneficial to the patient but occasionally because of associated myocardial involvement, the result may be less than hoped for and postoperative congestive heart failure may be a problem.

Intrapericardial Teratoma. Intrapericardial teratoma is a rare disease, recognized because of recurrent large collections of serous pericardial fluid in infancy. Angiography locates the teratoma as deforming the cardiac chambers and arising from the region of the root of the aorta. Surgicial excision may be curative. The main problem is recognizing this rare but curable disease.

Absent Pericardium. Anomalous absence of part of the pericardium can be recognized as a typical deformity of the cardiac contour on the chest x-ray. Occasionally, enough of the heart protrudes through the defect to allow interference with cardial function. Sudden death in this condition has been described and for this reason any recognized pericardial defect of more than minor size should be investigated to determine which structures are protuding. Surgical removal of the pericardium may be required.

Systemic Hypertension

JENNIFER M. H. LOGGIE, M.B.,B.Ch.

In the past decade it has become apparent that systemic hypertension is not uncommon in children and adolescents. A major problem in discussing management is that unless blood pressure is clearly abnormal by adult standards, we do not really know what constitutes hypertension in the child or teenager. Nor is it presently known whether treatment alters the long-term prognosis for adolescents, for example, who have sustained diastolic blood pressures ≥ 90 mm. Hg and who have primary or essential hypertension.

Since blood pressure rises from infancy through the teenage years, various definitions for hypertension have been proposed for children and adolescents. All are arbitrary; none has presently been sufficiently well tested to determine its validity. Some consider the young to have definite hypertension when their systolic and/or diastolic blood pressures are frequently between the 90th to 95th percentiles for age. Others consider hypertension to be present when either reading is frequently above the 95th percentile or greater than 2 standard deviations above the mean for age. In our clinic we, arbitrarily, classify youngsters as having borderline hypertension when their supine systolic and/or diastolic blood pressure readings are frequently or persistently between the 90th and 95th precentiles for age. We presume that those whose pressures are frequently above the 95th percentile do have hypertension but we rarely institute hypotensive drug therapy in patients with supine diastolic blood pressures below 90 mm. Hg. This is a conservative approach based primarily on our concern about the implications of initiating possibly lifelong therapy in growing youngsters when so little is known about the natural history of their problem.

Management of Labile and Borderline Hypertension. It is entirely unclear how youngsters with labile hypertension should be managed. A proportion of these patients appear to become normotensive over time without any specific intervention. After a youngster has been identified as mildly hypertensive on routine physical examination and referred to us, our approach has been to obtain several blood pressure readings over a three to six week period in order to obtain an idea of the average pressure. When circumstances permit, home blood pressure readings are obtained over a two to three week period instead. In order not to create undue anxiety, great care has to be taken in reassuring the patient and his parents and, in general, referral to a consultant is unnecessary.

Those patients whose average systolic and diastolic blood pressures tend to be usually below the 90th percentile during our initial observation period are thereafter seen at 3, 6 or 12 month intervals. Those found to have blood pressure readings persistently at or above the 90th percentile for age are carefully evaluated for other cardiovascular risk factors with special emphasis on the family history of cardiovascular disease and diabetes. We request that they not add salt to cooked food and avoid highly salted foods, providing them with a list of these. If they are overweight we recommend that they attempt to lose weight by both reduction in caloric intake and regular exercise. Whether these measures result in a lowering of blood pressure remains to be proved. Furthermore, in our experience, compliance with these recommendations is suboptimal among adolescents.

Management of Chronic Hypertension. Young adults who have diastolic blood pressure readings of 90 mm. Hg appear from actuarial data to have an increased cardiovascular morbidity and mortality. No study has yet shown conclusively, however, that treating adults who have diastolic blood pressure levels persistently between 90 and 104 mm. Hg improves their prognosis. Since there are no data regarding the prognosis for either treated or untreated hypertensive children and adolescents, we elect to treat them when their diastolic blood pressure is persistently ≥90 mm. Hg. Children are, moreover, considered as candidates for hypotensive drug therapy at lower levels of diastolic blood pressure if they show any evidence of target organ damage. Other important factors to weigh when deciding whether to initiate treatment include the race and sex of the patient, the family history of early death from hypertensive complications and the patient's levels of cholesterol, triglycerides and blood sugar.

In treating either acute or chronic hypertension, it is important when selecting antihypertensive drugs to know their time to onset of action and maximal effect, duration of action, sites of action and major side effects. Information of this nature has not been sought in systematic studies of these agents in the pediatric population but has been obtained from studies performed in adults. Table 1 summarizes relevant data about the more commonly used drugs and Table 2 outlines the sites of action of the available antihypertensive agents.

When selecting a particular drug regimen for a given patient one has to take into account the cause and possible mechanisms for the hypertension, the degree of blood pressure elevation, the age and usual life style of the patient, the likelihood of compliance in drug taking and the cost of individual drugs. In specific conditions where the mechanism for the elevation in blood pressure is fairly well understood, for example, catecholamine-secreting tumor or dexamethasone-suppressible and ACTH-dependent forms of hypertension, reasonably specific therapy is available. For the majority of patients with hypertension, particularly children and adolescents, in whom the mechanisms are not understood, drugs are selected empirically.

As in adults, in youngsters with mild to moderate hypertension it is reasonable to initiate therapy with a diuretic, to add one of the adrenergically acting drugs if an inadequate response is obtained and, if necessary, to add a vasodilator as a third agent. Each agent has to be titrated individually until an adequate effect has been observed, bothersome side effects supervene or the maximum adult dose has been reached. Since the hypotensive efficacy of

the diuretics has not been studied in youngsters, we do not increase the dose of these agents beyond that recommended for diuresis for their body size except when using furosemide in patients with varying degrees of azotemia.

In our experience it is difficult to make rational adjustments in drug dosage unless one has available a graph of blood pressure readings plotted against the drugs being administered. Clearly, if at maximum doses, one of the adrenergically active agents or one of the vasodilators is producing no effect, another agent should be substituted. If some effect is observed but the response is deemed suboptimal, an agent should be added that acts at sites different from those affected by the drugs already being administered. The diuretics should not, however, be discontinued because of lack of efficacy since it is now known that they potentiate the effect of the other hypotensive drugs and prevent the sodium and fluid retention that results when the other hypotensive agents, with the possible exception of propranolol, are used to lower blood pressure.

Home blood pressure readings are probably most useful to have when a child or teenager has severe hypertension necessitating frequent adjustments in therapy. However, one has to realize when instituting this measure that it may generate a great deal of anxiety or denial in both the parents and the patient.

When caring for the hypertensive youngster, one is obliged to offer advice not only about drug therapy but also about exercise and diet. Furthermore, teenage girls should be counseled about contraception. It is also important to warn all patients and parents about the interactions that can occur between, for example, some of the antihypertensive drugs and cold remedies containing pressor amines.

In our clinic, exercise is restricted only in patients with moderately severe or severe hypertension, patients with congestive heart failure or those taking guanethidine, a drug which produces post-exercise syncope. Because the effect of the diuretics can be overcome by a high dietary sodium intake, we do recommend that young hypertensive patients not add salt to cooked foods and avoid foods with a high sodium content, providing them with a simple written list of these. As for those with borderline hypertension, weight loss is encouraged when the hypertensive child or adolescent is obese.

Since oral contraceptives may produce or exacerbate hypertension, it has been our practice to recommend the insertion of an in-

TABLE 1. Initial Dosage, Course of Action and Major Side Effects of Commonly Used Drugs[*]

DRUG	SUGGESTED INITIAL DOSE		TIME TO ONSET OF ACTION	
	Oral	*Parenteral*	*Oral*	*Parenteral*
Reserpine (many trade names)	0.02 mg./kg./24 hrs. as a single dose (usually not >0.5 mg.)	0.02 mg./kg. I.M. up to 1 mg. total dose	Dose-dependent. Slow acting, i.e., days rather than hours	I.M. ± 2 hrs.
Methyldopa (Aldomet)	10 mg./kg./24 hrs. in 3-4 doses (usually not >250 mg./dose)	5-10 mg./kg. I.V. (30-60 min. infusion)	6+ hrs.	I.V. 3 hrs.
Guanethidine (Ismelin)	0.2 mg./kg./24 hrs. as a single dose	Not available	Dose-dependent—24 to 48 hrs. at low dosage	—
Hydralazine (Apresoline)	0.75 mg./kg./24 hrs. (usually not >25 mg.)	0.15 mg./kg./dose I.V. or I.M. (usually not >20 mg.)	30-60 min.	I.V.—may be immediate. I.M.—15-20 min.
Diazoxide (Hyperstat)	Not available for treatment of hypertension	4-5 mg./kg. I.V. (up to 300 mg.)	—	I.V. ± 1 min.

*Only methyldopa is approved for use in children by the Food and Drug Administration.

trauterine device for sexually active female adolescents. It is first explained to them that pregnancy may aggravate pre-existing hypertension so that childbearing should be carefully planned, with particular attention paid to the availability of good antenatal and postnatal care.

How frequently children and adolescents with drug-treated hypertension should be seen depends primarily on the severity of hypertension, the underlying cause, and the availability and reliability of home blood pressure readings. In general, once stabilized at a satisfactory level of blood pressure, in our clinic patients are seen every 6 to 12 weeks. At each visit a history is taken that is directed primarily toward eliciting symptoms related to hypertension and side effects of drugs. The physical examination includes measurement of blood pressure in the supine and upright positions and assessment of target organ damage, including ophthalmoscopic evaluation. The laboratory tests which are ordered and their frequency also depend on the severity of hypertension, its underlying cause and the drugs being administered. Most of our patients have blood urea nitrogen, serum creatinine, uric acid and potassium, as well as urinalysis performed at least twice a year. In addition, an electrocardiogram and a roentgenogram of the chest are obtained every 12 to 18 months.

In our experience, particularly with asymptomatic adolescents, much time has to be spent at each visit eliciting information about compliance in drug taking and discussing the prescribed drugs. Finally, since the long-term effects of the chronic administration of antihypertensive drugs on growth are not known, careful attention is paid to all aspects of development.

Management of Hypertension Associated with Chronic Renal Failure. Many patients, young or old, who have chronic renal failure, appear to develop so-called volume-dependent hypertension. The key to blood pressure control in these patients lies in salt restriction and the judicious use of a diuretic such as furosemide. The thiazide diuretics become ineffective as renal function deteriorates. When conservative therapy fails, dialysis is frequently successful in controlling volume-dependent hypertension.

Those patients who have hypertension which is refractory to (or worsened by) diuresis or dialysis, have so-called renin-dependent hypertension. When this is severe and nonresponsive to hypotensive drugs, the patient may have to undergo nephrectomy before blood pressure can be controlled. Recently, however, the investigational drug minoxidil has been found effective in lowering blood pressure in many of these patients. Its usefulness in children with end-stage renal disease has been observed.

Management of Hypertensive Emergencies. Hypertensive encephalopathy, intracerebral hemorrhage, accelerated hypertension, malignant hypertension and acute left ventricular failure secondary to systemic hypertension all represent hypertensive

TABLE 1.   Initial Dosage, Course of Action and Major Side Effects of Commonly Used Drugs (Continued)

TIME TO MAXIMUM EFFECT		DURATION OF ACTION		
Oral	*Parenteral*	*Oral*	*Parenteral*	MAJOR SIDE EFFECTS
7-14 days	4-6 hrs.	Effect may persist for several weeks when treatment is discontinued	I.M. 10-12 hrs.	Flushing and drowsiness (parenteral); nasal stuffiness, bradycardia, depression, diarrhea.
± 8 hrs.	4-6 hrs.	8-12 hrs.	8+ hrs.	Drowsiness, irritability, emotional lability, postural hypotension, diarrhea, Coombs' positive hemolytic anemia.
2-7 days	—	When treatment is discontinued, full effect may persist 3-4 days. Blood pressure returns to pretreatment level in 1-3 wks.	—	Postural hypotension, post-exercise syncope, diarrhea, retrograde ejaculation, rising BUN.
± 2 hrs.	10-80 min.	1-6 hrs. (possibly longer)	1-4 hrs.	Tachycardia, headache, nausea, vomiting, rheumatoid and lupus syndromes.
—	Within 5 min. unless rebound occurs	—	6-12 hrs.	Burning at injection site, transient tachycardia, weight gain, edema, hyperglycemia, hyperuricemia.

emergencies requiring prompt intervention in a hospital setting. It is also urgent to lower blood pressure in the presence of a dissecting aneurysm, a rare event in the pediatric population. The commonest hypertensive emergencies that we have seen in children and teenagers are accelerated and malignant hypertension and hypertensive encephalopathy.

In general, we consider diazoxide,* administered as an intravenous bolus in less than 30 seconds, to be the drug of choice in treating hypertensive encephalopathy and accelerated or malignant hypertension. Our initial dose is usually calculated at 4 mg./kg. and subsequent doses are increased up to 10 mg./kg., depending upon the response obtained. With effective doses, blood pressure is usually reduced within a couple of minutes and the effect may persist for up to 12 hours. In an occasional patient, blood pressure will fall dramatically immediately after the administration of diazoxide and within 15 to 30 minutes rebound to the pre-treatment level. Without further therapy, over the next half hour there is then a decline in blood pressure to an acceptable level. Because of this phenomenon, we usually delay administration of a second, larger dose of diazoxide for at least an hour. If the initial fall in blood pressure in response to a given dose of diazoxide is clearly inadequate, however, a second, larger dose may be administered 30 minutes after the first.

It should be pointed out that when multiple doses of diazoxide are used, fluid retention and refractoriness to the drug occur. In order to prevent this, a diuretic, usually furosemide, should be given concomitantly. Patients with accelerated or malignant hypertension frequently have some impairment of renal function and, initially, when blood pressure is lowered, there may be laboratory evidence of increasing impairment. This is usually transient and does not contraindicate attempts to control blood pressure.

In unusual circumstances, when a child's hypertension has been refractory to diazoxide or other hypotensive agents, we have used an intravenous infusion of sodium nitroprusside with good response.* The concentration of drug used depends upon the size of the child and his fluid requirements, but we have usually initiated therapy by diluting 12.5 mg. of sodium nitroprusside in 250 ml. of 5 per cent dextrose in water. Blood pressure is measured on a minute-to-minute basis as the drug is titrated to effect a gradual reduction in pressure. In one patient, who had been receiving other antihypertensive drugs in high doses, a satisfactory hypotensive effect was obtained using between 0.3 and 1.2 µg./kg./min. The effective dose range in adults is considered to be 0.5 to 0.8 µg./kg./min. During prolonged use, particularly in patients with impaired renal function, thiocyanate levels should be moni-

---

*Manufacturer's warning: The safety of diazoxide injection in children has not been established.

*Manufacturer's warning: The safety of sodium nitroprusside in children has not been established.

TABLE 2.   Probable Sites of Action of
Antihypertensive Drugs

DRUG	SITES OF ACTION
Sympathetic Depressants	
Reserpine	Hypothalamus, vasomotor center, adrenergic nerve terminal
Methyldopa (Aldomet)	Vasomotor center, adrenergic nerve terminal
Guanethidine (Ismelin)	Adrenergic nerve terminal
Clonidine (Catapres)	Vasomotor center
Adrenergic Blockers	
Propranolol (Inderal)	Vasomotor center, beta-adrenergic receptor site
Phentolamine (Regitine)	Alpha-adrenergic receptor site
Phenoxybenzamine (Dibenzyline)	Alpha-adrenergic receptor site
Vasodilators	
Prazosin (Minipress)	Arteriolar smooth muscle
Hydralazine (Apresoline)	Hypothalamus, vasomotor center, arteriolar smooth muscle
Diazoxide (Hyperstat)	Arteriolar smooth muscle
Minoxidil	Arteriolar smooth muscle
Diuretics	
Thiazides	Kidney, arteriolar smooth muscle
Furosemide (Lasix)	Kidney
Ethacrynic Acid (Edecrin)	Kidney
Spironolactone (Aldactone)	Kidney
Ganglionic Blocking Agents	
Pentolinium (Ansolysen)	Sympathetic ganglion
Trimethaphan (Arfonad)	Sympathetic ganglion
Mecamylamine (Inversine)	Sympathetic ganglion

tored. If renal function is poor, it is important to know that the toxic metabolites of nitroprusside can be removed either by peritoneal dialysis or hemodialysis.

Whether diazoxide, sodium nitroprusside or a ganglionic-blocking agent is used in the emergency situation, therapy with oral antihypertensive agents should be initiated as soon as possible. In general, in the three emergencies discussed, we prefer not to administer parenteral reserpine or methyldopa because they are slower acting and can produce drowsiness or confusion, which may interfere with assessment of the patient's neurological status. We have not found parenteral hydralazine, on its own, particularly effective and it may produce sustained tachycardia, nausea, vomiting and headache.

It remains controversial in adults with acute intracerebral hemorrhage how rapidly the blood pressure should be lowered, and pediatric experience is even more limited. Theoretically, sodium nitroprusside may be the agent of choice since titration of dose can be undertaken on a minute-to-minute basis, both the onset and offset of effect are rapid, and somnolence is not a troublesome side effect. Acute left ventricular failure secondary to hypertension should be managed by the use of furosemide and prompt reduction in blood pressure with, for example, diazoxide.

In the absence of any signs of target organ damage or symptoms of hypertension, there is no clear absolute level of blood pressure that demands aggressive therapy with parenteral hypotensive agents in youngsters with chronic hypertension.

Management of Acute Transient Hypertension. Acute transient elevations in blood pressure occur with some frequency in association with a variety of childhood conditions. Whether hypotensive therapy is indicated seems to depend on the degree of blood pressure elevation and the particular disease process which is accompanied by hypertension. For example, in our experience, seizures develop with sufficient frequency in hypertensive patients with burns and hypertensive children with leukemia to warrant the early (diastolic blood pressure ≥ 100 mm. Hg) use of hypotensive agents. The mechanisms responsible for elevation of blood pressure in these conditions have not yet been elucidated so that choice of drug is arbitrary. We prefer, however, to avoid reserpine in stressed patients and those receiving corticosteroids, because of its potential for producing peptic ulceration.

Traditionally, the hypertension that may accompany acute poststreptococcal glomerulonephritis is also treated early, usually with a combination of parenteral reserpine and hydralazine. For many years we have used reserpine, 0.02 mg./kg. (up to 1 mg.) intramuscularly, as our initial dose rather than the usually recommended dose of 0.07 mg./kg. When hydralazine is also given, its dosage is calculated at 0.15 mg./kg. In our institution, diazoxide is reserved for severe hypertension accompanying acute glomerulonephritis, although its safe and effective use has been reported for milder hypertension accompanying this disease.

Management of Hypertension Secondary to Catecholamine-Secreting Tumors. Hypertension secondary to an excess of norepinephrine, produced either by a pheochromocytoma or, less commonly, by other neural crest tumors, can be successfully managed preoperatively by the administration of the α-adrenergic blocking agent, phenoxybenzamine. This agent gives smoother control of blood pressure than phentolamine, which is shorter acting. Tachycardia or arrhythmia, if present, can usually be successfully treated with propranolol given orally, but use of this drug in the absence of alpha-blockade may aggravate hypertension. It has been our practice to continue both phenoxybenzamine and propranolol up to the time of surgery in order to minimize intraoperative cardiovascular complications.

An occasional patient with pheochromocytoma may not respond to phenoxybenzamine or may become refractory to its effect. In this circumstance, use of the investigational drug, alpha-methyl-para-tyrosine, may be indicated.

New Oral Hypotensive Drugs. Propranolol, prazosin and clonidine have been approved recently for use in the treatment of hypertension in adults but not in children. Propranolol has already been used extensively for the treatment of hypertension in adults both here and abroad, and it is apparently also being used with increasing frequency in the management of hypertensive children. Its mechanisms and sites of action remain to be elucidated but it appears that this agent may lower blood pressure irrespective of whether plasma renin activity is low, normal or high. In this institution, propranolol has been reserved for use in patients not responding to other agents with which we have more familiarity. It has also been administered as the initial drug of choice to a few highly selected patients (Wilms' tumor, renal artery stenosis, accelerated hypertension secondary to dysplastic kidneys). In addition, it is used with some frequency to treat hypertension developing after renal transplantation. Our limited, short-term experience is that propranolol is often effective and appears relatively free of troublesome side effects. We usually initiate therapy with a dose of 1 mg./kg./day, administered in four divided doses every six hours.

In studies in adults, clonidine has been found to be similar to α-methyldopa in terms of both efficacy and side effects. Abrupt cessation can, however, result in a marked rebound in blood pressure which is associated with tachycardia. For this reason, we have been unwilling to prescribe clonidine for the relatively noncompliant patient population followed in our clinic.

Prazosin hydrochloride, a new vasodilator, has had limited testing in this country in adults.

Published reports seem to indicate that it has fewer side effects when given either acutely or chronically than does hydralazine. A "first-dose" phenomenon of faintness, hypotension and tachycardia has, however, been reported to occur in approximately 1 per cent of those receiving it. Preliminary data suggest that prazosin may be of value in treating hypertension associated with renal failure.

Hypotension

GEORGE BENZING, III, M.D.

The purpose of this presentation is to provide an approach to the treatment of hypotension and shock without regard to specific etiology. Although hypotension is a manifestation of shock in some patients, the blood pressure of others may be normal. These latter patients may have very low cardiac outputs for weight but maintain a normal blood pressure because of a marked increase in systemic vascular resistance. This clinical picture may be recognized by a low urinary output and the physical appearance of "shock." The physician should attempt to assess the major cause of shock from the standpoint of therapy. Some of the major types of shock include depletion of the circulating blood volume, cardiogenic, septic, and neurogenic. Characteristic features of patients in shock are the lack of an adequate blood pressure and/or cardiac output to meet the metabolic needs of the body. In some instances the cardiac output must be in excess of "normal" to meet the metabolic needs. Thus treatment must encompass this concept.

Since the frequencies of different etiologies of hypotension vary with age, the mode of treatment may be varied with age. Because the range of normal blood pressures for children of different ages varies, no single systolic, diastolic, or mean blood pressure can be specified as indicative of hypotension for all children. From observations of the care of pediatric patients the two most frequent errors in dealing with hypotension are failure to make the diagnosis because of infrequent recording of blood pressure and delay in the institution of appropriate treatment. When hypotension occurs in a hospitalized patient immediate consultation should be sought from physicians who frequently manage patients in shock.

MANAGEMENT OF ACUTE HYPOTENSION

Since hypotension is life-threatening the immediate response should be to summon the aid of four or five trained personnel, preferably physicians. One of the physicians assumes the role of overall manager with input from all assistants.

When blood pressure is unattainable or the systolic pressure is less than 30 or 40 mm Hg, cardiac massage is begun while treatment is instituted. Repeated measurements of blood pressure are made when the spontaneous heart rate exceeds 80 to 120 beats per minute depending on the age of the patient. One person suctions the patient's nasopharynx to remove any secretions, mucus or vomitus and then begins face mask ventilation with 100 per cent oxygen. The chest is inspected for inflation and for the presence of breath sounds bilaterally. While ventilation is performed, the second person starts an intravenous line in the most accessible peripheral vein. As soon as the intravenous line has been established 2.0 mEq. of sodium bicarbonate solution per kg. should be given as a bolus. Then plasma, one third normal saline solution or whole blood, whichever is readily available, is administered; 5 to 20 ml./kg. is infused by syringe. Meanwhile, the third person has computed the amount of bicarbonate to administer, the volume of fluid to be given, and drugs to be given. This same person records serially heart rate, blood pressure, urinary output, bicarbonate and medications given, and volume of fluid administered.

The fourth person takes the patient's blood pressure by cuff technique every one to two minutes as the fluid is administered and thereafter. If the blood pressure is restored to normal with 5 ml./kg. of fluid volume then the patient is observed by repeated blood pressures. If no improvement in blood pressure is obtained then up to 20 ml./kg. is given intravenously. If blood pressure is not restored by volume expansion, the physician may conclude that the contractile state of the heart is inadequate or the peripheral vascular resistance is unduly low or both. Cardiac contractility may be improved by the use of a positive inotropic agent. The above steps should be accomplished within 10 to 15 minutes.

We have tried the use of isoproterenol, norepinephrine, phenylephrine, epinephrine and dopamine* in the initial treatment of patients with hypotension. From experience in pediatric patients the use of epinephrine has been observed to be superior to other catecholamines in the great majority of instances based on responses of heart rate, blood pressure, urinary output and ultimate recovery. Although dopamine causes less change in systemic vascular resistance and preferentially

increases renal blood flow, many patients with severe hypotension do not obtain a satisfactory rise in blood pressure but do respond to epinephrine.

Five ml. of 1:1000 aqueous epinephrine is added to a 250 ml. bottle of 5 per cent dextrose solution. It is preferable to insert an administration set with an infusion rate readout capability (IV-Ometer). If the intervening tubing is filled with a nonepinephrine solution, the infusion should be run as fast as possible until the epinephrine solution enters the patient's vein. In the emergency situation, for most pediatric patients from the newborn age to age 18 years, one may infuse this epinephrine solution in the range of 1 to 30 ml./hr. according to age. The rate of infusion of epinephrine is guided primarily by the response of the patient's blood pressure. Giving a large dose of epinephrine too rapidly may cause cardiac arrhythmia, including ventricular fibrillation, and is not recommended.

In most children we start the infusion at a rate of 10 ml. per hour and increase by 2 to 5 ml. per hour each 5 minutes until an adequate response is obtained. We have noted that attempts to calculate precise amounts of epinephrine and volume of intravenous solution under emergency conditions result in delay in treatment. The recommended dose of epinephrine is 0.1 to 1.0 μg./kg./min. After the patient has become normotensive the concentration of epinephrine is changed to fit within desired intravenous fluid requirements but without a change in dose of epinephrine administered to the patient per minute. The response to the drug may require five minutes and is manifest by an increase in heart rate and blood pressure. Electrocardiographic monitoring of the patient is performed for heart rate and arrhythmia. Since peripheral infusion of epinephrine causes local ischemic necrosis of the skin, a central venous infusion line is established by cut-down as soon as possible. Administration of the epinephrine solution is continued via this route for maintenance of blood pressure.

If respiratory support is necessary nasotracheal intubation is performed by an anesthesiologist or by the most experienced physician and intermittent positive pressure ventilation instituted whenever convenient in the course of above treatment. Blood is obtained by arterial puncture or from the central venous line before starting the epinephrine for blood gas analysis. A urinary catheter is inserted and hourly urinary output recorded.

If the conscious level of the patient is not restored, the blood sugar level is estimated by test stik method and confirmed by laboratory

---

*Manufacturer's note: The safety and efficacy of dopamine in children have not been established.

measurement. If the blood sugar is estimated to be less than 50 mg./100 ml., 1 to 2 ml./kg. of 50 per cent glucose solution is administered intravenously followed by infusion of a 10 per cent solution.

The house staff of a pediatric service should be so trained that this type of organized approach becomes automatic. If the approach is chaotic it could lead to complications, such as pulmonary edema and fluid "pouring" out of the endotracheal tube with compromise of the patient's ventilation.

MANAGEMENT OF A GRADUAL DECLINE IN BLOOD PRESSURE

When in the course of a patient's illness there is a successive gradual decline in a patient's blood pressure and hourly urinary output decreases to below acceptable levels, 5 to 10 ml. of plasma per kg. is given over 15 minutes. If no increase in blood pressure is observed dopamine is suggested for its effect on contractility of the heart and renal perfusion. A dose of 5 to 30 μg./kg./min. is usually sufficient to attain an improvement in blood pressure.* However, if no significant change occurs within 20 minutes of the onset of its infusion, an epinephrine infusion should be substituted for dopamine.

In some instances restoration of blood pressure to normal by an inotropic agent may not result in an adequate cardiac output. Under these circumstances the use of a vasodilating agent, such as sodium nitroprusside, may be advisable. Because of the complexity of the problems of patients being treated for hypotension a significant background of expertise in the use of vasodilating agents is mandatory before the institution of treatment.

In those centers where suitable facilities, expertise and equipment exist, a Swan-Ganz catheter with an inflatable balloon at its tip is inserted via a peripheral vein and advanced to the pulmonary artery. This catheter allows for pulmonary artery blood sampling and measurement of pulmonary artery wedge pressure (PAW). Since the wedge pressure usually approximates left atrial pressure, PAW measurement is used as a guide to filling pressure of the left ventricle. In hypotensive shock, left and right atrial pressure may vary significantly so that central venous pressure measurements are of little value in estimating left atrial pressure. In the treatment of hypotension, PAW pressure is increased to 15 to 17 cm. of water by transfusion of fluid. Experience with the use of these catheters in children is limited

and should only be used when careful observation is available.

FOLLOW-UP MANAGEMENT

After blood pressure has been restored, the patient is placed on continuous monitoring for heart and respiratory rate. Blood pressure is recorded every 15 minutes with gradual extension to 1 hour. Hourly urinary output is recorded and used as an important guide to the adequacy of cardiac output. It should be appreciated that clear solutions will not remain in the circulating blood volume for more than 1 to 2 hours. Therefore plasma or blood is given to maintain the circulating volume within 1 to 2 hours after the initial effort to restore blood pressure. When urinary output falls, extra volume is administered intravenously and the dose of epinephrine or dopamine increased.

The electrolyte replacement and the volume of maintenance fluids are guided by the chemical determinations on the patient's blood, by maintenance fluid requirements and by fluid losses.

When the patient's condition has improved, the epinephrine or dopamine infusion is gradually tapered over 6 to 12 hours. It should be appreciated that catecholamine infusions cause hyperglycemia which does not require treatment and resolves as the drug is withdrawn.

From experience the use of a "crash cart" that contains the necessary materials for the treatment of hypotension is highly desirable. House physicians should routinely assess hospitalized patients on routine medical care for potential development of hypotension. These selected patients are monitored closely on the floor or transferred to the intensive care unit. By following urinary hourly output we treat patients with declining urinary output by volume expansion so as to prevent the development of hypotension.

In summary, the approach to the problem of hypotension begins by physician education, by preparation of "crash carts" and by constant triage of hospitalized patients. Obviously prevention of hypotension is the best approach. When hypotension is diagnosed aggressive treatment is the keystone of success.

Peripheral Vascular Disease

WARREN G. GUNTHEROTH, M.D., *and*
D. EUGENE STRANDNESS, Jr., M.D.

Peripheral vascular disorders of whatever cause will present with similar findings on initial inspection: obstructed veins will result in markedly reduced arterial flow, and the results

---

*Manufacturer's note: The safety and efficacy of dopamine in children have not been established.

of arterial spasm may be identical to those of permanent arterial obstruction at the time of onset. Therapy, however, varies from minimal medical treatment to amputation, requiring a thoughtful approach to diagnosis as well as to selection of treatment.

PERIPHERAL ARTERIES: VASOACTIVE DISORDERS

Raynaud's Disease. Raynaud's phenomenon is a vasospastic disorder of fingers and toes with a characteristic sequence of pallor, cyanosis and rubor. Criteria for the diagnosis of Raynaud's disease are excitation of the vasospastic disorder by cold or emotion, bilaterality, absence of gangrene and absence of an underlying primary disease.

Therapy should be conditioned by the generally favorable prognosis of Raynaud's disease. Surgical sympathectomy is rarely, if ever, indicated in the primary disorder. If the symptoms are bothersome, selection of a warm, dry climate is helpful but not mandatory. Clothing selection should be directed toward conserving body heat rather than just covering the affected extremities; our studies show that cold applied directly to the affected extremity is less likely to produce vasospasm than is general body cooling. The clothing should not be tight-fitting; hard-finish, tightly woven material is essential to block wind, and bulky woolen clothing is necessary for insulation against cold. In adolescent girls, a program of increased physical exercise is probably beneficial in reducing susceptibility to cold.

Medications have not been successful in eliminating Raynaud's phenomenon in our patients, but they have reduced the severity and frequency of episodes in every instance. Although several similar drugs may be equally effective, we have used tolazoline (Priscoline), a direct-acting agent that substantially increases flow in vasospastic vessels without generalized flushing or hypotension. The beginning dose is 0.5 mg./kg. four times a day. (Adult dosage is begun at 25 mg. four times a day and may be increased to 50 mg. six times a day.) The major precaution in the use of tolazoline is in patients with gastritis or ulcers, since the medication stimulates gastric secretions. In addition to tolazoline, reserpine has been useful in small doses, 0.1 to 0.25 mg. daily by mouth.* (We do not believe that the statistics linking breast cancer and reserpine are strong enough to discontinue use of this valuable drug.)

Chilblains (Pernio). Apparently invoked by cold exposure, chilblains involve itching, localized erythema, and sometimes blisters, occurring over the dorsum of the proximal phalanges of fingers and toes, and over the heels and lower legs. It is said that this is a disorder of children in cool, damp climates, but oddly, we have not seen this problem in Seattle. The disorder is more of a nuisance than a threat to life or limb. Treatment during the acute phase consists of antipruritic medications and a soothing ointment in a lanolin-petrolatum base. Management outlined under Raynaud's disease should be considered for the more persistent cases.

Acrocyanosis. This is probably more common than Raynaud's disease, but the overlap of acrocyanosis with the normal response to cold is greater than in Raynaud's. In acrocyanosis there is a more generalized response of the entire extremity in a glove or stocking pattern, and there is usually only unremitting cyanosis, without the pallor and rubor phases of Raynaud's. Ulcerations are rare, and therapy is rarely required except for cosmetic reasons. When required, therapy is the same as for Raynaud's disease.

Livedo Reticularis. Livedo reticularis and cutis marmorata are even milder peripheral vascular responses to cold, with net-like patterns of cyanosis in arms and legs. Therapy is not usually required, but the general comments pertaining to Raynaud's disease would apply to these conditions.

Erythromelalgia. Although the number of cases of erythromelalgia is smaller than that of Raynaud's disease, the symptoms are so much more debilitating that therapy must be considered briefly. Erythromelalgia presents as a peripheral hyperreactivity to heat, the counterpart to reaction to cold in Raynaud's disease. The hot, swollen and tender hands and feet are extraordinarily unpleasant, and have led to suicide in a young adult in our hospital. Therapy should be directed toward physical factors as well as medication. Cooling of the body in general, as well as cool soaks to the affected extremities, brings some degree of relief. Ephedrine has been effective in some instances, 0.5 mg./kg. every 4 to 6 hours (average adult dose, 25 mg.), preferably with a tranquilizer or a sedative.

Aspirin is definitely worth trying on a regular basis (every 4 hours), not only for its analgesic effects but also because there are indications that endogenous bradykinin may be involved.

Other authorities have suggested that erythromelalgia is a form of "peripheral migraine," and that release of serotonin is re-

---

*Although this use of reserpine is not included in the manufacturer's instructions, this schedule has been found effective.

sponsible. Accordingly, they have suggested antiserotonin medications, such as cyproheptadine.* The adult dose is 4 mg. three times daily, increased as necessary up to eight times daily. For children, an average dose is 0.08 mg./kg. Curious side effects of the drug are stimulation of appetite and drowsiness, both of which may be desirable in some instances.

Causalgia. Although a deep wound with injury to a major nerve trunk leading to "major causalgia" is easily diagnosed, forms of minor causalgia often elude prompt and effective treatment by masquerading as primary vascular disorders. Unilateral vascular disorders, particularly when associated with exquisite tenderness, swelling and abnormal perspiration, should suggest post-traumatic sympathetic dystrophy, a form of minor causalgia. The vascular disorder is most often vasospastic, but we have successfully treated a boy with sympathetic dystrophy resembling unilateral erythromelalgia.

Therapy is the same regardless of the vascular disorder: paravertebral sympathetic blockade with injections of 1 per cent lidocaine. If the diagnosis is correct, subjective relief is striking and will last for several hours. Permanent improvement will depend on vigorous physical therapy, beginning at once under the effect of the block, continuing for days or weeks and usually requiring additional injections at intervals. It is imperative to interrupt the cycle of pain, disuse osteoporosis and so forth; exercise of the affected limb is the essential therapy. The main function of sympathetic blockade is to permit relatively painless exercise of the limb. Sympathectomy is rarely, if ever, indicated in the treatment.

PERIPHERAL ARTERIES: OBSTRUCTIVE DISORDERS

Trauma. The immediate goal of therapy for traumatic interruption of arterial flow is to prevent loss of tissue and limb. Continuity of the arteries must be restored, spasm relieved, intraluminal clots removed and prevented and tissue edema managed so that the arterial lumen is not compromised. None of these aspects of care may be neglected without jeopardizing the future growth of the limb and its function without claudication.

Restoration of adequate circulating blood volume is of primary importance, not only for the preservation of life but also to permit intelligent judgment of the state of the local circulation. Although actual gangrene is rare in children, a nonoperative approach to vascular in-

jury prolonged beyond 6 to 8 hours may lead to subsequent weakness and atrophy. Thus the ultimate function of the limb should govern the acute management, and early intervention by a skilled surgeon may be truely conservative. If the diagnosis of spasm is entertained, the period of nonintervention should be relatively brief, and the assumption tested by nonsurgical sympathetic block. Arteriography may be helpful in locating the site and extent of obstruction, but the use of a transcutaneous Doppler flowmeter is less traumatic and may be repeated at will.

Proper surgical technique will include scrupulous debridement; end-to-end anastomosis if adequate vessel length is available to avoid tension, and autogenous vein graft replacement otherwise; complete removal of distal clots; relief of arterial spasm; fasciotomy to control complications of edema and hematoma; and possible anticoagulation with heparin (see under Thrombophlebitis).

An increasingly frequent source of arterial problems is medical cannulation. Assisted ventilation in the neonate requires frequent arterial blood gases. Poor technique, or overly long use, may lead to embolic problems as well as occlusion. Left heart diagnostic studies via retrograde arterial catheterization have been found to produce leg shortening if the artery clots after the procedure. The instillation of heparin, 100 units/kg., in the arterial catheter is helpful, and these patients should be followed closely for arterial pulses and long term for leg growth.

Congenital Stenosis. Peripheral arterial stenosis rarely produces any definite signs or symptoms when it is congenital, reflecting the remarkable ability of youthful tissues to develop collateral circulation.

Arteritis. Inflammatory disease of arteries may occur locally or as part of a widespread disorder usually called polyarteritis. When smaller arteries are involved, a muscle biopsy is the only means of certain diagnosis. The most effective treatment is identification and removal of sensitizing drugs, infection or toxin, and in severe generalized arteritis, the use of steroids. Major vessel arteritis which obstructs may require bypass grafting, depending upon the site and adequacy of collateral circulation.

PERIPHERAL ARTERIES: FISTULAS

Trauma. It is quite possible that the most frequent cause of this disorder in the pediatric age group is needle puncture of the femoral vein by physicians. The treatment is obviously surgical, with proper caution that closure of

---

*This use of cyproheptadine is not mentioned in the manufacturer's directive.

the fistulous connection does not compromise the arterial lumen.

Congenital. Abnormal communications between small arteries and veins, particularly if extensive, pose difficult problems. Because of the extensive and diffuse nature of the fistulas, it is rarely possible to treat by surgical removal. Since these patients often develop edema and incompetence of the superficial veins, it is necessary to treat the patient with gradient support stockings to prevent stasis changes.

PERIPHERAL VEINS: THROMBOPHLEBITIS

This is rarely a pediatric problem, but its occurrence is attended by considerable risk to life if treatment is not prompt and effective. The aggressiveness required in the therapeutic approach depends on the extent of the thrombophlebitis, whether it is progressing in spite of medical therapy and whether pulmonary embolism has occurred.

Massive deep thrombophlebitis (phlegmasia cerulea dolens) involves the entire limb with edema, severe pain and cyanosis. The presence and quality of the pedal pulses depend upon the systemic blood volume and pressure and the degree of edema. In some cases, there may be associated arterial spasm which can reduce peripheral arterial flow as well. Thrombectomy, once considered effective, should not be attempted unless there is a question of limb viability. Venous ligation or plication is performed just below the renal vein but is indicated only in those patients with pulmonary embolism that recurs while on adequate anticoagulant therapy. The use of fibrinolytic agents, such as urokinase or streptokinase, to promote clot lysis and resorption cannot be recommended at this time.

Venous thrombosis of the major deep veins is treated with bed rest, elevation, heat and intravenous heparin. It is now recommended that heparin be given by continuous intravenous infusion to maintain either the whole blood clotting time to 2 to 2.5 times baseline values or the activated partial thromboplastin time of 50 to 80 seconds. It is mandatory to use an infusion pump to avoid fluctuations in the rate of administration.

Oral anticoagulant, such as sodium warfarin, is started when the status of the limb is satisfactory; the prothrombin time should be maintained at twice the normal control. The duration of therapy has not been settled but for venous thrombosis alone, six weeks is probably adequate. However, for massive iliofemoral venous thrombosis and/or pulmonary embolism, therapy is best continued for 3 to 6 months.

If there is any edema in the limb with ambulation, it must be controlled, preferably with tailored, pressure gradient stockings from the level of the foot to the upper thigh.

SMALL VESSEL DISORDERS

Frostbite. Rapid rewarming with moderately warm water (40 to 42° C.) should be promptly initiated if the extremity is still frozen or cold. However, for those situations in which the physician may be consulted by radio or telephone, and the patient is still remote from hospitalization, rewarming should not be undertaken unless all danger of refreezing is eliminated. The duration of rewarming required will depend on the depth to which the tissue is frozen; if there is through and through freezing, rewarming of the deeper layers may require over an hour.

The subsequent care requires fastidious hygiene of the injured extremity for a lengthy period; extirpation or amputation should be delayed since surprising recovery is characteristic of frostbite injuries. Daily care should include gentle cleansing, avoidance of pressure or even light contact, bed rest and analgesics until the acute inflammation has subsided. After that stage, physical therapy is essential to gradually restore full range of motion; whirlpool baths may aid in this.

Purpuric Disorders. Small vessel thrombosis may occur with a normal platelet count (nonthrombocytopenic purpura) or with a low platelet count (thrombocytopenic purpura). The treatment varies according to the underlying disorder. The most dramatic forms of purpura are those that are progressive, causing a consumptive coagulopathy. Treatment, therefore, is anticoagulation with heparin.

Disseminated Intravascular Coagulation and Purpura Fulminans

JAMES J. CORRIGAN, JR., M.D.

Disseminated intravascular coagulation (DIC) is an acquired coagulopathy characterized by intravascular consumption of plasma coagulation factors (fibrinogen, factors II, V, and VIII) and platelets and is frequently associated with a hemorrhagic diathesis and occasionally microthrombosis. DIC has been reported in a variety of human diseases including the entity purpura fulminans. Purpura fulminans or post-infectious gangrene is an acute form of necrotizing vasculitis often triggered by a preceding infection such as streptococcal disease, varicella, rubeola, vaccinia, and probably other infectious agents.

The onset of DIC may be sudden and of short duration (e.g., septicemia), sudden and prolonged (e.g., purpura fulminans), or insidious and chronic (e.g., giant hemangiomas, malignancies). It cannot be overstated that the importance of the treatment of the syndrome is the proper therapy for the underlying primary disease. After appropriate therapy has been directed toward the underlying disease, the next aim, especially in the patient who is bleeding, is the replacement of the coagulation factors and/or platelets to hemostatic levels. Depending on the need, this may be by the use of platelet concentrates (one concentrate per 5 kg. body weight), fresh frozen plasma (15 cc./kg.), or cryoprecipitate. Cryoprecipitates contain both factor VIII and fibrinogen. In our institution, there is 300 mg. of fibrinogen and 100 units of factor VIII per bag of cryoprecipitate. In calculating the dose for replacement of fibrinogen, 100 mg./kg. should provide hemostatic levels. The frequency of administration of any or all of these products will depend upon the severity of the depletion and the responsiveness of the underlying disease process. Although it has been suggested by other investigators that replacement therapy should not be given to patients with DIC unless they are heparinized, our experience and that of others suggests that this does not actually occur in the majority of patients treated in the above manner.

In some patients, however, the treatment of the underlying disease may be inadequate or too slow, replacement therapy may not be effective, or the clinical setting may be such that the third aim of management must be considered, that is, medically interrupting the DIC with anticoagulation. Heparin has been considered the drug of choice in view of its rapid onset of action, potent anticoagulating activity, and ease of regulation and neutralization. For interrupting DIC, heparin can be used on either a continuous or intermittent intravenous schedule. On the intermittent schedule, 50 to 100 units/kg. should be given intravenously immediately and repeated every four hours. Blood for coagulation studies to evaluate the effect of this therapy should be drawn on the fourth hour (immediately preceding the next heparin injection) to eliminate the possibility of heparin interfering with the test. Since the partial thromboplastin time and prothrombin time will usually be abnormal in DIC, they cannot be relied upon to judge the effectiveness of the anticoagulation. Specific factor assays are more desirable for judging both effectiveness and duration of therapy. Although controlled studies on the use of heparin in DIC are few, data suggest that heparin has been clearly beneficial in pediatric patients with acute promyelocytic leukemia, giant hemangioma, and purpura fulminans. In purpura fulminans, heparin is recommended strongly and has been shown to reduce the morbidity and mortality associated with this disease. In purpura fulminans, there have been reports on the clinical usefulness of dextran solutions. Dextran 6 per cent solution in saline or water is administered, 600 mg./kg., over a period of two to four hours daily for two days, and then every two to three days. Low molecular weight dextran (Dextran 40) may also be used. The dose of the 10 per cent solution is 10 ml./kg. every 12 hours for the first two days, then daily. The dextran should be employed until there is adequate healing. General treatment of shock, anemia, infection, renal failure, debridement, skin grafting, and amputations is performed as the clinical picture dictates. Corticosteroids have been used, but are not generally recommended. Recovery has also been reported in single case reports following hyperbaric oxygenation. Although DIC disappears when there is a removal or reduction in size of a giant hemangioma, anticoagulation may be necessary in some cases to abolish a hemorrhagic diathesis.

There are a great number of disease states in which DIC is presumed to be operative, but the value of heparin in either correcting the DIC or influencing the total clinical course is not established. Such pediatric conditions as bacterial infections, hemolytic-uremic syndrome, thrombotic thrombocytopenic purpura, renal homograft rejection, a variety of neonatal diseases, viral, rickettsial and fungal diseases, and so forth, fall into this category.

In certain clinical settings, heparin will be useless because of the event that elicited the coagulopathy. The best example is snake bite. Some snakes, such as the rattlesnake in this country, have a thrombin-like material in the venom. Thus hypofibrinogenemia may be seen. However, the material is not thrombin and cannot be eliminated with heparin. Antivenom is the treatment of choice in this disorder.

The treatment of DIC with other agents such as platelet inhibitors, fibrinolytic activators, and dextran are presently investigational and no general recommendations can be made.

COMPLICATIONS

Bleeding is the most common and most significant complication of heparin therapy. Although the frequency of heparin-induced bleeding in documented cases of DIC appears low, it must be realized that it does occur, even at a time when laboratory data suggests that DIC is being brought under control. Bleeding due to heparin excess can be controlled by neutralization with protamine sulfate, 1 mg./100 units of heparin. Give half the calculated protamine dose intravenously (slowly) initially. Check the resultant partial thromboplastin time. If it remains prolonged, administer the remainder. (Excess protamine is also an anticoagulant.) Bleeding can also be controlled by eliminating the next injection of heparin. Once the clotting time is within normal limits, reinstitute anticoagulation with a 10 per cent reduction in dose. Circulatory overload and transfusion hepatitis also may be complications of treatment of disseminated intravascular coagulation. Hypervolemia, as seen in cardiac failure or renal shutdown, is a contraindication for dextran. Excessive doses of dextran may produce hemorrhagic states. Rarely anaphylactic reactions have been experienced with both heparin and dextran. There is no indication for antifibrinolytic therapy and agents such as epsilon aminocaproic acid are contraindicated in patients with DIC.

Rheumatic Fever

EDWARD L. KAPLAN, M.D., *and*
LEWIS W. WANNAMAKER, M.D.

The management of patients with acute rheumatic fever is directed toward making them comfortable, preventing and treating complications, educating them about the disease and especially preventing recurrences.

Except perhaps in overwhelming rheumatic pancarditis, no treatment is available which will definitely alter the basic disease process. Therefore, establishment of a well-documented diagnosis should not be clouded or precluded by premature institution of therapeutic measures. Penicillin or other antibiotics will suppress or destroy bacteriological evidence of streptococcal infection; antibiotics should not be prescribed until several throat cultures have been taken in an attempt to recover the precipitating infectious agent, group A streptococci. Aspirin or steroids will suppress the development of clinical signs essential in arriving at a sound diagnosis, which must be based primarily on an unequivocal expression of one or more of the major manifestations of the revised Jones criteria (Circulation, *32*:664, 1965).

ERADICATION AND PREVENTION OF RECOLONIZATION BY GROUP A STREPTOCOCCI

This is the most specific form of management available. After several throat cultures have been taken, patients should be given an eradicating course of penicillin (unless allergic to the drug), regardless of whether the throat culture reveals the presence of group A streptococci. The throat culture is merely a diagnostic aid, and one assumes that the infecting agent is still present (perhaps in small numbers or deep in the lymphoid tissue), whether or not it can be demonstrated. Eradication of group A streptococci will not alter the course of the disease process at this stage, but it will be helpful in interpreting future throat cultures.

The eradicating course of penicillin should be followed by prompt institution of continuous prophylaxis, since nosocomial streptococcal infections occur in hospital settings and recurrences have been observed in these situations. Monthly intramuscular injections of benzathine penicillin G offer the best protection and are preferred in high risk patients: those with residual heart damage, all patients during the first few years after an acute attack, those who are likely to have frequent contact with streptococcal carriers or infections and those who are not likely to take oral medication regularly. Oral drugs of proven value for prevention of colonization ("secondary" prevention) by group A streptococci include penicillin, sulfadiazine, and perhaps erythromycin. Resistance to sulfadiazine used for secondary prophylaxis has not appeared to be a problem in recent years, but erythromycin resistance, although rare, may be becoming somewhat more prevalent. A urine test is available for monitoring compliance in patients for whom oral penicillin has been prescribed. Our recommendations for antibiotic dosages for both treatment of streptococcal infections and prevention of recurrences are those of the American Heart Association (Circulation, *55*:51, 1977).

Some physicians choose to culture all members of the patients' family at the time of diagnosis and treat all positives to attempt to remove group A streptococci from the environment.

MANAGEMENT OF CLINICAL MANIFESTATIONS

General Principles of Suppressive Therapy

Aspirin should be given in sufficient doses to control symptoms, but in doses which will avoid side effects as much as possible. The dose can usually be titrated clinically, but determination of the serum salicylate level is often helpful in establishing an effective dose.

High dose and prolonged steroid therapy can be dangerous and is not required, although some variations from conventional schedules may be needed in certain patients.

Bed rest need not extend beyond the period of fever or active inflammation. As soon as the acute symptoms have abated and the acute phase reactants (sedimentation rate, C-reactive protein) are returning to normal, the patient may be allowed gradually increasing ambulation. Of course, patients with congestive heart failure require bed rest.

Arthritis. The differential diagnosis of arthritis in the age group most likely to get rheumatic fever is extensive. It is often difficult in the early stages of the rheumatic diseases to differentiate arthralgia from arthritis. For these reasons, therapy should not be initiated until the nature of the joint disease is clarified.

In the patient with only arthritis, or arthritis associated with mild carditis, we prefer to use salicylates rather than steroids. If the patient is extremely uncomfortable before the diagnosis is firmly established, one may use an appropriate dose of an analgesic such as codeine (without aspirin) to alleviate pain. Aspirin, 90 to 120 mg./kg./day in 4 equally spaced and divided dosages, will usually provide an optimum blood salicylate level (15 to 25 mg./100 ml.). In patients whose symptoms are not controlled or who exhibit toxicity (tinnitus or hyperventilation), the dose may need to be adjusted depending upon the results of serum salicylate determinations. In most patients with the arthritis of acute rheumatic fever, the joint findings will subside within 12 to 24 hours following initiation of salicylate therapy. If improvement is not rapid the physician should question either the dose of aspirin or the diagnosis. Seldom are corticosteroids needed for the patient presenting with only arthritis.

In the patient whose clinical manifestations are limited to arthritis, aspirin can be continued at the initial dosage for 7 to 10 days depending upon the erythrocyte sedimentation rate and the clinical course. Rather than stop the salicylate suddenly and perhaps precipitate a "flare" or "rebound," the dose can be reduced by half and continued as long as there is evidence of inflammation (elevated erythrocyte sedimentation rate). Usually this dose is continued for 3 or 4 weeks, but therapy must be individualized depending on the progress of the patient.

Patients with only arthritis usually feel better quickly after salicylate therapy is started, but we keep them at bed rest until there is a return of the sedimentation rate toward normal, and then keep them at restricted activity for an additional 2 or 3 weeks. While on restricted activity, the salicylates may be stopped if the patient remains asymptomatic, and his normal level of activity may then be gradually resumed. Since the arthritis of acute rheumatic fever is short-lived and does not leave sequelae, there usually is no need for physical therapy.

Carditis. At one time it was thought that treatment for the carditis of acute rheumatic fever had two goals: to limit and suppress the inflammatory process and to prevent the development of chronic rheumatic valvular heart disease. Now, since there is little evidence that the treatment of acute carditis with any form of anti-inflammatory therapy will prevent the development of rheumatic valvular heart disease, therapy is directed at suppressing the inflammatory response.

Those patients with evidence of carditis who do not develop cardiomegaly or congestive heart failure are often treated with salicylates alone. The doses are similar to those suggested above for arthritis, but the patients are usually treated at least 3 or 4 weeks with a full dose of salicylates, 90 to 120 mg./kg./day, and for at least 6 to 8 additional weeks with a reduced dose, approximately 60 mg./kg./day. In the patient with minimal carditis the physician must plan the duration of therapy, taking the patient's clinical findings (heart rate, crispness of heart sounds, stabilization or disappearance of murmurs, and temperature) and laboratory data (erythrocyte sedimentation rate, C-reactive protein) into account. It is prudent to occasionally check serum salicylate levels during the course of therapy.

The development of cardiomegaly with or without other evidence of congestive heart failure is felt by many physicians to be an indication for corticosteroid therapy. It has been the impression of some physicians that the clinical response in this group of patients is better when steroids are given than when salicylates alone are used. The suspected benefits of steroids in treating the acute carditis of rheumatic fever should not be confused with the lack of any definite evidence supporting their effectiveness in preventing the development of rheumatic valvular heart disease.

Several regimens for steroid therapy have been used. We suggest *prednisone* in a dose of 2.5 mg./kg./day divided in two doses. At the same time, one may also choose to initiate salicylate therapy (see doses above). As soon as there is evident improvement in the cardiac status with clinical stabilization (usually requiring about 14 to 20 days of steroid therapy), the tapering of steroids should be started, leaving the salicylates at their initial level to reduce the likelihood of "rebound." Tapering of the steroid dose usually can be safely and satisfactorily accomplished over a period of 4 to 7 days. Salicylates may need to be continued for one to three months following discontinuation of steroids, again depending on the clinical and laboratory findings. During the time of active carditis with or without heart failure, it is best to restrict the patient's activities.

In children with significant congestive heart failure, the use of cardiac glycosides and/or diuretics is also indicated (see page 136). Salt restriction may be necessary. Some patients with acute carditis are unusually sensitive to the cardiac glycosides, and smaller digitalizing doses may be indicated—for example, a *total* digitalizing dose of digoxin of 0.02 to 0.03 mg./kg. In teenagers or adults the dose may require further modification. For oral diuretics many physicians prefer spironolactone, 2 to 3 mg./kg./day in divided doses, because of its potassium sparing qualities, although the thiazide drugs (chlorothiazide, 20 to 40 mg./kg./day divided in 2 doses) or oral furosemide are usually adequate. For infants and children the dose of oral furosemide is usually 2 mg./kg. as a single dose which may be repeated in 6 to 8 hours. In severely ill patients who need rapid diuresis, furosemide in a dose of 1 mg./kg. given intravenously is usually effective.

Patients with arthritis do not require bed rest for any reason other than early joint discomfort. In contrast the primary justification for bed rest in patients with carditis is to reduce cardiac output, imposing less work on an inflamed heart which may also be working less efficiently because of a hemodynamic defect such as mitral insufficiency.

The patient with only mild carditis (with or without evidence of arthritis) will usually require 2 to 4 weeks of bed rest before laboratory and clinical evidence of a resolution of the inflammatory process becomes clear. After release from bed rest patients usually are kept at home with restricted activity for another 2 to 3 weeks. They may then be allowed to resume normal activity gradually over the next month. It should be emphasized that continual observation of the cardiac status and monitoring for evidence of inflammation must be carried out. Some patients recover earlier than others and the clinician must always individualize the plan of therapy.

In the patient with evidence of more serious cardiac involvement (cardiomegaly or congestive heart failure) the same principles hold true except that the recovery period is usually significantly longer. For example, the patient with congestive heart failure may require several months of bed rest followed by another period of 4 to 6 months of restricted activity. Clinical observations and laboratory data must be used to determine the duration of bed rest and modified activity.

Chorea. Although self-limited, Sydenham's chorea can be disabling during the acute stage of the disease. In addition to the choreiform movements, there is often significant emotional instability which may not be immediately obvious to the family or medical personnel. Therapy is directed toward making the patient more comfortable and reducing the period of confinement.

There is no completely satisfactory pharmacologic agent to treat Sydenham's chorea. Many have been used. Phenobarbital has been used with mixed success. The usual sedative dose for children is 3 to 5 mg./kg./day in 4 divided doses. The barbituates may excite some patients and the physician should be aware of this possibility.

Diazepam, a benzodiazepine derivative, is the initial drug of choice of many neurologists. The oral dose for children ranges from 0.1 to 0.8 mg./kg./day in 3 or 4 divided doses.* The dose may be increased as tolerated. If the symptoms persist, some choose to add haloperidol (see below).

The phenothiazine drugs have been used successfully and are the drugs of choice for many physicians. *Chlorpromazine* has been effective, but the physician must remain alert for signs of toxicity. An initial oral dose of 1 mg./kg. is given and is followed by increasing the dose by 0.5 mg./kg. at each succeeding dose (chlorpromazine is usually given every 12 hours) until the choreiform movements are controlled or until signs of toxicity appear. When using chlorpromazine, signs of dyskinesia should be watched for. Baseline liver function tests should be obtained before initiating therapy, during therapy and for a period of time after therapy is stopped. Rarely agranulocytosis has been noted and it should be watched for. In many instances the drug may need to be given for only several weeks. However, it is not unusual for the drug to be required for several months or even for a longer period of time. When the physician is ready to discontinue the medication, it should be done gradually.

Recently the butyrophenones have been suggested by neurologists for the care of some refractory patients with Sydenham's chorea. One of these, haloperidol, has been used in starting doses of 0.5 to 3.0 mg., 2 or 3 times a day in adults and gradually increased by 0.5 to 1.0 mg./day until there are no longer choreiform movements present or the patient

---

*Manufacturer's precaution: Oral diazepam is contraindicated in children under 6 months of age because of lack of clinical experience.

shows evidence of toxicity, such as rigidity or oculogyric crises. In children the initial dose has been 0.25 mg. The use of this drug has not been officially approved in the pediatric age group; before it is used, careful evaluation of the patient by a neurologist should be carried out. Following the control of symptoms, it is recommended that the dose of haloperidol be reduced until the patient is on the minimal dose sufficient to curtail symptoms. If haloperidol is used it should be only with caution and careful surveillance as severe toxic effects have been occasionally reported.

In patients with moderate to severe chorea, bed rest is indicated until symptoms are curtailed to prevent the possibility of the patient's injuring himself. It may be necessary to pad the bed to prevent injury. A darkened and quiet room is often recommended. It is common to maintain pharmacologic agents until symptoms are well controlled (usually after 2 to 4 weeks of therapy, but it is not uncommon for the disease to last several months) and then to reduce the dosage gradually.

"Secondary" antibiotic prophylaxis for prevention of recurrences should be given even to those patients with only pure chorea.

CHRONIC RHEUMATIC FEVER

Most attacks of acute rheumatic fever subside completely after 4 to 6 months. However, there are rare patients with evidence of continuing rheumatic inflammatory activity who meet criteria for having chronic rheumatic fever (activity for more than 8 months). Because most of these patients will exhibit continuing evidence of carditis, they require prolonged anti-inflammatory therapy, usually with steroids and/or aspirin. Often, continuous therapy for congestive heart failure is required. Steroids (in the above mentioned doses) are used. Alternate-day steroid therapy (twice the daily dose given every other day) has been tried in some patients with acute rheumatic fever and the incidence of side effects has been reported to be reduced. The efficacy of alternate-day steroid therapy, however, has not yet been proved in well controlled studies. Bed rest is an essential part of treatment of chronic rheumatic fever.

It should be emphasized that this condition is rare enough to make it essential that the physician be certain of the diagnosis before therapy is continued.

COMPLICATIONS

Prevention of Bacterial Endocarditis. Patients with acquired or congenital structural anomalies of the heart and great vessels are at risk to develop bacterial endocarditis. Most patients with rheumatic heart disease who develop this complication do so, not in the acute stage of rheumatic fever, but later when they have established valvular disease. Nevertheless, the risk of endocarditis should be taken into consideration even during the acute phase of the disease and the proper means taken to prevent its occurrence.

The patient's dental hygiene may need attention, though not necessarily in the acute phase of the disease. Appropriate antibiotic prophylaxis for all dental procedures and surgical procedures on infected or contaminated tissues is recommended (the most recent recommendations by the American Heart Association appear in Circulation, *56*: 139A, 1977). Patients receiving oral penicillin for secondary rheumatic fever prophylaxis may have penicillin-resistant viridans streptococci in their oral cavities; therefore patients on oral penicillin require special consideration for bacterial endocarditis prophylaxis (for details see American Heart Association recommendations).

Arrhythmias. First degree heart block is rather common in patients with acute rheumatic fever and usually requires no specific therapy. Second degree heart block occurs less frequently. The presence of second degree or greater heart block may be an indication for steroid therapy if the patient is not already on steroids. Rarely, second degree heart block will progress to complete heart block. Atropine has been used successfully in some cases of complete heart block during the acute phase of rheumatic fever. This is based upon the suggestion that a vagal stimulus is important in the etiology of heart block in patients with rheumatic fever. The rare patient with complete heart block and bradycardia who is refractory to atropine may be a candidate for pacemaker therapy. Other arrhythmias such as sinus bradycardia have been noted, but they seldom require specific therapy.

Emotional Support of the Patient and Education of the Family. Anxiety is almost always present in children with acute rheumatic fever even if they have only arthritis, but especially if there is chorea or carditis with congestive heart failure. Much of this anxiety is a reflection of the concern they see in their parents and, in some cases, in the physicians and nurses caring for them. While the emotional overlay seldom requires pharmacologic therapy, we feel that the time of the initial diagnosis is an excellent opportunity to begin to educate the family and the patient regarding the extent, implications and possibility of control of his or her disease. This often will allay the anxiety. This discussion not only should include information about the relationship of streptococcal infections to rheumatic fever—with emphasis on secondary prophylaxis—but should also include an outline of what changes, if any, might be required in the patient's life style. In our experience the earlier this is begun, the better understanding the family has and the better the compliance with secondary prophylaxis.

6

Digestive Tract

Diseases and Injuries of the Oral Region

HARVEY A. ZAREM, M.D.

CLEFT LIP

The primary problem with a congenital cleft of the lip is appearance. An infant can function effectively with a cleft lip: it is not a cause of difficulty in feeding or a failure to thrive and it is not associated with otitis media as is cleft palate. Some plastic surgeons repair cleft lip in the newborn, but the majority of craniofacial teams in the United States prefer to close the cleft lip at approximately 3 months of age, when a child tolerates general anesthesia with less risk than does the newborn. There is no contraindication to postponing operative repair of the lip if there are extenuating circumstances. Subsequent to primary repair of the lip, secondary procedures are often necessary between 4 and 6 years of age to correct scar irregularities and to correct the invariable nose asymmetry.

CLEFT PALATE

Cleft palate presents several problems in contrast to cleft lip. Some infants can feed readily despite a cleft of the palate, but some infants do have difficulty with suction. A long, soft lamb's nipple is often effective. When the mother has learned to feed the infant patiently, the infant will thrive. If an infant fails to thrive, it is unwise to attribute failure to thrive to a cleft of the palate.

Children with clefts of the palate have a high incidence of otitis media even in the neonatal period. Some otologists have recom-mended that all children with clefts of the palate undergo routine myringotomy with insertion of polyethylene or stainless steel tubes to maintain patency of the drum. Early diagnosis of otitis media and early treatment with decongestants and antibiotics have prevented hearing loss.

The major problem associated with a cleft of the palate is difficulty in speech. In the past decade, with improved techniques of closing the palate and with use of pharyngeal flaps, there seems to have been a dramatic improvement in the quality of speech of patients with clefts of the palate.

Most palatal closures are done at age 18 months. At this time the child is old enough to tolerate the operative procedure safely and yet is young enough that speech patterns have not developed. Following closure of the palate, the family should be advised to enunciate clearly and speak deliberately to the child in order to encourage good speech habits. If there is inadequate closure of the soft palate to the pharynx (velopharyngeal competency) several measures may be considered.

A prosthodontist may make a speech bulb that will mechanically aid in closure of the space between the soft palate and the pharynx—a temporary measure to encourage development of the pharyngeal musculature. When a significant defect exists which has not improved with appropriate speech therapy, a pharyngeal flap has been effective in closing the defect and in improving speech. Problems associated with pharyngeal flaps are inadequate size of the flap (and therefore inadequate speech improvement), denasal speech, and nasal airway obstruction.

A child born with a unilateral cleft of the

169

lip and palate may expect a normal life pattern with the quality of operative correction of the deformities that are available today. The child with a bilateral cleft lip and palate, however, presents a significant number of developmental deformities that may produce problems even with excellent dental and surgical care. The midportion of the upper jaw (premaxilla) is prominent in infancy, but hypoplasia of the maxilla at puberty is the ultimate problem. The adolescent child who has had a bilateral cleft of the lip and palate is likely to have problems of deformity because of the hypoplasia of the maxilla, and nasal deformity associated with the bilateral cleft lip and palate is a persistent problem. Although judicious operative repair and sophisticated orthodontia have greatly improved the outcome of these problems at puberty, the child with bilateral cleft lip and palate usually has significant facial problems that require extensive orthodontic and operative reconstruction.

Routine tonsillectomy and adenoidectomy should not be carried out in the child who has had a repair of a cleft palate. Frequently the hypertrophic adenoids occlude the pharynx and thereby aid speech by minimizing velopharyngeal incompetency. Concern must also be applied to the child who has a submucous cleft. Frequently a child with a submucous cleft (which can be recognized by the bifid uvula, the thin blue midline in the soft palate, and a lack of a nasal spine with notching of the posterior border of the hard palate in the midline) has adequate velopharyngeal closure until a tonsillectomy and adenoidectomy have been carried out. Prior to recommending such an operative procedure, it is necessary to ascertain that the soft palate is normal.

MACROGLOSSIA

The term macroglossia is often applied to any condition in which the tongue appears to be large for the mouth. Occasionally the diagnosis is made when, in fact, the problem is a small mandible. The primary concern in macroglossia is airway obstruction as in the Pierre Robin syndrome. Most instances of macroglossia are due to lymphangioma of the tongue. In early infancy, the tongue appears to be normal but it is larger than normal. As the child grows, the small reddish blue cystic areas and papillomatous protruberances on the tongue make the diagnosis obvious. In a small number of patients, macroglossia may be the result of type 2 glycogen storage disease. There is dispute as to the proper management of macroglossia, but excising a portion of the tongue from the midline as well as the border of the tongue in a fleur de lys fashion effectively reduces the size of the tongue and has greatly reduced malocclusion, open bite, and drooling, which have accompanied extreme macroglossia when associated with lymphangioma.

PIERRE ROBIN SYNDROME

Robin originally described a syndrome which included cleft palate, macroglossia (large tongue) and micrognathia (retruded mandible). The primary significance of the syndrome was the fear of glossoptosis, the danger that the child could die from asphyxiation by "swallowing his tongue." Recognition of this syndrome is controversial. Many patients do not have the cleft palate. Awareness of the danger of glossoptosis in the first 6 to 8 months of life and recognition that the mandibles in the majority of patients with Pierre Robin syndrome develop normally by adolescence and require no orthognathic surgery are important therapeutic considerations. The difficulty in breathing is readily treated by placing the child on the abdomen or by pulling the tongue forward. When the syndrome is suspected and there have been episodes of airway obstruction, definitive treatment by suturing the tongue forward to the mandible is indicated. The success of the operative procedure is excellent in experienced hands. In Great Britain it is common to maintain the child with prone position until the neonatal period has passed and the danger of glossoptosis is no longer present. This is feasible with selected families or with hospitalized children, but it is not as definitive as the Beverly Douglas procedure of suturing the tongue forward to the mandible.

UNUSUAL CLEFTS

Although by far the most common clefts on the face involve the upper lip and palate, numerous other clefts may occur. Median upper lip clefts with absence of the nose have occurred, but these are usually associated with microcephaly and are incompatible with life. Lateral and oblique clefts of the face occur rarely. The clefts can extend from the oral commissure to the ear, or from the mouth to the base of the nose to the eye. Recognition of these clefts can sometimes be difficult because they may be subtle in infancy. There is no immediate treatment indicated and ultimate treatment should be deferred until development of the face is more nearly complete (approximately 2 to 4 years of age.) There is usually more extensive involvement than is immediately apparent in the infant, and there is often a significant lack of tissue requiring extensive reconstruction.

TONGUE-TIE

A significant number of infants are born with a short frenulum extending from the tongue to the central incisor area of the mandible. The majority of these children are asymptomatic. If the child can protrude the tongue, such as in licking a lollipop, the likelihood of tongue-tie affecting speech is minimal. However in significant tongue-tie, it is appropriate to release the tongue surgically. "Snipping" the tongue-tie is usually inappropriate since a definitive procedure with Z-plasty and extension of the length of the frenulum is necessary. When the band is extremely thin, simple "snipping" may be effective.

MACROSTOMIA

The diagnosis of macrostomia is occasionally missed because it is associated with underdevelopment of the mandible. The distance between the midline of the upper or lower lip and the oral commissure is greater on the affected side than on the normal side. It is commonly associated with the first and second brachial arch syndrome and with hypoplasia of the entire half of the face including the ear, the temporal muscle, masseter muscle, parotid gland, zygoma, and mandible. In addition, brachial cleft sinuses are often associated. The macrostomia can be closed by Z-plasty. The management of jaw deformity and hemifacial hypoplasia is a complex issue and should be deferred until development of the jaw and eruption of the teeth.

JAW DEFORMITIES

Micrognathia. Micrognathia may occur separately or in association with other syndromes such as Pierre Robin syndrome or hemifacial microsomia (first and second brachial arch syndromes). A significant number of micrognathias occur as hereditary features which are not necessarily a specific syndrome. Unless extreme, jaw development deformities are usually not apparent until the child is 5 to 6 years of age. The child should be evaluated by an experienced orthodontist, who is most capable of assessing dental and jaw development. The majority of the children who require operative correction are deferred until full dental eruption, usually at age 18 or older. Severe facial deformities due to extreme jaw abnormality are treated at varying ages, depending on dentition.

Macrognathia (protruded mandible or prognathism) is also a deformity which is not readily apparent until the child is 5 to 6 years of age. It is characterized by an obtuse angle between the ramus of the mandible and the body of the mandible, and often an open bite. As in micrognathia, the diagnosis, evaluation and treatment are sophisticated and the patient should be evaluated by an orthodontist.

Bony Overgrowth of Jaws. A number of disorders are not common but present a problem of diagnosis and treatment with overgrowth of either the maxilla or mandible. Overgrowth of the jaw may be the result of anteriovenous fistula, which is usually apparent by the increased prominence of the vessels, by a bruit in the external carotid and its branches to the involved area, and by the increased warmth of the soft tissues. The management of an arteriovenous fistula involving the mandible or maxilla is difficult. The disease is invariably progressive. Patients may have dramatic episodes of bleeding which require blood transfusions. Frequently it is necessary to ligate the external carotid artery to control the bleeding, but the ultimate treatment is radical excision of the involved parts. This decision is difficult since the surgery and the deformity are extensive; however, once the diagnosis is established and the course of progression of the arteriovenous fistula and progressive risk of serious hemorrhages have been declared, definitive treatment should be instituted.

A number of patients with neurofibromatosis, either local or diffuse as in von Recklinghausen's syndrome, have involvement of the face. Overgrowth of the soft tissues and of the bones on the involved side of the face are the consequence. There is increased bulk of maxilla and/or mandible with gingival hypertrophia and displacement of the teeth. Management is by excising the offending tissues and sculpturing the tissues to correct the deformity. To "cure" the disease would entail an extensive operative procedure with removal of many normal structures and is never advisable. The course of this disease depends on the progression and the age of onset of symptoms. The earlier the age of onset and the more rapid the course in youth, the worse the prognosis. Hemifacial hypertrophy, with enlargement of all of the facial structures (including jaw and teeth) unilaterally, presents a similar picture but is without the soft tissue neurofibromata.

Fibrous dysplasia of the jaws is an unusual condition involving the mandible and/or maxilla, which is enlarged because of the fibrous and noncalcified tissue within the bone. The presence of this entity is often not evident until late childhood, but it is usually self-limited when the child reaches puberty and growth ceases. This disorder must be recognized to avoid a misdiagnosis and radical excision of tissues. Contouring bone to reduce the deformity can be done in order to tide the child over until puberty and skeletal maturation. In some instances the excess bone that had been excised will recur, and this must be appreciated by the family before operative management of children with fibrous dysplasia of the jaws is undertaken.

Orofacial dysostosis is a congenital anomaly expressed in the oral region by alveolar clefts, tongue clefts, cysts of the upper lip and supernumerary teeth associated with anomalies of the hand and mental retardation.

Infantile cortical hyperostosis, or Caffey's disease, is a self-limiting disease of children seen with onset of fever, soft tissue swelling, and periosteal new bone formation of the mandible. It occurs most commonly in the neonatal period (2 to 4 months of age) and could be mistaken for osteomyelitis of the mandible. The clavicles are often involved and the x-ray picture is one of increased density on the surface of the bone due to new bone formation with overlying brawny induration of the soft tissues. In the mild cases no treatment is necessary except to maintain comfort of the patient, but in the severe cases treatment with corticosteroids is indicated. It is recommended that the steroid dosage be continued over several months because exacerbations have occurred with early withdrawal of steroids.

TRAUMA

The majority of injuries about the oral region are minor and do not necessitate hospitalization. For the occasional severe injury, the most immediate dangers are exsanguinating hemorrhage and airway obstruction owing to loss of control of the tongue or to the blood. Most bleeding can be stopped by direct pressure.

If a child has eaten solids or liquids within 4 hours prior to the injury, it is generally not wise to consider general anesthesia except in dire circumstances. Emptying time of the stomach is prolonged after injury, so that the time lapse following an injury is often not reliable for judging a safe period. The majority of injuries about the mouth and face can be repaired using local anesthesia if some sedation is given and if the manner of the treating physician and parents is calm. Once the area is anesthetized, the majority of children relax and even doze during the repair.

Anesthesia about the face is often accomplished either by direct infiltration of Xylocaine 1 per cent with epinephrine 1:100,000 or by regional nerve blocks. The entire upper lip can be anesthetized by injecting the infraorbital nerve, and the lower lip can be anesthetized by injecting the mental nerve. These simple nerve blocks are effective and once the area is anesthetized the child is usually cooperative.

Prior to the days of antibiotics, surgeons were cautious of closing any wounds that had occurred four or more hours prior to treatment. Today, it is appropriate to close all facial wounds that are not overly contaminated despite the fact that more than four hours may have elapsed from the time of injury to the time of treatment. In animal bites or severe contamination, the use of tetanus toxoid, antibiotics and judicious closure initially or closure secondarily (within several days of the injury) are appropriate. It is rarely advisable to allow a wound of the face or oral region to heal secondarily because of the resulting scar deformity. If a wound were closed when the degree of contamination was underestimated, examination daily would allow the treating surgeon to open the wound at the first sign of infection and prevent a serious consequence.

A major portion of wounds seen in children in the emergency room are puncture wounds of the lower lip from the incisors. This wound lacerates the mucosa, the lower lip musculature, and the skin. This "through-and-through" wound is best cleansed with saline irrigation after local anesthesia and closed primarily. Small wounds may be closed with sutures in the mucosa and in the skin, but large wounds that are through-and-through should be closed in layers to include fat and muscle. Nonabsorbable soft suture material (preferably silk) should be used in the mouth when it is feasible to remove the sutures postoperatively.

Absorbable sutures cause inflammation in the mouth and synthetic sutures such as nylon are stiff and extremely uncomfortable to the sensitive mucosa of the mouth. Closure of the muscle may be accomplished by absorbable sutures (Dexon, Vicryl, or catgut), and closure of the skin should be effected with nonabsorbable sutures such as a nonreacting fine (6-0) nylon which can be removed. In the rare instances in which it is felt that the sutures cannot be removed from the skin, nonabsorbable synthetic sutures such as Dexon or Vicryl are acceptable but only as second choices to the nonreactive synthetic fine nylon. Sutures on the skin of the face should be placed very close to the edge of the wound to avoid suture marks. They should also be removed approximately 4 to 5 days following the injury. The wounds can be supported after suture removal with an adhesive porous tape such as Steri-strips or Clearon. These paper tape closures will remain on the skin for approximately 5 to 7 days if left dry.

When the laceration about the lip extends across the mucocutaneous juncture (the white line between the vermilion of the mucosa and the white skin), care must be taken to align the fragments of the juncture. This is best done with the aid of magnifying loupes by aligning the fine white "roll" that is apparent due to the thick sebaceous glands at the juncture. A small malalignment is conspicuous. When there is a significant loss of mucosa, it is often advisable to excise the wound in a V fashion and close the wound primarily. When there has been a loss of mucosa, such as a dog bite, it is necessary to consider rotating a mucosal flap from the adjacent lip mucosa, a mucosal graft, or occasionally a tongue flap. Injuries in which there is a significant loss of tissue of the lip are difficult and the reconstruction is complex to restore mucosa, muscle, and skin. Sometimes it is best to close the wounds in a simple fashion and to defer extensive reconstructive procedures. When the immediate treating physician is not adequately experienced, it is always wisest to do a simple wound closure.

In general, it is preferable for the patient to have definitive wound repair at the time of the initial injury. If one allows the wounds to heal initially without definitive repair, scarring must be corrected secondarily. There are often circumstances (such as associated injuries, lack of available facilities and personnel, and the general condition of the patient) which may dictate secondary procedures rather than extensive primary repair. Secondary procedures, which include mucosal flaps, cross-lip flaps, and tongue flaps, should only be undertaken by an experienced surgeon.

Lacerations of the tongue are usually a problem because of extensive bleeding. The bleeding can be controlled by large sutures. The suture material should be a silk because it is soft and relatively nonreacting, but this must be done only in the child who will cooperate to allow removal of the sutures.

On all significant injuries of the mucosa of the mouth, including lips, gingiva, tongue soft palate, and pharynx, several steps have resulted in diminished infection and improved results. The child should be kept on a clear liquid diet for a minimum of three days and preferably seven days. A clear liquid diet consists of transparent liquids without particles. This prevents food particles from entering the wound as a nidus for infection. It is difficult to convince the family of the child that this diet is compatible with health and well being.

After solid foods have been resumed, it is wise to rinse the mouth after each meal with plain water or a milk salt solution (a quart of warm water in which has been dissolved one teaspoon of table salt and one teaspoon of baking soda). Frequent washing of the mouth and irrigating of the wounds in this manner have resulted in excellent wound healing. The use of antibiotics in these wounds is variable. Most surgeons agree that the use of an antibiotic for five days is safe and has resulted in a diminished incidence of wound infection and inflammation.

In all significant lacerations about the mouth, the treating physician should be aware of possible injury to the parotid duct and facial nerve. Parotid duct injury, if not recognized, can result in parotid secretions into the tissues, or in a parotid fistula, which are difficult to manage and often require secondary procedures. If, on the other hand, the injury to the parotid duct is recognized at the time of the trauma, repair of the duct is simple and effective, best accomplished under general anesthesia in the young child.

Injuries to the facial musculature or to the facial nerve should be appreciated prior to treatment, especially prior to the administration of local anesthetics. The child should be asked to activate all of the facial muscles of expression and asymmetry should be carefully noted. If the injury to the facial nerve occurs anterior to a vertical line through the lateral canthus of the eye, the likelihood of recovery of function without surgical repair of the nerve is excellent. However, if the injury occurs proximal to this line, which is proximal to the anterior border of the masseter muscle, it is wise to undertake a search and repair of the nerve. This must be done under general anesthesia with magnification and with microsurgical instruments.

Electrical burns of the mouth are unusual. They usually occur when a toddler places the juncture of an electrical appliance and of an extension cord in the mouth. The saliva acts as a conductor and causes an electrical burn. Severe electrical burns can result in loss of major portions of the upper and lower lip and gingiva, and even injury to the tooth buds and mandible. Fortunately, the majority of these injuries involve only the lips and oral commissure. Electrical injuries to the midportion of the upper and lower lip usually heal without severe deformities.

The treatment of the electrical injury to the lip must be definitive. Immediately after the injury, the degree of trauma is usually not evident. The child should be given sedation, antibiotics, and the family must watch the child carefully. Late bleeding from the labial artery can be dramatic and, if it occurs, does so between 5 and 7 days following injury. Parents are instructed to watch for bleeding and, if it occurs, to pinch the lip between the fingers and to bring the child to the emergency room immediately.

The majority of surgeons prefer to treat electrical burns with antibiotic therapy and to allow secondary healing. If a deformity occurs at a later date, reconstruction is undertaken electively. The primary reason that this has been a chosen course is that it is often difficult to determine the extent of loss of tissues in the early post-injury phase. About three weeks following the injury, the degree of tissue loss is usually evident. If a significant portion of the upper or lower lip at the commissure has been lost, restoration of the bulk of the lip using the tongue as the source of muscle and mucosa can be done as a tongue flap at 3 to 4 weeks post-injury. This procedure must be carefully executed but it is effective in extensive electrical burn injuries of the oral commissure.

Salivary Tumors

BURTON F. JAFFE, M.D.

Of all salivary tumors in children, parotid tumors are the most common, submaxillary tumors are very uncommon, and minor salivary gland tumors in the mouth are almost nonexistent. At each site, however, benign tumors far outnumber malignant tumors.

Parotid tumors in children are benign in at least 90% of cases. When a parotid mass occurs at birth, or within a few months of life, it is almost always a benign hemangioma or lymphangioma. These are both diffuse, soft bulging masses overlying the preauricular and ascending ramus of mandible areas. Because involution of these masses occurs frequently, reassurance to the parents and observation are the cornerstone of management. However, if the masses do not respond in a typical manner, surgical intervention may be indicated. Specifically, surgical removal is contemplated if the hemangioma progressively increases in size, if sudden hemorrhage into the tumor occurs, or if rapid growth occurs, raising the suspicion of a malignant lesion. In these cases, a superficial parotidectomy with removal of the subcutaneous tumor mass is accomplished with isolation and preservation of the facial nerve. Low dose radiation therapy for a benign lesion is not justified in view of possible late-occurring secondary malignancies.

If a tumor mass develops in the parotid in late infancy or childhood, the most likely tumor is a benign mixed tumor. These are slow growing tumors with clinical well defined margins, ranging in size from a tiny mass to a few centimeters in diameter. They are painless, immobile, and nontender. A superficial parotidectomy should be performed as the biopsy and as the definitive surgical cure.

About 10 per cent of all parotid tumors in children are malignant, and these may even be present in the newborn. Clinically, they are rapid growing and sometimes painful. If facial nerve paralysis accompanies a parotid tumor, the tumor is typically malignant. Retrograde sialography is helpful to rule out benign conditions. When a malignancy is suspected, an open biopsy is indicated.

The most common malignancies of the parotid are mucoepidermoid carcinomas, acinic cell carcinoma, and sarcomas (such as mesenchymal tumors, rhabdomyosarcomas, and undifferentiated tumors). Total parotidectomy is the treatment of choice. Radiation therapy and chemotherapy must be considered in each case and individualized care is predicated on tumor type, rate of tumor growth, and tumor extent. In general, the mucoepidermoid carcinomas carry a favorable prognosis, whereas the sarcomas have a poor prognosis.

Submaxillary tumors are usually benign mixed tumors and occur in older children. A malignant tumor is suspected only because of very rapid growth. In either case, total submaxillary gland removal is indicated as a diagnostic biopsy. Radiation therapy may be decided upon after the type of malignancy is determined.

Recurrent Parotitis

BURTON F. JAFFE, M.D.

Recurrent attacks of parotitis may occur unilaterally or bilaterally, and may flare up 1 to 25 times per year. Examination reveals a swollen, tender, firm parotid gland with little or no expressible saliva. Bimanual palpation of the parotid duct rules out a palpable stone or mass in the duct. If stones are not encountered, and parotitis has occurred one or two times, I treat symptomatically with analgesics (Tylenol, 300 to 1200 mg./day), one glass of fluid every hour while awake, local heat (10 minutes per hour), and antibiotics (penicillin, 50 mg./kg./day up to a maximum of 250 mg. four times daily). The patient is instructed not to eat citrus fruits or spices which stimulate the gland, giving more pain and swelling.

Usually the recurrent parotitis is due to a decreased formation rate of saliva, increased viscosity of saliva, and a decreased flow or stasis in the ductal system. The sequence of events leading to chronic recurrence of parotitis is decreased secretion of saliva, retrograde infection, low-grade ductal infection, metaplasia of ductal epithelium, and obstruction (mucous plugs, stricture, calculus).

When the child has three or more bouts of parotitis, I first consider systemic disease, since recurrent parotitis can be the early stage of Sjögren's syndrome. A dry mouth and dry and itchy eyes might be present. The neck is palpated for an enlarged thyroid; skin lesions indicative of collagen diseases are sought; and the history and presence of arthritis is determined. Examination by slit lamp may reveal keratoconjunctivitis. Blood tests for collagen diseases are indicated.

Sialography will determine the status of the duct and the parenchymal tissue of the parotid glands. The duct may reveal a stricture which can be dilated or a calculus which can be removed. In older or cooperative children, dilatation or removal can be carried out under local anesthesia, but in younger or uncooperative children, general anesthesia is required. If dilatation fails to control recurrent parotitis, a superficial parotidectomy may be indicated, depending on the rate and severity of the attacks.

Parotid parenchymal changes show a progression from a "lifeless" tree pattern due to atrophy of acinar tissue, to minor ectasia of acinar structures, to major ectasias, and culminate in cystic degenerative changes.

A superficial parotidectomy is clearly indicated for cystic degeneration, and may be indicated in lesser pathologic states if the recurrence rate is high and the discomfort severe. One or more calculi in the gland also mandates a superficial parotidectomy.

Superificial parotidectomy requires identification, isolation, and preservation of the facial nerve during the removal of the gland. The duct is included with the specimen to avoid future disease in the duct. For bilateral disease either concomitant or staged excision is required.

The pathological specimen may reveal lymphoepithelial islands with absent acinar tissue, consistent with Mikulicz's disease. Sjögren's disease is documented if two of three of the following occur: dry eye, dry mouth, or connective tissue disease. Even if no systemic disease is found, a repeat physical examination and blood tests are performed annually to detect collagen diseases.

Thyroglossal Duct Cysts

BURTON F. JAFFE, M.D.

Classically, the thyroglossal duct cyst is a mass occurring in the midline of the neck between the chin and the larynx. It ranges from 2 mm. to a few centimeters in diameter. In 80 per cent of children the mass is asymptomatic except for the cosmetic deformity present. Surgical excision is indicated.

In 10 per cent of children the cyst becomes secondarily infected during an upper respiratory infection. It enlarges in size, becomes tender, and may present as a fluctuant abscess. Penicillin, 50 mg./kg./day in three or four divided doses (not to exceed 250 mg. four times daily) for one to two weeks, is indicated. Application of local heat once an hour for 10 minutes throughout the day hastens resorption. If the infection fails to respond in a few days, needle aspiration is performed, the aspirate is cultured and sensitivity is determined. After the infection resolves, surgical excision is indicated.

In 10 per cent of children the cyst ruptures from the abscess, or an incision and drainage is performed, producing a chronic draining sinus. A culture is obtained and penicillin (as described above) is used to control the primary infection until the sensitivity report is available. Later, surgical excision is required.

The cyst typically has a tract that extends through the hyoid bone and then courses through the base of the tongue to the foramen cecum. As many as 12 ducts have been seen histologically in the base of the tongue. Correct surgical excision requires removing the body of the hyoid bone and a core of muscles in the base of the tongue. Surprisingly, the postoperative course is benign and no dysphagia, speech problems, or cosmetic problems occur. Recurrences result from unexcised persistent ducts.

Branchial Arch Cysts and Sinuses

BURTON F. JAFFE, M.D.

The human embryo has four well-developed arches and a fifth arch that is poorly defined. Each arch may give rise to a cyst or a tract.

Branchial Arch Cysts. These cysts may flare up concomitantly with acute upper respiratory infection and present with pain, tenderness, and erythema. Clinically, the appearance is similar to cervical adenitis or a suppurative node. Treatment with systemic antibiotics for gram-positive bacteria (pencillin, 50 mg./kg./day up to 250 mg. four times a day), hot soaks, and analgesics are indicated. Once the infection has subsided, surgical excision is indicated.

Often the cysts gradually and painlessly enlarge, creating concern because of a cosmetic problem or parental fear of malignancy. Clearly, surgical excision is also indicated.

The first branchial arch cyst may appear at any point below the pinna or in the submaxillary triangle. The second branchial arch cyst will appear along the anterior border of the sternocleidomastoid muscle from the level of the hyoid bone to the lateral border of the thyroid cartilage. The second cyst is the most common arch anomaly. The third cyst occurs rarely and presents in the lower third of the neck along the anterior border of the sternocleidomastoid muscle. Cysts may appear at any age, although 5 to 15 years are most frequent ages for development.

Surgicial excision requires care and knowledge of the embryology. The first cyst has a close relationship to the facial nerve which must not be traumatized. The second cyst may have a fistulous tract medially ascending in the neck, coming between the external and internal carotid arteries, lateral to the hypoglossal and the glossopharyngeal nerves, passing beneath the styloglossus muscle, and entering the pharynx at the supratonsillar fossa. Failure to remove this tract in its entirety will lead to a recurrent cyst.

Branchial Arch Sinuses. A tiny pinpoint opening in the skin of the neck, present from the time of birth, indicates the existence of a sinus. Many sinuses end blindly in the neck tissues, and may drain intermittently with upper respiratory infections. Antibiotic therapy (penicillin, 50 mg./kg./day up to 250 mg. four times a day), is indicated first, but surgical excision is the treatment of choice. Most external sinuses do not drain and are considered to be only a cosmetic problem, and are excised under general anesthesia. The first branchial sinus typically approaches the cartilage of the external auditory canal, and rarely will extend into the ear canal.

Some sinuses may communicate from the skin to the pharynx and are called fistulas. For example, a branchial fistula enters the supratonsillar fossa, this fistula drains saliva, so that early detection occurs and early surgical excision in infancy is advocated.

Disorders of the Esophagus

KATHRYN D. ANDERSON, M.D.

ESOPHAGEAL ATRESIA WITH TRACHEOESOPHAGEAL FISTULA

The importance of early diagnosis of esophageal atresia with tracheoesophageal fistula cannot be overemphasized. The infant born with discontinuity of the esophagus is at risk from pulmonary complications: (1) overflow of saliva and/or feeding from the proximal esophageal pouch into the trachea and (2) reflux of gastric contents through the lower esophageal segment into the tracheobronchial tree. Unless recognized and treated promptly, life-threatening pneumonitis is a consequence. Transfer to a tertiary pediatric care facility is most safely accomplished with the infant propped at an angle of 45° and the upper esophageal pouch intermittently decompressed by gentle suction. The position of the infant is maintained following arrival, and the upper esophageal pouch is then placed on constant sump suction with a No. 10 Replogle tube. This requires occasional irrigation with 1 ml. of saline to maintain patency.

The timing of definitive treatment depends on several factors. For the full-term infant without pulmonary complications or associated anomalies, early division of the tracheoesophageal fistula and primary repair of the esophagus without a preliminary gastrostomy are recommended. For infants with low birth weight or with evidence of pneumonia, primary repair is best delayed. A gastrostomy, using a No. 12 to 14 Malecot catheter, is performed under local anesthesia. Suction is maintained on the upper pouch and the infant is treated with antibiotics until the clinical condition permits a repair of the esophageal atresia.

Primary repair of the esophagus can be accomplished by a transpleural or retropleural approach. The latter approach minimizes heat loss during the procedure. It is also advantageous should an anastomotic leak occur, since the infant seems to tolerate a confirmed infection in the retropleural mediastinum better than empyema which may follow transpleural repair. Following the repair, a chest tube or drain is positioned near the anastomosis and placed to straight drainage or waterseal. In the early postoperative period, nasoesophageal catheter suction may be necessary if the infant cannot swallow his saliva. Careful pulmonary toilet is maintained. It is important that the catheter used for tracheal suctioning be pre-measured to prevent injury to the esophageal anastomosis. For several days, the infant is maintained on intravenous fluids, after which the gastrostomy can be used for feeding. The gastrostomy tube must be suspended no more than four inches above the infant; this will prevent gastric dilatation and reflux into the healing esophagus. Glucose water, 10 to 15 ml. every two hours, is given through the gastrostomy initially and followed by formula feeding. It is especially important to maintain the infant in a propped (45°) position to avoid reflux into the lower esophageal pouch. Antibiotics, started preoperatively, are continued for a full 10 days (ampicillin, 100 mg./kg./24 hrs., and gentamicin, 6 mg./kg./24 hrs.). Seven to ten days postoperatively, a contrast swallow using thin barium is carried out. If esophageal integrity is confirmed, the chest tube can be removed safely and oral feedings begun.

For the small, premature infant or the infant in whom the diagnosis has been delayed and who is referred with severe aspiration pneumonitis, a staged approach is indicated. (1) Gastrostomy and limited right thoracotomy with retropleural fistula division provides a time interval during which pulmonary toilet and antibiotics are employed. Later, a transpleural esophageal anastomosis is performed. (2) An alternative to thoracotomy is proximal gastric division which can be performed simply. Each gastric pouch is drained by a gastrostomy catheter. This effectively isolates the gastrointestinal tract from the tracheobronchial tree and while the small upper pouch is drained, the lower pouch can be used for feeding. Since distention of the lower pouch will cause secretion into the upper pouch, it is important to perform the gastric division high in the fundus. Esophageal reconstruction is performed when the clinical state of the infant permits. Subsequent reanastomosis of the stomach is readily accomplished when the infant is ready for oral feedings.

Esophagoscopy with inspection and calibration of the anastomosis may be carried out in three to six weeks. Esophageal dilatations are not done routinely, but reserved for established strictures in the infant who is choking on feedings. Currently, the survival rate in uncomplicated esophageal atresia with tracheoesophageal fistula is excellent (90 per cent). Appropriate staging procedures for the premature infant or the infant with pneu-monia have resulted recently in greater salvage, and have limited the persisting mortality to infants with those associated anomalies which are incompatible with life.

ESOPHAGEAL ATRESIA WITHOUT TRACHEOESOPHAGEAL FISTULA

Esophageal atresia without tracheoesophageal fistula accounts for 10 per cent of the infants with this anomaly. The finding of a blind upper pouch associated with the absence of air in the gastrointestinal tract confirms the diagnosis of isolated esophageal atresia. Suction of the upper pouch is established and gastrostomy is carried out for feeding purposes. Thoracotomy is contraindicated in infants with confirmed isolated esophageal atresia since the intrathoracic portion of the esophagus is insufficient to permit primary esophageal anastomosis.

Among the alternatives for the treatment of isolated esophageal atresia are: cervical esophagostomy, bringing the esophageal pouch out to the skin of the left side of the neck thereby establishing a salivary fistula, and gastrostomy. The infant's nutrition is maintained by gastrostomy feedings until a weight of approximately 20 pounds is attained. It is important to associate the gratification of hunger with oral feedings during the interim period; if this is neglected, oral feeding is difficult for the infant to learn after esophageal substitution. For this reason, gastrostomy feedings are accompanied by oral feedings which are evacuated from the salivary fistula. An alternative approach involves bougienage of both the upper and lower pouches with mercury-filled dilators in an attempt to bring the two esophageal ends closer together. If this is performed daily from birth for approximately six weeks, a primary repair can sometimes be accomplished and there is no need for a substitution procedure. This procedure warrants further clinical trial.

Interposition procedures using various segments of the colon, brought through the left chest or retrosternally, have been used extensively but may be complicated by marginal blood supply at the upper anastomosis, redundancy, and by ulcers or stricture due to gastric reflux into the interposed colon. Recently, gastric tube interposition has been employed and has proved effective. Adequate blood supply is assured and length has not been a problem. Normal growth and development has been confirmed following either of these procedures.

ESOPHAGEAL STRICTURES

Lye Burns. The accidental ingestion of corrosive cleaning agents remains an important cause of esophageal stricture in the toddler. Children in this age group gulp liquids, often without tasting them and, therefore, the absence of burns in the anterior portion of the mouth or on the tongue does not exclude serious esophageal involvement. Patients suspected of ingesting a caustic agent should be evaluated by esophagoscopy within 24 hours of injury. While under general anesthesia, a careful examination of the posterior pharynx and larynx is carried out. The esophagoscope is then inserted and the esophageal mucosa examined. Typical findings of caustic burns are a whitish coagulum on the surface surrounded by inflamed mucosa. Because strong alkali is extremely hygroscopic, it becomes firmly attached to the moist mucosal surface; damage by protein coagulation can, therefore, proceed to involve the entire thickness of the esophagus, making it vulnerable to perforation. Therefore no attempt is made to examine the damaged esophagus in its entire length, once proximal involvement is determined. Soon after endoscopy, a baseline barium swallow is carried out to assess the extent of injury. Antibiotics are started (ampicillin, 100 mg./kg./day) and given parenterally until oral or gastrostomy feeding is begun. The role of steroids in retarding the development of strictures has not been determined in a prospective fashion. If this modality of treatment is elected, the children receive prednisolone, 2 mg./kg./day intramuscularly, followed by prednisone, 2.5 mg./kg./day orally, or by gastrostomy for a total of three weeks, with gradual tapering of the dose.

For mild burns with noncircumferential mucosal damage, oral feedings are resumed when the child recovers from anesthesia. Citrus juices and carbonated liquids are excluded. For those children with circumferential burns or extensive involvement of the esophagus, a gastrostomy is performed. A string is passed down the esophagus, brought out through the nose and gastrostomy, and the ends tied together. Gastrostomy feedings are given as necessary if the child is unable to swallow. After three weeks, barium swallow and esophagoscopy are repeated in all children. Gentle dilatation is carried out at this time. Graded mercury dilators are used to dilate the esophagus from above. For the severely burned esophagus, linked Tucker dilators are attached to the previously placed string and drawn retrograde through the esophagus.

Dilatation is continued only to the point where the esophagus is felt to "grab" the dilator. The time interval between dilatations depends on the severity of the developing stricture and may be necessary twice weekly for the severely injured esophagus. Serial evaluation by barium swallow and esophagoscopy at three-monthly intervals for one year is recommended. As long as progress is made, dilatations are continued gradually increasing the time interval between dilatations until the child sustains improvement or is asymptomatic, i.e., is on a regular diet for at least six months. The length of strictures is difficult to define by barium swallow because streaming of barium distal to the narrowed area can be misleading. A roentgenogram obtained following the insertion of a barium-filled Penrose drain into the esophagus will outline more precisely the extent of involvement. Short strictures may benefit from the local injection of steroids. Triamcinolone (total 1 ml./40 mg.) is injected into each quadrant of the stricture under direct vision.

If no progress is made with esophageal dilatations and swallowing function remains impaired, esophageal substitution is performed. A reverse gastric tube has been employed with advantage in recent years. Traditionally, the colon has also proved a satisfactory esophageal substitute.

Congenital Esophageal Stenosis. Most stenoses of the esophagus are secondary to gastroesophageal reflux. This problem is considered in detail in another section. True congenital esophageal stenosis is rare but occurs as a web or a diaphragm, usually at the junction of the middle and distal third of the esophagus. Recurrent aspiration and dysphagia are the characteristic symptoms. The diagnosis is made by barium swallow and confirmed by esophagoscopy. Dilatation is performed by the passage of a filiform catheter through the aperture of the web, and this is used as a guide to dilators of progressively larger circumference until the obstruction is relieved. If repeated dilatations fail to establish an adequate lumen, a direct surgical approach is indicated. Thoracotomy and excision of a mucosal web with reconstruction of the esophagus or resection of the stenotic area with end-to-end anastomosis is performed. Postoperative care is identical to that outlined after primary esophageal anastomosis for atresia.

ACHALASIA

Achalasia is characterized by abnormally constricted muscle at the gastroesophageal junction with consequent megaesophagus. It is rare in children; when it occurs it is characterized by malnutrition, dysphagia and pain. The surgical procedure of choice is the Heller esophagocardiomyotomy in which a longitudinal incision through the fibromuscular layers of the lower esophagus and upper fundus of the stomach is performed, releasing the muscular constriction without entering the lumen. The myotomy is combined with a crural repair or a more formal antireflux procedure such as the Nissen fundoplication to avoid postoperative gastroesophageal reflux.

Hiatal Hernia

(Partial Thoracic Stomach)

IVO J. CARRÉ, M.D.

When considering the management of this disorder it is of the utmost importance that due regard be taken of its variable evolutionary pattern and relatively benign prognosis. A rational approach to therapy can only be formulated by relating therapeutic results to the expected outcome in the absence of treatment. Failure to do so has been one of the major factors responsible for the continuing controversy regarding the relative merits of conservative versus surgical management. In an early study of *untreated* patients I was able to identify two major clinical groups based on symptomatic progress (Arch. Dis. Child., *34*: 344, 1959).

Group I consisted of patients who, having vomited persistently from the early weeks of life, showed unmistakable evidence of clinical improvement between 3 and 9 months of age—an improvement which appeared to be related to the introduction of spoon feeding and a semisolid diet. Vomiting diminished gradually and had ceased in just over 50 per cent by 12 months and in almost all by 2 years of age. Those followed up to adult life have remained virtually asymptomatic; in some, however, a partial thoracic stomach has remained demonstrable on fluoroscopy. This clinical group represented about two thirds of all children referred to hospital with symptoms attributable to a partial thoracic stomach.

Group II comprised the remaining one third. The clinical progress of these children during the early weeks of life was indistinguishable from those in the previous group. Later, however, they showed no evidence of clinical improvement during the introduction of a semisolid diet. The majority suffered from troublesome vomiting and dysphagia up to 4 years of age and often much longer before they too became symptom-free. About one in

seven of this group, or approximately 5 per cent of all patients, developed an esophageal stricture. Unfortunately, there appears to be no means of identifying these latter patients from their early clinical history.

CONSERVATIVE MANAGEMENT

The fundamental basis of conservative management is postural therapy. This consists of nursing patients in a sitting posture with the trunk inclined at an angle of at least 60 degrees to the horizontal. The aim is to reduce gastroesophageal reflux and assist clearance of regurgitated gastric juice from the terminal esophagus thereby decreasing the risk of esophagitis and of aspiration pneumonia.

In my experience infants in group I respond relatively quickly to postural treatment, almost all becoming virtually symptom free within 3 months of starting therapy. When such treatment is started in early infancy about three quarters of the group II children will also respond, though much more slowly. Should the start of therapy be delayed until after 12 months of age only about one third of these group II patients improve. It is important to stress that these therapeutic results apply only if conservative postural therapy is adequate and strictly applied along the lines to be described. A large number of conservatively treated patients have now been followed into adult life. Although a partial thoracic stomach has remained demonstrable in some, all have remained in excellent health.

To maintain infants in a sitting posture of at least 60 degrees, it is important that they be nursed in an infant-sized chair or harness. This posture should be maintained throughout the 24 hours with obvious permissible intermissions for feeding, changing of diapers and play. It is particularly important that this upright position be maintained during the night, when gastric secretions are neither diluted nor buffered by milk feeds. At this time also salivation almost ceases and the frequency of swallowing is greatly reduced. As a result the neutralizing effect of swallowed saliva is lost and clearing of the lower esophagus of refluxed gastric juice is impaired owing to reduced esophageal peristalsis. Lesser degrees of propping achieved by using pillows or by placing blocks under the head of the crib are of no detectable value; maintaining an infant upright for half an hour or so after feeding is equally useless. These totally inadequate measures should never be equated with postural therapy.

The assessment of an individual patient's progress and response to therapy is derived from a composite analysis of many factors such as vomiting frequency, the occurrence of hematemeses, dysphagia, weight gain, anemia and pulmonary infections, radiological findings (occasionally) and esophagoscopic observations (rarely). In practice, the frequency of vomiting provides by far the most useful single clinical guide to progress during infancy. Parents should therefore always be asked to keep a record of vomiting episodes; each day on which vomiting occurs is termed a "vomiting day." In general a reduction of over 50 per cent in the frequency of vomiting days within 3 months of starting treatment can be accepted as a satisfactory response.

Postural treatment should be continued as long as there is measurable clinical improvement. This may mean continuing such measures for months, as the response to therapy is usually a gradual one, particularly in the case of group II patients. Brief relapses, often occasioned by an upper respiratory tract infection, are not of themselves an indication for discontinuing this type of treatment.

Except possibly for an initial brief period in hospital, patients who are otherwise well are treated at home and kept under regular hospital out-patient review to enable progress to be evaluated. Prematurity and low birth weight are not contraindications to postural therapy should the diagnosis of a partial thoracic stomach be established in the newborn period. Treatment should be instituted as soon as the diagnosis is confirmed, though these small patients will need to be kept in hospital for a longer initial period.

Medical personnel with little experience of this problem occasionally view postural therapy with foreboding. The belief that maintaining a baby in an upright posture will result in skeletal deformities, such as scoliosis, can be discounted on the basis of long-term follow-up results. A slight flattening of the vault of the skull which may occur in infants started on therapy before 3 months of age is no longer noticeable by 2 years.

Frequent small feedings (2 to 3 hourly) will often contribute to a reduction in vomiting especially in small infants. No alteration to the formula is necessary and breast feeding should not be discontinued unless contraindicated for some other reason. If bottle-fed, the addition to the formula of a thickening agent such as a carob seed preparation (Nestargel) can constitute a valuable supplementary measure. It is important to stress that to be effective, any such agent must always be added to milk feedings in the recommended maximum concentration. In some infants this may cause frequent, loose, gelatinous stools, necessitating

temporary withdrawal of this form of treatment. The value of antacid preparations is difficult to assess, but there are theoretical reasons for giving alkali, both for its neutralizing property and its capacity to increase gastroesophageal sphincteric tone. This may be given as Gaviscon, which in the stomach forms a viscous antacid demulcent gel which floats on the stomach contents. When reflux occurs this bland material will thus tend to be regurgitated into the esophagus ahead of other gastric contents. Atropine derivatives are to be avoided since they reduce gastroesophageal sphincteric pressure. Oral supplements of iron may be necessary to correct anemia.

Occasionally, particularly during early infancy, previously undiagnosed patients may present at the hospital acutely ill and in need of emergency treatment to combat dehydration, electrolyte and acid base imbalances, anemia and aspiration pneumonia. Appropriate therapy is indicated in these circumstances.

SURGICAL TREATMENT

Accurate evaluation of surgical therapy has been hampered in the past by the multiplicity of surgical procedures employed and the failure of authors to relate long-term results to the patient's initial clinical state and age at operation. Hiatal repair operations of the type originally devised by Allison have proved disappointing, and in recent years these have been largely superseded by antireflux operations based on a Nissen fundoplication procedure. At present this would seem to be the operation of choice for the few patients with a partial thoracic stomach and no esophageal stricture who require to be treated surgically.

CHOICE OF THERAPY

Patients Under 18 Months of Age with No Esophageal Stricture. In view of the excellent long-term results obtained with conservative medical management, especially when started in early infancy, there is no justification for subjecting patients of this age to surgical procedures without having first assessed the response to an adequate period of postural therapy. All patients of this age should be treated by postural means regardless of their clinical group, even though the majority of those over 9 months will belong to group II. Postural treatment as outlined above is instituted for a period of at least 3 months and longer provided there is continuing clinical improvement. Treatment is discontinued only after the patient has been asymptomatic for at least 6 weeks. If there is no significant improvement after 3 months' therapy (less than a

50 per cent reduction in vomiting days) then a fundoplication is advised. In fact few patients in this category require surgery.

Patients Over 18 Months of Age with No Esophageal Stricture. Postural therapy is much more difficult to carry out efficiently in these older and more active children. Results are also much less satisfactory. However, since an occasional child will respond to conservative management even at this age, an initial period of postural treatment should be tried. If within 3 months there is no obvious reduction in either vomiting or dysphagia the patient should be referred for fundoplication.

Patients with Esophageal Stricture. It is important to appreciate that most reflux esophageal strictures are capable of resolution. An irreversible fibrous stricture is fortunately relatively uncommon and is only rarely encountered under 2 years of age. Every effort must be made to conserve the esophagus, for no other form of conduit can adequately replace it; even an esophagus with residual scarring and a degree of permanent narrowing is preferable to an intestinal replacement.

Initial therapy should consist of an antireflux operation, preferably a fundoplication, combined with esophageal dilations as necessary. Only when these measures have manifestly failed should more radical surgery be contemplated. Most surgeons in these circumstances would probably advocate esophageal resection and a colon transplant or possibly a gastric tube replacement. Both procedures are beset with complications, and long-term results tend to be disappointing. A fundic patch operation as described by Thal combined with an intrathoracic Nissen type fundoplication may well prove to be a preferable alternative.

CHALASIA

Gastroesophageal incompetence with no anatomical abnormality is relatively uncommon, and compared with a partial thoracic stomach is a much less frequent cause of vomiting in infancy. The response to conservative therapy as outlined above is uniformly satisfactory with eventual complete clinical and radiological recovery.

Vomiting

FREDERICK H. LOVEJOY, JR., M.D.

Vomiting is one of the most common initial signs of illness seen in all pediatric ages. It may indicate a mild and short-lived disease, such as motion sickness or vomiting on an emotional basis, or a severe and potentially life-threatening disease, such as meningitis or a malignancy. Further, vomiting may be brief and self-limited as occurs with simple infectious gastroenteritis. It may also follow a protracted course as seen with chronic renal failure or malignancies. In all instances, vomiting should be viewed as a sign of significant disease and a strong indication for determining an underlying cause. Removal of the underlying cause is often curative, as with vomiting from an intermittent volvulus, from uremia and renal failure due to an underlying anomaly of the urinary tract, or from hyperammonemia secondary to an enzyme deficiency in which limiting protein intake is therapeutically effective. Simply stated, treat the cause, not the vomiting.

Vomiting in the child is most commonly due to simple gastroenteritis, whereas in the infant it is most often related to methods of feeding. Antiemetics generally contribute little and often incur significant risks. Certain indications do exist for antiemetics but these drugs always must be used under medical supervision with close attention to dose and potential side effects. In all instances, the physician must be alert for complications secondary to vomiting. The greatest hazard in infants is aspiration pneumonia with its potential for respiratory arrest. Dehydration is a second hazard of increasing concern in the younger the child.

The differential diagnosis for vomiting includes: (1) obstruction anywhere along the entire length of the gastrointestinal tract; (2) inflammation in any body organ; (3) metabolic derangements involving carbohydrate, protein or fat metabolism; (4) causes of increased intracranial pressure; (5) middle ear disease and motion sickness; (6) endogenous toxins such as those found in renal or hepatic failure; (7) exogenous toxins such as are seen with iron and salicylate poisoning; (8) malignancies; (9) adverse effects of medications and radiation therapy; and (10) postoperative vomiting. In all instances, an etiology for vomiting must be assiduously sought prior to recommending any therapy.

APPROACH TO THERAPY

A rational approach to vomiting in the neonate involves consideration of its many predisposing factors including swallowed air during feeding, gastroesophageal reflux, abnormal concentration or amount of formula, errors in methods of burping, inadequate hole size in the feeding bottle and nasal obstruction. The infant should be burped before, during and after feeding, and for a period of one to two hours should be kept in a sitting position. When placed in the crib, the prone position is preferable to supine position. Both upright and prone positions place air rather than food in the upper part of the stomach, thus reducing the likelihood of aspiration of stomach contents. Formula that is often too concentrated is irritating and may induce vomiting. Conversely, formula that is too dilute will necessitate a large intake to satisfy the infant, with increased hazards of vomiting and aspiration. In both instances a formula change often stops the vomiting. The hole in the nipple of the feeding bottle should be sufficiently large to permit the feeding to be delivered in no more than 20 to 30 minutes. For nasal obstruction, a bulb syringe to remove secretions, saline nose drops 15 minutes before feeding, and frequent rest periods during feeding often decrease the frequency of vomiting. In the breast fed child, attention to the method of feeding may be all that is required to determine the cause of vomiting.

In all other ages, the initial approach to the management of vomiting involves stopping all oral feedings. In the infant, clear fluids are then reintroduced as sugar water in small frequent feedings, followed, when tolerated, by half strength and then full strength formula. In the older child, clear fluids are best offered in the form of sweetened tea, bouillon, cola or ginger ale (shaken to remove carbonation) in small frequent feedings. Once tolerated, dry toast and crackers may then be introduced, followed by a bland and then normal diet. In all instances careful assessment of the state of hydration is needed to determine the necessity of intravenous replacement therapy. Because most simple vomiting is self-limited, antiemetics are not necessary.

DRUG THERAPY

In order to understand drug therapy, it is necessary to appreciate how various stimuli affect the vomiting center and induce emesis, and how medications arrest this process. Stimuli are relayed from peripheral sites to the chemoreceptor trigger zone and then to the vomiting center. Peripheral sites include the gastrointestinal tract (simple infectious vomiting), the labyrinth via the eighth nerve and cerebellum (motion sickness) and the cerebral cortex (vomiting on an emotional basis). Antiemetic drugs exert their effects on these pathways, phenothiazines by acting on the chemoreceptor trigger zone, nonphenothiazine antiemetics by acting on the chemoreceptor trigger zone or vestibular apparatus, antihistamines and anticholinergics by decreasing excitability of pathways originating in centers of the labyrinth, and barbiturates by operating at a cortical level.

Certain phenothiazines, prochlorperazine (Compazine) in the piperazine group and chlorpromazine (Thorazine) and promazine (Sparine) in the aliphatic group, act as effective antiemetic agents. The phenothiazines are the most potent of the antiemetics but also have a high incidence of side effects. They are best reserved for severe, short-term vomiting including radiation sickness, endogenous toxins, malignancies and following surgical procedures. They are not effective for motion sickness. The recommended dosages are prochlorperazine,* 0.4 mg./kg./day orally or rectally in 4 divided doses or 0.2 mg./kg./day intramuscularly in divided doses, and chlorpromazine,† 2 to 4 mg./kg./day orally or rectally in 4 divided doses, or 1.5 to 2 mg./kg./day intramuscularly in 4 divided doses. All phenothiazines, especially those in the aliphatic group, cause drowsiness and sedation. The phenothiazines, particularly the piperazine group, also induce extrapyramidal tract signs which are highly disturbing to parents and patients, and are often confused with other disease entities. Other severe, though uncommon, side effects of the phenothiazines include cholestatic jaundice, thrombocytopenia, granulocytopenia, dermatitis and hypotension. Phenothiazines should not be used if signs and symptoms suggest early Reye's syndrome or other hepatic disorders.

Nonphenothiazine antiemetics, including trimethobenzamide and diphenidol, are less effective than phenothiazines, are more expensive but have less side effects. They should be reserved for less severe instances of vomiting such as with infectious gastroenteritis and postoperative emesis. They are not effective for motion sickness. Dosages are trimethobenzamide (Tigan),‡ 15 mg./kg./day orally or rectally in 3 to 4 divided doses, and diphenidol (Vontrol),§ 5 mg./kg./day orally or rectally in 3 to 4 divided doses. The major side effect of nonphenothiazine antiemetics is sedation.

---

*Manufacturer's precaution: Prochlorperazine is not recommended for children under 20 pounds or 2 years. In children with acute illness or dehydration, use only under close supervision.

†Manufacturer's precaution: Chlorpromazine should not be used in children under 6 months except where potentially life-saving.

‡Manufacturer's precaution: Injectable form of trimethobenzamide (Tigan) is not recommended for children. Tigan suppositories are not recommended for premature or newborn infants. Since the suppositories contain benzocaine, they should not be used in patients known to be sensitive to this or similar local anesthetics.

§Manufacturer's precaution: Oral form of diphenidol (Vontrol) is not recommended for use in infants under 6 months or 25 pounds. Intravenous or subcutaneous administration is not recommended in children of any age.

Antihistamines are used for mild vomiting and are specifically effective for *motion sickness*. Indications for their use include vomiting caused by middle ear disease, labyrinthitis, radiation sickness, malignancies and antineoplastic drugs. Commonly used antihistamines include diphenhydramine (Benadryl), 5 mg./kg./day orally or rectally in 2 to 3 divided doses, and dimenhydrinate (Dramamine), 5 mg./kg./day orally or rectally in 2 to 3 divided doses. The latter medication is used most commonly for motion sickness. Side effects of these drugs are infrequent and include drowsiness, sedation and anticholinergic effects.

Anticholinergic drugs (atropine and scopolamine) are also effective antiemetics but their short duration of action and high incidence of side effects limit their general use. Barbiturates, 7 mg./kg./day in 2 divided doses, are used mainly in electroencephalographic proven abdominal epilepsy. Attacks of vomiting due to migraine will respond to ergotamine tartrate, 1 to 2 mg. sublingually, repeated in a half hour if necessary. Finally, initial information suggests the effectiveness of marijuana for treatment of vomiting associated with childhood malignancies.

Constipation

WILLIAM M. MICHENER, M.D.

Physicians caring for children have always been considered experts in toilet training and in the management of the disorders of elimination: diarrhea and constipation. A child with symptoms of acute diarrhea is considered ill and the physician accepts the challenge in management. Unfortunately, the child with symptoms of constipation is often received far less enthusiastically by the physician. In fact, the mother who has a problem with a child with constipation is frequently given minimal support and advice that often has little scientific validity. These children may well become the adults with chronic gastrointestinal complaints and therefore merit our concern and care.

No doubt constipation is a problem related to dietary factors and emotional stresses. Much has been written in the past few years concerning the relationship of constipation to dietary patterns in the United States. The highly refined, low fiber foods eaten by Americans produce a small intraluminal volume that directly decreases intestinal motility. This fact has been documented by comparing our eating and bowel habits with those of many Africans. The overwhelming preoccupation of parents with toilet training and stool production in this country has created an emotional environment that certainly contributes to the increased incidence of constipation in children. For some unexplained reasons, "a stool a day" is mandated by many parents from their children. If the parents note a departure from this routine, they manifest a variety of behavioral patterns. Punitive toilet training, artificial attempts to produce stooling, and various abnormal dietary approaches are developed within a family. The child's reaction to these attempts is often one of "fecal withholding" and in some cases this begins a lifelong habit of an abnormal elimination pattern—constipation.

The physician's role begins when the child is brought by the parents to the office for evaluation of constipation. Initially, if the child can talk, the history of the child's bowel habits should be obtained from the child. The parent, usually the mother, invariably will add her own interpretation of events. An accurate description of the frequency of stooling, the volume and consistency of the stool, changes from a preexisting pattern, and the presence of abnormal constituents such as blood, mucus, or undigested food in the stool, will help determine if the child is indeed constipated. Often the history is helpful in ruling out organic causes of constipation. A history of painful defecation or blood on the outside of the stool associated with painful defecation will point to an anal fissure as the probable cause. A careful history from the child alone and the parent alone will often indicate emotional stress or family conflict as a possible precipitating factor. A careful dietary history must be obtained. Often this is best obtained from the child in diary form over a period of one week.

The physical examination is also essential for the evaluation. Normal growth and development usually eliminate suspicion of an organic disease. Careful palpation of the abdomen for fecal masses, tenderness, hyperactive bowel sounds, gaseous distention and pain must be done. Examination of the external anal area for evidence of irritation, fissure, and injury, as well as a rectal examination for evaluation of sphincter control and the presence or absence of strictures, is necessary. The presence of fecal material in the rectum provides important information in differentiating physiologic constipation from congenital aganglionosis of the colon (Hirschsprung's disease). Mention must be made by barium x-ray examination of the colon. Most children with constipation have no organic disease. Therefore, the yield of positive results from barium examination is quite small. Most parents and physicians, however, find it reassuring to rule out organic causes of disease.

When a barium enema is given, attention must be paid to the cleansing following the enema. Children who are not adequately prepared may have stool present in the bowel; barium mixed with this stool produces a barium-stool mixture similar to cement which hinders management of physiologic constipation. Several cleansing enemas following the barium study should always be performed.

PHYSIOLOGIC PRINCIPLES OF MANAGEMENT

The goals of any therapy program are to attempt to allow the colon to perform its integrated responses that result in defecation. The primary regulators of the rate of transit of alimental contents are the pressure-receptor responses to intraluminal volume. Fortunately, the intraluminal volume contents are the most easily available for regulation.

1. The physician must give a clear and easily understood explanation of the physiology of colon emptying to the child and to the family. Subjects covered must include mechanism of evacuation, abnormal and normal stool patterns, childhood attitudes toward the bathroom, the importance of proper position during defecation (knees flexed upon the abdomen with the feet on a firm surface), and how the various activities of a family in the home can affect these patterns. Simple thoughts, such as how five members of a family can use a single bathroom, are necessary to ensure complete understanding. On subsequent visits this information should be reemphasized.

2. Exploration into the dietary habits of the family is necessary. It is important to indicate to the mother that the physiologic form of carbohydrates used in this country is constipating. Ingestion of natural colonic stimulants such as prunes, raisins, indigestible foodstuffs such as leafy vegetables, berries and fruits, and whole-grain cereals is necessary. This can be accomplished easily by the addition of bran to the regular cereals ingested by children. Milk and milk products are probably the only minimally constipating foods that children consume and therefore inquiry into excessive ingestion of these foodstuffs should be made.

3. The use of nondietary aids as a helpful means in effecting normal function is acceptable and necessary in the management of some cases. The following agents are useful:

a. Hydrophilic bulking agents. These can often increase the water content of stool approximately 10 per cent and therefore the intraluminal volume. As already mentioned, bran is effective. Semisynthetic cellulose compounds such as Metamucil are useful. One teaspoon in a glass of water in the morning is effective. Complex carbohydrates such as those found in unrefined dark Karo syrup and malt soup extracts (Maltsupex) act in the same manner as bran. These indigestible and hydrophilic compounds absorb water and increase bulk with a resultant increase in transit time by the gastrointestinal tract.

b. Stool softeners. Mineral oil is a basic agent. It is palatable and inexpensive and if used appropriately, complications are minimal, if any. The stool is made almost semiliquid so that it passes with ease and, in fact, is difficult to hold back. The dose of mineral oil varies. Enough is given to produce the desired result. Usually 1 to 2 oz. is given per day for the first month, every other day for the second month, and every third day for the final month. The dose is reduced if mineral oil leaks from the rectum. Dioctyl sodium sulfosuccinate is also useful. The mechanism of action in this compound is that of a synthetic surface lubricating agent.

c. Stimulant cathartics such as cascara, saline solution and castor oil are effective but should be used infrequently. They cause stomach cramping and often persistent diarrhea. Bisacodyl (Dulcolax), a polyphenolic laxative, probably stimulates mucosal chemoreceptors, which in turn stimulate the myenteric ganglia. These agents are effective but seldom needed.

SPECIFIC CONSTIPATION PROBLEMS

The Neonate with Constipation. Classically, this is the child brought to the pediatrician with a history of "straining." The mother describes the drawing up of legs, physical straining, and what is interpreted as irritability just prior to passing a stool. Occasionally, the passing of small pellet-like stools is also described. In this infant and in the newborn as well, congenital aganglionosis of the colon must be ruled out. The hallmark features are delayed passage of meconium in the newborn period associated with abdominal distention. If effective rectal dilatation occurs in the newborn nursery, the child may be discharged and in one or two weeks the mother calls the physician because of the absence of stooling. This child must be evaluated further by physical examination and barium studies. Usually, the symptoms previously described relate to immature gastrointestinal function. The addition of 5 to 10 cc. of dark Karo syrup to the feedings will often provide effective stimulation. Maltsupex will also work in this manner.

The Toddler with Constipation. In his second year of life, the child has a variable stool pattern. Looseness and firmness of stools are often noted in the same patient. If the firmness of stool begins to dominate the pattern, an illness, car trip, or visit away from home necessitating the use of new toilets may contribute to a sudden fecal withholding pattern. This pattern is relatively easily transformed into a serious constipation syndrome. The passing of a large stool associated with straining and the production of an anal fissure will augment the whole cycle. The intensity and quality of maternal intervention, which are based on her attitudes concerning child rearing and toilet training and the social and cultural pressures exerted upon her, will determine the course of this problem. The physician also plays an important role in the future of this patient. Failure to treat the condition properly will produce a longstanding problem of rectal inertia and often toilet phobia with resultant long-term emotional effects.

Usually removal of the fecal mass and attempts to keep the rectum empty are necessary. A pediatric Fleet enema and the oral ingestion of mineral oil in the manner described accomplishes this. There is no lack of bulk in this syndrome and no obstruction to outflow. Chronic distention is present and propulsive action is decreased. Sensation of fullness is decreased because of the constant state of distention. When the colon is empty, reeducation can begin. The child is encouraged to use the toilet after each meal in a relaxed and enjoyable manner. Reeducation of the family attitudes toward bowel function is necessary. The physician should provide a supportive role and every two or three weeks see the child to give maximal encouragement. The addition of raisins, prunes, fruits and fruit juices to the diet is usually helpful. When the problem is successfully controlled, the family should be cautioned about the ease with which relapse may occur during episodes of illness, family travel and emotional stress.

Fecal Soiling and Severe Constipation. The exact mechanism by which simple constipation becomes severe is unknown. There is no doubt that if simple constipation is recurrent or becomes chronic, an emotional complex can develop that is detrimental to the development of the child. For example, if an anal fissure becomes chronic and each episode of stooling is painful, fecal withholding is natural and deliberate. As the stool bulk becomes great, "overflow soiling" occurs and the child has constant dirtiness and odor of stool. Abdominal pain secondary to cramping and distention are present. The child is rejected by his peers and this adds significantly to the overall emotional stresses confronting the child. As

mentioned before, the initial approach is to evacuate the colon totally and attempt to allow the colon to reduce in size and begin reflex contractions. Effective management is often difficult. The child must become motivated to success.

Often an abnormal child-parent relationship is fully established and the physician must assume a dominant position. Frequent visits to the office by the child are required so that the physician can continue to give reassurance, support, and direct management. Parents must be reassured that with patience, success will occur. If the problem is rigidly established and difficulties in school are already evident, psychological help is frequently advantageous. Along with the psychological approach, basic bowel management support is necessary. If a fecal bolus cannot be prevented from accumulating in the colon, failure will occur. Therefore, a program that includes periodic emptying of the colon (an enema once a week, mineral oil in sufficient dosage to ensure passage of stool), dietary management to ensure effective intraluminal volume, and adequate time in the bathroom is necessary to ensure success. The psychological approach is built upon a basic bowel management program. Again it should be emphasized that even with success, the relapse rate in children who have had longstanding constipation is significant and families must understand the mechanism of bowel evacuation so that relapse can be prevented.

Chronic Nonspecific Diarrhea of Childhood

WILLIAM M. MICHENER, M.D.

From birth to school age, children have varied patterns of stooling. Those with increased fecal frequency are often thought by their parents to have diarrhea. The child aged six months to four years often has a stool pattern that changes periodically. These children have increased stool frequency with stools described as loose, containing mucus and food, and frequently watery. Examination of these children indicates normal growth and development patterns. The question posed to the physician by the mother is, "Why does my child always have diarrhea?"

This syndrome has often been defined as chronic nonspecific diarrhea or irritable colon of childhood. The child should be thriving vigorously, have normal growth and development patterns, and no evidence of dehydration, malabsorption, or secondary maldigestion deficiencies. The only abnormality is increased stool frequency interpreted by the parent as diarrhea.

Some observers have noted the onset of this stool pattern with assumption of the upright position. The majority of these children are in the second year of life and not yet toilet trained. Careful clinical assessment of the patient with chronic nonspecific diarrhea is important. A thorough history, as in most gastrointestinal diseases, will usually establish the diagnosis. Attention to growth records is important. The patient's growth pattern should be normal and show no change. Inquiry into the living conditions, urban or rural, eating habits of the family, and whether other members of the family have a similar stool pattern is mandatory. No abdominal distention, visible peristalsis, or palpable masses are present. The stool is loose, often foul-smelling, contains mucus, and bowel movements can occur as often as four or five times each day. The presence of undigested food particles is not uncommon.

Laboratory assessment of the child with this problem should be minimal. Examination of the stool for the presence of food and mucus, stool culture for enteric pathogens, and a stool pH (pH <6 suggests disaccharide intolerance) are usually all that is required. This may be done on an ambulatory basis. If hospitalization is necessary, the feeding of a regular diet and collection of a 72-hour stool for fecal fat excretion will usually be sufficient evaluation. Often hospitalization of a child with this problem will be revealing in that he or she may not pass a stool for several days.

There is no specific therapy for this condition. Careful counseling and reassurance of the parents are usually adequate. Repeated demonstration that the growth and development pattern of the child and his physical examination are normal, and one or two follow-up visits emphasizing height and weight measurements are also reassuring to the family.

Intractable Diarrhea of Infancy

WILLIAM M. MICHENER, M.D.

In infants usually younger than three months a syndrome of protracted severe diarrhea of unknown etiology labeled "intractable diarrhea of infancy" may occur. These infants are often admitted to the hospital with an admission weight below birth weight, severe dehydration and malnutrition, and often are close to death. Many inner-city and American

Indian children have been described. Frequently, they have been hospitalized several times and appear to have had diarrhea since birth. The mortality rate until the advent of total parental nutrition was almost 100 per cent. Severe malnutrition at this early age has profound effects on the growth and development of the child. For this reason, vigorous aggressive therapy is usually indicated. Evaluation of these cases has been frustrating and usually yields no specific etiologic factors. The infant in a weakened condition also tolerates extensive examination poorly.

The usual supportive measures for any child with severe dehydration and acidosis are instituted. Following correction of abnormal body chemistry determinations, e.g., fluid volume and blood volume, simple diagnostic procedures can be performed. The stool should be checked for the presence of reducing substance, acid pH, and qualitative assessment for fat. Blood and stool cultures will indicate any enteric pathogens; usually these patients do not have enteric pathogens as the cause of their problem.

The goal of therapy in intractable diarrhea of infancy is to support the infant through the long period of nutritional replacement. In most cases, this will require three to six weeks, depending upon the initial severity of the disorder. Sufficient fluids must be given intravenously to maintain body weight initially while results of the simple tests are being evaluated.

In those patients whose clinical condition seems to improve rapidly, a trial of oral alimentation is indicated. Dextrose water in small quantities, i.e., 15 ml. every two hours, with gradually increased amounts each day will indicate whether the damaged intestinal tract can tolerate oral alimentation. Careful regulation of the volume and frequency of feeding is absolutely necessary. If after 48 to 72 hours of dextrose water feedings no increase in stooling has occurred, a change to a readily absorbed formula, such as Pregestimil or Cho-Free, is indicated. Pregestimil is a nutritionally balanced formula with casein hydrolyte as the nitrogen source. Cho-Free is a nutritionally balanced soy bean formula. Either formula should be initiated at a 10 kcal./oz. strength. Again small volumes, 1 to 2 oz. every three to four hours, should be given. These infants are extremely sensitive to increased volumes of feedings, and stooling will increase if excessive feedings are administered. During the period of oral alimentation, intravenous fluid and electrolyte should be administered to equal 150 ml./kg. of body weight every 24 hours.

Unfortunately, most infants with severe

intractable diarrhea cannot tolerate oral alimentation this quickly. Therefore, a central venous catheter should be inserted early so that total parenteral nutrition can be given. A solution of 20 per cent glucose and 3 to 4 per cent amino acid should be administered to give 150 ml./kg./24 hr. and 125 cal./kg./24 hr. A weekly infusion of 10 ml./kg. of whole blood will provide trace elements. The intravenous fat emulsion Intralipid is also helpful. Aseptic care of the catheter insertion site and careful attention to the technique of hyperalimentation are mandatory for success with this mode of therapy. Usually, three to four weeks of therapy are required to allow the body to replace its nutritional stores, regenerate intestinal epithelium and allow the child a significant gain in weight. Before hyperalimentation is discontinued, oral feedings should begin. With the same techniques as described, dextrose. water followed by Cho-Free or Pregestimil, first in dilute and controlled small volume feedings, will allow the gut to be retrained. As the oral alimentation program is instituted, the rate of parenteral alimentation is decreased proportionately. Usually, four to six days of overlap is beneficial to the patient.

Following the institution of a successful full-strength oral alimentation diet, the infant should receive this diet for four to six weeks before attempting to determine the possible cause of the diarrhea. If he continues to gain weight and develop well, a gradual change to regular diet over three months can be attempted. Since no specific etiology has been found in this syndrome, in most cases investigation of the recovering child is probably not indicated.

Preoperative and Postoperative Care of Patients Undergoing Gastrointestinal Surgery

STEPHEN L. GANS, M.D.

Preoperative Care.   General preparation for gastrointestinal surgery in all instances includes correction of any depletions, such as fluid and electrolytes, whole blood or blood components, vitamins and nutritives.

Preparation of the bowel itself depends on the site of the lesion (proximal or distal) and the presence or absence of an acute inflammatory process or obstruction. In the patient undergoing gastric or upper intestinal surgery and who is without inflammation or obstruction, simply withholding feedings for eight hours (in the neonate, four hours) is adequate;

a nasogastric tube is placed in the stomach before induction of anesthesia.

When acute inflammation is present, peristalsis is diminished or has ceased and fluid and air collect in the bowel, much the same as in the presence of a true mechanical obstruction. Under these circumstances the bowel should be decompressed by passing a nasogastric tube into the stomach as soon as the condition is known. This is best accomplished by using as large a tube, well lubricated and with several holes cut near its end, as will pass through the nares a measured distance into the stomach. The tube should be connected to intermittent suction and should be irrigated every two hours with a measured amount of normal saline (10 mg. in the neonate, 15 or 20 in the older child) to ensure patency, and its position adjusted if the irrigating fluid is not returned. A tube that is not working is more harmful than no tube at all. It should not be plugged while the patient is being transported for x-rays or to the operating room. Small infant feeding tubes are not adequate for gastric decompression.

Before elective lower intestinal surgery the patient should be placed on a liquid diet for three days. Fecal residue in the colon is removed by warm normal saline enemas during the same period of time. This procedure should be the responsibility of experienced personnel. Retained stool makes surgery more difficult and more dangerous. There is some evidence that the addition of antibiotics to the bowel preparation or systemically is helpful, but this proposal is not universally accepted. Cultures of the stool before surgery and of the bowel lumen intraoperatively may be helpful if postoperative infection occurs.

When an indwelling bladder catheter is a necessary adjunct to the surgical procedure, this is best introduced in the operating room where sterile conditions are more secure.

Postoperative Care.   Only aspects of postoperative care pertaining to the gastrointestinal tract are discussed here; other features of general supportive treatment are covered elsewhere.

We strongly recommend that all tubes, drains and postoperative enemas be managed under the direction of a member of the operating team who knows the details of the operation and who is in a position to assess the condition of the bowel and security of any suture line.

The first basic need is effective decompression of the stomach and intestines until normal peristalsis is present and an anastomosis is patent. The use of a nasogastric tube in the manner described under Preoperative

Preparation is satisfactory in most instances of short duration. Suction or gravity drainage should continue until good peristalsis is audible and flatus is passed or, when there is an anastomosis, at least three days. When long-term decompression is anticipated and critical, gastrostomy should be considered at the time of surgery. This procedure and its management are discussed elsewhere.

Feedings may be started when decompression is discontinued. Progress is made from clear liquids to low residue diet to full diet for age as quickly as is tolerated by the patient.

In the absence of mechanical or neostomal obstruction, failure of the gastrointestinal tract to move gas along in normal fashion after 72 postoperative hours suggests adynamic ileus. Treatment consists of prolongation of decompression by the previously described methods, attention to possible deficiencies in fluids, electrolytes, blood or its components, and treatment of infection, respiratory problems, and any other complications. If there are signs of sepsis, compromise of intestinal viability, leakage or abscess, prompt surgical intervention is indicated.

Finally, in catastrophic problems involving the bowel, when it will not function properly over a considerable period of time, much benefit can be derived by the use of total intravenous nutrition while permitting the intestines to recover.

Differences of opinion exist as to either the value or possible complications from the routine use of antibiotics following gastrointestinal surgery. Believing that the greatest harm comes from going to either extreme, we suggest the following. Cultures should be made at surgery from free peritoneal fluid and from any open intestinal lumen. Antibiotics should not be used routinely for most gastric and upper intestinal surgery, but should be more commonly considered for lower bowel surgery. When suppuration is present in the peritoneum, when excessive contamination complicates the procedure, when questionably viable bowel remains in the peritoneal cavity or when a suture line is considered to be insecure, antibiotics should be used.

Ileostomy. Ileostomy is commonly used in the treatment of ulcerative colitis, but it is also sometimes used in the neonate for such conditions as necrotizing enterocolitis, meconium ileus, atresia of the ileum or Hirschsprung's disease involving the entire colon. A small plastic collecting bag is glued to the skin around the ileostomy at the time of surgery. This not only assists in measuring the output, which at times is copious, but also protects the surrounding skin from the irritating effects of ileostomy discharge.

When removing the pouch, cement solvent should be used to prevent the irritative trauma to the skin which occurs if the bag is pulled off. Gum karaya powder is then dusted on the skin and the excess blown away after two minutes, or gum karaya washer is applied. If properly fitted and applied, the bag will adhere to the abdomen for a period of at least 24 hours without any damage to the skin or stoma and will be accident-proof during that time.

Skin irritation is an ever-present threat and occurs in varying degrees of severity. There are many ways to cope with this problem, but all of them depend on the degree of meticulousness with which the patient is treated. Should any portion of the skin present a red, wet surface, dust gum karaya powder on it and blow away the residue. The bag can be applied right over the powdered area. Karaya gum washers will prevent many of the skin problems that arise.

Persistent raw areas or shallow ulcers present a more difficult problem, because an appliance will not adhere properly to this kind of skin. Meticulous cleansing and drying and the use of aluminum hydroxide gel in combination with karaya may be helpful. A neglected ileostomy may be a torturous thing. Sometimes it is necessary to place the patient in the prone position on a Bradford frame so that all discharges from the intestine flow directly into a pan underneath until healing is accomplished.

Although most children with ileostomies can eat a normal diet, some may experience difficulties with certain foods. In general, low residue diets are tolerated the best: lean meats, liver, hard boiled eggs, cottage cheese, rice, gelatin, simple sugars, cooked cereals, orange juice, clear soups and some cooked vegetables. It is advisable to avoid or use great care with the following: cabbage, turnips, corn on the cob or whole kernel corn, onions, nuts, raisins, coconut, berries with seeds, highly spiced or seasoned foods and large amounts of candy or sweets, especially chocolate.

Complications are better avoided than treated. Fistulas are usually the result of faulty application or fitting of the bag. Most strictures occur at skin level and respond to gentle daily dilatation with the finger. Minor degrees of prolapse or herniation may be controlled by the wearing of an elastic girdle over the appliance. More severe strictures, prolapse or herniation may require surgical revision. Obstruction may be due to edema or may result from eating large amounts of high residue foods. Irrigation with warm normal saline using a soft rubber bulb syringe or Foley catheter will bring relief.

Accustoming a child to the presence of an ileostomy and its care is a task of patience and forbearance. However, in most instances children respond in a manner that most adults would do well to emulate. Local ileostomy clubs are a source of great technical aid and psychologic encouragement.

Colostomy. Colostomy is used as a temporary bowel-decompressing or stool-diverting arrangement in infants or children with aganglionic megacolon, ectopic or imperforate anus or other anorectal anomalies, atresia or stenosis of the colon or severe injuries to the anus or lower bowel. There are many different types of colostomy, and the site and type will depend on the location and nature of the lesion being treated as well as on the definitive or reconstructive procedures planned for the future.

Many surgeons recommend a waiting period of 24 or more hours before opening the colostomy, but we have had no complications, particularly in the newborn with relatively sterile stool, as a result of making this opening immediately at the time of surgery. A plastic bag with a hole cut in its double-faced adhesive backing is worked over the colostomy and glued to the abdominal wall. This is kept in place until it starts filling with stool. Gas can be permitted to escape by pricking the bag with a pin. This transparent bag permits one to measure fluid or blood loss and to observe viability of the colostomy and onset of function without having to change dressings. It also seals fecal drainage from a nearby incision and helps prevent skin irritation.

The plastic bag may be discarded and replaced every day or when full. When the incision is healed and the stools are becoming formed, the plastic bag can be replaced by a strip of petrolatum gauze over the bowel end and covered with an ordinary diaper. Some parents prefer to use adherent plastic bags more or less permanently, as with an ileostomy. Others simply handle the colostomy as an "abdominal anus" by using the usual cleansing and diapering techniques.

Care of Bowel and Stoma. Satisfactory results are brought about by widely differing methods. In many infants, no special handling is necessary, particularly if the colostomy is to be present for a short time only. In others, the skin quickly becomes irritated or breaks down unless meticulous care is given. This can be controlled through diet, irrigations or local skin therapy, singly or in combination. Constipating or low residue diets, depending on age, will prevent constant soiling with its resulting irritation. Irrigation of the bowel thoroughly once daily or every other day, combined with the above mentioned diet, may result in no intervening spontaneous stools, thus allowing the skin to heal. The best local therapy is cleanliness. Acid soaps and a very dilute vinegar solution are better than alkaline soaps and tap water. Zinc oxide ointment should be applied for minor irritation; antimonilial (Vioform), antibacterial (neomycin) or anti-inflammatory (hydrocortisone) preparations should be used when indicated.

Occasionally the skin becomes inflamed because of bag adhesives or adhesive solvents, or by traumatic adhesive bag removal. Under such circumstances this method should be discarded, or at least the cement or solvent changed.

Tincture of benzoin painted over the area regularly will toughen the skin. A drying lotion (calamine) will help relieve itching. Bleeding from the stoma or mucocutaneous junction is common and can be easily controlled by applying a layer of petrolatum over the bleeding surface. More serious bleeding may require cauterization or electrocoagulation.

Stricture usually occurs at the skin level. This is not ordinarily a problem in the infant with soft stools and a temporary colostomy. In others, gentle daily dilatations will open the aperture to a satisfactory size. If it does not, surgical removal of a circle of skin and resuture of the mucosal margins are easily accomplished maneuvers.

Pylorospasm

HARRY MEDOVY, M.D.

Pylorospasm is to a large extent a diagnosis of exclusion. The description of Ellis appears to be the most acceptable: "Pylorospasm is a term applied to a group of hypertonic infants showing infrequent explosive vomiting without visible gastric peristalsis and in whom no pyloric tumor is palpable." One might add that a gastric x-ray series fails to show evidence of significant pyloric obstruction. Spence classes pylorospasm with "neuromuscular disorders of organ function" and compares it with congenital laryngeal stridor, colonic dysfunction of the spastic constipation type and adynamic ileus of the newborn. Symptoms are often present from birth and rarely persist beyond the fourth month.

Since infants suspected of this disorder rarely come to surgery, and gradual recovery is the rule, the pathophysiology can only be surmised. Whether these cases are in fact atypical or mild examples of pyloric stenosis or whether they represent a disorder of neuromuscular function is not known.

General Treatment. Once other causes of vomiting in this age group are excluded by history, examination and if necessary radiologic study, the parents should be reassured about the self-limited nature of the problem. All the details of the infant's feeding should be reviewed, including quality and quantity of feedings, frequency, prefeeding and postfeeding positioning and maternal attitudes.

The following points should be stressed in maternal counseling: (1) a quiet environment; (2) in bottle-fed babies a nipple with an opening large enough to ensure that the feeding can be completed without undue effort and in a reasonably short time; (3) the baby held as for breast feeding with interruptions of the feeding at least once for burping, and then positioning in the crib on the right side with the head of the crib elevated.

Frequent weighing should be discouraged on the basis that weight gain is likely to be irregular in any event; a poor weight gain one week may be followed by a substantial gain the following week. Frequent checking of the weight by the mother may only add to her anxiety. The baby should be re-fed if a considerable portion of a feeding is vomited within half an hour of receiving it.

Drug Treatment. *Drug treatment should be avoided if possible.* Discussion of feeding and child rearing techniques and counseling of the mother as indicated above, usually make drug treatment unnecessary. Occasionally sedation of the infant and the use of anticholinergic drugs may be indicated. Used in proper dosage with careful attention to signs of toxicity (drowsiness, flushing, rapid pulse, high fever), they minimize vomiting and ensure reasonable rest for infant and mother. If signs of toxicity appear, one or two doses should be omitted, and then treatment restarted.

Phenobarbital, 8 mg., may be given before the first, last, and mid-day feedings in the form of the elixir. The dose or the timing may be altered to ensure a restful but not oversedated infant.

The addition of anticholinergic drugs, which inactivate acetylcholine, thus blocking transmission of impulses from the parasympathetic nerve to the end-organ, is thought to give more satisfactory results. The trend has been to use products made of a combination of phenobarbital with methscopolamine (Don-natal Elixir), 0.5 to 0.75 ml. The recommended dose is given before each feeding and may need to be increased or decreased in any particular infant under one year of age, depending upon the amount of sedation produced by the phenobarbital, which is included in this product.

Prognosis. The prognosis for recovery is excellent, and recurrence unusual once the symptoms are controlled. Treatment may need to be maintained for 2 to 4 weeks, occasional cases giving trouble as late as 4 months of age.

Pyloric Stenosis

KATHRYN D. ANDERSON, M.D.

Progressive, projectile, nonbilious vomiting in a 4 to 12 week old infant is characteristic of pyloric stenosis. While pyloric stenosis is more common in males and in first born children, it also occurs in females. When the diagnosis is made soon after the onset of vomiting, the infant's state of hydration will be near normal, as will the serum electrolytes. Surgery in this group can be performed safely without prolonged preparation and with minimal morbidity. In infants whose diagnosis has been delayed, some degree of dehydration and hypochloremic, hypokalemic alkalosis will be present. In severely neglected cases, this is compounded by increased potassium loss in the urine and also by paradoxical urinary hydrogen ion excretion. Correction of the metabolic deficits is mandatory prior to surgery. An infant depleted from prolonged vomiting requires maintenance fluids plus replacement estimated upon the extent of dehydration. In addition, he will need supplementary sodium and potassium chloride to correct the metabolic alkalosis.

For the severely dehydrated infant, an initial fluid load of 360 ml./m^2 of dextrose and one third normal saline is given over a 45 minute period (20 to 30 cc./kg. over 45 minutes). This will establish urinary flow and potassium replacement can then begin safely. Electrolyte and fluid deficits are then corrected by administering 5 per cent dextrose in normal saline with added potassium (2 to 4 mEq./kg.) over a 24 hour period. Serum electrolyte determinations every six hours and urine output with specific gravity measurements are used to make adjustments in the fluid and salt replacement. Colloid, provided as albumin, 1 gm./kg., or Plasmanate 20 ml./kg., administered over a four hour period, may be required for the infant with severe volume depletion and peripheral collapse. Nasogastric drainage is instituted and thorough aspiration of the stomach just prior to the induction of anesthesia minimizes the risk of vomiting and aspiration. A Ramstedt-Fredet pyloromyotomy is the surgical procedure of choice.

Postoperative Care. The nasogastric tube can usually be removed immediately following pyloromyotomy and oral feeding commenced after six hours, according to the following regimen: glucose water (15 ml.) each hour for two hours followed by half-strength formula (30 ml.) every two hours for a total of six to eight feedings. The concentration of the formula is then increased to full-strength but the volume is restricted to 30 ml. given every two hours for a total of eight to twelve feedings. If these feedings are well tolerated, the diet can be liberalized until the infant's normal feeding schedule is resumed. Intravenous fluids are discontinued at this time. The infant is discharged 24 hours after resumption of normal feedings.

For the nursing infant, the baby is put to the breast after two feedings of glucose water and allowed to nurse five minutes at each breast every two hours, gradually increasing the length of time of nursing. It is not unusual for these infants to vomit once or twice during the first few postoperative feedings. This is probably the result of irritation of the gastric mucosa by retained gastric secretions. This can be alleviated by gentle lavage of the stomach with a few milliliters of saline. Persistent vomiting is extremely unusual and, following surgery for pyloric stenosis, normal feeding and rapid weight gain can be anticipated.

Peptic Ulcer

KATHRYN D. ANDERSON, M.D.

Infants and children usually present with complications of acid-peptic disease. This is especially true in the newborn period when gastrointestinal hemorrhage or perforation may be the first indication of peptic ulceration of the stomach or duodenum. In the newborn, gastrointestinal hemorrhage is best treated with nasogastric lavage using small quantities of normal saline. The saline is not chilled to avoid cooling the infant. Vitamin K, 1 to 5 mg., is given intramuscularly, and the hematocrit is monitored closely, replacing the blood as necessary, using a base figure of 10 cc. of whole blood per kilogram. Surgery is reserved for those infants who do not respond to these measures after 24 hours or in whom bleeding exceeds replacement. When surgical intervention is required, the findings are usually multiple superficial gastric erosions. Bleeding is controlled by suture ligature of the bleeding points. Vagotomy and pyloroplasty or other drainage procedures are rarely necessary and would be reserved for serious recurrent hemorrhage.

Another important complication of gastrointestinal ulceration in the newborn is perforation. These infants present with abdominal distention, respiratory distress, and radiographic evidence of free air under the diaphragm. For the infant with severe respiratory distress from massive pneumoperitoneum, aspiration of the intraabdominal air can be performed simply and safely by insertion of a No. 20 needle in the supraumbilical area just to one side of the midline. After resuscitation with intravenous fluids, usually dextrose and Ringer's lactate and antibiotics (ampicillin, 100 mg./kg./24 hours, and gentamicin, 6 mg./kg./24 hours), surgical repair is undertaken. Duodenal perforation is usually found on the anterior wall and is readily closed with interrupted, nonabsorbable suture. Postoperatively, nasogastric suction, antibiotics and parenteral fluids are continued for four to five days until the perforation is presumed to be healed.

In older children with peptic ulceration, the symptoms are often vague. Characteristically, the child suffers from chronic abdominal pain, often worse at night, which may or may not be relieved by food ingestion. A barium study will show a duodenal ulcer crater or deformity of the duodenal bulb, and there may be some element of gastric outlet obstruction. The role of gastroscopy in the diagnosis of peptic ulcer in children is increasing. Once the diagnosis is confirmed, the child is placed on a bland diet with frequent feedings including a nighttime snack, and magnesium or aluminum hydroxide antacids (such as Maalox), 10 to 30 ml. one hour after meals and every two hours during the day and at bedtime. Cimetidine, a histamine-receptor antagonist, is a potent inhibitor of acid secretion and currently is being used in clinical trials. This drug may soon prove to be a first-line agent in the management of patients with hypersecretion of acid and peptic ulcer disease. After six to eight weeks of therapy, a regular diet may be resumed but spicy foods should be avoided initially. Repeat contrast study is performed and will usually show healing of the ulcer. Antacids are discontinued once the patient is asymptomatic, and resumed only for recurrence of the symptoms.

Indications for surgery in the older children with peptic ulcer are: (1) Perforation which not uncommonly presents as a surgical emergency in a patient with no previous ulcer symptoms. Radiographic evidence of free air under the diaphragm is confirmatory. After appropriate fluid resuscitation and parenteral antibiotics, surgery is indicated. Perforations on the anterior duodenal wall are closed with nonabsorbable sutures and a portion of the omentum is used to reinforce the suture line. (2) Massive gastrointestinal hemorrhage which cannot be controlled by nasogastric suction, replacement of blood loss, and iced saline lavage of the stomach. (3) Intractability over many months with no demonstrable healing on repeat gastrointestinal series.

Gastrectomy is not advised in children as a definitive surgical treatment of peptic ulcer. Vagotomy and pyloroplasty are usually adequate to control the disease and avoid the malnutrition which may be a consequence of gastrectomy. For small children, the pedicle pyloroplasty is the preferred technique. Highly selective vagotomy has not been extensively evaluated in children but may well lessen the need for drainage procedure.

Gastritis

KATHRYN D. ANDERSON, M.D.

Gastritis results from the ingestion of a variety of agents readily accessible to toddlers. Medications such as ferrous sulfate cause acute chemical gastritis. Superficial erosions of the gastric mucosa are a consequence of chronic aspirin ingestion. Strong alkalis found in commercial drain cleaners do their major damage in the esophagus. Rapid passage through the esophagus into the stomach may cause edema, pylorospasm, and antral ulcerations. Outlet obstruction may develop as a long-term complication. Stress ulcers, presenting as hematemesis, may occur in seriously ill and burned patients.

Gastritis is usually self-limited and readily controlled by dietary restriction and antacids. The treatment for hematemesis, secondary to gastric erosions, is similar to that for peptic ulcer. Gastric lavage is instituted and antacids are instilled hourly through the nasogastric tube or given orally during waking hours. Frequent small feedings and antacids are continued until the child is asymptomatic. When surgery for control of gastrointestinal hemorrhage caused by acute ingestion or stress ulcer is required, oversewing of ulcerations combined with vagotomy and pyloroplasty is recommended.

Malformations of the Intestine

LUCIAN L. LEAPE, M.D.

NEONATAL INTESTINAL OBSTRUCTION

Regardless of etiology or exact anatomic location of the obstruction, intestinal obstruction of the newborn requires prompt therapy. A nasogastric tube of sufficient caliber (12 to 16 Fr.) should be inserted and placed on continuous suction to decompress the stomach and prevent further abdominal distention. A major cause of postoperative morbidity is aspiration pneumonia secondary to vomiting of gastric contents. Intravenous fluids are indicated if the patient is dehydrated, but transfer for definitive therapy should not be delayed for this purpose. All require operation urgently, within hours, at a properly equipped neonatal center. The patient must be kept warm during transfer and should be accompanied by an experienced nurse or physician.

Preoperative preparation is directed toward restoring vascular volume, fluid deficit, and electrolyte imbalance before induction of anesthesia. If the patient is severely dehydrated and shows evidence of shock (poor peripheral perfusion, low urine output, tachycardia, or hypotension) infusion of colloid (plasma or 5 per cent albumin solution), 20 cc./kg. in 5 to 10 minutes, is indicated. The amount of crystalloid to be given is dictated by the clinical condition, but if there has been no intake in the past 24 hours or more, it is safe to infuse one half normal saline in an amount equivalent to the daily maintenance fluid volume (100 cc./kg.) over a four to six hour period. Other electrolytes are given as indicated by serum chemical determination. Arterial blood gas analysis will indicate the degree of acidosis which should be corrected by infusion of sodium bicarbonate. Antibiotics (penicillin and kanamycin or gentamicin) should be given if there are signs of perforation, infarction or sepsis. In these cases, resuscitation must be rapid and operation carried out as soon as possible, preferably within one to two hours. If the patient has uncomplicated intestinal obstruction and is stable, four to six hours may be used profitably in correcting fluid and chemical imbalance. It is mandatory that blood volume be adequately restored and that there is good evidence of organ perfusion prior to induction of anesthesia.

Operative correction usually entails either intestinal anastomosis or performance of a colostomy. Most patients will benefit by insertion of a gastrostomy which, in addition to providing more satisfactory gastric and intestinal decompression, spares the infant obstruction of the nasal passage. When feedings are begun gastrostomy permits careful monitoring of gastric emptying, prevents vomiting, and makes possible controlled feeding if the infant is unable to suck or swallow. Careful attention to intravenous fluid and electrolyte replacement is mandatory in the immediate postoperative period. In addition to appropriate replacement of fluid and electrolyte losses (nasogastric drainage, ileostomy drainage, etc.), most of these patients benefit from daily albumin infusions for two to three days to replace the protein loss in the obstructed gut.

Prophylactic antibiotics, penicillin and kanamycin or gentamicin, given at the time of operation and for 24 hours postoperatively, are probably of value in decreasing postoperative sepsis, although this has not been proved and many surgeons do not use them. If there is perforation or peritonitis a full therapeutic course of antibiotics should be given for 7 to 10 days.

The major postoperative complications that should be sought are pneumonia, sepsis, and recurrent obstruction. A small percentage of patients need re-operation for adhesive or functional obstruction. Unless there is a loss of significant length of intestine, most of these patients do well and have no long-term sequelae after discharge from the hospital.

Duodenal Atresia. Because of the high level of obstruction, these patients present with vomiting early and thus the diagnosis is usually made before extensive dehydration. Diagnosis is made by upright x-ray of the abdomen; contrast studies are not necessary. Preoperative preparation is as indicated above. The operation consists of direct duodenoduodenostomy. A significant number of these babies are premature and approximately half of them have significant associated anomalies which should be searched for in the postoperative period; 30 per cent have down syndrome.

Jejunoileal Atresia. Most of these patients require extensive preoperative resuscitation because of dehydration and electrolyte imbalance. at operation it is important to resect massively dilated proximal bowel since it will not function even when the obstruction is relieved. An alternative is to do a "tailoring" procedure reducing the diameter of the bowel to permit more effective peristalsis and more accurate anastomosis. End-to-end anastomosis is preferred.

These patients are notoriously slow to "open up" and effective intestinal function may not be resumed for three to four weeks. Parenteral nutrition should be started early in the postoperative period before further depletion occurs.

Malrotation. The prime danger in malrotation is bowel infarction secondary to volvulus of the midgut. Many patients do not have a volvulus and present only as duodenal obstruction which may be partial or complete. Lysis of the peritoneal bands completely relieves the obstruction.

If volvulus is present (noted by characteristic x-ray findings and abdominal distention in addition to evidence of high intestinal obstruction) operation is urgently required in the hope of reducing the volvulus prior to the onset of gangrene. Rapid fluid resuscitation is necessary. At operation, the twisted bowel is rotated to relieve the obstruction and peritoneal bands are lysed. Obviously necrotic bowel must be resected. In some cases the viability of the intestine is not clearly evident. Resection should not be carried out, but a "second look" operation should be performed within 24 to 48 hours at which time the viability of intestine can be more accurately assessed and only the minimal amount necessary removed.

If the entire midgut is infarcted, with no viable intestine distal to the ligament of Trietz, survival is impossible and parenteral nutrition should not be instituted. If, however, there is 15 cm. or more of small intestine, total parenteral nutrition over an extended period of time may permit hypertrophy of the intestine and eventual adequate enteral function.

Meconium Ileus. Unless the patient has signs of peritonitis, a mass, or incipient intestinal gangrene, nonoperative treatment should be tried first. After suitable fluid and electrolyte resuscitation, Gastrografin enema is administered. Because of its hypertonicity, this substance stimulates the shift of fluid through the mucosa into the intestinal lumen, thus loosening the inspissated meconium. The amount of fluid transfer can be sufficient to cause shock. Accordingly, fluid must be administered intravenously at the same time the enema is being carried out in the ratio of 6 ml. for each 1 ml. of contrast material. Often more than one enema is required, although 6 to 12 hours should be allowed to elapse between them. If Gastrografin enema therapy is not successful, operation is indicated.

At operation, it is sometimes possible to perform enterotomy and evacuate the inspissated and sticky meconium by irrigation with N-acetylcysteine, 2 per cent (*not* 20 per cent). If all of the obstructing meconium cannot be removed, a "T" ileostomy is performed to permit distal irrigation and proximal decompression in the postoperative period. Markedly dilated or compromised segments of bowel should be resected.

In addition to the usual postoperative measures, these patients will require pancreatic enzyme supplementation when formula feedings are begun. They are particularly prone to develop pneumonia which should be prevented by vigorous pulmonary physiotherapy, mist, etc. The diagnosis of cystic fibrosis must be confirmed by sweat test.

The vast majority of these patients survive operative treatment of meconium ileus, but this group of patients typically has severe cystic fibrosis and later succumb to pulmonary complications. A significant fraction never leave the hospital.

Meconium Plug.   Barium enema which is diagnostic is usually also therapeutic in this condition. If not, repeat enema with Gastrografin may sufficiently loosen the meconium to permit normal evacuation. It is important that these patients be carefully observed for development of normal bowel action following relief of the obstruction. Persistent evidence of obstruction requires operative intervention. Because of the risk of Hirschsprung's disease and cystic fibrosis, probably all patients with meconium plug syndrome should subsequently have a rectal biopsy and sweat test.

Hirschsprung's Disease.   See page 198.

MECKEL DIVERTICULUM

Rectal bleeding is the symptom that most commonly brings the patient with a Meckel diverticulum to the doctor. The amount of bleeding may be significant—several ounces or more, but seldom causes shock. Blood is bright red or maroon, rarely tarry. Other patients present with signs of intestinal obstruction due to volvulus about a Meckel diverticulum or intussusception. Occasionally there is a diverticulitis with localized pain or perforation leading to peritonitis. In the absence of these latter symptoms, which require urgent surgery, attempts should be made to confirm the diagnosis of a meckel diverticulum by barium enema or small bowel contrast study, both of which, unfortunately, have a low yield. Since bleeding is due to ulceration caused by acid produced by ectopic gastric mucosa, ^{99m}Tc pertechnetate scan may demonstrate uptake of the isotope in the gastric mucosa (if the amount of gastric mucosa exceeds 2 cm². in area).

Initial treatment is directed toward resuscitation if necessary. Massive bleeding requires transfusion; patients with intestinal obstruction or peritonitis require fluid resuscitation. operative treatment is urgently indicated for patients with obstruction, peritonitis or continuing hemorrhage once resuscitation is carried out. In the usual case, bleeding is less massive and does not require transfusion. In these, surgical exploration is indicated if the diverticulum is demonstrated radiologically or by isotope study, and in patients who have recurrent episodes of bleeding sufficient to significantly depress the hematocrit, even in the absence of a specific diagnosis.

Operation consists of excision of the diverticulum with transverse closure of the intestine, making sure to completely remove all the abnormal tissue. Sometimes segmental resection and end-to-end anastomosis are required. If there is volvulus or intussusception, these are treated in the usual manner, resecting the diverticulum and any compromised bowel.

Postoperatively these patients require no special care other than that for any patient operated on for intestinal obstruction.

Since the incidence of Meckel diverticulum is approximately 2 per cent and only 4 per cent of these will develop a complication, elective removal in the asymptomatic patient or "incidental" removal at the time of surgery for other conditions is not indicated.

DUPLICATIONS AND CYSTS OF THE INTESTINE

Duplications (or enterogenous cysts) may occur at any level of the gastrointestinal tract from pharynx to rectum. Obstructive symptoms predominate, although the presence of ectopic gastric mucosa in an intestinal duplication may lead to acid-peptic erosion and bleeding. The combination of a palpable abdominal mass, intestinal obstruction and guaiac-positive stools should suggest duplication. [99m]Tc pertechnetate scan may be positive if there is ectopic gastric mucosa.

Operation is indicated in all of these patients, and may be urgently necessary because of obstructive symptoms. Preoperative preparation consists of blood and fluid replacement as indicated. The objective of surgical treatment is to remove the duplication cyst if possible. In difficult anatomical situations a "window" procedure may be satisfactory in which the common wall between the duplication and the main lumen of the intestine is opened to permit adequate drainage. This is particularly indicated in long duplications in which resection of an extensive length of intestine would be required for removal. If gastric mucosa is present, resection must be carried out to prevent later bleeding. Postoperatively, these patients require the usual care of anyone undergoing intestinal resection.

Mesenteric cysts are usually asymptomatic except for the presence of a soft mobile mass. Generally, they can be enucleated or opened, and intestinal resection is seldom necessary.

OMPHALOCELE AND GASTROSCHISIS

Omphalocele is a large hernia into the umbilical cord in which the abdominal viscera are covered only by a thin peritoneal sac. In gastroschisis, there is a full-thickness defect and no sac to cover the eviscerated intestines which become engorged and edematous. Immediately after discovery at birth the sac or exposed intestines should be covered with warm, sterile, saline-soaked gauze sponges and the lower half of the infant placed in a plastic bag to prevent heat loss which can be considerable. If the intestines are exposed, they should be supported in such a way as to prevent angulation and compromise of circulation. A nasogastric tube should be promptly placed to prevent gaseous distention of the intestine.

Omphalocele is an emergency and requires immediate surgical treatment. Nonoperative treatment with Mercurochrome has been recommended in the past, but has a higher mortality than surgical correction and requires two to three months of continuous hospitalization.

Operation consists of reduction of the intestinal contents with fascial and cutaneous closure, and gastrostomy. If this is impossible, a prosthetic "chimney" can be constructed to extend the capacity of the peritoneal cavity. This is reduced in size daily, stretching the abdominal wall, while simultaneously permitting shrinking of the edematous intestines. In 7 to 10 days it is removed and complete fascial closure is accomplished.

Postoperatively, these patients may require ventilatory support, especially if the abdominal closure is tight. Antibiotics are administered if the intestines were exposed. Parenteral nutrition is necessary to maintain positive nitrogen balance until the intestinal tract resumes function, often two to three weeks. Some degree of intestinal obstruction is common, but usually resolves with time. Accordingly, re-exploration should not normally be contemplated before three weeks.

Significant other congenital anomalies are frequently found, particularly in the cardiovascular and genitourinary systems. They are less common with gastroschisis than omphalocele, where they account for much of the mortality associated with this condition. Incisional hernias are also common, but usually can be repaired without significant risk when the child is several months of age.

DIAPHRAGMATIC HERNIA

Bochdalek diaphragmatic hernia is one of the most urgent surgical conditions of the newborn. Diagnosis is usually made shortly after birth when the characteristic findings are noted on a chest x-ray taken because of severe respiratory distress. It is important that an *upright* film be obtained to avoid confusion with congenital pulmonary cysts.

Initial treatment consists of insertion of a nasogastric tube of adequate size (12 to 14 Fr.) which is placed on continuous suction to prevent further gastric and intestinal distention. Oxygen is administered via endotracheal tube to maintain ventilation. Care must be taken to avoid excessive pressure which easily ruptures the dysplastic lung. Sodium bicarbonate, 3 mEq./kg., is administered intravenously to combat acidosis which is often severe and uncorrectable until the hernia has been corrected.

Operation is indicated in all of these patients, and time is of the essence. The baby should be transferred immediately to a pediatric surgical center for definitive treatment. Transfer should not be delayed in misguided attempts to correct acid-base imbalance, put in an arterial or venous catheter, etc. *The most common cause of preoperative death in these patients is delay in operative treatment.* The patient should be transferred with physician or experienced nurse administering oxygen and maintaining nasogastric suction, while keeping the baby warm.

Upon arrival at the receiving center, the baby should be taken immediately to the operating room where further preoperative resuscitative efforts can be carried out in a controlled environment. If the patient's condition permits, the pH should be elevated to 7.2 or better and blood gases improved by carefully controlled ventilation. The baby should be warmed to normal temperature before operation.

Operation consists of reduction of the hernia and closure of the defect in the diaphragm, which may be accomplished by either the abdominal or thoracic route. Gastrostomy is performed.

Postoperatively most of these patients need ventilatory assistance and constant monitoring by experienced personnel. They may need frequent administration of bicarbonate as well as volume expanders. The lung must be allowed to inflate slowly over a period of several days, without endotracheal pressure or pleural suction. Because the lungs are hypoplastic, there is a significant hazard of contralateral pneumothorax. Balancing the position of the mediastinum by regulating intrapleural pressure will prevent overdistention of the opposite lung during this period.

Outcome in large measure depends on the degree of pulmonary hypoplasia. Paradoxically, patients who are operated on earliest have the poorest survival rate since they have the most severe degree of pulmonary insufficiency, hence their early symptoms. Associated anomalies, particularly patent ductus arteriosus, coarctation of the aorta, and atrial septal defect, are common and should be sought in the postoperative period.

Eventration of the diaphragm, though not actually a hernia, may mimic diaphragmatic hernia in radiologic and clinical aspects. There is marked hypoplasia of the muscle of the diaphragm which becomes attenuated and stretched. Phrenic nerve paralysis produces a similar physiologic and radiologic picture. In the newborn, either of these conditions may produce severe respiratory distress because of the paradoxic motion of the diaphragm and the mobility of the mediastinum. Diaphragmatic plication is curative and should be carried out in symptomatic infants.

Hernia of the foramen of Morgagni, or retrosternal herniation, is rare and usually asymptomatic unless incarceration occurs. Surgical repair should be carried out when the diagnosis is made and cure is to be expected.

POLYPS AND TUMORS OF THE GASTROINTESTINAL TRACT

Colonic polyps are one of the more common causes of blood in the stool of children. Such bleeding is usually painless, typically red streaking on the outside of the stool, although occasionally occurring in larger amounts with clots. It is unusual for such bleeding to be severe enough to cause an alteration in the hematocrit. Because these are almost invariably *juvenile* polyps, having no malignant potential, extensive treatment is not indicated. Barium enema confirms the presence of one or several polyps in the colon. Removal of those within the reach of the sigmoidoscope should be carried out if they are symptomatic. Higher polyps should be disregarded unless they cause persistent significant bleeding or serve as lead-points for intussusception. Colonoscopic removal is usually possible and open operation is rarely necessary. The majority of these polyps will ultimately slough, so in the absence of symptoms no treatment is indicated.

Familial polyposis is an inherited malignant disease in which the polyps are numerous and adenomatous in nature. Malignant change is certain to occur and is sometimes seen before the teens. Accordingly, total colectomy is recommended after the age of ten. Semiannual barium enema and colonoscopy should be carried out in any in whom surgery is delayed. Subtotal colectomy in which the ileum is anastomosed to the rectum can be used as a temporizing measure in patients in whom rectal polyps are few in number and are easily removed at sigmoidoscopy. If the rectum is retained, semiannual sigmoidoscopy and fulguration of any new polyps must be carried out. Ultimate proctectomy and ileostomy may well be necessary. In some patients an endorectal pull-through of the Soave type has been successful, but frequently there are difficulties in bowel control due to the ileo-anal anastomosis.

Lymphoma is the other primary tumor of the intestinal tract that is not rare in childhood. Although resection should be carried out, it alone is seldom curative. These patients benefit by multi-drug chemotherapy and radiation therapy which should be instituted promptly. Since a significant fraction develop leukemia if chemotherapy is withheld, many oncologists favor a treatment regimen similar to that for lymphatic leukemia, using vincristine and cyclophosphamide.

Rare tumors of the gastrointestinal tract which have been described at all ages, from the neonate on, include leiomyoma, embryonal sarcoma, neurofibroma and carcinoma of the colon. Since these are all exceedingly rare, treatment must be individualized, but usually involves resection and subsequent chemotherapy. In childhood, tumors not infrequently act as lead-points of intussusception, and should be particularly suspected if intussusception occurs in a child over one year of age.

Foreign Bodies of the Gastrointestinal Tract

LUCIAN L. LEAPE, M.D.

Ingestion of foreign bodies is common and seldom serious. Three generalizations apply: (1) Almost all ingested foreign bodies will pass through the intestinal tract without difficulty, regardless of age of the child; therefore patience is indicated and usually rewarded. (2) No foreign body should remain in the esophagus for more than 24 hours. (3) There is no substance known, food or medication, that will hasten or make safer the transit of a foreign body through the intestine.

If ingestion of a foreign body is suspected by the history, x-rays of the chest, including the pharynx, should be obtained. This will usually demonstrate a foreign body in the esophagus or stomach. If none is seen, then an abdominal film is indicated. If the foreign body is non-radiopaque, judicious use of thin contrast barium swallow is indicated to determine if an object is stuck in the esophagus.

If an esophageal foreign body is smooth in contour, it can usually be pushed into the stomach by passage of a soft rubber catheter or, under fluoroscopic control, removed by careful, premeasured inflation of a Foley catheter balloon distal to the object which is then extracted as the catheter is removed. The patient should be positioned on his side with the head down to prevent accidental aspiration of the foreign body or vomitus. Failure of this technique should lead to immediate esophagoscopy. If the foreign body is sharp (safety pin, nail, etc.) the catheter method should not be used and immediate esophagoscopy is indicated. If there is a history of prior esophageal surgery or stricture, esophagoscopy and dilatation are usually indicated. The presence of a stricture is suggested if meat or food become impacted since this is a rare occurrence in patients with a normal esophagus.

Foreign bodies of the stomach require no specific treatment and these patients do not require hospitalization. There is no need to limit diet or activity. All stools should be examined. A useful method is to drape cheese-cloth over the toilet bowl, under the seat, and then wash the stool away with hot water. If the foreign body is not recovered, abdominal x-rays should be repeated at weekly intervals. The parents should be instructed to bring the child back at any time if he develops pain, vomiting or fever.

Operative removal is indicated for foreign bodies that fail to leave the stomach in three weeks. Gastroscopy with the flexible fiberoptic endoscope is usually successful. General anesthesia is indicated in the young child. Operative extraction is indicated for those which cannot be removed by gastroscope or foreign bodies which pass into the small intestine and fail to advance after a week. Operation is indicated promptly if the patient develops signs of penetration or perforation—pain, fever, ileus, or signs of peritoneal inflammation.

It is to be emphasized that well over 90 per cent of patients with foreign bodies in the stomach will not require operative treatment, regardless of size or shape of the foreign body.

Intussusception

LUCIAN L. LEAPE, M.D.

There are three distinct forms of intussusception, each with its own pitfalls in diagnosis: idiopathic, lead-point, and postoperative. In *idiopathic* intussusception (probably secondary to enteric viral infection) the typical age of onset is the last half of the first year of life. These babies typically (but not always) have intermittent sharp abdominal pain and bloody or "currant-jelly" stools. A mass may be palpable. With time they develop vomiting and distention. *Lead-point* intussusception may occur at any age, and can be due to a Meckel diverticulum, intestinal polyp, enterogenous cyst, Henoch-Schönlein purpura, or cystic fibrosis. Symptoms of intestinal obstruction predominate and bleeding is less common. *Postoperative* intussusception is the most insidious; it occurs as early as two days after major surgery or as late as two weeks. (Pain or rectal bleeding is rarely noted.) Unlike the other forms of intussusception, it is usually difficult to feel a mass, in part because of the recent incision. The diagnosis is suspected in the patient who has persistent or progressive vomiting or increasing gastric aspirates.

Since 95 per cent of intussusceptions are ileocolic or colocolic, barium enema is usually diagnostic. Hydrostatic reduction should be attempted and is successful in approximately 80 per cent. Ileoileal and ileocolic intussusception are more difficult to diagnose and are rarely reducible by barium enema.

The details of hydrostatic reduction by barium enema are important. It should be done under fluoroscopic control in a well hydrated patient who has undergone appropriate intravenous fluid resuscitation. The barium container should not be elevated above three feet, and external compression is to be avoided. Usually the intussusception reduces with ease, but the radiologist must note free reflux of barium well into the ileum to ensure complete reduction. If the first attempt is not successful, evacuation should be permitted and a repeat study done in 30 minutes or so. Several attempts may be necessary. If barium enema reduction is successful, symptoms disappear and the patient frequently falls asleep. All patients should be kept for 12 to 24 hours after reduction to make sure it has indeed been successful.

Barium enema reduction is contraindicated if there are signs of gangrenous bowel, shock, severe distention or dehydration. In these cases, urgent preparation is necessary so that a corrective operation can be carried out before there is gangrene of the intestine. The usual preoperative fluid resuscitation is in order. Operative treatment of intussusception is also indicated for the failures of hydrostatic reduction and in patients with an obvious lead-point.

At operation, manual reduction by taxis (pressure, not traction) will be successful in some patients in whom hydrostatic reduction failed. In others, resection of the irreducible intussusception will be necessary. If there is a lead-point, resection is indicated to prevent recurrence. End-to-end anastomosis is preferred to an exteriorization resection of the Mikulicz type. Postoperatively these patients respond to the usual care for patients following intestinal resection. If manual reduction is successful, the patient may run a low grade fever for one to two days postoperatively.

Hirschsprung's Disease

WILLIAM K. SIEBER, M.D.

Hirschsprung's disease is a congenital anomaly characterized by partial to complete, acute or chronic low intestinal obstruction caused by absence of intramural ganglion cells in the distal alimentary tract. The aganglionosis may involve only the rectum or it may extend proximally to varying levels and may involve the entire alimentary tract. There is little correlation between the extent of aganglionosis and the severity of symptoms. The diagnosis is suggested by the clinical findings, reinforced by barium enema studies and definitively established by histological study of a full thickness rectal biopsy.

When Hirschsprung's disease is suspected, surgical consultation for diagnosis and treatment should be promptly obtained. Nonsurgical treatment is ineffective. Treatment with cathartics and smooth muscle stimulants such as methacholine (Mecholyl) may be harmful by promoting fatal enterocolitis. Older children with moderate chronic constipation as the only symptom may respond to enemas administered daily or every second or third day. Since the rectum is inactive, impactions are high and may require the use of detergent retention enemas, dioctyl sodium sulfosuccinate (Colace), one part in three parts of saline, followed by a saline cleansing enema in 12 hours. The dangers of rectal perforation and water intoxication from enemas are well documented. Enemas should be isotonic. Fecal impactions are avoided by the use of preparations which

tend to keep the stools soft such as Zymenol or psyllium hydrophilic mucilloid (Metamucil).

In infancy, acute colonic (90 per cent) or low bowel obstruction (10 per cent aganglionosis coli) requires emergency relief by enterostomy in the normally innervated intestine just proximal to the aganglionic intestine. Frozen section control of the placement of the enterostomy requires the service of a pathologist familiar with the appearance of intramural ganglion cells in infants. The colostomy is done as a loop colostomy or as a divided colostomy with the proximal end brought up to function as a single lumen, the distal end being closed and returned to the peritoneal cavity. When the aganglionic segment is short and involves only the rectum, a right transverse loop colostomy is done. An emergency colostomy is indicated to prevent the development of enterocolitis, a frequently lethal complication in infancy. A colostomy is done preliminary to definitive surgical treatment in the newborn; in symptomatic infants up to 6 months of age; and in older patients with long-standing symptoms associated with a grossly distended colon and poor general health. Definitive surgical treatment is deferred until the infant is approximately 1 year of age or in an older child until general health improves and colonic impactions are completely removed. This usually takes 6 months.

Preparation for definitive surgery includes mechanical emptying of the colon with enemas and a clear liquid diet.

Definitive surgical treatment involves the resection of the aganglionic intestine and re-establishment of the continuity of the alimentary tract. This is currently done by one of three abdominoperineal procedures—the Swenson, Duhamel or Soave procedure.

The Swenson procedure is the original and the time-tested standard procedure. In this operation, the aganglionic intestine is freed and removed to within 1½ cm. of the pectinate line anteriorly, and includes a sphincterotomy of the internal anal sphincter posteriorly. The normally innervated intestine is then brought down and anastomosed to this remaining rectal stump.

In the Duhamel procedure, the aganglionic intestine is resected down to the rectum. The rectum is sutured closed but left in place. A recto-rectal channel is developed, and the normally innervated intestine pulled through this channel and through an incision in the posterior rectal wall 1 cm. above the pectinate line. One-half of the circumference of the distal rectum is then anastomosed to the posterior one-half of the pulled-through normally innervated intestine. The anterior one-half of the pulled-through colonic wall is opposed to the posterior one-half of the retained rectum. Clamps are placed intraluminally to remove this common wall, thus resulting in an end of the colon to posterior wall of rectum anastomosis. Variations of the Duhamel procedure involve differences in the type of crushing clamp or suturing method used. When long segments of aganglionosis are present the Martin procedure in which a long side-to-side anastomosis of the pulled-through intestine and the distal aganglionic colon is done is now the preferred procedure.

In the Soave procedure (the endorectal pull-through procedure), the mucosa is removed from the rectum down to the skin of the anus. Normally innervated intestine is then pulled through the resultant muscular cuff and anastomosed either directly as in the Swenson procedure (Boley) or in delayed fashion as a two stage procedure (Soave) to the anal skin.

The operative mortality associated with these procedures is negligible and the initial result in all is very good. At the present time the personal experience of the operating surgeon should determine the best procedure for the individual patient. My preference at this time is the Duhamel procedure preceded by a right transverse colostomy.

Enterocolitis may occur as a serious complication of Hirschsprung's disease. The sudden abdominal distention, disinterest in nursing, vomiting and foul diarrhea terminate in high fever with dehydration and may cause death within 24 to 48 hours. When enterocolitis is suspected, intravenous fluids, gentle copious saline rectal irrigations and gastric suction followed by decompression by colostomy may be life-saving. Enterocolitis may first appear after a colostomy has been done for obstruction or it may appear as long as 6 to 8 years after an uneventful definitive procedure. The Swenson procedure is, in our experience, more likely to be followed by enterocolitis than are the other procedures.

Short segment Hirschsprung's disease, in which only the lower rectum is aganglionic, has been treated by transluminal rectal myectomy by Lynn. This procedure is actually an extension of full thickness rectal biopsy. Personal experience with this procedure has been limited and disappointing.

Ulcerative Colitis

JEAN F. PERRAULT, M.D., *and*
GUNNAR B. STICKLER, M.D.

Treatment programs for inflammatory bowel diseases are mainly symptomatic since the cause is not known. But there are some regimens which have proved to be effective, as we will point out.

GENERAL MEASURES

A good relationship between the physician and the patient and his family remains the cornerstone of therapy. The patient and the patient's family should understand as much as possible about the disease itself and the extent of personal involvement necessary so that changes in drug therapy or the possibility of surgery will not be unexpected.

Because the value of diet has never been demonstrated in ulcerative colitis and the patient already has many preoccupations because of his disease, adherence to a strict diet would be an added burden; however, bulky foods should be restricted during a moderate attack (hematochezia added to diarrhea and abdominal pain), or nothing should be taken by mouth during a severe attack (symptoms of a moderate attack plus fever, nausea and vomiting, and severe diarrhea), at which time the parenteral administration of fluids may be necessary. Unless a child has a lactase deficiency, or is suspected of having such a deficiency, the use of milk should not be restricted.

When the diarrhea is severe, serum electrolyte levels should be checked occasionally, because hypokalemia can lead to weakness or more severe complications. Anemia can accompany hematochezia, especially when the hematochezia is severe, or can be the result of the chronic disease; in the former, the use of iron supplements such as ferrous sulfate, 150 to 300 mg./day, is justified. In either situation, blood transfusion may be needed if the hemoglobin level decreases to less than 9 gm./dl. Sulfasalazine (formerly salicylazosulfapyridine) also can cause anemia, either because of hemolysis or because of folate malabsorption; in hemolysis, the medication must be stopped, whereas in folate deficiency the adding of folate, 1 mg. daily, should be sufficient to maintain an adequate level of folate.

Whereas anticholinergic drugs probably have no place in the treatment of ulcerative colitis, antidiarrheal agents offer some help. Because of the possibility of toxic megacolon, the patient must be instructed to stop their use completely, or at least not to increase the dosage, if his symptoms are aggravated with fever and abdominal pain. We prefer to use diphenoxylate hydrochloride,* 2.5 to 5 mg.,

---

*Manufacturer's precaution: Diphenoxylate hydrochloride (Lomotil) is contraindicated in children under 2 years of age. Lomotil should be used with special caution in young children due to the variable response in this age group. In children 2 to 12 years of age, use Lomotil liquid. Do not use Lomotil tablets for this age group.

three or four times daily (not exceeding 10 mg./day) for children less than 12 years old or 8 mg./day for children less than 8 years old. Because atropine is added to diphenoxylate to prevent abuse, atropine toxicity could develop in children, even at the suggested doses.

MEDICAL TREATMENT

The goal of any treatment is to eradicate the disease, but in ulcerative colitis, the goal is more modest; short of surgery we plan only on arresting an acute attack and then preventing or limiting recurrences. To this goal, two agents have been useful: sulfasalazine and steroids.

Sulfasalazine. Sulfasalazine (Azulfidine)* contains both sulfapyridine and 5-aminosalicylic acid. Although still not known, the mechanism of action could involve an effect on the bacterial flora, an anti-inflammatory effect, or an antiprostaglandin effect. The use of this drug should be advocated mainly for (1) treatment of an attack that is acute mild or moderate but not severe and (2) maintenance therapy to prevent recurrences. Although the results can be slow to manifest, both the symptoms and the mucosal changes respond to a dosage of 1 to 2 gm. four times a day. This dosage should be continued for four to six weeks after disappearance of the symptoms and then be gradually reduced to a maintenance dosage. For maintenance therapy, a dose of 1 to 2 gm./day is effective in limiting recurrences of attacks. Like other investigators, we have noticed a rapid recurrence of the symptoms and mucosal changes when the medication was stopped within a year after an acute attack. The use of sulfasalazine probably should be continued indefinitely if this low dosage is well tolerated.

Sulfasalazine should not be given to patients who are allergic to sulfonamides or who have significant liver disease. Its use also implies that the patient be observed carefully for possible complications, such as anemia, agranulocytosis, dermatologic reactions, and others, which fortunately are rare. Interestingly, these reactions, as well as the more common nausea, vomiting, and headache, seem to be more prevalent if the serum levels of sulfapyridine (one of the two components of sulfasalazine) are greater than 50 μg./ml. Decreasing the dosage or starting at a low dose before reaching the suggested dosage should avoid most of the adverse effects.

Steroids. Being more powerful agents,

steroids are accompanied by more frequent and severe side effects, and their use is restricted to patients with an acute severe episode or with an acute moderate attack not relieved by sulfasalazine. Steroids also can be used in the latter situation if extracolonic manifestations are present, such as eye, skin, or joint involvement. Corticotropin, cortisone, and other steroid preparations have been used, but we do not see any advantage of these over the use of prednisone.

During the first four weeks, a total of 30 mg. of prednisone, given in one or two doses daily, is adequate, with a gradual decrease in the dose to zero during the next four to six weeks. If no significant response is noted during that time, surgery should be considered. During the last weeks of steroid treatment, sulfasalazine should be started and continued for maintenance therapy (in some instances adding sulfasalazine in therapeutic doses to the steroid regimen at the beginning of treatment might be of added benefit). Steroid treatment has *no* place in maintenance therapy. However, the use of steroids for only six to eight weeks should help control most of the effects of the colitis and cause no side effects. If the patient requires surgery during steroid treatment, the surgeon should be aware of possible hypertensive and convulsive complications.

Steroid Enemas. Steroid enemas also have a place in the treatment of ulcerative colitis, but mainly when the patient has tenesmus (frequent and painful urge to empty the rectum which produces nothing or only small quantities) or mild distal disease. Hydrocortisone-retention enemas (100 mg. of hydrocortisone in 60 ml. of isotonic saline) can be administered through a squeezable bottle or can be dripped into the rectum. The cost is reduced if the patient prepares the solution at home. The solution should be retained in the rectum for at least 1 hour. Foam solutions are now available if the liquid cannot be retained adequately. One dose a day is usually sufficient, given in the morning if the symptoms are more troublesome during the day, otherwise given in the evening. The steroid-retention enemas should not be given more than twice daily, and the treatment should last only two weeks. Because of the possible significant absorption of the steroid, the enemas should be reduced in frequency over another week and then stopped completely; the child is subject to the side effects of steroids, although experience suggests that not much hydrocortisone hemisuccinate and hydrocortisone acetate are absorbed.

Intravenous and Elemental Nutri-

---

*Manufacturer's precaution: Sulfasalazine is contraindicated in children under 2 years of age.

tion. Total parenteral nutrition and elemental diets have the theoretic advantage of "putting the colon to rest" while replenishing the caloric deficit often encountered. This does not treat the primary problem, and the intravenous method is not without significant risks, although the elemental diet often cannot be taken in sufficient quantity because of its unpalatability and because its high osmolarity may increase the diarrhea. The main advantage of these diets is in preparing the patient for surgery, especially if malnutrition is already present, and a better postoperative course seems to accompany their use.

More Recent Measures. Disodium cromoglycate has been tried, and this compound may be helpful in preventing recurrences, the rationale being that acute exacerbations of ulcerative colitis might be mediated by a type I hypersensitivity reaction, which can be blocked by this agent. The studies have been done in adults only, and the results seem encouraging, but larger groups of patients need to be studied.

SURGERY

Indications. Once the colon and rectum have been resected, there is no more disease, but the alternative of an ileostomy may be taxing to the young patient. Indications for surgery are (1) toxic megacolon, (2) no response to medical management, (3) stunting of growth, and (4) a risk of carcinomatous changes.

Severe symptoms persisting after eight weeks of prednisone therapy, massive bleeding, or continued blood and protein loss in spite of full medical treatment are valid reasons for surgery; if the lesion is confined to the distal colon, longer medical management should be tried (but usually the symptoms are not as severe in distal disease). Surgery may afford significant benefits to the young patient who has growth failure secondary to disease, especially if the surgery is done before puberty. "Prophylactic" proctocolectomy for possible carcinomatous changes is often not accepted by either the patient or the treating physician, especially if the patient is doing well. However, one must consider that the incidence of carcinoma is almost 20 per cent per decade after the first 10 years of colitis in patients who have the onset of their disease in young age with pancolitis and fairly active disease. This increase should be convincing enough to indicate the need for early surgery, especially because carcinomatous changes in ulcerative colitis are very difficult to detect. The decision is more difficult for patients who have less severe involvement from colitis.

Procedure. The only satisfactory operation is total proctocolectomy, either in one or two stages. Although the Koch pouch (continent ileostomy) seems favorable for the adult patient, it probably is not to be recommended yet for the younger patient. Although treatment centers present the Koch pouch operation as the best procedure developed so far, many patients develop complications. So, for pediatric patients, it might be best to have the conventional ileostomy; if after more years of follow-up, the patients who had the Koch pouch tolerate it well and have no complications, then those who had a simple ileostomy will have the choice of continuing with the ileostomy or of having their simple ileostomy changed into a Koch pouch.

In any patient who requires surgery, preoperative contact with an enterostomal therapist or a patient with an ostomy can be beneficial, because many questions can be answered this way. Contact with an "ostomy association" after the surgery also can be helpful to the patient.

Surgical Complication. Besides the usual postoperative morbidity, patients who are still taking steroids at the time of surgery may experience severe hypertension (peak of 170 to 180 mm. Hg systolic and 110 to 120 mm. Hg diastolic) accompanied by seizures during the first 72 hours after the surgical procedure (this also can occur in patients with Crohn's disease who undergo surgery). Fluid retention may be a contributing factor. Seizures are controllable by the intravenous administration of diazepam or phenobarbital, while appropriate steps are being taken to maintain the blood pressure below 150/100 mm. Hg; the use of steroids has to be continued for some time because of the risk of adrenal insufficiency.

COMPLICATIONS OF ULCERATIVE COLITIS

Toxic Megacolon. Although relatively infrequent, especially in the pediatric age group, toxic megacolon can occur, being more frequent in the patients taking anticholinergic or antidiarrheal medications or after a barium enema. The immediate steps in treatment are to (1) allow decompression by nasogastric suction, (2) maintain fluid-electrolyte balance through the intravenous route, (3) continue close observation by frequent examinations and abdominal films, and (4) obtain an early surgical consultation. Parenteral nutrition should be considered in patients who are already debilitated.

Steroid therapy with intravenously administered hydrocortisone should be started or continued in each patient, but there is a risk of silent perforation with subsequent peritonitis. Antibiotic coverage with penicillin and gentamicin also should be added.

If the symptoms have not abated after 48 hours, or if perforation occurs, the patient should undergo surgery; colectomy or proctocolectomy can be done as a primary procedure.

Liver Disease. Different forms of liver involvement are encountered, but fortunately these do not all lead to chronic liver damage. If the liver is chronically damaged either by primary sclerosing cholangitis or by cirrhosis, it usually follows a course independent of the colitis, and treatment, including proctocolectomy, is often unrewarding. In primary sclerosing cholangitis, steroids and antibiotics can be tried, but generally surgery on the biliary tree is needed to allow decompression. If there is chronic active hepatitis, steroid therapy can halt the progression, but generally, cirrhosis eventually develops. Some selected patients who had resection of the colon before cirrhosis developed had evidence of histologic regression of the lesion when the lesion was rebiopsied three to seven years after surgery.

Arthritis. Fleeting symptoms in the peripheral joints and ankylosing spondylitis are the main problems, and each behaves differently. The former usually occurs during exacerbations of the colitis and responds to treatment of the colitis itself, although bed rest and salicylates are of added benefit; it is rarely deforming. The ankylosing spondylitis is more chronic and persists even though the colitis might be under control; the damage will be permanent. Treatment is mainly symptomatic, with salicylates and appropriate physiotherapy. Some patients will present with only roentgenographic evidence of sacroiliitis, and this requires no specific therapy.

FOLLOW-UP

Follow-up is important (every year, every six months, or more frequently if necessary) because exacerbations are frequent, treatment needs to be supervised regularly, and complications, including carcinoma, can develop at any time. If sulfasalazine is used, a blood count should be done twice a year to check on the possibilities of anemia, either hemolytic or macrocytic, and of agranulocytosis. Barium enema and proctosigmoidoscopic examinations should be done every two years. Colonoscopy is not done routinely in all patients with colitis, but everyone with a colonic stricture

should undergo colonoscopy and the stricture should be biopsied regularly. Follow-up needs to be arranged with a colleague once the patient reaches adulthood.

Crohn's Disease

JEAN F. PERRAULT, M.D., and
GUNNAR B. STICKLER, M.D.

Whereas ulcerative colitis is limited to the colon and involves mainly its mucosa, Crohn's disease can affect the entire alimentary canal from mouth to anus and is a transmural process. Because the course of Crohn's disease is unpredictable, therapy is difficult to evaluate. Even surgical procedures, such as resection of all apparently affected tissues, does not ensure complete cure. Thus our approach to therapy is slightly different from that in ulcerative colitis, even though the drugs used are essentially the same. In Crohn's disease, we first want to answer the following four questions.

1. How extensive is the disease?
2. Is the patient sick enough to warrant any form of therapy?
3. Does the patient have any complications such as failure to thrive, fistulas, abscess, or extraintestinal manifestations?
4. Is surgery appropriate for the type of involvement?

GENERAL MEASURES

A close relationship between the physician and the patient and family is important. Office visits and visits to the hospital will be frequent, and confidence in all areas is important: the patient's confidence that the disease can be controlled, the physician's confidence that his advice will be accepted, and general confidence that the medications will be used judiciously.

When partial obstruction occurs, low-residue diets should be used. Otherwise, high-protein, high-caloric foods should be emphasized. The use of milk should be encouraged, except if there is lactose deficiency, and daily vitamin supplements are suggested. Vitamin B_{12} may be needed when the distal ileum is involved; the serum level should be checked regularly, especially if the patient has macrocytic anemia. If the level is low, intramuscular injections of vitamin B_{12}, 50 μg. for four consecutive days (unless a Schilling's test is done), followed by monthly injections of 50 to 100 μg., will compensate.

The patient can have microcytic anemia because of chronic blood loss or poor iron absorption if the disease extends proximally or can have normocytic anemia because of chronic disease or a combination of iron and vitamin B_{12} deficiency. When iron is needed, ferrous sulfate, 300 mg. once or twice a day orally, can be given. Blood transfusions are sometimes necessary, especially when the hemoglobin level is less than 9 gm./dl.

Because of the nature of Crohn's disease, elemental diets and total parenteral nutrition have better applications in Crohn's disease than in ulcerative colitis. Elemental diets can be of great help in partial obstruction, fistulas, or anal disease because of their low residue; half-strength diets should be tried first. Flavors can be added to increase the palatability of the diet, but these increase the osmolarity even more. Their use in the short-bowel syndrome or in patients with ileostomies should be checked carefully because these agents can increase the frequency of diarrhea owing to their osmotic effect.

Total parenteral nutrition is useful because it allows the bowel "to rest," thus allegedly permitting subsidence of the inflammatory process and closure of fistulas. However, in our experience, although we noted these effects during total parenteral nutrition administration, we also noted recurrences soon after the return to a more normal alimentation. In spite of its many side effects, total parenteral nutrition has permitted replenishment of nutrition in malnourished patients and has been an excellent preoperative preparation.

Certain selective patients who have either total intestinal involvement or the short-bowel syndrome are instructed in "home total parenteral nutrition"; however, it implies a permanent connection with a large venous channel and daily manipulations of sterile solutions, with 8 to 10 hours of intravenous drip. Thus cooperation of the patient and family, strict adherence to instructions, and a fairly large investment for the material are required. This technique could become more widely available as more experience is gained.

Pain, whether visceral or parietal, can be troublesome and merits attention. Cramping abdominal pain is usually the most frequent symptom and is related to obstruction. After edema and inflammation of the bowel subside, fasting or a low-residue diet can offer relief, but the pain may persist even when the patient is fasting. If pain continues, a non-narcotic pain reliever should be used, after which codeine tablets and even injections of meperidine or pentazocine may be required; however, use of these latter agents should be limited because of the danger of addiction, especially in chronic disease. Anticholinergic agents do not add any benefit.

The diarrhea in Crohn's disease is different from that in ulcerative colitis because it can result from several mechanisms. When the diarrhea is secondary to inflammation, as in granulomatous colitis, diphenoxylate hydrochloride, 2.5 to 5 mg. three or four times a day (not exceeding 10 mg. and 8 mg. a day in children less than 12 and 8 years old, respectively), can be used; tincture of opium is an alternative. The same precautions apply as with ulcerative colitis. These medications do not affect the primary process itself. When the diarrhea accompanies malabsorption, restriction of long-chain triglycerides can help. If bile salt diarrhea is present, as with resection of less than 100 ml. of ileum, leading to bile salt malabsorption, cholestyramine,* 2 to 4 gm. before each meal, is a better choice. The further loss of bile salts (because of their binding to cholestyramine) may lead to mild steatorrhea, but the severity of the diarrhea will be decreased.

Steroids. As in ulcerative colitis, prednisone alone is as effective as other forms of steroid preparations; and because it can be used orally, prednisone has an advantage. The indications for steroid use are not clear-cut but include (1) systemic manifestations such as fever and loss of weight, (2) significant diarrhea that is nonresponsive to the usual measures, (3) blood or protein loss and malabsorption, (4) partial obstruction, (5) either extensive involvement prohibiting surgery or postsurgical recurrence, and (6) growth failure. All of these indications warrant a trial of prednisone, 30 to 40 mg. daily. The preliminary results of the National Cooperative Crohn's Disease Study (NCCDS), available for part I of the study, i.e., control of actively symptomatic disease during four months of high-dose treatment (Gastroenterology, 70:938, 1976), suggest that prednisone, in a dosage of 0.25 to 0.75 mg./kg., was significantly superior to placebo. The population was mainly an adult one, but the results should be applicable to children.

If the patient is too ill to take the medication orally, therapy can be started with intravenously administered hydrocortisone, 50 to 100 mg. every six to eight hours, until the patient can tolerate an oral intake. The duration of treatment is varied, and the clinical response, including biochemical parameters, serves as a titrating index. Because of the known side effects of steroids, the duration of treatment should be as short as possible, but

---

*Manufacturer's precaution: The dosage of cholestyramine has not been established for infants and children.

two to four months of therapy may be needed. Some patients may need to be treated for two or three years, but most patients have some evidence of side effects by this time. As usual, gradual tapering of the dose proportional to the length of treatment is required before therapy is stopped completely.

The response is not predictable, and whereas some patients will show rapid, dramatic improvement, others progress inexorably and develop many complications, and still others relapse soon after the dose is tapered.

Steroid enemas are used less often in Crohn's disease than in chronic ulcerative colitis because rectal involvement is less frequent in Crohn's disease. But when they are needed, as in Crohn's colitis with rectal disease, the dosage is the same as that used in ulcerative colitis (see p. 200).

Sulfasalazine. Sulfasalazine is frequently used in Crohn's disease, either during the acute stages or as maintenance therapy, but its efficacy has never been convincingly demonstrated. The NCCDS has supplied more than anecdotal results. Their preliminary report suggests that the four-month use of sulfasalazine,* 1.0 gm./15 kg./day, is superior to placebo in controlling actively symptomatic disease; no data are available for maintenance therapy, however. For definitive results, the study will require more patients and a longer period of observation.

Azathioprine. Reliable evidence for or against the use of this agent is lacking, although isolated reports have suggested that azathioprine can arrest inflammation and close fistulas; however, a preliminary report by the NCCDS shows no advantage of azathioprine over placebo.

Other Drugs. A few reports, based on data from very few patients, have suggested that other drugs such as metronidazole and dapsone are useful, but we have not substantiated the efficacy of these agents.

SURGICAL TREATMENT

The diversity of the populations studied, the different procedures and surgical techniques used, and the frequency of incorrect diagnoses have all contributed to widely dispersed opinions. However, two facts remain: (1) surgery is vital in the treatment of many patients and (2) even if all diseased tissues seem to have been resected, the patient cannot be assured of complete cure. The indications for surgery are no different from the

ones defined for ulcerative colitis, except that the threat of carcinomatous changes is not as pronounced in Crohn's disease, although patients with involvement of the small bowel and colon are at a higher risk of developing carcinoma of the colon.

Acute Ileitis. Acute ileitis may be secondary to Crohn's disease (*Yersinia* infection probably is more frequent), but because recovery generally occurs within a few months, resection should not be done. However, if acute ileitis is diagnosed at surgery, incidental appendectomy can be done unless the cecum is involved; if the cecum is involved, appendectomy can lead to fistulization.

Chronic Ileitis. Accepted surgical indications are complete obstruction, partial obstruction not responding to treatment, perforation or abscess, fistulous tract formation, failure of growth and delayed puberty, and persistent systemic manifestations. Extensive disease, previous extensive resections, or inadequate medical trial are relative contraindications. Surgery usually involves resection with anastomosis. Bypass alone is less favored because it does not reduce the rate of recurrence (as reports first suggested) and because complications may arise in the bypassed segment.

Ileocolitis. Toxic megacolon is also a surgical indication when the colon is involved. If the small bowel is affected more than the colon, the surgical procedure generally involves resection and anastomosis, whereas if the colon is primarily involved, the procedure of choice is ileocolostomy or ileostomy with resection.

Colitis. Controversy exists as to the course of patients who had surgery for Crohn's colitis, whether proctocolectomy with ileostomy, ileorectostomy, or some other procedure. Although some reports have minimized the risk of recurrences after surgery, others have emphasized that almost 50 per cent of surgical patients can expect a recurrence proximally, with the possibility of having to undergo reoperation. In our experience, Crohn's colitis does not behave much differently from Crohn's disease of other parts of the gastrointestinal tract.

Morbidity after surgery is relatively high, primarily from the disease process itself and from the malnutrition that accompanies it, and hypertension with or without seizures may occur early during the postoperative stage. The use of steroids preoperatively may not influence the rate of complications. Fluid and electrolyte management should be checked closely; total parenteral nutrition can be of great help postoperatively.

---

*Manufacturer's precaution: Sulfasalazine is contraindicated in children under two years of age.

COMPLICATIONS

As with ulcerative colitis, Crohn's disease can be associated with extraintestinal manifestations, and their management can present problems.

Perianal Disease. Perianal disease is a frequent accompaniment in Crohn's disease, generally with Crohn's colitis, and can be the source of frustrations; its chronicity is notorious. Fissuring and fistulous formations can occur but these generally cause relatively few symptoms and should be left untreated because they eventually disappear if the primary disease is controlled. However, they can lead to a miserable existence, and then a more aggressive, usually surgical, approach can be taken. A direct attack or stool diversion has been used, but neither has achieved overwhelming success, and after each, a long healing period is to be expected.

Perianal and perirectal abscesses are accompanied by toxicity and sharp pains; drainage relieves the symptoms within hours. After the treatment of abscesses, a long healing period is to be expected.

Malabsorption. Because the small bowel is often involved in Crohn's disease, malabsorption problems are frequently present, compounded by fistulous tracts, blind loop formation, or surgical resections, which all lead to more severe malnutrition. Also, there is always the possibility of the short-bowel syndrome, and this could complicate the treatment of the malabsorption.

If significant steatorrhea is present, the intake of fat should be decreased to 40 or 50 gm./day. If calories need to be added, medium-chain triglycerides, given in the form of an oil, can be used; 1 tablespoon of the oil contains about 120 calories. Because of bile salt depletion, the use of medium-chain triglycerides is especially valuable when more than 100 cm. of ileum have been resected. If there is bacterial overgrowth of the small bowel, a short course of ampicillin, 250 mg. two to four times a day, or of lincomycin,* 30 mg./kg./day for 7 to 10 days, is useful (in older children, tetracycline can be used). At times, these short courses may need to be repeated at monthly intervals.

Bile salt deficiency, steatorrhea, and poor nutrition may lead to deficiency of the fat-soluble vitamins (A, D, E, and K). Hypocalcemia, at times accompanied by tetany or

bone disease, needs close attention. Vitamin D preparations, 10,000 I.U. daily, should be tried, often with a course of calcium supplements, all given orally; calcium lactate is best absorbed, but other calcium salts also are effective. Because increased fat excretion leads to increased loss of calcium, calcium should be given between meals. If symptomatic hypocalcemia occurs, intravenous treatment may be necessary. The serum calcium level should be checked not only to verify a response to the therapy but also to prevent hypercalcemia, which can occur if the doses of calcium are too high or when the primary disease is being controlled. If improvement does not occur, the doses of calcium might need to be increased. At times, hypomagnesemia is also present and may lead to resistance of the treatment of the low calcium level, until the magnesium level is restored to normal. (Note, the low magnesium is not due to low calcium but results from the same causes that lead to low calcium.)

Because hypoprothrombinemia may occur but not be apparent, the status of the vitamin K-dependent factors (Factors II, VII, IX, and X) should be checked by means of a prothrombin time before any diagnostic or surgical procedure is considered. If the prothrombin time is elevated and a procedure is to be done or a coagulation abnormality is apparent, phytonadione, 2.5 to 10 mg., should be given intramuscularly, otherwise 5 to 10 mg. daily of an oral vitamin K preparation would be adequate.

Nephrolithiasis. Two types of renal stones can develop: uric acid stones and calcium oxalate stones. Uric acid stone formation is facilitated by dehydration and acidic urine; a high-output ileostomy can be a common cause of this problem. Oxalate stones are usually found in patients with steatorrhea, whose intake and absorption of oxalate is increased.

In uric acid stone formation, treatment (as well as prevention) includes rehydration and addition of alkali to keep a urine pH between 6.0 and 6.5. In calcium oxalate stone formation, restriction of long-chain triglycerides and oxalates in the diet is required. In either type, urologic manipulations might be necessary in the acute situation.

Other Complications. Other complications, which include joint and liver involvement, are similar to those found in ulcerative colitis. Eye and skin involvements are also found in both conditions, and the oral use of steroids is then suggested because the inflammatory bowel disease is usually active when these complications are seen.

---

*Manufacturer's warning: Until further clinical experience is obtained, lincomycin is not indicated in the newborn.

Necrotizing Enterocolitis

JOHN C. LEONIDAS, M.D., *and*
ROBERT T. HALL, M.D.

Necrotizing enterocolitis is a serious and often lethal disease of newborn infants characterized by ischemic necrosis of the gastrointestinal tract which may lead to perforation and peritonitis. Prematurity, perinatal complications (especially asphyxia), respiratory distress syndrome, sepsis, indwelling umbilical vessel catheters, exchange transfusions, hyperosmolar or high caloric formula feedings seem to be significant predisposing factors. The incidence of the disease varies in neonatal intensive care units, and has been reported to occur in 1 to 7.5 per cent of all neonatal admissions.

Early symptoms include temperature instability, usually hypothermia, poor feeding and gastric retention. Abdominal distention, decreased bowel sounds and lethargy are also usually present. There may be decreased volume of stools or diarrhea. Stools are frequently blood-streaked. Vomiting occurs and may be bile-stained or brownish and guaiac-positive. Deterioration is manifested by apnea, pallor, hyperbilirubinemia, oliguria and bleeding diathesis, and local signs of peritonitis such as abdominal tenderness and resistance, erythema and edema of the anterior abdominal wall or palpable masses. Radiographic findings of ileus, pneumatosis intestinalis, gas in the portal vein and increased peritoneal fluid or pneumoperitoneum are of great diagnostic value.

Treatment is started as soon as the disease is suspected and prior to confirmation of the diagnosis. Oral and gavage feedings should be discontinued and a nasogastric tube placed for decompression. Intravenous fluid and electrolyte solutions are administered to maintain balance and replace losses. Cultures are obtained (including blood, cerebrospinal fluid and urine) and broad spectrum antibiotics given, preferably ampicillin, 150 mg./kg./24 hours, and gentamicin, 3 to 5 mg./kg./24 hours, or kanamycin, 15 mg./kg./24 hours. Antibiotic therapy should be modified depending on culture results and prevailing resistance patterns of organisms.

The patient should be examined frequently (at least every 4 to 6 hours), if possible by the same team of physicians. Roentgenograms of the abdomen in the supine and upright or left lateral decubitus positions are obtained at the same time. Laboratory studies to be performed frequently include hematocrit, white blood count and differential, platelet count, serum bilirubin, albumin, BUN, electrolytes, blood pH, blood gas determination, glucose, partial thromboplastin time and prothrombin time. Urine volume and specific gravity are quantitated and daily weight measured to assist in management of fluid balance.

Topical administration of antibiotics by gavage has been advocated with apparently good results. Kanamycin or gentamicin has been used in doses 2 to 3 times that of the parenteral dose. The antithrombotic action of low molecular weight dextran also has been advocated as beneficial. Dextran 40 is given as a 10 per cent solution intravenously in doses of 10 ml./kg. every 6 hours for 48 hours. Total parenteral nutrition is a valuable modality of treatment, especially in patients whose slow improvement makes prolonged withdrawal of oral feedings mandatory.

With the supportive medical management described above most patients treated early in the course of the disease will show clinical improvement and disappearance of pneumatosis intestinalis usually within 48 to 72 hours. With continuing improvement and disappearance of radiographic abnormalities, oral feedings may be carefully instituted after 10 days, at which time all other measures are also terminated.

The results of this medical management have been generally successful, with a 70 per cent to 90 per cent survival rate without the need for operation. The overall prognosis has markedly improved from an early survival rate of 30 to 40 per cent to 50 to 80 per cent including patients treated medically and surgically. The reasons for improved prognosis are twofold: awareness of the disease leads to early recognition and institution of medical therapy in the early stages; and there has been a significant refinement of indications for surgical treatment, from the early recommendation that only those with overt bowel perforation should be operated upon. The result is that at present fewer patients are subjected to operation but a greater number survive. Indications for surgical management vary, but the following are considered reasonable: (1) radiographic evidence of perforation (pneumoperitoneum); (2) sudden clinical deterioration with shock and respiratory insufficiency, and clinical signs of peritonitis; (3) radiographic manifestations of bowel necrosis and peritonitis, such as persistently dilated isolated loops of bowel or significant amounts of peritoneal fluid (under the circumstances preoperative paracentesis of peritoneal fluid and culture is recommended), and (4) persistent metabolic acidosis not responding to appropriate therapy, or signs suggestive of disseminated intravascular coagulation such as sudden drop in platelet count or lengthening of partial thromboplastin time or prothrombin time. Failure to improve clinically or radiographically within 48 hours has also been proposed as an indication for operation.

Surgical treatment consists of resection of necrotic bowel, unless the extent is such that it precludes survival. Depending on the situation, an end-to-end or end-to-side anastomosis may be performed or the bowel exteriorized in the form of enterostomy. Survival is approximately 60 per cent in recent years. Survivors of medical or surgical management may develop strictures, usually colonic. Resection and anastomosis is performed with good results.

Recent experimental work indicates that formula feedings enhance the effect of hypoxia on the mucosa of the gut and precipitate enterocolitis, whereas breast milk may prevent the development of the disease. Controlled clinical data are not available at this time to confirm these experimental observations.

Purulent Peritonitis

J. J. TEPAS, M.D., *and*
J. ALEX HALLER, JR., M.D.

Intelligent management of peritonitis in children requires a basic understanding of the nature and intensity of the pathophysiologic changes that occur. Generalized peritonitis or inflammation of the visceral and parietal peritoneum is characterized by fluid sequestration and intestinal dysfunction. Since the peritoneum is a semipermeable membrane equal to 20 per cent of body surface area, inflammation can produce enormous fluid losses both as visceral edema and intraperitoneal exudate. The relative hypovolemia and dehydration thus produced will present as dry mucous membranes, oliguria, hyperthermia and, when severe, hypotension.

The most common causes of peritonitis are inflammatory diseases of bowel, which, as they progress and spread, produce a thickened peritoneal surface that can extend to any contiguous organ or structure. Intestine, being most extensively invested by peritoneum, usually manifests the greatest dysfunction in the form of transmural inflammation and edema resulting in loss of both propulsive and absorptive function. Adynamic ileus, with its intraluminal, transmural and serosal fluid accumulation, produces abdominal distention,

anorexia, nausea and, often, vomiting. Parietal peritoneum is likewise involved and causes an inflammatory irritation to overlying abdominal musculature which presents as localized pain and tenderness, and eventually may result in generalized abdominal wall rigidity.

Progression of intestinal disease often leads to perforation with bacterial contamination. When this occurs, the inflamed peritoneum serves as a large absorptive surface for both bacteria and endotoxins. Voluminous contamination will often overwhelm this absorptive capacity resulting in accumulation of necrotic, purulent material and abscess formation. The intermittent bacteremias and endotoxemia thus produced result in spiking fevers and, in some circumstances, complete cardiovascular collapse.

Advanced generalized peritonitis will then manifest itself in the form of a critically ill, catabolic, dehydrated child with a history of anorexia, nausea and vomiting, whose abdomen is distended, tender, rigid and markedly painful to touch in the area of greatest parietal peritoneal involvement.

Appropriate therapy must provide adequate circulatory volume, decompress inflamed intestine and restore normal homeostasis. A central venous line and urinary catheter are absolutely essential since the effect of initial fluid therapy is best demonstrated by restoration of adequate perfusion pressure and maintenance of urinary output of at least 1 to 2 cc./kg./hr. Ringer's lactate, 10 to 20 mg./kg/hr., will provide adequate fluid resuscitation, as it most closely approximates the slightly hypotonic extracellular fluid loss occurring within the abdomen. Colloid, as either Plasmanate (10 ml./kg.) or albumin (0.5 to 1.0 gm./kg.), can be used to restore oncotic pressure, but should be used cautiously, as the administered protein will traverse damaged capillaries and may actually increase fluid sequestration in inflamed tissues.

A large sump nasogastric tube (16 to 18 French) must be placed to decompress the in-inflamed, atonic gut. High fever is most efficiently treated by Tylenol suppositories (120 mg.), supplemented, when necessary, by cold intravenous solutions and a cooling blanket.

Initial antibiotic therapy is based upon the assumed type of infection suspected to be present. Continuing antibiotic therapy is based upon the organisms which are identified in primary cultures. The majority of patients present with a mixed polymicrobial infection which requires both aerobic and anaerobic coverage. Clindamycin, 20 to 30 mg./kg./day, and gentamicin, 5 mg./kg./24 hr., have recently been shown to be most effective both in treatment of initial sepsis and prevention of later abscess formation. Since clindamycin has not been used extensively in infants, it can be replaced by chloramphenicol sodium succinate, 50 to 100 mg./kg./day, in these patients; the dosage for newborn infants is 25 mg./kg./day.

Surgical intervention should take place when resuscitative measures have restored homeostatic mechanisms to as near normal as possible. Operative therapy should correct or remove the source of contamination, debride necrotic tissue and, when appropriate, provide adequate drainage. Aerobic and anaerobic cultures, as well as Gram stains, must be done on an aspirate of peritoneal fluid to guide later antibiotic therapy.

Discrete, walled-off abscess cavities are drained with soft rubber catheters or Penrose drains. Generalized purulent peritonitis requires gentle debridement with copious irrigation. Drainage of the peritoneal cavity has not been shown to be of benefit in preventing postoperative abdominal abscess, and may, by allowing entry of opportunistic organisms, contribute to recurrent abscess formation. Both intraoperative and postoperative lavage of the peritoneum with antibiotic solutions has recently been recommended as effective in preventing abscesses. There remains, however, considerable controversy over both techniques and choices of antibiotic.

Postoperative care includes maintenance of proper hydration, continuation of nasogastric suction until signs of normal bowel peristalsis return, effective antibiotic therapy, and close observation for signs of recurrent sepsis. In cases where extensive bowel involvement or severe inflammatory disease are encountered, normal bowel function may take weeks or months to return. Under these circumstances, parenteral nutrition should be employed to provide enough calories to reverse catabolism and allow proper healing.

Although treatment of peritonitis in children is similar to that of adults, certain disorders frequently encountered in children may require modification of this therapy. An unusual variety of monomicrobial, hematogenously induced peritonitis, termed *"primary peritonitis,"* can occur in very young children and in uremic patients. The offending organism is usually hemolytic streptococcus, pneumococcus or *Staphylococcus aureus*. It is appropriately treated by either aqueous penicillin, 50,000 to 100,000 units/kg./8 hr. intravenously, or methicillin, 100 to 400 mg./kg./day intravenously.* Diagnosis must be

confirmed by demonstration of positive cocci on Gram stain of peritoneal aspirate. Operative intervention is usually unnecessary, as long as objective improvement occurs within 48 hours of beginning treatment. Antibiotics should be continued until the patient is afebrile for at least 48 hours.

Secondary purulent peritonitis is much more commonly encountered in children and represents a polymicrobial, mixed bacterial infection. Acute perforated appendicitis is the best example of this and is the most frequent cause of secondary peritonitis in children. Appendectomy is usually the correct surgical therapy; although in children who present with a discretely walled-off abscess, simple drainage with interval appendectomy six to eight weeks later should be considered.

Finally, consideration must be given to the peritonitis associated with perforation from necrotizing enterocolitis. This is also a mixed polymicrobial infection; it occurs in stressed infants who, by nature of their tenuous physiologic state, require extended intensive care and are often colonized by atypical resistant organisms that proliferate in hospital environments. Methicillin, ampicillin (150 mg./kg./day), and gentamicin presently appear most effective against these organisms, although chloramphenicol must also be considered, since some of these infants ultimately succumb to sepsis from anaerobic organisms despite otherwise proper management.

Idiopathic Unconjugated and Conjugated Hyperbilirubinemias

M. MICHAEL THALER, M.D.

CHRONIC NONHEMOLYTIC UNCONJUGATED HYPERBILIRUBINEMIA

Gilbert's Disease. The clinical importance of this common disorder—approximately 1 per cent of the general population is affected—lies in the frequency with which it is mistaken for hepatitis or a hemolytic condition. The only findings are mild scleral icterus, vague abdominal complaints and occasional weakness. The unconjugated fraction of serum bilirubin is persistently elevated, varying be-

---

*Manufacturer's precaution: The number of instances in which methicillin has been administered intravenously to infants and children is not large enough to permit specific intravenous dosage recommendations.

tween 2 and 6 mg./100 ml. The patient may become visibly jaundiced during periods of stress, fasting or illness, and the serum bilirubin may double. These pigment levels are not dangerous, and treatment with phenobarbital, 3 to 5 mg./kg./day, is rapidly effective. Prognosis is excellent.

Crigler-Najjar Syndrome. In contrast to Gilbert's disease, the serum bilirubin in Crigler-Najjar syndrome is elevated to potentially toxic levels. The hyperbilirubinemia in this condition must be treated without interruption throughout life, as the patient's condition may deteriorate suddenly and irreversibly during viral infections or other illnesses. Serum bilirubin concentrations in excess of 20 mg./100 ml. are reached during the first week after birth. Repeated exchange transfusions and phototherapy are necessary at this time to prevent brain damage. In the past, most patients succumbed from kernicterus in infancy or childhood; those who survived were severely retarded. New therapeutic approaches hold the promise of improving this gloomy outlook considerably.

The syndrome is recognized in two therapeutically distinct forms. Patients in whom the serum bilirubin cannot be reduced with phenobarbital are classified as type I or nonresponders. Type II patients are those in whom the serum bilirubin can be maintained at 3 to 10 mg./100 ml. with 3 to 10 mg./kg./day of phenobarbital. Type I patients are currently being managed with phototherapy. We have followed a child with this form of Crigler-Najjar syndrome for nearly 6 years, beginning in early infancy. He has been treated with phototherapy, currently with blue fluorescent light from 10 high-intensity 20-watt T-12 Special Blue lamps (Westinghouse), applied for 8 to 12 hours nightly. The serum bilirubin has stabilized at 13 to 16 mg./100 ml.

This patient has developed normally, is of above-average intelligence and has always had excellent health. However, at 2 years of age, the bilirubin gradually increased to nearly 20 mg./100 ml., despite frequent replacement of bulbs (the Westinghouse lamps are adequate for at least 10,000 hours of continuous phototherapy) and prolongation of exposure periods. This upward trend was reversed with cholestyramine, 4 to 8 gm. daily.* The rationale for this treatment was the observation, previously made in jaundiced rats, that significant amounts of unconjugated bilirubin

were excreted in the bile during phototherapy. The unconjugated pigment may re-enter the circulation from the small intestine, and blood levels may rise because production of bilirubin increases with age. Cholestyramine, an insoluble and indigestible resin, binds unconjugated bilirubin and prevents its reabsorption from the intestinal lumen. The therapeutic combination of light and cholestyramine should be further evaluated in other patients with type I Crigler-Najjar syndrome.

FAMILIAL CONJUGATED HYPERBILIRUBINEMIA

Dubin-Johnson Syndrome. This rare inherited deficiency in excretion of organic anions by the liver causes mild to moderate elevations of serum bilirubin, most of which is direct-reacting. The diagnosis may be suspected on the basis of a positive family history and is confirmed by liver biopsy. The liver cells are filled with a dark melanin-like pigment which is concentrated in centrilobular regions. No specific treatment is available, but prognosis is excellent. Patients should avoid fasting, excessive exercise and alcohol ingestion.

Rotor Syndrome. This condition is in all respects similar to the Dubin-Johnson syndrome and may represent a milder form of the same disorder. A point of differentiation may be the absence of pigmentation in the liver of a patient with the milder condition. No treatment is necessary.

IDIOPATHIC BENIGN RECURRENT CHOLESTASIS

This mysterious chronic illness occurs more commonly in female children and adults than in males, and it may surface in teenage girls during pregnancy. The characteristic episodes of severe jaundice and pruritus are occasionally precipitated by intercurrent illness, but are usually spontaneous in onset. Each attack may persist for several months, and is followed by symptom-free intervals of up to several years. Excessive fatigability and steatorrhea due to biliary insufficiency are common features. In addition to markedly elevated serum bilirubin and bile acid levels, BSP clearance is delayed. Other standard indices of liver function are almost invariably normal. Percutaneous liver biopsies reveal severe cholestasis, most marked in central regions of lobules, and occasional small inflammatory infiltrates in peripheral lobular regions. The serum bilirubin may reach 20 mg./100 ml., but this represents no danger to the brain, as most of the pigment is conjugated.

Treatment of cholestatic episodes consists of phenobarbital, 5 to 10 mg./kg./day, and cholestyramine, 8 to 12 gm./day. Each agent

---

*Manufacturer's note: A dosage schedule for cholestyramine has not been established for infants and children.

may be used alone, but the combination is more effective. Relief from pruritus is usually obtained within a few days, while jaundice clears more slowly. Steroid therapy has been successful in shortening attacks of cholestasis in occasional patients, whereas others have failed to respond to high doses of prednisone or dexamethasone. Attacks may be aborted with phenobarbital administered as soon as weakness and pruritus appear in a child known to have the disease, but treatment of any kind is usually unnecessary during symptom-free periods.

Despite its chronicity (more than 26 episodes in a single patient have been described), the disease has an excellent prognosis, and patients are generally without symptoms between attacks.

IDIOPATHIC INTRAHEPATIC CHOLESTASIS

This poorly defined condition usually becomes apparent in the neonatal period and is characterized by prolonged conjugated hyperbilirubinemia and bile acidemia without other hepatic abnormalities. Biopsies of the liver reveal inspissated bile and occasional inflammatory infiltrates. This type of cholestasis usually clears without treatment after several months. The recovery process can be accelerated with phenobarbital, 5 to 10 mg./kg./day, which relives pruritus in the older infant and may facilitate elimination of bilirubin and bile acids in bile.

The long-term outlook is favorable. However, occasional infants with idiopathic cholestasis may eventually develop chronic liver disease indistinguishable from hypoplasia of the intrahepatic bile ducts. In these cases, treatment with phenobarbital and cholestyramine may be indicated, as described for Benign Recurrent Cholestasis.

Cirrhosis and Tumors of the Liver

M. MICHAEL THALER, M.D.

CIRRHOSIS

Chronic liver damage may occur with several metabolic disorders (such as galactosemia, alpha-l-antitrypsin deficiency, cystic fibrosis, Wilson's disease), biliary malformations (such as choledochal cyst, intrahepatic and extrahepatic biliary atresia) and in association with drugs (such as antimetabolites, phenytoin, thiouracil, chlorpromazine, tetracycline, erythromycin, phenothiazine). The outcome of hepatic complications may be influenced by specific treatment of the primary disease. However, liver damage in these disorders and in instances of chronic liver disease from unknown causes (cryptogenic) may progress to cirrhosis, an intractable process characterized by a circle of inflammation→cell death→fibrosis→regeneration→vascular insufficiency→cell death. Once cirrhosis becomes established, management should be directed toward: (1) maintenance of optimal nutrition, (2) prevention of intercurrent infections and anemia, and (3) treatment of complications associated with portal hypertension and hepatocellular failure. The three major complications of cirrhosis are ascites, upper gastrointestinal bleeding, and hepatic encephalopathy.

Nutrition. The exact role of nutrition in childhood cirrhosis remains poorly understood. However, children with biliary insufficiency due to severe hepatocellular damage often absorb dietary fat and fat-soluble vitamins (A, D and K) poorly. Caloric and vitamin deficiency may contribute to retarded growth, lack of stamina, anemia, bleeding tendency, and reduced resistance to infections. An adequate protein intake may also play a positive role in liver regenerative processes and in maintenance of hepatic protein synthesis (mainly albumin).

The general aim in children with cirrhosis uncomplicated by ascites or encephalopathy is the provision of a diet with sufficient calories and essential nutrients to maintain growth and to prevent specific deficiencies. Such a diet should not be rigid, should cater to individual tastes, and should be monitored with a planned program of regular follow-up visits, including a careful evaluation of dietary intake, physical examination and liver function tests.

A diet containing at least 1.5 gm. of protein per kilogram, excluding fatty foods, is usually well tolerated. In advanced cases, medium-chain triglycerides (Progestimil) may be added to ensure adequate caloric intake. Vitamins A and D are administered daily (2 to 3 times normal requirements) and one vitamin K tablet (5 mg.) is taken twice weekly. Severe pruritus may be controlled with cholestyramine (Questran),* 8 to 15 gm. daily. In patients with partial biliary obstruction due to intrahepatic ductile hypoplasia, phenobarbital, 5 mg./kg./day, may stimulate biliary secretion and improve pruritus and jaundice.

---

*Manufacturer's note: A dosage for cholestyramine has not been established for infants and children. This use is not mentioned in the manufacturer's instructions.

Treatment of Complications

Anemia. Mild to moderate anemia occurs in a majority of children with cirrhosis. Hypersplenism, expanded blood volume, decreased erythropoiesis, blood loss due to hypocoagulability and thrombocytopenia, or due to gastrointestinal hemorrhage from esophageal varices or duodenal ulcer, and increased red cell fragility are among contributory causes of anemia in cirrhosis. Stools should be tested for blood, and serum analyzed for iron and iron binding capacity. When significant blood loss occurs, the deficit is replaced with fresh blood and vitamin K (1 to 3 mg.) is administered intramuscularly. Iron deficiency is treated with oral iron preparations.

Infection. Infection in a cirrhotic child is a serious complication, since systemic spread to lungs and meninges is not uncommon. Cultures of blood, urine and ascitic fluid should be obtained promptly and the infection treated with appropriate antibiotics.

Hemorrhage. Gastrointestinal bleeding in cirrhotic patients is complicated not only by their depleted general condition but also, specifically, by impaired synthesis of clotting factors, thrombocytopenia or hypersplenism and circulating fibrinolysins. Other complicating factors include excessive reabsorption of ammonia from the breakdown of blood in the intestine, electrolyte abnormalities such as hyponatremia and hypokalemia, as well as the severe metabolic alkalosis associated with the latter. Correction of these abnormalities has a direct bearing on prevention of coma and eventual survival and, therefore, must be considered as an integral part of the emergency management of bleeding.

An adequate airway should be maintained and oxygen administered when necessary. Transfusions of fresh whole blood are given to maintain blood volume, to ensure adequate tissue perfusion and to elevate levels of circulating coagulation factors and platelets. Stored blood and transfusions of platelets can be used when fresh blood is unavailable. Fluid and electrolyte balance should be managed parenterally. This is also a convenient route for the administration of vitamin B complex and vitamin K. Venous pressure should be measured frequently, and a urinary catheter may be necessary for close surveillance of urinary output.

Measures for the prevention of hepatic coma should be instituted in all cases of gastrointestinal bleeding in the presence of severe hepatic decompensation. Cathartics and enemas are administered repeatedly to remove blood from this source. Liquid neomycin is given orally, 2 to 4 gm./24 hours, or by enema, in an effort to suppress the production of ammonia by bacterial enzymes. Blood can also be aspirated from the stomach through a lavage tube.

A patient with advanced liver disease may bleed at sites other than esophageal varices. Because the treatment of hemorrhagic peptic ulcers or gastritis or other lesions differs from the aggressive procedures employed in intractable esophageal bleeding, the site of bleeding should be located as soon as the patient has been given transfusions. Such an examination is best accomplished with endoscopy by a skilled operator. This procedure should not be attempted by one who uses an endoscope only occasionally. The diagnosis can be established with a high degree of accuracy, especially if the varices continue to ooze blood, or a clot is visible.

In preparation for endoscopy, the stomach is lavaged with ice water. This simple procedure occasionally slows or stops esophageal bleeding. When bleeding esophageal varices are demonstrated, the following measures are taken. Vasopressin (or posterior pituitary extract) is administered intravenously over a period of 10 minutes in doses of 10 to 20 units in 25 ml. of saline to reduce portal venous pressure.* Effective pharmacologic dosages are evidenced by an increase in blood pressure and diarrhea. If the response is positive, the treatment can be repeated at hourly intervals. Because coronary artery disease is not a problem in children, vasopressin therapy is less dangerous than balloon tamponade, particularly if the patient is monitored with electrocardiograms, and coronary dilators such as amyl nitrite are kept on hand.

When all else fails and massive life-threatening bleeding continues, the use of a balloon tube (Sengstaken-Blakemore tube) becomes necessary. The gastric balloon is inserted and then inflated to at least 300 ml. volume in older children (smaller volumes may be sufficient in infants), fitted against the esophageal hiatus, and held in position with the use of foam rubber under the nose. Additional traction is usually not required. If venous compression at the cardioesophageal junction controls the bleeding, inflation of the esophageal balloon may not be necessary. Otherwise, the esophageal balloon is inflated to approximately 30 mm. Hg and monitored with a manometer.

The administration of antibiotics and cathartics as well as removal of blood from the

---

*This use of vasopressin is not mentioned in the manufacturer's instructions.

stomach can be accomplished through the tube. There are great hazards involved in the use of the tube, especially the danger of massive pulmonary aspiration of vomitus, suffocation by an improperly positioned balloon and damage to the esophageal mucosa. Fatal complications in about 20 per cent of intubated patients have been reported from a medical center experienced in the use of the tube.

Although bleeding from esophageal varices usually can be controlled with these measures, portal shunting may become necessary in many survivors. This operation should be done on an elective basis. Other measures, such as total body hypothermia and sclerosing injections, are extremely difficult and relatively unrewarding. Portal decompression by means of thoracic duct drainage and extracorporeal portosaphenous anastomosis via the umbilical vein are still in the experimental stage, but appear promising.

Ascites. A combination of hypoalbuminemia, hyperaldosteronism and renal failure associated with impairment of liver function may result in retention of sodium and total body water, whereas portal hypertension appears to be mainly responsible for the localization of the excess fluid in the abdomen. Despite better understanding of mechanisms involved in the production of ascites, it is not known whether this condition represents a physiologic adjustment or a pathologic state. Therefore the mildest therapeutic measures are employed in order to limit dangerous accumulations of fluid. Therapeutic paracenteses should be avoided unless acute dyspnea develops. Approximately 50 ml. of fluid may be withdrawn for diagnostic purposes, especially to rule out peritonitis.

Sudden ascites can be precipitated during the course of chronic liver illness by intercurrent infections, hemorrhage or surgery. Obviously, these stresses are best avoided, and infections should be treated rapidly. Acute ascites is often reversed by limiting daily dietary sodium to between 300 and 500 mg. It is important that growing children on such a diet receive an adequate caloric and protein intake.

"Chronic" ascites, which is a reflection of progressive liver decompensation and portal hypertension, gradually results in discomfort, dyspnea and severe limitation of physical activity. In addition to the dietary management outlined, successful diuresis in these patients may be accomplished with combinations of diuretic agents and inhibitors of sodium-potassium exchange. Among the various types of diuretics available are thiazides, organomercurials, furosemide and ethacrynic acid. Agents that block the exchange of sodium for potassium include spironolactone (Aldactone) and triamterene (Dyrenium). The rationale for specific combinations of diuretic agents should be understood, because these drugs differ in their site of action in the renal tubule, in their response to factors that condition the diuretic effect and in their ability to produce hypokalemia.

We prefer thiazides to mercurials, because the latter are nephrotoxic, probably because of intracellular deposits of inorganic mercury. Furthermore, they are ineffective in the presence of hypokalemic alkalosis, which they eventually produce (intermittent acidification with acetazolamide is required to reverse this effect), and they are unavailable in oral preparation. Mercurial diuretics, however, do not cause the rapid loss of potassium associated with thiazides, furosemide and ethacrynic acid.

Treatment is initiated in the hospital. A dietitian prescribes salt-depleted proteins and starches, which augment caloric intake and make the diet more palatable, and vitamin supplements. In children with advanced cirrhosis, protein intake is limited to 1 gm./kg./day because of the danger of hepatic coma. The most useful diuretic combination is probably hydrochlorothiazide, 2 mg./kg./day in two doses, combined with spironolactone, 3 mg./kg./day. Dosages may be decreased or increased according to the diuretic response. A mean 24-hour weight loss of up to 1 pound is considered satisfactory.

Serum and urinary sodium and potassium levels should be determined daily, especially during the initial stages of therapy. Spironolactone reduces the need for potassium supplements. However, as much as 90 mEq. of potassium chloride may have to be added daily for the maintenance of blood potassium levels. Enteric-coated potassium chloride tablets should be avoided because of the danger of ulcerative obstructive lesions of the small bowel. If hypokalemia persists despite these measures, triamterene can be substituted or used with spironolactone, because the effect of these agents on potassium retention is additive.

Several weeks in the hospital are often required for relief of ascites and elaboration of a suitable maintenance regimen. Ascites can then be controlled at home with a low-sodium diet and intermittent diuretic therapy when weight gain becomes excessive. Children with chronic active hepatitis often require steroid therapy and potassium supplementation during exacerbations of the underlying pathologic process.

Most patients with ascites can be returned

to normal water and electrolyte balance. An occasional case of hepatic decompensation may be complicated by relative hyponatremia due to expansion of the vascular space by retained water, or by hypokalemia that is difficult to correct with potassium supplements. Renal failure may intervene spontaneously or as a result of intestinal hemorrhage. Diuretic therapy is contraindicated in such cases. Protein intake is reduced to counteract the rising level of blood urea nitrogen, fluid intake is restricted because of oliguria and water retention, and potassium intake is limited in the presence of hyperkalemia. Steroid therapy and mannitol injections may occasionally improve urinary output. The prognosis is extremely grave, and coma frequently intervenes.

Coma. Coma can be precipitated in a cirrhotic patient by infection, fluid imbalance, diuretic therapy, surgery or hemorrhage. Appropriate respective measures include antibiotics, correction of overhydration or underhydration, removal of diuretics and, obviously, avoidance of surgery and prevention of hemorrhage.

When the deleterious effects of ammonia were finally recognized, the management of hepatic encophalopathy shifted from the use of high-protein diets to avoidance of excessive protein intake. Nevertheless, the exact role of ammonia in inducing hepatic coma is still controversial, and controlled clinical trials involving factors such as dietary protein, antibiotic therapy and the possible toxicity of diuretics have not been published. Available results of single controlled studies suggest that arginine and sodium glutamate are not useful, nor is volume expansion during diuretic therapy effective in the prevention of renal failure and coma.

A therapeutic dilemma arises because protein restriction may spare the brain but further endanger the liver. Current therapy of hepatic coma is based on efforts to diminish production of ammonia by eliminating protein intake during the comatose period, cleansing enemas, and use of poorly absorbed antibiotics, such as neomycin, kanamycin or paromomycin, to control intestinal ammonia-producing bacteria. A daily oral dose of 2 to 4 gm. of neomycin is given during the acute period; smaller doses may be required for maintenance. Because neomycin is slightly absorbed, patients with renal failure may be exposed to the nephrotoxic effects of this drug unless carefully followed. Alternately, lactulose can be administered by nasogastric tube to reduce ammonia formation by bacteria (1 to 2 tablespoons 3 times daily). Other measures include control of renal ammonia by maintenance of normal potassium levels and avoidance of diuretics.

The usefulness of special amino acid mixtures intended to reverse amino acid abnormalities in plasma of patients with liver failure is currently under investigation.

Fluid replacement is provided with intravenous preparations of 10 per cent dextrose at maintenance rates of 1000 to 1500 ml./m²/24 hrs. Serum sodium and potassium levels are used as guides for electrolyte replacement. Sodium must be added with great caution because of reduced renal clearance, but potassium is often necessary in large amounts to prevent alkalosis and rapid production of ammonia.

Pulmonary infection, which may greatly complicate treatment of the comatose patient, should be prevented with a prophylactic antibiotic such as ampicillin.

Patients with uncomplicated chronic liver disease usually recover when treated in this manner, but those with progressive liver disease, renal failure or encephalopathy that develops after a shunt anastomosis usually do not recover.

Patients who recover from coma are placed on limited amounts of protein, beginning with 0.5 gm./kg., increasing gradually to 1.5 gm./kg., while the remainder of the caloric intake (100 calories/kg./day) is provided by carbohydrates. Vitamins are added to the regimen.

Removal of ammonia by hemodialysis and peritoneal dialysis has not been therapeutically effective. Cross-circulation with human volunteers or perfusion through isolated animal liver has been more successful. The best results in hepatic coma with fulminant hepatitis have been achieved with exchange blood transfusions. Whether this method can be applied to patients with cirrhosis complicated by encephalopathy remains to be determined.

TUMORS OF THE LIVER

Primary Tumors. *Benign tumors* originating in the liver include nodular hyperplasia of the liver, hepatocellular adenoma, mesenchymal hamartoma, cavernous hemangioma, and infantile hemangioendothelioma.

Nodular hyperplasia usually presents as an asymptomatic upper abdominal mass. Treatment may not be required in such cases. Portal hypertension may develop in others. When a simple nodule is found at laparotomy, excision of the tumor or involved lobe is indicated, and is usually followed by complete resolution of the hypertension. Multiple nodules cannot be removed.

Hepatocellular adenoma is extremely rare in childhood. This benign tumor may present as a silent mass producing pressure symptoms, as as an acute abdomen due to rupture or infarction of the tumor. Surgical removal is life-saving in the presence of these complications. In uncomplicated cases, the prognosis is excellent without treatment. Mesenchymal hamartoma may enlarge gradually or rapidly. Hamartomas are usually composed of solid and cystic elements which may be visualized by ultrasonic echography. Results of surgical excision are generally excellent.

Cavernous hemangiomas and hemangioendotheliomas are among the most common primary liver tumors of childhood. Approximately half are asymptomatic, whereas others may present with hepatomegaly, congestive heart failure or jaundice. Although these tumors are reportedly capable of spontaneous regression, this is a rare event in our experience. A solitary tumor can be excised with satisfactory results. However, most hemangioendotheliomas occur as multiple lesions and must be treated with a variety of generally unsatisfactory approaches. Radiation in repeated small doses (500 rads), corticotherapy (prednisone, 2 mg./kg. for several weeks) or ligation of the hepatic artery have been reported as successful in isolated cases.

Prognosis is largely dependent on control of associated congestive heart failure or hemorrhage due to thrombocytopenia.

Primary *malignant tumors* of the liver include hepatoblastoma, hepatocellular carcinoma, embryonal rhabdomyosacroma and undifferentiated sarcoma.

Hepatoblastoma usually becomes apparent in children under 2 years of age as a painless mass. Serum alpha-fetoprotein levels are often elevated and return to normal after successful surgical removal of the tumor. These lesions occur as a single mass in the majority of patients, and show preference for the right lobe. Early surgical excision of the affected lobe is essential for survival. While the prognosis must remain guarded for years in individual patients, numerous long-term survivals have been published.

Hepatocellular carcinoma is generally discovered after 3 years of age, and is mainly found in males. Chronic liver disease of metabolic or unknown origin (such as alpha-l-antitrypsin deficiency, glycogen storage disease, galactosemia, tyrosinemia, neonatal hepatitis) appears to predispose to the development of hepatocellular carcinoma, as does long-term therapy with anabolic androgen steroid hormones for aplastic anemia or Fanconi's anemia. Prognosis is uniformly poor, the only chance for long-term survival being early extensive surgical extirpation. Chemotherapy and liver transplantation may offer temporary relief, but the tumor usually recurs despite treatment with vincristine, cytoxan or 5-fluorouracil, even in patients receiving successful liver transplants.

Embryonal rhabdomyosarcoma is usually diagnosed under 5 years of age in a child with weight loss and progressive jaundice, a right upper quadrant mass, and epigastric pain. This tumor involves the extrahepatic bile ducts and may spread along the intrahepatic ducts. Prognosis is hopeless.

Undifferentiated sarcoma presents as a rapidly growing mass often associated with pain or fever and vomiting. The tumor is usually located in the right lobe. Lobectomy is the treatment of choice, supplemented by chemotherapy and radiotherapy. Prognosis is extremely guarded.

Metastatic lesions involving the liver include Wilson's tumor, neuroblastoma and gonadal tumors. Chemotherapy and radiation are applied to these tumors, as described in chapters dealing with these malignancies.

Portal Hypertension

SHEILA SHERLOCK, M.D.

Portal hypertension is nearly always due to obstruction to blood flow in the portal venous system. It can be divided into two main categories; presinusoidal, and sinusoidal or postsinusoidal. In the presinusoidal type of portal hypertension, the obstruction is in the main portal vein or in the portal vein radicles in the portal tracts. In the sinusoidal or postsinusoidal form of disease, the obstruction is at the level of the sinusoids, the central hepatic vein or in the main hepatic vein. This is the more prominent form in the cirrhoses. It is important to make the distinction. In the presinusoidal type of portal hypertension, hepatocellular function is intact, whereas in the second form, it is defective and liver cell failure is liable to be precipitated by hemorrhage.

In childhood the presinusoidal (extrahepatic) portal vein occlusion is more frequent. In the neonatal period, obstruction of the portal vein is usually secondary to umbilical sepsis. The infection spreads along the umbilical vein to the left branch of the portal vein and hence to the main portal vein. The portal vein may be obstructed by an abscess at the hilus of the liver following other neonatal infections. It may also follow an exchange transfusion through the umbilical vein.

In later childhood, infection is equally important, and conditions causing liver abscess, such as osteomyelitis and pylephlebitis following an appendix abscess or even a clinically missed appendicitis, must be included. Congenital anomalies of the portal venous system are exceedingly rare.

Congenital hepatic fibrosis is a rare form of intrahepatic presinusoidal portal hypertension. It is due to deficiency of terminal branches of the portal vein in the densely fibrotic portal zones of the liver. It is readily confused with cirrhosis.

Cirrhosis can be due to previous neonatal hepatitis, viral hepatitis, Wilson's disease, galactosemia, tyrosinosis or other metabolic liver disease or chronic active ("lupoid") hepatitis, and in many instances it is cryptogenetic. Postsinusoidal portal hypertension can follow toxic involvement of the central hepatic veins due to Senecio (Ragwort). Rarer causes of postsinusoidal portal hypertension in childhood include congenital valves and webs in the hepatic veins and vena cava and constrictive pericarditis.

Diagnosis and Investigation.   Treatment depends upon accurate localization of the site of obstruction and, if possible, knowledge of the cause.

Delay in diagnosis is usually due to failure to perform liver biopsy and splenic venography. In children these may be done under general anesthesia on the same occasion. The intrasplenic pressure is estimated at the same time, and this is used as a baseline for further serial determinations. It is also useful to confirm that portal hypertension is present. The splenic pressure may be normal if the portal-systemic collateral circulation is sufficiently great. If the spleen has already been removed, selective celiac or mesenteric angiography via the femoral artery may be done. The portal circulation is followed by exposing serial films, and the portal vein and portal-systemic collaterals are visualized in the venous phase of the angiogram.

There may be doubt whether to perform these special and rather complicated investigations in an apparently otherwise well child who has splenomegaly. They are virtually without risk and should be undertaken without delay once portal hypertension is diagnosed, even before hemorrhage has taken place. Knowledge of the anatomy of the portal system and the cause of the portal hypertension allows management to be rational and enables any surgical procedure to be tailored to the actual state of the portal system.

Management Before and Between Hemorrhages.   Apart from any treatment necessary for underlying cirrhosis, the child should be allowed to lead as normal a life as possible. He should attend ordinary school, and provided the spleen is not too large, games and physical education may be allowed. Particularly vigorous sports, such as football, must be forbidden. The child should not be allowed to become overly tired. The school principal should be informed of the situation, and the parents should not press the child to be overly competitive in either work or play.

Note should be taken of fecal color and the parents told to report if it becomes black. Hemoglobin estimations should be done if the child appears anemic or passes black stools. Oral iron treatment is given as required. The cirrhotic child requires occasional estimations of the prothrombin time, and intramuscular vitamin K_1 (5 mg.) may be useful from time to time.

Hemorrhage commonly follows an upper respiratory tract infection, and these should be avoided if possible and all necessary inoculations given. If infection develops, it should be taken seriously and broad-spectrum antibiotics given from the start. Drugs containing acetylsalicylic acid must be avoided.

Undue attention should not be paid to the platelet and leukocyte counts. Although both may be low, the effects on the patient are not definite. Multiple infections are unusual. Low values should not indicate splenectomy.

Management of Hemorrhage.   If the diagnosis is in doubt endoscopy should be done using a pediatric endoscope. If the technique has not been performed previously, an emergency percutaneous splenic venogram is performed.

If the patient is cirrhotic, hepatic precoma and coma may be precipitated by the hemorrhage. This should be anticipated by giving no protein by mouth, keeping the bowels moving freely, giving an enema if necessary and prescribing oral neomycin, 15 mg./kg. four times a day for 3 days. All types of sedation should be avoided. If the child has extrahepatic portal venous obstruction and normal hepatic function, there is virtually no danger of the development of hepatic precoma. The precoma regimen is therefore unnecessary, and sedation can be given as required. It is unusual for these patients to bleed before the age of 3 years.

Blood transfusion is usually necessary. In patients with extrahepatic portal obstruction, hemorrhages are likely to be multiple over years. The greatest possible care must be taken to preserve peripheral veins for further transfusions and to give absolutely compatible blood.

If liver cell function is adequate, the bleeding usually ceases spontaneously. If liver cell function is deficient and if the bleeding continues, I prefer to use vasopressin (Pitressin) intravenously, although this route is not recommended by the manufacturer. This drug lowers portal venous pressure by constriction of the splanchnic arterial bed, causing an increase in resistance to the inflow of blood to the gut. It controls hemorrhage from esophageal varices by lowering portal venous pressure. A large dose, 1 unit per 3 kg. of body weight, is given well diluted in 5 per cent dextrose intravenously in 10 minutes. Mean arterial pressure increases transiently, and portal pressure decreases for three-quarters to one hour. The stomach is aspirated every 30 minutes through a gastric tube, and control of hemorrhage is shown by the disappearance of blood from the aspirate and by serial pulse and blood pressure readings. Abdominal colicky discomfort and evacuation of the bowels, together with facial pallor, are usual during the infusion. If these are absent, it may be questioned whether the vasopressin is pharmacologically active. Inert material is the most common cause of failure. Regular vasopressin injections may be repeated in 4 hours if bleeding recurs, but efficacy decreases with continual use. The ultimate failure of vasopressin to control terminal hemorrhage reflects hepatocellular failure rather than improper method of treatment.

The value of vasopressin is its simplicity of use. In an emergency it can even be used in the home. Special nursing and medical care are not essential. The short duration is obviously unsatisfactory, and the side effects are unpleasant even if short-lived. However, this dosage is necessary to achieve an adequate reduction in portal pressure.

If vasopressin fails to produce the desired effect, the Sengstaken trilumen esophageal compression tube is used. A special small-sized tube is available for pediatric use. A rubber tube is inflated in the esophagus at a pressure of 20 to 30 mm. Hg, slightly greater than that expected in the portal vein. Another balloon is inflated in the fundus of the stomach. The third lumen communicates with the stomach. The tube is passed relatively easily if the pharynx is well anesthetized. When the tube is in position, traction has to be exerted and this causes difficulty. Too little traction means that the gastric balloon falls back into the stomach. Too much traction causes discomfort, with retching, and potentiates gastroesophageal ulceration.

The compression tubes are very successful in controlling bleeding from esophageal varices. They do, however, have many complications. They should not be left inflated longer than 24 hours. Their use should be part of a plan of management culminating either in surgery or in withdrawal of the tube and conservative treatment if the patient's condition is too poor. Complications include obstruction of the pharynx with consequent asphyxia, aspiration pneumonia and ulceration of pharynx, esophagus and fundus of the stomach. The tube is not well tolerated by the patient. Skilled nursing is required for supervision of the patient while the tube is in position.

Emergency surgery is rarely necessary. If bleeding does not cease or if it recurs and active intervention becomes essential, the best surgical method is probably transhepatic sclerosis of the portal and splenic vein tributaries feeding the varices. In patients having normal liver function, and in whom the splenic venogram or mesenteric angiogram has shown a portal or superior mesenteric vein of adequate caliber, a portacaval or mesocaval shunt may be performed. Emergency shunt surgery has a high mortality rate if the patient has cirrhosis, and if possible should be avoided in these circumstances.

Elective Surgery.   Prophylactic surgery is not indicated. The patient must have bled from varices before operation can be considered. The choice of procedure depends largely upon the state of the portal venous system as revealed by splenic venography or selective splanchnic angiography. If the portal vein is patent and of adequate caliber, end-to-side portacaval anastomosis is the most satisfactory procedure. In experienced hands this operation carries a low mortality rate of less than 5 per cent. Because of vein size, the operation can rarely be undertaken before the age of 10 years. It carries a small risk of shunt encephalopathy. In children this is particularly small, and in the presence of a normal liver, e.g., obstruction to the portal vein at the hilus of the liver, the chances are almost nonexistent. In the presence of cirrhosis, the possibility varies with the degree of underlying damage to the liver. The operation should not be performed in the presence of jaundice, ascites or a past history of hepatic coma.

Splenorenal anastomosis may be considered in portal venous occlusion if the splenic vein is of adequate size. It is less efficient than a portacaval anastomosis, because the shunt is small and often occludes. The danger of postshunt encephalopathy, however, is very small.

Superior mesenteric vein–inferior vena caval shunt is used to treat portal hypertension in patients who have occlusion of the portal and splenic veins, making neither available for anastomosis. The vena cava is transected just proximal to the junction of the two iliac veins, and the distal segment is ligated. The proximal segment is then anastomosed to the side of the intact superior mesenteric vein. Sometimes an intervening Dacron graft is used and the superior mesenteric vein and inferior vena cava so anastomosed side to side. Failures may be due to superior mesenteric vein thrombosis, and the mortality rate is about 10 per cent. This operation, provided it is done by an experienced surgeon, provides a better chance of improvement in patients with extrahepatic portal venous obstruction than do the various local attacks on esophageal or other varices.

Direct attacks on the varices and on various dangerous collaterals are numerous and rarely of long-lasting benefit. They include splenectomy, transection of the esophagus, partial and total gastrectomy and partial esophagectomy. In general, they are not to be recommended. Patients with extrahepatic portal venous obstruction rarely die of exsanguinating hemorrhage. Conservative management usually helps them over the acute episode. Bleeding becomes more infrequent as time allows for the opening of collateral vessels to the renal and lumbar veins. Ultimately, portal pressure may decrease. This possibility may be lessened with repeated operations and removal or transection of such benign collaterals. The operative and postoperative mortality rate of the local operations on varices in a cirrhotic patient with borderline liver function is high, and the ultimate benefit doubtful.

Chronic Active Hepatitis

SHEILA SHERLOCK, M.D.

Active chronic hepatitis is diagnosed by the continuation for longer than 6 months of fluctuant hepatocellular jaundice with transaminases increased more than five times normal and gamma globulin levels usually elevated to more than twice normal. Hepatic histology, obtained by needle biopsy, shows cellular, largely mononuclear, infiltration with active septa passing inwards from the portal zone isolating groups of live cells which show piecemeal necrosis.

The condition is not one of single causation. In infants and children it may be associated with persistence of hepatitis B antigenemia, autoimmune features (high titer of smooth muscle antibody), other virus infections such as cytomegalovirus and rubella, and

Wilson's disease. Alpha-l-antitrypsin deficiency must also be considered, but usually produces a more cholestatic picture. Before treatment is commenced, therefore, it is important to assess the serum biochemical changes and hepatic histology by needle biopsy. More detailed investigations include hepatitis B antigen, smooth muscle antibody, antibody levels against cytomegalovirus and rubella and serum ceruloplasmin levels together with urinary copper excretion before and after penicillamine. The eyes must be examined with a slit lamp for Kayser-Fleischer rings in an attempt to exclude Wilson's disease. If necessary, the copper content of the liver biopsy may be measured. Serum alpha-l-antitrypsin values are noted.

If specific causes, such as Wilson's disease, can be excluded, then immunosuppressive therapy, usually with prednisolone, must be considered. The indications for such treatment are not clear-cut, but if the serum transaminase levels are increased five times and gamma globulin levels are more than twice elevated, steroid therapy should be given. Liver biopsy findings of piecemeal necrosis with inflammation and bridging necrosis between portal zones and central areas are also indications. The initial dose is 0.4 mg./kg. of prednisolone for 2 weeks. This is then reduced to a maintenance dose of 0.2 mg./kg.

Twenty per cent fail to respond, deteriorate, develop hepatocellular failure and die. In such patients a trial of higher doses of prednisolone (0.8 mg./kg.) is worth considering. Prednisolone usually must be used for at least 6 months. Attempts are made to withdraw therapy when serum bilirubin, transaminase and, if possible, gamma globulin levels are normal. Relapses follow discontinuation of treatment in about a half, usually within 6 months of stopping, and necessitate reinstitution of the drug.

Retardation of growth may be a problem in those less than 10 years old and in these children alternate day therapy with prednisolone 0.4 mg./kg. every other day must be considered. This may minimize the effects of corticosteroids on growth. Alternatively, if complications such as facial mooning, obesity, growth retardation or diabetes are a problem, then prednisolone (0.15 mg./kg.) may be combined with azathioprine (1 mg./kg.). Azathioprine alone gives less satisfactory results than when prednisolone is used.* Corticosteroid therapy is of particular value in preventing

---

*This use of azathioprine is not mentioned in the manufacturer's directions.

deaths during the first 2 years after diagnosis, when the disease is most active. Most patients, however, end with cirrhosis, a lesion which is irreversible. There are, however, plenty of examples where the disease has become inactive and the patients have survived 10 to 20 years.

Biliary Atresia

DAVID P. CAMPBELL, M.D.

The diagnostic evaluation of the persistently jaundiced infant should proceed with utmost haste, for surgical intervention before two months of age is indicated if the diagnosis of biliary atresia cannot be excluded. The old adage that exploration, operative cholangiogram and liver biopsy in the persistently jaundiced infant do more harm than good is no longer valid, for the risk of such a procedure is now considered minimal. More important, surgery now holds some hope for the infant with biliary atresia. The pediatrician's primary role in the persistently jaundiced neonate is, therefore, to rapidly rule out nonsurgical causes of jaundice, i.e., neonatal hepatitis, toxoplasmosis and CID. When biliary atresia cannot be ruled out with certainty, surgical referral is indicated. No extensive preoperative preparation is necessary prior to referral. One need only ascertain that the infant's prothrombin time is within normal limits. If the prothrombin time is prolonged, 5 mg. of vitamin K (AquaMephyton) should be administered intramuscularly and the value rechecked in 48 hours.

Operation in the infant with proven or suspected biliary atresia should start with an operative cholangiogram and liver biopsy through a small incision. If the diagnosis of biliary atresia is made, one should proceed with hepatic portoenterostomy under the same anesthetic. Although there is disagreement as to its value, Japanese and several American surgeons are reporting cure rates of 40 to 50 per cent with hepatic portoenterostomy. Before its development the cure rate for infants with biliary atresia was virtually nil. The operation of hepatic portoenterostomy is based upon evidence that biliary atresia is not a congenital abnormality but rather the result of a sclerosing inflammatory process of the biliary tree. Although distal extrahepatic bile ducts may be closed by this process early in its course, microscopic proximal extrahepatic and/or intrahepatic ducts may remain open in the area of the porta hepatitis. Hepatic portoenteros-

tomy attempts to connect such patent but often microscopic bile ductules with a loop of small bowel before they are also irreversibly sclerosed shut. Irreversible occlusion of these ducts usually develops by three months of age. The need to proceed with surgery before two months of age is therefore obvious.

Infants in whom a successful biliary-enteric anastomosis is constructed by hepatic portoenterostomy are at continued high risk for developing ascending cholangitis. Such cholangitis, if recurrent and uncontrolled, can cause postoperative occlusion of the intrahepatic ductules. Episodes of unexplained fever or fever plus an increase in serum bilirubin must therefore be assumed to be ascending cholangitis and treated accordingly. This requires hospitalization and high doses of parenteral antibiotics which are effective against the gram-negative organisms found in the gut. Ampicillin, 200 mg./kg./day given intravenously in four divided doses, is appropriate therapy.

Approximately 50 per cent of infants with biliary atresia will have no extrahepatic or intrahepatic ducts suitable for hepatic portoenterostomy even if operated on before two months of age. The prognosis is hopeless in such infants. Their postoperative care is actually the treatment of cirrhosis and portal hypertension, both of which are well covered in other sections. Infants with incorrectable biliary atresia and infants who have undergone unsuccessful hepatic portoenterostomy usually have a prolonged and miserable existence. Their parents need continued support from all concerned with the infant's care. Much can be done to improve the terminal course of such infants. Their lack of bile excretion into the gastrointestinal tract greatly compromises digestion, especially the digestion of fats. They best tolerate pre-digested formulas in which fats are in the form of medium chain triglycerides (e.g., Pregestimil). They should be placed on the water soluble forms of the fat soluble vitamins A, D, E and K: Aquasol A (vitamin A), Drisdol (vitamin D), Aquasol E (vitamin E), and Synkayvite (vitamin K). Despite regular oral administration of such vitamins, these infants will often require additional doses of parenteral vitamin K (5 mg. AquaMephyton intramuscularly) to maintain their prothrombin time within normal limits.

The final course of infants with incorrectable biliary atresia is one of gastrointestinal bleeding and sepsis. Because of the persistent danger of upper gastrointestinal bleeding, we caution parents against the use of aspirin or aspirin-containing compounds.

Choledochal Cyst

DAVID P. CAMPBELL, M.D.

Choledochal cyst is a rare aneurysmal dilatation of the common bile duct which causes obstruction to the flow of bile into the duodenum. The etiology is unknown. Choledochal cyst is much more common in the Orient than in the western hemisphere.

The infant or child with a choledochal cyst presents with intermittent abdominal pain, an abdominal mass and jaundice. Adequate treatment of choledochal cyst requires surgical intervention, for nonsurgical attempts at therapy carry a mortality approximating 100 per cent. The primary responsibility of the pediatrician therefore is to make or suspect the diagnosis and refer the patient for surgical exploration. The surgical treatment of choledochal cyst consists of constructing an unfettered pathway for bile to flow from the liver to the duodenum. This can be accomplished by constructing an anastomosis between the cyst and the small bowel or excising the cyst and performing an anastomosis between the common bile duct proximal to the cyst and a loop of small bowel. Postoperative morbidity and mortality after surgical correction of choledochal cyst are due primarily to ascending cholangitis, a common problem after biliary-enteric anastomoses. Children who have undergone surgery for choledochal cyst must therefore be watched closely for signs and symptoms suggesting ascending cholangitis. They should be treated with parenteral antibiotics whenever an episode of ascending cholangitis is suspected. The antibiotic used must be effective against the gram-negative organisms found in the small bowel and biliary tract. Ampicillin, 200 mg./kg./day, administered intravenously every six hours is recommended.

Diseases of the Gallbladder

DAVID P. CAMPBELL, M.D.

Cholelithiasis. Cholelithiasis and the often associated acute and chronic cholecystitis are rare entities in the pediatric age group. One should suspect a hemolytic disorder as the etiology. The diagnosis of cholelithiasis is made by oral cholecystogram. Intravenous cholangiography is only indicated in the child with an acute abdomen in whom cholecystitis is suspected. Children shown to have gallstones on cholecystogram should be referred to a surgeon for cholecystectomy, for the dissolution

of gallstones with drugs such as chenodeoxycholic acid is still in the experimental stage. No specific preparation is necessary prior to referral. The patient is instructed to follow a low fat diet prior to surgery because fats or fatty foods may trigger an attack of acute cholecystitis.

The morbidity and mortality of cholecystectomy in an otherwise healthy child are practically nil. Nonsurgical management of the child with gallstones will lead to recurrent episodes of cholecystitis and the possibility of being forced to operate on an emergency basis. Morbidity and mortality are markedly increased in such nonelective surgery.

Treatment of the child with acute cholecystitis consists of: (1) placing the bowel at rest by eliminating oral intake and providing intravenous fluids and nasogastric suction; (2) antibiotics—ampicillin, 100 mg./kg./day intravenously in four divided doses; and (3) analgesics—meperidine (Demerol), 2 mg./kg./ every 4 hours as needed. Cholecystectomy should be carried out as soon as the definitive diagnosis is made.

Diseases of the Pancreas

DAVID P. CAMPBELL, M.D.

Pancreatitis. Acute pancreatitis is a rare cause of abdominal pain in the pediatric age group. The diagnosis is confirmed by elevated serum or urine amylase levels. One should rule out mumps, steroids, and trauma as causes of the pancreatitis. The treatment of acute pancreatitis (except when secondary to trauma) is nonoperative. Therapeutic efforts are aimed at placing the exocrine pancreas at rest, replacing third space fluid losses and providing pain relief. The exocrine pancreas is placed at rest by withholding oral intake, aspirating the stomach with a large bore nasogastric tube, and administering anticholinergics at regular intervals (atropine, 0.2 mg. to 0.4 mg. intramuscularly every four to six hours). These measures eliminate gastric distention and diminish the flow of foodstuffs and gastric acid into the duodenum, all of which stimulate pancreatic secretion. Adynamic ileus, always present with acute pancreatitis, is also treated by the above measures.

Acute pancreatitis is accompanied by large losses of fluids, colloids, and electrolytes into the retroperitoneal space, bowel wall, and bowel lumen. One must therefore be sure to carefully monitor and replace such losses. Calculated losses are best replaced with Ringer's lactate solution and maintenance fluids given as 5 per cent dextrose in 0.2 normal saline + 20 mEq./liter of potassium chloride. Daily infusions of albumin or plasma may also be necessary to maintain an adequate intravascular volume. Blood transfusions should be administered to keep the hematocrit above 30 per cent. Serum calcium levels must be followed closely and small doses of calcium gluconate, 5 to 10 mEq., administered by the intravenous route if the calcium level drops below normal levels. Meperidine (Demerol), 2 mg./kg. intramuscularly every four hours as needed, or 1 mg./kg. intravenously every two hours as needed, should be used for pain relief. Morphine is contraindicated for pain relief in pancreatitis for it is known to cause spasm of the sphincter of Odi. The use of antibiotics in acute pancreatitis is controversial. Their use is probably only indicated in fulminating cases of hemorrhagic pancreatitis where there is significant pancreatic necrosis and a high probability of abscess formation. The medical therapy of acute pancreatitis should continue until the patient is relieved of abdominal pain and tenderness and serum amylase levels are well on their way toward normal.

Traumatic Pancreatitis. Pancreatitis secondary to trauma is a surgical problem. In the pediatric age group the etiology may be a penetrating wound but is more commonly a blunt abdominal injury. The immobile nature of the pancreas accounts for its vulnerability to blunt trauma. It is firmly fixed in the retroperitoneal space anterior to the vertebral column over which it can be easily fractured. Continued abdominal pain, tenderness, fever, and ileus after blunt abdominal trauma should arouse suspicion that there is a pancreatic injury. The diagnosis can usually be confirmed with a serum or urine amylase determination. Acute pancreatitis secondary to trauma requires referral to a surgeon for definitive care which entails exploration, drainage, and possible resection. Preoperative and postoperative treatment is as outlined above for acute pancreatitis with special emphasis being given to adequate replacement of fluids, colloids, and electrolytes.

Pseudocysts. The child with a pancreatic pseudocyst usually presents with abdominal pain, fever, and ileus two to three weeks after an episode of pancreatitis or abdominal trauma. An upper abdominal mass can often be palpated and the diagnosis is confirmed by the radiographic demonstration of such a mass and an elevated serum amylase.

The treatment of a pancreatic pseudocyst is surgical drainage. Preoperative therapy consists primarily of assuring an adequate intravascular volume. Intravenous fluids and blood transfusions are often necessary. At operation the pseudocyst is preferably drained into the stomach or a loop of small bowel. External drainage, however, is sometimes necessary. The postoperative care of the child undergoing drainage of a pseudocyst entails elimination of oral intake, nasogastric suction and intravenous fluids until bowel function returns. One must be sure to provide for maintenance fluids in addition to replacing third space losses and nasogastric tube losses. Daily weights and strict measurements of intake and output are essential to calculate such losses.

Hypoglycemia. The medical treatment of hypoglycemia is well covered in a previous section. There is an occasional rare infant in whom idiopathic hypoglycemia cannot be controlled by medical measures, and in whom pancreatic resection is indicated. The diagnosis of islet cell hyperfunction (hyperplasia or adenoma) should be confirmed by blood insulin levels before such resectional therapy is considered. Pancreatic resection should be carried out without delay once the need is ascertained, for permanent brain damage may occur with continued episodes of hypoglycemia. The primary role of the pediatrician in the infant or child requiring resectional therapy is to maintain adequate blood sugar levels prior to surgery. Control of hypoglycemia secondary to islet cell hyperplasia requires a subtotal resection of the pancreas, i.e., removal of the entire tail and body of the pancreas. It is a surprisingly simple procedure in the pediatric age group. Intraoperative and postoperative management require continued careful monitoring of blood sugar levels and appropriate correction of hypoglycemia with intravenous glucose solutions. It is not at all uncommon for hypoglycemia to persist for several days after resectional surgery. An occasional child with islet cell hyperplasia does not respond to subtotal pancreatectomy and requires total pancreatectomy.

Surgical exploration in the older child with hypoglycemia must include a careful search for an islet cell adenoma, usually found in the body or tail. However such tumors are rare. Preoperative diagnosis is usually not possible. Islet cell adenomas may be multiple, so a subtotal pancreatectomy is indicated when one is found in the body or tail. An adenoma located in the head of the pancreas is treated by local resection alone.

Cystic Fibrosis

CARL F. DOERSHUK, M.D., *and*
ROBERT C. STERN, M.D.

Successful treatment of cystic fibrosis requires awareness of its protean manifestations. This includes appreciation of the great individual variability in age of onset and severity of involvement in the various organ systems. Although the prognosis is steadily improving (up to 50 per cent cumulative survival rate beyond age 25 years), cystic fibrosis remains an ultimately fatal condition. Since the condition is chronic and many organs are involved, care is complex and requires a team effort to coordinate the services of many medical specialists along with experienced physical and respiratory therapists, nurses, technicians and many others. In view of these considerations, it is advisable that, whenever possible, patients receive most of their care at centers in which the necessary comprehensive approach is feasible.

Pulmonary infection and obstruction result in most of the morbidity and over 90 per cent of the mortality. The exact pathogenesis of the pulmonary lesion remains unclear; however, diagnosis before irreversible pulmonary damage has occurred appears important for improving the prognosis. Almost all patients have some degree of chronic pulmonary obstruction and/or infection including *Staphylococcus aureus* and gram-negative organisms including *Pseudomonas aeruginosa*. Success in therapy depends heavily on a long-term plan of frequent evaluation and control of the pulmonary disease. At the same time it is also necessary to evaluate and appropriately treat the other physical manifestations and, insofar as possible, alleviate or avoid psychologic, social and financial problems. The national network of regional Cystic Fibrosis Centers has proved increasingly effective in providing the base to accomplish this difficult task. Most Center Directors are also available for phone consultations from other physicians.

At our center, all patients are seen at regularly scheduled visits, usually at 4 to 6 week intervals. At each visit the interval history and physical examination are made by an experienced physician and a deep throat swab, after forced cough or a sputum sample, is obtained for culture and susceptibility studies. Emphasis is placed on detecting changes in the cough history, sputum production and pulmonary examination, and in determining whether growth (especially weight gain) has occurred. Irritability and decreased activity and/or appetite can also be early indicators of increasing pulmonary infection. Routine chest roentgenograms are obtained 1 to 2 times yearly and pulmonary function tests 2 to 4 times yearly or more often if indicated.

Hospitalization following initial diagnosis is virtually always necessary to allow proper patient-family education and institution of therapy. This affords the opportunity to repeat the sweat test (pilocarpine iontophoresis with quantitative chloride analysis), obtain gastrointestinal-pancreatic tests, evaluate pulmonary status and educate the family about the disease and the significance of autosomal recessive inheritance, as well as to initiate the treatment measures that will be continued at home. The patient is hospitalized for as long as required to gain optimal control of the pulmonary involvement and achieve steady weight gain. This may take only a week or up to several months. Re-hospitalizations, usually for a minimum of 14 days, are used whenever the pulmonary disease or the patient's general condition does not respond to the outpatient measures. Pulmonary deterioration can be acute but more often reflects slow progression. Intravenous antibiotics are used during each such hospitalization (see Antibiotic Therapy).

As in any chronic condition, prevention of complications and complicating diseases (e.g., rubeola, influenza, pertussis) is important. Routine immunizations are essential including administration of influenza vaccine annually. Most of our patients have fewer acute respiratory illnesses than their normal siblings and influenza has been unusual.

PULMONARY THERAPY

Because the basic defect remains unknown, treatment is empirical and symptomatic. Although some aspects of therapy are controversial, the effect of the overall program including close supervision, continuity of care, aggressive intervention, and an optimistic outlook is more important than minor variations in individual measures. Individual measures should not be judged with the anticipation that each measure will be effective for all patients.

Intermittent Aerosol Therapy. Intermittent aerosol therapy can be used either to deliver medications in small amounts to the lower respiratory tract or to deliver bulk water to the same area. Better delivery and potentially better deposition occur with mouth breathing than with nasal breathing. A relatively brief period of therapy of 10 to 20 minutes is employed, either before or after

Supported in part by grants AM 08305 and HL 13885 from the National Institutes of Health.

segmental postural drainage or both. Intermittent positive pressure breathing is not required for this therapy to be successful and is often contraindicated in cystic fibrosis because of possible aggravation of the obstructive lesion.

INTERMITTENT MEDICATION AEROSOL THERAPY. This form of therapy is used to deliver 2 to 4 ml. amounts of decongestant, bronchodilator, antibiotic, mucolytic, and/or anti-inflammatory agent. Our basic aerosol is 1/8 per cent phenylephrine (Neosynephrine R) in 10 per cent U.S.P. propylene glycol (by volume) for a decongestant effect in almost all patients beyond infancy. This aerosol is used 2 to 4 times daily prior to segmental postural drainage. For bronchodilation, isoproterenol 1:200 strength is added in a dosage of 0.01 ml./kg. to a maximum of 0.5 ml. for those patients who exhibit bronchospasm clinically or by pulmonary function testing. Isoproterenol or isoetharine can be added up to 4 times daily as needed in chronic situations or up to every 2 hours for more acute attacks of bronchospasm.

Mucolytic agents (most commonly N-acetyl-cysteine and on occasion enzymes such as DNA-ase) can also be used for short periods to liquefy unusually tenacious secretions in selected patients. We use 2 to 4 ml. of 10 to 20 per cent N-acetyl-cysteine or 75,000 to 100,000 units of DNA-ase for 10 minutes with or after the decongestant aerosol and before segmental postural drainage, but we usually avoid long-term use because of their potential to act as irritants or allergens.

When infection is difficult to control or when bacteria are resistant to the available oral medications, aerosolized antibiotics can be helpful. These can be added to the basic decongestant aerosol before postural drainage, but if time permits are best given afterwards in 1 to 1.5 ml. of saline. We use colistimethate, gentamicin, or tobramycin in a dosage of 20 mg. per aerosol or carbenicillin in a dose of 1 gm. per aerosol 2 to 4 times a day in home therapy and frequently in the hospital in conjunction with intravenous therapy.* For patients with gastrointestinal intolerance to semi-synthetic penicillins, methicillin in a dosage of 1 gm. per aerosol can be effective. Methicillin by aerosol also can be helpful in controlling or eliminating *Staphylococcus aureus* when used in conjunction with related agents orally.

A small compressor-driven nebulizer, such as the Bennett twin-jet, is usually used for aerosol therapy. The choice of compressor depends on durability and local availability. We use the oil-free DeVilbiss 501 compressor for home therapy, or a 110, 12 and/or 220 volt travel kit (MEFSCO, Cleveland, Ohio) for those desiring more flexibility. Intermittent positive pressure is not required. The aerosol unit should be cleaned daily, rinsed and allowed to air-dry after each use.

Once the patient is over 6 to 7 years of age, inhalation by mouth breathing should be encouraged. Occasional breath holding during inspiration can increase deposition. The patient's position should not restrict diaphragmatic breathing during aerosol administration. As with any form of inhalation therapy, irritation or intolerance must be looked for and the therapy discontinued if either is suspected.

DIRECT INHALATION THERAPY. Inhalation from an ultrasonic nebulizer is used for 10 to 20 minute periods prior to postural drainage to deliver bulk water to the lower respiratory tract. One fourth normal saline is nebulized. Direct inhalation therapy can follow the decongestant aerosol and precede segmental postural drainage.

Antibiotic Therapy. Infection and the resulting injury and permanent damage play a major role in the progression of the pulmonary lesion of cystic fibrosis. The goals of antibiotic therapy are reducing the intensity of infection as completely as possible and minimizing and delaying the progression of pulmonary infection as long as possible.

Usage, duration of therapy and choice of antibiotic are complicated. The infection is usually low grade, it is difficult to differentiate colonization from infection, and the usual guidelines for acute infection, such as acute onset, fever, tachypnea and pleuritis, are usually absent. Increasing cough or sputum production, development of night cough or paroxysms, increasing irritability or inactivity, less than anticipated weight gain or weight loss must be considered along with changes in the chest examination, chest roentgenograms and/or pulmonary function tests.

Patients range from those with minimal or quiescent pulmonary involvement and normal cultures to those with chronic symptoms and signs and a heavy growth of a variety of pathogens. As a result, duration and intensity of antibiotic treatment also vary from an intermittent short course of one antibiotic to continuous treatment with one or more antibiotics for a particular period. Since it is usually difficult to achieve effective drug levels in respiratory tract secretions, especially with oral

---

*This use of colistimethate, gentamicin, carbenicillin, and tobramycin is not mentioned in the manufacturer's indications. The dosage of tobramycin in newborn infants is not well established.

therapy, antibiotic therapy is best used in conjunction with respiratory physical therapy and inhalation therapy measures which facilitate mucus removal (see Intermittent Aerosol Therapy).

In our experience, there is a lower incidence of symptomatic, acute respiratory illness in our patients than in their normal siblings. In addition, the school attendance of the patients is usually better than that of their siblings, except when pulmonary damage has become severe.

OUTPATIENT ANTIBIOTIC THERAPY. Most of our patients are seen at 6 week intervals and most then receive at least 2 weeks of some antibiotic therapy before their next appointment. Even apparently healthy patients frequently produce sputum during cough stimulated by a deep pharyngeal culture swab. Although *Staphylococcus aureus* and/or *Pseudomonas* or other gram-negative organisms are eventually dominant, these patients are also susceptible to common respiratory tract agents such as *Pneumococcus* and *Hemophilus influenzae* or para-influenza. When acute symptoms develop, antibiotic therapy should include appropriate therapy for these organisms. Acute symptoms may also be viral or, frequently, mycoplasmal in origin. For patients with acute symptoms superimposed on significant chronic disease, earlier and more intensive antibiotic treatment is indicated. For those with minimal chronic symptoms and/or chest roentgenogram abnormality, antibiotics might be withheld a few days to see if the presumed viral symptoms clear as anticipated. An increase of symptoms each time antibiotics are stopped is a strong indication that repeat courses of therapy or even continuous therapy are necessary. Alternatively, hospitalization may be indicated.

Prophylactic or low-dosage antibiotic therapy is not recommended because of the propensity for *Staphylococcus* or *Pseudomonas* organisms to develop resistance. We use minimum periods of at least 2 weeks of therapy at relatively high dosage (Table 1) of each agent as determined by the results of a throat or, if obtainable, a sputum culture and antibiotic susceptibility study alone with our evaluation of the other clinical information obtained at each visit. If the clinical response is inadequate, we subsequently change the therapy empirically.

As seen in Table 2, we treat *Staphylococcus aureus*, if recovered on culture, at least 2 weeks out of the next 6 week period. *Staphylococcus* can often be eradicated for significant periods of time. *Pneumococcus* and streptococcal organisms are treated similarly. *Hemophilus* is always treated in symptomatic patients and frequently is treated in quiescent patients who have not had a change in symptoms.

Antibiotic treatment of *Pseudomonas* is a recurring problem for the clinician. We place less emphasis on *Pseudomonas* in asymptomatic

TABLE 1. Oral Antimicrobial Therapy

ANTIMICROBIAL AGENT	ORAL DOSE PER DAY (MG./KG.)
Oxacillin	100–200
Cloxacillin	50–100
Dicloxacillin	30–50
Penicillin	30–50
Ampicillin	100–200
Amoxicillin	50–100
Cephalexin	50–100
Chloramphenicol	50–100
Tetracycline	50–100
Methacycline	10–15
Sulfonamides*	150–200
Novobiocin	30–50
Erythromycin	50–100

*Systemic sulfonamides are contraindicated in infants under 2 months of age.

TABLE 2. Indications for Antibiotic Therapy by Organisms Recovered on Culture*

ORGANISM	INFANT A	INFANT S	OLDER PATIENT A	OLDER PATIENT S	ORAL ANTIBIOTICS
Staphylococcus aureus	+	+	+	+	Methicillin, dicloxacillin, cephalosporins, novobiocin, erythromycin
Pneumococcus, Streptococcus, Group A	+	+	+	+	Penicillin, erythromycin
Hemophilus, untypable/type b	±	+	±	+	Tetracycline, ampicillin, chloramphenicol
Pseudomonas, mucoid or other	±	+	±	+	Ampicillin, tetracycline, erythromycin, chloramphenicol, novobiocin, cephalosporins, sulfisoxazole
Other gram-negative organisms	−	+	±	+	Sulfisoxazole, tetracycline, chloramphenicol, novobiocin, and others according to susceptibility

*A = asymptomatic, S = symptomatic, + = always treated, ± = occasionally treated, and − = usually not treated.

infants who are doing well since gram-negative organisms are frequently encountered in the respiratory tract of even normal subjects up to the age of 2. In symptomatic infants with cystic fibrosis not responding to antistaphylococcal or *Hemophilus* therapy, every effort is made to treat the *Pseudomonas* as well.

Often sulfisoxazole* is the only agent to which the *Pseudomonas* is susceptible in vitro especially in older patients and is used frequently in full dosage. In patients not responding to oral therapy, admission for 2 week periods of intensive intravenous antibiotics, physical and respiratory therapy is advised. Tetracycline is avoided as much as possible in children under 6 to 7 years. Chloramphenicol sodium succinate is frequently an extremely valuable antibiotic for treatment of *Pseudomonas* and is also effective against *Staphylococcus aureus*. We do not hesitate to use this drug for a 2 or 3 week course if less hazardous therapy is not effective.

In older patients with a productive cough, one or more colonial types of *Pseudomonas* including the mucoid form are often the only pathogens encountered. Full dosage antibiotic treatment is usually carried out for at least 2 weeks of each 6 week period. Patients with more advanced disease may require 4 weeks of therapy or even continuous therapy with one or more antibiotics against *Pseudomonas* and whatever other organisms are present to prevent progression of symptoms and further loss of pulmonary function.

INPATIENT ANTIBIOTIC THERAPY. When the response to optimal doses of oral antibiotics is inadequate, the patient is hospitalized for intravenous therapy along with increased inhalation therapy and segmental postural drainage 4 times or more daily. With the use of the "heparin lock" for intravenous therapy, the patient is free between infusions, and most ambulatory activities, including school or work, can be maintained.

A 21 gauge scalp vein needle with a resealing cap or an indwelling intravenous cannula with an attachment to allow intermittent use can be used. The former can be maintained for up to 10 days with rare evidence of irritation or local phlebitis. The intravenous heparin lock system is filled with a solution containing 10 units of heparin per ml. of normal saline between antibiotic infusions.

Patients hospitalized for intensive intravenous therapy often have a significant remission of symptoms and physical findings within 3 to 5 days. Since early relapse is common, we usually continue therapy to a minimum of 14 days of in-hospital therapy for each episode and advise readmission regardless of the period of remission if symptoms increase.

Antibiotics for intravenous use are determined from the results of sputum culture and susceptibility studies. We usually try to use two agents against *Pseudomonas*, such as carbenicillin, 300 to 500 mg./kg./24 hours administered every 4 hours, in conjunction with gentamicin, colistimethate, or tobramycin in an initial dosage of 7 mg./kg./24 hours administered every 8 hours to a maximum daily dose of 210 mg. Pharmacokinetic studies for gentamicin-tobramycin have indicated a relatively short half-life in many patients with cystic fibrosis and the total daily dose can then be increased while decreasing the interval between infusions. Toxicity is minimized if blood levels are monitored and peak levels are kept below 9 to 10 mg./liter.

In the hospital, an antistaphylococcal antibiotic is often added intravenously even if this organism was not present on the most recent culture, especially in patients with hemoptysis or those not responding as anticipated. Therapy should be guided by culture results. Response should be monitored clinically and changes made empirically if necessary. Toxic reactions to systemic antibiotics occur frequently and may necessitate a change.

The agents and dosages for systemic antimicrobial therapy are shown in Table 1. Antibiotics directed against *Pseudomonas* are frequently administered by aerosol as well.

Although some patients can learn self-administration (intramuscular or intravenous) of parenteral antibiotics at home, there are many drawbacks—the increased likelihood of missed doses, local reactions to repeated intramuscular injections, inadequate monitoring of blood chemistries, difficulty in insertion and maintenance of intravenous infusion and, in general, the inability to maximize therapy by use of combination parenteral drug therapy. We have limited home use of parenteral antibiotics to special circumstances.

Respiratory Physical Therapy. Respiratory physical therapy is probably most effective when employed along with inhalation and antibiotic therapy. Segmental postural drainage involves the use of 12 positions with clapping for 1 to 2 minute periods followed by vibrating during 5 exhalations.[2] With older patients who can cooperate, the exhalations are extended using pursed lips breathing to permit

---

*Manufacturer's precaution: Use of sulfisoxazole is contraindicated in infants less than 2 months of age (except in treatment of toxoplasmosis).

better emptying of the lungs. We instruct each family and/or each older patient in the use of all 12 positions at diagnosis even if there are no objective pulmonary findings. The use of each position is recommended at least once daily.

Segmental postural drainage is generally felt to facilitate the removal of secretions although there are, as yet, little data. Even older patients may require at least some assistance by another person to effectively drain all the segments. Patients with substantial bronchiectasis often find they need 3 to 4 sessions daily; other patients may remain stable with only 1 or 2. In school age children, it is frequently difficult to get in more than 1 or 2 sessions daily. We recommend that each segment be drained at least once daily in 1 or preferably 2 sessions (morning and evening are best). Localized mucus plugging may occur even in patients with little or no clinical evidence of active pulmonary infection. We recommend a minimum of 1 aerosol per day followed by 20 to 30 minutes of respiratory physical therapy so that all segments are treated regularly. Relatively asymptomatic patients require additional therapy during acute respiratory illnesses or with flare-ups of their pulmonary infection.

Infants and children can be treated most effectively on the therapist's lap. Use of a tilt board, pillows or folding therapy table* can facilitate this treatment for older patients. Clothing should be loose, and patient and therapist should be comfortable. If properly done, even vigorous clapping with cupped hands should not be uncomfortable. Coughing is encouraged after therapy to each segment and, if the cough is productive, the clapping and vibrating are repeated. This repetition is also recommended if any given segment is severely affected.

Many patients feel that mechanical percussors and vibrators are less effective than manual therapy. However, for patients living away from home or for adolescents seeking more independence, the use of a manual percussor† which can simulate clapping and vibration, can be effective in patients old enough (usually over 14 years of age) and strong enough to hold it. A vibrator with vertical oscillation such as the Oster (Sr. and Jr. model) can also be used. We have not used these units or a large floor-model vibrator in the hospital be-

cause we believe the manual therapy to be more effective.

Respiratory physical therapy may contribute to or prolong episodes of hemoptysis and therefore may have to be modified (see Hemoptysis).

Breathing exercises aimed at improving lung mechanics have not been emphasized since they are time-consuming and we have seen little evidence of their continued use at home. Physical activity and forced deep breathing, which frequently result in significant expectoration of mucus, should be encouraged along with a regular program of exercise to maintain muscle mass and general well being. The activities most helpful for mucous clearance remain undefined; however, swimming and jumping rope are usually available and appear effective.

Mist Tent Therapy. The conflicting reports about mist tent therapy may, in part, be due to differences in equipment, solutions, patient selection, other therapy, and cleaning of equipment. Consequently, strict observation of details is important. We use mist tent therapy overnight in the home treatment program in many patients and during periods of hospitalization to add bulk water to the lower respiratory tract or to ensure adequate humidification. A pneumatic type nebulizer or an ultrasonic unit can be used to generate an adequate mist with a mean particle size of 1 to 2 microns. Ultrasonic units are quiet and usually have a large water output but are more easily contaminated by potential pathogens including *Pseudomonas*, and are harder to maintain and clean. The choice of ultrasonic units is best determined by availability of service. The pneumatic type is less readily contaminated but requires a source of compressed air that makes for more noise than an ultrasonic unit. A relatively small tent should be used so that the mist is more dense.

In the ultrasonic units, the solutions most commonly nebulized include 5 per cent U.S.P. propylene glycol by volume in distilled water, a dilute (approximately one fourth normal) saline solution or, in some centers, distilled water alone. In the pneumatic units, 10 per cent U.S.P. propylene glycol by volume in distilled water is used. The solution must be sterile and free from organic matter to minimize bacterial growth.

Proper cleaning is essential. In the home, we recommend nebulizing a 2 per cent acetic acid solution through the ultrasonic nebulizer and tubing and thorough washing, rinsing and drying every other day. For the pneumatic nebulizer, twice weekly washing and rinsing

---

*Available through the Cystic Fibrosis Foundation, 3091 Mayfield Rd., Cleveland Heights, Ohio 44118; or some units of the Knights of Pythias.

†International Therapeutics, Inc., Dallas, Texas 75235; or Southwest Medical Manufacturing, 5635 Yale Boulevard, Dallas, Texas 75206.

are recommended with special attention to the jet portions. Burrs or irregularities increase the chance of contamination. All nebulization equipment is cleaned and gas sterilized every other day in our hospital.

A few patients do not tolerate mist, as evidenced by discomfort, difficult breathing or, occasionally, wheezing. This therapy is usually employed only during sleeping hours but can be used longer during periods of increased symptoms. Total therapy time should be limited to 20 hours per day. Cooling of the tent or of the room is advisable during hot weather. Small, durable, oil-free, diaphragm-type compressors are available for pneumatic nebulizers. During the day these compressors can also be used for aerosol administration. Tank-type compressors may become contaminated with molds and are not recommended.

Mist tent therapy can be helpful for patients of any age with substantial sputum production or productive coughs. We are not presently recommending mist tent therapy for asymptomatic patients or most young infants.

Allergy and Bronchodilator Therapy. Allergies occur in patients with cystic fibrosis at least as often as they do in the general population. Most commonly encountered are allergic rhinitis and bronchospasm. The allergy symptoms may not be severe, may be atypical or may masquerade as symptoms of cystic fibrosis. Pulmonary function tests before and after a bronchodilator, nasal smears, sputum cytology and peripheral blood counts can be helpful diagnostically.

When allergy is suspected, judicious use of antihistamine and/or bronchodilator therapy may provide symptomatic relief. Antihistamines and decongestants may thicken or dry respiratory secretions and thus are used for brief periods and as infrequently as possible. With bronchospasm, both oral and aerosol bronchodilators can be useful (see Aerosol Therapy). Oral theophylline dosage is usually in the range of 15 to 20 mg./kg./24 hours. In problem cases, theophylline blood levels should be used to adjust dosage and the newer medications such as cromolyn sodium (for use in children over five years of age) or aerosol corticosteroid or atropine may deserve a trial. Skin testing and careful history taking may be helpful. Avoidance of possible irritants or allergens is the cornerstone of successful allergy control. Air conditioning and the use of an electronic air cleaner should also be considered.

We have added dexamethasone, 0.1 to 0.2 ml. per aerosol two or three times a day, to the aerosol in patients with otherwise uncontrollable chronic bronchospasm. Beclomethasone (Vanceril)* delivered by pressurized cartridge may be a useful alternative to dexamethasone in an asthmatic patient with cystic fibrosis. Recently, atropine, 0.1 ml./kg. per aerosol, has been found effective in adult patients with bronchospasm.

Corticosteroids. Oral corticosteroids have no place in the routine care of patients with cystic fibrosis. Occasionally a patient with sufficient allergies and symptoms is encountered in whom aerosol corticosteroids may be useful (see Allergy and Bronchodilator Therapy). Also, on occasion, an infant with cystic fibrosis will present with severe bronchospasm or develop this problem during treatment. The addition of hydrocortisone, 5 to 10 mg./kg./24 hours intravenously, or prednisone, 1 mg./kg./24 hours orally, to the other forms of therapy may be successful. These patients may also benefit from aerosol corticosteroid. Every effort must simultaneously be made to control infection and eliminate potential allergens or irritants from the infant's environment.

We have occasionally used topical nasal corticosteroid spray in an effort to prevent the recurrence of nasal polyps. Four of our patients have required prolonged oral corticosteroid therapy for conditions unrelated to cystic fibrosis without apparent worsening of pulmonary status.

Expectorants. Systemic drugs that clearly assist with the physical removal of secretions from the respiratory tract are not available. Iodides and glycerol guaiacolate in safe systemic doses have not been shown to increase water secretion into the tracheobronchial lumen or to change the rheologic properties of the secretions. Similarly, clinical improvement with these agents has not been demonstrated. Unsatisfactory side effects, such as goiter formation with prolonged use of iodides, have been well documented and are not rare. Patient hydration may improve mucous clearance and should not be overlooked in therapy.

Bronchoscopy and Lavage. Bronchoscopy is indicated for treatment of atelectasis and mucoid impaction and for investigation of hemoptysis. Treatment of obstructive airway disease may sometimes include tracheobronchial suctioning or lavage. The flexible fiberoptic bronchoscope has made endoscopy simpler and better tolerated but has limitations in smaller patients.

Bronchopulmonary lavage has been performed by a variety of techniques ranging

---

*Manufacturer's precaution: Insufficient data exist with respect to administration of beclomethasone to children under 6 years of age.

from the instillation of a few milliliters of saline or mucolytic agent through a bronchoscope to the use of many liters through a double-lumen endotracheal tube. We have infrequently used general anesthesia and the rigid bronchoscope or the Carlens double lumen tube for lavage. The size of the Carlens tube limits its use to patients at least the size of a 12 year old (150 cm. tall).

Our technique involves the use of a small (3.5 mm.) fiberoptic bronchoscope to guide a cuffed endobronchial catheter into a lobar or mainstem bronchus. The bronchoscope is removed once the catheter is in place and the balloon inflated. After ventilation with 100 per cent oxygen for several minutes, saline is run into the lung through the catheter. Volumes of 200 to 400 ml. are alternatively infused (by gravity, with the reservoir 30 to 40 cm. above the lung) and withdrawn. Usually a total volume of 3 to 7 liters is used, with recovery of all but about 200 ml. N-acetylcysteine is often added (30 to 90 ml. of 20 per cent Mucomyst/liter) and antibiotics (according to results of in vitro susceptibility testing of the patient's sputum culture), usually gentamicin or colistin, 80 to 150 mg./liter, are added to the final liter of lavage solution. The indications for any type of lavage procedure have not been clearly defined, are currently made on an individual patient basis, and lack convincing evidence for sustained benefit.

Tracheal Catheter. Without, and even with, intravenous antibiotics, it is difficult to achieve bactericidal levels against gram-negative organisms in tracheobronchial secretions. Although inflammation increases the permeability of the tissues, increasing infection results in high DNA levels in the secretions due to bacterial and cellular debris. DNA inactivates many antibiotics, rendering therapy less effective. Usefulness of aerosol antibiotic may be limited by uneven ventilation, thus resulting in inadequate deposition in more severely affected areas.

Another approach has been to use a large-bore, 16 gauge needle to penetrate the cricothyroid membrane to allow insertion of a small polyethylene catheter through which antibiotics and/or mucolytics can be directly instilled into the trachea. Such a catheter can be used for up to 1 or 2 weeks. Although this technique provides a direct route to the airways, it is not satisfactory for long-term therapy and direct instillation of liquid is not well tolerated without some degree of prior topical anesthesia which has to be repeated each time.

Tracheostomy plays no role in the long-term management of patients with cystic fibrosis although a previously tracheotomized patient who has a permanent tracheostomy is occasionally encountered.

TREATMENT OF PULMONARY COMPLICATIONS

Pneumothorax. Unilateral pneumothorax, occasionally under tension, is increasingly common in teenage and young adult patients. If the pneumothorax is stable and less than 5 to 10 per cent, the patient is admitted for observation. Severe pleuritic pain may necessitate one of the definitive treatments described below.

Pneumothorax greater than 10 per cent or any tension pneumothorax requires definitive treatment. Because of the extremely high rate of recurrence with closed thoracostomy treatment alone, we perform a sclerosing procedure (pleurodesis or open thoracotomy with plication of blebs, apical pleural stripping and basal pleural abrasion) with the first occurrence. In virtually every case, this approach should be carried out within a day of diagnosis.

In patients over 10 years of age, chemical pleurodesis with Atabrine is performed by instilling 100 mg. in 50 ml. of saline into the chest tube daily for 3 days beginning on the first day of the pneumothorax. Occasionally the third dose is not administered if the prior development of high fever, chest pain, or pleural effusion indicates that sufficient pleural reaction has already occurred. Tetracycline pleurodesis is performed using 100 to 250 mg. of tetracycline hydrochloride. Following each instillation, the chest tube is clamped, and the patient is rotated through head down, flat and head up positions, to allow contact with the entire pleural surface.

Open thoracotomy through a small incision is also useful as a primary procedure, and is essential if chemical pleurodesis fails to achieve resolution or is followed by recurrence of pneumothorax. Aggressive treatment of pulmonary infection with intravenous antibiotics is begun on admission. Rapid resumption of chest physiotherapy is essential. If pneumothorax is bilateral, a unilateral closed thoracotomy with chemical pleurodesis is indicated regardless of the percentage of collapse. Chemical pleurodesis should be completed on one side before being initiated on the other.

Atelectasis. Lobar atelectasis, even if asymptomatic and discovered on routine chest roentgenogram, warrants aggressive therapy and usually hospital admission. Intravenous antibiotic therapy should begin immediately (see Antibiotic Therapy). Postural drainage is increased to the affected lobe. If there is no improvement in chest roentgenogram within 5 to 7 days, bronchoscopy is indicated for examination and aspiration of a mucus plug if one is seen. The lobe can then be lavaged with a small amount of saline or dilute N-acetyl cysteine (Mucomyst). If there is minimal or no improvement within a few days the procedure may be repeated.

Occasionally, the atelectasis does not resolve despite very intensive therapy and bronchoscopy. The patient may then be discharged with continuation of the added postural drainage to the affected area. Lobectomy should not be done since resolution of the atelectasis may still occur within the next several weeks or months. Less commonly, the atelectasis never resolves and future therapy is then determined by the patient's course. If the lobe appears to become totally fibrosed, its function is lost but it should not be a threat to the remainder of the lung. On the other hand, if there is evidence that this area is a source of infection or if the patient is incapacitated by systemic symptoms (e.g., fever, anorexia) or by unrelenting cough or sputum production, lobectomy may be necessary.

The role of intermittent positive pressure breathing or blow bottles in the treatment of this complication is unclear. Intermittent positive pressure breathing carries with it the risk of iatrogenic pneumothorax and should be used with caution.

Hemoptysis. Many patients have occasional blood-tinged sputum or hemoptysis of small amounts (less than 20 ml.). Treatment need not be changed but a repeat culture should be obtained to ensure that antibiotic coverage is appropriate. Some patients who do not show *Staphylococcus aureus* on sputum culture may nevertheless respond to the addition of antistaphylococcal therapy. Frequent hemoptysis of small volumes of blood necessitates admission and treatment in the same manner as described for massive hemoptysis.

Massive hemoptysis (total blood loss exceeding 250 to 500 ml. within 24 hours) requires hospitalization for observation and intensive treatment of infection. A blood sample for cross-match should be obtained on admission but transfusion is usually not indicated unless there are blood pressure changes or unless the patient has lost 15 per cent of his estimated blood volume. Intravenous antibiotic therapy should be instituted immediately and includes the use of antistaphylococcal drugs even if cultures do not reveal *Staphylococcus aureus*. Chest physical therapy is discontinued until 12 to 24 hours after the last bleeding episode and is reinstituted in stages beginning with position-

ing and progressing through gentle clapping, vibrating and, finally, full therapy. All patients with massive hemoptysis should receive vitamin K orally or by intramuscular injection.

With continuing hemoptysis, fiberoptic or rigid bronchoscopy may show which lobe is bleeding and an emergency lobectomy may then be considered. Lobectomy should be avoided if at all possible, both to preserve potentially useful pulmonary tissue and because it is often quite difficult to be absolutely sure that the bleeding site has been determined. Patients with active hemoptysis are very frightened and need continued reassurance that the bleeding will stop. Supplemental oxygen, most likely by nasal cannula, may be helpful. Medical personnel should avoid urging the patient not to cough since in most cases coughing is uncontrollable when there is blood in the airway. The containers into which the patient is expectorating should be changed frequently.

Allergic Aspergillosis. Allergic aspergillosis is suspected when a patient with cystic fibrosis becomes acutely worse with wheezing, dyspnea and increased overinflation, especially if asthma has not been present previously. The diagnosis is supported by the appearance of localized infiltrates on chest roentgenogram and the recovery of *Aspergillus* from sputum or tracheal aspirate culture. The patient may have multiple serum precipitins to *Aspergillus*. *Aspergillus* recovered from cultures should be assessed for in vitro susceptibility to amphotericin B (Fungizone) and newer systemic antifungal agents including 5-fluorocytosine (Ancoban).

Treatment is directed at eradication or suppression of *Aspergillus* together with intensive bronchodilator therapy. Aminophylline is given orally in adequate doses to achieve therapeutic blood theophylline levels. Aerosol bronchodilator (e.g., isoproterenol) is also indicated. Systemic corticosteroid (e.g., prednisone) and aerosol corticosteroid (e.g., dexamethasone or beclomethasone) are also useful in severe cases. Aerosol administration of amphotericin B in a dosage of 5 to 10 mg. in each aerosol will aid in clearing *Aspergillus*.* Amphotericin B given by aerosol may increase bronchospasm and should be given in conjunction with aerosol corticosteroid and bronchodilator. Systemic treatment with amphotericin is rarely necessary; if the organism is sensitive to 5-fluorocytosine, and the patient has not responded to other therapy, a trial with this agent may be justified. Allergic aspergil-

---

*This use of amphotericin B is not mentioned in the manufacturer's instructions.

losis is usually a self-limited illness and truly long-term treatment is not necessary. Recurrence is rare.

Hypertrophic Osteoarthropathy. Fortunately symptomatic hypertrophic osteoarthropathy is rare. When it does occur and causes bone pain, edema and joint effusions, symptomatic treatment is all that is available. These patients usually respond to aspirin or acetaminophen, but more potent analgesics may be necessary. Intensive treatment of the pulmonary lesion may decrease the severity of symptoms. Some patients claim that various medications including sulfisoxazole, other antimicrobials and vitamins seem to aggravate these symptoms but there are no objective data.

Acute Respiratory Failure. A severe viral illness may result in acute respiratory failure in patients with preexisting widespread pulmonary disease. Influenza or measles are particularly apt to do this. These patients can usually regain their previous status and are given all available intensive therapy. Intravenous antibiotic treatment begins on admission. Right heart failure, if present, is treated with intravenous digitalization, intravenous diuretics and low salt diet (see Right Heart Failure).

Postural drainage is essential but treatments may have to be spread over a longer time period; occasionally it is best to do a few positions every 3 to 4 hours. This therapy should be given around the clock. Supplemental oxygen may have to be increased during treatments. Endotracheal or bronchoscopic suction may be useful and may be repeated daily.

Oxygen should be administered to raise the arterial Po_2 above 50 mm Hg if possible. A rising Pco_2 may necessitate intermittent positive pressure breathing therapy or even prolonged periods of ventilator assistance. Recovery may be very slow and does not usually begin until after the acute viral illness has started to resolve. As the patient improves, reduction in therapy becomes possible. Ventilator assistance is gradually decreased; FiO_2 is gradually reduced; postural drainage sessions can be longer and less frequent. Intensive intravenous antibiotic therapy and postural drainage should be continued for at least 2 weeks after supplemental oxygen is no longer necessary.

Chronic Respiratory Failure. Chronic respiratory failure is an occasional problem in teenagers and young adults and may precede heart failure by quite some time. The patient should reduce salt intake and report edema,

upper abdominal pain and extreme fatigue. Prophylactic digitalization has been suggested but its efficacy has not been demonstrated. Similarly, the effective use of nightly low-flow oxygen therapy to forestall heart failure has not been reported in cystic fibrosis.

In-patients should be given sufficient oxygen to raise the arterial Po_2 above 50 to 55 mm Hg if possible. Occasionally, hypercapnia prevents the use of optimal FiO_2 concentrations. These patients are generally not benefited by continuous ventilator assistance and only rarely by intermittent positive pressure breathing with intensive therapy. Most patients improve sufficiently with antibiotic therapy to be discharged after gradual weaning from supplemental oxygen. An occasional patient may require low flow oxygen therapy at home.

Right Heart Failure. Patients with long-standing advanced pulmonary disease, especially those with severe hypoxemia (i.e., arterial Po_2 below 50 to 55 mm Hg), often develop overt right heart failure. Aggressive in-patient antibiotic treatment of pulmonary infection as previously described is important although the use of carbenicillin may be hazardous because of its relatively high sodium content. The concurrent administration of probenecid (Benemid), 500 mg. 4 times a day, may allow the use of a lower dose of carbenicillin.* These patients cannot be stabilized without some restriction of salt intake although eventually this may be liberalized to a "no added salt" (usually 2 gm. sodium/day) diet. Oxygen therapy by nasal cannula or mask is usually indicated with a minimal goal of raising the arterial Po_2 above 50 mm Hg within the constraints imposed by the loss of the hypoxic respiratory drive with worsening hypercapnia.

Diuretic therapy is extremely important especially in the acute management of these patients. Furosemide (Lasix), 1 mg./kg. administered intravenously, may be required at 24 to 48 hour intervals initially. Safeguards against potassium depletion may include diuretics such as triamterene (Dyrenium) or spironolactone (Aldactone). Digitalis may be useful as well, particularly in those patients who also have evidence of left heart failure.

In refractory cases, a 3 week course of tolazoline (Priscoline), 1 mg./kg./dose every 12 hours by slow intravenous injection, has often been effective. During tolazoline treatment, every effort is made to maintain arterial oxygen saturation at or above 90 per cent. Me-

---

*Manufacturer's note: The use of probenecid is contraindicated in children under 2 years of age.

chanical measures to prevent reaccumulation of fluid (e.g., SuppHose or custom fitted Jobst Stockings) may be helpful.

GASTROINTESTINAL THERAPY

Pancreatic Deficiency. Exocrine pancreatic deficiency causes some degree of digestive difficulties in over 85 per cent of patients. Meconium ileus, the earliest manifestation, is discussed elsewhere. Replacement therapy is the cornerstone of treatment. Pancreatic enzymes (e.g., Cotazym, Viokase, Panteric, etc.) are given with meals. The dose is empiric and based on stool history, appetite and other symptoms of malabsorption including abdominal pain and irritability. Most patients can be adequately controlled with a dose of 1 to 6 enzyme capsules per meal and 1 or 2 with snacks. We consider the dose to be adequate if stools can be reduced to 2 or 3 a day and are not excessively greasy, and if the patient is not troubled with excessive gas or abdominal pain. Some patients with daily crampy pain or excess flatus may obtain relief with the use of simethacone (Silain).

The dose of pancreatic enzymes required seems to increase with age initially, but some teenagers and young adults may have a decrease in their requirement for this therapy. Pancreatic enzymes are given in applesauce to infants and young children.

Some patients require a modified low fat diet although other patients can eat a normal diet with the exception of being unable to tolerate the fat load of whole milk. Enzyme replacement therapy is best distributed throughout the meal but may be sufficiently effective when taken either right before or after eating. When treatment with pancreatic enzymes alone is unsuccessful, the addition of bile salts (e.g., Accelerase, Cotazym B, etc.) is often effective. Young infants with cystic fibrosis do not utilize soy protein well and may develop anasarca if it is used. Supplemental vitamins, including 50 to 100 units of vitamin E, are given.

If reasonable pancreatic replacement therapy is used, nutrition should be adequate unless the cachexia caused by chronic pulmonary infection interferes. It is extremely important to recognize that anorexia secondary to pulmonary infection cannot be consciously overcome by the patient and that attempts by parents or physician to force the patient to consume more calories will be unsuccessful and lead to unnecessary friction.

In our experience, medium chain triglycerides (MCT oil) add another unpleasant feature to the patient's day. Anabolic steroids have been used for short periods in cystic fibrosis patients who do not have a clear reason for not gaining weight, but their long-term efficacy has not been established.

Meconium Ileus. Meconium ileus, the most common cause of intestinal obstruction in the newborn period, allows immediate diagnosis of cystic fibrosis in the approximately 10 per cent of patients with this complication. Gastrografin enema with penetration of the contrast medium into the area of obstruction is occasionally successful in drawing water into the bowel and flushing out the inspissated material. When this treatment is not successful, surgery is necessary. Similarly, surgery is needed for those patients in whom meconium ileus is associated with volvulus or atresia. Standard surgical approaches (e.g., Mikulicz or Bishop-Koop procedures) are described elsewhere.

All patients suspected of having had meconium ileus on the basis of radiologic studies and/or surgical findings should be treated as having cystic fibrosis until pilocarpine sweat testing is possible at 3 to 6 weeks of age. Pancreatic enzyme replacement and vitamins together with appropriate pulmonary treatment should begin immediately. Nutrition is extremely important and parenteral nutrition should not be delayed if oral feedings are not possible for a prolonged period after surgery. Meconium peritonitis after perforation requires intensive broad spectrum antibiotic treatment.

Meconium Ileus Equivalent, Intussusception, and Constipation. Patients with cystic fibrosis who require pancreatic replacement therapy with meals rarely have bowel movements less often than once every 24 hours. When increasing accumulation of fecal material at the ileocecal valve causes partial or complete obstruction (meconium ileus equivalent), stool frequency decreases and the patient may interpret this change as indicating that the enzyme dose is too high. In this situation, however, pancreatic replacement should continue as before and the patient should take laxatives and/or stool softeners (milk of magnesia, Colace, mineral oil). Enemas are sometimes helpful; however, the enormous capacity of the colon in this disease makes it unlikely that a self-administered enema will reach the ascending colon or caecum. In some patients, oral N-acetyl cysteine (Mucomyst) may be helpful (1 teaspoon 4 times a day).

Intussusception, usually ileocolic, may occur at any age in patients with cystic fibrosis and often follows a one or two day history of "constipation." If intussusception is suspected, the patient should be admitted and scheduled for emergency Gastrografin enema. Gastrografin is hydrophilic and, if the enema reaches the terminal ileum, will draw water into the bowel and flush out the inspissated fecal material. Thus, an intussusception may be diagnosed and treated by the Gastrografin enema. Contrast studies with barium should be avoided because of its tendency to aggravate constipation. In some cases in which an intussusception is diagnosed radiologically but reduction is not accomplished, a Gastrografin enema under general anesthesia may be successful. If not, anesthesia is continued and a laparotomy performed. If the problem is recurrent, mineral oil (1 tablespoon once or twice a day, but not near bedtime) can be continued for long periods with success. Repeated episodes of intussusception may necessitate laparotomy and caecectomy. These patients should receive intravenous fluids in large amounts during and after Gastrografin contrast studies. After reduction of suspected intussusception, the patient should be observed closely for compromised bowel or volvulus.

Biliary Cirrhosis. Symptomatic hepatic disease occurs in about 2 to 4 per cent of patients. Portal hypertension with esophageal varices, hypersplenism and/or ascites may result from the characteristic biliary cirrhosis. Cellular hepatic function usually remains adequate. The acute management of bleeding esophageal varices includes nasogastric suction and iced saline lavage. If necessary, catheterization of a celiac artery and infusion of pitressin is performed as for other patients with this complication.

Recurrence of bleeding episodes may necessitate a shunting procedure. This type of surgery may have to be postponed, if possible, to allow the vessels to attain adequate size for effective anastomosis. All patients with bleeding esophageal varices are likely to eventually require portal-systemic shunting. Splenectomy and splenorenal anastomosis result in the relief of hypersplenism and reduction of portal blood flow, as well as an effective shunt. This procedure has proved satisfactory in many patients. Portacaval anastomosis may also be used. If splenectomy is indicated to relieve hypersplenism, a "prophylactic" splenorenal shunt is performed even if esophageal varices have not been demonstrated or have not yet bled.

All patients with acute variceal bleeding should be given vitamin K by intramuscular injection. Intravenous vitamin K has resulted in anaphylactic reactions in cystic fibrosis and this route should not be used. Vitamin K

treatment may subsequently be continued orally. Ascites is best managed conservatively initially with a low sodium diet forming the mainstay of treatment. Diuretics may be necessary. Again, these patients usually require a shunting procedure.

Obstructive jaundice which occurs infrequently in newborns with cystic fibrosis probably requires no specific therapy. A rare patient with symptoms secondary to portal hypertension may have progression to hepatocellular failure. This complication should be treated as it is in other patients with severe cirrhosis.

Rectal Prolapse. Rectal prolapse occurs in patients with poorly controlled pancreatic deficiency and is often associated with moderate or severe pulmonary infection. Repeated coughing paroxysms, with their associated rise in intraabdominal pressure, occur fairly frequently in cystic fibrosis and the absence of cough may partially explain the rarity of rectal prolapse in other malabsorptive diseases such as celiac syndrome.

The prolapsed rectum is usually easily replaced manually by continuous gentle pressure with the patient in the knee-chest position. If the prolapsed portion has become edematous and is not easily reduced, it should be wrapped in gauze and compressed slowly to force out fluid prior to another attempt at reduction. Sedation may be helpful. Following reduction, an ordinary bottle nipple with the end cut off can be inserted into the rectum and the gluteal folds taped closed around it to prevent an immediate recurrence. Usually the more difficult the reduction, the more likely that the edema in the bowel will delay recurrence.

Patients with recurrent rectal prolapse should be treated with larger doses of pancreatic enzymes. Enzymes should be spaced throughout the meal rather than taken prior to or after eating. Dietary fat should be reduced as much as possible. In addition to these measures, a low roughage diet may be helpful to reduce stool volume. Pulmonary infection may also require added attention including intensive treatment with intravenous antibiotics.

Patients may continue to have rectal prolapse despite all medical measures and require a surgical approach (e.g., a rectal "sling" of Silastic placed around the rectum and just below the skin) to provide the support necessary to prevent recurrent prolapse.

Pancreatitis. Pancreatitis, often recurrent, is a rare complication of cystic fibrosis and occurs almost exclusively in those patients who have not had digestive symptoms. Treatment is symptomatic and includes analgesia and often intravenous fluids and nasogastric suction. When the acute attack has resolved, the patient is advised to avoid fatty foods and alcoholic beverages. We have seen patients whose attacks appear to be precipitated by tetracycline on some occasions but not invariably. Tetracycline is a valuable antibiotic in the home management of the pulmonary infection in cystic fibrosis and may have to be tried again in these patients regardless of the risk of aggravating pancreatic symptoms. Prolonged elevation of the serum amylase may occur and need not prolong hospitalization.

OTHER THERAPY

Salt Depletion. Sweat salt losses can be high on hot summer days, in athletes who do not have an opportunity to eat or drink during prolonged periods of exertion, and in infants who cannot communicate their need for salt. Prevention is all important. Patients and families should be warned about the possibility of excessive salt loss and should anticipate the problem. Supplemental salt (e.g., 500 to 1000 mg. 4 times a day) may be necessary on hot days especially in warmer climates. Infants who present with hyponatremic dehydration may require large volumes (10 to 15 ml./kg.) of normal saline to reestablish an adequate circulating volume.

Hyperglycemia. Extensive pancreatic fibrosis with destruction of the islets may lead to hyperglycemia. If blood glucose levels are only moderately elevated and urine glucose losses are not excessive, no treatment is necessary. With more marked elevation of blood glucose, urine calorie losses become significant and, in addition, there is the theoretical possibility that glucose may spill over into the sputum and aggravate pulmonary infection. Oral antidiabetic agents are not usually effective in cystic fibrosis related hyperglycemia. Diabetic acidosis is rare in these patients. Patient education and initiation of insulin treatment is necessary. Patients with severe pulmonary disease, especially those with a history of right heart failure, must be started on treatment cautiously lest the sudden disappearance of osmotic diuresis precipitate acute heart failure. Because of the exocrine pancreatic deficiency and associated malabsorption, strict dietary control of hyperglycemia is virtually impossible and should not be attempted. The patient should be reassured that this complication is different from diabetes mellitus and does not seem to be associated with the same complications.

Nasal Polyps. Nasal polyps are a recurring problem in 10 to 20 per cent of patients with cystic fibrosis. Prophylactic treatment with corticosteroid-containing nasal drops or spray has not been shown to prevent recurrence. Allergy skin testing and possibly hyposensitization may be helpful in those patients with allergic symptoms and/or a strong family history of allergy. Surgical removal is indicated if the polyps completely obstruct the nose and force the patient to become a mouth breather, if they produce a large amount of mucus which is a threat to the lungs or an inconvenience to the patient, or if intranasal infection, particularly with *Pseudomonas*, does not respond to other treatment. For patients whose pulmonary status is reasonably good, polypectomy may be performed easily with either general or local anesthesia depending on preferences of surgeon and patient. For patients with severe pulmonary disease, local anesthesia should be used if at all possible. Repeated polypectomy entails increased risk because of the possibility of injury to the optic nerve and the increasing incidence of substantial blood loss. Nasal polyps may disappear spontaneously and patients with many recurrences may inexplicably stop developing polyps.

Reproductive Problems. Delayed sexual maturation, often associated with short stature, occurs fairly frequently in association with cystic fibrosis. Although many patients have severe pulmonary infection and/or poor nutrition, delayed puberty also occurs in those with otherwise mild disease. The lack of information about the pathophysiology of this problem makes rational treatment impossible. Some females seem to respond to estrogen-progesterone cycling with growth and breast development. Males are almost always azoospermic because of anatomic interruption of the vas deferens. A rare patient may have normal sperm counts and a few well documented fathers have been reported.

Although females probably have reduced fertility, many pregnancies have been reported. All women with cystic fibrosis who are having regular menses should be considered to be fertile. Pregnancy presents several potential risks. Many antibiotics have not been shown to be safe in pregnancy (e.g., polymyxins including colistin and aminoglycosides including gentamicin, tobramycin, and amikacin); other antibiotics entail known risks and should be avoided if possible (e.g., tetracycline, chloramphenicol). Systemic treatment with penicillin derivatives, sulfisoxazole, and cephalosporins may be used.

All patients with cystic fibrosis should receive counseling concerning sexual development and potential reproductive problems. Although the optimal age for such counseling varies considerably, it should usually be completed early in high school.

Surgery. All minor surgical procedures, including dental work, should be performed under local anesthesia if possible. When general anesthesia is required for elective surgery, stable patients whose pulmonary status is good or excellent can be admitted the day prior to surgery. These patients do not usually require any change in antibiotic therapy. Patients with moderate or severe pulmonary infection should usually be admitted for a course of intensive antibiotic treatment prior to surgery. Up to 2 weeks of preoperative treatment may be necessary. All patients should receive one aerosol and postural drainage treatment on the morning of surgery before they are taken to the operating room. Patients with marginal pulmonary function may benefit from introduction to positive pressure therapy prior to surgery. All patients admitted for emergency surgery should have one aerosol and postural drainage treatment prior to anesthesia. It is also advisable to start intravenous antibiotic therapy.

If possible, anesthesia should be administered by or under the supervision of a senior anesthesiologist with extensive experience with children with pulmonary disease. Total anesthesia time should be kept to a minimum. After induction, all patients should have direct laryngoscopy and tracheal suctioning before endotracheal intubation. In some cases a small amount of saline can be instilled into the trachea to liquefy secretions to facilitate suctioning. This can be repeated during the procedure and immediately after surgery endotracheal suctioning should always be performed prior to terminating anesthesia. Frequent monitoring of blood gases is necessary in patients with severe pulmonary disease but is unnecessary in stable patients with good or excellent pulmonary status. Bacteriologic study of tracheal secretions obtained at surgery may be crucial in postoperative management.

After surgery, postural drainage treatments should be reinstituted as soon as possible (usually within one or two days) and gradually intensified until full clapping and vibration are being done. For most surgical procedures, vigorous therapy is possible by the 5th to 7th postoperative day. Intravenous antibiotics are continued for a minimum of 10 postoperative days. Further adjustments in antibiotic treatment should be made as soon as endotracheal aspirate culture results are available. Early ambulation and intermittent deep breathing are important. An incentive inspirometer can be very helpful in encouraging patients to breathe deeply. This instrument can also be used in conjunction with aerosol therapy.

Although respiratory failure certainly increases anesthesia and surgical risks, we have not had operative deaths or anesthetic complications in such patients. Intermittent positive pressure breathing or full ventilator assistance may be needed transiently in patients with severe pulmonary disease and respiratory failure.

SPECIAL CONSIDERATIONS FOR THORACIC SURGERY. Following open thoracotomy for treatment of pneumothorax, lobectomy or other procedure, the general measures described above also apply. The chest tube rapidly becomes the greatest single obstacle to effective pulmonary therapy after thoracic surgery and should be removed as quickly as possible. We have generally been able to remove the tube by the first or second postoperative day. Wound infections with *Pseudomonas* or *Staphylococcus aureus* are extremely uncommon. When they do occur, local irrigation with an appropriate antibiotic is indicated. Thoracic surgical procedures should be performed through the smallest possible incision.

PSYCHOLOGY

Cystic fibrosis, because of the involvement of the patient's parents in home care and their great concerns about prognosis, places a tremendous strain on the entire family. Every effort must be made, beginning with the initial counseling sessions following diagnosis, to minimize secondary gain from illness and to allow the patient to realize his full potential. Parents should be encouraged to delegate responsibility to the patient as early as the child's maturity allows. For example, as soon as the child is old enough to get the pancreatic enzymes and take them, the parents should no longer check up on or pester the patient to take medication. Similarly, the patient should measure the aerosols as soon as possible, keep track of dwindling drug supplies and gradually take over in giving the history at interval visits to the physician. By 12 years of age, many patients should be seeing the doctor alone and be well on the way to achieving true independence in self care. The technique of self-administered postural drainage can be taught to most patients by the mid-teens. Other aspects of counseling including the area of reproductive problems are discussed above. Realistic information about prognosis is always necessary for realistic planning.

As with other chronic illness, the 24 hour availability of the physician is important, not only for the proper care of medical problems, but also to indicate continued commitment to the patient. At interval visits, all aspects of the patient's life must be intermittently examined: What is the school attendance and how is the patient doing scholastically? How are peer relationships and extracurricular activities being pursued? How is the family coping with the illness? Can the physician help by contacting a social agency or social worker?

If physical health deteriorates and forces the patient to abandon work or career goals, the continued interest and help of the physician is critical if a spiral of depression, decreased cooperation with treatment and eventual total apathy is to be prevented.

For the majority of patients started on comprehensive treatment before the advent of irreversible pulmonary changes, the short and intermediate term prognosis is excellent. These patients should be encouraged to plan their careers as if they had a normal life expectancy. They should of course continue to use common sense and not plan to work in an environment which is likely to be detrimental to their lungs, e.g., chemical factories, coal mines, etc. Most of these persons are maintaining excellent work productivity with normal attendance records.

References

1. Doershuk, C. F., Reyes, A. L., Regan, A. G., et al.: Anesthesia and surgery in cystic fibrosis. Anesth. Analg., *51*:413, 1972.
2. Lough, M. D., Doershuk, C. F., and Stern, R. C. (eds.): Pediatric Respiratory Therapy. Chicago, Year Book Medical Publishers, Inc., 1974.
3. Stern, R. C., Boat, T. F., Doershuk, C. F., et al.: Course of ninety-five patients with cystic fibrosis. J. Pediat., *89*:406, 1976.
4. Stern, R. C., Pittman, S., Doershuk, C. F., et al.: Use of a "heparin lock" in the intermittent administration of intravenous drugs. Clin. Pediat., *11*:521, 1972.
5. Stern, R. C., Stevens, D. P., Boat, T. F., et al.: Symptomatic hepatic disease in cystic fibrosis: Incidence, course, and outcome of portal systemic shunting. Gastroenterology, *70*:645, 1976.
6. Wood, R. E., Boat, T. F., and Doershuk, C. F.: Cystic fibrosis—State of the art. Am. Rev. Resp. Dis., *113*:833, 1976.

Malabsorption Syndromes and Intestinal Disaccharidase Deficiencies

JAY A. PERMAN, M.D., *and*
JOHN B. WATKINS, M.D.

The definition of malabsorption syndrome has now advanced beyond the clinical description of a child with poor growth, distended abdomen, and frequent foul-smelling, greasy stools. Our therapeutic approach is based upon current knowledge of the physiology of gastrointestinal function and the pathophysiology of disease states. Since numerous proprietary formulas are available, defects of intestinal function may now be specifically treated. Proper therapy thus requires that an accurate diagnosis be made when possible. When referral to specialized centers is indicated to confirm or establish a diagnosis, the rationale for such a referral will be stated. Modalities and duration of therapy are indicated and commonly occurring difficulties in management are discussed.

INTRALUMINAL PHASE

Disordered Lipolytic Phase and Pancreatic Insufficiency. Isolated disorders of lipolysis due to pancreatic insufficiency are most commonly due to cystic fibrosis. Far rarer are children with pancreatic insufficiency as in the Shwachman-Diamond syndrome or secondary to surgery, recurrent pancreatitis, or other acquired states. Both protein and fat absorption are affected by pancreatic insufficiency, and in infancy use of a formula with partially hydrolyzed protein and medium chain triglycerides, such as Portagen or Pregestimil, may be helpful (Table 1). Pancreatic enzyme replacement, the dosage of which must be individualized, is only partially successful and steatorrhea usually persists, equaling between 10 and 20 per cent of intake. A reduction in fat intake to 2 gm./kg./day may help control the balance between absorption and excretion and reduce symptomatology. Additional bicarbonate therapy has been useful in some children with cystic fibrosis.

Disordered Micellar Phase. Fat malabsorption may occur in conditions associated with disruption of the enterohepatic circulation of bile acids and in the presence of liver disease. To solubilize fat soluble vitamins, long chain fatty acids and cholesterol, intraluminal bile acids must be present above a certain concentration termed the "critical micellar concentration." In the absence of sufficient concentration of bile acids during meals, steatorrhea often exists. Clinically, this occurs most commonly as the result of ileal resection or disease. (Conditions in which ileal disease or multiple resections have reduced the mucosal absorptive surface in addition to creating a bile acid losing syndrome are discussed in the section on short bowel syndrome).

In patients with ileal dysfunction, bile acid concentrations are often normal in the morning after an overnight fast, but diminish throughout the day. Similarly, the stooling pat-

TABLE 1. Infant Formulas*

FORMULA	CALORIES/ 100 ml.	PROTEIN TYPE** (gm./100 ml.)	CARBOHYDRATE TYPE** (gm./100 ml.)	FAT (gm./100 ml.)	Na (mEq./L)	K (mEq./L)	Ca (mEq./L)	P (mEq./L)	IRON (ml./L)	OSMOLARITY (mOsm./L)
Human	67	1.2 Lactalbumin Casein	7.0 Lactose	3.8	7	14	17	9	1.5	133
Whole cow's milk	67	3.3 Casein Lactalbumin	4.8 Lactose	3.7	25	35	60	62	1.0	362
Regular infant formulas										
Similac with iron	67	1.5	7.3 Lactose	3.6	12	20	30	26	1.0 / 12.0	262
Similac 13 Cal.	43	1.2	4.5 Lactose	2.4	10	15	25	21	1.0	155
Similac 24 with iron	80	2.2 Casein Lactalbumin	8.4 Lactose	4.3	15	27	42	42	15	310
Premature	80	2.2	9.1 Sucrose Lactose	4.1	14	23	63	37	.4	358
Enfamil with iron	67	1.5	7.0 Lactose	3.7	12	18	27.5	27.5	1.4 / 12.0	262
"Humanized" formulas										
SMA	67	1.5 Lactalbumin Casein	7.2 Lactose	3.6	7	14	21	21	12.0	272
PM 60/40	67	1.5	7.5 Lactose	3.5	7	14	17	10	2.6	275
Soy based formulas										
Prosobee	67	2.5	6.8 Sucrose,† corn syrup solids	3.4	18	19	40	31	12.0	233
Isomil	67	2.0 Soy Protein‡ Isolate	6.8 Sucrose, corn syrup solids	3.6	13	18	35	29	12.0	202
Cho-Free	39	1.8	0 Add glucose	3.5	17	25	47	47	8.4	No glucose 131 / Glucose 355
Special formulas										
Portagen	67	2.4 Caseinate	7.8 Sucrose, corn syrup solids	3.2§ (MCT)	14	22	32	28	12.0	211
Nutramigen	67	2.2 Casein¹¹ Hydrolysate	8.8 Sucrose Starch	2.6	14	17	32	28	12.0	397
Pregestimil	67	2.2 Casein Hydrolysate	8.8 Glucose Starch	2.8 (MCT)	14	17	32	28	12.0	539
Pedialyte	20	0	5.0 Glucose	0	30	20	4	0	0	325

*Formula composition may undergo change without notice, and inspection of label is essential.

**Upper ingredient is present in greater abundance.

†Corn syrup solids are hydrolysates of corn starch containing varying mixtures of glucose, maltose, tri- and higher saccharides.

‡Soy protein isolates are methionine fortified.

§MCT = medium chain triglycerides with adequate essential fatty acids. MCT oil for oral use, 1 gm. of fat/ml., 9 cal./ml.

¹¹Casein hydrolysates contain 60 per cent free amino acids.

tern is often normal in the morning but becomes loose and watery as the day progresses due to colonic water secretion induced by malabsorbed bile acids.

Therapy consists of redistributing the dietary fat load, usually heaviest in the afternoon and evening, more evenly throughout the day to take advantage of bile acids synthesized the previous night. Use of medium chain triglycerides and finally a moderate reduction in fat intake may be necessary. Cholestyramine, a resin which nonspecifically binds bile acids, may be exceedingly helpful in controlling the diarrhea associated with ileal resection but should not be used indiscriminately.* We generally use 250 mg./kg./day as an initial dose, divided equally between the morning and noon meal and omitted in the evening. The dose may then be increased up to 10 to 12 gm./day. Constipation, malabsorption of fat soluble vitamins and, rarely, metabolic acidosis may result; vitamin replacement therapy may be indicated. Folic acid deficiency has been reported on long-term therapy, and in such cases we administer folic acid, 1 mg./day. Deficient bile acid concentrations also occur in the presence of severe liver disease or cholestasis as seen in children with neonatal hepatitis or biliary atresia. In children with steatorrhea secondary to liver disease, addition of medium chain triglycerides, control of the load of fat in the diet, and addition of vitamins are the most useful forms of therapy.

Bacterial Overgrowth. Stasis within the small bowel may result in contamination of the lumen by colonic-type flora. Because bacteria often possess enzymes capable of deconjugating bile acids, which renders them ineffective in forming micelles, fat malabsorption may occur. Treatment is ideally directed toward eliminating the underlying cause of contamination. Structural abnormalities such as chronic volvulus, adhesions, blind loops or strictures may be amenable to surgical correction provided large resections can be avoided. Other disorders such as immunodeficiency syndromes and motility abnormalities are less amenable to correction; thus, the bacterial overgrowth itself must be treated.

Neomycin has been used in the past but is now avoided because it may exacerbate malabsorption by complexing bile acids or injuring the intestinal mucosa. Older children may be treated with oral tetracycline, 50 mg./kg./day. In infants, we use oral kanamycin for 1 week periods. Alternatively, penicillin, which has

---

*Manufacturer's note: A dosage for cholestyramine has not been established for infants and children.

antimicrobial action against anaerobes, has been used successfully. Repeated courses of antibiotics (such as 2 weeks each month) may be necessary if the underlying cause of overgrowth persists. Carbohydrate malabsorption is often observed in these conditions and appropriate dietary modification may be necessary. (See following section on carbohydrate intolerance.)

MUCOSAL PHASE

Disorders of Intestinal Function— Specific Defects. Disorders of the intestinal mucosa may affect absorption of all three classes of nutrients or in some cases be specifically restricted to substrates of a single class. Specific carbohydrate malabsorption occurs most commonly and its treatment is discussed first.

MONOSACCHARIDE INTOLERANCE. Specific monosaccharide intolerance due to deficiency of the carrier for glucose and galactose is an extraordinarily rare condition characterized by diarrhea and dehydration after ingestion of formulas containing glucose or galactose in any form. Thus intolerance to almost every dietary carbohydrate is demonstrated early in the neonatal period. Treatment consists of elimination of all dietary carbohydrates with the exception of fructose, which is absorbed by a mechanism other than glucose.

Far more common is secondary monosaccharide intolerance, which frequently occurs in infants after intestinal surgery or gastroenteritis. Because bacterial overgrowth has been associated with the pathogenesis of monosaccharide intolerance after surgery, this possibility must be considered, evaluated and treated if found (see section on Bacterial Overgrowth). In the absence of bacterial overgrowth, intolerance to monosaccharides is usually self-limited. A carbohydrate-free formula such as Cho-Free (see Table 1) is useful during this period.

Dextrose monohydrate may be added in increasing amounts as tolerance to glucose improves; 6 tablespoons per 26 ounces of Cho-Free (at 1:1 dilution) yields a 20 cal./oz. formula. We have often found it more convenient to add carbohydrate as honey, which is essentially glucose and fructose, although a small amount of sucrose is present. Cho-Free becomes a 20 cal./oz. formula containing 6.4 per cent carbohydrate when 3 tablespoons of honey are added to 26 ounces of formula. We suggest beginning with Cho-Free containing 1 to 2 per cent of added carbohydrate. One must be aware that in the absence of added carbohydrate, sugar-free formulas are low in calories per ounce; thus, if glucose cannot be added in a reasonable period of time, either total or supplemental intravenous hyperalimentation may become necessary.

DISACCHARIDE INTOLERANCE–LACTASE DEFICIENCY. Malabsorption of lactose, the disaccharide present in human or cow's milk, may occur frequently as a secondary deficiency after acute gastroenteritis and chronic gastrointestinal disorders (such as celiac disease), in a majority of the world's population after the first five years of life, or rarely at birth (congenital). Symptoms include abdominal bloating, nausea, cramping, and especially in the younger age group, diarrhea. Therapy in infancy, during which time lactase deficiency is almost always secondary and hence transient,

requires elimination of all dairy products from the diet. We use sucrose-containing formulas such as Isomil or ProSobee (see Table 1).

Parents should be instructed to identify lactose-containing prepared food by reading labels. If the formula being used contains adequate amounts of calcium, supplementation of this mineral is not necessary. However, in the older age group, supplementation with calcium is suggested. In addition riboflavin may also require supplementation in the diet. In using the lactose-free diet it is important to stress to the child and his parents those foods which may be included in the diet as well as those which are to be excluded (Table 2).

Duration of secondary lactase deficiency is variable, lasting from weeks to months. At

TABLE 2. Lactose-Free Diet

FOODS ALLOWED	FOODS AVOIDED
Lactose-free formulas listed in Table 1, fruit juices, carbonated beverages, Kool-Aid, cocoa without added milk solids, nondairy cream or milk substitutes, coffee, tea	Milk (fresh, evaporated, condensed, dried, butter), frappés, ice cream soda, "Great Shakes," Instant Breakfast
French, Italian or Vienna bread. Homemade french toast without added milk. Unkneaded biscuits, saltines, graham, oyster, soda crackers, Triscuits	Breads, rolls, biscuits, muffins made with or enriched with milk solids (hamburger and frankfurter buns), pancakes, waffles, doughnuts and pop-tarts
All types of cereals	Check all commercial breakfast and baby cereals
Jell-O, water ice, popsicles, fruit pie (pie crust made without butter or regular margarine), tapioca, homemade cornstarch pudding or junket made with fruit juice or milk substitute	Cakes, cream pie, cookies made with milk, ice cream, milk ice, sherbet, custard, commercial pudding mixes
Milk free cookies such as fig bars, gingersnaps, lemonsnaps	
Kosher margarine, lard, vegetable oil, cream substitutes such as Coffee Rich or Coffee Mate	Butter, margarine, sour cream, whipped cream, salad dressing made with milk, mayonnaise
All types of fruits	
All types of meat, fish and poultry	Creamed meats, gravies, processed or canned meats such as luncheon meat, sausage, hash, frankfurters unless 100 per cent pure meat, commercial hamburgers
Eggs	All kinds of cheeses
All potatoes or substitutes (macaroni, rice and spaghetti)	Potatoes mashed with milk or butter
Clear soups, broth	Creamed soups
Limit amount of sweets for good dental hygiene: sugar, jam, jellies, syrups, honey, candies such as gum drops, butterscotch, Canada mints, Planter's Jumbo Block, Good n' Fruity, Dots, Neco Wafers, Mason's Black Crows	Candies made with milk chocolate, butter or cream, butterscotch
All kinds of vegetables	Vegetables in butter or creamed sauce
Mustard, relish, catsup, salt, pepper, spices, peanut butter, gravy without added milk or cream, potato chips, pretzels, pickles, olives	Yogurt

some point, therefore, a decision must be made to return the child to a lactose-containing diet. Conventionally, this may be done by clinical trial, such as addition of foods which contain small amounts of lactose (hard cheeses or cottage cheese). Breath hydrogen determination following lactose administration detects nonabsorption and thus may be useful in assessing recovery of lactase activity. Identification of lactase deficiency in older healthy children requires removal of milk and other lactose-containing foods to the extent necessary for elimination of symptoms. Lactose intolerance in the healthy child is not a disease; therefore, inclusion of lactose-containing foods in the diet in amounts which cause few or no symptoms will not adversely affect the child.

SUCRASE-ISOMALTASE DEFICIENCY. Intolerance to sucrose produces the same symptoms described for lactase deficiency. Congenital deficiency of the brush border enzymes sucrase and isomaltase occurs rarely as an autosomal recessive disorder. Accordingly, a family history of chronic diarrhea in infancy or intolerance to fruits is helpful. Affected children generally grow well but have persistent diarrhea. Diagnosis is achieved by tolerance test, mucosal biopsy with enzyme determination or by a specific breath test. Referral for confirmatory diagnosis is thus appropriate.

Sucrose (table sugar) and sucrose-containing foods must be eliminated from the diet of sucrase-deficient infants and toddlers to avoid severe diarrhea (Table 3). Either glucose or the artificial sweeteners may be used. Formulas containing sucrose must of course be avoided. Breast fed infants should not experience difficulty until solids containing sucrose are administered. Occasionally, medications in the form of syrups contain sucrose; these may produce diarrhea and thus should be avoided. Interestingly, starch, which requires isomaltase

TABLE 3. Sucrose Restricted Diet

FOODS ALLOWED	FOODS AVOIDED
Milk, unsweetened evaporated milk and cream	Sweetened condensed milk and formulas containing sucrose
Asparagus, broccoli, Brussel sprouts, cabbage, cauliflower, celery, chard, chicory, cucumber, lettuce, mushrooms, spinach, tomatoes, bamboo shoots, radishes and potatoes (0.3 gm./100 gm.)	Peas, dried beans, lentils, turnips, parsnips and other vegetables not listed in foods to include or those not tolerated
Grapes, fresh cherries, dried Kadota figs, blackberries, cranberries, currants, (red and white), lemon, loganberries and medium ripe strawberries (0.3 gm./100 gm.)	Those not on the list of fruits to include or those not tolerated
Fried, hard cooked, soft cooked and poached eggs	
Fresh meat, fish and ham	Check all commercially prepared meats and fish
All cheeses	
Bread (homemade), spaghetti and macaroni (without sugar)	Breakfast cereals, wheat germ, rice and bran
Butter, margarine, cooking oil, lard and salad dressing (oil and vinegar)	Mayonnaise, salad dressing (French, Roquefort, Thousand Island)
Cocoa (unsweetened), coffee, tea, vegetable juice and "special" eggnog (see recipes)	Malted milk, milk shake, Kool-Aid, pop
Salt, pepper, gravy, spices, herbs and vinegar	Olives, pimiento and pickles (sweet and sour)
Chicken and beef broth, boullion and consommé	
Glucose (dextrose) and artificial sweeteners	Sugar (cane, beet, granulated, powdered, brown), jam, honey, jelly, candy, molasses, maple syrup and frosting
Homemade cake, cookies, ice cream using glucose (see recipes), gelatin tapioca and diabetic chocolate	Commercially prepared pies, cookies, cakes, diabetic products (unless mentioned elsewhere), ice cream, sherbet and any food prepared with sugar
	Salad dressing, pickles, chutney and medicines made up in syrup

to facilitate the breakdown of oligosaccharides, is usually well tolerated despite deficiency of the enzyme.

As the child becomes older, he usually becomes tolerant to larger amounts of sucrose. Hence, by clinical trial his diet may be liberalized to just below the threshold of symptoms. Secondary sucrase deficiency, similar to transient lactase deficiency, may occur in association with other disorders affecting the integrity of the intestinal mucosa. Dietary modification is as for congenital sucrase-isomaltase deficiency. Prolonged dietary restriction is generally unnecessary; recovery of sucrase activity may be evaluated by breath hydrogen analysis, intestinal biopsy or by clinical trial.

Disorders of Mucosal Function— Generalized Defects. CELIAC DISEASE. This disorder, best described by the term "gluten-sensitive enteropathy," is induced in susceptible individuals by dietary gluten. Histologically, it is characterized by flattening of intestinal villi, and clinically it is associated with malabsorption. The diagnosis should never be made on clinical grounds alone. Histological confirmation of an intestinal lesion is essential and referral to a center equipped to make the diagnosis is appropriate. The therapy requires lifelong commitment to a gluten-free diet. Because this is expensive and difficult, the child without celiac disease who recovers coincidentally with the institution of a gluten-free diet and is thus presumed to have gluten-sensitive enteropathy has been done a disservice!

Celiac disease should be suspected whenever there is good evidence for malabsorption. Specifically, this includes weight loss with or without deceleration in growth velocity, unresponsive iron deficiency, acquired carbohydrate intolerance and finally persistent diarrhea. However, it is important to note that malabsorption may be present without a characteristic history of diarrhea. A quantitative 72 hour fat collection is a good screening tool and is often effectively completed in the home.

Treatment consists of complete withdrawal of all gluten from the diet (Table 4). Foods containing wheat, rye, oats, buckwheat or barley and their derivatives must be excluded. Flours made from rice, soy bean, corn, potato and gluten-free wheat starch are permissible. It is important to read labels since many commercially prepared foods include gluten-containing flours.

Ingredients which should raise suspicion include starch, emulsifiers, stabilizers, cereals, hydrolyzed vegetable proteins, flour, bran, farina and wheat germ. Until manufacturers uniformly list ingredients, any products whose ingredients are unclear should be avoided. Caution is also required in eating restaurant-prepared meals. It is important to emphasize that despite restrictions the affected child can and should have a well balanced diet with representatives from each of the "four basic food groups":

1. *Milk group.* Three or more glasses for children. Initially, in the first three to four weeks, a lactose-free diet may be indicated to hasten improvement of diarrhea. Lactase activity present in the brush border returns with mucosal recovery; thus lactose may be gradually reintroduced provided no exacerbation of diarrhea or symptoms occurs.

2. *Meat group.* Two or more servings. Luncheon and preserved meats must be 100 per cent pure.

3. *Vegetables and fruits.* Four or more servings.

4. *ALLOWED bread and cereals.* Four or more servings. It should be noted that gluten-free bread is not therapeutic per se.

Gluten-free recipes are available from:

French, A. B.: Low Gluten Diet with Tested Recipes. Ann Arbor, Michigan, University Hospital.
Sheedy, C. B. and Keifetz, N.: Cooking for Your Celiac Child. New York, Dial Press, Inc., 1969.
Wood, M. N.: Gourmet Food on a Wheat-Free Diet. Springfield, Illinois, Charles C Thomas, 1967.

Specific vitamin and mineral deficiencies must be corrected. The newly diagnosed patient is frequently iron-deficient; therapeutic dosages of oral iron are indicated in this situation. Folic acid supplementation may also be required for the initial months of treatment, as may fat soluble vitamins K and D. Rickets, although now rare in untreated celiac disease, requires therapeutic dosages of vitamin D.

Institution of a gluten-free diet results in resolution of symptoms within weeks. Subjective improvement, specifically resolution of apathy and irritability, may result within a few days after gluten withdrawal. Abdominal distention, diarrhea and muscle tone show progressive improvement.

Steroids are not indicated except in the child with celiac disease who presents with severe diarrhea, dehydration and weight loss—so-called "celiac crisis." Associated abnormalities may include hypoproteinemia, hypokalemia, hypocalcemia, hypomagnesemia, hypoprothrombinemia, acidosis, paralytic ileus and intraluminal fluid accumulation. Vigorous fluid, electrolyte and colloid replacement in addition to prednisone, 2 mg./kg./day, are indicated.

Lifelong adherence to a gluten-free diet is indicated despite the possibility of prolonged periods free of overt symptomatology in later childhood while ingesting gluten. Return of the adolescent to a gluten-containing diet will result in recurrence of the flat intestinal villus

TABLE 4. Gluten-Free Diet

FOODS ALLOWED	FOODS AVOIDED
Chocolate, tea, coffee (from fresh ground), carbonated drinks, cocoa (no wheat flour added), and all milk	Instant coffee containing wheat; postum, beer, ale, malted drinks
Corn pone, spoon bread, soy bean wafers, rice bread and corn bread made without wheat	All breads and all cereals except those allowed, baking powder biscuits, zwieback, pretzels, gluten bread, pancakes, waffles, all crackers, rye crisps
Corn cereals, hominy cornstarch, potato flour, rice cereals and rice tapioca	
Corn flour and rice flour	Wheat flour, bread flour, all purpose flour, cake flour, pastry flour, self-rising whole wheat, rye, buckwheat, barley, cracked wheat, graham, flour-wheat germ, bran, farina, cracker meal, bread crumbs, cake mixes and cookie mixes
Beef, lamb, pork, veal, liver, chicken, turkey, duck, cod, mackerel, haddock, tuna, crab, oysters, shrimp, clams, sardines, all cheeses, meat frankfurters made without bread crumbs, cracker crumbs, wheat or rye flours	Croquettes, fish or meat patties or loaves made with bread crumbs, cracker crumbs, or wheat flour. Meat products containing wheat such as frankfurters, cold cuts and sausages.
Any fruits Any vegetables	
Gelatin, ice or sherbet, custard, cornstarch pudding, homemade ice cream, junket, rice pudding and tapioca pudding	Cakes, cookies, pie, donuts, commercial ice cream, ice cream cones, prepared mixes and prepared puddings
White or sweet potatoes and rice	Noodles, macaroni, spaghetti and dumplings
All clear and vegetable soups, cream soups thickened with cream, cornstarch or potato flour	All canned soups, cream soups unless made at home without wheat
All eggs	
Butter, margarine, corn oil, olive oil, French dressing, pure mayonnaise, Spry, Crisco, other animal and vegetable fats and oils	Commercial salad dressings
Honey, syrups, jellies, jams, candies made without wheat products, white or brown sugar and corn syrup	Commercial candies containing cereal products
Nuts, olives, pickles, pop corn, Fritos, potato chips and chocolate	Pretzels, sauces and gravies thickened with wheat flour

lesion. Certainly older children require continued physician support in adhering to this diet.

TROPICAL SPRUE.   Frequently presenting with symptoms and signs of gluten-sensitive enteropathy, tropical sprue should be considered if patients have been in endemic areas, even on short trips. Treatment with tetracycline, 50 mg./kg./day (maximum 1 gm./day), for a period of at least 6 months is effective. Improved nutrition is essential; folic acid supplementation in some cases may be specific therapy. In addition, vitamins and mineral supplementation, including iron, calcium and magnesium, may be required.

GIARDIASIS.   This is a parasitic infestation capable of producing an intestinal lesion with concomitant malabsorption. Infection is ac-

quired through the ingestion of cysts, most commonly from contaminated water supplies. The diagnosis may be made by examination of the fresh stool, particularly during acute infection. In chronic cases diagnosis by stool examination is unrewarding; duodenal intubation and/or touch preparation of an intestinal mucosal biopsy produces the highest diagnostic yield.

Therapy with quinacrine (Atabrine) tablets is effective in the following dosages: 8 mg./kg./day in three divided doses for 5 to 7 days. Metronidazole (Flagyl), while often used in the treatment of giardiasis, has not been approved for such usage in children. Recent reports of oncogenesis and mutagenesis associated with this drug dictate avoidance of its use in children for the treatment of giardiasis.

IMMUNE DEFICIENCY STATES. Giardiasis is often found in association with immune deficiency states. Other associated factors which possibly contribute to malabsorption in immune deficiency are bacterial overgrowth and disaccharidase deficiency. Giardiasis and bacterial overgrowth may be treated specifically as indicated previously. Appropriate dietary management, as previously discussed, will alleviate symptoms associated with disaccharide intolerance. Specific therapy of the immune deficit, which may result in an improvement of the gastrointestinal manifestations, such as gamma globulin, fresh frozen plasma and colostrum, are helpful in specific instances.

ALLERGIC GASTROENTEROPATHY (EOSINOPHILIC GASTROENTERITIS). This disorder, which may be associated with structural villus change, is characterized by eosinophilia, chronic diarrhea, abdominal pain, gastrointestinal blood and protein loss, and often allergic manifestations. Referral to a pediatric gastroenterologist is appropriate when this condition is suspected, as diagnosis may be established by a mucosal biopsy of the stomach and the intestine. Therapy is begun with a milk-free diet, particularly when the diagnosis is made in an infant who has been on cow's milk protein. Prednisone, 1 mg./kg./day, is occasionally beneficial and may be indicated for prolonged periods.

TRANSPORT PHASE

Intestinal Lymphangiectasia. Because dietary triglyceride is dependent on lymphatic transport for delivery to the blood stream, impedance of intestinal lymphatic flow due to a congenital abnormality or secondary obstruction may result in fat malabsorption. More prominent, however, is the generalized luminal loss of protein from dilated lymphatics, resulting in hypoalbuminemia and hypogammaglobulinemia as well as lymphopenia. Unless the obstruction is amenable to surgical correction, therapeutic efforts must be directed to reducing engorgement of dilated lymphatics, thus reducing leakage of proteins. This may be achieved by significantly restricting long chain fat and substituting medium chain triglycerides (MCT) which are absorbed by the portal circulation. Formula fed infants require preparations containing MCT (such as Portagen or Pregestimil). Older children require a high-protein diet containing MCT as the major fat component (Table 5). One tablespoon of MCT oil contains 115 calories; this preparation may be mixed with juices, used as a dressing, or used in cooking or baking.

TABLE 5. Diet Containing Medium Chain Triglycerides as the Major Fat Component

FOODS ALLOWED	FOODS NOT ALLOWED
Milk substitute, skim milk, skim milk powder, include 1 pint daily if no milk substitute is taken*	Whole milk, full cream milk powder, cream, yoghurt, condensed and evaporated milks, ice cream
Dry skim milk, cottage cheese	All other cheeses
Lean meats and fish cooked without fat or fried in MCT oil; makes sauces and gravies with allowed foods only	Fish or meats cooked with fat or oil; fish canned in oil; fatty meat, such as pork, ham, bacon; commercially prepared meats, such as sausages, pies, salami
Egg white; include a maximum of 1 egg daily	Extra egg yolk
MCT oil, MCT margarine; if MCT margarine is not available, a maximum of 3 teasp. butter or table margarine may be used daily	Extra butter or table margarine; all other fats and oil
All vegetables; potatoes may be plain, boiled, mashed with skim milk or roast; potato chips made with MCT oil	Vegetables cooked in other oils or fat; potatoes cooked in other fats or oils
All fruits, fresh, stewed or canned; fruit juices	Avocado pear
All plain white, brown or wholemeal unsliced breads without added milk	Breads containing milk
Flour, corn flour, rice, spaghetti, macaroni, pasta, sago, barley, semolina; Corn Flakes, Wheat Flakes, Puffed Wheat and Rice Bubbles	Oatmeal, wheatgerm; check all breakfast cereals
Jelly, fruit gels, meringues; puddings, cakes and biscuits using special recipes	Commercial pastry, puddings, cakes and biscuits
Sugar, jam, jelly, honey, syrups, barley sugar, glucose and boiled sweets; yeast extracts	Chocolates, butterscotch; check all other commercial sweets; all nuts
Clear soups, soup cubes, meat extracts	Canned and packet soups, cream soups
Coffee, tea, cocoa powder, fruit juices, soft drinks, cordials	Chocolate and caramel milk flavorings
Salt, pepper, herbs, spices, essences, mustard, vinegar, tomato ketchup, tomato sauce, pickles, chutney	Mayonnaise, commercial salad dressings

*Depending on the milk substitute used, vitamin and mineral supplementation may be needed and should be individually prescribed.

SHORT BOWEL SYNDROME

Therapy of short bowel syndrome (resection of varying lengths or regions of small intestine) requires use of a number of modalities discussed in previous sections. Intraluminal phase defects may occur for a variety of reasons: (1) gastric hypersecretion frequently associated with small bowel resection alters duodenal pH, thereby preventing optimal action of lipase on fat as well as conversion of zymogens into active proteolytic enzymes; (2) occurrence of bacterial overgrowth, particularly likely if the ileocecal valve has been removed, may result in deconjugation of bile acid leading to defective micellar solubility; (3) ileal resection may result in malabsorption of bile acids leading to a choleraic enteropathy, thus depleting the bile salt pool; and (4) depletion of bile acids may further compromise the newborn who, even in health, has a contracted bile salt pool with increased losses of fat.

Associated with malabsorption of fat are deficiencies of the fat soluble vitamins D and K. The complexing of calcium to malabsorbed fats may result in calcium depletion and may in turn lead to hyperoxaluria due to inadequate luminal binding of oxalate by calcium. Furthermore, malabsorption of magnesium parallels malabsorption of calcium. Also occurring within the lumen is the possible matabolism of protein by bacteria, thus leading to hypoalbuminemia.

Mucosal phase defects may occur due to toxic injury secondary to gastric hypersecretion or bacterial overgrowth. Carbohydrate malabsorption is thus likely. Furthermore, a combination of rapid transit and decreased absorptive surface due to resection may impair absorption of specific nutrients. Upper small bowel resection may result in iron deficiency due to loss of absorptive sites, and terminal ileal resection may affect vitamin B_{12} levels.

Therapy thus requires an awareness of the many pathophysiologic mechanisms potentially present and requires knowledge of the extent and the region of small bowel resection. Diet therapy may be achieved through a variety of methods, all requiring meticulous attention to osmolarity and rate of administration. Small, dilute feeds of a protein hydrolysate formula containing MCT to which dextrose may be added in gradually increasing amounts starting with 1 gm./100 ml., should be used initially (such as sugar-free Pregestimil). Alternatively, Modular Formula (Ross) described by Klish et al. (J. Pediat., 88:948–52, 1976) may be tailored to individual requirements by adding specific carbohydrates and fats to the sodium caseinate base. With increasing tolerance to carbohydrates, the infant may be weaned to protein hydrolysate formulas, such as regular Pregestimil or, if sucrose can be tolerated, Nutramigen.

The infant with short bowel who is intolerant to oral feeds by bolus may be tolerant to continuous nasogastric infusion of a protein hydrolysate formula or an elemental diet such as unflavored Vivonex. We begin with one-half strength Vivonex at a rate of 50 ml./kg./day. Supplemental fluid is given intravenously. If tolerance to this strength and rate is demonstrated as evidenced by decreased stool rate and absence of reducing substances in the stool, the volume is increased over a 3 day period until a maintenance rate of 165 ml./kg./day is achieved. With demonstration of tolerance, intravenous infusion may be discontinued and the infant advanced to two-thirds strength formula providing 110 cal./kg./day. Following a period of stabilization, during which stool frequency and reducing substances in stools decrease at this strength and in which weight gain occurs, the infant may be gradually weaned to bolus feedings of one-half strength Pregestimil or Nutramigen. Simultaneous reduction of the elemental diet should be achieved. Eventually, advance to full-strength formula feedings can occur. If, despite these modalities, intractable diarrhea and failure to gain weight persist, total parenteral nutrition becomes necessary.

Bacterial overgrowth, if present, should be eradicated as previously discussed. Cholestyramine may be of value if choleraic enteropathy is present. Evidence of iron deficiency should be sought and treated parenterally if indicated. Vitamin B_{12} should also be given parenterally, particularly in the absence of ileum (100 μg. intramuscularly monthly). Vitamins D and K may be required in increased amounts if the feeding used is inadequate or if steatorrhea is present. Monitoring serum calcium and magnesium levels is also necessary, especially in the presence of fat malabsorption. Antacids have been used in adults with short bowel syndrome to counter the effects of hypersecretion.

Although the child with small bowel resection frequently becomes less of a management problem with age, continued vigilance for generalized or specific malabsorption defects must be maintained.

Disorders of the Anus and Rectum

JOHN H. SEASHORE, M.D.

Anorectal Malformations. Low anomalies usually can be managed by local perineal procedures in the neonatal period. *Anal membranes* are incised or ruptured at the bedside. Once or twice daily dilatations are necessary for several weeks. *Anal stenosis* is treated by the same program of dilatation. A gloved, well lubricated finger is the safest and best dilator, but if the opening is initially too small for a finger, graded Hegar dilators can be used. *Covered anus* in either sex is treated by perineal anoplasty. Dilatations are started on the tenth postoperative day and continued for four to five weeks. The prognosis for continence in all these groups is excellent.

Children with *ectopic perineal anus* have anterior displacement of the anus away from the normally positioned external sphincter but are generally continent. Some degree of stenosis is usually present and can be treated by dilatation. In girls, perineal hygiene may be a problem because of accumulation of stool in the vestibule. In this situation, or if soiling is a problem in either sex, anoplasty is indicated.

Female infants who have fistulas into the distal (subhymenal) genital tract may be more difficult to manage. If the fistula is in the area of the posterior fourchette and clearly passes subcutaneously to the anal dimple (*anovulvar fistula*), perineal anoplasty is done. Fistulas higher in the vestibule commonly have a more cephalad course and may be intimately adherent to the posterior vaginal wall (*rectovestibular fistula*). The fistula is dilated to allow normal stooling, and at about six months of age the fistula is closed and the distal rectum mobilized and transposed to its normal location. At this age, there is less risk of injury to the posterior vaginal wall or perineal musculature.

Infants who appear to have low anomalies by the presence of an external fistula but who have unusual or complex anatomy are treated by colostomy in the neonatal period. An example is a male with rectobulbar fistula and hypospadias, so that both urine and meconium are passed from a single scrotal or penile shaft orifice. Definitive repair is performed at six months to a year of age when the precise anatomical relationships can be more clearly defined by radiological studies and at the operating table. If there is doubt as to the nature of the anomaly in a neonate, it is always preferable to do a colostomy initially. There is no place for blind perineal dissection in hopes of finding a low anomaly amenable to local repair.

Neonates with *high anorectal malformations* are treated by double-barreled transverse colostomy. Before discharge the distal colon is irrigated with saline to evacuate meconium and allow free egress of colonic secretions through the mucous fistula. At about six months of age or when the infant weighs 6 to 8 kg., the anatomical relationships in the pelvis are defined by barium studies through the mucous fistula. Voiding cystogram may be helpful in some patients.

Anal reconstruction is started through a sacroperineal approach. The puborectalis muscle is identified and a tunnel created through it to the perineum. If a rectourinary or rectovaginal fistula is present, it is divided under direct vision. Occasionally the rectum has descended close enough to the perineum to allow completion of the pull-through from the posterior approach. More commonly it is necessary to close the sacral incision, turn the patient over and perform a laparotomy to mobilize the distal colon so that it will reach the perineum without tension. The rectum is passed through the puborectalis muscle and sutured to a cruciate incision in the perineum at the site of the external sphincter fibers. Daily dilatations are started on the fourth postoperative day and continued for several weeks. The colostomy is closed two to three weeks after pull-through if healing has been satisfactory.

The relationship of anorectal malformations to the urinary tract and the incidence of urinary tract abnormalities are of paramount importance. All children with anorectal malformations should have an intravenous pyelogram. Since renal concentrating ability is poor in the neonatal period, we prefer to do a renal scan as a screening test and defer the pyelogram for three to six months. Children who require preliminary colostomy have a pyelogram just before the definitive pull-through procedure to detect abnormalities which can be corrected at the same operation and as a baseline should urinary tract complications develop postoperatively.

Major symptomatic urinary tract anomalies may need to be corrected more urgently than the anorectal malformation. Urinary tract infection due to a neurogenic bladder or anatomic abnormality is not uncommon, but infection related solely to the rectourinary fistula is rare if a totally diverting colostomy has been done. Occasionally, a large rectovesicular fistula leads to pooling of urine in the defunctionalized colon. Infection due to stasis or hyperchloremic acidosis from reabsorption of urinary chloride through the colonic mucosa may result. Early operation to divide the rectourinary fistula may be necessary.

In the best of hands, only about one-half to two-thirds of children who have high anorectal malformations have good to excellent results, and even in this group, several years of careful management may be necessary. Children who have less than good results are challenging problems, but can often be managed by some combination of dietary manipulation, stool softeners, habit toilet training, anal dilatation and rectal irrigations. Muscle transplant procedures have had only limited success in correcting incontinence. Optimal results may not be achieved for 10 to 15 years. A few patients will be served best by permanent sigmoid colostomy after other methods of treatment have failed.

Anal Fissures. Fissures are treated by warm baths and liberal doses of mineral oil. Kondremul, an emulsified preparation of mineral oil, is more palatable than plain oil. Dosage ranges from 1 to 2 teaspoons a day for infants, to 3 to 4 tablespoons a day in older children. The dose is adjusted to keep stools soft and well greased but without pure oil oozing out of the rectum. Mineral oil is continued for a week or two after the fissure heals.

Perianal and Perirectal Abscess and Fistula. Superficial abscesses are incised and drained under local anesthesia, but deep perirectal abscesses should be opened under general anesthesia to ensure adequate drainage. *Anal fistulas* which persist after drainage of an abscess are opened throughout their length, taking care to identify and open the anal or rectal end of the fistula. The lining of the sinus tract is curretted and the wound is packed open and allowed to granulate. Fistulas which appear de novo in early infancy are usually subcutaneous anal fistulas and may resolve spontaneously. If they persist more than three to four months, they should be opened and allowed to granulate.

Prolapse. Rectal prolapse is managed best by identifying and treating the underlying cause, most commonly cystic fibrosis. Prolapse is often a result of frequent passage of hard or bulky stools and can be treated with large doses of mineral oil. Prolapse in infants in diapers sometimes can be controlled by tight strapping of the buttocks after reducing the prolapse. Children who are toilet trained should be encouraged to use appropriate size potty chairs to provide proper support for the buttocks and a firm platform for the feet. Patience is indeed a virtue in the management of rectal prolapse. As long as the prolapse is reducible and not progressive, watchful waiting is indicated since the prolapse may resolve spontaneously or with the conservative measures outlined above. If the condition is progressive or does not resolve, a variety of operations are available but none is totally satisfactory.

Polyps. Gastrointestinal polyps are discussed elsewhere but are mentioned here since nearly half of all colonic polyps are within reach of the sigmoidoscope. Rectal polyps present with bleeding or prolapse, and often can be palpated by digital examination. Their presence and location are confirmed by proctoscopy in the awake child. Over 95 per cent of rectal polyps in children are of the juvenile type; excision is indicated primarily to relieve symptoms. Polypectomy is usually done under general anesthesia using an operating sigmoidoscope and an electrocautery snare to control bleeding from the stalk.

Pruritus Ani. This common problem usually can be controlled by good hygiene and avoidance of local irritation. If itching is persistent it is worthwhile to examine a fresh, early morning rectal swab for the presence of pinworms, which can be treated by a single dose of mebendazole (Vermox).*

Foreign Bodies. Most rectal foreign bodies pass spontaneously. The most common foreign body encountered in children is a broken rectal thermometer. More harm may be done by vigorous rectal examination and proctoscopy than by the glass fragments, so it is best not to attempt removal unless the fragments fail to pass or the child has persistent symptoms. Large impacted foreign bodies should be removed; general anesthesia may be necessary to achieve adequate relaxation and dilatation of the anus.

Trauma. Cursory examination often fails to reveal the full extent and complexity of anorectal injuries. The rectum is so short, especially in infants, that sticks, rectal thermometers and other pointed objects may cause intraperitoneal perforation. Unrecognized extraperitoneal perforations can also have serious consequences. The urinary tract and, in girls, the vagina, may be involved. Careful

---

*Manufacturer's precaution: Mebendazole has not been studied extensively in children under 2 years of age; therefore, the risk/benefit should be considered in the treatment of children under 2 years of age.

examination under general anesthesia may be necessary to assess the full extent of injury. If gross or microscopic hematuria is present, an intravenous pyelogram and/or voiding cystogram is done preoperatively. Rectal perforations and lacerations are repaired as accurately as possible. Pararectal drains are placed if there has been extensive contamination of the extraperitoneal pelvis. Most patients who have major rectal injuries require temporary loop colostomy to divert the fecal stream while the wounds heal. Urinary tract injuries are repaired if possible and suprapubic urinary drainage is established.

7

Blood

Anemias of Iron Deficiency, Blood Loss, Renal Disease and Chronic Infection

JOHN N. LUKENS, M.D.

IRON DEFICIENCY ANEMIA

The treatment of iron deficiency is two-fold: replenishment of body iron and correction of the factor or factors responsible for the deficiency state. Both aspects of management are necessary if recurrence is to be prevented and if occult disease is to be identified.

Iron Replacement. Iron can be given orally, intramuscularly, or intravenously. Oral iron is the safest, least expensive form of treatment, and is as effective as parenterally administered iron. There is no indication for the intravenous infusion of iron in children.

The treatment of choice for iron replenishment is ferrous sulfate. Ferrous gluconate and ferrous fumarate, while as effective, are more expensive. Numerous other iron salts, with and without adjuvants, are marketed with claims for improved palatability, enhanced absorption, or fewer side effects. Most of these preparations are therapeutically inferior to ferrous sulfate and all are more expensive. Enteric coated tablets and sustained release capsules should be avoided, as they ensure transit of iron beyond the site of maximal absorption. Convenience in the administration of ferrous sulfate is facilitated by the availability of several preparations: pediatric "drops" for infants and small children (each 0.6 ml. contains 15 mg. of elemental iron), an elixir for toddlers (each 5 ml. contains 30 mg.

of elemental iron), and tablets for older children (each tablet contains 60 mg. of elemental iron).

Iron is given in a dose of 5 mg./kg./day (25 mg. of ferrous sulfate/kg./day) to a maximum dose of 180 mg./day. More iron does not effect a more rapid recovery. The daily dose is divided into three portions and given with meals. Gastrointestinal intolerance to iron given in this manner is rarely encountered. Reversible staining of teeth is seen in all children taking oral iron; its absence is a clue of non-compliance.

Subjective improvement may be noted within a day or two after starting iron therapy: irritability is less prominent, spontaneous activity increases, pica is corrected, and appetite returns. A reticulocytosis, inversely proportional to the initial hemoglobin concentration, is noted within three to five days. Reticulocytes are maximal (5 to 10 per cent) at 5 to 10 days. The rate of hemoglobin rise is a function of the magnitude of anemia. The more severe the anemia, the greater the daily increment in hemoglobin concentration. Approximately 18 days following initiation of therapy, the hemoglobin reaches a level midway between the initial value and that which is normal. Irrespective of the severity of anemia, approximately two months are required to achieve a normal hemoglobin concentration. Full doses of iron are continued for two to three months after correction of anemia in order to provide iron reserves. Suboptimal response to iron most commonly reflects failure of iron administration, inadequate dosage, or use of an iron preparation which is poorly absorbed. Less frequently, a coexistent infection compromises marrow response to iron or ongoing blood losses obscure an appropriate marrow response. Although some deficient children have a paradoxical and reversible decrease in iron absorption, treatment failure is rarely the result of malabsorption.

Iron tablets should be dispensed in bottles equipped with safety caps. Parents are instructed to ensure inaccessibility of the tablets to small children. Because of their relatively low iron concentration, liquid preparations pose little or no risk of accidental iron poisoning.

Parenteral iron therapy is painful, expensive (relative to oral therapy), and attended by a slight but measurable risk of hypersensitivity reaction. The rate of hemoglobin rise is no greater than with iron given by mouth. Nevertheless, the intramuscular injection of iron is indicated in the face of steadfast noncompliance, inflammatory bowel disease, iron malabsorption, and intractable blood loss. Iron dextran (Imferon) is the preparation with which there is greatest experience. It contains 50 mg. of elemental iron per ml. The requisite dose may be calculated as follows:

$$\text{Iron needed (mg.)} = \text{Weight (kg.)} \times \\ \text{Desired Increment Hgb (gm./dl.)} \times 2.5$$

An additional 10 mg. of iron per kg. is given in order to assure an iron reserve. The calculated volume is given over a period of several days so as not to exceed volumes of 2 to 3 ml./day. Care is taken to deliver the preparation deep into the upper outer quadrant of the buttock. The skin and subcutaneous tissue are retracted laterally prior to insertion of the needle in order to avoid staining of the skin.

Because the response to iron is prompt and predictable, the transfusion of blood is rarely indicated. It is reserved for children whose anemia is of such severity as to produce frank or impending cardiac decompensation. In this setting, sedimented red blood cells are given as a modified exchange transfusion. Patient blood is replaced with packed red cells in 10 to 20 ml. increments. The volume of the exchange need not exceed 20 ml./kg.

Correction of Predisposing Factors. Of paramount importance is the identification and correction of factors which precipitated the iron deficiency state. Approximately 50 per cent of infants with severe iron deficiency anemia have a milk-induced enteropathy associated with occult loss of blood into the gut lumen. Most of these infants have been maintained on large volumes of whole cow's milk from early infancy. Therapeutic doses of iron, given without modification of milk consumption, fail to "turn off" the intestinal leak. In contrast, the loss of red cells and plasma proteins is effectively arrested by the substitution of a soybean formula or a heat-treated cow's milk preparation for fresh milk. Unless corrected, ongoing blood losses may obviate iron replenishment or predispose to recurrence of the deficiency state. When occult blood loss is suspected or documented in children less than five years of age, an evaporated milk preparation or a nonmilk-based formula is substituted for whole cow's milk for a span of several months.

Since milk is a poor source of iron, curtailment of milk consumption is required for all infants with nutritional iron deficiency. Nutritional counseling is provided for those of high school and college age. Search for occult disease is necessary when dealing with unexplained iron deficiency.

BLOOD LOSS ANEMIA

The management of blood loss anemia is dictated by the magnitude of hemorrhage and by the interval which has transpired since the blood loss. The needs of infants and children who have sustained massive, acute hemorrhages are different from those of patients who have experienced chronic or remote bleeds.

Acute Blood Loss. It is not until 20 per cent or more of the blood volume is lost that disturbances in circulatory dynamics occur. As a result, no therapy is required for blood losses unattended by alterations in vital signs unless recurrence of bleeding is anticipated. With losses of 30 to 40 per cent of the blood volume, all the signs and symptoms of shock are observed: peripheral perfusion is poor, the skin is moist and cool, the blood pressure and central venous pressure are low, and the heart rate is accelerated. These physical findings are of far greater value than is the hemoglobin concentration in assessing the need for therapy. Since several hours are required for plasma volume expansion, the magnitude of acute blood loss is not betrayed by alterations in the hemoglobin concentration.

The immediate need is an expansion of the blood volume, best accomplished with whole blood. If the urgency of the situation obviates the delay inherent in obtaining properly cross-matched blood, plasma or a plasma protein solution (Plasmanate) may be infused until blood is available. Approximately 20 ml./kg. of the most readily available product is given by rapid intravenous infusion. The need for subsequent infusions can best be assessed by monitoring the central venous pressure. The initial transfusion is followed by repeat infusions of 10 ml./kg. until a measurable central venous pressure is obtained and peripheral circulation is restored.

If massive volumes of blood are lost, the blood infused must be fresh in order to prevent a "washout" of platelets and selected clotting factors. Blood stored for more than 48 hours is deficient in platelets and in factor VIII. In general, coagulopathy resulting from massive blood transfusion is encountered only if more than the estimated blood volume of the recipient is replaced in a 24 hour period.

Chronic or Remote Blood Loss. The signs and symptoms of chronic or remote blood loss are those of anemia rather than hypovolemia. Because blood loss imposes a drain on iron, the anemia may have all the morphologic and biochemical hallmarks of iron deficiency.

Anemia is usually well compensated. Because volume overload is a potential problem, blood is not given. Congestive heart failure secondary to severe anemia is best managed with a small exchange transfusion (20 ml./kg.). The use of sedimented red cells instead of whole blood facilitates rapid correction of anemia and permits creation of a volume deficit. If erythropoiesis is limited by the availability of iron, a therapeutic course of iron is given (see preceding section).

ANEMIA OF RENAL DISEASE

The anemia associated with mild renal failure is not attended by significant symptoms or physiologic disturbances and requires no treatment. In contrast, the anemia associated with severe and protracted renal failure seriously limits the effectiveness of therapy. Although hemodialysis is a satisfactory substitute for the excretory function of the kidney, it has no influence on renal erythropoietic function. The primary factor responsible for anemia in chronic renal disease is deficient erythropoietin elaboration. Since erythropoietin is not available for clinical trials, treatment of the anemia is symptomatic rather than substantive.

The cornerstone of therapy for the anemia of chronic renal disease is blood transfusion. The indication for transfusion is based on a patient's symptoms rather than on an arbitrary level of hemoglobin concentration. Since transfusions enhance the hepatitis risk, contribute to iron overload, and suppress erythropoiesis, they should be avoided in the absence of symptoms. Most active children experience no significant symptoms until the hemoglobin drops below 7 to 8 gm./dl.; some tolerate hemoglobin levels of 5 to 6 gm./dl. remarkably well. If dictated by symptoms, blood is given as sedimented red cells (approximately 10 ml./kg.). Frozen, deglycerolized red cells are used for children who are potential transplant recipients so as to avoid sensitization to tissue antigens. If the symptoms attributed to anemia are corrected, transfusions are repeated as symptoms recur. In the absence of symptoms, the hemoglobin concentration is allowed to fall until it stabilizes at approximately 5 gm./dl.

Iron deficiency is a common complication of chronic hemodialysis when there is no transfusion requirement. The deficiency results from loss of blood to the dialysis apparatus. For this reason, therapeutic amounts of iron are given to dialysis patients who do not require transfusion therapy. Because folate is dialyzable, reserves of this essential nutrient may also be exhausted. Folate-limited erythropoiesis is easily prevented by giving 1 mg. of folic acid (pteroylglutamic acid) daily.

ANEMIA OF CHRONIC INFECTION

A wide variety of chronic infectious, inflammatory, and malignant states are associated with a mild anemia having well defined morphologic, kinetic, and biochemical features. The anemia is relatively mild and nonprogressive. Rarely is the hemoglobin concentration less than 8 to 10 gm./dl. The significance of the anemia is its disclosure of a major primary disease. Therapeutic efforts should be focused on the underlying disease rather than on the anemia itself. If anemia is so severe as to justify blood transfusion, additional pathogenetic mechanisms (such as iron deficiency) should be sought.

Aplastic and Hypoplastic Anemia

BLANCHE P. ALTER, M.D.

Proper therapy for bone marrow failure requires specific diagnosis. Diseases which are acquired must be distinguished from those that are congenital, and pancytopenias from failures of single cell lines. This discussion is restricted to those disorders in which pancytopenia or anemia is associated with decreased bone marrow cellularity, and in which infiltrative diseases such as leukemia have been ruled out.

ACQUIRED APLASTIC ANEMIA

Acquired aplastic anemia (pancytopenia) occurs at any age, and may be caused by toxins or by infections such as hepatitis; half the cases are classified as idiopathic. The most commonly associated toxins include ionizing radiation, alkylating agents, antimetabolites, and antibiotics used for chemotherapy. In some cases, removal of these agents may lead to return of bone marrow function. Agents which occasionally lead to pancytopenia in an idiosyncratic fashion have included chloramphenicol, benzene (e.g., airplane glue), sulfonamides, arsenicals, quinacrine, anticonvulsants, phenylbutazone, and gold. Some of these agents, in particular chloramphenicol, also lead to a dose-dependent depression of bone marrow function, which responds to withdrawal of the drug. Any toxic chemicals or drugs which might be potential causes for aplastic anemia should be eliminated from the patient's environment.

Severe aplastic anemia must be distinguished from moderate pancytopenia, because the immediate prognoses are different. Moderate cases may recover spontaneously or with drug therapy. Severe aplasia is defined as pancytopenia in which the granulocyte count is below 500/mm³, platelet count below 20,000/mm³, and corrected reticulocyte count below 1 per cent. In addition, the bone marrow aspirate and biopsy show hypocellularity, with below 25 per cent of the normal amount of cellular elements. The majority of children whose disease meets these criteria do not survive; over half die within the first six months after diagnosis. Because of the high risk of early mortality, these children should be considered candidates for bone marrow transplantation.

Bone Marrow Transplantation. Upon diagnosis of severe aplastic anemia, the patient should be placed in a laminar flow room, or isolated with reverse precautions, in order to decrease the risk of infection from outside sources. HL-A typing should be performed on the patient, parents, and siblings. If an HL-A match is found the patient should be referred to one of several centers capable of bone marrow transplant therapy. Identical twins are ideal candidates for bone marrow transplants. Although transplantation is risky and is still being developed, the outcome of early transplantation in severe aplastic anemia appears to be much better than with conventional management (see below). Transplantation is usually performed within 2 to 3 weeks of diagnosis. During that interval, patients are treated with prednisone, 10 mg./m²/day, which is used for its action in decreasing the bleeding tendency. Supportive transfusions are kept to a minimum and are restricted to single unrelated donors in order to decrease potential sensitization of the recipient to donor antigens.

Frozen washed packed red cells are used for severe anemia (hemoglobin below 6 gm./100 ml.), single donor platelets for bleeding, and white cell transfusions for severe infections. Infections are treated aggressively with appropriate antibiotics or antimycotics.

If there is an HL-A identical potential bone marrow donor, but transplantation is declined, the donor can then be used as a source of HL-A matched blood products.

Treatment with Drugs. Cases in which bone marrow transplantation is not done require proper supportive care (see below), and may be treated with drugs. In addition, children with moderate aplastic anemia may respond to these therapeutic agents. Glucocorticoids have only a minor role in the management of the aplastic patient. They do not appear to stimulate hematopoiesis, and in large doses may increase the risk of infection. They can be used in small doses to decrease the bleeding tendency. Prednisone is given at 0.25 to 0.5 mg./kg./day. In addition, prednisone may have a role in counteracting the effect of androgens on the acceleration of bone growth. Currently a collaborative study is under way which compares the outcome of transfusion, no androgens, or androgen therapy in severe aplastic anemia. The study presently indicates that androgens offer little benefit in severe aplastic anemia.

Early use of androgen therapy employed sublingual methyltestosterone, or testosterone propionate, 1 to 2 mg./kg./day. More recently, the oral androgen of choice has been oxymetholone, 3 to 6 mg./kg./day. A complication which may be related to 17α-methylated androgens such as oxymetholone has been liver disease. Cholestatic jaundice has been seen, which usually disappears when the androgen is stopped. Rare cases of usually benign hepatic tumors have been reported, as have cases of peliosis hepatis. Androgens which are not methylated in the 17α position can be used, such as 19-nortestosterone decanoate (nandrolone decanoate). These are given at 3 to 5 mg./kg. intramuscularly once a week, with cold compresses and good pressure for several minutes to prevent bleeding in thrombocytopenic patients.

In cases in which hematologic response has been thought to be due to androgens, such response takes at least two to three months, but usually much longer. The transfusion requirement declines, hemoglobin begins to rise and, months later, granulocytes appear. Platelets are the last element to respond, and often never return to normal levels. Most patients who have been thought to respond to androgen therapy can eventually discontinue medications when the hemoglobin reaches 12 gm./100 ml., although occasionally patients require the androgen, and relapse when it is stopped. Side effects of androgen therapy are those of virilization, characterized by hirsutism, deepening of the voice, enlargement of genitalia, acne, fluid retention, hypertension, and weight gain. Bone growth rate is accelerated, but the epiphyses fuse early, and thus the final height may be short.

Supportive Care. Bleeding is the most important complication of severe aplastic anemia, followed by infection, with anemia third. If small doses of prednisone (0.5 mg./kg./day) do not suffice to prevent bleeding, platelet transfusions must be employed. Platelet concentrates should be prepared from single donors. After bone marrow transplant, the donor's platelets can be used. The aim is to maintain a platelet count above 10,000/mm³ and the patient free from bleeding. One unit of platelet concentrate provides an increment of 10,000 platelets/mm³ per m². The number of platelet transfusions should be kept low, because sensitization will occur. If the latter develops, HL-A compatible platelets must be sought. In females, menses should be suppressed by the use of oral contraceptives, but breakthrough bleeding may occur. These agents are unnecessary if the patient is on androgen therapy. Drugs which impair platelet function, such as aspirin, should be scrupulously avoided. Soft toothbrushes, electric razors, and stool softeners such as Colace are used to decrease potential bleeding problems.

Efforts should be made to avoid infections. Patients should be kept out of the hospital as much as possible; when hospitalized, laminar flow or reverse isolation techniques should be utilized. Skin hygiene is maintained by Betadine bathing. Good dental care is important. If the patient has an infection, cultures of every possible source should be obtained, including blood, sputum, urine, stool, skin, and sometimes spinal fluid and bone marrow, for aerobes, anaerobes, fungi, and tubercle bacilli. Treatment of gram-positive and gram-negative organisms should be initiated with intravenous cephalothin and gentamicin until culture results are available. Enteric sources should be suppressed by the use of oral nonabsorbable antibiotics, including gentamicin, vancomycin, and Mycostatin. Rectal temperatures are not taken, and the rectal area is kept clean and free of fissures. If infection is life-threatening, white blood cells can be prepared with continuous flow centrifugation or filtration; 1 to 2.5×10^{10} granulocytes are given daily for at least 4 to 7 days.

Prior to any transfusions, complete blood typing is done in order to minimize the chance for sensitization to minor blood group antigens and to enable identification of antibodies should they develop subsequently. Frozen packed red blood cells are used to decrease the risk of sensitization to HL-A and white cell antigens and to reduce the chances of hepatitis, cytomegalovirus, or toxoplasmosis. If frozen blood is not available, packed red cells should be used to prevent volume overload. Leukopacs or washed red cells can be used to decrease the chance of reactions to white cells in the transfusions. The hemoglobin should be maintained between 7 and 10 gm./100 ml. for comfort and to keep the patient out of heart failure. Complications of multiple transfusions include sensitization to red cells, white cells, or HL-A antigens, febrile reactions, and transfusion reactions. If the patient survives long enough, iron overload is a potential problem.

Splenectomy is no longer thought to be therapeutic in aplastic anemia, except in patients with documented hypersplenism. The potential benefits of this operation must be balanced against the risk of overwhelming sepsis occurring in a splenectomized patient with no granulocytes who is on androgen and glucocorticoid therapy. Prophylactic penicillin, 125 to 250 mg. twice daily, is used to prevent pneumococcal sepsis.

There is as yet no specific cure for severe acquired aplastic anemia. While bone marrow transplantation appears to be promising, it is complicated and risky and only available for those patients with appropriately matched donors. Successful management of both transplanted and nontransplanted patients depends on the excellence of supportive care for bleeding, infection, and anemia, so that the patient survives these early complications until the transplant is engrafted, the disease remits spontaneously, or androgens have the opportunity to be effective.

CONGENITAL APLASTIC ANEMIA

In congenital aplastic anemia associated with characteristic physical abnormalities, termed Fanconi's anemia, the onset of pancytopenia usually occurs between ages 4 and 11, although it can begin at birth or as late as the third decade. Treatment depends on the symptoms. If bleeding is the problem, it may be controlled with low doses of prednisone, 0.25 to 0.5 mg./kg./day. Anemia may respond to androgen therapy as outlined above for acquired aplastic anemia. Problems with infection due to low white counts usually are not seen early in the course of these patients as outlined above for acquired aplastic anemia.

Those patients whose hemoglobin and perhaps other blood counts rise on androgen treatment usually relapse if the drug is stopped. Often the high doses which are employed initially can be decreased to a maintenance level. Because patients with this disease often do respond initially to androgens, bone marrow transplant is not considered until or unless the patient is refractory to a variety of androgen preparations. By this time, multiple red cell and platelet transfusions have been given, leading to sensitization and thus increasing the challenge of bone marrow transplantation. As this technique becomes more readily available, patients with Fanconi's anemia should be considered for transplant before they have been sensitized by multiple transfusions. However, many patients will do well on androgen or sometimes on no treatment for long periods of time, and the ultimate outcome of this disease remains unpredictable.

Other forms of congenital or familial aplastic anemia are those in which several family members have pancytopenia, but lack the physical abnormalities which characterize Fanconi's anemia. The treatment for these patients is the same as for others with pancytopenia: consideration for bone marrow transplant coupled with proper supportive care and androgen trial. Another form of congenital disease is amegakaryocytic thrombocytopenia, in which low platelet counts at birth do not improve, and which progresses to aplasia. The approach is as outlined above.

CONGENITAL PURE RED CELL APLASIA

This disease, commonly known as Diamond-Blackfan anemia but originally termed congenital hypoplastic anemia, begins in infancy or early childhood and is characterized by anemia only. The bone marrow shows a marked depression in erythroblasts with an otherwise normal appearance. At least 80 per cent of the children with this disorder respond dramatically to treatment with prednisone. Initial therapy is 2 mg./kg./day given in 3 or 4 divided doses. The reticulocyte count will rise within one to three weeks, and the hemoglobin will also rise. Although the hemoglobin may not reach normal levels, the transfusion requirement will disappear. When the hemoglobin has reached 10 gm./100 ml. or has plateaued, the prednisone dose is changed to 4 mg./kg. as a single dose on alternate days, and then tapered over several weeks. The aim is to maintain a hemoglobin above 10 gm./100 ml. Often these children can be tapered to 5 or 10 mg. of prednisone every other day. Some patients require much higher doses and a compromise is reached between hemoglobin

level and prednisone dose. A hemoglobin above 8 gm./100 ml. is sufficient to prevent symptoms of anemia if the prednisone dose is too high otherwise. The mild anemia will raise the level of diphosphoglycerate and promote oxygen release from hemoglobin. Thus a low hemoglobin level will be tolerated.

The major long-term side effect of prednisone has been growth retardation. In some children, prednisone can be given three days a week or even once a week. Some patients can be treated daily for one week out of every three, with less growth retardation. This regimen is not effective in those whose reticulocyte response occurs slowly. Patients who fail to respond to prednisone may respond to prednisolone in equivalent doses. The side effects of high-dose corticosteroids include obesity, moon facies, buffalo hump neck, hypertension, diabetes and growth retardation. Other side effects of long-term steroids have been occasional cataracts which have not been progressive, and osteoporosis.

Patients who fail to respond to steroids can be given a combination of steroid and androgen, as described above for aplastic anemia. Rarely, responses have been seen. As in aplastic anemia, splenectomy has been useful only if severe hypersplenism occurred, and deaths from overwhelming sepsis have occurred following this operation.

Children who do not respond to steroids can be supported by transfusions with all the precautions outlined above. Since their white blood cell and platelet counts are normal (the latter may even be elevated), their major problem is anemia and chronic transfusions. This leads to all the potential complications given above, particularly iron overload. Chelation with intramuscular desferrioxamine is the only treatment currently available, but more effective or alternative routes for desferrioxamine are becoming established.

Bone marrow transplantation has theoretical application in resistant cases, although there has been reluctance to submit a child with normal white cells and platelets to total marrow ablation. As in Fanconi's anemia, patients are usually not considered for transplant until they have been multiply transfused and probably sensitized. As the results of transplantation improve, this approach may change.

Rare spontaneous remissions can occur, either after several years of transfusion (16 in one case) or following prednisone therapy.

ACQUIRED PURE RED CELL APLASIA

Rarely, cases have occurred due to autoimmune hemolytic anemia. These may respond to prednisone, immunosuppressants, or splenectomy. Cases have also been reported due to drugs such as anticonvulsants. These may improve upon removal of the drug. The adult form of red cell aplasia is often due to a serum inhibitor of erythropoiesis, although this has not been demonstrated in children. These patients usually fail to respond to prednisone, but may do well on immunosuppressants such as cyclophosphamide, often combined with splenectomy.

TRANSIENT ERYTHROBLASTOPENIA OF CHILDHOOD

These children have red cell aplasia, sometimes following a viral illness. The onset is often later than in children with Diamond-Blackfan anemia. Children with the transient disease recover spontaneously, requiring transfusion only if the hemoglobin is below 6 gm./100 ml. If prednisone is used because of the concern that the child has Diamond-Blackfan anemia, the response may be dramatically swift, with elevation in reticulocytes within a week, and rapid restoration of a normal hemoglobin level. This level is maintained when the steroid is discontinued, which can be done rapidly since therapy should be continued for only 2 or 3 weeks.

THE FUTURE

New forms of treatment may develop from current studies in which red cell aplasia and pancytopenias are being investigated for serum or cellular factors which inhibit erythropoiesis and hematopoiesis. If antibodies or "killer cells" are etiologic in these disorders, better modes of immunosuppressive therapy can be designed.

Megaloblastic Anemia

BERTIL E. GLADER, Ph.D., M.D.

Megaloblastic anemias in children are relatively uncommon. Most cases are due to folate deficiency. Rarely vitamin B_{12} deficiency is responsible. The causes of folate deficiency include inadequate diet, decreased absorption due to intestinal disease, drug-induced inhibition of dietary folate absorption (phenytoin, phenobarbital), increased folate utilization (hemolytic anemias), and drug-induced inhibition of folate metabolism (methotrexate, pyrimethamine). The causes of vitamin B_{12} deficiency include dietary insufficiency (rare), absence or abnormality of gastric intrinsic factor, abnormal absorption of the vitamin B_{12}-intrinsic factor complex due to previous small intestinal surgery or lack of intestinal receptors

(rare), and inherited abnormalities of vitamin B_{12} transport proteins.

In certain areas of the world, disorders such as kwashiorkor produce megaloblastic anemia associated with multiple deficiencies. In the United States, however, megaloblastic anemia generally is due to specific deficiencies in folate or vitamin B_{12}. The metabolism of these two vitamins is interrelated, however, and this must be considered when therapy is instituted. Large doses of vitamin B_{12} may correct the hematologic problems due to folate deficiency. Conversely, large doses of folate may correct the hematologic disturbances due to lack of vitamin B_{12}. Folate, however, will not correct the neurologic problem associated with vitamin B_{12} deficiency.

In cases of suspected folate deficiency, a therapeutic trial can be instituted with 50 to 100 μg. of folate per day orally. This dose produces a prompt reticulocytosis in cases of folate deficiency, but is without effect in patients with vitamin B_{12} deficiency. Once the response to folate is established, full therapeutic dosages of folate (0.5 to 1.0 mg. per day orally) are employed. These doses are in large excess of the adult minimal daily requirement (50 μg./day). Commercially available preparations include tablets (0.5 and 1.0 mg.) and an elixir (1.0 mg./ml.). Parenteral preparations also are available but are used only under conditions where the underlying pathology prevents using oral folate. Even in patients with severe malabsorption, folic acid tablets generally correct the anemia. The therapeutic response to folic acid is heralded by reticulocytosis which is maximal in 4 to 7 days.

The duration of therapy depends on the underlying pathology. In patients with chronic hemolytic disorders, folate should be continued throughout life. In cases of dietary insufficiency or malabsorption, folate should be continued for 3 months after the hemoglobin returns to normal and the underlying problem is rectified. Megaloblastic anemia due to inhibition of dietary folate (polyglutamate) absorption responds rapidly to folic acid (monoglutamate) therapy. There is no need to discontinue offending drugs such as phenobarbital or phenytoin. Children receiving drugs which are folic acid antagonists (methotrexate, pyrimethamine) occasionally develop megaloblastic anemia. In these cases the antagonism can be overcome by folinic acid, one 5 mg. tablet daily.

Patients with suspected vitamin B_{12} deficiency are given a therapeutic trial with 25 to 100 μg. of vitamin B_{12}. This dose corrects the hematologic problem due to this vitamin deficiency, but will not correct the defect in folate-deficient patients. The reticulocyte response to this therapy is similar to that noted in folate deficiency. Once a definite response is noted, monthly vitamin B_{12} injections (200 to 1000 μg.) are started and continued throughout life.

Megaloblastic anemia develops insidiously, and children with folate or vitamin B_{12} deficiency frequently are anemic out of proportion to their clinical symptoms. This relative lack of symptomatology occurs because of intraerthrocytic and cardiovascular compensatory adjustments to the slow decrease in hemoglobin. In view of this physiological adaptation and because the response to appropriate therapy is rapid, blood transfusions rarely are necessary. The indications for red blood cell transfusions are infection or incipient heart failure. For unknown reasons the bone marrow frequently is refractory to hematinic therapy during infections. When transfusions are indicated, packed red blood cells should be given at a very slow rate (2 ml./kg./hr.).

Failure of specific vitamin therapy to achieve a complete hematologic response may indicate other coexisting problems such as iron deficiency. The lack of any response to folate or vitamin B_{12} may indicate the wrong diagnosis. Consideration then should be given to the other rare causes of megaloblastic anemia, including those due to primary bone marrow failure.

Hemolytic Anemia

PHILIP LANZKOWSKY, M.D.

A diagnosis of hemolytic anemia may be suggested by the family history, the development of anemia following exposure to drugs, the presence of splenomegaly, anemia, reticulocytosis, or by the red cell morphology of a blood smear. The first step in the investigation of hemolytic anemia is to confirm that hemolysis is occurring. Additional tests should then be carried out in order to determine whether the hemolytic anemia is due to corpuscular (membrane, hemoglobin or enzyme) or extracorpuscular (immune or nonimmune) defects. Following this the precise cause of the hemolytic anemia has to be determined.

CORPUSCULAR HEMOLYTIC ANEMIAS

Membrane Defects

Hereditary Spherocystosis. In the newborn, hereditary spherocytosis may present with unconjugated indirect-reacting hyper-

bilirubinemia, anemia, reticulocytosis, spherocytosis on the blood smear, a negative Coombs' test and frequently a positive family history. During this stage, an *exchange transfusion* might be required if the unconjugated bilirubin level approaches or exceeds 20 mg./100 ml. Occasionally, conjugated direct-reacting hyperbilirubinemia might occur in the newborn with hereditary spherocytosis (as well as in other causes of congenital or acquired hemolytic anemia). This occurs when the amount of bilirubin being conjugated exceeds the cell's excretory capacity. Histologic studies have shown hepatocellular necrosis and giant-cell transformation. The cause of the cellular damage is unknown but anemia and hypoxemia have been implicated. Its recognition is important and no treatment is required as it is a self-limiting condition.

During the first year or so of life continuous hemolysis may not be compensated for by increased marrow activity sufficient to maintain the hemoglobin level, and the hemoglobin level may fall to levels lower than 7.0 gm./dl. Under these conditions *leukocyte depleted red cell transfusions* may be required.

Splenectomy in hereditary spherocytosis is carried out in order to prevent crises of transient erythroblastopenia, persistent hyperbilirubinemia, hyperhemolytic crises, the formation of gallstones and its complications and rarely hemochromatosis. It should be done before 10 years of age since the incidence of gallstones increases considerably after 10 years of age. The precise age of splenectomy in any individual patient may vary depending upon the briskness of the hemolytic disease. In general, splenectomy is avoided in the first 5 years of life because of the increased risks at younger ages of overwhelming post-splenectomy infection.

Continuous unconjugated hyperbilirubinemia and excessive hemolysis during the first years of life might be an indication for early splenectomy since the continuous load of bilirubin may result in the formation of gallstones early. Early splenectomy might avoid the additional need for cholecystectomy for cholelithiasis in these cases. A cholecystogram should always be carried out before splenectomy to exclude the presence of asymptomatic gallstones. Following splenectomy, children should be maintained on prophylactic penicillin, 250 mg. twice daily, in order to prevent overwhelming post-splenectomy infection.

Erythroblastopenic crises occur in hereditary spherocytosis prior to splenectomy occasionally following viral infections. During these crises the hemoglobin may rapidly fall in a matter of a day or two to extremely low and even dangerously low levels requiring leukocyte depleted packed cell transfusions. Since this may happen to a number of siblings in the same family at the same time, once an erythroblastopenic crisis occurs in one member of the family, other members with hereditary spherocytosis (nonsplenectomized) should be kept under close hematologic surveillance. Following the crises, there is increased red cell formation and supplementary folic acid is required to prevent temporary megaloblastosis.

Prophylactic *folic acid,* 5 mg./week orally, should be given to all patients with chronic hemolytic disease because of the rapid red cell turnover leading to increased folic acid requirements.

Hereditary Elliptocytosis. Only 10 per cent of patients with elliptocytosis have evidence of clinical hemolysis, and treatment for the morphologic findings of elliptocytosis without evidence of hemolytic disease is not required. Indications for transfusion, splenectomy and prophylactic folic acid in the treatment of elliptocytosis with hemolytic anemia are the same as for hereditary spherocytosis.

Hereditary Stomatocytosis. A few syndromes have been associated with this morphologic finding, but few patients have benefited from splenectomy. Some patients require periodic transfusion in early childhood because of anemia.

Infantile Pyknocytosis. This is a transient hemolytic anemia in the newborn associated with the presence of unconjugated hyperbilirubinemia, anemia, pyknocytes in the blood smear, reticulocytosis and splenomegaly. It is a self-limiting disorder due to both corpuscular and extracorpuscular factors. Treatment of this condition is exchange transfusion when the level of unconjugated indirect-reacting bilirubin reaches 20 mg./100 ml. during the newborn period.

Enzymatic Defects

More than 20 different red cell enzyme deficiencies have been described and 18 of them have been associated with acute or chronic hemolysis. They may present in the newborn period as a Coombs' negative hemolytic anemia with marked unconjugated indirect-reacting hyperbilirubinemia necessitating exchange transfusion (e.g., glucose-6-phosphate dehydrogenase, 6 phophogluconic dehydrogenase, glutathione peroxidase, 2,3-diphosphoglycerate mutase, hexokinase, glucosephosphate isomerase, triosphosphate isomerase and pyruvate kinase) or may present later as a nonspherocytic hemolytic anemia.

The severity of hemolysis in the neonate varies with the specific enzymatic defect (qualitative and quantitative), with gestational age, exposure to certain drugs or chemicals and with intercurrent infections. Some infants with red cell enzyme deficiencies do not exhibit manifestations during the neonatal period.

If the nonspherocytic hemolytic anemia due to red cell enzyme deficiency is associated with significant anemia and/or hyperbilirubinemia, a splenectomy may be required. Although improvement may follow splenectomy the degree of improvement varies with the enzyme deficiency and from patient to patient with the same enzyme deficiency. Since G-6-PD and pyruvate kinase deficiency are by far the commonest causes, they are singled out for more detailed comment.

G-6-PD Deficiency. The most common enzymatic defect is G-6-PD deficiency, a sex-linked disorder. The disorder noted in blacks (A-variant) is milder than in Caucasians (B-variant). G-6-PD deficiency produces an acute hemolytic anemia which is usually drug-induced and the Caucasian variant may be associated with a chronic nonspherocytic hemolytic anemia. Hemolysis may occur without drug exposure in such diverse conditions as viral pneumonia, diabetic acidosis and hepatitis. Hemolysis is usually self-limited, but if the hemoglobin falls to low levels transfusion therapy may be required. In an acute hemolytic episode a blood transfusion from a donor with normal G-6-PD activity is indicated and the offending drug should be removed. Hydration and urinary output should be monitored because of marked hemoglobinuria and the potential for renal shutdown.

Pyruvate Kinase Deficiency. The clinical severity of this disorder varies from an extremely mild hemolytic anemia to a severe disorder that makes the patient transfusion-dependent. Neonatal manifestations are frequent and severe, including death in utero from hydrops fetalis to severe unconjugated hyperbilirubinemia requiring an exchange transfusion. If repeated red cell transfusions are required because of chronic nonspherocytic hemolytic anemia, splenectomy may significantly ameliorate the severity of the hemolytic anemia and decrease or eliminate the transfusion requirement.

Hemoglobin Defects

Congenital Erythropoietic Porphyria. This is a rare inborn error of porphyrin metabolism and heme synthesis. Clinically photosensitivity, hemolytic anemia and splenomegaly occur. Treatment consists of protection from the sun and the avoidance of drugs such as phenobarbital, which may precipitate or aggravate the metabolic disorder. Splenectomy may be required when symptomatic hypersplenism occurs.

EXTRACORPUSCULAR HEMOLYTIC ANEMIA

Immune Hemolytic Anemia

Autoimmune Hemolytic Anemia. Autoimmune hemolytic anemia might be idiopathic or secondary to a number of conditions. Treatment is directed toward the hemolytic anemia and the underlying disease when such a disease is identified. When hemolytic anemia is drug-induced, cessation of drug therapy will correct the hemolytic anemia. In connective tissue disorders corticosteroid therapy for the hemolytic process may be all that is necessary. If the underlying condition is an ovarian cyst, teratoma or dermoid, surgical treatment is indicated. Treatment of underlying hematologic disease or lymphoma may require chemotherapy and radiotherapy.

Autoimmune hemolytic anemia may be associated with warm- or cold-acting antibodies. *Warm antibodies* (IgG 7S) are active at 37° C., attach to erythrocytes, are usually present in serum and frequently are panagglutinins or Rh specific. They are detected by gamma Coombs' serum and usually occur without an underlying process. They generally respond well to therapy and have a more favorable prognosis. *Cold antibodies* (IgM, 19S), on the other hand, are active below 32° C., attach complement to erythrocytes and are frequently I or i specific. They are detected by nongamma (anti-complement) Coombs' serum and usually are associated with an underlying disease process. Occasionally both IgG and complement coat the red cells. They are detected by broad spectrum Coombs' serum and usually occur when an underlying disease process is present.

The following parameters should be carefully monitored in all cases of autoimmune hemolytic anemia: hemoglobin level, reticulocyte count, Coombs' test, haptoglobin level, urine for hemoglobinuria, and splenic size.

Autoimmune Hemolytic Anemia Due to Warm Antibodies. This illness can be severe and life-threatening and the hemoglobin level may rapidly fall to very low levels. The clinician has to cope with a rapidly dropping hematocrit and an absence of compatible blood allowing safe transfusions. In this urgent setting rapid and appropriate decisions are necessary in order to develop a plan of treatment. Blood transfusions, steroids and splenectomy are the most important modalities of treatment.

BLOOD TRANSFUSIONS. Before blood transfusion the specificity of the antibody should be determined in order to aid in donor selection. An attempt to elute antibody from the patient's red cell should be made so that it may be tested against a panel of donor erythrocytes by the indirect antiglobulin technique. If a specific antibody is identified, compatible donors may be selected. However, the antibody usually behaves as a panagglutinin and reacts with all donor cells tested and no totally compatible blood can be found. When this occurs, cross-match donors known to be compatible with the patient's major blood group and Rh type and select those donors whose erythrocytes show the least agglutination in the patient's serum. Thereafter, a biological cross-match should be done by transfusing a small volume of blood and carefully monitoring the patient for one or two hours for signs of increased hemolysis (hemoglobinemia or hemoglobinuria or profound fall in hemoglobin level). If no reaction ensues, transfusion should proceed. Washed, packed red cells should be used for transfusions after plasma and leukocytes have been removed from the blood. The volume of transfused blood should be of sufficient quantity to relieve any cardiopulmonary embarrassment caused by the anemia.

Heroic efforts at correcting the hemoglobin to normal levels should not be attempted; only small amounts of serologically incompatible blood should be used at any one time. This will prevent adverse effects should the transfused blood be rapidly destroyed. In our experience the use of such poorly matched blood is made relatively safe by doing the biological cross-match, transfusing relatively small volumes of blood at a given time and the concomitant use of high dosage corticosteroid therapy. Often the hemolytic process is brisk and transfusions might be required as frequently as 8 to 12 hourly.

CORTICOSTEROID THERAPY. This is the mainstay of treatment of autoimmune hemolytic anemia. There appears to be no selective benefit of the various corticosteroid preparations. Hydrocortisone, 240 mg./day in divided doses, should be administered intravenously, or prednisone, 60 mg./day, should be employed orally before the transfusion is started. In children under 4 years of age the hydrocortisone dosage should be reduced to 160 mg./day, and prednisone dosage to 40 mg./day. This high dosage corticosteroid therapy should be maintained for several days if the hemolytic process is very active. Thereafter, corticosteroid therapy in the form of prednisone should be slowly tapered over a 3 to 4 week period. The dose of prednisone should be tailored to maintain the hemoglobin at a reasonable level and when the hemoglobin stabilizes, the corticosteroids should be discontinued.

The following schedule of steroid therapy has been found to be useful in our hands. Initially, either hydrocortisone, 240 mg./day intravenously, or prednisone, 60 mg./day, is used. As soon as a demonstrable response (clinically, hematocrit, reticulocyte count) is observed, the dose of prednisone is reduced by 15 mg./day every week. Recurrence of hemolysis using this type of regimen is usually gradual and readily recognized. The corticosteroid dosage should then be increased and more gradual reduction attempted. While the response to therapy is sometimes dramatic, hematologic improvement may not become evident before the third or fourth day, with a median response of 7 days.

Eighty per cent of patients with the idiopathic form of the disease have a favorable response. The onset of the response is commonly heralded by a transient paradoxical rise in reticulocyte count, followed by a gradual rise in hematocrit and hemoglobin and a fall in reticulocyte count and other signs of hemolysis. Lack of response for 21 days should be considered a steroid failure and other modalities should be considered. Responses after 21 days are occasionally observed but are incomplete and usually require persistent high dosage corticosteroids to maintain a marginal response. The Coombs' test may remain persistently positive for months in the absence of clinical evidence of hemolytic anemia. A persistently positive Coombs' test in an asymptomatic patient is not an indication to continue corticosteroid therapy.

SPLENECTOMY. Splenectomy may be beneficial in some patients. Splenectomy is indicated if the hemolytic process continues to be brisk despite high dosage corticosteroid or is nonresponsive to corticosteroid therapy for three to four weeks, and frequent packed cell transfusions are necessary to maintain a reasonable hemoglobin level. The results of splenectomy are usually beneficial but unpredictable. Although by no means absolute, children with marked splenic and little hepatic sequestration of ^{51}Cr-labeled erythrocytes have warm compared with cold antibodies, a palpable spleen, and incomplete antibodies are more likely to respond favorably to splenectomy.

ANTIMETABOLITES. Azathioprine, 6-mercaptopurine, chlorambucil and cyclophosphamide have been used with variable success but their use has not been completely evaluated nor are there any studies to indicate preference of the immunosuppressive agents. This type of therapy should only be used in patients refractory to steroids and splenectomy. The incidence of a good response with cytotoxic drugs is about 45 per cent.

Thymectomy has been resorted to in desperate cases of autoimmune hemolytic anemia with some success. *Heparin* has been useful in some patients but its value as a practical measure of therapy remains uncertain.

The treatment of autoimmune hemolytic anemia requires skill and judgment as to the frequency of transfusions and the time of splenectomy in any individual case.

Autoimmune Hemolytic Anemia Due to Cold Antibodies. This disease may be idiopathic but is more frequently seen in conjunction with infections such as mycoplasma and less commonly with lymphoproliferative disorders. Although present in high titers, they rarely cause clinical hemolysis unless active in the physiologic temperature range. Treatment consists of control of the underlying disorder. Transfusions may be necessary and again identification of compatible blood may prove difficult. Warming of the blood to 37° C. during administration by means of a heating coil or water bath is indicated to avoid further temperature activation of antibody. There are efficient "in-line" blood warmers (McGaw Water Bath, Fenwall Dry Heat Warmer) available today designed to deliver blood at 37° C. to the patient. Unmonitored or uncontrolled heating of blood is extremely dangerous and should not be attempted. Red cells heated too much are rapidly destroyed in vivo and can be lethal to the patient.

If the anemia is severe, a trial of *cytotoxic drug therapy* is appropriate. Alkylating agents such as cyclophosphamide and chlorambucil may be capable of lowering the titer of cold agglutinins and, less commonly, reduce the degree of hemolysis. Corticosteroids have not been demonstrated to be effective, although we have had occasional success with this treatment. *Plasmapheresis* is a valuable approach in the management of autoimmune hemolytic anemia due to cold antibodies and is a method to reduce the level of cold agglutinins. If the blood is obtained at 37° C., with the patient's arm warmed by hot pads, the warm unit can be separated quickly by centrifugation and the red cells can be returned to the patient through an efficient in-line blood warmer.

Paroxysmal Nocturnal Hemoglobinuria. Paroxysmal nocturnal hemoglobinuria is a rare disease characterized by a defect of red cell membrane protein resulting in intravascular lysis of red cells leading to hemoglobinemia, hemoglobinuria and hemosiderinuria coupled with deficient and defective hematopoiesis. It may present as a hemolytic anemia and hemoglobinuria exacerbated during sleep, a chronic unexplained hemolytic anemia or as an aplastic or hypoplastic anemia with or without leukopenia and/or thrombocytopenia. The diagnosis is made by the acid Ham or the sucrose lysis test.

Treatment in this condition consists of transfusion with washed erythrocytes as needed to maintain an adequate hemoglobin level. Prednisone in high doses, 60 mg./day, can ameliorate hemolysis abruptly by means which are not clear. The dose should be rapidly reduced to the dose needed to maintain adequate hemoglobin levels or to prevent hemolysis. Beneficial effects have been reported with the use of warfarin sodium (Coumadin) derivatives for thrombotic episodes but they do not alter hemolysis. Androgen therapy has been recommended for the marrow hypoplasia. Iron therapy for the accompanying iron deficiency is recommended but it may precipitate bouts of increased hemolysis.

Paroxysmal Cold Hemoglobinuria. In this condition hemoglobinuria recurs upon exposure to cold or the patient may have a chronic mild hemolytic anemia without influence by cold exposure. This may accompany viral exanthems such as measles, mumps, chickenpox and infectious mononucleosis, and rarely syphilis. The diagnosis is made by the demonstration of the presence of the Donath-Landsteiner antibody which is an IgG cold-reacting antibody with the unique ability to lyse red cells directly, an action mediated by complement and one which explains the hemoglobinuria and hemoglobinemia. The autologous cold-warm hemolysins of paroxysmal cold hemoglobinuria reacts with all human red cells except the rare blood type Tj (a-). The patient should be kept in a warm environment and pre-warmed packed cell transfusions should be administered when required. In the usual case in which the antibody for paroxysmal cold hemoglobinuria shows anti-Tj[a] activity, the use of Tj (a-) red cells should correct anemia without risk of lysis. Frozen-thawed red cells are optimal for this task because there is no accompanying native plasma with its content of naturally occurring anti-Tj[a] antibodies. Prednisone appears to benefit patients with autoimmune paroxysmal cold hemoglobinuria.

Nonimmune Hemolytic Anemia

This group of conditions is due to extracorpuscular causes of hemolytic anemia in which the antiglobulin (Coombs') test is negative. Those caused by various infections, drugs and underlying hematologic disease respond to the treatment of the underlying condition, as well as the necessary acute supportive care.

Traumatic Hemolysis. Mechanical hemolysis secondary to prosthetic heart surgery may require surgical repair or replacement of the prosthesis. Iron deficiency anemia may develop when long-standing iron loss in the urinary tract has occurred.

Hemolytic-Nephropathic Syndrome. The management of renal failure is the most important element in treatment, and peritoneal dialysis is invaluable in the treatment of renal failure. Peritoneal dialysis may be required daily for several weeks in severe cases. Transfusions of platelet concentrates and packed red cells are indicated as adjuncts in therapy for severe thrombocytopenia with bleeding manifestations and in order to correct marked anemia. In patients with clear-cut clinical and laboratory evidence of disseminated intravascular coagulation, heparin has been advocated but it should only be used in those cases in which progressive disseminated intravascular coagulation can be demonstrated. We have recently observed beneficial results from aspirin, 1 gr. per year of age daily and dipyridamole, 2 mg./kg. orally daily.* These drugs impair platelet function by inhibiting platelet aggregation and have resulted in a rise in the platelet count in 24 hours in some cases. Recently hyperuricemia has been observed to be present in the hemolytic-uremic syndrome, and when uric acid levels are high allopurinol may be employed. If the patient is on dialysis the uric acid levels return to normal following dialysis.

Thalassemia

ANDREAS ATHANASIOU, M.D., *and*
THOMAS F. NECHELES, M.D.

The thalassemia syndromes are a heterogeneous group of genetically determined hypochromic anemias characterized by a quantitative inability to synthesize the protein portion of the hemoglobin molecule. The clinically significant forms can be classified into the β

---

*This use of dipyridamole is not mentioned in the manufacturer's directive.

(beta) and α (alpha) forms depending upon the specific polypeptide chain that is deficient. Each of these variants can be further subclassified into minor (heterozygous) and major (homozygous) forms. Clinically recognizable intermediate forms are occasionally seen, the vast majority of which represent the βδ variant of the disease. Hemoglobin H disease is related to the α-thalassemia variant. Although most commonly associated with people of Italian or Greek ancestry, thalassemia is not uncommon in Southeast Asia, the Middle East, India and Africa, and scattered cases have been reported in Northern Europe.

β-Thalassemia Minor. This is usually a subclinical syndrome with hemoglobin levels 1 to 3 grams below the normal level for age, often associated with a mild reticulocytosis. Clinical attention should be focused on the differentiation from other hypochromic anemias and on genetic counseling of the affected individual. Individuals with thalassemia minor are refractory to iron therapy, and the prolonged administration of iron-containing hematinics can be potentially harmful. The mild anemia sometimes observed in these patients is asymptomatic and cannot be held responsible for chronic fatigue. Aggravation of the mild anemia is usually associated with pregnancy and infection, the former by placing an increased stress on the erythropoietic system and the latter by suppressing erythropoiesis. Even with pregnancy the hemoglobin concentration rarely drops below 8 or 9 gm./100 ml. and transfusions are virtually never required. The genetic predictability of the disease on the basis of its simple mendelian inheritance makes genetic counseling a powerful tool in the prevention of homozygous disease.

Thalassemia Major (Cooley's Anemia, Mediterranean Anemia). This is a severe erythroblastic anemia requiring, in the great majority of patients, repeated transfusions for survival. Anemia is usually noted in the second portion of the first year of life and the patient frequently requires the first transfusion at this time. It is important to obtain a pretransfusion blood sample for complete blood typing, including the minor subgroups. If possible, blood typing of patient and both parents should be carried out at one of the major blood grouping laboratories. Information obtained at this time may prove to be invaluable at a later date when minor group incompatibilities complicate transfusion therapy. The use of washed-packed or frozen red cells may often circumvent the allergic and febrile reactions presumably due to antibodies against leukocytes and plasma proteins. Common practice

has been to transfuse blood at the hemoglobin level at which the patient develops shortness of breath, fatigue and tachycardia. After the initial transfusion, additional blood is not given until hemoglobin level drops to about 1 gm./100 ml. above this level (usually in the neighborhood of 7 to 8 gm./100 ml.).

During the last 8 to 10 years the practice of maintaining the hemoglobin at a level of about 10 gm./100 ml. by regular transfusion, usually every 3 to 4 weeks, has been evaluated by many major medical centers throughout the world. The aim of such treatment is directed toward minimizing the effects of ineffective erythropoiesis as related to skeletal changes and growth and development, as well as to improving the general well-being of the affected individual. Patients maintained on such a program show increased exercise tolerance, improvement in cardiovascular function and, in the younger child, marked improvement in growth and development. Most patients treated with such an intensive transfusion program are able to lead a relatively normal life. A problem inherent in this approach is the accumulation of excessive iron deposition in vital organs and the development of generalized hemochromatosis usually in the latter part of the second decade of life. It is estimated that in a 10 year period of intensive transfusion therapy, more than 50 gm. of elemental iron are offered for excretion and storage, not counting increased amounts of iron absorbed by the gastrointestinal tract. The excretory capacity of the kidney in thalassemic patients is no more than 3.5 gm. during the same time period, an amount about 10 times that seen in normal individuals.

Irreversible congestive heart failure often associated with arrhythmias, polyendocrine deficiencies and malabsorption constitute the hallmarks of hemochromatosis associated with chronic hypoxia. The development of congestive heart failure is an ominous sign and the usual supportive measures including digitalis and diuretics are only palliative. At least 50 per cent of patients are dead within a year after the onset of cardiac symptomatology.

The pathophysiology of the multiple endocrine deficiencies is as yet not clear and the management difficult. Hypogonadism is usually the first to appear, with low estrogen and testosterone levels. Replacement therapy with estrogens and testosterone appears justifiable although clinical information regarding the efficacy of such an approach is unclear and mostly anecdotal. Growth retardation with normal growth hormone levels in the serum has been linked to somatomedin deficiency, a hormone generated in the liver. Replacement therapy with this hormone has not been tried thus far. Variable deficiencies of the adrenal-pituitary axis are seen; they are likely to be subclinical and treatment is not usually required. The vast majority of thalassemics develop abnormal glucose tolerance during the course of their disease, and a large number of them manifest frank diabetes mellitus. Diabetes is usually insulin-dependent; large doses are often required and optimal control of the disease is at times difficult. Pancreatic exocrine deficiency is manifested by symptoms of malabsorption. Pancreatic enzyme preparations (Viokase, 4 tablets before meals) and dietetic manipulations usually provide symptomatic relief.

Liver function abnormalities are seen in the majority of hemochromatotic thalassemics, and liver biopsy often reveals early cirrhotic changes. Caution should be exercised in dealing with hepatotoxic medications and agents, and periodic liver function tests are advisable.

The use of desferrioxamine B and DTPA as chelating agents on a daily intramuscular basis, originally thought to be promising, did not significantly postpone the onset of symptomatic hemochromatosis, and mortality patterns remained essentially unchanged. Ascorbic acid alone, given by mouth, increases iron excretion only marginally. More intensive desferrioxamine B regimens using continuous intravenous infusion are currently under investigation. There is preliminary evidence that prolonged chelation therapy can improve cardiac and liver function.

Congestive heart failure may be seen in the younger child who inadvertently receives too much blood too rapidly. (In general, individual blood transfusion in young children should be limited to 10 ml. packed red cells per kg. of body weight administered over a four hour period). Congestive failure under these circumstances usually responds rapidly to the administration of digitalis and/or diuretics, and in itself carries no poor prognosis. Another cardiac complication frequently seen in thalassemia major is pericarditis. The cause is unknown and the treatment is entirely supportive. Most episodes are self-limited but recurrences are frequent. The use of adrenocortical steroids appears to offer no distinct benefit and the side effects in terms of increased osteoporosis and increased susceptibility to infection outweigh any beneficial effects. Pericardiocentesis should be carried out whenever an effusion is sufficiently large to cause hemodynamic symptoms, and may at times be life-saving. The advent of hypertransfusion programs may have reduced the incidence of this complication.

Splenomegaly usually becomes prominent during the first decade of life and may lead to several complications: mechanical displacement of the stomach with anorexia and abdominal discomfort, and hypersplenism with a progressive increase in transfusion requirements frequently associated with mild thrombocytopenia and at times leukopenia. Splenectomy at this time usually reduces the frequency of necessary transfusions and corrects both thrombocytopenia and symptoms of mechanical displacement. Splenectomy is not, however, without hazards. A number of well documented studies suggest that patients with thalassemia major who are splenectomized are unusually susceptible to serious infections. These infections, often penumococcal, are characterized by an extremely rapid course with about 50 per cent mortality within 24 hours after the onset of symptoms. It thus appears justifiable to place such patients on prophylactic antibiotic therapy (penicillin G or erythromycin) and to treat high fevers of unknown origin more vigorously than in nonsplenectomized individuals. Since fatal infectious episodes have been observed as long as 10 years after splenectomy, antibiotic prophylaxis should extend indefinitely.

Patients with severe chronic hemolytic anemias, including the ineffective erythropoiesis of thalassemia, often develop borderline folic acid deficiency and, at times, frank megaloblastic changes. This is characterized by reticulocytopenia and falling hemoglobin levels. Folic acid supplementation (5 mg./day orally) is therefore useful in the long-term management of these patients. Cholecystitis and cholelithiasis occur in about 20 to 25 per cent of patients with thalassemia major. The diagnosis may be overlooked because of the atypical age group involved. However, pain in the right upper quadrant associated with increasing jaundice and acholic stools should provide sufficient evidence to initiate further diagnostic studies. Cholecystectomy is warranted in patients with radiologically demonstrable stones, and exploration of the common duct may be indicated particularly because these patients may have "sludge" in addition to discrete stones. Other complications of chronic hemolysis such as chronic leg ulcers, generalized osteoporosis, and maxillary overgrowth with orthodontic deformity are also frequently observed in patients with thalassemia major. These complications appear to respond best to an increase in the mean hemoglobin level, although longstanding deformities may become irreversible.

Careful cooperation among a number of subspecialties is essential for the optimal care of these patients. Especially important is careful orthopedic and dental follow-up. Social service and psychiatry often have definite roles to play in helping the patient and his family cope with this chronic illness which requires constant medical care.

α-**Thalassemia.**   Although often clinically indistinguishable from β-thalassemia minor, α-thalassemia is more likely to pose diagnostic problems due to the absence of the characteristic elevation in Hb A_2 seen in β-thalassemia minor. Alpha-thalassemia is especially prevalent in Orientals and blacks, although cases have been reported in Greece, Italy and other Mediterranean countries. The degree of anemia and morphologic changes is usually milder in black populations. Anemia of any significance is found only when additional factors such as pregnancy or infection complicate the picture. Occasionally α-thalassemia trait may present as neonatal jaundice. Only rarely are exchange transfusions indicated; the criteria for this procedure are the same as for neonatal jaundice due to isoimmunization. Homozygous α-thalassemia results in the formation of γ_4 tetramers (Hgb. Barts) and is incompatible with extrauterine life. Such infants are stillborn with the classic findings of hydrops fetalis but without evidence of isoimmunization. There is no treatment at present and genetic counseling represents the only means of prevention.

Hemoglobin H Disease.   In this form of α-thalassemia, a relatively large proportion (10 to 20 per cent) of the circulating hemoglobin consists of tetramers formed from normal β chains (β_4= Hgb H). This variant of α-thalassemia is probably due to the interaction of two different genetic events which parenthetically form the basis of the phenotypic variations of the α-thalassemic syndromes. Persons with hemoglobin H disease exhibit a degree of anemia that is intermediate between that found in thalassemia minor and in beta-thalassemia major. They usually do not require transfusions and are able to carry on normal activities. However, they may be susceptible to many of the complications of a chronic hemolytic process, including an increased incidence of cholelithiasis. Splenomegaly may be marked, and in the patient with the moderately severe anemia or in one who shows signs of secondary hypersplenism (thrombocytopenia), splenectomy may be of distinct benefit.

Hemoglobin H is an unstable hemoglobin and is quite susceptible to oxidative denaturation. Drugs with oxidant properties such as sulfonamide derivatives, nitrofurantoin (Furadantin) and high doses of salicylate may lead to acute hemolytic episodes. Since hemoglobin H disease is also characterized by increased erythropoiesis, folic acid supplementation (5 mg. daily) may be of value in preventing megaloblastic anemia.

Transfusion Reactions to Blood Products

RONALD G. STRAUSS, M.D.

Blood products should be prescribed for patients only when clearly indicated. Even with modern blood banking techniques, adverse reactions accompany approximately 10 per cent of transfusions. *Immediate* reactions are caused by either immune (hemolysis or a febrile, allergic syndrome) or nonimmune mechanisms (infusion of infected products, air embolization and volume overload). *Delayed* reactions include immunization to blood products (thus providing the basis for an immediate reaction in subsequent transfusions), hemosiderosis and infections with serum hepatitis virus, cytomegalovirus, toxoplasma and Epstein-Barr virus. The remainder of this discussion will be directed primarily to the management of immunologically-mediated, immediate reactions.

Immediate reactions are those that occur during or shortly after completing the transfusion. Since they can be fatal, the first therapeutic measure is to recognize and treat them promptly. In many instances patients who receive blood products are seriously ill, and the underlying disease may mask a transfusion reaction. Suspect a reaction if the clinical picture is suddenly complicated by anxiety, flushing, tachycardia and tachypnea, pain in the chest, back and extremities, urticaria, pruritus, edema, dyspnea with laryngeal or bronchospasm, cyanosis, hypotension, fever, delirium, bleeding and renal failure. Temporarily halt all transfusions, but keep the intravenous line open. Management is then divided into immediate measures taken for all patients and those employed for specific reactions.

IMMEDIATE MEASURES FOR ALL PATIENTS

1. Symptoms and signs, particularly life-threatening ones, require prompt treatment. Patients exhibiting signs of severe disease should receive 0.3 ml. of 1:1000 epinephrine

subcutaneously, diphenhydramine (Benadryl), 1 mg./kg. intravenously, not exceeding 50 mg. per dose, and hydrocortisone, 100 mg. intravenously. If the patient is in shock, give up to 10 ml. of 1:10,000 epinephrine slowly intravenously. If no response is apparent within 5 to 10 minutes, repeat the doses of epinephrine and hydrocortisone. Patients with mild to moderate symptoms can be given oral prednisone, 2 mg./kg., diphenhydramine, 1 mg./kg., and aspirin in the usual antipyretic doses.

2. Make a presumptive diagnosis upon which to base further evaluation and treatment. If the transfused blood product contains erythrocytes, particularly if the patient has not had repeated transfusions previously, consider a hemolytic reaction. Confirm that the blood being infused was cross-matched with and was intended for the recipient. Examine the patient's plasma and urine for the presence of free hemoglobin. If the erythrocytes have been mismatched or if a hemolytic reaction seems likely, proceed as outlined in the section below. The possibility of an allergic reaction to plasma components or leukocytes is increased in patients who have received several preceding transfusions, although a hemolytic reaction still must be considered. An allergic reaction is the diagnosis of choice in recipients of blood products containing small numbers of or lacking erythrocytes such as plasma components and platelet or leukocyte concentrates. Details of management of allergic reactions and special problems that arise with component therapy can be found in the following section.

3. The decision must be made to resume or to permanently discontinue the transfusion. A hemolytic reaction is always an indication to stop the transfusion; whereas in allergic reactions it is usually completed, providing the symptoms and signs can be reasonably controlled. Allergic reactions occur most frequently in patients who need blood components repeatedly, and it is expensive and impractical to discard all products that elicit a reaction. Obviously, any transfusion should be permanently discontinued if bacterial contamination is likely.

MEASURES EMPLOYED FOR SPECIFIC REACTIONS

Immediate hemolytic reactions occur in recipients whose blood contains preformed antibodies against donor erythrocytes. Regardless of whether hemolysis is intravascular (mediated, in most instances, by a complement-fixing antibody directed against antigens in the ABO system) or extravascular in the reticuloendothelial system, free hemoglobin will appear in the plasma and urine as soon as the hemoglobin-binding proteins are saturated and provides the key to diagnosis. If the incompatibility is recognized before this relatively serious phase, the transfusion is stopped and no further treatment is necessary. The most severe disease, however, is characterized by shock, renal failure and intravascular coagulation. The crucial aspects of management are to treat hypotension and prevent renal injury.

1. Stop the transfusion and arrange for diagnostic studies as they will be necessary to monitor therapy (plasma and urine hemoglobin, serum haptoglobin and indirect bilirubin, culture of recipient blood and the transfused product, stained smear of the latter for bacteria, platelet count and coagulation studies including fibrinogen, fibrin monomer and fibrin degradation products). The diagnosis is confirmed by documenting the presence of hemolysis and incompatibility, i.e., the presence of antibody in recipient blood directed against donor cells. Occasionally hemolysis may be due to the passive administration of large amounts of antibody in the donor plasma directed against recipient erythrocytes. Rarely, a delayed (4 to 14 days posttransfusion) hemolytic reaction characterized by a positive direct Coombs' test occurs in a recipient in whom no antibody was detected in the original cross-match. Presumably the recipient was sensitized previously and forms antibody rapidly via a secondary immune response. Obviously, the patient suffering a severe reaction must be treated before the results of all diagnostic studies are available.

2. Maintain the systolic pressure above 100 mm. Hg and the urinary output at about 100 ml./hour with intravenous fluids. Infuse mannitol,* 1 gm./kg. (not to exceed 20 gm. per dose), as a 20 per cent solution during the first 30 to 40 minutes. Continue with fluids containing sodium, 25 to 50mEq./liter, and potassium, 20 mEq./liter, at a total intake of 3000 ml./m²/ 24 hours. Initially the sodium should be given as sodium bicarbonate ($NaHCO_3$) to alkalinize the urine, later as sodium chloride. Restrict fluids at any time signs of circulatory overload appear, and institute therapy for acute renal failure if urinary output is inadequate after 2 hours of therapy. When renal shutdown occurs before fluid therapy can be started, give a bolus infusion of mannitol, 0.3 gm./kg., as a 20 per cent solution over 10 minutes. If the urinary output is increased by this trial, administer fluids as outlined above; if not, treat as if the

---

*Manufacturer's precaution: Dosage requirements for mannitol for patients under 12 years of age have not been established.

patient is in acute renal failure. Blood transfusions should be avoided until the etiology of the reaction is identified, but compatible erythrocytes can be given for severe anemia or persistent shock.

3. Intravascular coagulation with consumption of fibrinogen, platelets and other labile clotting factors should be treated *if active bleeding is present.* Give a bolus of heparin intravenously, 100 units/kg., and repeat this dose as a bolus every 4 hours or as a continuous infusion (preferably as the latter). Active intravascular clotting generally abates with the cessation of brisk hemolysis and the treatment of shock. Criteria for the duration of heparin therapy may not be clear-cut, but consider discontinuing it when bleeding ceases, fibrin monomer is no longer detected in the blood, hemoglobinemia diminishes or the concentration of coagulation factors approaches normal values. In addition to heparin, replace clotting factors such as fibrinogen and platelets to halt bleeding. Clear evidence does not exist to prove that treating laboratory evidence of intravascular coagulation is necessary in patients who are not bleeding.

Most *allergic reactions* are mediated by antibodies directed against plasma proteins or leukocyte antigens, and thus can accompany the infusion of nearly every blood product. They occur most commonly in patients receiving repeated transfusions for chronic diseases such as constitutional anemia, hemophilia and aplastic anemia. Aspects regarding management of the acute symptoms and the decision to resume or discontinue the transfusions were discussed in the section on immediate measures. Preventive treatment is also important. Unsensitized patients who are likely to receive multiple transfusions should be treated initially with purified components in an attempt to avoid exposure to plasma and leukocyte antigens, e.g., use frozen erythrocytes to treat patients with aplastic anemia rather than packed red cells prepared in the usual fashion. Prepare patients with a history of allergic transfusion reactions with diphenhydramine (Benadryl), 1 mg./kg. orally, 1 to 2 hours before the transfusion is to be given, and attempt to remove irrelevant proteins and leukocytes from the desired component.

Unusual reactions to blood components have become more frequent and will be discussed briefly.

1. Immediate allergic reactions occur commonly in patients with hemophilia and other coagulation disorders, particularly if the clotting factor is replaced with whole plasma. Treat the active reaction as outlined in the section on immediate measures and attempt to prevent reactions. Centrifuge the plasma to remove leukocytes and platelets; use purified factors and prepare the patients with diphenhydramine. Two additional complications may arise. One is a hemolytic reaction in which recipient erythrocytes interact with antibody acquired passively, e.g., type A or B recipients receiving plasma from type O donors that contains large quantities of anti-A or B. The resulting hemolysis is generally not severe if recognized promptly, and the only treatment is to provide clotting factor replacement prepared from type-specific plasma. The other is intravascular coagulation and/or thromboembolic disease triggered by concentrates of the vitamin K dependent factors (II, VII, IX and X). These preparations contain activated clotting factors and should be avoided in patients with liver disease and in newborn infants. It has been recommended for the present time to supplement these concentrates with heparin, 5 to 10 units/ml., and to use them only when directly indicated.

2. Bleeding can be controlled by platelet transfusions in some disorders characterized by either thrombocytopenia or platelet dysfunction. Repeated transfusion of platelets from random donors results in recipient immunization to donor histocompatibility (HL-A) antigens and loss of platelet effectiveness. Frequently, satisfactory post-transfusion function can be restored by infusion of HL-A matched platelets, although not all sensitized recipients benefit from this maneuver. In addition, immunized patients may suffer immediate allergic reactions. Leukopenia, which may be severe in patients with poor marrow reserve, can also follow platelet infusions into sensitized recipients. The precise mechanism of this last reaction is unclear, but is probably related to either the formation of platelet antigen-antibody complexes with the leukocytes involved as "innocent bystanders" or to the presence of antileukocyte antibodies, produced as a response to the leukocytes that contaminate platelet concentrates. Manage acute allergic reactions with drugs as outlined under the immediate measures section. An improvement in post-transfusion increments and platelet function can be obtained in some sensitized recipients if platelets are prepared from HL-A matched donors and centrifuged to remove the majority of contaminating leukocytes. Eventually it may be possible to prevent sensitization by employing highly purified platelets that are washed to eliminate unbound plasma proteins and given only to well matched recipients.

3. A similar situation exists with leukocyte transfusions, although the immunologic mechanisms involved are even less well defined. The allergic syndrome is undoubtedly related in part to sensitization to HL-A or specific leukocyte antigens. There is evidence, however, that cell damage as a result of collection techniques may contribute. Efforts are being made to correct these problems and to investigate the importance of donor-recipient matching. Treat allergic reactions as they arise or attempt to prevent them with drugs as indicated in previous sections.

Hemolytic Diseases of the Newborn

STEPHEN R. KANDALL, M.D., *and* AARON R. RAUSEN, M.D.

The term "hemolytic disease of the newborn" (HDN) is usually reserved for those instances of an increased rate of red cell destruction during the first month of life due to maternal alloimmunization. Many other conditions are also associated with hemolytic disease in the newborn period: (1) congenital red cell enzymopathies, e.g., glucose-6-phosphate dehydrogenase and pyruvate kinase deficiencies; (2) red cell dysmorphisms, e.g., spherocytosis; (3) infections, either bacterial, viral, protozoal, spirochetal or parasitic; (4) exogenous drug administration, e.g., water soluble vitamin K in large amounts; (5) disseminated intravascular coagulation; and (6) uncommon metabolic disorders, such as galactosemia and osteopetrosis. In many, but not all, of these conditions, hyperbilirubinemia and anemia coexist in the neonatal period; a multiplicity of tests, including type and Coombs' test, peripheral blood smear, enzyme quantitation, and serologic titers, is required to establish the precise etiologic diagnosis. Although in this discussion management is restricted primarily to HDN caused by maternal alloimmunization, the general principles of management of anemia and hyperbilirubinemia also apply to the other diagnostic categories.

Administration of Rh antibody shortly after delivery to the mother at risk has markedly reduced the incidence of Rh-HDN. ABO HDN is now more common; it is usually less severe and rarely causes intrauterine death or hydrops fetalis. Less common maternal antibodies causing HDN include Rh4 (hr' or c), K1 (Kell), and Rh3 (rh" or E). The natural occurrence of anti-A and anti-B antibodies explains the development of ABO HDN in incompatible first pregnancies; production of anti-Rh and other antibodies is dependent on prior maternal exposure such as a previous sensitizing pregnancy or prior blood transfusion.

Proper management of non-ABO HDN is based on collaboration between obstetric, pediatric, blood bank and clinical chemistry personnel. Care of identified at-risk mothers should be restricted to medical centers equipped for total management of mother, fetus and neonate.

ANTEPARTUM CARE

Blood Typing. Routine ABO and Rh typing should be performed early in pregnancy to determine those expectant mothers who are type O, Rh negative, or both. Testing of fathers, although helpful in certain circumstances, is not routinely performed. ABO HDN occurs with type O mothers and type A or B babies; Rh-associated HDN occurs with Rh negative mothers and Rh positive babies. Routine screening for Rh (D) and other antibodies should be carried out early in the pregnancy. When such antibodies are found, serial titration may assist in the management of the pregnancy. History of a previously affected offspring should alert the obstetrician to possible alloimmunization, and should prompt a complete workup for maternal antibodies.

Amniocentesis. In pregnancies complicated by Rh sensitization, amniocentesis should be performed when maternal titers exceed 1:16. Since 1961, serial spectrophotometric analysis of the amniotic fluid has proved of great help in management of such pregnancies. Amniocentesis, the withdrawal of amniotic fluid through a needle under sterile conditions, is an outpatient procedure; technical aspects of the procedure are beyond the scope of this discussion. Complications of amniocentesis, including bloody taps, placental trauma, and fetomaternal hemorrhage, have been markedly lessened by ultrasonic localization of the placenta and fetal parts.

Five to ten cc. of amniotic fluid are withdrawn and protected from the light to avoid photooxidation of bilirubinoid pigments. Amniotic fluid contaminated by blood or meconium gives misleading results and is discarded. After centrifugation, one of several methods is employed to quantitate bilirubinoid pigments in the amniotic fluid. The most widely used method involves the determination of the optical density of the fluid over the range from 520 to 360 nm. in a continuous recording spectrophotometer. The optical density peak at 450 nm. is compared with that of the "expected slope" at that wavelength, and a ΔOD_{450} derived. Severity of

Rh-associated erythroblastosis fetalis correlates with the rate of fetal red cell hemolysis and therefore to the rate of bilirubin production, as reflected in the ΔOD_{450}. Additional tests on amniotic fluid, including the bilirubin: protein ratio and quantitation of anti-Rh antibody, appear to be of value in enhancing the predictive accuracy of amniotic fluid analysis in determining severity of Rh HDN in the fetus. Serial amniocenteses are therefore of great value in determining the state of fetal compromise due to hemolysis, and have major impact on the planned date of delivery.

Fetal Management. Obstetric management is based on a decision as to whether continued intrauterine existence is more favorable to the fetus than delivery and management ex utero. Accelerated fetal hemolysis may lead to severe anemia, tissue hypoxia, congestive heart failure, and death in utero. Prematurity, on the other hand, may be complicated by hyaline membrane disease, increased susceptibility to infection and the need for special nutrition. The reasonable statistical correlation between amniotic fluid analyses and fetal hemolysis allows assessment of fetal jeopardy. Mild fetal hemolysis will allow delivery at between 38 and 40 weeks. Moderate involvement usually leads to delivery at between 35 and 38 weeks of gestation. This critical decision should be aided by assessment of fetal lung maturity by the "shake test" or by lecithin:sphingomyelin ratio performed on amniotic fluid. If the fetus is severely affected, and 34 weeks of gestation or greater, delivery should be carried out promptly. If the fetus is severely affected and under 34 weeks of gestation, intrauterine intraperitoneal transfusion may be considered, despite the risk of the procedure. Hazards of fetal transfusion include premature labor, rupture of membranes, amnionitis, and fetal death. This procedure should only be performed by skilled, experienced personnel. Should labor ensue, preparations for care of the baby must be made immediately. Intrauterine transfusion invalidates the interpretation of subsequent amniocenteses. Serial transfusions are therefore usually done 1 to 2 weeks after the initial procedure and every 3 weeks thereafter until delivery is effected at approximately 34 weeks of gestation.

Maternal Plasmapheresis. Recent reports suggest that intensive maternal plasmapheresis antenatally can significantly reduce Rh antibody levels in those mothers carrying highly sensitized Rh(+) fetuses. This procedure alone or in combination with intrauterine transfusion appears to increase the survival rate of otherwise severely involved fetuses with Rh HDN.

Maternal Administration of Promethazine. Animal and preliminary human studies have suggested that administration of large doses of promethazine to the mother during pregnancy may ameliorate Rh erythroblastosis fetalis. Documentation of neonatal immunoincompetence following maternal administration of promethazine has contributed to extreme caution regarding its use.

CARE AT BIRTH

The delivery and care of an infant affected with Rh hemolytic disease should take place in a medical center with expertise in such problems. Since the clinical condition of the infant can only be suspected before delivery, preparations must be made for the birth of a severely affected newborn. In severe cases, care of the infant is provided by as many as four or five people skilled in management of this condition. Hyperbilirubinemia, though almost always present at birth, is not the major immediate concern. Rather, the management of anemia, asphyxia, shock, cardiac failure and ventilatory insufficiency forms the focus of delivery room efforts. The key to a successful outcome is *preparedness*.

Respiratory therapy, ranging from airway suctioning and provision of an increased ambient oxygen concentration to endotracheal intubation and positive ventilation, should be managed by one person. Two other persons are primarily responsible for procedures performed on the umbilical cord, e.g., cutdown on artery, vein, or both, sampling of bloods, measurements of intravascular pressures, and administration of fluids, such as whole blood, packed cells, and plasma expanders. A fourth person may monitor systemic blood pressure externally, and be responsible for handling of specimens, preparation of additional medications, etc. All necessary equipment (such as endotracheal tubes, ventilatory equipment, paracentesis tray, exchange transfusion set) should be available immediately and all necessary medications available in syringes prior to delivery.

At the time of birth, cord blood is sent immediately for type and Coombs' tests, total and direct bilirubin, hemoglobin concentration, hematocrit, reticulocyte count, blood smear, and platelet count. If the infant is not severely compromised, he should be stabilized and rapidly transported to the neonatal special care unit. If the infant is severely affected, the hematocrit should be determined immediately, as decisions must be made in the delivery room. Under a radiant heater, ventilatory status is assessed rapidly, both clinically and with blood gas confirmation via an umbilical artery catheter. Endotracheal intubation and ventilation with oxygen is usually carried out in severely compromised infants. Abdominal paracentesis or even thoracocentesis to remove fluid will occasionally be necessary to improve ventilation.

Assessment of the infant's cardiovascular status is aided by direct intraarterial and venous pressures in conjunction with careful interpretation of the clinical condition. Most commonly, the severely affected infant is hypovolemic, manifested by pallor, reduced peripheral pulses, and poor capillary filling. Interpretation of arterial blood pressure reading must always be correlated with clinical appearance, since peripheral vasoconstriction associated with hypovolemia may cause an elevation of arterial pressure. Symptomatic anemia (hemoglobin concentration less than 8 gm./100 ml. or hematocrit less than 24 per cent) with hypovolemia (mean aortic blood pressure less than 40 mm. Hg., or clinical evidence of poor tissue perfusion) may be treated initially with a small simple transfusion of packed red cells. If anemia and normovolemia coexist, a limited exchange transfusion with either whole blood or packed red cells will raise the hemoglobin level safely. Hypervolemia is less common than originally thought. Umbilical venous pressure values may be spuriously elevated in the face of abdominal ascites and are not necessarily a valid determining factor for defining hypervolemia. In severely compromised newborns, initial phlebotomy may be deleterious; if done for clinical evidence of hypervolemia, intravascular pressures are monitored carefully. In patients further compromised by cardiac failure, intravenous digoxin should also be considered. It is preferable, if possible, to infuse solutions into the umbilical vein rather than the umbilical artery. Once the infant is stabilized, he should be transported to the neonatal special care unit.

CARE AFTER BIRTH

Exchange Transfusion

Criteria. Despite the introduction of new methods, exchange transfusion remains the cornerstone of treatment for significant hyperbilirubinemia. The decision to perform an exchange transfusion after birth is based on the level of unconjugated bilirubin in the serum. Methods for determination of "albumin-binding capacity" or "free bilirubin" have not been sufficiently tested to permit their routine use as the absolute criterion for exchange transfusion. Although one may statistically predict the need for treatment based on cord bilirubin level, rate of rise subsequently, and assessment of the rate of red cell hemolysis, the eventual peak serum bilirubin level will vary from individual to individual. The often quoted level of 20 mg./100 ml. of indirect bilirubin as an indication for exchange transfusion applies only to healthy term newborns without significant perinatal problems other than hemolysis.

Guideline levels of total bilirubin, when the direct-reacting fraction is less than 1.5 mg./100 ml., are presented in Table 1. Values are given according to weight in infants with an uncomplicated neonatal course, and in infants with a course complicated by specific problems believed to increase the risk of kernicterus. These problems include: (1) prematurity (less than 37 weeks of gestation), (2) birth asphyxia (5 minute Apgar score less than 7, or documented acidemia in cord blood), (3) hypoxemia (Pao_2 less than 50 mm. Hg. after neonatal stabilization) (4) metabolic acidemia at any time (pH less than 7.25), (5) hypothermia (rectal temperature under 35°C. for greater than 4 hours), and (6) neurologic deterioration possibly attributable to hyperbilirubinemia. Since tiny premature infants often have many of these problems, and susceptibility to kernicteric brain damage in this group is high, exchange transfusions are often performed at levels under 10 mg./100 ml. (Table 1).

Selection of Blood. Donor red cells should be compatible with hemagglutinins in the mother's plasma, and donor plasma should be compatible with the infant's red cells. Selection of compatible red cells often necessitates packing these cells and using plasma which is ABO compatible with the infant's red cells. We prefer citrate-phosphate-dextrose (CPD) blood over acid-citrate-dextrose (ACD) blood be-

TABLE 1. Guideline Levels of Total Bilirubin* by Weight Which Indicate Exchange Transfusion

<1000 GM.	1000–1250 GM.	1250–1499 GM.	1500–2000 GM.	2001–2500 GM.	2500 GM.
Normal infant with erythroblastosis					
10	13	15	17	18	20
Infant at-risk for kernicterus					
8	10	13	15	17	18

*When the direct-reacting fraction is less than 1.5 mg./100 ml.

cause of its more physiologic pH. Heparinized blood, when used, must be neutralized at the end of the exchange transfusion with protamine sulfate; it also may produce elevated levels of free fatty acids, which may compete with bilirubin for albumin-binding sites. Banked whole blood should be less than five days old, and preferably less than three days old. Reconstituted blood is also acceptable.

Some of the complications of exchange transfusion are due to the blood used for the procedure. Old stored blood may induce hyperkalemia and acidosis. Other metabolic problems include hypocalcemia, hypomagnesemia, and hypernatremia. Blood from heavy smokers usually has a high concentration of carboxyhemoglobin, which may raise the infant's carbon monoxide level acutely. Transmission of hepatitis, syphilis, cytomegalovirus, and malaria through donor blood has also been described. In the rare baby with immunoincompetence, white cells in the exchange transfusion blood may cause a graft-versus-host reaction. This has also been reported in normal fetuses receiving mid-trimester intrauterine transfusions.

Technique of Exchange Transfusion. This procedure should be performed or supervised by experienced personnel, since its mortality can reach 1 per cent, the major contribution to this mortality rate being small, sick premature infants who are clinically unstable. We prefer to use the umbilical vein route, even if an umbilical artery catheter has already been inserted. Exchange transfusion through a femoral vein is hazardous and should be discouraged. Before beginning the procedure, the infant should be stabilized clinically under a radiant warmer, and the stomach emptied to minimize the risk of aspiration. In acutely ill babies, the procedure may have to be performed at their care station. All infants should have careful continuous monitoring of heart rate and respiration. Equipment required for suctioning and resuscitation should be checked and readily available. Disposable exchange transfusion equipment (Pharmaseal Laboratories, Glendale, California) should be used, and the blood warmed by an in-line coil passing through a warmer (Fenwal Laboratories, Morton Grove, Illinois) before entering the baby.

The umbilical cord area is washed with povidone-iodine solution, and the periumbilical area covered with sterile drapes. A 5-French or 8-French catheter is inserted into the umbilical vein and passed to the first point at which blood can be easily infused and withdrawn. Routinely, we do not confirm the posi-

tion of the catheter radiographically before beginning the procedure. The first aliquot of blood removed from the baby is labeled "preexchange blood" and sent for determination of bilirubin concentration, hemoglobin concentration, and hematocrit. An equal volume of donor blood is then given to the baby, and the procedure continues, with exchange of aliquots not exceeding 10 per cent of the infant's circulating blood volume. Estimates of blood volume average 85 ml./kg. in term infants, but may be as high as 105 ml./kg. in small, premature infants. A double-volume exchange removes approximately 85 per cent of the infant's original red cell population. In small infants, the donor unit may be divided into two packs, saving the second half for a possible second exchange transfusion. A second unit of blood should not be used in the course of one exchange transfusion, even in macrosomic infants, in whom one unit of blood is not sufficient to accomplish a complete two-volume exchange.

In order to prevent administration of low-hematocrit blood at the end of the procedure, the plastic donor blood bag is laid on its side or compressed mechanically with the outlet facing upward. We routinely administer calcium during the procedure when using citrated blood (1 cc. of 10 per cent calcium gluconate per 100 cc. of blood exchanged in term babies; 0.5 cc. of 10 per cent calcium gluconate per 50 cc. of exchanged blood in premature infants). If the infant has a metabolic acidemia and is clinically unstable, we may elect to buffer the donor blood to a pH of 7.3 with the addition of sodium bicarbonate or THAM. One might alternatively obtain arterial blood gases at intervals during the procedure and infuse bicarbonate as indicated.

The procedure should take between 45 and 90 minutes, depending on the size of the infant. We do not delay during the procedure for equilibration of intravascular and extravascular bilirubin pools. One should stop the procedure if the infant displays significant alteration in vital signs or a change in color. The last specimen should be clearly labelled "postexchange blood" and sent for determination of bilirubin concentration, hemoglobin concentration, hematocrit, and type and crossmatch, in preparation for another exchange transfusion. We do not administer albumin to the infant or add albumin to the donor blood prior to beginning the procedure. Prophylactic antibiotics are not prescribed routinely, but may be administered when multiple exchange transfusions are required.

Postexchange Management. After the

exchange transfusion is completed, the infant is carefully monitored until stable. Vital signs are taken frequently, and the umbilical area is observed for bleeding. Hemorrhage may be due to local factors, postexchange thrombocytopenia, or a more serious condition, such as disseminated intravascular coagulation. Because of the risk of hypoglycemia, stable infants are fed soon after the exchange transfusion. Once oral dextrose is taken well, formula feedings are begun promptly. Alternatively, one may elect to maintain an intravenous infusion of glucose until carbohydrate homeostasis is achieved.

Although a two-volume exchange transfusion will usually immediately reduce the serum bilirubin by about 50 per cent, equilibration from extravascular sites will produce a rise in this value once the exchange is completed. Serial bilirubin determinations should be obtained after an exchange transfusion every four hours until the bilirubin has peaked and begun to drop. Hemoglobin and hematocrit levels should also be monitored periodically since postexchange anemia is common. Since this anemia frequently becomes most marked after discharge from the hospital, provisions for follow-up of the patient must be made.

Although exchange transfusion has been performed for many years and its attendant mortality risk is quite low, significant complications, particularly in inexperienced hands, continue to occur. Aside from complications due to donor blood, the procedure itself carries its own risks. These dangers include hypothermia and hyperthermia of the infant, complications from catheter placement (embolic phenomena, arterial spasm, thrombosis, arrhythmias from inadvertent intracardiac placement), infection (local, hepatic phlebitis, sepsis), bowel infarction or perforation, necrotizing enterocolitis, acute changes in vital signs due to blood volume shifts, and possible late-appearing portal vein thrombosis with portal hypertension. It is obvious, therefore, that the risks should always be balanced against the benefits for the individual infant considered for this procedure.

Phototherapy. Visual light in the 420 to 470 nm wavelength range photo-oxidizes bilirubin into compounds which are water-soluble and bile-excretable. These breakdown products, although held to be nontoxic, have not been completely identified in vivo. Questions have arisen regarding the effects of phototherapy on many metabolic functions, and its efficacy in prevention of bilirubin encephalopathy has not been established. We do not use this treatment on a routine basis, but

do employ it when exchange transfusion is not feasible or felt to be unduly hazardous. Examples include abdominal surgery, umbilical cord anomalies, and suspected necrotizing enterocolitis. Since data culled from small, premature infants suggest a significant morbidity from exchange transfusion, we are also using phototherapy early in the management of sick infants weighing under 1500 gm., especially those requiring ventilator support. Adjunctive phototherapy is also considered in those infants requiring multiple exchange transfusions due to severe hemolysis, although phototherapy may be inadequate in the face of severe hemolysis. Phototherapy without a complete workup to establish the cause of hyperbilirubinemia is condemned.

Phenobarbital. Phenobarbital is one of many agents, although the only one used clinically, that stimulates development of microsomal enzyme systems within the liver. The drug is most effective when given to the mother late in pregnancy and continued after birth in the neonate. Although some studies have suggested an effect in lowering bilirubin levels in infants of sensitized mothers, we do not routinely use this treatment modality.

Substances Which Alter Enterohepatic Reabsorption of Bilirubin. Agar and activated charcoal have been shown to reduce serum bilirubin levels when given early in life. This is believed to be the result of reduced reabsorption of bilirubin from meconium in the bowel, with a lowered bilirubin load presented to the liver for conjugation. Various studies have suggested that this mechanism may play a major role in some causes of neonatal hyperbilirubinemia, but its contribution in hemolytic states has not been well defined. We do not employ this therapy at the present time.

Sickle Cell Anemia

JANE F. DESFORGES, M.D.

PREVENTIVE MEASURES

The ideal treatment of any disease is prevention or, at least, prevention of its manifestations and complications. In sickle cell anemia, there are a number of steps to consider in young children to avoid some of the morbid and even mortal consequences of this disease. Because sickling is exacerbated by decreased Po_2, acidosis, and dehydration, special attention should be given to dealing with any of these factors as quickly as possible in the course of an associated illness. Situations which may result in any of them should be avoided. Air travel, for example, involves a decrease in Po_2 since cabins are not pressurized to sea levels, and should be avoided. The parents should be made aware of these special hazards and both parents and child should understand that he must drink frequently in hot weather and during games and athletics.

In early childhood the presence of splenomegaly provides a circulatory hazard which, under adverse environmental conditions, results in trapping of sickled cells with abrupt sequestration of a large pro ortion of the red cell mass. Such an episode may occur without evident cause, but may also be precipitated by hypoxia. This sequestration crisis may be fatal, and when it does occur, its treatment should be immediate and vigorous, with transfusion of packed red cells, hydration and administration of oxygen. Whether or not dehydration has played a role in its pathogenesis, special attention should always be given to fluid intake since the kidney is unable to conserve water effectively in sickle cell disease. Therefore, an intravenous solution of hypotonic saline, 10 to 20 ml./kg., is started immediately and given the first hour while awaiting blood from the blood bank. This may paradoxically increase the hematocrit by releasing red cells from the spleen.

Children with sickle cell anemia are especially subject to overwhelming sepsis and consequent death. The infection that occurs appears to be related to functional asplenia and autosplenectomy which occurs in patients with homozygous hemoglobin S. This susceptibility to sepsis is less likely in the heterozygote states of SC and S thalassemia. The frequency of this complication is greatest in young children and is seldom a problem in teenagers and adults. From the age of about six months to eight years, the subjects are at risk for overwhelming sepsis with a relatively small number of organisms, pneumococcus being most common, *Hemophilus influenzae* next, and a variety of other organisms being occasional offenders. One may choose to give oral penicillin daily as prophylaxis against pneumococcus, or ampicillin, which is effective in infections with either pneumococcus or *H. influenzae*. The problem of developing infection with resistant organisms exists and one must balance the likelihood of this as well as the untoward side effects of the drugs against the risk of no prophylaxis.

Another approach to prevention of these two infections is vaccination. Polyvalent vaccine against pneumococcus should soon be available and vaccine against *H. influenzae* is presently under study. Pneumococcus vaccine is given at the age of one year and that for *H. influenzae* at 18 months. There is as yet no study to document the efficacy of this approach in children with sickle cell disease. However, since their ability to respond to antigen by antibody response is not reduced, one can assume that their response would be appropriate and that the incidence of death with overwhelming sepsis would be decreased.

One may choose simply to watch the child carefully, and to encourage the parent to bring the child to the physician whenever there is fever. Such a patient should promptly be treated with ampicillin while cultures are awaited. In the critical age group, this is actually necessary with or without more specific prophylactic procedures. There is at present no study to determine which approach is most effective in preventing death due to overwhelming sepsis in this group of patients.

Preventive measures are also in order to avoid deficiency of folic acid due to increased marrow activity. In a child with the increased demands of growth and a diet of undetermined quality, increased erythropoiesis may deplete supplies of folate and result in a superimposed megaloblastic state. Therefore, it is wise to give children 1 mg. of folic acid daily. Whether this is actually necessary can be challenged, but it may prevent folic acid deficiency which occasionally occurs under these circumstances.

Not the least of the preventive measures is psychological support. The child should be encouraged to participate in activities which he enjoys and every effort must be made to have him maintain school work with his peers. Parents need support in dealing with the recurrent episodes of illness and encouragement regarding the potential of their child to become a productive and happy adult.

At the same time, the family and the patient, too, should be made aware of special risks. Situations in which Po_2 may decrease should probably be avoided. Pregnancy is complicated by morbidity and mortality in sickle cell disease, and the teenager should know this before making any decision regarding reproduction.

TREATMENT OF SPECIFIC PROBLEMS

The chronic anemia of this disease does not need treatment, and since transfusions provide only transient benefit and contribute to iron overload, potential for hepatitis, and possibility of developing immune antibodies to donor cells, chronic transfusion therapy has no place. However, besides the acute sequestration syndrome, which requires immediate transfusion, and secondary megaloblastic state, which responds to folic acid, one may see an increased degree of anemia due to transient aplasia of the erythroid organ, the "aplastic crisis." This is often associated with infection, which may be viral and very mild, itself. Because of the short life span of sickle cells, extreme anemia develops in a short time and it may be necessary to support with transfusion until the marrow regenerates, a time interval of 7 to 10 days as a rule. Transfusion should achieve at least the chronic values of hemoglobin and hematocrit for the patient, and it is practical to transfuse to achieve values of at least 7 gm. per 100 ml. to allow some leeway for continuing aplasia.

Emphasis on the complications of iron-loading in patients with hemolytic anemia is so great that one may forget these patients may have nutritional iron deficiency in infancy just as their siblings do. In this setting, routine iron therapy is appropriate and will relieve that degree of anemia for which iron lack is responsible.

The complications of sickle cell disease which make it unique among hemolytic syndromes are a consequence of vaso-occlusive disease. Pain crises, presumably due to resultant ischemia, occur unpredictably and with varying frequency. Minor episodes are easily managed at home with analgesics, rest and attention to hydration. Aspirin may be given every four hours, 40 to 325 mg. depending on the child's size. Acetaminophen, 60 to 325 mg. every four hours, may also be used. Even if the patient is G-6-PD deficient, aspirin may be used since the patient's red cell population is young and therefore more resistant to drug toxicity. Moreover, the drug may be injurious to cells with G-6-PD deficiency only when given in high doses.

Episodes of pain severe enough to require narcotics, associated with fever, or presenting diagnostic problems such as an acute abdomen, require hospital admission for more intensive study and treatment. The diagnostic dilemma is complicated by the propensity of patients with sickle cell anemia to develop gallstones as well as to sequester sickled cells in the liver to produce hepatomegaly and jaundice. All of these complications must be considered in evaluating abdominal pain in these patients. In the presence of fever, associated infection should be considered a possibility and after appropriate cultures, antibiotics should be given. If the pain appears to be due to a surgically remediable cause, special precaution during and after surgery are indicated.

The major risk of surgery in these patients is related to the possibility of transient hypoxia and/or acidosis, both states being associated with an increased potential to sickling. In elective surgery, one can prepare the patient by transfusion with normal red cells to maintain a hematocrit of 35 for approximately a month. This allows the disappearance of the original population of SS cells and suppression of further production of these cells. The patient, then, is no longer prone to sickling. In urgent situations, one can transfuse to achieve a normal hematocrit, but this will not eliminate the possibility of vaso-occlusive complications due to the remaining SS cells. Therefore, the possibility of sickling induced by low Po_2 and acidosis remains. During anesthesia, maintenance of adequate Po_2 and normal pH can be accomplished effectively; however, in the postoperative period when aeration may be depressed, diaphragms high, and/or lungs atelectatic, sickling may complicate the picture. It is imperative at this time to maintain a good airway and proper ventilation. Even in uncomplicated cases of sickle cell anemia, Po_2 is lower than normal because of prior lung damage or shunting. To minimize hypoxia superimposed by the postoperative state, oxygen should be administered.

As the child grows older, infection remains a complication of the disease but its character changes. Overwhelming sepsis is no longer a special risk. Instead these children are prone to local infection, especially osteomyelitis. There appears to be a susceptibility to salmonella, and any hint of this is an indication for numerous blood cultures and special bone films. Without an organism evident, differentiation from simple bone infarct may not be immediately possible. However, a continuing febrile course and x-ray evidence of intracortical fissuring with early diaphyseal involvement of bone are points favoring osteomyelitis. Before treating, however, the organism must be identified, even if direct sampling is necessary to obtain this. Staphylococcus osteomyelitis may be treated with parenteral oxacillin,* 300 to 400 mg./kg./day every six hours for four to six weeks; often immobilization of the part for several weeks beyond that time is necessary. Salmonella may be treated with intravenous ampicillin,* 50 mg./kg. every six hours, if the organism is sensitive. However, it may be necessary to treat with chloramphenicol sodium succinate at a dose of 100 mg./kg./day, despite its propensity for suppressing

---

*These high dosages have been found to be safe and effective in this life-threatening situation.

erythropoiesis. In this situation, hemoglobin and reticulocyte count are monitored closely and if anemia progresses, the child is treated as in aplastic crisis.

MANAGEMENT OF SPECIFIC ORGAN DAMAGE

Infarction of tissue in any organ is a hazard in sickle cell anemia. Therefore specific organ failure may require management. Uremia, for example, is one complication of the disease and renal transplant may be considered in this form of irreversible renal failure. Besides the usual problems of maintenance on dialysis and at transplant, attention must be given to the continuing propensity for sickling, and prior to surgery, exchange transfusion should be carried out. Another complication of the disease, aseptic necrosis of the hip, may also eventuate in major surgery. If hip replacement is to be carried out, again preparation should include exchange transfusion.

Pulmonary complications are multiple and result in some chronic functional impairment. On this background, the development of any acute respiratory syndrome requires prompt treatment. While the differential diagnosis of infection versus thrombosis and infarction cannot always be made, any possibility of infection should be treated promptly with antibiotics after appropriate cultures are taken. In young children, pneumococcus and *H. influenzae* should be considered possible agents and treatment given for both with ampicillin.

Microvascular occlusion may be associated with venous thrombosis. This is not treated with anticoagulants since the source is not embolic and the thrombus itself is limited by the time symptoms are evident. The possibility of hemorrhagic complications in this disease outweighs any known benefits of anticoagulant treatment. In any case of respiratory problems associated with sickling, however, oxygen should be administered to minimize hypoxia and consequent aggravation of the sickle state.

In general, the treatment of infarction of organs is unsatisfactory short of the replacements mentioned above. There is, as yet, no therapy available or even ready for clinical trials which can reverse the microvascular sludging induced by sickled cells, nor has there yet been demonstrated an effective prophylaxis against sickling. One can only treat each event as one would in any other patient, but with great caution to treat infection early and vigorously, to maintain adequate fluid balance and avoid dehydration and to prevent acidosis and hypoxia.

Who should follow the patient? The physician who follows children with sickle cell disease is committed to personal care of the child in a continuum. He must understand the pathophysiology of the disease and be prepared for any of the myriad of clinical manifestations. The patients should be seen every 8 to 10 weeks during early childhood or more often if the parents seem insecure about dealing with the problem. Each visit should provide some lesson for the parents in managing the child's illness and its ramifications. Most important, the physician must be geographically and psychologically close enough to the family so that the parents will report any problem promptly and will be able to take the child to the physician conveniently at any time. If the pediatrician or family physician takes on the responsibility, he should have a hematologist available for consultation. If the hematologist becomes the primary physician he must be prepared to provide for all of the medical needs of the child. These patients are potentially the most diverse and complicated medical cases and require all the skills of a committed, sophisticated and compassionate physician.

Polycythemia

JAMES A. WOLFF, M.D.

Recognition of the physiologic characteristics of polycythemia is essential to a discussion of its treatment. Polycythemia is defined as an abnormal increase in red cell mass in relation to body weight. Increased concentrations of erythrocytes and hemoglobin may result from a decreased plasma volume, producing a relative polycythemia, a situation not encountered as a chronic process in childhood. In the pediatric age group polycythemia results from conditions characterized by insufficient delivery of oxygen to the tissues, particularly cyanotic heart disease with shunting of blood from right to left, pulmonary disease, or a decreased environmental oxygen.

In the newborn, increased blood viscosity when the hematocrit is greater than 65 per cent may be responsible for a variety of symptoms. These include plethora, cyanosis, respiratory difficulty, hyperbilirubinemia, hypoglycemia, hypocalcemia, thrombocytopenia and seizures. Simple phlebotomy may aggravate these symptoms unless the infant is hypervolemic, a condition difficult to document. Therefore if the newborn is symptomatic, a partial exchange transfusion, replacing whole blood with fresh frozen plasma, should be performed. The venous hematocrit in such circumstances should be reduced to 60 per cent or slightly less. The following formula for calculation of the volume of the exchange transfusion is useful:

Exchange volume (ml.) =
$$\frac{\text{Blood volume} \times (\text{observed Hct} - \text{desired Hct})}{\text{Observed Hct}}$$

Reduction of hematocrit in asymptomatic babies with polycythemia is more controversial. We recommend intervention only in those infants whose venous hematocrit is 75 per cent or greater. The same formula for calculation of replacement volume is used.

Infants or children with congenital heart disease who have arterial oxygen desaturation may experience disability because of "relative anemia," characterized by a low hemoglobin level in relation to a polycythemic red cell count. As a result of increased need for iron, a state of iron-deficiency occurs, evidenced by microcytosis and hypochromia of the erythrocytes and a low mean corpuscular volume. Administration of iron results in a rise in hematocrit, return to normal red cell morphology and clinical improvement. Following iron therapy, a rise in hematocrit above 75 per cent with consequent increased viscosity may result in return of symptoms. Exchange transfusion, as described above for the symptomatic polycythemic neonate, may also be carried out as a temporizing proceeding in iron-treated infants with cyanotic congenital heart disease who again become symptomatic or in those not iron-deficient but symptomatic as a result of increased blood viscosity due to a very high hematocrit level, if the underlying congenital cardiac malformation is not amenable to surgical repair or palliation.

Polycythemia secondary to abnormal hemoglobin with increased oxygen affinity is almost always asymptomatic and requires no treatment.

Leukopenia, Neutropenia and Agranulocytosis

JAMES A. WOLFF, M.D.

Leukopenia refers to an absolute decrease of total peripheral white blood cell count. At any age it is defined as a total circulating white cell count of less than 4000/cu. mm. Recent studies have shown that blacks and certain other ethnic groups normally may have total white cell counts that are slightly lower. The commonest cause of leukopenia is infection and its management is not considered here. Other forms of leukopenia are characterized by a decrease in circulating neutrophils.

Agranulocytosis strictly refers to an absolute decrease in all granulocytes, neutrophilic, eosinophilic and basophilic, in the presence of normal red cell and platelet levels. By common usage distinction of agranulocytosis from neutropenia has disappeared.

Neutropenia is generally defined at any age as an absolute neutrophil count of less than 1500/ cu. mm. The majority of cases are due to either decreased production or to accelerated destruction of neutrophils. A few instances have been reported to result from a combination of these two mechanisms. Pseudoneutropenia has been described, in which there is a disproportionate percentage of cells in the marginating pool, although the total neutrophil pool is normal. These children, as might be expected, have normal resistance to infection.

The majority of cases of neutropenia encountered in clinical practice result from drug administration, or radiation therapy, usually as a consequence of decreased production of neutrophils. Neutropenia caused by decreased production less commonly is encountered as a hereditary disorder, in association with pancreatic insufficiency, agammaglobulinemia or dysgammaglobulinemia, and intermittently in the condition known as cyclic neutropenia. Increased destruction of neutrophils occurs with splenomegaly from various causes. A benign form of chronic neutropenia in early childhood, presumably due to increased destruction of neutrophils, is unassociated with severe infection and tends to be self-limited.

The management of neutropenia in the pediatric age group is concerned primarily with protection from infection and treatment of established infection in children who have become neutropenic as a result of drug administration or irradiation or in those who are neutropenic because of blood dyscrasias. Although neutropenia is defined as a total granulocyte count of less than 1500/cu. mm., incidence of infection is not increased until the absolute neutrophil count falls below 1000/cu. mm. When the total neutrophil count is 500/cu. mm. or less, defense mechanisms are so severely impaired that the incidence of severe infection rises sharply. The many studies carried out in recent years concerning a protected environment for neutropenic subjects have shown contradictory results. Because bacterial infections in such individuals are due overwhelmingly to endogenous organisms, it is not surprising that various methods of enforcing "reverse precautions" have not proved successful. Indeed, the use of gowns and masks by family members and attendants frequently results in inadequate examination and supervision of the neutropenic child. Careful handwashing and exclusion of individuals with apparent infection have been as effective in preventing infection as more cumbersome precautionary techniques. Laminar flow rooms, which divert air particles in the room away from the patient, are used whenever available.

If neutropenia develops when the child is at home, management outside the hospital should be encouraged unless fever ensues, as the possibility of exposure to infection is usually greater in the hospital than at home. Rectal thermometers should be avoided because irritation of the rectal mucosa may serve as a portal of entry for endogenous bacteria. Likewise, venipunctures for blood withdrawal, when easily performed, are preferable to capillary punctures, as the latter not infrequently lead to localized infection in the neutropenic patient with subsequent dissemination of microorganisms. Neutropenia in an afebrile patient should not be considered an indication for antibiotics because inappropriate therapy may lead to resistance of microorganisms. When presumptive infection occurs in the course of a neutropenic episode, evidenced by a rise in temperature, hospitalization for the ambulatory child should be accomplished at once.

When fever occurs in the child whose absolute neutrophil count is 1000/cu. mm. or less, cultures should be obtained immediately from all possible sites of infection. These should include bacterial and fungal and, if possible, viral cultures of the throat, blood, urine and cerebrospinal fluid. In the presence of severe neutropenia, clinical evidence of meningitis may be lacking, making lumbar puncture mandatory. In addition, cultures should be obtained from any detectable localized areas of infection. X-rays of the chest are indicated even when clinical signs of pneumonia are absent.

After cultures have been obtained antibiotic therapy should be started immediately for the neutropenic child with fever. Intravenous administration is essential, although the choice of appropriate antibiotic agents is less clearly defined. There is some evidence that gentamicin alone, which has a wide spectrum against gram-negative organisms, may not be effective in eradicating infection with *Pseudomonas aeruginosa* in the neutropenic patient. A combination of gentamicin, 5 mg./kg./day in 3 equal doses every 8 hours, and oxacillin, 200 mg./kg./day in 6 equal doses every 4 hours, or a combination of gentamicin in the same dosage and cephalothin, 150 mg./kg./day in 6 equal doses every 4 hours, protects the patient against possible gram-negative and gram-positive organisms. If the type of infection is ascertained from pre-treatment cultures or from daily cultures thereafter, appropriate specific therapy should be substituted.

In those patients whose fevers defervesce in the first 4 days of treatment but in whom all cultures remain sterile, antibacterial therapy should be continued for a period of 7 days, and in those with pneumonia or sepsis for 10 to 14 days. The first recommendation is based on studies which indicate that cessation of therapy after 4 days results in a relatively high mortality. If fever persists for 4 days, in the absence of positive cultures, a third antibiotic not used in the initial combination, such as carbenicillin, 400 mg./kg./day in 6 equal doses every 4 hours, should be added and further search for an organism carried out. If no response occurs in one week with triple drug treatment, all antibiotics should be discontinued and a further search for the cause of the infection initiated. At this time consideration of antifungal therapy is appropriate.

Because neutropenic patients in most instances are immuno-incompetent, the possibility of infection with opportunistic organisms, particularly *Pneumocystis carinii*, must be constantly kept in mind. If chest films show evidence of pulmonary infiltrates, an attempt to obtain material for identification of infection, either by lung aspirate or lung biopsy, should be carried out. Trimethoprim-sulfa (20 mg. of trimethroprim and 100 mg. of sulfamethoxazole per kg. per day in 4 equal doses every 6 hours by mouth) has been shown recently to be a useful agent against *Pneumocystis carinii* and probably is as effective as pentamidine. Therefore identification of pneumocystis should be immediately followed by institution of trimethoprim-sulfa therapy. If improvement has not occurred within 72 hours, pentamidine, 5 mg./kg./day intramuscularly, should be substituted. Pentamidine must be used with precaution because it may produce renal toxicity, hypoglycemia or abscess formation at the site of injection.* A positive fungal culture from the blood or lung is an indication for appropriate antifungal treatment.

A number of recent studies have attempted to evaluate the role of granulocyte transfusions in the prevention and treatment of infection in neutropenic patients. These investigations have utilized granulocytes ob-

*Pentamidine is an investigational drug and can be obtained only from The Center for Disease Control, Atlanta, Georgia.

tained from buffy coats of multiple donors, by single-donor continuous-flow centrifugation leukapheresis and by filtration leukapheresis. In the majority of these trials, donors and recipients were matched for major red cell type and less often were screened to rule out leukocyte toxicity. In most studies HL-A tissue histocompatibility has not been a requirement for donor selection.

Several controlled studies have now shown that granulocyte transfusions shortened the febrile period and increased the number of short-term survivors in neutropenic patients with fever and presumed or documented infection. Some evidence exists that at least 4 daily granulocyte transfusions are necessary to show a difference in outcome between the treated and the control groups. Neutropenic children with persistence of fever or infection for several days after initiation of antibiotic therapy should be considered candidates for daily granulocyte transfusions. Granulocytes from single donors obtained by continuous-flow centrifugation or filtration leukapheresis should be used when possible. Although results of controlled trials of multiple donor buffy coat granulocyte transfusions have not been reported, they should be tried if other methods of collection are not available.

Splenectomy has been advocated in the past for selected patients with chronic neutropenia. Primary splenic neutropenia for which splenectomy is said to have produced cure has been described in the adult but not in children. Neutropenia associated with some degree of pancytopenia secondary to splenomegaly, in conditions such as storage diseases or portal hypertension, does not require splenectomy because there is rarely an increased incidence of severe infection in these patients from the neutropenia itself.

Although androgenic steroids have been shown to be therapeutically effective in some children with aplastic anemia, there is no evidence that their use is beneficial in the various forms of chronic neutropenia. Corticosteroids, although beneficial for children with congenital hypoplastic anemia when given early in life, have not proved useful for the treatment of chronic congenital neutropenia or other forms of chronic neutropenia. For infants with the rare Kostmann type of congenital neutropenia, bone marrow transplantation should be considered whenever a compatible donor can be obtained, as the mortality in this condition is extremely high, even though no reports have appeared to date concerning bone marrow transplants in this disease.

Acute Leukemia

CAROLE G. H. HURVITZ, M.B. Ch.B.

ACUTE LYMPHOCYTIC LEUKEMIA

The outlook for children with acute leukemia has improved remarkably in recent years. Such a child need no longer be regarded as one whose case is hopeless, but rather since the majority of children can be expected to survive longer than five years, he or she should reap the benefits of optimal medical care, and cure—not palliation—should be the goal.

The term acute lymphocytic leukemia is used to include acute lymphoblastic, acute stem cell, acute undifferentiated leukemia, and includes all cases which cannot be diagnosed definitely as myeloid or monocytic or containing Auer rods.

Complete remission means the complete absence of demonstrable leukemia by any clinical or laboratory tests. The bone marrow should contain less than 5 per cent lymphoblasts and less than 40 per cent lymphocytes and lymphoblasts combined. There should be normal erythroid, myeloid and megakaryocytic maturation other than that reduced by chemotherapeutic toxicity. In complete remission there is no evidence of organ infiltration or CNS leukemia. Central nervous system leukemia occurs when there are any leukemic cells identifiable in the cerebrospinal fluid. All specimens of CSF should be examined by cytocentrifuge to identify the presence or absence of leukemic cells.

The treatment of leukemia can be divided into three phases. During the first phase a remission is obtained by destroying the bulk of leukemic cells rapidly using specific drugs. Early in remission craniospinal prophylaxis is given to prevent CNS leukemia; this constitutes the second phase. The third phase consists of maintenance therapy to maintain the patient in remission for a variable length of time using a combination of chemotherapeutic agents with the purpose of eradicating all leukemic cells or reducing the leukemic cell population to a minimum level sufficient to be handled by the body's own immunologic mechanisms. The reader should understand that the treatment methods described below are examples of what constitutes optimal treatment at the time of writing of this article but could be entirely different one year hence. Treatment of childhood leukemia should therefore, whenever possible, be carried out in cooperation with a trained pediatric hematologist who is up to date with the latest treatment and regimens.

Drugs Used. The common chemotherapeutic agents have certain properties which make some more useful for inducing a remission and others more useful for maintaining it. The dosages listed below are examples only and must be varied according to the drug regimen being used.

PREDNISONE (Corticosteroid). Its major function is to produce lysis of lymphocytes and lymphoblasts. The exact mechanism is unknown. The major side effects are Cushing's syndrome, water retention, muscle wasting, hypertension, hyperphagia, electrolyte disturbances, immunosuppression, diabetes mellitus, gastrointestinal ulceration and osteoporosis. The usual dose is 40 to 60 mg./m²/day orally in three divided doses for 4 to 6 weeks for induction.

VINCRISTINE (Natural Alkaloid). Specific action is to inhibit synthesis and processing of molecular RNA precursors. It disrupts the microtubules during mitosis, being a powerful inhibitor of mitosis, specifically inhibiting the passage of cells through metaphase. The primary toxicities consist of peripheral neuropathy with loss of deep tendon reflexes, paresthesias, extensor weakness and frank paresis. Alopecia, constipation, ileus, hypertension and hypernatremia due to inappropriate secretion of antidiuretic hormone are also complications. Usual dose is 1.5 mg./m² intravenously per week for 4 to 6 weeks for induction. Dosage must not exceed 2 mg.

L-ASPARAGINASE. Extracted from *E. coli*, L-asparaginase is an enzyme that catalyzes the hydrolysis of L-asparagine to L-aspartic acid, thereby depleting the cells of L-asparagine. Leukemic cells require large amounts of L-asparagine. Some inhibitory effect on RNA polymerase activity has been noted. This is an investigational agent available only from the National Cancer Institute. Optimal dose is not yet known.

METHOTREXATE. Methotrexate is a synthetic antimetabolite of folic acid causing inhibition of purine and pyrimidine synthesis. The final result is inhibition of DNA synthesis leading to cell death. The major side effects are bone marrow suppression, mucosal ulceration, pneumonitis, vomiting, abdominal cramps and diarrhea, and hepatic fibrosis. Usual dose is 15 to 30 mg./m² weekly intravenously, orally or intramuscularly, depending on other drugs used.

6-MERCAPTOPURINE. This synthetic derivative of guanine inhibits DNA synthesis. The major side effects are diarrhea, mucosal ulceration, alopecia, megaloblastic anemia and depressed immune response. Usual dose is 50 to 90 mg./m²/day orally, depending on other drugs being used.

CYCLOPHOSPHAMIDE. This synthetic alkylating agent primarily inhibits DNA synthesis; however, RNA synthesis and protein are also damaged. The major side effects are bone marrow suppression, alopecia, mucosal ulceration and hemorrhagic cystitis. Frequently used dosages are 2.5 to 5.0 mg./kg./day orally or 10 mg./kg./day orally or intravenously for 7 to 10 days. The dosage varies according to other drugs being used.

CYTOSINE ARABINOSIDE. Cytosine arabinoside must be phosphorylated in vivo to the active form. It inhibits formation of DNA and also prevents reduplication. The major side effects are bone marrow suppression, nausea and vomiting and alopecia. Usual dose is 120 mg./m²/week intramuscularly for remission maintenance. The dosage is dependent upon other drug combinations.

DAUNORUBICIN AND ADRIAMYCIN. These drugs belong to the class of anthracycline antibiotics. Both agents appear to exert their cytotoxic action through intercalation with DNA thereby inhibiting polymerases. Major side effects are bone marrow suppression and cardiac arrest. Usual dose for both drugs is 50 mg./m²/week intravenously every 1 to 3 weeks. This must be varied according to other drugs used. Daunorubicin is an investigational agent.

Induction of Remission. Using a combination of vincristine and prednisone, a remission can be obtained in over 90 per cent of children with acute lymphocytic leukemia. The method we currently employ is as follows: prednisone, 40 mg./m²/day for 28 days; vincristine 1.5 mg./m² (not to exceed 2 mg.) is given intravenously each week for 4 weeks. We also add L-asparaginase, an investigational agent, although there is insufficient evidence as yet to conclude that its addition is beneficial. The dose we use is 6000 units/m² intramuscularly for 9 doses. Prior to initiating therapy, the following studies are carried out: complete blood count, sedimentation rate, platelet count, CRP, T and B cell levels, skin tests including PPD histoplasmosis, coccidioidomycosis, chest x-ray and serum uric acid.

At 28 days following initiation of therapy, bone marrow aspiration and spinal tap are performed. If the patient is in complete remission he proceeds to craniospinal prophylaxis and maintenance therapy. If he is not in remission, he may have an unusual form of leukemia requiring other chemotherapeutic agents.

Other supportive measures during induction therapy include treatment of infections (discussed later), transfusions of red cells and platelets, and increased fluid intake, especially if large masses of tumor or very high white count are present. In these patients allopurinol, 200 mg./m² orally in 2 or 3 divided doses daily, is also given for five to six days.

Central Nervous System Prophylaxis. Central nervous system leukemia can be effectively prevented in three ways: by cranial irradiation combined with intrathecal methotrexate; by craniospinal irradiation; and by intrathecal methotrexate alone. The method we prefer is to administer 2400 rads (2000 in infants) to the cranium over 15 days. Methotrexate, 12.5 mg./m², is given intrathecally once a week simultaneously with the radiation and afterwards for a total of 6 doses. Methotrexate without preservative is used. It is diluted in preservative-free saline or can be diluted in the patient's cerebrospinal fluid, so that approximately 1 mg. of methotrexate per cc. is given and the same amount of CSF is removed. This is infused via the intraspinal needle without aspirating in the presence of a free flow of spinal fluid. If the tap is bloody it is preferable to defer the methotrexate injection for a few days. Older patients are advised to remain supine for a few hours following the injection. Headache and pleocytosis occasionally accompany the intrathecal injections although they are well tolerated on the whole. Using this method of treatment, the incidence of central nervous system leukemia has been reduced from an incidence greater than 75 per cent to less than 5 per cent for children surviving longer than 2 years.

Maintenance Therapy. For maintenance therapy we use 6-mercaptopurine, 75 mg./m²/day orally, and methotrexate, 20 mg./m² orally once a week, adjusting the dosage for toxicity while giving the maximum tolerated therapy. The aim is to keep the total neutrophil count above 1500 cells per cu. mm. Vincristine, 1.5 mg./m², is given once a month intravenously, and prednisone, 40 mg./m² orally, is started on the same day and continued for 5 days and then stopped. Patients are continued on this regimen for 3 to 5 years unless they relapse, although the vincristine and prednisone pulses are frequently discontinued after 12 months in continuous complete remission.

Bone marrow examinations are performed every 3 or 4 months in order to detect an early relapse or significant toxicity, and complete blood and platelet counts are done every month. They often need to be performed more frequently. Evaluation of liver function is performed every 3 to 4 months along with the bone marrow by means of serum SGOT, SGPT, alkaline phosphatase. Spinal tap should be performed at least twice a year to monitor for central nervous system relapse.

Specific Toxicities. Virtually all the chemotherapeutic agents used in the treatment of leukemia cause bone marrow suppression to a variable extent. This leads to anemia, neutropenia with overwhelming infection and thrombocytopenia. If the total granulocyte count falls below 1500 cells per cu. mm., the dosage of chemotherapy is halved. If the count falls below 1000 the chemotherapeutic agents ars withheld until the count has risen above 1500 cells per cu. mm.

Corticosteroids are associated with weight gain, hypertension, hyperphagia and increased susceptibility to infection.

Alopecia is associated with vincristine, cyclophosphamide, Adriamycin, daunorubicin and radiation. The alopecia resolves when the drugs are withdrawn but the patient may need a temporary wig or hairpiece and should receive encouragement to purchase one.

Nausea and vomiting are associated with cyclophosphamide, Adriamycin, daunorubicin and cytosine arabinoside, and can be alleviated by the judicious use of chlorpromazine (Thorazine) or prochlorperazine (Compazine) tablets or suppositories. Thorazine is given in a dose of 0.5 mg./kg. every 6 hours orally. The dose of Compazine is 0.1 mg./kg. orally every 6 hours. A larger dose is given for rectal routes.

All of the agents are immunosuppressive, and infection with unusual organisms is frequent, particularly infections with *Staphylococcus aureus*, *Pseudomonas*, fungi, *Pneumocystis carinii* and cytomegalovirus.

Mouth ulcers are common with methotrexate and resolve when the drug is withdrawn. If the drug is continued in the presence of mouth ulcers, ulceration of the entire gastrointestinal tract can occur.

Following craniospinal irradiation, many children develop a syndrome consisting of somnolence, fatigue, low-grade fever, dizziness and nausea. There may be pleocytosis of the cerebrospinal fluid. The syndrome typically occurs about 6 weeks following irradiation, is self-limiting and regresses spontaneously over 3 to 15 days. Parents should be warned that this may occur.

Duration of Therapy. At the present time it is not known precisely how long it is necessary to continue maintenance therapy. There are indications that the relapse rate following cessation of therapy at 3 years is the same as that at 5 years. Large studies are currently evaluating this.

There are several reasons for wishing to stop treatment even though the patient is doing well: these agents are immunosuppressive and carry the risk of fatal infection; furthermore, long-term chemotherapy carries the risk of sterility, infection, damage to vital organs such as the liver and lungs, and the possibility of neocarcinogenesis. There is also the fear that these agents may suppress without totally eradicating the leukemic cells and a resistant clone may develop.

GENERAL SUPPORTIVE CARE

Treatment of Infections. Any patient with an absolute neutrophil count of less than 1000 is at increased risk of bacterial infection. The risk is markedly increased when the neutrophil count falls below 500 cells per cu. mm. Patients are at particular risk from the following organisms: *Staphylococcus aureus, Pseudomonas, E. coli, Klebsiella* and fungi. Patients with suppressed cellular immunity (which includes most patients on chemotherapy) or in relapse are at risk for fungal and protozoal infections, particularly *Candida, Pneumocystis carinii* and viral infections such as those caused by cytomegalovirus.

High fevers in a neutropenic patient should alert one to the possibility of serious infection and cultures should be taken immediately of blood, urine, throat and nasopharynx, and the patient placed on broad spectrum antibiotics pending specific culture results. We have found the combination of methicillin and gentamicin to be highly effective for this purpose. Methicillin is given at a dosage of 100 mg./kg./day in 4 doses and gentamicin, 5 mg./kg./day in 4 divided doses. If the presence of *Pseudomonas* is confirmed or strongly suspected, carbenicillin in a dose of 200 to 500 mg./m² is added. Patients below 5 years of age should also receive coverage for *Hemophilus influenzae.* Ampicillin and carbenicillin can be used for this. Carbenicillin and gentamicin should not be mixed in the same bottle or syringe. If blood cultures are positive, the patient is treated for 10 to 14 days with the antibiotic to which the organism is sensitive. If cultures are negative but the patient appears to respond to the antibiotics, it is probably well to continue for a complete 10 to 14 days of therapy. If there is no improvement after 5 to 7 days it would appear that the antibiotics are not helping and they should be discontinued.

INTERSTITIAL PNEUMONITIS. This is a frequent complication of patients both in relapse and remission. The differential diagnosis includes bacterial infection, *Pneumocystis carinii,* cytomegalovirus, other virus, drug toxicity, leukemic infiltration and radiation toxicity. It is estimated that approximately 50 per cent of interstitial pneumonitis in patients in remission is due to *Pneumocystis carinii.* The diagnosis can be made by needle aspirate or open lung biopsy and the material stained by methenamine silver stain (Gomori's). The material can also be stained for bacteria and fungi. Two antibiotics are known to be effective for the treatment of *Pneumocystis carinii.* Pentamidine isethionate, 4 mg./kg./day intramuscularly for 14 days, is effective in 70 to 80 per cent of cases. The agent is associated with severe toxic reactions including abscess and necrosis at the site of injection, nephrotoxicity and alteration in liver function. Pentamidine isethionate is manufactured under the name of Lomidine by May and Baker Ltd., Degenham, England. It is investigational and available in the United States only through the Center for Disease Control in Atlanta, Georgia. The new drug combination trimethoprim-sulfamethoxazole, manufactured under the name of Bactrim or Septra, has been shown in preliminary studies to be as effective as pentamidine. It has the obvious advantages of less toxicity and greater availability. The recommended dosage is 20 mg. of trimethoprim and 100 mg./kg./day of sulfamethoxazole in 4 equally divided doses. The treatment is continued 10 to 14 days.

Supportive care of the patient with oxygen, respirator care if necessary and monitoring of blood gases during the course of the interstitial pneumonitis is important.

CHICKENPOX AND MEASLES. Patients with leukemia are highly susceptible to chickenpox and frequently die if they contract it. All patients should be warned to avoid it unless they have previously had chickenpox. If a leukemic patient who is susceptible is exposed to chickenpox, he should if possible receive zoster immune globulin, 5 ml. intramuscularly within 48 hours. This agent is in short supply and is available only from the Center for Disease Control, which may be reached directly by telephone requests: day—(404) 633-3311; night—(404) 633-2176. Varicella can also be effectively prevented by infusion of fresh or frozen plasma at a dose of 10 cc./kg. from patients recently convalescing from herpes zoster. Patients exposed to measles who have not been previously vaccinated should receive specific immune globulin.

BLOOD COMPONENT THERAPY. Anemia can be treated with packed red cells at a dosage of 10 cc./kg. packed red cells over 3 hours. This can be calculated to increase the hemoglobin approximately 3 gm. This may be repeated after an interval of 6 hours. Since after repeated transfusions febrile reactions and crossmatching difficulties arise, it is advisable to use frozen packed red cells when possible.

Platelet concentrates are used in thrombocytopenia. Our practice is to transfuse platelets when the count is less than 20,000 or if there is bleeding. Four to six packs per m^2 can be estimated to increase the platelet count to greater than 50,000, which should be sufficient to prevent serious bleeding. Platelets from one or two single donors, especially HL-A compatible, prolong the patient's responsiveness to transfused platelets.

In severely neutropenic patients with overwhelming infections not responding to broad spectrum antibiotic therapy, granulocyte transfusions are available in the larger centers. These are time-consuming to obtain and cause severe febrile reactions in most patients.

EMOTIONAL AND PSYCHOLOGIC SUPPORT

The importance of an ongoing relationship between the patient and family and physician cannot be overemphasized and here the primary physician's true role lies, be he the general practitioner, pediatrician or pediatric hematologist.

It is our practice to initially explain the diagnosis with complete honesty to the family. We attempt to explain to the fullest of their comprehension all that is known about the disease at the present time, including the good or bad prognostic features of their child's case. It is stressed that no doubt exists regarding the diagnosis and they are warned that they will question the diagnosis once the child is well and in remission. Parents are encouraged to ask questions freely, especially in the early days, and they are encouraged to write down their questions to save for future meetings. After the initial discussion we always keep an optimistic attitude and encourage them to do the same. We encourage them to continue in as usual a way as possible, not only for their sake but also for the child's.

Where the child is concerned, we attempt to be as honest about the disease as is reasonable and we encourage children to ask questions and answer them to the best of their comprehension. Always the positive and optimistic aspects are emphasized since we need their cooperation in what is frequently a tedious and at times unpleasant experience. The child is encouraged to continue his school and regular activities unless real sickness keeps him away. Fortunately, during remissions most children are well and are able to continue their daily pursuits in a completely normal fashion.

Children, when confronted with the knowledge of a serious illness, will frequently ask, "Am I going to die, doctor?" This is usually a request for the reassurance that this is not so, and although the naked truth may be a currently popular course, it does little to comfort and sustain the patient. The physician should be sure he understands the implications before answering such a question in the affirmative. Every patient has the need and the right to hope and it is the job of the physician to help him to this end to the fullest.

Wherever possible, even in a busy hematology clinic, every effort should be made to give each patient a "personal" and concerned physician. In this way parents are encouraged to bring problems about spouse, siblings, finances and other matters before a major crisis develops. Specific psychiatric counseling is generally not necessary when there is a good patient-physician relationship and open lines of communication exist between them, although such counseling is frequently helpful and necessary to support the medical and nursing staff. Many patients gain comfort from sharing their concerns with others in the group setting. Above all, the role of the physician is to give genuine support, comfort and hope to the family.

PROGNOSIS

Generally, using methods outlined previously, it is estimated that between 50 and 70 per cent of children with acute lymphocytic leukemia will be in continuous remission at 5 years, and it is reasoned that a certain percentage, perhaps 20 to 30 per cent in all, will remain in remission indefinitely. It is also evident that certain characteristics allow one to prognosticate on an individual child's outlook in that those children tend to have a more favorable outcome who have initial white blood counts less than 20,000, are between two and seven years of age, have a small celled lymphoblast and do not have central nervous system or mediastinal disease. The patient with a white blood count greater than 50,000 with a mediastinal mass tends to be older, to have early onset of central nervous system disease, an earlier relapse rate and a poorer prognosis. In fact, it is possible that the patient with a very high initial white blood count should be regarded as a different entity requiring different therapy. Several clinical trials are under way to evaluate this.

ACUTE MYELOGENOUS LEUKEMIA

This form of acute leukemia accounts for approximately 10 to 15 per cent of cases of childhood leukemia and encompasses acute myelogenous, acute monocytic and acute myelomonocytic. The diagnosis is made only when there is a definite myelogenous differentiation of the leukemic blast cell and if Auer rods are present.

The outlook for acute myelogenous leukemia is far less favorable than that for acute lymphocytic leukemia, and the average remission time, although improving, is only about 12 months. Because of the poor prognosis the patient with acute myelogenous leukemia is best treated in a center where the latest drugs and regimens are available. Presently there are several therapeutic regimens under study but none is worthy of particular recommendation.

The method we currently employ is as follows. Again the reader is reminded that this is an overview of one form of currently acceptable treatment regimen. Improved methods may have been developed since this writing.

On the first day of treatment vincristine, 1.5 mg./m², is given intravenously once. Prednisone is given for 4 days at a dose of 40 mg./m² orally in three divided doses. Daunomycin, 30 mg./m², is given intravenously for 3 days. Cytosine arabinoside is given at a dose of 25 mg./m² intravenously every 8 hours for 12 doses, and 5-azacytidine, 50 mg./m², is given twice a day by intramuscular injection for 8 days. Daunorubicin and 5-azacytidine are investigational agents and can be obtained only from the National Cancer Institute. Cyclophosphamide at a dose of 25 mg./m² can be given intravenously every 8 hours for 12 doses as an alternative to 5-azacytidine. Studies are currently under way to evaluate which of these two and other regimens are better.

The above cycle is repeated every 28 days for 4 or 7 courses as tolerated. If at that time the patient is in remission he is maintained on the following regimen: 6-thioguanine, 75 mg./m²/day orally for 10 days, cytosine arabinoside, 75 mg./m², and 5-azacytidine, 100 mg./m², are given intravenously for the first four days of each cycle. Vincristine, 1.5 mg./m², is given intravenously on the first day of each cycle. An alternative regimen utilizes cyclophosphamide at a dosage of 75 mg./m²/day intravenously for the first 4 days in place of cytosine arabinoside. This cycle is repeated every 28 days. Drug dosage must be modified for toxicity.

Various clinical trials are under way to evaluate the adjuvant use of immunotherapy including BCG and allogeneric leukemic blast cells, but their effectiveness is yet to be evaluated.

Central nervous system prophylaxis and general supportive measures are the same as those included under the heading of Acute Lymphocytic Leukemia.

The treatment of erythroleukemia (di Guglielmo's) and histocytic leukemia is similar to that described above for acute myelogenous leukemia.

Neuroblastoma

THOMAS F. NECHELES, M.D.

Neuroblastoma is one of the more frequent solid tumors encountered in the pediatric age group. In contrast to several of the other childhood malignancies, however, survival in disseminated neuroblastoma has changed little in the past several decades despite the use of a number of chemotherapeutic agents. This is particularly important in that, in contrast to Wilms' tumor, for example, many children (67 percent) with neuroblastoma have disseminated disease at the time of diagnosis.

Prognosis (and therapy) of neuroblastoma is based on the age of the patient and extent of disease at time of diagnosis. Thus, proper evaluation of the patient is crucial. The clinical workup should include complete physical examination, x-rays of the long bones, vertebrae, skull and chest, an intravenous pyelogram, and bone marrow aspiration. Laboratory evaluation should include complete blood counts and evaluation of liver and renal function. Measurement of urinary catecholamine levels is of particular importance, not only as an aid in establishing the diagnosis, but also in following the response to therapy. Over 85 per cent of children with neuroblastoma have elevated urinary excretion of VMA and/or HVA at the time of diagnosis. Information gained from the diagnostic evaluation is used to stage the patient. The staging system devised by Evans et al. (Cancer, 27:374, 1971) is outlined in Table 1 and is now almost universally accepted. Additional factors such as tumor histology, location of the primary tumor, and degree of lymphocytosis have been related to prognosis but do not appear to be as well defined as the age of the patient and extent of disease (stage) at the time of diagnosis. The choice of modalities is thus based on these two factors.

In children with obvious widely disseminated disease (Stage IV), a histological diagnosis can be established by a simple biopsy. All

TABLE 1. Staging of Neuroblastoma	
Stage I	Tumor confined to the organ or structure of origin
Stage II	Tumor extending beyond organ or structure of origin but not crossing the midline. Ipsilateral lymph nodes may be involved.
Stage III	Tumor extending beyond the midline
Stage IV	Distant metastases involving skin, liver, bones, bone marrow, or distant lymph nodes
Stage IV-S	Patients under 1 year of age who would otherwise be Stage I or II but who have remote disease confined to one or more of the following sites: liver, skin or bone marrow without radiographic evidence of bony lesions

TABLE 2. Curative Radiation Doses°

AGE (MONTHS)	TOTAL TUMOR DOSE (RADS)
Birth to 12 months	1800
13 to 18	1800 to 2400
19 to 30	2400 to 3000
31 to 40	3000 to 3500
41+	3500 to 4000

*Dosages recommended by Radiotherapy Committee, Cancer and Acute Leukemia Group B.

other children should be surgically explored, not only to determine the extent of disease, but also to evaluate resectability. In those patients with localized disease, the tumor should be removed in toto if possible. This is rarely possible in children with Stage III disease, particularly since in many cases the tumor involves the celiac axis. In all cases, however, the surgeon should place clips around the margin of the tumor to aid the radiotherapist in the proper placement of treatment portals and also to guide in the later evaluation of response. Although several groups have recently suggested "second-look" operations following radiation and/or chemotherapy, the clinical results reported to date (as well as our own experience) do not appear to justify this procedure. Occasionally a patient presents with evidence of neurological impairment secondary to spinal cord compression. The treatment of choice is immediate decompressive laminectomy, although surgical removal of the complete tumor is rarely possible, even with two-stage operations.

The role of radiation therapy remains controversial. Although the tumor appears to respond rapidly to even relatively low doses of radiation, local recurrences are frequent, indicating that residual nests of tumor cells may be quite radioresistant. Nonetheless, current practice is to give radiotherapy to the tumor bed in patients with Stages II and III disease. The total dose varies somewhat with age of the patient, and current recommendations are outlined in Table 2.

Whether postoperative radiotherapy in this group of patients contributes to increased long-term survival has not, as yet, been established by appropriate control studies. In contrast to the uncertainty of the curative role of radiotherapy in patients with limited disease is the use of radiotherapy for palliation in pa-

tients with widespread disease. Even single doses of 300 to 500 rads can relieve local discomfort in patients with retro-orbital or bony lesions and can often contribute significantly to the "quality of survival" in children who have disseminated neuroblastoma. Utilization of such relatively low-dose localized radiotherapy is particularly important in children with compromised bone marrow reserves in whom higher doses or more extensive fields would compromise the use of aggressive chemotherapy. Reappearance of localized disease can be treated with similar doses. In children whose bone marrow reserves appear to be adequate, longer disease-free intervals can be obtained using higher doses. Retro-orbital or bony disease of the calvarium can be controlled with total doses of 2400 to 3000 rads to the entire calvarium. Similar doses can be given to lesions of the long bones or vertebrae, especially if pathological fractures are a possibility. Although such doses control local disease for reasonable periods, they should be considered palliative since they do not appear to extend overall survival.

Neuroblastoma responds to a wide variety of chemotherapeutic agents. Responses have been reported with vincristine, cyclophosphamide, doxorubicin hydrochloride (Adriamycin), daunorubicin, nitrogen mustards, and dimethyltriazeno-imidazole-carboxamide (DTIC).* In many cases, complete tumor regression has been observed and urinary catecholamine levels returned to normal. Despite this, the tumor has ultimately reappeared in a majority of cases suggesting the existence of nests of tumor cells resistant to each of these agents. Conventional chemotherapy consists of a combination of vincristine (1.5 mg./m^2 weekly for four weeks) and cyclophosphamide (10 mg./kg. every other day for 10 days). This cycle is repeated at 12 week intervals. Care must be taken to avoid hemorrhagic cystitis secondary to cyclophosphamide by maintaining adequate urinary flow. Children's Cancer

*Daunorubicin and DTIC are investigational drugs not yet approved by the Food and Drug Administration.

TABLE 3.   Recommended Treatment of Neuroblastoma

STAGE	AGE	SURGERY	RADIATION	CHEMOTHERAPY
I	<1 yr.	Complete excision	None	None
	>1 yr.	Complete excision	+	None
II	<1 yr.	Complete excision	+	Vincristine + cyclophosphamide
	>1 yr.	Complete excision	+	Vincristine + cyclophosphamide
III	<1 yr.	Removal of as much as possible	+	Vincristine + cyclophosphamide
	>1 yr.	Removal of as much as possible	+	Vincristine + cyclophosphamide + Adriamycin
IV	<1 yr.	Biopsy	*	Vincristine + cyclophosphamide + ½ dose adriamycin
	>1 yr.	Biopsy	*	Vincristine + cyclophosphamide + Adriamycin
IV-S	<1 yr.	Removal of primary if possible	None	Vincristine + cyclophosphamide

*Palliation only.

Study Group has observed increased efficacy with the addition of DTIC (200 mg./m² for 5 days with each cycle). Cancer and Leukemia Group B, in a pilot study, has observed an increased response rate with the addition of Adriamycin (20 mg./m² for 3 days every second monthly cycle). Although the response rate (complete plus partial responses) was increased, the survival of those patients who did respond was no better than those who responded to vincristine and cyclophosphamide alone. All of these chemotherapeutic regimens are toxic in terms of nausea, vomiting and myelosuppression, especially in patients with bone marrow invasion. Neutropenia and/or thrombocytopenia in such patients does not, however, contraindicate further therapy. Current recommendations for therapy, based on age of patient and stage of disease, are outlined in Table 3.

The natural history of neuroblastoma has continued to intrigue clinicians. The rare cases of spontaneous remissions, especially in very young infants, the histological evidence of maturation in some tumors, and evidence for specific antitumor lymphocyte sensitization in many patients all suggest a definite host immunological response to the tumor. In light of this evidence, several centers have undertaken trials of adjuvant immunotherapy in patients with disseminated disease. At least one of these pilot studies has reported improved survival in a limited number of children. This approach is still investigational but may in the near future contribute to an improved salvage rate for children with disseminated neuroblastoma.

As is evident from this discussion, neuroblastoma is a complex tumor which responds only poorly to conventional combination therapy. Median survival for children with widespread disease is less than a year and has not significantly improved in the past decade. It is therefore strongly recommended that children with this disease be referred, whenever possible, to comprehensive cancer care centers for evaluation and, wherever appropriate, that newer investigational agents and techniques be utilized.

Hemorrhagic Disorders

THOMAS F. NECHELES, M.D., *and*
EUGENE M. BERKMAN, M.D.

Bleeding episodes frequently present as medical emergencies and one is often tempted to jump in immediately with therapy. If the patient shows signs of cardiovascular decompensation or bleeding into a vital organ, this may be unavoidable but there is always sufficient time to draw appropriate samples to establish a diagnosis. Emergency replacement therapy will depend upon the type of bleeding encountered: hypovolemia with cardiovascular embarrassment requires volume expansion and red cell transfusion, while bleeding into vital organs associated with petechiae may indicate the need for platelet concentrates. Soluble clotting factors are usually transfused when needed as fresh frozen plasma. Cryoprecipitate is used as a source of fibrinogen and/or factor VIII. Commercial lyophilized factor VIII and IX concentrates are used almost exclusively in patients with hemophilia A and B.

In the presence of disseminated intravascular coagulation (see below) heparin therapy may be advisable before transfusion of clotting factors. Only rarely is there insufficient time to examine a smear of the peripheral blood to evaluate the numbers of platelets as well as the presence of fragmented red cells (schistocytes). Once the possibility of DIC has been eliminated, plasma products can be used as indicated. However, a definite etiologic diagnosis is needed for specific therapy, possible prophylactic treatment, and to discuss prognosis and genetic aspects with the patient and his family.

The hemostatic mechanism consists of three components: the plasma clotting factors, platelets and the vascular system. Defects in each component can, in general, be either congenital or acquired. Many of the latter are secondary to other underlying disease processes, and these must be treated, if possible, before the long-term integrity of the hemostatic system can be restored.

COAGULATION DISORDERS

Emergency Therapy. If faced with a bleeding patient with an abnormal prothrombin time (PT) or prolonged partial thromboplastic time (PTT) in the absence of significant thrombocytopenia or schistocytes on the peripheral blood smear, one can assume to be dealing with a disorder of the plasma clotting factors and, in the absence of other information, infusion of fresh frozen plasma is the treatment of choice. The usual dose is 10 ml./kg., which can be repeated every 8 to 24 hours as symptoms indicate. Usually the laboratory is able to establish a definitive diagnosis before a second infusion becomes necessary.

Minor bleeding episodes, such as prolonged epistaxis or bleeding following dental extraction, can often be controlled by local measures and do not require plasma infusions. Pressure packs with thromboplastic agents

such as Oxycel supplemented with a few drops of a concentrated solution of Adrenalin (1:100 strength) will often suffice. By avoiding the use of nonspecific plasma therapy, one can often establish an exact diagnosis in a much shorter time and allow the use of specific replacement therapy, if necessary, as well as alleviate the normal anxiety in the patient and his family.

Classic Hemophilia (Factor VIII Deficiency). The congenital deficiency of factor VIII is inherited as a sex-linked recessive trait. Patients with this disease are classified as mild, moderate or severe depending upon the level of factor VIII present. Patients with known factor VIII deficiency are best treated with concentrates containing high levels of factor VIII activity (see Table 1); fresh frozen plasma may be used initially if concentrate is not available but is at best only a second choice.

Replacement therapy can be used as treatment of acute bleeding episodes, in patients having major surgery or dental procedures, or as long-term prophylaxis to prevent most bleeding episodes. Acute bleeding episodes are most often manifested as bleeding into a closed space such as a joint, or bleeding into soft tissues. Less frequently, major bleeding episodes occur. All require prompt attention. For minor bleeding episodes our usual course is to give a rapid infusion of one of the factor VIII concentrates in a quantity calculated to be sufficient to elevate plasma levels to 30 per cent or more. We use the formula

$$\text{Expected level (in \% of normal)} = \frac{\text{AHG units administered}}{\text{Body weight (in kg.)} \times 0.4}$$

TABLE 1. Blood Products Useful in the Treatment of Bleeding Disorders

PREPARATION	MAJOR FACTOR(S)	VOLUME	USUAL REGIMENS* Initial	USUAL REGIMENS* Maintenance	HALF-LIFE OF MAJOR FACTOR(S)
Fresh frozen plasma	All	200 ml.	10 ml./kg.	5 ml./kg./6 hr.	12–24 hr.
Cryoprecipitate	Factor VIII and fibrinogen	10 ml.	10 ml./5kg.	10 ml./5 kg./12 hr.	12 hr.
Factor VIII concentrate†					
Hyland	Factor VIII	7 ml.	25 units/kg.	12 units/kg./12 hr.	12 hr.
Courtland	Factor VIII	25 ml.	25 units/kg.	12 units/kg./12 hr.	12 hr.
Armour	Factor VIII	25 ml.	25 units/kg.	12 units/kg./12 hr.	12 hr.
Cutter	Factor VIII	10 ml.	25 units/kg.	12 units/kg./12 hr.	12 hr.
Parke-Davis	Factor VIII	10 ml.	25 units/kg.	12 units/kg./12 hr.	12 hr.
Factor IX concentrate‡ Cutter	Factor IX (II,VII,IX,X)	10 ml.	50 units/kg.	25 units/kg./24 hr.	24 hr.
Hyland	Factor IX (II,VII,IX,X)	30 ml.	50 units/kg.	25 units/kg./24 hr.	24 hr.

Fibrinogen is no longer recommended for clinical use.

*This suggested dose schedule should be modified by the clinical response of the patient and by the results of detailed laboratory studies.

†Contains approximately 250 units of factor VIII.

‡Contains approximately 500 units of factor IX.

to calculate the dose. A simple slide-rule calculator is available from Hyland Laboratories for this calculation.

If therapy is prompt, a single outpatient infusion may suffice for an early hemarthrosis. For the advanced hemarthrosis, if the patient is to be treated as an outpatient, as many patients with joint or soft tissue bleeding are, therapy is repeated at 24 hour intervals at the full dose.

If bleeding is severe, as in the case of gastrointestinal hemorrhage or the fracture of a major bone, the level of factor VIII must be maintained at 30 to 60 per cent at all times and the interval between injections may be shortened to 8 hours. Therapy is best monitored by the use of factor VIII levels done immediately prior to the injection of the next dose. However, since factor VIII determinations are rarely available when one needs them, a return of the PTT to within the normal range indicates a level of at least 25 to 30 per cent and is usually sufficient for monitoring purposes.

In the case of bleeding into a joint or soft tissues, therapy for 1 or 2 days usually suffices; progress is evaluated by measurements taken at clearly marked points (we usually instruct the parent to mark, with a ballpoint pen, the place on the joint or extremity where measurements using a tape are made). Bleeding from a wound, into the gastrointestinal tract, or around the site of a fracture usually requires more prolonged therapy which may range from 7 to 10 days or more.

Patients having major surgery or major dental work must have hemostatic levels during the period of risk, i.e., until primary wound healing occurs. The dosage required depends to some extent upon the amount of bleeding encountered, but if the preparation has been adequate, bleeding should be minimal. The usual course is to infuse sufficient concentrate immediately prior to surgery to raise the circulating level to 100 per cent (as calculated by the above formula) and repeat one-half the initial dose at 12 hour intervals. Close cooperation with the surgical staff is essential, especially to ensure that proper monitoring is carried out and that subtle signs of bleeding are not overlooked. Using this program, it is possible to perform major surgery, when indicated, in patients with severe hemophilia.

Long-term prophylactic therapy is a relatively recent development in the treatment of hemophilia. Such therapy was not possible prior to the widespread introduction of the commercial concentrates and was facilitated by the development of home therapy, parents or patients giving concentrate on a predetermined schedule. Initial fears of an increased incidence of sensitization have proved unfounded. The aim of most such programs is to maintain a minimum factor VIII level of 10 per cent, a level sufficient to prevent most bleeding episodes. Therapy is individualized for each patient but most programs prescribe 250 to 500 units of concentrate every 2 or 3 days. Such prophylactic therapy does not, of course, preclude the prompt administration of additional AHF for acute episodes.

The selection of patients suitable for inclusion in such a program presents some problem. In general, such therapy is necessary in a limited number of patients who are having frequent severe bleeding episodes with major disability. Placing a patient on a prophylactic program does not release the physician of his supervisory responsibilities. Hopefully, there will be fewer visits for acute bleeding episodes, but initially at least, the patient must be carefully monitored with repeated factor VIII levels to determine the optimal schedule for administration of the concentrate and, once the patient is regulated, his physician must pay continued attention to the ancillary care of the hemophiliac (see below).

Although it is possible to have the patient visit the physician at regular intervals to receive prophylactic infusions, in most patients a considerable advantage is gained if the patient or his family (or a visiting nurse) can administer the concentrate at home. This obviates the necessity for office or hospital visits with attendant patient travel and waiting. Teaching the patient or his family may not be easy, but patience and understanding will overcome more normal fears. The help of a skilled nurse-practitioner in this area may be invaluable.

Inhibitors appear in about 5 to 10 per cent of all patients with classic hemophilia and apparently are unrelated to the number of prior infusions. These inhibitors are probably antibodies specific to factor VIII activity and clinically are characterized by a reduced or absent response to otherwise adequate infusions of factor VIII concentrate. The appearance of circulating inhibitors of factor VIII requires re-evaluation of the proper management of the patient. First we determine if the inhibitor is "inducible," i.e., if an infusion of factor VIII activity will call forth an anamnestic response—a secondary rise in antibody (inhibitor) activity following the infusion. If the inhibitor is not inducible and of low titer, it is usually possible to treat with factor VIII infusions. The dose may need to be increased and given more frequently to achieve hemostasis. If the inhibitor is inducible the patient is treated for minor bleeding episodes with local measures (ice packs, immobilization, pressure dressing), and the use of factor VIII is avoided.

On the other hand, in life-threatening situations several courses are available and depend on the inhibitor titer at the time of the bleed. In the absence of factor VIII infusion inhibitor titers fall slowly and may be low or absent at the time of the emergency.

1. If the inhibitor titer is low an infusion of factor VIII concentrate, enough to "swamp" the inhibitor and provide therapeutic levels of factor VIII activity, may be possible. Immunosuppressive therapy may be given at the time of the initial infusion in an attempt to delay or prevent the anamnestic response. Cyclophosphamide* is the most widely used agent and is given in large doses (10 to 20 mg./kg. intravenously). Plasma exchange may be used in conjunction to lower circulating inhibitor titers.

2. If a high-titer inhibitor is present infusion of factor IX concentrate may be effective in achieving hemostasis. Factor IX concentrates contain variable amounts of activated clotting factors and have been used successfully in patients with factor VIII inhibitors. Thrombotic episodes have been reported as a complication of factor IX therapy as well as increases in inhibitor titers to factor VIII.

3. The clinical effectiveness of an activated prothrombin complex (Auto-Factor IX, Hyland) in several hemophiliacs who had high concentrations of inhibitors has also been reported. This material appears to be effective in patients otherwise refractory to therapy with standard factor IX concentrates. However, because of the nature of the material, thrombotic complications represent a significant potential risk and further clinical trials must be carried out. At present, this material is an investigational agent, not released for general use, and can be obtained only by special application from Dr. Aaron Josephson, Travenol Laboratories, Chicago, Illinois. It cannot be overemphasized that the use of this material should be considered experimental at present and should be used only for life-threatening bleeding in patients with high-titer antibody levels otherwise refractory to therapy and in clinical settings where adequate laboratory monitoring facilities are available.

4. The use of porcine or bovine factor VIII is still another possible therapeutic approach. The molecule may not be inactivated by the circulating inhibitor due to differences in antigenic determinants. In vitro tests may

give a hint but are not completely reliable for indicating the usefulness of either material. A clinical trial gives definitive data, but since these materials are derived from a different species, specific antibodies will probably develop and limit the long-term use of such products. The use of these products should be considered experimental.

The use of the above mentioned approaches should be sufficient to tide most hemophiliacs with inhibitors over the most severe bleeding episodes. These procedures, however, require close cooperation between a clotting laboratory, the blood bank and the clinician.

Various ancillary measures have been proposed at one time or another in the therapy of hemophilia. Some of them, such as the use of peanut oil in the preventive therapy of bleeding episodes, have been thoroughly discredited. Others, such as the use of epsilon aminocaproic acid to control clot breakdown and thus further utilization of circulating factor VIII, may be of value. The use of steroids (prednisone in a dose of 2 mg./kg./day for 5 days) in hemarthrosis to suppress the inflammatory response and possibly impede the development of interarticular fibrosis is probably of some value, but definitive proof is still lacking. Controlled studies in this area are difficult to carry out, since well defined endpoints are usually lacking.

All too often the problems of patients with hemophilia are treated in the emergency room as a series of disconnected acute episodes and there is little or no long-term continuity of care. A patient with hemophilia has a chronic disease similar in many respects to diabetes mellitus. Long-term survival without major disability is now a practical goal but depends upon close cooperation between a number of specialty services all attuned to the particular problems of this disease.

Hemarthrosis frequently requires orthopedic consultation with the preparation of bivalve casts and possibly the use of sleeping splints to help correct contractures. Once the acute bleeding episode is past, the physical therapist is called in to begin exercises to the affected joints, first passive to maintain or regain mobility and then active exercises to strengthen muscles around the affected joint. Continuous exercises are prescribed to maintain the stability of the joint and to prevent, as far as possible, further bleeding episodes.

Preventive dental care is also essential since extensive dental work almost invariably requires hospitalization and prolonged concentrated therapy. Of particular importance is

*This use of cyclophosphamide is not mentioned in the manufacturer's instructions.

the avoidance, if possible, of intramuscular injections. This is especially true in dental care, where the use of local anesthesia (nerve blocks) is contraindicated, unless appropriate replacement therapy is administered. Antibiotics and preoperative medications should be given orally. One should give intramuscular injections at a site that is suitable for direct application of pressure and one is able to apply such pressure for at least 10 minutes. Thus, routine immunizations should be given with care and, in the severe hemophiliac, preferably at the time when factor VIII concentrates are being administered.

Attention to the social aspects of this problem are also important. The ultimate goal is to ensure that these boys will develop into healthy functional adults. Group therapy, as practiced on an informal basis by organizations such as the National Hemophilia Foundation (25 West 39th St., New York) and its regional and local chapters, is helpful especially in reassuring the parents that other families can live with this problem. Social service follow-up is helpful in ensuring that families are aware of the resources available in the community for schools, transportation, vocational advice and training, and blood replacement, if necessary.

The physician must also be prepared to spend considerable time with the growing boy explaining the disease, the therapy, and the precautions which are necessary. The boy must be given the opportunity to ask questions and discuss his problems. The necessity for avoiding contact sports such as football and basketball should be pointed out and reasons given. The physician can also advise on the use of items such as padded plastic head protectors, especially during the age period where the child is active but before he is old enough to understand the importance of avoiding head injuries. Genetic counseling, both to the parents and ultimately to the patient, is quite important and occasionally may require the services of a specialist in this field. Close continuous cooperation between the physician, the patient and his family is necessary to achieve a happy and essentially normal childhood and adolescence.

Finally, a major cause of trouble for the hemophiliac is the use of drugs which interfere with platelet function and make the bleeding tendency more severe. These drugs are listed in Table 2. Percodan and Darvon compound, both of which contain aspirin, are often given for joint pain in hemophilia, with disastrous results. No bleeder should receive any of the drugs listed in Table 2.

TABLE 2.   Drugs Known to Interfere with Platelet Function

Aspirin*
Glycerol guaiacolate (found in many cough preparations)
Phenacetin
Butazolidin
Phenothiazides (especially prochlorperazine, chlorpromazine, promazine, and cyproheptadine)

*A large number of commercial "cold" preparations contain aspirin. For a current list see New Engl. J. Med., *291*:711, 1974.

Von Willebrand's Disease. This is a congenital bleeding disorder affecting platelet aggregation and factor VIII synthesis. It is inherited as an autosomal dominant and thus both boys and girls are affected. Clinical symptoms are usually mild, and many affected individuals are diagnosed only through family studies. Problems are usually limited to mucous membrane bleeding, particularly epistaxis and bleeding following dental extractions. Occasionally major trauma or surgical procedures can be followed by excessive bleeding. Hemarthrosis is rare.

A major cause of clinical problems in patients with von Willebrand's disease is epistaxis. Although the nosebleeds are usually mild, they often recur with sufficient frequency to lead to a severe iron deficiency anemia. Pressure or nasal packing is usually sufficient to stop the bleeding, but recurrence is common. The application of a few drops of concentrated Adrenalin (1:100) to the pack may be useful in stopping the bleeding.

Occasionally, however, infusions are required. Cryoprecipitate or fresh frozen plasma immediately augments the circulating factor VIII level and, in addition, serves as a precursor for endogenous factor VIII production. The usual initial dose is 1 bag of cryoprecipitate/10 kg. or 10 ml./kg. of fresh frozen plasma. This dose is usually repeated at 24 hour intervals if necessary.

Factor VIII concentrates are not used in von Willebrand's disease, since they will correct factor VIII levels but not the bleeding time. Patients with von Willebrand's disease are prone to iron depletion because of repeated mucous membrane bleeding and should be placed on iron supplementation (ferrous sulfate, 6 mg./kg./day) when indicated.

Factor IX Deficiency (Christmas Disease). Clinical features are similar to those of mild to moderate classic hemophilia (factor VIII deficiency). Inherited as a sex-linked recessive characteristic, Christmas disease is one of the more common of the congenital bleeding disorders. Differentiation from classic hemophilia is important because concentrates useful in the therapy of the latter are of no value in Christmas disease. Factor IX is present in refrigerated, fresh frozen and lyophilized plasma. The initial dose of any of these plasma preparations is 10 ml./kg. but, because of the longer half-life of factor IX, the dose needs to be repeated only at 24 hour intervals.

Concentrates of factor IX (plus factors II, VII and X) are available (Konyne, Cutter Laboratories; Proplex, Hyland Laboratories) for the treatment of bleeding episodes or for operative replacement therapy.

The dose of concentrate sufficient to achieve plasma levels of 50 per cent is roughly one vial (500 units) per 10 kg. body weight. Major and minor bleeding episodes are treated as in factor VIII deficiency, but infusions are repeated at 24 hour intervals due to the longer biological half-life of factor IX. Long-term prophylactic therapy in patients with factor IX deficiency has not, in our experience, been found necessary but certainly is feasible. The indications are similar to those in factor VIII deficiency. The use of these preparations may be associated with an increased risk of hepatitis, but this is a hazard common to many products prepared from pooled plasma, not unique to factor IX preparations. Thrombotic complications have also been reported by others.

Factor XI (PTA) Deficiency. This rare autosomal dominant disorder in its clinical symptomatology resembles mild to moderate hemophilia. No concentrates are currently available, and bleeding manifestations are treated with infusions of fresh plasma. The biological half-life of factor XI is 24 hours, so infusions are repeated at 24 to 36 hour intervals.

Factor I (Fibrinogen) Deficiency. Fibrinogen deficiency is a rare autosomal recessive disorder comparable in clinical severity to mild hemophilia. Bleeding manifestations usually follow severe trauma, but epistaxis is also said to be common. Most episodes can be controlled with local measures including pressure packs and the use of topical Adrenalin. Massive bleeding, bleeding into inaccessible sites, or preoperative preparation for surgery requires infusions. Cryoprecipitate or factor VIII is fibrinogen-rich and is the therapy of choice. Concentrates of human fibrinogen are also available but their use is not, at present, recommended because of a very high risk of hepatitis.

Factor II (Prothrombin) Deficiency. This is another rare autosomal recessive bleed-

ing disorder similar in terms of clinical severity to mild hemophilia. Prothrombin is present in fresh plasma or fresh frozen plasma, or in bank blood which is less than 72 hours old, so replacement therapy is not difficult. It is also present in adequate amounts in factor IX concentrates (Konyne or Proplex), but these preparations should not be used due to the high risk of hepatitis. Since factor II has a half-life of 72 hours, the infusion need not be repeated as frequently as in factor IX deficiency.

Factor XIII Deficiency. In this rare autosomal recessive disorder, the hemorrhagic manifestations may not become evident until 24 to 48 hours following formation of the initial clot. Patients proved or suspected of having this deficiency must therefore be observed for 3 or 4 days following a bleeding episode or infusion therapy to ensure that the clot does not break down and bleeding resume. Most bleeding episodes can be managed with local measures. Replacement therapy requires the use of fresh frozen plasma given at 24 to 48 hour intervals. There is no concentrate presently available for the treatment of bleeding due to factor XIII deficiency.

ACQUIRED BLEEDING DISORDERS

Vitamin K Deficiency. Probably the most common acquired bleeding disorder is due to a deficiency of the factors (II, VII, IX and X) which are dependent upon vitamin K for their synthesis. The underlying deficit may be nutritional, due to liver dysfunction, or secondary to medications. Nutritional defects include dietary deficiency, malabsorption or prolonged diarrhea. Liver dysfunction includes the immature liver of the newborn (and especially the premature infant), obstructive jaundice and parenchymal liver disease. Drugs may interfere with the action of vitamin K (such as the Coumadin derivatives) or may interfere with its synthesis by the intestinal flora and absorption (such as some antibiotics).

In those patients in whom the bleeding defect is due to a deficiency of vitamin K, correction of the prolonged prothrombin time can usually be achieved with a single intramuscular dose of 1 to 2 mg. of vitamin K_1 (Mephyton), which will usually begin to act within 4 to 6 hours. However, the prothrombin time may continue to be prolonged for 24 to 48 hours. The administration of vitamin K_1 even intravenously, therefore, cannot be depended upon to treat serious acute bleeding episodes but must be supplemented by the administration of the appropriate factors in the form of fresh frozen plasma. The factor IX concentrates (Konyne or Proplex), which also contain adequate amounts of factors II, VII and X, should not be used because of their risk of hepatitis.

A lack of response to low doses of parenteral vitamin K usually indicates some degree of liver impairment, and repeated doses, except in rare instances, do not lead to an improvement in the response and may indeed lead to hemolysis and jaundice in susceptible individuals. The frequent practice of administering repeated high doses of vitamin K to patients with bowel surgery or liver disease is unjustified.

The treatment of bleeding in patients with liver disease is complicated by the multiple disorders which are frequently found. Not only is there a decrease in the vitamin K–dependent coagulation factors, but thrombocytopenia is frequently present (sometimes, but not always, due to hypersplenism) and vascular abnormalities (such as esophageal and gastric varices) are common. Acute bleeding episodes are best treated with fresh frozen plasma as a source of soluble clotting factors. The presence of thrombocytopenia mandates the use of platelet concentrates to control thrombocytopenia bleeding episodes. Disseminated intravascular coagulation often complicates liver disease.

Fibrinolysins. Circulating fibrinolysins are an extremely uncommon cause of bleeding in children. Those that do occur are usually associated with a malignancy such as promyeloblastic leukemia, where breakdown of the malignant cell is thought to release fibrinolytic activators. Extracorporeal perfusion during open heart surgery is also thought to produce some fibrinolytic activity, although this is usually minor.

An abnormality of the euglobulin-lysis time associated with clinical signs of bleeding never justifies a trial of epsilon aminocaproic acid (EACA or Amicar), since the fibrinolysis may be secondary to DIC. If heparin therapy produces no improvement, EACA may be added. EACA should not be given to an unheparinized bleeding patient. A loading dose of 70 mg./kg. is followed by 15 mg./kg. every 8 hours until bleeding ceases.

EACA should be used with caution and trepidation in the face of urinary tract bleeding, since inhibition of the normal urinary fibrinolytic mechanisms may lead to acute urinary tract obstruction by blood clots. It may be reiterated that clinically important circulating fibrinolysins are uncommon in pediatrics and treatment with EACA is rarely indicated.

Inhibitors. Circulating inhibitors to one of the normal coagulating factors usually appear secondary to repeated replacement therapy such as in factor VIII or factor IX deficiency; roughly 5 to 10 per cent of all patients eventually develop this complication. The spontaneous occurrence of circulating inhibitors has also been observed in patients with systemic lupus erythematosus, malignancy, rheumatoid arthritis and dermatitis herpetiformis. The inhibitor may be directed against any one of a number of the coagulation factors and is an IgG or IgM immunoglobulin. Treatment is seldom required. Prednisone is sometimes of value in these cases. Long-term therapy with immunosuppressive drugs appears to be more successful with spontaneous inhibitors than in treating the inhibitors found in hemophilias. There are, however, no controlled studies on the use of immunosuppressive drugs. Plasma exchange and infusion of activated clotting factor are possible therapeutic maneuvers.

PLATELET DISORDERS

Idiopathic Thrombocytopenic Purpura. ITP is an acute, usually self-limited disease in childhood, frequently following infections but just as frequently with no apparent antecedent illness. Acute thrombocytopenia is frequently associated with few or no symptoms and children appear to tolerate very low platelet counts for prolonged periods of time. Acute bleeding episodes, when they occur, can be catastrophic and prior to the advent of the use of corticosteroids, a significant number of children died of acute intracranial hemorrhage. It is usually possible to prevent this complication by judicious use of corticosteroid therapy, but since most children with ITP never experience such bleeding episodes, the selection of patients for therapy is sometimes difficult.

In general, however, children with platelet counts above 20,000 to 25,000/mm^3 do not have spontaneous bleeding manifestations, and counts above 50,000/mm^3 are sufficient to support normal hemostatic mechanisms even in the face of severe trauma including surgery. Therapy can therefore safely be limited to those children with platelet counts below 20,000 or in whom surgery cannot be deferred. This platelet count is not an absolute level, and frequently children whose platelet count is much lower can go for prolonged periods without problems; retinal hemorrhages, retinal petechiae and petechiae in the posterior oropharynx, however, are suggestive of increased susceptibility to central nervous system hemorrhage.

Children who have severe thrombocytopenia (platelet counts of less than 20,000 to 25,000/mm³), but who do not have clinical signs of a severe bleeding diathesis, are usually treated with prednisone in a dose of 2 mg./kg. given once a day by mouth. There is no objective evidence that corticosteroid therapy either shortens the recovery phase or increases the effectiveness of the circulating platelets, but it appears that steroids reduce the bleeding tendency in thrombocytopenic children, perhaps by reducing capillary fragility. Prednisone therapy is usually continued until the platelet count rises to levels above 100,000/mm³ and the dose is then rapidly tapered and discontinued. A slight (25 per cent or less) transitory drop in the count is seen in some patients but rarely is sufficient to require resumption of steroid therapy.

Acute bleeding episodes, such as severe gastrointestinal and genitourinary bleeding, or signs of impending bleeding, such as retinal petechiae and hemorrhages, are treated with platelet concentrates. The use of platelet concentrates is controversial since the recovery of transfused platelets may be poor and platelet survival is markedly reduced. A definite, albeit temporary, hemostatic effect may be achieved if sufficient numbers of platelets are given frequently enough because of the kinetics of the antigen antibody reaction.

Seventy-five per cent or more of all children with acute ITP recover in 6 months or less. The percentage is probably higher, but many children with acute ITP undoubtedly never come to the attention of the physician and recover spontaneously. That small group of children who fail to recover in 6 months can be divided into two groups: those who never respond to steroid therapy and those who have a profound drop in platelet count when steroid therapy is discontinued.

The latter group usually responds when therapy is reinitiated. One again starts with a dose of 2 mg./kg./day and, when the platelet count again rises, the dose is tapered to a level which is just sufficient to maintain the count. This dose is maintained until the platelet count rises or problems (gastrointestinal symptoms, growth failure, hypertension) arise from continued steroid therapy.

Most clinicians will wait 6 to 18 months before considering splenectomy, but this decision must be tempered by the clinical condition of the patient. If the patient is stable and requires little or no therapy, the decision can be put off for two years or more; if, on the other hand, the child requires large doses of corticosteroids to maintain his platelet count in a range found necessary to avoid bleeding episodes, and particularly if this dose is associated with serious clinical side effects, splenectomy may have to be carried out before 6 months are up.

Finally, in the rare child who fails to respond to steroid therapy and who has continued bleeding manifestations controlled only by the frequent administration of platelet concentrates, splenectomy may have to be carried out very early in the clinical course.

The majority of children with ITP who come to surgery respond to splenectomy. This is particularly true of those individuals who initially responded to corticosteroid therapy. Patients who fail to respond to surgery are usually considered candidates for immunosuppressive therapy, particularly with azathioprine (Imuran).*

Thrombocytopenia in the Newborn. This condition may be due to the passive transfer of maternal antiplatelet antibody to perinatal sepsis, to hemolytic disease of the newborn, to congenital leukemia, or to congenital aplastic anemia. The most common cause appears to be perinatal sepsis, such as rubella, toxoplasmosis, cytomegalovirus, syphilis or neonatal bacterial infection. The decrease in platelet count is usually moderate and rarely results in hemorrhagic complications. Platelet concentrates can be used if bleeding problems occur, but primary therapy should be directed, when possible, to the underlying infection.

The thrombocytopenia frequently found associated with severe hemolytic disease of the newborn is usually thought to be due to sequestration of platelets within an enlarged spleen. Exchange transfusions may accentuate the drop in platelet count. Although hemorrhagic manifestations are rare, when they do appear they may be treated with platelet concentrate transfusions.

Neonatal thrombocytopenia due to the passive transfer of maternal antiplatelet antibody is rare but may occur in mothers who have, or who have a history of, ITP or systemic lupus erythematosus. Isoimmunization against antigens specific to platelets as well as to the more generally distributed HL-A antigens may also occur. Since the maternal IgG has a relatively long half-life in the fetal circulation, thrombocytopenia may persist up to 4 to 6 weeks. These infants present with skin and mucosal bleeding manifestations at, or shortly after, birth. Intracranial hemorrhages are more common in this age group than in the older child and are a leading cause of mortality

---

*This use of azathioprine is not included in the manufacturer's indications for this drug.

in neonatal thrombocytopenia. Because of this hazard treatment may need to be aggressive. In isoimmune thrombocytopenia use of "washed" maternal platelets is an appropriate treatment. One unit of platelets per 7 kg. can be expected to elevate the platelet count to safe levels and can be repeated as needed to control the bleeding manifestation. Thrombocytopenia due to passive transfer of maternal auto anti-platelet antibody may be alleviated by exchange transfusion which decreases the amount of circulating antibody. Prednisone in a dose of 2 mg./kg. may increase "vascular integrity" but is usually ineffective in the treatment of thrombocytopenia due to passively transferred antibody.

Neonatal thrombocytopenia may also, in rare instances, be the presenting sign of congenital aplastic anemia or congenital leukemia. The amegakaryocytic thrombocytopenia in congenital aplastic anemia may be present for a variable period of time before a decrease in granulocytes or red cells becomes evident. Both aplastic anemia and congenital leukemia are diagnosed by examination of the bone marrow. Basic therapy should be directed against the underlying disease but the immediate management of bleeding manifestations usually requires the use of platelet concentrates.

Secondary Thrombocytopenia. There are a number of disease entities which can present with bleeding manifestations and thrombocytopenia. Some of these, such as sepsis, have already been mentioned. A few others deserve comment. Thrombocytopenia has been associated with the administration of several drugs, the most noteworthy of which is quinidine, although other drugs have, at times, been implicated. In at least some instances the drug plays the role of a haptene in an antigen-antibody reaction. Withdrawal of the drug results in a prompt increase in the platelet count; the use of platelet concentrates or corticosteroids is rarely necessary.

Cyanotic congenital heart disease can also be associated with a mild thrombocytopenia but is usually not the cause of bleeding problems; the thrombocytopathy associated with this entity (see below) is probably of greater clinical significance. Thrombocytopenia can also be caused by sequestration of platelets in a giant hemangioma. Interestingly enough, the platelet count may respond for a time to corticosteroid therapy. This is usually only of temporary benefit and if the thrombocytopenia is symptomatic, surgical resection may be needed.

Splenomegaly is still another cause of secondary thrombocytopenia; occasionally the degree of splenic sequestration may be sufficient in itself to indicate the need for splenectomy. Finally, several congenital disorders may be associated with thrombocytopenia. Chief among these is the Wiskott-Aldrich syndrome, in which the hemorrhagic manifestations may be the presenting clinical aspect. Although splenomegaly is frequently present, splenectomy is not indicated in this disorder. Bleeding manifestations are frequently episodic and appear to be alleviated by short courses of prednisone. Administration of platelet concentrates is indicated only for serious hemorrhages.

Platelet Concentrates. Platelet concentrates represent the most useful form of replacement therapy in the treatment of most forms of thrombocytopenia (with the thrombocytopenia of DIC a notable exception). Improvements in the techniques of collection and preservation have enhanced recovery and survival of transfused platelets. Storage at room temperatures (between 20 and 24° C.) rather than 4° C. allows platelet concentrates to be kept for several days rather than 24 hours. Because of the small volume, platelet concentrates are the treatment of choice in severe thrombocytopenia with hemorrhage.

One unit of platelet concentrate per 7 kg. of body weight will raise the platelet count significantly in the absence of platelet antibodies or abnormal sequestration (such as in an enlarged spleen). Since the platelets often stick to the vascular endothelium, exact predictions of increase in counts are not possible. The best end point is the cessation of bleeding. The effective half-life of transfused platelets is about 4 days and thus, in the absence of severe bleeding, platelet transfusions can be spaced at appropriate intervals.

Prophylactic use of platelet transfusion is not widespread. The main deterrent to prophylactic use is the eventual development of isosensitization and refractoriness. The use of HL-A compatible donors can be life-saving in the thrombocytopenic patient who has become sensitized. Antigenic systems unique to platelets appear to be a less common cause for isoimmunization. In the patient who has become sensitized, as evidenced by poor platelet recovery following transfusion and shortened survival, in the absence of ITP or hypersplenism, the use of family donors may lead to an increase in the clinical benefit derived from platelet transfusions.

Functional Platelet Defects (Thrombopathy). The primary disorder in this group of syndromes is a defect in the aggregation of platelets, defined as an in vitro defect in ADP-, epinephrine- or collagen-induced aggregation. The platelet count is usually normal but the bleeding time is prolonged. The congenital forms of this syndrome are quite common. The patients may have an increased susceptibility to bruising with a tendency to bleed excessively with epistaxes and menorrhagia. These individuals usually require no therapy except at surgery or other trauma. The acquired form of platelet dysfunction is usually seen in association with uremia, use of certain drugs, or in cyanotic congenital heart disease, where the platelet dysfunction appears to be more significant than the mild thrombocytopenia which may also be present.

These patients do not appear to have serious hemorrhagic tendencies, and an increased incidence of prolonged epistaxis appears to be the major clinical manifestation of this syndrome. However, it appears prudent to correct the abnormality, as far as possible, prior to major surgery. Prednisone (0.4 mg./kg./day by mouth) given for 3 days prior to surgery may improve the bleeding time in some patients but does not appear to affect the in vitro aggregation abnormalities.

VASCULAR DEFECTS

Congenital Defects. Hereditary disorders of the vascular component of the hemostatic system are quite uncommon. The best known of these is hereditary hemorrhagic telangiectasia, in which multiple telangiectasias scattered throughout the mucous membranes and gastrointestinal tract may lead to recurrent epistaxes or gastrointestinal hemorrhage. The bleeding is usually controllable by local measures and transfusions are rarely indicated, but the patients frequently become iron deficient and iron supplementation is often indicated. In the Ehlers-Danlos syndrome, easy bruisability is due to a poor collagen substructure of the vascular bed. There is no effective treatment other than the avoidance of trauma.

Acquired Defects. Scurvy in the past was a common cause for vascular purpura but is now quite infrequent in this country particularly because of vitamin C supplementation of most commercial infant formulas. The major bleeding manifestations are hemorrhages into the skin following even the slightest trauma. In children, subperiosteal hemorrhages with bone tenderness are quite typical. Treatment consists of 50 mg. of ascorbic acid given four times a day for a week. Maintenance therapy (50 mg./day) can then be continued for another 3 months.

Septic thrombi can be mistaken for petechiae but occur in the absence of thrombocytopenia or other bleeding manifestations and are usually slightly tender to palpation. The causative organism can frequently be cultured from the thrombus by careful aspiration. Treatment is directed against the underlying infection.

Anaphylactoid purpura (Henoch-Schönlein or allergic purpura) is thought to be a hypersensitivity reaction, related to acute nephritis, in which there is a diffuse acute inflammatory reaction around the capillaries and small arterioles. It is relatively common in children and should be distinguished from acute ITP, which it may resemble. In anaphylactoid purpura, however, the petechiae and ecchymoses are typically distributed over the buttocks, lower extremities and face with few on the trunk, and the platelet count is normal. Scalp edema and joint involvement may be prominent.

The uncomplicated case requires no therapy and recurrences are uncommon. There are two possible complications, however, which require therapy. The most common is colicky abdominal pain related to vasculitis and edema of the bowel wall. This may be accompanied by vomiting, diarrhea, and gastrointestinal hemorrhage. In the occasional patient, the gastrointestinal involvement leads to intussusception and perforation which require surgical intervention. Because of this hazard, children in whom the abdominal symptoms are prominent are best treated with a short course of prednisone (2 mg./kg./day by mouth) which is continued until there are no fresh skin lesions.

Most children with allergic purpura show some degree of microscopic hematuria and proteinuria during the acute stages of the disease. In a majority of patients these abnormalities rapidly resolve and there is no evidence of residual renal damage. In about 5 to 10 per cent, however, urinary abnormalities persist beyond 6 months and eventually evolve into a picture indistinguishable from chronic nephritis and end-stage renal disease. If this is recognized early enough, the use of immunosuppressive therapy (azathioprine or cyclophosphamide) appears to be associated with subsidence of signs of active disease and stabilization of renal function. Because of the possibility of persistent renal involvement, children who have had an episode of anaphylactoid purpura should have a routine urinalysis at 6 and 12 months following the acute episode.

The Immunodeficiency Disorders

RICHARD A. GATTI, M.D.

Treatment of patients with immunodeficiency disorders can be divided into two categories: that which is aimed at correcting the primary or basic disorder and supportive treatment of problems that derive secondarily from an immunodeficient state. The second category thus includes general recommendations for treatment of patients with transient and secondary immunodeficiencies. In patients in whom supportive treatment is often inadequate for long-term care, it is of utmost importance to correct the basic immunologic disorder as soon as possible.

Planning therapy for patients with primary immunodeficiency disorders depends heavily upon the findings of an immunologic analysis of that patient. In general, an attempt should be made to determine whether the perturbation is primary or secondary and whether it is most pronounced in the B- or T- compartment, i.e., humoral (HI) or cell-mediated (CMI) immunodeficiency. The preliminary work-up should include: (1) skin testing to antigens such as mumps, Candida, streptokinase/streptodornase, and tetanus toxoid (CMI), (2) Schick testing (HI); (3) isohemagglutinin titers (HI); (4) quantitative serum immunoglobulins, including IgE (HI); (5) B/T lymphocyte levels (HI, CMI); and (6) in vitro stimulation of lymphocytes by phytohemagglutinin (CMI). Specialized laboratories can, of course, measure many other parameters if the clinical status of the patient so warrants. A significant proportion of patients with severe combined immunodeficiencies have now been recognized to lack certain enzymes in their lymphocytes, such as adenosine deaminase, and nucloside phosphorylase. It is also important to establish whether there is a family history of similar immunodeficiencies and whether a pattern of inheritance exists.

CORRECTION OF BASIC DISORDER

Because the primary immunologic disorders have historically represented deficiencies rather than excesses, most forms of therapy presently represent attempts to replace missing components.

Humoral Immunodeficiency. Progress thus far has allowed replacement of serum immunoglobulins by only two methods. Immune serum globulin U.S.P. (ISG) replaces serum IgG but contains little IgM, IgA or IgE. No attempt should be made to restore IgG levels to normal—a level of 300 mg./100 ml. is adequate for minimizing recurrent bacteria infections. This can usually be attained in children with an initial intramuscular dose of 1.5 ml./kg. followed by half that dose every month. In older children requiring larger volumes of ISG, a total of up to 10 ml. can be injected weekly into each buttock. To minimize discomfort, we add a small amount of local anesthetic (less than 1 ml./20 ml. of ISG) and redirect the injecting needle after delivering 5 ml. to any one site. We follow the IgG levels at first on a monthly basis and then annually if the patient is responding to therapy. Reactions to intramuscular ISG are uncommon, but do occur. They are usually mild and may be characterized by gastrointestinal symptoms, joint pains, back pain, dyspnea and syncope shortly after injection. Aqueous epinephrine should be readily available whenever gamma globulin is injected.

Plasma infusion (20 ml./kg.) has been utilized whenever gamma globulin therapy is not adequate for reducing the frequency of bacterial infections, especially chronic progressive pulmonary infections. Plasma therapy for such patients should be combined with a program of aggressive pulmonary hygiene and semiannual pulmonary function tests. There is an ever-present danger of exposing the patient to hepatitis, an infection which is often fatal to patients with hypoimmunoglobulinemia. This can be minimized by pre-testing the plasma for hepatitis B antigen and by changing plasma donors as infrequently as possible.

Cell-Mediated Immunodeficiency. The first successful reconstitution of an infant with DiGeorge syndrome, the prototype of cell-mediated immunodeficiency, was accomplished in 1968 by transplanting fetal thymus. This experience has since been successfully repeated and the transplant recipients remain immunologically normal; their development is frequently limited, however, by cardiac and/or neurologic abnormalities which often accompany the syndrome. They must also continue to receive replacement therapy for their hypoparathyroid state; we used dihydrotachysterol. Thymus for transplantation is obtained from an aborted fetus of 12 to 16 weeks. It is implanted within the sheath of the rectus abdominis muscle. Following successful transplantation, no further immunotherapy is necessary; the patient's T-cell compartment is, in some way, induced to develop. Improvement of in vitro lymphocyte responses to phytohemagglutinin have been documented within hours after transplantation, with return to full function over a period of days to weeks. (A modified form of thymus transplantation is discussed below).

The rationale for transplanting thymus in DiGeorge syndrome was based on the absence of this organ in these infants. The rationale for using transfer factor or thymus extract to treat patients with other forms of cell-mediated immunodeficiencies is less definitive. Transfer factor is an extract from lymphocytes which transfers cell-mediated immunity, such as delayed hypersensitivity skin testing to a specific antigen. A nonspecific component of cell-mediated immunity is also transferred by such extracts. To avoid the limitations of transferring only a single person's immunity, transfer factor is usually prepared from pooled lymphocytes. Although it is still an investigational drug in the United States, transfer factor preparations are being prepared and tested at many centers throughout the world and have been used to treat hundreds of patients. A significant number of patients with chronic mucocutaneous candidiasis appear to have improved dramatically following a combination of antifungal therapy and transfer factor administration. In patients with Wiskott-Aldrich syndrome, eczema often clears shortly after transfer factor therapy is initiated, but this effect is transient; a few patients have also experienced fewer recurrent infections. Ongoing trials suggest that transfer factor may also have a role as an immune stimulant for certain cancer patients. Adverse reactions are few; they include transient leukopenia and a slight risk of hepatitis. In general, the results of transfer factor therapy have been less exciting than originally expected.

Extract of calf thymus (thymosin) is a very recent addition to the armamentarium of the clinical immunologist. Preliminary results are encouraging although the effect of thymosin appears limited to reconstitution of the T-compartment. In patients with ataxia-telangiectasia, T-cell parameters improved in all of six patients so treated. In several patients with Wiskott-Aldrich syndrome, eczema has cleared and fewer infections are experienced. An attempt to predict which patients would be helped by thymosin, by in vitro incubation of this preparation with the candidate's lymphocytes, has proved of some prognostic value. As with transfer factor, there are few theoretical dangers to the patient and adverse reactions have been mild.

Severe Combined Immunodeficiency Disease (SCID). In 1968, the rationale for treatment of infants with SCID was to replace a hematopoietic stem population with bone marrow cells which would be capable of differentiating into immunocompetent lymphocytes under the influence of the patient's own central lymphoid organs. Prior to this time, numerous attempts to reconstitute such patients with thymus transplantation had uniformly failed. Bone marrow transplantation successfully and permanently reconstitutes both T and B compartments as evidenced by approximately 40 long-term survivors over the past nine years. The major limitation to this approach is the ever-present and poorly understood danger of a graft-versus-host reaction—a rather uniform syndrome of high fever, a morbilliform rash, hepatosplenomegaly (with elevated serum liver enzymes) and anemia followed by pancytopenia and death within two weeks of the initial insult. (Treatment of graft-versus-host disease is discussed below). The insult derives from transplanting histoincompatible lymphocytes or their precursors to a patient who lacks the ability to reject histoincompatible cells. For this reason, successful bone marrow transplantation for SCID has been limited almost entirely to infants fortunate enough to have a sibling who matches for the major histocompatibility genes on chromosome 6. Matching is determined in two ways: (1) HLA serology and genotyping of the family and (2) mixed leukocyte culture reactions between the potential donor and recipient. In the latter studies, little or no response between the cells indicates histocompatibility and acceptability for a bone marrow transplant. Recent developments in this area, however, portend a final breakthrough in HLA-D typing which promises to allow identification of potential histocompatible donors beyond the immediate family.

Meanwhile, for infants with SCID but without a histocompatible sibling, numerous innovative approaches have been tried. Transplantation of fetal liver offers the availability of an uncommitted stem population which also has the potential to develop tolerance to its new host, the histoincompatible patient. Since 1975, seven patients with SCID have been successfully reconstituted with fetal (8 to 16 weeks) liver transplants. In two of these, however, reconstitution was limited to the T-compartment. Fetal thymus transplantation, preceded by transfer factor administration, has also resulted in reconstitution of the T-compartment in several SCID patients; the remaining B-compartment deficiency can then be treated with ISG.

Recently, Hong and coworkers have allowed thymus remnants, removed during cardiac surgery, to remain in culture for several weeks. During this time, lymphocytes egress from the thymus, leaving behind an "empty" organ which is much less apt to be rejected or to produce graft-versus-host disease. When similar thymus preparations have been transplanted between allogeneic (mismatched) rabbits, little or no rejection reaction against this tissue has been observed. The cultured thymic preparation is injected intraperitoneally through an indwelling catheter. This approach has been successful in restoring both T- and B-compartments in six patients with SCID. The mechanisms by which this reconstitution is accomplished are unclear.

Enzyme Replacement. Several patients with combined immunodeficiency and ADA deficiency have improved following transplantation of frozen irradiated packed red cells (15 ml./kg. in infants; it may be necessary to first remove a similar amount of the patient's blood). The half-life of transfused enzyme ADA approximates one month. These transfusions have restored immunologic functions; the patients have remained free of infection and are developing normally.

Transcobalamin II Deficiency. Several families have been identified in which infants develop severe granulocytosis, thrombocytopenia and megaloblastic anemia accompanied by malabsorption syndrome, agammaglobulinemia and absence of serum transcobalamin II. After an injection into one infant of vitamin B_{12} (1 mg. intramuscularly each week), the fetal vitamin B_{12} binding-protein, transcobalamin III, appeared and Ig levels rose to normal. Family studies suggest that this disorder is transmitted as an autosomal recessive trait.

Immunostimulants. The rationale for the use of immunostimulants in the treatment of patients with immunodeficiencies does not differ greatly from the use of transfer factor or thymosin; an attempt is made to boost whatever immune function the patient has. BCG has been used in this way for more than a decade in attempts to help cancer patients. It is more effective locally than systemically, but overall results of recent clinical trials are discouraging. BCG has been responsible for several deaths when administered as a vaccination to patients with severe combined immunodeficiency. Perhaps for this reason, it has not been used as an immunostimulant in patients with immunodeficiency. *Corynebacterium parvum* has received attention recently as an immunostimulant, again primarily in cancer patients. After weekly intravenous administration, rises in diphtheria antibody titers as well as in the levels of serum IgG have been observed. However, its administration is associated with high fevers, severe nausea, vomiting and chills, making it rather impractical for routine use. Levamisole, originally introduced as an antihelmintic, shows great promise as an immunostimulant. Still an investigational drug also, various dose schedules are being evaluated. Experience with this preparation in patients with immunodeficiency is as yet limited and efficacy will no doubt depend upon the underlying pathology of each patient. Patients with rheumatoid arthritis, aphthous stomatitis and herpes simplex infections appear to improve following administration of levamisole. Clinical trials have, thus far, associated levamisole with leukopenia, unusual sensitivity to odors and taste, headaches, myositis, irritability and several other symptoms. However, it appears that many of these symptoms may have been related to excessively high doses used in early studies.

COMPLICATIONS

Recurrent Infections. The spectra of microorganisms which most commonly affect patients with B- or T- compartment deficiencies, or patients with chronic granulomatous disease, are described in detail in a previous edition. (Current Pediatric Therapy, Edition 6, 1973). Although the fact remains that patients with humoral immunodeficiencies suffer primarily from infections with extracellular pyogenic bacteria and *Pneumocystis carinii,* there is increasing evidence that these patients do not combat viral infections effectively either. Numerous workers have documented prolonged viral excretion in patients with hypogammaglobulinemia (polio, hepatitis, ECHO, adeno, herpes, cytomegalo, measles, rubella) and in Wiskott-Aldrich syndrome (papova). We recently described a subset of patients with hypoimmunoglobulinemia who develop a chronic progressive panencephalitis which is invariably fatal after two to four years. Onset of the complication may be delayed for many years after initial diagnosis of the immunodeficiency. Boys are more commonly affected than girls and preliminary evidence suggests that patients typing for HLA-B7 may be more susceptible to this complication than others with immunodeficiency but without HLA-B7. We recommend an annual spinal tap for such patients to check for pleocytosis in the cerebrospinal fluid. No specific therapy is available at present although we have tried in one patient—steroids, *C. parvum,* levamisole, plasma infusion and cultured thymus transplantation—all to no avail.

Pneumocystis carinii infections are characterized by an insidious onset of dyspnea with mild fever and cough; a marked eosinophilia has been noted in some patients with congenital hypoimmunoglobulinemia. Open lung biopsy is the most effective approach to a definitive diagnosis although this is not always advisable due to other clinical considerations. Recent studies suggest that cotrimoxazole or trimethoprim-sulfamethoxazole (Septra or Bactrim) is effective in the treatment of *Pneumocystis carinii* and is associated with fewer side affects than pentamidine (the latter is available only from the National Disease Control Center, Atlanta, Georgia). Two hundred mg. of trimethoprim/m²/day in three divided doses (in combination with sulfamethoxazole) has been associated with a remarkable decrease in the number of infectious complications of patients suffering with chronic granulomatous disease. We supplement such therapy with 3 mg. of folinic acid per os every two weeks to prevent secondary folic acid deficiency; however, limited studies by others suggest that this may not be necessary. The use of other antimicrobial agents in the treatment of patients with immunodeficiency disease does not differ significantly from the principles outlined elsewhere in this volume.

Gastrointestinal Complications. *Giardia lamblia* is found frequently in patients with humoral immunodeficiency. Symptomatic patients can be treated with metronidazole (Flagyl), 10 mg./kg./day, in divided doses for 10 days. Patients with IgA deficiency may suffer from food intolerance as well as *Giardia lamblia* infection. In these patients, a search should be made for autoantibodies to intestinal wall antigens as well as determination of B-cell antigens common to patients with celiac disease. Occasionally patients with severe combined-system deficiencies have been found to suffer from protein-losing enteropathies secondary to either an inflammatory process or to a fistula between lymph channels and the duodenal lumen. In the former, gut biopsies demonstrate flattened villi with dilated lacteals. Lymphangiograms reveal grossly dilated lymphatic ducts and nodes; this has been confirmed by direct inspection. Hypocalcemic tetany often accompanies this syndrome and must be treated aggressively with administration of calcium gluconate. A medium-chain triglyceride diet may reverse protein-losing enteropathy after a period of several months with return to normal of serum Ig, lymphocyte levels and other parameters. Eventually this diet can often be discontinued leaving the patient symptom-free. The therapy of patients with specific food intolerance is discussed elsewhere in this volume.

Autoimmune Disorders. Patients with selective IgA deficiency often suffer from autoimmune diseases such as systemic lupus erythematosus, rheumatoid arthritis or thyroiditis. Vitiligo associated with IgA deficiency may also have an autoimmune etiology. Chronic sinopulmonary infections are common among IgA deficient patients and one wonders whether some of the frequent gastroenteritis may be secondary to repeated courses of antibiotics. It is also conceivable that recurring insults to bowel mucosa may precipitate the formation of some of these autoantibodies. A peculiar stippling of the cornea (appreciated best by slit-lamp examination) has been described and may be responsible for impaired vision in some patients with selective IgA deficiency. Patients with various types of complement deficiencies appear to develop a form of systemic lupus erythematosus which is occasionally characterized by negative lupus erythematosus preparations.

Malignancy. The incidence of cancer among children with certain types of immunodeficiency is approximately 1000 times higher than that among the general pediatric population. Patients with ataxia-telangiectasia and Wiskott-Aldrich syndrome have the highest incidence (approximately 1 in 8 develops a malignancy before death); however, an increased malignancy has been reported for every major form of primary immunodeficiency disease. While most of these malignancies are lymphoid, nonlymphoid tumors have also been reported with considerable frequency. IgA deficient patients and patients with the thymoma-immunodeficiency syndrome actually suffer more from epithelial than from lymphoreticular cancers. Recent evidence indicates that the incidence of malignancy is also higher among the families of patients with ataxia-telangiectasia.

CONTRAINDICATED TREATMENT

Blood Transfusion. Transfusion of blood products can be a very dangerous procedure for patients with immunodeficiency disease. As alluded to above, when live histoincompatible lymphocytes are transfused (as in an ABO-matched but HLA-mismatched blood transfusion) into a patient who lacks cell-mediated immunity, these lymphocytes may produce a graft-versus-host reaction which is uniformly fatal. Treatment of this complication, once the rash appears, has been difficult. Some reports claim that the reaction can be reversed with antithymocyte globulin (ATG); however, others using the very same ATG preparation have not been successful in confirming this result. Steroids have been ineffective. The treatment of choice at present remains ATG which can be obtained only in limited supply and as an investigational drug. If blood products are required for a patient with severe cell-mediated immunodeficiency, the well-oxygenated blood should be irradiated with 3000 R prior to administration. For unforeseen emergencies, we routinely store several units of frozen Rh negative, group O blood which has been irradiated prior to freezing. The charts of patients requiring only irradiated blood are tagged to indicate that such blood is being held for them in the blood bank.

When frequent platelet transfusions are necessary for a patient with Wiskott-Aldrich syndrome, HLA-matched platelets should, if possible, be used to reduce the risks of sensitization. The in vivo survival of such platelets is also thought to be greater than that of non-HLA-matched platelets. When a patient is a potential candidate for bone marrow transplantation, every effort is made to avoid presensitizing that patient with any blood products.

Patients with selective IgA deficiency, especially those with levels of IgA close to zero, often have antibodies against IgA. When such patients receive IgA-containing plasma or blood, they may experience anaphylactoid shock. If blood transfusion is required, washed packed cells can be utilized. Such patients are encouraged to wear Medic-Alert wrist bands indicating their diagnosis and a telephone number where more information will be supplied, including a warning to avoid IgA-containing blood products.

Immunizations. Many of the infants who died in previous years from vaccinia gangrenosa suffered from severe combined immunodeficiency. Because smallpox vaccination is no longer performed routinely in the United States, such cases are now rare. BCG vaccination can also prove fatal to these patients. Such problems can generally be avoided by postponing immunizations involving live microorganisms until after six months of age, since by this time a history of frequent infections will usually raise the suspicion of immunodeficiency. As a general rule, patients with suspected or proven immunodeficiency disease should not receive immunization with live viruses.

8

Spleen and Lymphatic System

Management of Patient after Splenectomy

LOUIS K. DIAMOND, M.D.

The syndrome of overwhelming post-splenectomy infection deserves separate consideration inasmuch as its course, especially its speed of progression, is far different from that usually seen in individuals with intact spleens. (What is said here about the postsplenectomy syndrome applies equally well to congenital absence or to hypoplasia of the spleen, and to certain functional aplasias of the spleen, e.g., in some sickle-cell anemias.) Necessary are constant alertness to the danger of the occurrence of the syndrome, early recognition of its onset and prompt specific treatment. The frightening speed of the spread of infection is characterized by progression from a slight sore throat and malaise at onset to coma and death from bacteremia, septicemia and meningitis within 12 to 18 hours. The causative organism is most commonly the pneumococcus, less often *Hemophilus influenzae* and, rarely, the meningococcus. All of these organisms have a distinctive carbohydrate capsule and multiply very rapidly. Splenic function is thereby important as an inline blood filter and as a processor of antibody production on first contact with one of these bacteria.

Management is as follows:

1. When the average responsive child of about 3 years of age or older complains that he feels ill or develops a sore throat, a headache or nausea followed by vomiting, the parents should be impressed with the need to notify the physician promptly. Within the first hour or two from onset of symptoms, in conjunction with the physical examination, the nasopharynx and blood should be cultured for bacteria and, unless a diagnosis of some other illness seems likely, the patient should be started on antibiotic therapy. Ampicillin is the drug of choice because of its general effectiveness against the pneumococcus, as well as the influenza bacillus and the meningococcus. The dosage should be at the maximum level for the size of the patient, probably 250 mg. every 4 hours for the first 24 hours and then every 6 hours until recovery is evident. Intravenous administration is indicated when bacteremia or meningitis is likely, or confirmed, or if oral medication cannot be tolerated. If the causative organism is identified as the pneumococcus, aqueous penicillin may be used (see Pneumococcal Infections).

If the family physician is not able to see the patient within a few hours to assume full responsibility, it is advisable for the parents to be instructed to start ampicillin treatment to guard against the possibility of uncontrolled pneumococcal infection. Occasionally, if a viral infection is the cause of the illness, the patient may receive ampicillin unnecessarily for 48 hours; nevertheless, this is far preferable to failure to treat a pneumococcal invasion if it is actually occurring.

2. For the child under 3 years of age, or sometimes even an older child who cannot be trusted to complain or otherwise indicate when a sore throat or other early symptoms of an upper respiratory infection have their onset, it is safer to use prophylactic ampicillin medication routinely from the time of splenectomy. For prophylactic treatment, a schedule of 125 mg. of ampicillin twice daily should protect against infection with pneumococcus or the other organisms responsible for the syndrome under discussion. If sensitivity to ampicillin

develops, one of the other antibiotics which combat these particular organisms should be used.

3. When a postsplenectomy patient develops signs of serious infection, such as high fever, chills, severe headache, stiff neck, drowsiness or coma, it is imperative that a diagnostic workup be performed promptly and treatment started simultaneously. In addition to the complete physical examination, a white blood count and differential should be obtained; swabs of the nasopharynx should be cultured for organisms, followed by cultures of the blood and spinal fluid. The spinal fluid should be smeared on a glass slide and examined immediately while routine analysis is being carried out. With pneumococcal meningitis, the spinal fluid may appear relatively clear yet contain many organisms which can be recognized easily by a Gram stain. Treatment for suspected bacteremia and meningitis should be vigorous and comprehensive. Ampicillin should be administered intravenously in full dosage. For hypovolemia and dehydration from fever, sweating and vomiting, parenteral fluids containing glucose should be given intravenously. To combat possible adrenal hemorrhage (Waterhouse-Friderichsen syndrome), corticosteroids, blood, plasma or albumin infusion may be indicated.

A new approach to the much desired protection against pneumococcal infection in the asplenic individual consists of the use of polyvalent pneumococcal vaccines for immunization. This should induce specific antibodies in about 2 weeks to 2 months after subcutaneous injection. Such immunization is best given at least 1 to 2 weeks before splenectomy to patients in whom the operation can be scheduled in advance, or as soon after splenectomy as possible if the operation has been done without such preliminary preparation. This protective immunization against the common types of pathogenic pneumococci should materially diminish the hazard of overwhelming postsplenectomy infection and improve the prognosis for the spleenless individual.

Disorders of the Spleen

HOWARD A. PEARSON, M.D.

CONGESTIVE SPLENOMEGALY AND HYPERSPLENISM

The venous flow from the spleen may be obstructed at the level of the splenic or portal veins or within the substance of the liver producing splenic congestion and ultimately splenomegaly. Liver diseases which cause destruction of hepatic cells and subsequent fibrosis include postnecrotic cirrhosis, galactosemia, cystic fibrosis, biliary atresia, alpha-1 trypsin deficiency and schistosomiasis. Omphalitis, either primary or following umbilical vein cannulation, may lead to portal or splenic vein thrombophlebitis with subsequent obliteration. Congenital anomalies of the portal vein may also cause venous obstruction with secondary splenomegaly.

The clinical manifestations of this condition are those of an enlarged spleen. In addition, the enlargement of the spleen from any cause may be associated with excessive destruction of the formed elements of the blood, resulting in hemolytic anemia, thrombocytopenia and neutropenia—alone or in combination—the so-called hypersplenic state.

Peripheral pancytopenia of varying degrees of severity is present, but the bone marrow shows active hematopoiesis. Although the peripheral neutrophil and platelet count may be quite low, infection and bleeding are unusual. This may be because the enlarged spleen may sequester blood cells without actually destroying them. In response to obstruction, portal venous pressure increases and a network of collateral circulation develops through the short gastric, esophageal and hemorrhoidal veins. These vessels become enormously enlarged and tortuous. Massive upper gastrointestinal bleeding from thin-walled, easily traumatized esophageal varicosities may be the first clinical manifestation of congestive splenomegaly.

Therapy of acute hemorrhage is directed at restoration of blood volume and correction of red cell loss. Emergency surgical intervention is rarely indicated during the first bleeding episode. With supportive treatment, the bleeding almost always stops spontaneously, and many years may intervene between bleeding episodes. Sengstaken tubes are of limited use in children.

The treatment for congestive splenomegaly involves determining the anatomic site of venous obstruction. Portal pressure is measured, and injection of radiopaque dye into the spleen permits visualization of the splenic and portal vein. In older children this may be done percutaneously.

When only the splenic vein is obstructed, splenectomy is curative. In cases with extensive involvement of the portal vein or in instances in which intrahepatic obstruction secondary to cirrhosis is present, splenectomy may correct the hematologic abnormalities. However, it will not relieve, and may actually aggravate, the hemorrhagic consequences of portal hypertension. Portacaval anastomosis, which is preferable to splenorenal shunting in the young child, may be indicated when repetitive bleeding has occurred from esophageal varices. Successful relief of portal hypertension by shunting procedures may result in decreased splenic size and resolution of a depressed blood count.

Splenic Cysts.   Two types of splenic cysts have been described. Pseudocysts, which occur after trauma or infarction, have no epithelial lining and are filled with necrotic blood and tissue. The rare epidermoid cysts contain clear fluid and are lined with stratified columnar epithelium. A diagnosis of splenic cyst can be made by isotopic scanning or sonographic techniques. Splenectomy is indicated.

Rupture of the Spleen.   Traumatic injury to the spleen may result from a hard blow to the left side or flank, such as may occur in automobile accidents or contact sports. When the spleen is enlarged, particularly when the enlargement is acute as in infectious mononucleosis or in the infant with erythroblastosis, rupture may occur after relatively minor trauma. Although laparotomy and splenectomy have been strongly recommended in the past, some surgeons are currently attempting to preserve the spleen in selected cases.

Splenectomy.   Excision of the spleen is performed for a variety of indications including splenic rupture, removal of cysts or tumors, as part of a staging procedure for Hodgkin's disease, and as therapy for hematologic conditions associated with excessive destruction of red cells (hereditary spherocytosis, autoimmune hemolytic anemia) or platelets (chronic idiopathic thrombocytopenic purpura).

Postsplenectomy Infection.   Absence or removal of the spleen is associated with an increased risk of severe, overwhelming and often fatal pneumococcal and H. influenzal sepsis and meningitis. The magnitude of risk varies depending upon both the age of the patient at the time of splenectomy and the reason for which the operation is performed. The risk is quite low when the operation is performed for traumatic rupture, hereditary spherocytosis or idiopathic thrombocytopenic purpura, much greater in thalassemia major and Hodgkin's disease, and extraordinarily high in the Wiskott-Aldrich syndrome. The risk is increased in all categories in younger infants and children. It should be emphasized that postsplenectomy infection has occurred at all ages, regardless of the indication for splenectomy. Because of these risks, splenectomy should only be performed for pressing indications and, when possible, should be delayed until at least five to six years of age.

Prophylactic oral peninillin, 250 mg. twice daily, has been advocated after splenectomy, but there are no data to assess the effectiveness or necessary duration of this prophylaxis. In the future, immunization with polysaccharide vaccines against pneumococci and *H. influenzae* may be of benefit.

Lymphangitis

TERRY YAMAUCHI, M.D.

Lymphangitis is an inflammation of the lymphatic system draining an area of suppuration. It is manifested in the form of painful red streaks which radiate proximally from the infected site and is a sign of spreading infection. The regional lymph nodes are also often involved.

Streptococci are the most commonly associated bacteria. Erysipelas is the most obvious form of lymphangitis. Although streptococci are not often recovered from skin lesions, initial therapy should be aimed at eradication of this organism. Treatment involves incision and drainage of localized infection, elevation and antibiotics. Local heat in combination with analgesics may be of value for symptomatic relief. Penicillin remains the most effective antibiotic in the treatment of streptococcal infections. In the child under 10 years of age, phenoxymethyl penicillin in doses of 400,000 units every six hours by mouth should be used. Older children should receive larger doses, up to 800,000 units per dose. For the penicillin-sensitive individual, erythromycin, 50 mg./kg./day in four divided doses orally, is effective. Therapy should be continued for 10 days. In the toxic child with high temperature and rapid progression of lesions, systemic penicillin G in doses of 50,000 to 100,000 units/kg./day should be administered.

Staphylococci can also produce lymphangitis and, if suspected, should be treated with a penicillinase-resistant penicillin, dicloxacillin, 50 mg./kg./day in four divided doses orally.* In severe infections methicillin or cephalothin, 100 mg./kg./day in four divided doses intravenously, is indicated.†

Tetanus prophylaxis should be considered in any child with lymphangitis. If tetanus im-

---

*Manufacturer's note: Experience with dicloxacillin in the neonatal period is limited, therefore dosage for the newborn is not recommended.

†Manufacturer's note: Clinical experience with the intravenous use of methicillin in infants and children is too limited to permit intravenous dosage recommendations.

munization is not adequate, tetanus toxoid, 0.5 cc. or human tetanus immune globulin, 250 units should be administered.

Recurrent lymphangitis, although rare, does occur in patients with lymphedema. These few patients may benefit from long-term antibiotic prophylaxis. Penicillin is the drug of choice, either benzathine penicillin G, 1.2 million units intramuscularly once a month, or phenoxymethyl penicillin in amounts of 400,000 units four times a day orally 5 to 7 successive days each month. For the penicillin-sensitive individual, erythromycin can be substituted for phenoxymethyl penicillin.

Lymph Node Infections

TERRY YAMAUCHI, M.D.

Lymph node infections in children often are difficult to diagnose and treat. Bacterial lymphadenitis is usually associated with a primary focus. If the primary infection is treated vigorously with debridement and antibiotics, the lymph node involvement will resolve. However, if there is no well delineated site other than the lymph node, which may be covered by tense, erythematous, tender skin, and if the lymph node is large and fluctuant or the child toxic, therapy needs to be directed at the infected node itself. Treatment should include incision and drainage or aspiration and appropriate antibiotics. Any material obtained by drainage or aspiration should be cultured to demonstrate the etiologic agent. The microorganisms most commonly recovered from these infections are *Streptococcus pyogenes* and *Staphylococcus aureus*, and antibiotic therapy should be aimed at their eradication. In streptococci infections, penicillin is the drug of choice and a dose of 200,000 to 400,000 units every six hours by mouth for 10 days is usually adequate treatment. In the penicillin-sensitive individual, either cephaloxin or erythromycin, 50 mg./kg./day in four divided doses for 10 days, may be used.

Staphylococcus aureus may be a more common cause of lymph node infection in the infant under one year of age. Since the majority of staphylococci isolated from these infections are resistant to penicillin, therapy should include anti-penicillinase antibiotics. Dicloxacillin,* 25 mg./kg./day orally, or methicillin,† 100

mg./kg./day intravenously in four divided doses, are the drugs of choice. The spectrum of these antibiotics includes streptococci and therefore provides appropriate antibiotic coverage for the two most common pathogens in this disease process. Although resolution of the infected lymph node is often quick and 10 days of antibiotics will usually be sufficient, more lengthy treatment may be necessary with larger, suppurative lymph nodes.

Lymphadenitis is most easily recognized in the cervical lymphatic system; however, inflammation of nodes in the axilla and inguinal region is not uncommon. Treatment is the same regardless of the location.

On rare occasions lymph node infections may be caused by microorganisms other than the previously mentioned gram-positive bacteria. In the western and southwestern portions of the United States, plague is still a consideration in the etiology of lymphadenitis. *Yersinia pestis* can be treated with streptomycin, 20 to 40 mg./kg./day in two doses intramuscularly, or chloramphenicol sodium succinate, 50 mg./kg./day intravenously in four divided doses for 10 days.

Tularemia is also a cause of lymph node inflammation usually in association with a cutaneous ulcer or ocular infection. Streptomycin, 20 to 40 mg./kg./day in two doses intramuscularly for 7 to 10 days, will usually lead to rapid resolution.

Lymphadenitis may also be seen in a number of viral infections such as measles and infectious mononucleosis. Lymph node involvement will diminish as the viral infection resolves. Treatment is symptomatic and aimed at relieving fever and discomfort.

Chronic inflammation of the lymph nodes may be caused by atypical strains of *Mycobacterium*. For these infections a combination of antituberculous agents plus surgical excision of the involved lymph node provides optimal therapy. The recommended drug treatment is a combination of isoniazid, 10 to 30 mg./kg./day in two doses orally, and ethambutol,* 15 to 20 mg./kg./day orally, or para-aminosalicylic acid, 300 mg./kg./day in three doses orally. Treatment with two drugs should be continued for one year after complete healing of the excision wound. Cat-scratch disease may also cause lymph node enlargement and will usually resolve without medical intervention. If the node involvement is prolonged or the swelling causes discomfort, surgical excision is indicated.

---

*Manufacturer's note: Experience with dicloxacillin in the neonatal period is limited; therefore dosage for the newborn is not recommended by the manufacturer.

†Manufacturer's note: Clinical experience with the intravenous use of methicillin in infants and children is too limited to permit intravenous dosage recommendations.

---

*Ethambutol is not recommended in children under 13 years of age.

Lymphedema

ERIC W. FONKALSRUD, M.D.

Idiopathic primary lymphedema that produces swelling of the extremities in infancy and childhood may be congenital (13 per cent), which is present at birth, or lymphedema praecox (87 per cent), which usually first appears in early adolescence. When congenital lymphedema is hereditary (uncommon), it is designated Milroy's disease. Although the exact pathophysiology of congenital lymphedema has not been clearly defined, it is believed that the superficial lymphatic network is hypoplastic or absent and is therefore unable to effectively transport lymph, which then pools in the subcutaneous fat until the oncotic pressure of the tissue exceeds the superficial venous osmotic pressure and venous decompression occurs. Whereas lymphedema praecox is almost invariably a disorder of the superficial lymphatics, congenital lymphedema may also involve the subfascial lymphatics and displace bones and tendons. Congenital lymphedema most often involves the dorsum of the foot and rarely extends above the knees but is occasionally present in the upper extremities. Children with congenital lymphedema of the upper extremities frequently have lymphatic abnormalities in other areas of the body, particularly the external genitalia, and often intestinal lymphangiectasia with protein-losing enteropathy. Lymphedema praecox usually involves one or both lower extremities often extending up to the groin, is three times more common in females, and rarely, if ever, involves the hand and arm.

Acquired lymphedema may result from wide resection of inguinal or axillary tissues, or following radiation of these areas. In contrast to primary lymphedema in which the lymphatics are hypoplastic, in acquired lymphedema, the subcutaneous lymphatics are usually markedly distended and lymphangitis commonly occurs.

Cosmetic deformity and swelling of the foot which make wearing of shoes difficult and uncomfortable are the initial complaints of most children with primary lymphedema. Lymphangitis is very uncommon. Obesity appears to accelerate the limb swelling due to lymphedema praecox. Lymphangiograms, which are usually technically unsuccessful and difficult to perform, are not helpful in most children with primary lymphedema. Arterio-grams and venograms are almost invariably normal in children with primary lymphedema and are not necessary as a part of the workup. Roentgenograms of the bony structures of the hands and feet in patients with congenital lymphedema may show wide separation of the metacarpal or metatarsal bones. The overlying skin is usually normal in both congenital lymphedema and lymphedema praecox.

Nonoperative measures are recommended for congenital lymphedema during the first 2 years of life, since the majority of children will experience a decrease in severity of the lymphedema compared with general body growth. Elastic support stockings or bandages are usually of little benefit for congenital lymphedema. For severe congenital lymphedema, staged subcutaneous lymphangiectomy may provide a very significant reduction in the bulk of the extremity and improve function. The modified Kondolean procedure in which full thickness skin flaps are used generally provides an excellent functional and cosmetic result. Full thickness or split thickness free skin grafts have generally been unsatisfactory in the management of childhood primary lymphedemas.

In adolescents with lymphedema praecox, considerable benefit may result from the use of above knee form-fitting elastic stockings. Full extremity inflatable compression units may provide transient improvement in limb swelling for a few hours; however, it is generally not practical for the majority of children. Exercise appears to promote lymphatic drainage from the extremities and should be encouraged. Diuretics have no place in the management of congenital lymphedema or lymphedema praecox. Prolonged extremity elevation may reduce the swelling in lymphedema praecox, although it is rarely feasible. Lymphedema praecox does not appear to improve with age in the majority of patients.

In children with moderate to severe lymphedema praecox, staged subcutaneous lymphangiectomy under general anesthesia and tourniquet control may significantly reduce the swelling of the extremity. Prolonged postoperative elastic bandage support is recommended. Wound healing is usually excellent and infection is uncommon. Autologous blood transfusions are recommended if blood replacement is necessary. Omental transposition operations have been unsuccessful in the management of primary lymphedemas in childhood.

Lymphangioma

ERIC W. FONKALSRUD, M.D.

Lymphangiomas are malformations or hemartomas of the lymphatic system of non-neoplastic origin. They may occur almost anywhere in the body, but are most often found in the neck, axilla, tongue, trunk, mediastinum, and retroperitoneal areas. Lymphangiomas may be classified into three groups: lymphangioma simplex, consisting of small capillary-sized lymphatic channels; cavernous lymphangioma, consisting of dilated lymphatic vessels, often with fibrous adventitia; and cystic lymphangioma or hygroma, composed of endothelium-lined cysts of varying size.

Lymphangiomas and hygromas are believed to originate from a sequestration of the primitive embryonic lymphatic anlage although they probably also represent areas of localized lymphatic stasis caused by congenital absence or blockage of regional lymphatic channels. Lymphatic malformations are believed to enlarge without the formation of new tissue as a result of fluid accumulation that causes distention of existing endothelial lined lymphatic spaces. It is unlikely that lymphangiomas represent proliferating neoplasms, as suggested by the infrequency of their growth during childhood and the rare coincidental occurrence of malignant lesions in the involved areas.

Lymphangiomatous cysts and channels are filled with serous fluid that may contain lymphocytes and occasional neutrophils. Groups of hyperplastic lymph nodes often occur in close proximity. Vascular capillaries and cavernous spaces are frequently interspersed with, or adjacent to, the lesion; when the vascularity is extensive, the lesions may be called hemolymphangiomas. When irritation or infection has been minimal, the walls are thin and delicate.

Although cystic hygromas may appear clinically different from cavernous lymphangiomas, there is no clear dividing line between the two. In general, the larger cystic lesions occur in close proximity to the large veins and lymphatic ducts, for example, in the neck and axilla, whereas lymphangiomas are usually located on the trunk, in the tongue, or in the extremities. Different macroscopic and microscopic forms of lymphangioma may occur in different parts of the same lesion. Lymphangiomas occur with equal frequency in male and females. Approximately 90 per cent are diagnosed before the age of 18 months, and they rarely appear after the age of 5 years.

The most common initial complaint is the presence of a mass or lesion that has gradually enlarged. Rapid expansion may be produced by hemorrhage or inflammation, usually in infancy, and may cause respiratory distress if the lesion is located in the neck or thorax. Hygromas usually are located in the neck, most commonly in the posterior triangle. They tend to transilluminate unless filled with blood. Hygromas rarely involve the skin and usually infiltrate around muscles, vessels, and nerves rather than through them. Lymphangiomas of the tongue, trunk, and extremities generally infiltrate adjacent muscle and may produce small cystic lesions of the overlying skin. Both lymphangiomas and hygromas may extend into the upper mediastinum through the thoracic outlet

TREATMENT

Surgical excision is the only consistently effective method of management. Since spontaneous regression is rare, observation of large or unsightly lymphangiomas for prolonged periods does not appear justified. Repeated aspiration, injection of sclerosing solutions, and radiation therapy have in general been of limited value. Operation in small infants should be avoided when possible to minimize the risk of injury to vital structures. Complete excision of the lesion should be performed when feasible; however, in occasional patients, staged resection may be required. Staging is usually necessary for lymphangiomas of the tongue, floor of the mouth, and chest wall, in which deep muscular infiltration commonly occurs. Cavernous lymphangiomas and cystic hygromas may in most circumstances be excised safely during the first several months of life. Keen judgment must be exercised to avoid permanent injury to nerves and other vital structures during resection of such malformations. Occasionally repeated aspiration or injection of sclerosing solutions may be helpful in managing residual hygromas that are in close proximity to vital structures. True malignant degeneration into lymphangiosarcoma has never been documented prior to the age of puberty and therefore radical resection should not be undertaken.

Lymphangiomas in the parotid gland may be managed most effectively by parotidectomy during the first several months of life with care taken to identify and preserve the facial nerve.

Lymphangiomas of the tongue and frequently the floor of the mouth should be excised during the first few months of life, preferably in multiple stages. The lesion usually involves the anterior and mid portion of the tongue and may be removed by resection of the tip with partial debulking of the mid portion of the tongue to provide adequate function for speech.

Although rare, lymphangiomas have been reported to occur within the liver, spleen, pancreas, bone, intestine, and may be a source of chylous effusions within the abdomen or thorax.

Intestinal lymphangiectasia is characterized by dilated intestinal submucosal and subserosal lymphatics, protein-losing enteropathy, hypoalbuminemia, hypoproteinemic edema, and lymphopenia. The condition may be mild or severe, and transitory or chronic. Diarrhea is the most common initial manifestation. Vomiting frequently occurs and growth retardation is often present. Many patients will have associated peripheral lymphedema of one or more extremities. The diagnosis may be confirmed in severe cases by gastrointestinal roentgenograms or by jejunal mucosal biopsy. Specific treatment with a high-protein, low-fat diet with added medium-chain triglyceride has been helpful in alleviating symptoms in most patients. Surgical resection has little merit in the management of intestinal lymphangiectasia, which is usually a diffuse condition. Chylous peritoneal effusions may be present with intestinal lymphangiectasia as well as with lymphangiomas involving the retroperitoneal tissues.

Non-Hodgkin's Lymphoma

NORMA WOLLNER, M.D.

Non-Hodgkin's lymphoma in children, regardless of primary site, histologic type or age, is a disease that progresses rapidly, with dissemination to bone marrow and central nervous system. Treatment should be instituted on an emergency basis as soon as the disease distribution is determined and the patient is staged. All patients, with the exception of those with initial bone marrow or central nervous system involvement, are treated for two years. Those with bone marrow or central nervous system involvement at the time of diagnosis are treated for three years. Treatment is multidisciplinary and includes chemotherapy, surgery and radiation therapy.

CHEMOTHERAPY

The LSA2L2 protocol, in use since 1971 for pediatric patients, consists of three phases: induction, consolidation and maintenance.

Induction. Day 0: Cyclophosphamide, 40 mg./kg. or 1200 mg./m^2 intravenously by single push. Intravenous hydration with a multielectrolyte solution is started 24 to 48 hours prior to cyclophosphamide, or 4 hours in extreme emergencies. The hydration (a) avoids hemorrhagic cystitis by keeping the urine diluted to a specific gravity of 1.010 or less; (b) avoids renal shutdown due to increased load of tumor breakdown and hyperuricemia; and (c) replaces fluid loss by emesis resulting from administration of cyclophosphamide. The drug should be given early in the morning, or, if it has been given at night, the patient should be awakened every 2 hours to void. Allopurinol and an antiemetic are also given prior to cyclophosphamide.

Day 3: Start prednisone, 2 mg./kg. or 60 mg./m^2 orally in three divided daily doses for a total of 28 days, and then taper it to zero over a period of 5 to 7 days. Give vincristine, 1.5 to 2.25 mg./m^2, by intravenous push. Patients should be given a mild cathartic 24 to 48 hours before the vincristine in order to avoid constipation. The total single dose of vincristine should not exceed 2.5 mg. Start and continue preferably with the higher dose unless there is severe toxicity such as jaw pain, trismus, sore throat, tingling and numbness of fingers and toes, and abdominal pain, distention or severe constipation. In these cases decrease subsequent dosage to about 0.25 mg./m^2 less than that originally given.

Day 5: Methotrexate, 0.25 mg./kg. or 6.25 mg./m^2 intrathecally.

Day 10: Second dose of vincristine, 2 to 2.25 mg./m^2.

Day 12: Daunomycin,* 2 mg./kg. or 60 mg./m^2 intravenously by single push. The urine may become red from the medication.

Day 13: Second dose of daunomycin, 2 mg./kg. or 60 mg./m^2.

Day 17: Third dose of vincristine, 2 to 2.5 mg./m^2 intravenously.

Day 24: Fourth dose of vincristine, 2 to 2.5 mg./m^2 intravenously.

Day 29: Methotrexate, 0.25 mg./kg. or 6.25 mg./m^2, intrathecally.

Day 31: Methotrexate, 0.25 mg./kg. or 6.25 mg./m^2 intrathecally.

This completes the induction phase. At this time a bone marrow aspiration is performed to evaluate response. For those with initial bone marrow involvement, complete remission should be achieved. Marrow should be normal in others. Also, it is at this stage of treatment that all initially abnormal tests (x-

---

*Daunomycin, an investigational drug, is available from the National Cancer Institute.

rays or scans) are repeated to assess clinical and radiologic response.

Consolidation. This should begin two days after the second intrathecal methotrexate injection, or on day 33.

(1) Cytosine arabinoside, 5 mg./kg. or 150 mg./m², to be given early in the morning. Blood counts are taken daily. When bone marrow depression occurs (white blood cell count under 1500, platelets less than 150,000), the drug is stopped. It is restarted when the white count is over 1500 and platelets over 150,000 at the same dose.

(2) Thioguanine, 2.5 mg./kg. or 75 mg./m² orally, 10 to 12 hours after the injection of cytosine arabinoside. This drug is to be discontinued at the same time as cytosine arabinoside, when bone marrow depression occurs. Toxic reactions include nausea, vomiting, fever, rash and conjunctivitis. The nausea and vomiting can be treated with antiemetics and hydration. Fever can be abated with acetominophen, and the rash is to be treated with Benadryl every 8 hours.

(3) L-asparaginase, 2000 I.U./kg. or 60,000 I.U./m² intravenously, daily for a total of 12 injections. This drug is to be started on the day after the last injection of cytosine arabinoside. The patient should be observed for 1 hour after the administration of the drug, and daily for the advent of anaphylactic reactions (urticariform rash, angioneurotic edema, severe chest pain and difficulty in breathing, petechial hemorrhage, cyanosis). These should be treated on an emergency basis by discontinuing the drug and giving Benadryl and hydrocortisone intravenously, with epinephrine subcutaneously if necessary. An anaphylactic reaction terminates this phase of treatment. Other manifestations of toxicity may be nausea, vomiting and headache, but these are not contraindications for continuation of therapy.

(4) 24 hours after the last dose of L-asparaginase, the patient should receive methotrexate, 0.25 mg./kg. or 6.25 mg./m² intrathecally; this dose is repeated 2 days later.

(5) 1,3-bis (2-chloroethyl)-1-nitrosourea (BCNU),* 2 mg./kg. or 60 mg./m², is given intravenously 3 to 5 days after the second intrathecal injection of methotrexate. Bone marrow aspiration is repeated at this time.

After the induction and consolidation phases are completed, rest for one week and then start the maintenance phase.

Maintenance. This phase consists of 5-day cycles of different drugs with a rest period of 7 to 10 days between cycles.

FIRST CYCLE. Thioguanine, 10 mg./kg. or 300 mg./m² orally at night for 4 consecutive days. On the fifth day cyclophosphamide, 20 mg./kg. or 600 mg./m², is given intravenously with hydration.

SECOND CYCLE. Hydroxyurea, 80 mg./kg. or 2400 mg./m² orally at night for 4 consecutive days. Daunomycin, 0.5 to 1.0 mg./kg. or 15 to 30 mg./m², is given intravenously on the fifth day. In the first course of the maintenance phase use 0.5 mg./kg. or 15 mg./m² of daunomycin, increasing the dose to 1.0 mg./kg. or 30 mg./m² in the following course. If tolerated well, the higher dose is used thereafter.

THIRD CYCLE. Methotrexate, 5 mg./day orally for 4 days, followed by BCNU, 1 to 2 mg./kg. or 30 to 60 mg./m² intravenously (average dose tolerated is 30 to 45 mg./m²).

FOURTH CYCLE. Cytosine arabinoside, 5 mg./kg. or 150 mg./m² intravenously for 4 days, to be followed on the fifth day by intravenous vincristine, 1.5 mg./m².

FIFTH CYCLE. Two intrathecal injections of methotrexate, 0.25 mg./kg. or 6.25 mg./m², are given two days apart. Bone marrow aspiration is repeated at the end of this cycle. The total dosage of daunomycin should not exceed 500 mg./m². If the patient has received radiation therapy to the mediastinum, the total dosage of daunomycin should not exceed 350 mg./m².

These cycles are repeated every 7 to 10 days. In disease stages I, II and III, treatment is continued for a total of two years. For patients with stage IV disease or with initial bone marrow or central nervous system involvement, treatment is continued for three years.

FOLLOW-UP AND EVALUATION. All patients should be completely evaluated at the end of the induction phase. If some tests remain positive or questionable with no evidence of clinical disease, the abnormal tests should be repeated in 1 month. If there continues to be no clinical evidence of disease activity, all initially abnormal tests will be repeated again at the end of the treatment.

If the primary site is mediastinal, chest x-rays are to be taken monthly for the first year and every two months for the second year. In all other patients, chest x-rays are obtained every 6 months, or more often if clinically indicated. An electrocardiogram should be obtained every 6 months, or more often if abnormal. If radiation therapy has been given to the mediastinum, even though the total dosage of daunomycin has not exceeded 350 mg./m²,

---

*BCNU is an investigational drug.

an EKG should be obtained every 2 or 3 months until therapy is completed.

In stages I, II and III, bone marrow aspiration should be done monthly for 6 months after completion of therapy. Lumbar punctures are to be performed every 2 months for the first 6 months. In stage IV, bone marrow aspirations are carried out monthly during the first year after cessation of therapy, every two months in the second year, every 4 months in the third year, and twice in the fourth year. Bone marrow examination is not necessary after the fourth year. Spinal taps are performed every 2 months during the first year and then at the time of each bone marrow aspiration in the following years.

RADIATION THERAPY

Radiation therapy to a bulky area of disease (5 cm. or larger) is given if the disease is localized to one area and is not near marrow-producing sites. The total dosage should be 4000 rads in 4 weeks. Therapy is to be started either concomitantly or within 2 or 3 days after the injection of cyclophosphamide.

Mediastinum.   In patients with a primary mediastinal site whose chest x-ray does not show regression greater than 25 per cent, 2000 rads in 2 weeks should be given starting on the third day of chemotherapy. Dosage may be increased to 3000 rads in 3 weeks if reduction in tumor size is slow or if there is still residual disease after 2000 rads. If the initial response to chemotherapy has been good, radiation therapy may be delayed until the third injection of vincristine in the induction phase. Total dosage to be given is 2000 rads. If the pleura is involved, the entire lung and pleura are given 1400 rads while the radiation therapy to the mediastinum is being administered.

Intestines.   If the primary site is bowel, no radiation therapy is to be given until the third vincristine injection in the induction phase, when repeat surgical exploration will be performed in order to determine the amount of residual disease. If no residual disease is found, no radiation therapy is given. If residual disease is found and is surgically removable without spillage, no radiation therapy is given. If residual disease is found and is not resectable, metallic clips are placed around the tumor and radiation is given to this area alone, totaling 2000 to 3000 rads in 2 to 3 weeks, depending on the size of the tumor.

If the primary intra-abdominal disease is in the liver or spleen, radiation is given to the entire epigastrium so as to include both organs. It is administered at the time of the third vincristine injection in the induction phase. The dosage should not exceed 2000 rads in 2 weeks.

In patients presenting with widespread disease, and in whom hepatic and splenic involvement is a manifestation of disseminated disease, radiation is directed at the liver and spleen as well as to other bulky sites of disease.

Ovary.   In primary ovarian lymphoma, radiation is given to the pelvis and the para-aortic nodes, after the healthy ovary has been moved out of the radiation field. The total dose is 2000 to 2500 rads.

Nasopharynx.   All patients with primary nasopharyngeal disease should receive 4000 rads, even if the lesion measures less than 5 cm. If the base of the skull or a peripheral cranial nerve is involved, these should be included in the radiation portal. Radiation therapy should begin at the time of the first vincristine injection. If neck nodes are involved, radiation is directed to both sides of the neck.

Paravertebral Nodes.   If paravertebral masses are present, even though the size of the lesion is less than 5 cm. and the myelogram and neurological examination fail to show any epidural involvement, patients should receive radiation therapy. Recurrence of disease at these sites is a serious complication. The total dosage should be in the range of 3000 to 4000 rads over a 3 to 4 week period. Radiation therapy is begun at the time of the first vincristine injection during induction.

Bone.   Primary bone lesions should receive 6000 rads to the entire bone shaft. If possible, one or both epiphyses should be spared. If there are multiple bone lesions, the area with the largest lesion (presumably the oldest lesion) will receive 4500 to 6000 rads and the other areas 2000 rads. Radiation therapy is to begin at the time of the first dose of vincristine in the induction phase of chemotherapy.

Central Nervous System.   If a patient has evidence of CNS involvement at the time of diagnosis, 2400 rads should be directed to the entire skull over a 2½ to 3 week period, starting at the time of the first vincristine dosage in the induction phase. Additional dosages of intrathecal methotrexate may have to be added between the third and fourth dosages of vincristine, until cell count or the protein returns to normal and cytology is negative.

Subcutaneous Lymphoma.   In the case of primary subcutaneous disease or subcutaneous metastases, radiation therapy should be given to the entire skin by electron beam once a week for 4 to 6 weeks, at 400 rads per dose. This form of radiation therapy will not interfere with the scheduled chemotherapy and should be started at the time of the first vincristine injection of the induction phase.

Peripheral Nodes.   All areas with disease masses 5 cm. or larger should receive radiation therapy. If the disease involves lymph nodes, above and below the diaphragm, the same technique used with Hodgkin's disease should be applied. Since chemotherapy is given at the same time, the total dosage should not exceed 2000 rads in 2 weeks. If the lower neck, supraclavicular and mediastinal nodes are involved, radiation therapy should be given to both sides of the neck, the supraclavicular nodes bilaterally, and to the mediastinum. The entire mediastinum is irradiated and not "postage stamped."

Bone marrow involvement in any of these situations should not be regarded as a deterrent to "curative" radiation.

SURGERY

The role of surgery is mainly diagnostic, either at the time of initial diagnosis or at any time during treatment when there is a question of recurrence.

9

Endocrine System

Hypopituitarism

SOLOMON A. KAPLAN, M.D.

The method of treatment depends upon the nature of the disease and which pituitary hormones are affected. Successful therapy can only be achieved if the nature of the defect is properly ascertained. Adequate and careful testing must first be performed to determine which hormonal functions are disturbed and which require replacement therapy. The testing must yield precise information on the capacity of the pituitary gland to secrete growth hormone (GH), adrenocorticotropic hormone (ACTH), thyroid stimulating hormone (TSH), follicle stimulating hormone (FSH), luteinizing hormone (LH), prolactin and vasopressin. Testing for other hormones such as melanocyte stimulating hormone and vasotocin is rarely required in pediatric practice and these will not be dealt with here. In addition, if hormonal abnormalities are suspected or proven, the nature of the underlying cause must be ascertained, such as tumor (e.g., craniopharyngioma), histiocytosis, granuloma, trauma, anorexia nervosa, vascular insufficiency, and so on.

In the absence of a clearly defined organic lesion which itself needs therapy, hormonal therapy may be the only form of treatment necessary. Idiopathic processes, insofar as they affect the anterior pituitary, are now considered as often being hypothalamic in origin. They comprise isolated or multiple hormonal deficiencies. For example, a patient may suffer from isolated growth hormone deficiency or from combined deficiency of growth hormone, thyroid stimulating hormone, adrenocorticotropic hormone, luteinizing hormone, and fol-

licle stimulating hormone. Any combination of deficiencies may occur as may isolated deficiency of any hormone. Vasopressin deficiency itself may also occur as an isolated finding or in combination with anterior pituitary insufficiency.

THERAPY FOR GROWTH HORMONE (GH) DEFICIENCY

Two factors are of paramount importance in considering the effectiveness of GH therapy. The first is species specificity which requires that humans receive GH only from human or anthropoid sources. The only practical source for GH is pituitary material obtained at autopsy. The complex human GH molecule has not been synthesized in the laboratory in quantities sufficient for therapeutic purposes. The amount of GH available for treatment thus remains seriously limited. The second consideration is that, with few exceptions, GH administration effectively increases growth for sustained periods of time only in those few children whose growth retardation is caused by GH deficiency. With occasional exceptions it is apparent that only children with GH deficiency benefit from therapy with GH.

Human GH is administered by intramuscular injection generally in dosage of 2 to 3 I.U. three times weekly* (1 mg. is approximately 1 I.U.). Optimal dosages have not been determined, largely because limited supplies of growth hormone have limited extensive, well controlled, therapeutic studies. The response may be better if doses higher than 2 to 3 I.U. are used. Generally, the response is better in

---

*This therapy is still considered experimental and can only be carried out under a specific approved research protocol.

the earlier months of treatment. The response is also generally better when treatment is given to younger children in whom growth increments in excess of 10 cm. per year may be seen. Although treatment may be beneficial at any time prior to epiphyseal fusion, it tends to be less effective in older children.

Administration of GH results in some increase in skeletal maturation but, generally, advance in height age is equal to, or greater than, acceleration of skeletal age. The ultimate height achieved is therefore as great as that to be anticipated from the growth potential estimated from the delay in skeletal age. Failure of anticipated enhancement of growth rate with therapy may be ascribed to one of several causes:

1. If the diagnosis of GH deficiency is incorrect and shortness of stature is the result of other factors, GH administration will generally be ineffective.

2. As mentioned above, with passage of time, therapy tends to become less effective. This deteriorating response may be the result of development of antibodies to GH. It is apparent, however, that such antibodies are rarely neutralizing and little correlation exists between development of these antibodies and diminution of growth response.

3. Generally, the growth response tends to be less marked in subjects with pituitary tumors than in those whose hormonal deficiency is of the idiopathic type.

4. If TSH deficiency coexists with GH deficiency, adequate growth will not occur unless thyroid hormone is administered in addition to GH. A collaborative study report suggests that if thyroid hormone and cortisone are administered concomitantly with GH, epiphyseal maturation may be accelerated excessively. Thus, thyroid hormone should not be part of the treatment regimen unless the existence of hypothyroidism is established. Even if hypothyroidism is not present prior to therapy with GH, diminution in thyroid function may occur after GH therapy is initiated. For this reason it is important to monitor thyroid hormone levels in the blood at regular intervals after beginning GH therapy, even if thyroid function is normal when treatment is started. If the level of thyroxine in the blood falls to subnormal levels, and particularly if the growth rate also decelerates sharply, thyroid hormone should be administered in addition to GH.

5. Administration of ACTH or glucocorticoids tends to diminish responsiveness to GH even if the subject suffers from deficiency of ACTH. Generally, there is little clinical evidence of adrenal deficiency in subjects with hypopituitarism, even if ACTH deficiency is demonstrable by laboratory testing. It is recommended that the patient with ACTH and GH deficiency receive only GH therapy but that he be observed carefully to determine if adrenal insufficiency develops. ACTH or glucocorticoids should be administered only if signs or symptoms of adrenal insufficiency develop. Hypoglycemia may be a sign of ACTH deficiency and if subnormal blood glucose levels are not corrected by GH treatment, administration of cortisone or one of its analogs may be necessary.

THERAPY FOR THYROID STIMULATING HORMONE (TSH) DEFICIENCY

In cases of deficiency of thyroid function due either to hypothalamic dysfunction (TRH deficiency) or pituitary dysfunction (TSH deficiency) the therapy of choice is thyroid hormone. L-thyroxine is preferred over desiccated thyroid or tri-iodothyronine. The biologic potency of thyroid extracts varies significantly, whereas that of synthetic L-thyroxine is constant. Use of tri-iodothyronine may result in high and widely fluctuating levels of this hormone in the blood. One dose of L-thyroxine given daily produces sustained levels of both thyroxine and tri-iodothyronine in the plasma. The dose of L-thyroxine is generally found to be about 2.5 μg./kg./day in the adolescent and about 7.5 μg./kg./day in the infant. A rough approximation for all ages is about 100 μg./m^2/day. In all cases, however, appropriate dosage should be determined by monitoring plasma thyroxine concentrations (and plasma thyrotropin levels in cases of primary hypothyroidism).

THERAPY FOR ADRENOCORTICOTROPIC HORMONE (ACTH) DEFICIENCY

In ACTH deficiency, administration of glucocorticoids is generally the simplest and most effective therapy. ACTH and its derivatives are generally less desirable because they have to be administered by injection. The dosage of glucocorticoids used in subjects with secondary hypoadrenocorticism is generally equivalent to that used in subjects with primary adrenal insufficiency (for details the reader is referred to the section on Adrenal Disease). Generally, glucocorticoids are administered orally 2 or 3 times daily, 5 to 15 mg./m^2 per day of cortisone equivalent. To obviate growth impairment, the smallest dose of glucocorticoid which counteracts symptoms of hypoadrenocorticism is used. Therapy with mineralocorticoids is usually unnecessary but should the need arise, fludrocortisone (Florinef), 0.05 to 0.1 mg. orally per day, may be used.

GONADOTROPIN DEFICIENCY

With isolated growth hormone deficiency, puberty is usually delayed and therapy for gonadotropin deficiency need not be undertaken until it is clear that neither time nor administration of growth hormone will produce gonadotropin secretion. When it is clear that permanent gonadotropin deficiency exists a choice must be made between therapy with gonadotropins, androgens or estrogens.

Gonadotropin Therapy. Gonadotropin therapy is potentially more effective than therapy with androgenic steroids because it may result in stimulation of spermatogenesis or oogenesis. Androgenic steroid therapy can produce only those effects which normally result from elaboration of testosterone and do not include spermatogenesis or oogenesis. Gonadotropin therapy, however, has the disadvantage of having to be administered by intramuscular injection. Two kinds of preparations are available:

1. Human chorionic gonadotropin (HCG) produces effects largely by virtue of its luteinizing hormone (LH) type of action. It is administered by intramuscular injection two or three times weekly in dosage of 500 to 2000 I.U. per injection. Dosage and frequency of injection are determined by response of the patient.

2. Treatment with HCG by itself will not produce spermatogenesis, however. When promotion of fertility is considered desirable, injections of human menopausal gonadotropin (HMG), marketed as Pergonal, will be necessary. This material, prepared from the urine of post-menopausal women, has an action comparable to FSH (follicle stimulating hormone).

Androgenic (Anabolic) Steroid Therapy. Patients with hypothalamic (or pituitary) hypogonadism who also have GH deficiency should undergo therapy with GH initially. If GH is not available androgenic steroids may be used to promote growth. It is not clear if long-term therapy with testosterone will ultimately impair capacity for spermatogenesis but no solid evidence has been advanced that this occurs. In the prepubertal child with GH deficiency, gonadotropin deficiency is a normal physiological state and no means are at hand yet for predicting if gonadotropin or releasing factor deficiency will ultimately develop. The prepubertal child with GH deficiency, for whom GH is not available, may be a suitable candidate for therapy with androgenic (anabolic) steroids.

The dose must be carefully chosen, however, to obviate acceleration of skeletal age in excess of height age. Frequent checks of the skeletal age must be made (3 to 4 times yearly) to determine if adverse effects have been produced. In addition, a search must be made for other undesirable effects, such as pubic hair growth, penile or clitoral enlargement, facial hair growth, etc. In my opinion, anabolic steroids are all more or less equally androgenic when therapeutic dosages are used. Claims that a particular anabolic steroid is less likely to advance skeletal age generally have not been substantiated.

In the prepubertal child with GH deficiency, methyl-testosterone, 2.5 to 5 mg. daily, may be administered sublingually or orally.* Absorption is about twice as complete via the sublingual route. If untoward signs or symptoms do not develop, the dose may be increased gradually, but the prepubertal child should rarely receive more than 5 mg. sublingually or 10 mg. orally. Other anabolic steroids may be used in equivalent dosage.

When the normal age of puberty is reached, puberty may be delayed in the child with GH deficiency. When it is determined that permanent gonadotropin deficiency exists and (for reasons given above) it is elected to use long-term therapy with androgenic steroids, rather than gonadotropins, full replacement doses may be used (25 to 50 mg. daily of an oral preparation such as Oreton). More convenient may be the administration of 200 mg. testosterone enanthate of cyclopentyl-propionate by intramuscular injection once every 2, 3, or 4 weeks depending on the patient's response.

Estrogen and Progestin Therapy. Because estrogens tend to accelerate epiphyseal fusion in doses necessary to promote sexual development in patients with hypogonadotropic hypogonadism, treatment with estrogens should be deferred until growth retardation is no longer a serious problem. If estrogens are administered before adequate growth has occurred, careful attention must be paid to epiphyseal development and the minimum dosage used which is compatible with maximum growth potential. Numerous estrogen preparations are available. Ethinyl estradiol, 20 to 50 μg., may be given daily for 3 to 6 months and then cyclical therapy may be instituted to induce regular menses. The above dose of ethinyl estradiol is given from day 1 to 23 of each calendar month. From day 16 to 23 a progestational agent (e.g., Provera 2.5 to 10

---

*This use of methyl-testosterone is not mentioned in the manufacturer's instructions.

mg. daily) is taken also. It is advantageous to have the patient follow such a regimen and to have regular menses. In this way irregular or intermenstrual bleeding may have the same significance as the harbinger of malignancy in the genital tract as it has in the woman with normal hypothalamic pituitary function. Eventually, attempts at induction of fertility may be made with administration of combinations of preparations of FSH and LH as outlined above.

VASOPRESSIN DEFICIENCY

Vasopressin deficiency may be transitory (e.g. following removal of a pituitary tumor) or partial. Generally, however, once established it is permanent. Once the diagnosis is established treatment may consist either of administration of vasopressin or of other agents which are unrelated structurally to vasopressin.

Vasopressin Therapy. Vasopressin is generally administered by intramuscular injection or nasal insufflation (it has not been approved for intravenous use). The preparation used for intramuscular injection is pitressin tannate suspended in oil (5 units/ml.). This material produces antidiuretic activity for 36 to 72 hours. The usual dosage for children and adolescents is 2.5 to 5 units administered every other day. Infants often require smaller doses. The dosage varies with the individual subject and must be adjusted to his needs. The suspension must always be warmed and shaken vigorously before use to ensure that the small volume of the active principle is well mixed with the vehicle. A stable aqueous preparation of lysine vasopressin (Diapid) is also available. This material, dispensed in plastic compressible containers, is insufflated into either one or both nostrils as often as 3 to 6 times daily. Frequency of administration and number of insufflations per administration must be determined for each individual. The frequency with which this agent needs to be administered must be considered in weighing its advantages over pitressin, given by injection.

In recent years a newer synthetic preparation, 1-desamino-8 D-arginine (Desmopressin, Minirin, DDAVP), has been used in Europe and elsewhere for treatment of diabetes insipidus. This synthetic analog of vasopressin is administered by nasal inhalation and has the advantage that it need be administered only once or twice every 24 hours. The preparation has been tested in the United States and at the time of writing the Food and Drug Administration is considering the question of its release in this country. The most frequently used dosage is 2.5 to 10 μg. (0.025 to 0.1 ml.) twice daily.

The dose used is determined by the individual response of each patient. The manufacturer supplies an insufflation device which is efficient and easy to use. We have used this preparation in children as young as 2 years and believe it is clearly the preparation of choice in the treatment of diabetes insipidus.

Chlorpropamide Therapy. Chlorpropamide, administered orally, may be useful in some children with diabetes insipidus.* Used widely as an oral hypoglycemic agent, it also appears to sensitize the renal tubules to the action of circulating vasopressin. It may be effective, then, in those subjects in whom small quantities of vasopressin can still be secreted by the neurohypophysis. The major advantage of chlorpropamide therapy is the ease of administration, but occurrence of hypoglycemia may seriously limit its usefulness. It has been suggested that the initial dose be 250 mg./m^2 day, in three divided doses. The dosage may be then increased or decreased depending on the occurrence of untoward symptoms. Initial adjustment of dosage should probably be carried out under carefully controlled conditions such as in a hospital.

Unusually Tall Stature in Adolescent Girls

FELIX CONTE, M.D.

Physicians who treat children and adolescents are sometimes faced with the problem of tall stature in females. Psychosocial pressures from peers as well as the anxiety of well-meaning parents bring the child to the physician for help. They and their parents seek assurance that their final mature height will not be "excessive" and ask for therapy directed at stopping growth. An open discussion with the child and parents about the risk-benefit ratios of therapy may suffice to dissuade them from pharmacologic therapy. In some cases, psychiatric consultation may help to allay the anxieties of the child and parent about relatively tall stature. In extreme cases of tall stature and in those patients who are not helped by psychiatric consultation, the physician may then be faced with the decision of either treating the child or refusing to do so because of the risk-benefit ratio.

Tall stature may be defined mathematically as greater than 2.5 standard deviations above the mean in height for age which,

---

*Manufacturer's warning: Chlorpropamide should not be used in juvenile diabetes.

in adult females in the United States in the 1970's, is 162.8 ± 6.8 cm. and makes 179.8 cm. (5'11") 2.5 standard deviations above the mean. However, being too "tall" is a subjective phenomenon based on parental size, career goals, and real or imagined psychosocial pressures.

The evaluation of the tall child should be directed toward ruling out pathologic causes of tall stature, such as pituitary gigantism, Marfan's syndrome, homocystinuria, and cerebral gigantism. To this end, a history including parental height and age of puberty, the growth pattern of the child as assessed from serial measurements of height, a complete physical examination, lateral skull x-ray, and a left hand and wrist x-ray to determine bone age according to the atlas of Greulich and Pyle, should be obtained. Utilizing the above information, one can attempt to predict mature height by the use of the "RWT" method (Pediatrics, 56:1026–1033, 1976) and the tables of Bayley-Pinneau (J. Pediat., 40:433–441, 1952). Applying both methods may make possible a more finite mature height prediction. However, in order to confirm the accuracy of the original forecast, serial predictions should be made.

Patients whose mature predicted height is greater than 180 cm. on serial determinations have been considered candidates for therapy with pharmacologic doses of estrogens, the rationale for which was first suggested by the fact that females and males with precocious puberty usually are short adults. The studies of Wiedemann and Schwartz have suggested that estrogens in large doses can suppress the production of somatomedin. Thus pharmacologic doses of estrogens may promote a decrease in growth rate by suppressing somatomedin, while epiphyseal maturation rapidly accelerates due to the effect of the estrogen, with the result being a decrease in mature height. However, the mean decrement in height in three recently published large series is only 3 to 4 cm., with a range from 0 to 10 cm. In any one patient, there can be no guarantee regarding final height. Therapy may be unnecessary, unphysiological, and possibly harmful from a somatic point of view, so that the patient and her parents should be realistically appraised of the expectations and side effects of this therapeutic adventure.

In the event that both physician and parents agree on estrogen therapy, written informed consent from the parents and child should be obtained. The candidate for therapy should have a mature height prediction greater than 180 cm. and have at least 6 cm.

growth potential before starting therapy. Although a greater response has been found in patients with younger bone ages, diminution in height can be obtained in the postmenarcheal female. A recent study indicates that therapy need not be started before a bone age of 11 to 11.5 years according to the Greulich-Pyle atlas. We concur with this point of view, but in girls with extreme tall stature it may be beneficial to start therapy at an earlier age.

Ethinyl estradiol, conjugated estrogen, and stilbestrol have all been utilized with approximately the same degree of success. There is no evidence at present that any one type of estrogen is more likely to be carcinogenic than any other. We have utilized conjugated natural estrogens (Premarin), 10 mg. by mouth daily for the first 21 days of the month and medroxyprogesterone acetate (Provera), 5 mg. on days 17 to 21, to facilitate menses.* Alternatively, ethinyl estradiol, 0.3 mg. by mouth daily for the first 21 days of the month, may be used with norethindrone, 5.0 mg. daily on days 17 to 21. Therapy is usually initiated with one-fourth of the estrogen dose the first week, increased by one-fourth dose per week so that the full dose is given in the second cycle. The progestin is given in full dosage on the first cycle.

The patient should be examined every three months, at which time the menstrual history, as well as pubertal changes and adjustments should be discussed. A complete physical examination should be performed including evaluation of the vagina, cervix and ovaries, palpation of the breasts, height and weight check. A bone age is obtained every six months.

Therapy may be discontinued when epiphyseal fusion has occurred at the hand and wrist (at a bone age of 15 to 16 years) and knees. In most patients, spontaneous menarche will ensue within two or three months after the last cycle. Fertility has been reported in many patients who have received this therapy for tall stature. After completion of treatment, these patients should be followed yearly on a prospective basis for evidence of the possible long-term untoward effects of pharmacologic estrogen and progesterone therapy.

Observed side effects from estrogen therapy include rapid pubertal maturation, weight gain, menarche, nausea, and mild hypertension. Other potential sequelae include

---

*This use is not listed in the manufacturer's instructions for Premarin, Provera, ethinyl estradiol, norethindrone, or stilbestrol.

thromboembolic episodes and an increased risk of coronary artery disease, liver tumors, and malignancies of the breast and genital tract. Wettenhall noted two patients in his series who developed ovarian cysts during therapy. Nausea may be transient and is amenable to antiemetic therapy and taking the medication with meals. The long-term effects and risks of pharmacologic doses of estrogens have not yet been assessed in the females treated.

Thyroid Disease

DELBERT A. FISHER, M.D.

The spectrum of thyroid disease in pediatric patients is broad, and the therapeutic decisions often controversial. Appropriate therapy usually is based upon precise diagnosis for which highly sophisticated in vitro and in vivo procedures are available. Treatment in the pediatric setting, however, is less precise, and rarely emergency oriented. Long-term considerations thus become important; concerns such as the early thyroid hormone dependency of the central nervous system, thyroid hormone requirements for normal somatic growth, the radiation sensitivity of the child's thyroid gland, and the long life expectancy of children.

NEWBORN GOITER

In areas of the world without endemic goiter, thyroid enlargement in the newborn indicates either compromised capacity to synthesize thyroid hormones or neonatal hyperthyroidism. Therapy must be directed to possible local obstructive effects of the goiter as well as the associated thyroid dysfunction. Maternal ingestion of iodides for treatment of asthma or thyroid disease, or maternal antithyroid drug treatment for hyperthyroidism may result in fetal goiter. On occasion the goiter can be very large, especially that due to iodine. If the airway is obstructed in the newborn with goiter, careful positioning with neck extension is appropriate with or without intubation. In severe cases, tracheostomy and/or subtotal thyroidectomy may be necessary.

Iodide-induced goiter in the newborn of a mother without hyperthyroidism or Graves' disease will spontaneously disappear within a period of two to three months. Remission can be hastened by administration of exogenous Na-1-thyroxine in a dose of 10 to 15 μg./kg./day for three months. It is important to document thyroid status in such infants by objective laboratory tests (serum thyroxine [T4], free T4 index, and TSH concentrations) before

therapy and one month after discontinuing thyroid medication to exclude the possibility of permanent hypothyroidism.

NEONATAL GRAVES' DISEASE

If a mother has Graves' disease or a history of Graves' disease, neonatal thyrotoxicosis is a possible diagnosis. Such infants may or may not have a large goiter at birth but usually have some enlargement of the thyroid gland. Because of transplacental passage of maternal antithyroid drugs and because the fetus converts T4 predominantly to the inactive metabolite reverse T3, the newborn with Graves' disease will usually appear euthyroid at birth. Thyroid function tests and careful follow-up of all newborns of mothers with Graves' disease or a history of Graves' disease are essential for early diagnosis. Therapy must be vigorous and includes sedatives and digitalization as necessary, and administration of a thionamide drug (propylthiouracil or methimazole) and/or iodides. The thionamides inhibit hormone synthesis; iodides potentiate this effect and, in addition, block thyroid hormone release. Adequate doses of both drugs are essential for most effective therapy. Propylthiouracil or methimazole should be administered in doses of 5 to 10 mg./kg./day or 0.5 to 1.0 mg./kg./day,* respectively, in divided doses at eight hour intervals. Strong iodine solution (5 per cent iodine and 10 per cent potassium iodide, 126 mg. of iodine per ml.) is given in doses of one drop (about 8 mg. iodine) every eight hours. If a therapeutic response is not observed within 24 to 48 hours, the dose of both drugs (iodides and thionamide) can be increased 50 to 100 per cent.

Propranolol hydrochloride also is useful in controlling sympathetic overstimulation and can dramatically reduce cardiac rate; the recommended dose is 2 mg./kg./day divided into two or three portions.† Treatment with digitalis should be discontinued when propranolol is given. Finally, adrenal corticosteroids acutely inhibit thyroid hormone secretion in Graves' disease, and these drugs can be useful in unusually severe cases. Minimal effective doses have not been established, but the usual 2 mg./kg./day anti-inflammatory dose of prednisone would seem appropriate.

The need for careful follow-up cannot be

---

*This dose of methimazole is higher than that recommended by the manufacturer but has been found to be safe and effective.

†Manufacturer's warning: Data on the use of propranolol in the pediatric age group are too limited to permit adequate directions for use.

overemphasized. In perhaps 10 to 30 per cent of infants prolonged or intermittent disease may ensue.

CONGENITAL HYPOTHYROIDISM

Congenital hypothyroidism is an important therapeutic problem in the newborn and small infant; diagnosis is difficult and delayed treatment can lead to irreversible mental retardation. The diagnosis may be suspected on the basis of results of newborn screening of blood T4 and/or TSH levels or from clinical suspicion. The hypothyroidism may be *primary* due to thyroid dysgenesis, an inborn defect in thyroid hormone metabolism, or goitrogen exposure, or it may be *secondary* due to a hypothalamic-pituitary disorder.

Treatment of primary hypothyroidism is accomplished by administration of replacement thyroid hormone. Several preparations are available including synthetic Na-1-thyroxine (T4), synthetic Na-1-triiodothyronine (T3), combinations of synthetic thyroxine and triiodothyronine in a 4:1 ratio, thyroid U.S.P., and thyroglobulin. Thyroid U.S.P. is a cleaned, dried, and powdered preparation of porcine or bovine thyroid gland previously deprived of connective tissue and fat. Thyroglobulin is the relatively purified porcine thyroid storage protein with a molecular weight approximating 700,000. Equivalent doses of the several preparations are Na-1-thyroxine, 100 μg. (0.1 mg.); Na-1-triiodothyronine, 25 μg. (0.025 mg.); T4 + T3, 50 to 60 μg. and 12.5 to 15 μg. respectively; thyroid U.S.P., 60 mg. (1 gr.); thyroglobulin, 60 mg. (1 gr.).

Of these preparations Na-1-thyroxine is the drug of choice. It is more uniform in its potency and absorption; it is easily measured in serum; and it provides physiological serum T3 levels since most of the circulating T3 normally is derived from T4 by monodeiodination in tissues. The dose of oral T4 for infants is 8 to 12 μg./kg./day. The usual total dose during the first six months ranges from 30 to 90 μg. (0.03 to 0.09 mg.) (Table 1). Approximately 50 to 75 per cent of the drug is absorbed so that the absorbed dose is less than the total dose.

In adults with hypothyroidism a rapid increase in metabolic rate may produce uncomfortable symptoms and cardiac decompensation if there is underlying cardiac disease. Therefore, treatment usually is begun with a small dose of hormone and the dose is increased gradually to optimal replacement levels. In infants, in contrast, it is important to achieve optimal replacement promptly in order to minimize the period of central nervous system thyroid hormone deficiency. The estimated total replacement dose is given orally from the first day of treatment. Some have advocated a relatively large intravenous priming dose of T4 to achieve normal circulating levels more rapidly. Ten to twenty μg./kg. of the intravenous preparation of Na-1-thyroxine can be injected intramuscularly daily for two days, after which oral medication can be substituted.

TABLE 1. Dose of Oral Na-1-Thyroxine for Replacement Therapy of Hypothyroidism in Infancy and Childhood

AGE	USUAL ORAL DOSE OF NA-1-THYROXINE	
	(μg./kg./day)	(range of dose, μg.)
1 to 6 months	8 to 12	30 to 90
6 to 12 months	6 to 8	50 to 100
1 to 5 years	4 to 6	75 to 150
5 to 10 years	3 to 5	100 to 200
10 to 20 years	2 to 3	100 to 250

Two to three weeks usually are required to observe the maximal effects from a constant dosage. In infants with severe hypothyroidism, this period may be more prolonged. In an occasional infant with a delayed diagnosis and severe disease associated with manifest or suspected cardiac disease a more gradual approach to optimal therapy over four to six weeks may be indicated. Overtreatment acutely produces tachycardia, excessive nervousness, disturbed sleep patterns, diarrhea and other findings suggesting thyrotoxicosis. Excessive dosage over a prolonged period of time may produce premature synostosis of the cranial sutures, undue advancement of bone age and osteoporosis.

Adequacy of therapy is judged, first, by clinical evidence of normal growth and development and lack of signs and symptoms of toxicity. Growth in length and weight should be plotted monthly during the first three months and at two to three month intervals thereafter during the first year. Bone age should be assessed at three months and at 6 to 12 months of treatment. Thereafter 12 to 24 month evaluations will suffice. Measurements of circulating hormone concentrations are essential to assess adequacy of treatment. Measurements of T4, TSH and, on occasion, T3 are helpful. Serum T4 levels should be adjusted to the upper two thirds of the normal range for age. At this time the serum TSH level should be normal (< 7 μU./ml) and the serum T3 concentration within the normal range for age.

If the hypothyroidism is *secondary*, due to hypothalamic-pituitary dysfunction, treatment with adrenal corticosteroids and growth hormone (GH) is necessary if deficiencies of

ACTH and GH are documented. Adrenal insufficiency may be manifest as failure to thrive and/or hypoglycemia in the neonatal period. GH deficiency also may contribute to hypoglycemia and may impair growth after three to six months.

HYPOTHYROIDISM IN CHILDHOOD AND ADOLESCENCE

Acquired hypothyroidism before five or six years most commonly results from delayed failure of the thyroid remnant in infants with thyroid dysgenesis, but inborn defects in thyroid hormone synthesis, ingested goitrogens, chronic thyroiditis or hypothalamic-pituitary disease may be involved. After five to six years the same spectrum of etiologies is involved, but hypothyroidism most commonly is due to chronic lymphocytic (Hashimoto's) thyroiditis. Surgery or radioiodine treatment also can result in hypothyroidism.

Irreversible brain damage is not a likely result of hypothyroidism acquired after two or three years of age. By this time central nervous system growth is largely complete. Delayed growth, however, may be marked, and most commonly is manifest as delayed tooth development and eruption, delayed skeletal growth and maturation, and linear growth retardation. Aberrations in pubertal development and menstrual irregularities are common. These manifestations are reversible with adequate replacement therapy. As in infants the treatment of choice is oral Na-1-thyroxine. The replacement dose on a body weight basis decreases progressively with age (Table 1). The dosage should be adjusted at two to four week intervals to a level which maintains the serum T4 concentration in the mid-range of normal together with normal T3 and TSH concentrations. In contrast to adults, it is not necessary in most children with hypothyroidism to increase the dose of replacement T4 gradually. Initial administration of the total daily estimated replacement dose will result in a gradual increase in serum T4 concentrations over a three to four week period. If cardiac disease is suspected more gradual replacement may be indicated.

Treatment of secondary hypothyroidism in childhood or adolescence may require simultaneous replacement with adrenal corticosteroids, growth hormone and gonadal steroid(s).

SUPPURATIVE THYROID DISEASE

Acute suppurative thyroiditis is rare in childhood. Infected thyroglossal duct cysts or thyroglossal duct remnants are more common. Therapy is directed to the offending organism(s) as well as the underlying embryological abnormality. Surgical drainage may be necessary. Definitive surgery is delayed and is conducted on an elective basis after resolution of the acute infection.

ACUTE-SUBACUTE NONSUPPURATIVE THYROIDITIS

This entity usually is referred to as subacute thyroiditis because the course runs several weeks to several months. The disorder is self-limited and of uncertain cause, although it seems likely that most cases are of viral etiology. There are local and systemic manifestations of the inflammatory process as well as a transient hypermetabolism due to release of thyroid hormones from the damaged follicular cells. There is no specific therapy; antithyroid drugs are of little benefit. Symptomatic treatment for the local and/or systemic discomfort is helpful. Patients with marked painful goiter have been treated with adrenal corticosteroids, but such therapy usually is not warranted. When hyperthyroid manifestations are marked, propranolol may be useful.

HASHIMOTO'S THYROIDITIS

Hashimoto's thyroiditis, or chronic lymphocytic thyroiditis, is an autoimmune disease most frequently involving only the thyroid gland. Occasionally, however, Hashimoto's thyroiditis is associated with other endocrine gland autoimmunity and deficiencies. These include the pancreas and diabetes mellitus, the adrenal gland with adrenal insufficiency, the parathyroid glands with hypoparathyroidism and, on rare occasions, the gonads with hypogonadism. Autoimmune gastritis with pernicious anemia and cutaneous moniliasis sometimes are associated. Treatment of all the endocrine gland deficiencies may be necessary. Most frequently, however, the disease involves only the thyroid gland and presents as a mild to moderate euthyroid goiter. The disease remits spontaneously in about one-third of children. The remainder gradually develop hypothyroidism. There is no specific therapy, but if the goiter is large, if the serum TSH concentration is elevated, or if the patient is clinically hypothyroid, replacement therapy with Na-1-thyroxine is indicated. Some physicians favor thyroxine treatment of all children with Hashimoto's thyroiditis to avoid mild, undiagnosed hypothyroidism.

NONTOXIC DIFFUSE COLLOID GOITER (SIMPLE GOITER; COLLOID GOITER)

Simple colloid goiter refers to a smooth, symmetrical enlargement of the thyroid gland in a euthyroid patient without detectable abnormality in thyroid function tests or thyroid autoantibody titers. It is most common during adolescence in females and has been referred to as adolescent goiter. The goiter usually disappears spontaneously and requires no treatment. Some prefer to prescribe thyroid hormone replacement therapy, particularly if the goiter is large.

JUVENILE HYPERTHYROIDISM

Chronic hyperthyroidism in childhood usually is due to Graves' disease, but less commonly can be associated with Hashimoto's thyroiditis, hyperfunctioning thyroid nodule(s) or, rarely, TSH hypersecretion. Treatment is directed to the thyroid hormone hypersecretion and the cause of the hyperthyroid state when possible.

Treatment of the hyperthyroid state may be accomplished with antithyroid drugs, surgery or radioiodine. Radioiodine treatment is not considered the approach of first choice in children. There is a 10 per cent incidence of permanent hypothyroidism during the first year after treatment and an additional 2 to 3 per cent incidence yearly thereafter. Thus 10 to 20 years post treatment about half of radioiodine treated patients will be hypothyroid. Projection of this figure suggests that hypothyroidism is nearly inevitable in children thus treated. Additionally, in contrast to adults, children after radioiodine therapy of thyrotoxicosis may have an increased incidence of thyroid malignancy, including both adenoma and carcinoma. The experience, however, is limited to date, both in terms of numbers of children treated and the duration of follow-up. Finally, the results are not uniformly good. About 10 per cent of children treated with radioiodine have experienced relapse and about 5 per cent have been operated upon subsequently.

Surgery has the disadvantages of a finite mortality, considerable morbidity, and a significant incidence of complications. These include recurrent laryngeal nerve damage with vocal cord paralysis and permanent hypothyroidism. The combined incidence of the latter problems has varied from 1 to 8 per cent in several reports, and probably averages 2 to 3 per cent in most clinics. In addition, there is a 25 per cent incidence of permanent hypothyroidism after 15 to 20 years. For these reasons, surgery is not usually considered the therapy of first choice.

Medical therapy with antithyroid drugs is considered the treatment of choice by most pediatric endocrinologists. Both propythiouracil (PTU) and methimazole are effective.

These are drugs of the thionamide class which act by inhibiting the organification of iodine and hormone synthesis by the thyroid gland. PTU also inhibits peripheral tissue conversion of thyroxine to triiodothyronine but this action is of lesser importance in therapy of thyrotoxicosis. Both drugs can produce skin rash, drug fever, agranulocytosis and rarely a collagen-vascular like reaction. Drug fever and rashes occur in 3 to 5 per cent of cases and disappear promptly on withdrawal of medication. Agranulocytosis occurs in 0.2 to 0.3 per cent and usually is observed during the first six to eight weeks of treatment. Agranulocytosis resolves upon drug withdrawal and administration of antibiotics.

Initial therapy is instituted with PTU, 5 to 7 mg./kg./day, or methimazole, 0.5 to 0.7 mg./kg./day, in three divided doses at about eight hour intervals. The dose is increased if improvement is not observed within two weeks. Nearly all patients will respond to PTU in doses of 10 to 15 mg./kg./day or methimazole in doses of 1 to 1.5 mg./kg./day.* However, an occasional patient may require as much as 20 mg./kg./day of PTU for control. Methimazole has a longer half-life than PTU and some patients will maintain effective blockade of thyroid hormone synthesis with once daily drug administration, particularly after remission has been induced. PTU often can be given in two daily doses.

In patients with severe disease or distressing cardiovascular symptoms, propranolol† is useful adjunctive therapy; 0.1 to 0.3 mg./kg. intravenously followed by 2 mg./kg./day orally in divided doses, or oral therapy alone has been utilized. The dose of propranolol can be increased to 4 to 6 mg./kg./day.

Potassium iodide in large doses potentiates the action of thionamide drugs and inhibits thyroid hormone secretion. The effect, however, is transient. Therapeutic doses for hyperthyroidism range from 2 to 4 mg./kg./day, usually given as strong iodine solution or a saturated solution of potassium iodide. The inhibitory effect on hormone synthesis and/or release usually persists 10 to 40 days. Thus potassium iodide is most useful for short-term treatment of severe disease and for preoperative preparation of patients for surgery.

After the patient has become euthyroid, which usually takes 30 to 90 days, the dose of

---

*This dose of methimazole is higher than that recommended by the manufacturer but has been found to be safe and effective

†Manufacturer's precaution: Data on use of propranolol in children are too limited to permit adequate directions for use.

medication can be reduced to 3 to 4 mg. of PTU/kg. or 0.3 to 0.4 mg. of methimazole/kg. Treatment must be monitored with measurements of serum T4 concentrations to ensure an adequate drug effect and avoid hypothyroidism. Measurements of serum T3 concentration often are useful when the clinical assessment and serum T4 measurement are in disagreement; on occasion the antithyroid medication will be adequate to inhibit T4 but not T3 secretion. Serum TSH measurements are helpful in assessing hypothyroidism.

It is possible in follow-up either to adjust the antithyroid drug dosage to maintain normal thyroid hormone levels or to continue a blocking dose which produces hypothyroidism and maintain the patient on exogenous Na-1 thyroxine in replacement doses. The duration of antithyroid drug treatment cannot be predicted and usually is considered long-term— one year or more. The rationale is that Graves' disease, like other autoimmune disorders, usually remits spontaneously. Drug treatment only maintains a euthyroid state as we await such remission. The remission rate approximates 50 per cent each two years. As a general rule, patients with continuing goiter not due to drug-induced hypothyroidism will experience exacerbation of hyperthyroidism if treatment is withdrawn. Also remission is not likely if the thyroid gland remains nonsuppressible.

At the end of one year, if the goiter has disappeared and the patient is euthyroid, treatment can be discontinued. Some physicians prefer to document suppressibility before drug withdrawal. Perhaps 30 per cent of patients will remain in remission off treatment after one year, and some feel that three months of treatment is adequate to define this group. The majority require long treatment; perhaps 25 per cent will require four or more years of treatment before remission occurs.

If drug toxicity ensues, the drug becomes ineffective for patient or pharmacological reasons, or if the goiter is large and unresponsive to a reasonable drug treatment regimen, alternative treatment may be considered. If an experienced thyroid surgeon is available, thyroidectomy may be preferable. Radioiodine is a viable alternative in the adolescent. It should be emphasized, however, that the physician threshold for abandoning medical therapy should be kept relatively high. These patients require frequent follow-up, support, and encouragement.

Graves' ophthalmopathy is common in juvenile patients, but usually is not severe. Lid retraction, lid lag, stare, and mild to moderate proptosis are seen, but severe infiltrative changes, severe proptosis and eye muscle weakness are rare. Thus specific treatment for ophthalmopathy is not usually necessary during childhood and adolescence. If periorbital edema should occur, the patient should sleep with the head of the bed elevated. Patients with diplopia should wear an alternating eye patch. If the eyelids fail to close properly a protective shield at school or while sleeping is useful. More severe disease requires consideration of adrenal corticosteroid treatment and/or surgery.

THYROID NODULES

Thyroid nodules in children are significant for three reasons: they may herald underlying thyroid disease, they may be hyperfunctioning nodules and produce hyperthyroidism, or they may represent carcinoma. In the first instance, the approach is to the basic disease, often Hashimoto's thyroiditis. Functioning nodules producing clinical and chemical thyrotoxicosis require treatment, and surgery is the most frequently employed and reliable therapeutic modality. Partial thyroidectomy is conducted with minimal risk of recurrent nerve or parathyroid gland damage. Functioning nodules not resulting in hyperthyroidism have a very low incidence of malignancy and can be followed without treatment. Nonfunctioning or "cold" nodules, those which do not concentrate radioiodine, are considered potentially malignant. The likelihood of carcinoma in a cold nodule in an otherwise normal thyroid gland approaches 40 per cent in children. Most of these are thyroid follicular cell neoplasms, but about 5 per cent are medullary carcinomas secreting calcitonin and can be identified with a serum calcitonin measurement with or without stimulation.

It is difficult to differentiate malignant and nonmalignant masses in the remainder of cases. Surgery is indicated if there is a prior history of therapeutic radiation to the head or neck, if the nodule is hard, if there is evidence of tracheal invasion (dysphagia, hoarseness or cough) or vocal cord paralysis, if adjacent lymph nodes are involved, or if there are distant metastases. If none of these malignancy criteria is present thyroid suppression with 0.2 to 0.3 mg. of Na-1-thyroxine daily can be employed. If over a period of four to six months the nodule grows, or if over a period of 12 months the nodule does not decrease in size, surgery is indicated. If the nodule decreases in size longer follow-up is in order. It is important to remember that thyroid follicular cell carcinomas in children are rather indolent neoplasms and do not require urgent treatment.

Parathyroid Disease

HAROLD E. HARRISON, M.D.

HYPOPARATHYROIDISM

Transient Physiologic Hypoparathyroidism. The treatment of this entity by addition of soluble calcium salts to the feedings is discussed in the section on Tetany (p. 345).

Congenital Absence of Parathyroids, Idiopathic Hypoparathyroidism and Surgical Hypoparathyroidism. The treatment of these disorders can be discussed together. In some older patients with surgical hypoparathyroidism (post thyroidectomy) there is sufficient residual parathyroid function that the principles of treatment of transient physiologic hypoparathyroidism are applicable. In these patients sequestration of phosphate in the intestinal tract may suffice to lower serum phosphate and permit the maintenance of serum calcium concentrations close to the normal range. The sequestrating agent may be calcium carbonate, calcium lactate or calcium gluconate.

For older children, calcium carbonate is the preferable drug since 40 per cent of its weight is calcium, whereas only 13 per cent of calcium lactate and 9 per cent of calcium gluconate is calcium. Five to 10 gm. of calcium carbonate powder per day as a suspension given in divided doses should be tried. The end point is reduction of serum phosphorus into the normal range for age (4.5 to 6 mg./100 ml.) and maintenance of serum calcium concentrations between 8.5 and 10.0 mg./100 ml. If these serum calcium concentrations cannot be achieved, it will be necessary to use activated sterol therapy as outlined below in the treatment of the total aparathyroid state.

Patients with congenital absence of the parathyroids or idiopathic hypoparathyroidism of childhood cannot be managed adequately by calcium salts and require treatment with pharmacologic doses of vitamin D or dihydrotachysterol to overcome the lack of parathyroid hormone. We prefer dihydrotachysterol now that it is available as a pure steroid. Dihydrotachysterol is more potent than vitamin D as a pharmacologic substitute for parathyroid hormone, but its most important advantage is its more rapid rate of inactivation in the body. Vitamin D is only slowly metabolized to inactive products and when given in pharmacologic doses is stored in body fat and circulates in high concentration in the plasma. It thus tends to be cumulative in its action and after months of therapy may cause hypercalcemia which persists for many weeks despite withdrawal of vitamin D treatment.

If hypercalcemia occurs during dihydrotachysterol treatment, cessation of treatment for 1 or 2 weeks usually results in elimination of the excess and then treatment can be resumed at a lower dose. The maintenance dose of dihydrotachysterol has to be individually determined. General guidelines are 0.05 to 0.1 mg. daily for infants, increasing to 0.5 mg. for older children. Adults are usually maintained on 0.5 to 1.5 mg./day. When therapy is initiated doses of five times the expected maintenance dose may be given daily for 3 to 5 days to obtain a more rapid initial effect with reduction to maintenance after this time.

The preparations of dihydrotachysterol are Hytakerol (Winthrop), available as a solution, 1 ml. = 0.25 mg., and crystalline dihydrotachysterol (Philips-DuPhar), available as tablets or in bulk as the crystalline material which can be dissolved in sesame oil to make a solution, 1 ml. = 1 mg. The latter is the most economical method of dispensing the drug, and hospital pharmacies can prepare the solution.

If dihydrotachysterol is not available, vitamin D_2 (ergocalciferol) can be prescribed in doses of 15,000 to 25,000 units/day (0.4 to 0.6 mg.) for infants and increasing up to 100,000 units/day (2.5 mg.) for older children and adolescents. For the smaller doses vitamin D_2 in propylene glycol (Drisdol, 1 ml. = 10,000 units) can be prescribed. For larger doses concentrates in capsule form (50,000 units per capsule) are available. The vitamin D can be given every other day or twice weekly if intermediate doses are needed.

All patients on dihydrotachysterol or vitamin D must have serum calcium concentrations monitored at weekly and biweekly intervals at first, and then the intervals can be extended as stable regulation is achieved. The serum calcium concentrations should be maintained in the low normal range of 8.5 to 9.5 mg./100 ml. Many patients can be maintained on dihydrotachysterol or vitamin D without supplementary calcium salts. If serum phosphorus levels remain high, calcium lactate or calcium carbonate can be added to the treatment to bring the serum phosphorus levels down and make possible reduction of the doses of dihydrotachysterol or vitamin D.

Occasionally patients are encountered who are relatively refractory to activated sterols or become refractory after having been responsive. The mechanism of this refractoriness is not completely understood. Some patients have steatorrhea as one of the manifestations of idiopathic hypoparathyroidism, leading to malabsorption of the orally administered fat soluble steroid. If very large doses of dihydrotachysterol are given along with the recommended amounts of calcium carbonate and the serum calcium brought back to normal the loss of fat in the stools is lessened, suggesting that hypocalcemia per se interferes with fat absorption. After such massive treatment, responsiveness to standard doses may return.

Other patients are hypomagnesemic, and magnesium deficiency alters responsiveness of serum calcium to treatment. Magnesium supplementation either as $MgSO_4$ intramuscularly (0.2 ml./kg. of 50 per cent $MgSO_4 \cdot 12\ H_2O$) twice daily or oral $MgCl_2$, 2 to 4 mEq./kg./day (0.2 to 0.4 gm./kg./day of the crystalline salt) in divided doses has in some instances resulted in increase of serum calcium concentration and better control on continued activated sterol treatment. The newer vitamin D metabolites 25-hydroxycholecalciferol or 1,25-dihydroxycholecalciferol may eventually be found to be useful in the treatment of hypoparathyroidism, but they are investigational drugs at present.

Associated Disorders. Idiopathic hypoparathyroidism is associated with other endocrinopathies, particularly adrenocortical insufficiency and less commonly hypothyroidism and diabetes. In young patients with hypoparathyroidism the possibility of adrenocortical insufficiency occurring at a later date must be kept in mind. One of the manifestations of diminished cortisol output may be increased sensitivity to activated sterols with hypercalcemia. Conversely treatment with cortisol or other potent glucocorticoids may increase the requirement for vitamin D or dihydrotachysterol to maintain normocalcemia.

Pernicious anemia due to loss of intrinsic factor can also be a complication of hypoparathyroidism and may present with neurological manifestations which may be mistakenly regarded as due to the hypocalcemia. Another of the problems seen in hypoparathyroidism is the ectodermal dysplasia which may be associated with severe moniliases of skin, nails and mucous membranes. This is difficult to eradicate and must be treated with local and oral mycostatin.

HYPERPARATHYROIDISM

Hyperparathyroidism in infancy and childhood is rare, but when it does occur it is usually a familial disorder with chief cell hyperplasia of the parathyroids as the underlying pathologic lesion. This may be congenital with obvious manifestations at birth, or the hypercalcemia may be detected later in childhood.

Hyperparathyroidism due to solitary adenoma of the parathyroid is much less likely to occur in children than in adults. This is of importance in the therapeutic approach. The definitive treatment of hyperparathyroidism is removal of the source of the excess parathyroid hormone. If this is an adenoma the operative therapy is excision of the adenoma, leaving the other functioning normal parathyroid glands. Although adenomas may be multiple, they are more likely to be single, and the surgical procedure is exploration of the areas where parathyroid adenomas may be found, including the mediastinum if necessary.

If the underlying process is chief cell hyperplasia of the parathyroids, removal of a single parathyroid gland or even three hyperplastic glands may be unavailing, as the remaining hyperplastic parathyroid tissue may continue to overproduce parathyroid hormone so that hypercalcemia may persist postoperatively. Two approaches are possible: one is to remove three of the four hyperplastic glands if they can be identified, leaving a metal clip on the fourth so that it can be readily located if a second operation is needed to remove the remaining parathyroid. The other is to do a total parathyroidectomy at the initial operations, being prepared to treat the subsequent permanent hypoparathyroid state as outlined above.

We have used this latter approach in an infant with severe congenital hyperparathyroidism with multiple fractures at birth. There was rapid remineralization of the bones postoperatively and the hypoparathyroidism has been easily controlled by standard treatment with dihydrotachysterol. Other members of the family have had removal of three hyperplastic parathyroids without amelioration of the hypercalcemia.

Hyperparathyroidism may present with a parathyroid storm—marked hypercalcemia with central nervous system manifestations including impaired state of consciousness and convulsions. The latter may be the result of hypertensive encephalopathy. Emergency treatment of the hypercalcemia is probably best accomplished by methods directed at increasing urinary excretion of calcium. This can be done by the intravenous administration of a calciuretic diuretic such as furosemide or ethacrynic acid,* 1 mg./kg. every 4 hours for two or three doses, and replacement of sodium and

---

*Manufacturer's note: Ethacrynic acid is contraindicated in infants until further experience has accumulated.

potassium lost in the urine by an infusion of two thirds Ringer's lactate solution and one third 5 per cent dextrose in water with KCl added in a concentration of 30 mEq./liter as soon as urine output is assured. This is given in a volume equal to the urine output.

Following initial reduction of the hypercalcemia, oral phosphate treatment should be added. A solution of sodium and potassium phosphate (Neutra-Phos) is given in divided doses to provide 1 to 2 gm. phosphorus per 24 hours (300 to 600 ml. of the standard Neutraphos solution). Parathyroidectomy should be done as soon as feasible following temporary reduction of the serum calcium. Salmon calcitonin (Calcimar) is effective in the treatment of acute hypercalcemia; 5 to 8 units/kg. are given intravenously or intramuscularly at 12 hour intervals until the serum calcium concentration is reduced. Other hypocalcemic agents such as mithramycin are not approved for children and it is not possible to outline a treatment regimen with these agents.

Adrenal Disorders

GEORGE E. BACON, M.D.

CONGENITAL ADRENAL HYPERPLASIA

Dehydration in salt-losing infants is treated with normal saline, or with 0.45 per cent saline and sodium bicarbonate if significant acidosis is present. Mineralocorticoid replacement is also necessary: desoxycorticosterone acetate (DOCA) administered intramuscularly is appropriate. In our experience, initial dose varies from 1 to as much as 5 mg./day, depending on the severity of the hyponatremia, and also on whether supplemental dietary sodium chloride (0.5 to 2 gm./day) is provided when oral feedings are begun.

Early glucocorticoid therapy consists of hydrocortisone, 20 to 30 mg./m^2/day in three or four divided doses, given intravenously, intramuscularly or orally, depending on the degree of illness. An alternative is the use of cortisone acetate, about 20 mg. intramuscularly every three days.

Once a salt-losing patient is stabilized, the dose of mineralocorticoid can be reduced gradually to a maintenance level of 1 to 2 mg./day of DOCA intramuscularly, or 0.1 to 0.2 mg./day of fludrocortisone acetate (Florinef) orally. We prefer the latter for use at home; it is more convenient and is effective if vomiting is not a problem. Reduction to maintenance occasionally requires up to several months, but may be achieved much more rapidly in some patients; this dose usually is satisfactory in-

definitely. It is frequently possible to discontinue salt supplements during this period as well.

Subcutaneous DOCA pellet (125 mg.) implants are favored instead of intramuscular or oral mineralocorticoids in some clinics. This program assures a constant source of steroid for periods varying from about 4 to 9 months, but hypertension may occur, and it is of course critical to determine when the pellet has dissolved.

Mineralcorticoid therapy is monitored initially with blood pressure measurements and serum sodium and potassium determinations. Subsequently, periodic observation for hypertension and clinical evidence of fluid retention or weight loss are usually sufficient. Older children are able to describe a craving for salt if the intake of sodium or mineralocorticoid is inadequate. In some cases it is possible to discontinue the mineralocorticoid during adolescence, but we do not generally advocate this approach.

Non-salt-losers and salt-losers both require chronic glucocorticoid therapy, but the optimum amount varies considerably from patient to patient. Difficulty may be encountered in determining a steroid dose which will suppress androgen secretion to normal without causing evidence of hypercortisolism. Hydrocortisone, 20 to 25 mg./m^2/day orally in at least three divided doses, is often satisfactory, but adjustments may be necessary.

Prednisone or prednisolone, 5 to 7 mg./m^2/day in two or three doses, is also acceptable, and has the advantage of a longer half-life. However, it has been suggested that some steroid analogs cause more growth suppression than the naturally occurring hormone. Also, the relative lack of salt-retaining activity may be disadvantageous. As a third possibility, intramuscular cortisone acetate can be continued during early infancy as described above.

Note that mineralocorticoids also exert some glucocorticoid effect. For example, 0.1 mg. of fludrocortisone is equivalent to about 1.5 mg. of hydrocortisone. This fact should be considered during infancy when the patient is small and the dose of mineralocorticoid may be relatively high.

Glucocorticoid therapy is continued throughout life and is monitored by measurements of height, weight, bone age, 24-hour excretion of urinary 17-ketosteroids or pregnanetriol, and observation for signs of inappropriate masculinization. Serum 17-hydroxyprogesterone determinations may also be useful, but interpretation depends upon the time of the sample in relationship to the previous dose of steroid.

The above recommendations concern the salt-losing and non-salt-losing forms of 21-hydroxylase deficient congenital adrenal hyperplasia, by far the most common types. In addition, congenital lipoid adrenal hyperplasia and 3-β-ol-dehydrogenase deficiency, both rare and frequently fatal, require treatment with mineralocorticoid and glucocorticoid. The hypertensive forms of congenital adrenal hyperplasia (17-hydroxylase and 11-hydroxylase deficiency), also infrequent, are treated with glucocorticoid only. An analog with less salt-retaining potency than hydrocortisone, such as methylprednisolone, is probably preferable. Adolescents with 17-hydroxylase deficiency may require sex hormone replacement as well.

Emergency Treatment. Glucocorticoid treatment should be increased two- or three-fold if a febrile illness occurs. Parents should also be instructed in the emergency use of an injectable hydrocortisone preparation if oral administration is not possible. A dose of 25 to 50 mg. intramuscularly every four hours is usually sufficient, but immediate medical attention should be sought.

Prior to surgery, we recommend cortisone acetate, 100 mg./m² in three or four divided doses, beginning 36 to 48 hours before the procedure. The relatively long half-life of this preparation provides adequate protection for two or three days following surgery.

If time does not allow the use of cortisone acetate, hydrocortisone, 100 mg./m²/day intramuscularly in four doses, may be substituted. This regimen is also appropriate for other forms of severe physical stress requiring hospitalization. Because of the salt-retaining effect of pharmacologic amounts of cortisone and hydrocortisone, an increase in mineralocorticoid during stress is often unnecessary.

Surgical Management. We recommend clitorectomy during the initial hospitalization for females with ambiguous external genitalia. However, if surgery is not performed, clitoromegaly will become less apparent with adequate medical treatment and growth of the patient. There is evidence that sexual gratification is not compromised following amputation of the clitoris, but some clinics prefer relocation and recession to assure preservation of sensitivity. Widening of the introitus at the time of clitorectomy is indicated, to reduce urinary retention, in patients with a urogenital sinus.

The optimum time for definitive vaginoplasty is controversial, but this procedure can be deferred until pubertal changes have occurred. Repair during the first few years of life may be less traumatic psychologically, but subsequent revision is often necessary.

Newborn infants with congenital adrenal hyperplasia ideally should be hospitalized in a tertiary care facility for definitive diagnosis, initial medical management, and surgery if necessary. Discharge usually is possible within two or three weeks. Thereafter, outpatient follow-up should include consultation with an endocrinologist. Clinical visits should occur about every three months during infancy, and one or two times per year thereafter.

HYPOADRENOCORTICISM

In general, the regimen for replacement of mineralocorticoid and glucocorticoid in salt-losing congenital adrenal hyperplasia is also suitable for children with primary adrenal insufficiency (Addison's disease). However, a smaller dose of glucocorticoid is often sufficient since suppression of adrenocorticotropic hormone (ACTH) is not as critical. An approximation of the physiologic cortisol production rate frequently proves adequate: 20 mg. of hydrocortisone/m²/day for the first few weeks of life, and 12 mg./m²/day thereafter in three divided doses.

The same dose of glucocorticoid is appropriate for children with hypoadrenocorticism secondary to ACTH deficiency. Because these children frequently have growth hormone deficiency as well, it is particularly important to avoid further growth inhibition due to excessive steroid. These patients generally do not require mineralocorticoid, since salt-retaining hormones can be produced independently of ACTH.

Likewise, children with hereditary adrenocortical unresponsiveness to ACTH may be treated with hydrocortisone as described above; mineralocorticoid is not necessary.

As in congenital adrenal hyperplasia, children with hypoadrenocorticism require increased amounts of glucocorticoid during periods of stress.

Acute adrenal insufficiency resulting from trauma or infection may be treated with isotonic saline and hydrocortisone, 2 mg./kg. intravenously immediately, and approximately 100 mg./m² intramuscularly daily in four divided doses, as needed thereafter.

CUSHING'S SYNDROME

Adrenal adenomas or carcinomas require surgical removal. Because of suppression of the contralateral gland, glucocorticoid should be provided preoperatively, and then tapered over a period of at least one month.

Pituitary tumors (such as chromophobe adenomas) are removed surgically if possible; the trans-sphenoidal approach has become popular.

Total adrenalectomy is probably the treatment of choice for children with adrenal hyperplasia and no demonstrable pituitary lesion. The cure rate is higher than with unilateral or subtotal adrenalectomy, but lifelong replacement with both glucocorticoid and mineralocorticoid, in addition to preoperative treatment, is necessary.

Pituitary irradiation has gained favor recently, but the advantages of this approach must be weighed against the possibility of resultant hypopituitarism in the growing child. This complication may not become evident for several years or more. The efficacy of pituitary irradiation can be assessed by the dexamethasone suppression test.

Drugs (o,p'-DDD, metyrapone, and aminoglutethamide) have been used, but responses are variable and side effects may occur. The management of Cushing's syndrome requires the expertise of an experienced endocrinologist and surgeon.

OTHER ADRENAL DISORDERS

Tumors producing excessive androgens, estrogens, or aldosterone are removed surgically. Patients are followed postoperatively with periodic serum and urinary measurements of the appropriate steroid. (The term acquired adrenal hyperplasia is sometimes applied to patients who have normal genitalia but develop excessive virilization during adolescence. Some probably have a mild form of 21-hydroxylase deficiency and may be treated with glucocorticoid but the condition may also be due to an adrenal tumor).

Hyperaldosteronism secondary to bilateral adrenal hyperplasia can be managed with spironolactone or by adrenalectomy. Isolated hypoaldosteronism (18-"oxidation" defect) is treated with mineralocorticoid: fludrocortisone acetate, 0.1 to 0.2 mg./day orally, should be sufficient in the presence of adequate dietary salt.

Pheochromocytomas, which commonly originate in the adrenal medulla, are treated surgically. Patients must be monitored closely because of the risk of a hypertensive crisis during the procedure, and the possibility of a dangerous decline in blood pressure in the immediate postoperative period. Thereafter follow-up includes urinary VMA determinations to assess the completeness of removal and to detect possible recurrence of the tumor at another site.

Endocrine Disorders of the Testis

THOMAS MOSHANG, JR., M.D.

Endocrine disorders due to testicular dysfunction will be manifested in childhood by abnormalities of sexual development. These abnormalities may be either problems of sexual differentiation in the newborn or abnormalities of pubertal development. Those disorders of the testes not associated with abnormalities of sexual development, such as infertility, will not in all likelihood be diagnosed during childhood.

TESTICULAR FAILURE

Failure of the testes to function during fetal life can produce a variety of clinical situations ranging from a child with a normal female phenotype but with 46XY chromosomes to a completely well developed male with bilateral cryptorchidism (anorchia). Failure of the testes postnatally results in sexual infantilism.

Fetal Testicular Failure. The fetal testis secretes at least two hormones, mullerian-inhibiting factor (probably a polypeptide) and testosterone, to cause male differentiation of the sexual organ anlage. Failure of the fetal testis before the 12th week of gestation can produce the pure gonadal dysgenesis syndrome or sexual ambiguity. The infant with the pure gonadal dysgenesis syndrome will certainly be reared as a female, whereas the child with sexual ambiguity is often reared as a female (see page 322). In this situation, exploratory surgery and removal of dysgenetic gonads should be performed. Any endocrine function of these dysgenetic testes at the time of puberty will probably be inappropriate for the gender assignment and therefore there is no reason to retain the gonads. Furthermore, dysgenetic or streak gonads in the presence of a Y chromosome have a propensity for development of gonadal tumors.

The anorchid male will often virilize spontaneously at puberty. This spontaneous development of secondary sexual characteristics is probably due to the presence of Leydig cells scattered along the spermatic cord. In this situation, no hormonal therapy is necessary for sexual development and none available for the infertility. However, the implantation of Silastic prosthetic testes into the scrotum should be considered for cosmetic and psychological reasons. If the anorchid patient does not spontaneously virilize, then androgen therapy should be instituted at age 12 to 13 years.

Sexual Infantilism. Adolescent development normally occurs around age 11 (testicular enlargement), with development of pubic hair at a mean age of 13.4 years. Delay of adolescent development several years later than mean age is often normal. However, testicular failure may be suspected upon finding small sclerotic testes even at a young age. The disorders causing testicular failure may be associated with elevated gonadotropins (primary hypogonadism), of which Klinefelter's syndrome is the most common, or with low levels of gonadotropins (hypogonadotropic hypogonadism). In primary testicular failure, gonadotropins may be elevated above normal ranges by 10 years of age but, conversely, low levels of gonadotropins at 10 to 12 years of age do not rule out primary testicular failure. Upon finding significantly elevated gonadotropins, androgen therapy can be instituted at age 11 or older.

The diagnosis of hypogonadotropic hypogonadism is often more difficult to establish unless associated findings such as anosmia (Kallmann's syndrome) or other pituitary hormone deficiencies are present. This difficulty is directly related to the fact that gonadotropin levels are normally low in children and remain low through the early teens, especially in those children with constitutional delay of growth and development. Although it is theoretically possible to use gonadotropins to treat hypogonadotropic hypogonadism, the present therapy is androgens. Injections of human chorionic gonadrotropin (HCG) will develop and maintain Leydig cell function but, since HCG is mainly LH-like in its activity, adequate spermatogenesis will not occur because the presence of FSH is necessary for spermatogenesis. FSH preparations are available as extracts of urine from menopausal women, but at present are approved only for use in the treatment of infertility in women. In those patients with hypogonadotropic hypogonadism secondary to hypothalamic dysfunction, as determined by positive LH and FSH responses to exogenously administered gonadotropin releasing hormone (GnRH), the use of synthetic GnRH for treatment is a real possibility for future consideration. In this latter disorder, GnRH would, theoretically, not only stimulate Leydig cell function but also stimulate spermatogenesis as well. Clinical trials using GnRH in patients with hypogonadotropic hypogonadism secondary to hypothalamic dysfunction are now in progress.

In those patients with growth hormone deficiency as well as gonadotropin deficiency, there is a rationale for use of both androgens and human growth hormone simultaneously for the treatment of the sexual infantilism. Growth hormone and testosterone are synergistic in their biological activities upon the development of accessory sexual organs as well as on linear growth.

Androgen Therapy. Androgens will adequately develop the secondary sexual characteristics in males with sexual infantilism, although testicular growth will be limited. Classically, the therapeutic regimen is to wait until age 12 or 13 and then to utilize testosterone either orally or intramuscularly to develop and then to maintain secondary sexual characteristics. However, since a change in growth rate heralds the onset of puberty by several years, there is a rationale for using low-dose androgens earlier if limited height potential and associated psychological problems are considerations in management.

The oral alkylated synthetic androgens, such as methandrostenolone (Dianabol) or oxandralone (Anavar), have been found to improve linear growth in patients with Turner's syndrome without the loss of height from premature epiphyseal fusion. These drugs, in low doses, are less virilizing than testosterone and therefore are useful in the younger age groups. Although the alkylated synthetic androgens have been implicated as etiologic agents of cholestatic jaundice as well as hepatic tumors, the incidence of such occurrences with low doses used over short periods is low. However, when these drugs are used for treatment of sexual infantilism in patients who also have limited growth potential, liver dysfunction should be monitored. If limited height potential is not a consideration, testosterone enanthate or cyclopentylpropionate, 100 to 200 mg. intramuscularly monthly, or methyltestosterone, 10 to 20 mg. sublingually daily, is strongly recommended. Testosterone enanthate or cyclopentylpropionate is used for chronic maintenance therapy.

Treatment Regimen for Low-Dose Androgens. Ages 10 to 12: The patient is treated with methandrostenolone, 0.04 to 0.05 mg./kg./day for 3 months, and then no treatment for 3 months. The cycle is repeated if clinically there are no signs of liver dysfunction or rapid virilization. Skeletal age and height predictions are appraised yearly. Liver function tests are performed during each cycle of therapy.

Ages 12 to 14: Fluoxymestrone, 10 to 20 mg. daily, is used for 4 to 6 months, and then no treatment for 4 to 6 months. Skeletal age and height predictions are monitored on a yearly basis. Liver function is also monitored.

If virilization is inadequate after one cycle of fluoxymestrone, use testosterone enanthate or cyclopentylpropionate, 100 mg. intramuscularly per month, increasing to 200 mg., or biweekly injections if necessary.

For chronic maintenance, testosterone enanthate or cyclopentylpropionate, 100 to 200 mg. intramuscularly monthly or biweekly, is used for long-term therapy.

SEXUAL PRECOCITY

Sexual precocity occurs much less often in the male than in females and, as a disorder in the male, is much more likely to have a diagnosable cause. The diagnosis of cryptogenic (or idiopathic) sexual precocity can be made only after careful evaluation to exclude possible primary etiologic diseases, including adrenal disease, Leydig cell tumors, hepatomas and central nervous system lesions. Precocious sexual development in the male is often less psychologically disconcerting, and therapy is indicated mainly because of the rapid rate of skeletal maturation and premature epiphyseal fusion.

Unfortunately, drug therapy using either medroxyprogesterone acetate or antiandrogens, such as cyproterone acetate, has had only variable success. Nevertheless, if advancement of skeletal maturation is rapid, and no treatable primary cause can be elucidated, it is worthwhile to try medroxyprogesterone acetate, 100 to 200 mg. intramuscularly at monthly or biweekly intervals. This drug is still considered to be investigational for treatment of sexual precocity and parents must be so informed. The theoretical possibility of infertility from prolonged medroxyprogesterone administration, although not yet documented in humans, must also be revealed to the parents. Finally, if therapy is initiated and there is a response with marked slowing of the skeletal maturation, treatment must be continued for many years.

Gynecomastia

JOHN S. PARKS, M.D., PH.D.

Gynecomastia, or enlargement of the male breast, is a normal feature of puberty. A majority of boys have some degree of subareolar breast budding during early puberty, coincident with increases in testicular size, penile length and the appearance of pubic hair. Parenchymal hyperplasia of the breast occurs in response to rising levels of testosterone and estrogens. The degree of breast development does not correlate well with estrogen levels.

Gynecomastia is also seen during iatrogenic induction of puberty with androgens such as methyltestosterone which cannot be converted to estrogens. The firm, easily palpable breast tissue is often tender and may be asymmetrical. In most boys, this subareolar "button" of tissue recedes within a few months. Even when there is visible breast enlargement, it usually disappears within two years. Management consists of recognizing and answering the adolescent's frequent concerns that the condition is unusual, that it represents a tumor, or that it will inevitably progress to full feminine breast development. Reassurance can be very helpful to the teenager with mild and transient gynecomastia. It is fair to tell him that the condition reflects rapid pubertal virilization.

Evaluation of boys with more severe gynecomastia requires a careful history and physical examination. Psychological consequences may be out of proportion to the degree of breast enlargement. Be alert for the boy who wears a heavy wool shirt in midsummer, sits with his shoulders hunched forward, shuns the beach and swimming pool, or feigns injury to avoid gym class. His needs will not be met by simple reassurance. It is seldom possible to elicit a history of teasing or of fear of rejection by girls on an initial visit. Even severely distressed boys tend to affect an attitude of nonchalance. The duration of gynecomastia is important. Breast enlargement which has persisted for more than two years is unlikely to show further regression. By this time the lobular and ductal tissue have usually been replaced by connective tissue and fat. A family history of persistent gynecomastia likewise implies a poor prognosis for regression. Gynecomastia may develop late in puberty during recovery from a severe illness or as a consequence of drug use. The most commonly implicated drugs are digitalis, reserpine, spironolactone, tranquilizers and marijuana. If there is a causal relationship, discontinuation of the drug will result in regression.

Physical examination should focus on the question of whether the other aspects of pubertal development are proceeding appropriately. Gynecomastia appearing after the newborn period but before the age of 12 years presents special problems. It may reflect congenital adrenal hyperplasia, precocious puberty, exposure to exogenous sex hormones or malignant tumors of the liver, adrenal or testis. Alternatively, unilateral breast enlargement may result from a local neoplasm, as in neurofibromatosis. Klinefelter syndrome is the most common and easily recognized abnormality associated with pubertal gynecomastia. The presence of testes which are abnormally small for the patient's degree of pubertal development should prompt the physician to obtain a buccal smear and/or lymphocyte karyotype for recognition of a 47 XXY chromosome constitution. The association of gynecomastia with hypospadias also dictates a complete endocrine evaluation. This combination of findings is observed in the 3β-hydroxysteroid dehydrogenase and 17 alpha-hydroxylase varieties of congenital adrenal hyperplasia, in enzymatic defects of testosterone synthesis and in several varieties of end organ resistance to the effects of testosterone. Appropriate medical treatment of these rare conditions depends upon precise diagnosis. Generalized obesity is an important finding for two reasons. First, some obese boys have abundant fatty breast tissue which does not represent true gynecomastia. This situation can often be markedly improved by weight reduction. Second, the penis in obese boys may be partially obscured by suprapubic fat. This physical finding should not be mistaken for hypogonadism.

Most families who seek advice about their son's gynecomastia start with the assumption that their son has a correctable hormonal imbalance. It must be explained in a patient and thorough manner that this is not the case. The vast majority of boys with troublesome gynecomastia have no other physical, genetic or hormonal characteristics which set them apart from their peers. There is no medical means of ameliorating the condition. The use of androgens, androgen antagonists and human chorionic gonadotropin is contraindicated. The only available treatment is surgical. The operation involves partial removal of breast tissue through a subareolar incision. Cosmetic results are usually quite acceptable when the operation is done by an experienced pediatric or plastic surgeon. Although it is a major procedure, it is in no sense comparable to a mastectomy for breast carcinoma or even to a reduction mammoplasty in a female. The criteria for surgical treatment include duration and degree of breast enlargement, psychological handicaps incident to the condition and realistic expectations on the part of the patient and his family.

Hermaphroditism and Intersex

JOHN S. PARKS, M.D., PH.D.

The birth of a child with ambiguous genitalia constitutes a true medical emergency. The physician's reaction to this event will have a profound impact upon the child and family.

In most instances, it is appropriate to tell the husband and wife, together, that the infant's genital development was not completed before birth and that tests will be required to determine whether it is a boy or girl. From the very first contact, it is essential to stress that the infant will be all boy or all girl and not a little bit of each. The terms hermaphrodite, pseudohermaphrodite and intersex should not be used in talking with parents. On the day of birth, it should be possible to set a timetable for obtaining and interpreting the tests required to arrive at a correct gender assignment. The time required is generally less than four days. More time may be required to arrive at a definitive diagnosis and to determine whether the condition poses a threat to the child's survival. Announcement of birth beyond the immediate family should be delayed until the issue of gender assignment is resolved.

Infants with ambiguous genitalia usually fit into one of three broad etiologic categories—the virilized genetic female, the undervirilized genetic male, and the infant with combined abnormalities of gonads and sex chromosomes. Since the appearance of the external genitalia is dependent primarily upon fetal exposure to androgens, infants in each category tend to have a similar external appearance. The genital tubercle may be large and resemble a penis or it may be small and bound down by chordee. The urethrolabial folds may be fused to form a penile urethra in a genetic female, or there may be varying degrees of hypospadias. Similarly, the labioscrotal folds may be completely or only partially fused. Two aspects of the physical examination are of practical importance. Palpation of two scrotal or inguinal gonads implies that the infant is a genetic male. However, if the penile structure is extremely small or malformed, the infant is best assigned a female gender regardless of chromosome constitution.

The first level of testing involves examination of a buccal smear for nuclear chromatin and for Y chromosome fluorescence. A genetic female will have a chromatin-positive buccal smear and no Y chromosome fluorescence. These tests have the advantage of speed. Results should be available in less than 48 hours. They have the disadvantage of being subject to misleading artifact in inexperienced laboratories. Lymphocyte karyotype analysis should always be done to verify the more rapid tests and to detect the presence of chromosomal mosaicism.

A female fetus may be virilized by androgens from three possible sources—maternal drug ingestion, a virilizing maternal tumor, and its own adrenal glands. Progestational agents, in the form of oral contraceptives taken after conception or as medications taken to forestall a threatened abortion, are now a rare cause of fetal virilization. Virilizing tumors of the ovary are even less commonly encountered, as they generally cause infertility. Exposure to androgens prior to 12 weeks of gestation produces labial fusion, and exposure at any time results in clitoral enlargement. There will be a positive history of drug ingestion in the one case and an elevated maternal testosterone level in the second. With either etiology, the infant's urinary 17-ketosteroid excretion will be normal and no medical treatment will be required.

Congenital adrenal hyperplasia is a much more common cause of virilization of the female fetus. This category of disease poses a threat to the infant's development and to her survival in addition to causing confusion regarding gender assignment. In 21 hydroxylase deficiency and in the less common disorders of 11 hydroxylase and 3β-hydroxysteroid dehydrogenase activity, urinary 17-ketosteroid excretion remains elevated. Differentiation from normal is possible after two or three days of age. Recently developed radioimmunoassays for serum 17-hydroxyprogesterone and 21-desoxycortisol may permit even more rapid diagnosis. Lifelong treatment with hydrocortisone or cortisone is required to prevent further virilization, to promote normal growth and skeletal maturation, and to permit normal feminine development at puberty. In the saltlosing varieties of adrenal hyperplasia, treatment is essential for survival beyond a week or two of age.

The virilized female infant invariably has normal ovaries and fallopian tubes and a normal uterus. She will have normal pubertal development and will be fertile. A female gender assignment is entirely appropriate. The enlarged clitoris tends to recede in prominence as the child grows. However, if the mother is troubled by the incongruity of a large clitoris, if there is a penile urethra, or if the appropriate gender assignment has been delayed for weeks or months, surgery may be indicated. Partial resection of the clitoral corpus with retention of the glans is preferred. Vaginoplasty may be required to establish continuity between the perineum and the upper vagina. If x-ray contrast studies indicate that this will be complex, the repair may need to be done in stages with the final vaginoplasty deferred until puberty.

The undervirilized male infant may have hypospadias, chordee and defective scrotal fusion, or he may have an extremely small penis with a phallic urethra and a normal scrotum. The first set of findings implies defective testicular synthesis of or end organ responsiveness to testosterone before the 12th week of gestation. Enzymatic defects affecting both adrenal and gonad include 3β-hydroxysteroid dehydrogenase and 17α-hydroxylase deficiencies. Both disorders may be recognized by abnormal patterns of urinary steroid excretion and both require treatment with hydrocortisone. There are at least two additional enzyme deficiency states which impair testicular androgen production without affecting adrenal function. Defects in end organ recognition of androgens include 5α-reductase deficiency and partial testicular feminization. On a practical level, the pediatrician should obtain urinary 17-ketosteroid measurements to exclude the potentially lethal 3β-hydroxysteroid dehydrogenase defect, and collect at least 5 ml. of serum for special studies such as luteinizing hormone, follicle-stimulating hormone and testosterone. A precise diagnosis is required for the purpose of genetic counseling and estimation of the risk of recurrence in future siblings. Decisions regarding gender assignment should be made with the consultation of a pediatric surgeon or urologist and should reflect a realistic opinion as to the potential for normal male sexual function. The penis which initially appears small may actually have chordee and be quite repairable.

The finding of an extremely small penis in an otherwise normal male infant implies failure of testosterone production after 12 weeks of gestation. Normal stretched penile length at birth is 3 to 5 cm. and a penis less than 1 cm. is termed a micropenis. The condition may result from incomplete development of the testes and be associated with anorchia. Alternatively, micropenis may indicate inadequate pituitary gonadotropin stimulation of the testis. In the former case, serum LH and FSH will be elevated and in the latter they will be low in relation to age-specific norms. Isolated gonadotropin deficiency together with a defective sense of smell is termed Kallmann syndrome. Gonadotropin deficiency may be accompanied by deficiencies of growth hormone, thyrotropin and ACTH. Every genetic male with a micropenis should be suspected of having anterior hypopituitarism. The occurrence of neonatal hypoglycemia should prompt complete evaluation of pituitary function.

Management of micropenis is controversial. There is no potential for surgical construction of a satisfactory penis. The usual practice is to assign a female gender. In this case, gonadectomy, diversion of the urethra and creation of a cleft between the labioscrotal folds are accomplished before two years of age. Estrogen replacement and construction of an artificial vagina at puberty will lead to an amenorrheic and infertile but otherwise normal female. In selected cases, the option of enhancing penile growth has been attempted. Testosterone cypionate, in a dosage of 25 mg., is given intramuscularly each two weeks for a total of two months.* If penile length does not approach the normal range by the end of this time, a female gender assignment is made. There are no studies of adult outcome in males treated in this fashion, but endocrinologists and urologists are quite familiar with the tragic situation of adolescent boys with a persistently tiny penis. Treatment with testosterone should not be attempted unless the pediatrician and a psychiatric consultant feel that the family will be able to tolerate a two month delay in the decision regarding final gender assignment.

Girls with Turner syndrome and boys with Klinefelter syndrome have abnormalities of sex chromosomes and gonads, but they do not have ambiguous genitalia. The girl with a missing or abnormal X chromosome deserves estrogen and progestin treatment beginning at age 13 to 15 years to promote breast development and cyclical menses. She will probably have a more dramatic adolescent growth spurt and enhanced adult stature if estrogen replacement is preceded by one or two years of treatment with low doses of an oral androgen. Some boys with 47 XXY Klinefelter syndrome will benefit from testosterone supplementation at puberty, whereas others will virilize quite well on their own.

Girls with testicular feminization and a 46 XY karyotype also have normal female genitalia at birth. They may be recognized during an operation for a palpable inguinal gonad, or the diagnosis may be made during an investigation of primary amenorrhea. Testicular function prior to the 12th week of gestation causes regression of müllerian structures, so that there is no uterus and no potential for menses or fertility. Gonads should be removed because of a potential for malignancy, and estrogen replacement is indicated.

Occasionally an infant will not fit these etiologic categories. Examples include 45X:46XY chromosomal mosaicism with mixed gonadal dysgenesis or an infant with a 46 XX karyotype, genital ambiguity, and a palpable gonad who probably has true hermaphroditism. In these instances, gender assignment should still be made on the basis of the appearance of the external genitalia. However, vaginography and laparotomy with inspection of internal duct structures and biopsy of gonads should be done before two years of age to establish a diagnosis and to clarify future management. Müllerian remnants should be removed in children with a male gender assignment to eliminate the possibility of menstruation at puberty. Gonads should be removed in the 46 XY or 45 XO:46 XY infant with a female gender assignment to prevent possible virilization at puberty.

Regardless of the nature of an error of genital development, certain management principles should be kept in mind. Following an initial phase of grief and resentment, the parents should be secure in the belief that their child is being raised in an appropriate gender. If they are secure in their approach to the child over his or her first two years, the child's sexual identity will be firmly established. The family's attitudes are much more important than chromosomes or hormones in determining outcome. Explanations should be introduced gradually and with a sensitivity to the family's capacity to understand and integrate information. The most common mistake is to flood the family or older child with explanations which would be more appropriate for a lecture to colleagues or medical students. It is best not to use gender-specific terms when the terms are at odds with the child's gender assignment. It is disturbing and unnecessary for a girl's family to hear of a male karyotype, a penis and testes. The same information can be conveyed using less specific terms. Surgical management is directed toward removal of incongruous structures at a fairly early age and, when necessary, enlarging or constructing a vagina at the age of puberty. Feminization at puberty may be accomplished by oral administration of ethinyl estradiol, 0.02 mg. each day. When cyclical menstruation is a goal, the estrogen is given for 21 days of a 28 day cycle and dydrogesterone or medroxyprogesterone may also be given in a dosage of 5 to 10 mg. per day from days 15 to 21 of the cycle. Pubertal virilization may be achieved with methyltestosterone, 10 to 20 mg. per day sublingually, or with intramuscular testosterone cypionate or testosterone enanthate given in doses of 100 to 400 mg. each month.

___

*The Food and Drug Administration has not approved a dosage range for the use of androgens in early infancy.

10

Metabolic Disorders

Infants Born to Diabetic Mothers

JOHN P. CLOHERTY, M.D., *and*
MICHAEL F. EPSTEIN, M.D.

Significant advances have been made in recent years in reducing the perinatal mortality in the offspring of women with diabetes mellitus. While general improvements in both obstetric and neonatal medical care have certainly influenced this better prognosis, as important are (1) a better understanding of the basic metabolic abnormalities in the mother and their effect on body composition and metabolic homeostasis in the developing fetus and (2) an early and increased involvement of the pediatrician in the care and planning for the fetus and neonate. This team approach has allowed the pediatrician to better anticipate, prepare for, and treat the specific risks to which the infant of the diabetic mother is exposed.

CLASSIFICATION

Planning for the care of the infant in the perinatal period is greatly aided by two classifications of maternal diabetes. White's classification (Clin. Perinatol., *1*:331–347, 1974) is used in deciding appropriate management, and when combined with Pedersen's Prognostic Bad Signs in Pregnancy (PBSP) (Diabetes, *23*:302, 1974), a more accurate prediction of outcome can be made (Table 1).

White's Classification of Maternal Diabetes

Class A— Chemical diabetes: positive glucose tolerance tests prior to or during pregnancy. Prediabetes: history of large babies (>4 kg.) or unexplained stillbirths after 28 weeks.

Class B— Medication-dependent, onset after 20 years of age, duration less than 10 years

Class C— C_1 Onset 10 to 19 years of age
C_2 Duration 10 to 19 years

Class D— D_1 Onset under 10 years of age
D_2 Duration 20 years
D_3 Calcification of vessels of the leg (macrovascular disease)
D_4 Benign retinopathy (microvascular disease)
D_5 Hypertension

Class E— Same as D with calcification of pelvic vessels

Class F— Nephropathy

Class R— Malignant retinopathy

Class G— Many reproductive failures

Class H— Diabetic cardiomyopathy

Pedersen's Prognostic Bad Signs in Pregnancy (PBSP)

Clinical pyelonephritis
Precoma or severe acidosis
Toxemia
"Neglectors" (women who would not cooperate with the treatment plan)

TABLE 1. Combination of White's and Pedersen's Classifications of Maternal Diabetes*

| WHITE'S CLASS | PERINATAL MORTALITY | |
	PBSP PRESENT	PBSP ABSENT
A B	17.1%	3.4%
C D E	26.7%	9.8%
F	37.5%	30.8%

*Modified from Pedersen, J., et al.: Assessors of fetal perinatal mortality in pregnancy. Diabetes, *23*:302, 1974.

MATERNAL-FETAL PROBLEMS

Diabetic women have normal fertility. In the first trimester there is an increased rate of spontaneous abortions, the incidence of these early losses varying with the diabetic classification: Class A, 5–10 per cent (not significantly different from the general population); Class B, 10 per cent; Class C, 24 per cent; Class D, 30 per cent; and Class E, 74 per cent. Episodes of hypoglycemia may occur in the first trimester but it is not known whether these are associated with fetal damage. In the second trimester there is increased insulin requirement sometimes associated with ketoacidosis and resultant high fetal mortality. In the third trimester the major problem is sudden unexpected fetal death. These deaths are sometimes associated with ketoacidosis, preeclampsia, or maternal vascular disease of the decidua and myometrium, but many are unexplained. Most diabetic pregnancies are associated with polyhydramnios. While this is usually not a sign of significant fetal anomaly as in the nondiabetic pregnancy, it may be associated with premature rupture of membranes and early labor. In classes A, B and C, the placenta and cord are usually large, but when vascular disease is present as in classes D, E and F, the placenta may be small and have multiple infarcts. The placenta has extramedullary hematopoiesis in diabetic pregnancies, and this observation may be helpful in the postpartum investigation of the etiology of late stillbirths.

PREGNANCY MANAGEMENT

Perinatal outcome improves with good metabolic control of maternal diabetes. The goal is to maintain maternal blood sugar in a range where glucosuria is less than 20 gm. a day. Diabetic mothers needing treatment beyond dietary control should receive insulin rather than oral agents which cross the placenta and may be associated with severe neonatal hypoglycemia if used near the time of birth.

Delivery is planned according to diabetic class with approximate goals (Class A, 38 to 40 weeks; Classes B and C, 37 weeks; Classes D and E, 36 weeks; and Classes F, R and H, 35 weeks) based on the incidence of fetal death in the various classes and the risks of immaturity in the prematurely delivered neonate. In the third trimester, urinary estriols are followed as an indicator of fetoplacental integrity.

Other tests have been used as indicators of placental function such as human chorionic gonadotrophin (HCG), human placental lactogen (HPL), estradiol, and progesterone. Ultrasonography is a noninvasive method of estimating gestational age and assessing fetal growth. Lecithin-sphingomyelin ratio (L/S) or shake test (New Engl. J. Med., *286*:1007, 1972) on amniotic fluid obtained by transabdominal amniocentesis can be utilized to predict pulmonary maturity. The oxytocin challenge test may predict impending fetal demise and/or the ability of the fetus to tolerate labor.

If the L/S ratio is favorable, delivery is usually accomplished on the planned date by induction of labor or cesarean section. If, however, the L/S ratio is immature and all indicators of fetal health are favorable, delivery should be postponed. Although the L/S ratio remains the best predictor of lung maturity, there have been reports of hyaline membrane disease in infants of diabetic mothers who had mature L/S ratios (2 to 1). While many of these reports may be colored by the inclusion of other respiratory conditions in the category of hyaline membrane disease, several have been well documented.

These apparent false positive tests may be due to the occasional presence of nonpulmonary or nonsurface active lecithin. Until this problem has been further studied by separation of this nonsurface active lecithin, it is best to use a higher L/S ratio for predicting pulmonary maturity in infants of diabetic mothers. The exact ratio should be individualized for each institution or laboratory for this group of patients.

A decrease in the rate of maternal weight gain, a fall in insulin requirement, a decrease in fetal activity, a fall in estriols, an unfavorable oxytocin challenge test or the appearance of preeclampsia may necessitate emergency delivery to prevent fetal demise even in the face of an unfavorable L/S ratio. Prior to and during the delivery there should be careful control of the mother's fluids and blood sugar to prevent hyperglycemia, hypoglycemia and acidosis. The delivery should be planned in cooperation with a pediatrician who is informed about the mother's status and the infant's maturity and who is present in the delivery room, able and equipped to care for the infant's problems.

INFANT PROBLEMS

The evaluation of the infant in the delivery room begins prior to the actual delivery. Immediately prior to opening the amniotic sac at the time of cesarean section, the obstetrician can obtain a sterile sample of amniotic fluid for culture, Gram stain, and L/S ratio or shake test when indicated. Once the baby has been delivered, a careful assessment using the Apgar score should indicate the need for any resuscitative efforts. The infant should be well dried and placed under a heat source, and careful attention should be paid to clearing the airway of mucus. The stomach is not suctioned at this point because of the risk of reflex bradycardia and apnea with pharyngeal stimulation. In the delivery room a screening physical examination for major congenital anomalies is performed, and the placenta is examined. A specimen of cord blood is obtained for glucose concentration to anticipate the reactive hypoglycemia associated with hyperglycemia at delivery.

In the nursery a more complete physical examination with special attention to the heart, kidneys and extremities is performed. Reports indicate a 56 per cent risk of significant hypoglycemia, 18 per cent risk of hypocalcemia, 35 per cent risk of hyperbilirubinemia, and a 34 per cent risk of polycythemia; therefore the following studies are performed:

Blood sugar: 1, 2, 3, 6, 12, 24, 36, 48 hours. Dextrostix* will be reliable if over 40. Readings under 40 should be checked rapidly by a clinical laboratory or by Ames Eyetone Instrument.*

Calcium: 6, 12, 24, 48 hours
Hematocrit: 1 hour, 24 hours
Bilirubin: 24, 48 hours and as indicated

SPECIFIC PROBLEMS IN INFANTS OF DIABETIC MOTHERS

Respiratory Distress. Infants of diabetic mothers have a roughly sixfold increased risk of hyaline membrane disease over infants of nondiabetic mothers of the same gestational age, independent of the method of delivery. Nevertheless, other causes of respiratory distress such as diaphragmatic hernia, pneumothorax, congenital heart disease, aspiration of meconium, transient tachypnea of the newborn and infection must also be considered in the differential diagnosis. Studies should include:

1. Obtaining gastric aspirate during the first hour of life after the baby has been stabilized. A polyethylene catheter with a mucus trap is used. The gastric aspirate is used for two tests: Gram stain for polymorphonuclear leukocytes and bacteria (5 polymorphonuclear leukocytes per high power field or the presence of bacteria is associated with infection); and gastric aspirate shake test to assess the amount of pulmonary surfactant in the newborn's lungs (New Engl. J. Med., 292:113, 1975). This test has been used to predict the risk of the development

of hyaline membrane disease and is done on gastric aspirates as follows:

Absolute alcohol, 0.5 ml., is added to 0.5 ml. of gastric aspirate in a 4 ml. glass tube, 82.0 by 10.25 mm. (as supplied new from the manufacturer).* The test tube, capped by the thumb, is vigorously shaken for 15 seconds and allowed to stand for 15 minutes. The test is then read:

Negative—no bubbles

1+—Very small bubbles in meniscus extending one third or less of distance around test tube (a magnifying glass is usually required to determine that these small bubbles are indeed bubbles as opposed to particles)

2+—Single rim of bubbles extending one third to all around the test tube (a magnifying glass is not necessary)

3+—Rim of bubbles all the way around the test tube, with a double row in some areas

4+—Double row or more of bubbles all the way around the test tube

The test is interpreted: 3+ or 4+—little chance of hyaline membrane disease; negative—high risk; 1+ or 2+—intermediate risk.

2. A chest x-ray to evaluate aeration, presence of infiltrates, cardiac size and position, the presence of pneumothorax and so forth.

3. Blood gasses—by umbilical, radial or temporal artery cannulation or by capillary method to evaluate gas exchange and the presence of right-to-left shunts.

4. Electrocardiogram and blood pressure measurements.

5. Cultures of the surface (nose, throat, ear canal, umbilicus and rectum), gastric aspirate, urine and blood. Spinal fluid should be included if the infant's condition allows.

THERAPY OF HYALINE MEMBRANE DISEASE. Proper therapy necessitates: adequate oxygen to maintain a PaO_2 between 50 and 70 mm. Hg; delivery of oxygen with continuous positive airway pressure (CPAP) by nasopharyngeal or endotracheal intubation when the FiO_2 requirement exceeds .40 to .60; use of assisted ventilation if the FiO_2 requirement exceeds .60 and if apnea spells or other evidence of respiratory failure is evident; monitoring blood pressure and giving adequate volume as fresh frozen plasma, 5 per cent albumin or blood to maintain normal pressure and perfusion; maintenance of normal fluid, electrolyte and nutritional requirements:

DAY	FLUID (cc./kg.)	GLUCOSE (gm./kg.)	PROTEIN (gm./kg.)	CALORIES (per kg.)
1	65	6.5	—	—
2	100	7.5	2	40
3	125	10	2.5	50
4	150	12	3	60

These fluids are given as water, dextrose and amino-acid preparations. After the first day, 3

---

*Ames Company, Division of Miles Laboratory, Elkhart, Indiana.

*Becton, Dickinson & Co., No. 4852 red stopper tube.

mEq./kg./day of sodium and 2 mEq./kg./day of potassium are required. The fourth day schedule will provide maintenance calories. If the infant is still given nothing by mouth after one week, extra calories in the form of parenteral lipid should be provided. Infants need 100 to 120 cal./kg./day for adequate growth. The range is dependent on whether the nutrients are taken by mouth or parenterally.

Use of antibiotics is individualized. Because of the difficulty in distinguishing infants with hyaline membrane disease from those with group B streptococcal pneumonitis, if there is any increased risk of infection (e.g., prolonged rupture of membrane), the infant is started on appropriate antibiotics after cultures are taken. If cultures are negative after 48 hours, antibiotics are stopped.

Especially with premature infants, a thermoneutral environment must be provided. This is most easily accomplished in servocontrolled incubators with the temperature probe on the anterior abdominal wall set to register approximately 36.5° C. Large infants being observed in incubators must be monitored closely to avoid overheating.

Hypoglycemia. Hypoglycemia is defined as a blood sugar under 30 mg. per 100 ml. in any infant regardless of gestational age whether associated with symptoms or not. Infants of diabetic mothers, if symptomatic from hypoglycemia, usually are quiet and lethargic rather than jittery. Other symptoms such as apnea, tachypnea, respiratory distress, shock, cyanosis and seizures may occur. If symptoms are present the infant is probably at greater risk for sequelae. The significance of hypoglycemia without symptoms is unclear but conservative management to maintain the blood sugar in the normal range appears to be indicated.

In our nursery, we begin to feed "well" infants of diabetic mothers by bottle or gavage with 5 cc./kg. of 10 per cent dextrose in water by one hour of age. Infants under 2 kg. should be given nothing orally and have parenteral sugar starting in the first hour of life. The larger infants can be fed hourly for 3 to 4 feeds until the blood sugars are stable. Feeds can then be given every 2 hours and then every 3 hours; as the interval between feeds increases, the volume is increased. If all goes well, by 12 hours of age the infant should be on 20 cal./oz. formula with extra dextrose added as needed. This method of rapid oral feeding will prevent or correct the hypoglycemia in most of these infants. If by 2 hours of age the blood sugar is low in spite of feeding or if feedings are not tolerated as indicated by large volumes of feeds retained in the stomach, more aggressive treatment is indicated to raise the blood sugar.

While readying the equipment for intravenous therapy, an initial step in treatment in the symptomatic infant is the administration of crystalline glucagon, 300 μg./kg. intramuscularly or subcutaneously, to a maximum dose of 1.0 mg. This will cause a rapid rise in blood sugar in infants who have good glycogen stores (not reliable in the smaller infants of classes D, E, F and others). This rise may last 2 to 3 hours and is useful until parenteral sugar can be administered.

The basic element in treatment, however, is intravenous glucose administration. This must be done through a reliable route. Administration of fluids via peripheral scalp vein or "butterfly" needles has several disadvantages. First, they may be difficult to place quickly in obese infants. Second, it may be difficult to maintain patency, raising the risk of frequent hazardous interruptions in the infusion. Third, because of the risk of infiltration and subsequent tissue necrosis, these infusion sites must be continuously observed (see below). On the other hand, the peripheral site is free of the infectious and vascular complications of the umbilical venous or arterial catheters. We use peripheral veins for treatment; however, in emergency situations with symptomatic babies, we have utilized umbilical venous catheters placed in the inferior vena cava above the diaphragm.

Specific treatment is determined by the baby's condition. If the infant is in distress (e.g., seizures or respiratory compromise), 0.5 to 1.0 gm. of glucose/kg. is given by intravenous push of 2 to 4 ml. of 25 per cent dextrose in water at a rate of 1 ml./min. For example, a 4 kg. infant would receive 8 to 16 ml. of 25 per cent dextrose in water over 8 to 16 min. This is followed by a continuous infusion of dextrose at a rate of 4 to 8 mg. of glucose/kg./min. The concentration of dextrose in the intravenous fluid will depend on the total daily fluid requirement. For example, on day one, the usual fluid intake is 65 ml./kg. or 0.045 ml./kg./min. Therefore, 10 per cent dextrose in water would provide 4.5 mg. glucose/kg./min. and 15 per cent dextrose in water would provide 6.75 mg. of glucose/kg./min. In other words, 10 per cent dextrose in water at standard intravenous fluid maintenance rates usually supplies sufficient glucose to raise the blood sugar above 30 mg. per 100 ml. However, the concentration of dextrose and the infusion rates are increased as necessary to maintain the blood sugar in the normal range.

If the infant is not symptomatic but has

blood sugars in the hypoglycemic range, an initial push of concentrated sugar need not be given. Rather, an initial infusion of 5 to 10 ml. of 10 per cent dextrose in water at 1 ml./min. is followed by the continuous infusion of glucose at 4 to 8 mg./kg./min. Blood sugars must be monitored carefully at frequent intervals after beginning intravenous glucose infusions to be certain of adequate treatment of the hypoglycemia and also to avoid hyperglycemia with the risk of osmotic diuresis and dehydration.

Parenteral sugar should never be abruptly discontinued because of the risk of a reactive hypoglycemia. As oral feeding progresses, the rate of the infusion can be gradually decreased, and the concentration of glucose infused can be reduced to 5 per cent dextrose in water. It is particularly important to measure blood sugar levels during this process of tapering the intravenous infusion.

Since the hypoglycemia of most infants of diabetic mothers responds to the above treatment, unresponsiveness or persistence (over 48 hours) should cause a search for other problems (i.e., infection, islet cell tumor, etc.). Hydrocortisone, 5 mg./kg./day intramuscularly in two divided doses, has been occasionally helpful. In our experience other drugs (epinephrine, diazoxide, growth hormone) have not been necessary.

Hypocalcemia. Hypocalcemia is often found in infants of diabetic mothers, and its incidence may be increased in the presence of other known causes of hypocalcemia.

First 3 days
    Maternal
        Toxemia
        Dietary deficiency of calcium
        Maternal hyperparathyroidism
    Intrapartum
        Asphyxia, prematurity
        Small-for-gestational age infants
    Postnatal
        Hypoxia, shock, sepsis, treatment with bicarbonate
After 3 days
    High phosphate diet (whole cow's milk), magnesium deficiency
    Hypoparathyroidism (check for thymus on x-ray)
    Renal disease
    Vitamin D deficiency or defect of vitamin D metabolism

Signs of hypocalcemia in the newborn are nonspecific and the classic Chvostek's sign and carpopedal spasm are helpful only if present. Irritability, jitteriness and seizures are more commonly the presenting symptoms. Treatment of hypocalcemia is associated with certain risks which can be minimized by attention to details:

Intravenous pushes of calcium can cause sudden elevation of serum calcium leading to bradycardia or other cardiac arrhythmias.

Extravasation of calcium solutions into subcutaneous tissues can cause severe tissue necrosis; therefore, calcium containing solutions should not be infused into a peripheral vein by a pump, except in unusual circumstances.

Calcium cannot be mixed with $NaHCO_3$ since this may lead to $CaCO_3$ precipitation.

Calcium can cause necrosis of liver if it is administered via an umbilical vein catheter which is in the portal system.

Calcium pushed into the aorta causes blanching of the bowel in laboratory animals and may be a factor in necrotizing enterocolitis; therefore, it should be given only by slow maintenance drip if an umbilical artery catheter is used.

If one routinely determines calcium levels as scheduled above, substantiated if necessary with electrocardiographic measurements of the Q-OTC or QT intervals, significant hypocalcemia can be anticipated and prevented. If hypocalcemia is not present by 48 hours of age, it will not usually occur. Treatment is usually started at calcium levels of less than 7 mg. per 100 ml. We prefer to use only one calcium salt (gluconate) for either intravenous or oral administration: 1 ml. of 10 per cent calcium gluconate = 100 mg. of calcium gluconate = 9 mg. of elemental calcium.

Infants with hypocalcemia (under 7 mg. per 100 ml.) without symptoms can be given maintenance calcium (45 to 90 mg./kg./day of elemental calcium) starting at the low dose (45 mg./calcium = 5 cc./10 per cent calcium gluconate) and increasing the dose as needed. Acute symptomatic hypocalcemia is treated according to the following formula: Extracellular deficit of calcium in mg. = normal serum concentration of calcium (i.e., 10 mg. per 100 ml.) − the measured or presumed serum concentration (e.g., 5 mg. per 100 ml.) × the extracellular volume.

Extracellular volume in a 4 kg. infant is 25 per cent of body weight or 100 cc. In the above example with a serum calcium of 5 mg. per 100 ml., the deficit is 5 mg. per 100 ml. or 5 mg./100 cc. Five mg./100 cc. × 1000 cc. = 50 mg. deficit or 5.5 cc. of 10 per cent calcium gluconate. This amount can be given slowly (1 ml./min.) intravenously with careful observation of the heart rate and the vein if a peripheral vein is being used. This dose is on the conservative side and can be repeated in 15 minutes if there is no clinical response. The maximum acute dose is 5 ml. of 10 per cent calcium gluconate for prematures and 10 ml. of 10 per cent calcium gluconate for term infants. Following the acute dose, maintenance calcium parenterally or by mouth should be given. A low phosphate milk should be used when oral feeds are started, and calcium can be added directly to the formula if necessary.

Milk	Ca (mEq./liter)	PO$_4$ (mEq./liter)
Breast	17	9
PM 60/40	17	12
Similac	32	29
Enfamil	29	27

Treatment of hypocalcemia is rarely necessary for more than 4 or 5 days unless other complications are present. During treatment calcium levels are monitored every 12 to 24 hours and the dose gradually tapered as indicated. By one week of age most infants of diabetic mothers maintain normocalcemia on regular formula or breast milk without supplements.

Rarely, hypocalcemia is associated with hypomagnesemia and will not respond unless the hypomagnesemia is treated. (Normal magnesium levels in the newborn are 1.2 to 1.8 mEq./liter or 2.4 to 3.6 mg./100 ml.). Treatment consists of administration of 0.1 to 0.2 ml./kg. of 50 per cent magnesium sulfate intravenously or intramuscularly, repeated if necessary every 12 hours, and addition of 3 mEq./liter of magnesium to maintenance fluids.

If despite adequate calcium supplementation and normal magnesium levels the infant remains hypocalcemic, a search for other causes of hypocalcemia must be started. If renal insufficiency or a defect in vitamin D metabolism is discovered, further treatment with phosphate chelators or vitamin D may be necessary.

Aluminum hydroxide gel [Al(OH)$_3$], which makes a nonabsorbable complex [Al$_2$(Po$_4$)$_3$] with phosphate, has been used in doses of 3 to 6 ml. per feeding in prolonged resistant cases. One ml. of Al(OH)$_3$ complexes 15 mg. of Po$_4$. Vitamin D in doses of 10,000 to 25,000 units/day of vitamin D or 0.5 to 1.5 mg./day of dihydrotachysterol has also been used.

Despite adequate treatment with calcium, glucose, and magnesium, many infants remain jittery. The etiology and consequences remain unknown, and we have not treated the jitteriness with sedatives.

Polycythemia. See p. 270.

Jaundice. Hyperbilirubinemia is diagnosed and treated as in any other infant.

Congenital Anomalies. The incidence of anomalies increases with increased severity of the diabetes by class. The most common cardiac defects are ventricular septal defects, transposition of the great vessels and coarctation of the aorta. Skeletal defects such as hemivertebra and sacral agenesis are also seen. Absence of one umbilical artery occurs in 3 to 5 per cent of infants of diabetic mothers.

Other. Other problems seen are renal vein thrombosis, small left colon syndrome, poor feeding, excess mucus, gagging, poor suck necessitating gavage feedings, and high gastric residuals.

Juvenile Diabetes Management

ROBERT KAYE, M.D.

At the time of onset of diabetes in the child, endogenous production of insulin is markedly reduced or almost absent. This is in marked contrast to the hypersecretion of insulin characteristic of the adult onset diabetic. The latter may be considered "insulin-resistant" diabetes whereas the disease in the child represents "insulin-deficiency" diabetes and indicates the need for exogenous insulin in treatment. Insulin deficiency affects the metabolism of carbohydrate, fat and protein as follows:

Carbohydrate Metabolism
  Decreased
    glucose uptake by tissues
    glycogen synthesis
  Increased
    glucose production (gluconeogenesis)
    glycogen breakdown (glycogenolysis)
    hepatic output of glucose
Fat Metabolism
  Decreased
    synthesis of triglycerides (lipogenesis)
    tissue uptake of circulating lipids
  Increased
    Triglyceride breakdown (lipolysis)
    ketone production
Protein Metabolism
  Decreased
    amino acid uptake by tissues
    protein synthesis
  Increased
    tissue protein catabolism
    amino acid conversion to glucose
    (gluconeogenesis)

The net effects of these changes are hyperglycemia and glycosuria; decrease in fat stores with weight loss, ketonemia and acidosis; and wastage of body protein due to uncontrolled gluconeogenesis. Water and electrolyte deficits result from the solute diuresis initiated by glycosuria and may compromise whole body perfusion with failure of the peripheral circulation. Reduced renal perfusion reduces H^+ excretion and augments the acidosis initiated by ketonemia. The process proceeds to a fatal outcome unless reversed by treatment with insulin, water and electrolytes. There is evidence that juvenile diabetes is associated with hypernormal secretion levels of glucagon and with concurrent insulin deficiency constitutes a bihormonal disease. Glucagon excess, by virtue of its gluconeogenic, lipolytic and glycogenolytic effects, compounds the metabolic derangements of insulin deficiency.

While exogenous insulin is life-saving to the juvenile diabetic, it is usually ineffective in preventing the microangiopathic and macroangiopathic complications which produce significant morbidity after 15 to 20 years and the reduction of the life expectancy of the juvenile diabetic by about one-third. There is abundant evidence relating the appearance and progression of these complications to the imperfect metabolic control achieved by current treatment. By monitoring the blood glucose of juvenile diabetic patients at frequent intervals throughout the day, it is clear that normal glycemic excursions are not accomplished even with multiple injections of regular insulin before meals and at bed-time. Utilizing constant intravenous infusions of insulin at varying rates for the period of food ingestion, between meals and during sleep, a close approximation of normal blood glucose concentration may be achieved. Others maintain that unless the insulin delivery system reproduces the initial rapid phase of insulin secretion followed by a secondary slow rise and decline as seen in the normal, glycemic control cannot be accomplished.

It is hoped that the above brief review will provide a rational basis for the treatment of the diabetic child and a realization of the limitations of currently available treatment regimens. The following provides support for adopting a rather lenient approach to management of the patient and indicates the need for seeking potentially more effective modes of treatment such as the mechanical or artificial pancreas and pancreas transplantation.

DIAGNOSIS

Diabetes in the child is usually diagnosed following days or weeks of increased frequency of urination, striking thirst and weight loss of varying degree depending on the duration of symptoms. Increased intake of food is less frequently observed. Enuresis appearing in a previously continent child is not uncommon as an early symptom. When early symptoms are unrecognized, a more profound metabolic disturbance supervenes with dehydration, ketonemia and acidosis, impaired peripheral circulation and depression of consciousness—diabetic ketoacidosis. With current levels of awareness of the significance of early diabetic symptomatology, a positive diagnosis of diabetes is usually made before progression to the ketoacidotic state.

When the presence of diabetes is suspected because of the above symptoms, and supported by a positive test for glucose in the urine, the diagnosis can be established by determination of a markedly elevated blood glucose concentration. Determinations of blood glucose concentration, in symptomatic patients, under fasting or postprandial conditions will usually so far exceed the range of normal that glucose tolerance tests are unnecessary for further confirmation. Diagnostic values for the glucose tolerance test based on analysis of whole blood by the glucose-oxidase method are:

Time	mg/dl
Fasting	110 or more
1 hr.	180
1½ hr.	160
2 hr.	140

The dosage of glucose recommended for tolerance testing is:

0 to 18 mos.	2.5 gm./kg.
1½ to 3 yrs.	2.0 mg./kg.
3 to 12 yrs.	1.75 gm./kg.
7 to 12 yrs.	1.25 gm./kg. (max. 100 gm.)

A number of chemical agents or hormones may impair glucose tolerance. Among these are oral contraceptive agents, salicylates, nicotinic acid, thiazide diuretics and sympathomimetic drugs such as phenylephrine. Hyperglycemia may be a feature of stress (burns, trauma and infection). Decreased glucose tolerance is associated with potassium deficiency and endocrine abnormalities: acromegaly, hyperadrenocorticism, thyrotoxicosis, neuroblastoma and pheochromocytoma.

TREATMENT

Hospitalization of the newly diagnosed diabetic child has a number of advantages. The parents have much to learn in preparation for assuming the care of the child at a time when their ability to assimilate the required information is impaired by their upset feelings consequent to the realization that their child's illness will be a lifelong problem. Parents are encouraged to verbalize their concerns and these are dealt with realistically. Most families have the emotional and intellectual resources to cope with the additional burden which diabetes adds to their family situation. During the hospitalization, it is the responsibility of the dietitian to explain the basics of the American Diabetes Association Exchange System of dietary prescription. The nurse teaches the technique of insulin measurement and injection and reinforces the physician's explanation of the metabolic alterations of diabetes and how they are modified by treatment.

DIET

The author recommends the "free diet" with limited use of concentrated carbohydrate in dietary management of juvenile diabetics. This practice has a number of advantages for the patient, his parents and the physician. The prescription of caloric intake for an individual patient is based on data obtained from measurement of the average intake of groups of healthy children comparable in age and weight. The caloric intake of the group from which the average is derived may vary widely above or below that of the caloric needs of an individual in the group. Most diabetic children at the time of diagnosis are not obese and therefore may be assumed to have an intact "caloristatic" mechanism enabling them to self-regulate caloric intake to correspond with caloric requirements. Obese children, on the other hand, lack this mechanism, and restricting them to a diet more equivalent to their expected caloric needs is appropriate.

At the time of initial treatment of diabetes a diet is prescribed for the child in terms of total calories, distribution among carbohydrate, protein and fat and the quantity to be given at the three major meals and at snacks in mid-morning, mid-afternoon and at bed-time. Calories are estimated from the following table:

Age (yr)	Calories/kg/24 hr.
½ to 1	120 to 100
1 to 3	100 to 90
4 to 6	90 to 80
7 to 9	80 to 70
10 to 12	70 to 60
13 to 15	60 to 50
16 to 18	50 to 40

Protein provides 15 per cent of the total calories; carbohydrate, 50 per cent and fat, 35 per cent. The calories are distributed as follows: 2/11 at breakfast, 3/11 at lunch and supper and 1/11 at each of 3 snacks.

The diet is outlined to the parents using the exchange system in order to provide them with a guide for offering a nutritious and varied diet. The parent is informed that the diet is prescribed as an approximation which will be increased or decreased depending on its capacity to meet the child's satiety needs. Parents are encouraged to permit the child's appetite for good quality food at meal times to regulate his intake and not to require that the same caloric quantity be ingested each day. In this way, increases in caloric intake with growth and activity occur automatically, and the necessity for repeatedly changing the dietary prescription as the child grows is obviated.

All too often, children are seen whose parents are vainly attempting to force adherence to a diet prescribed for the child 2 to 3 years earlier and which has not been increased, commensurate with growth, during the interval. Use of the free diet avoids much of the strain which attends the parents' attempt to enforce adherence to a diet which fails to satisfy the child's appetite and which makes him prone to sneak unauthorized extras with its attendant guilt and fear of doing harm to himself.

INSULIN

Insulin is a polypeptide of molecular weight 5800 derived from a precursor, proinsulin, synthesized by the beta cells of the pancreas. Prior to secretion into the blood, proinsulin is enzymatically cleaved to insulin and a connecting peptide, C-peptide. The latter can be measured in body fluids where its presence serves as a "marker" of continued endogenous insulin secretion. Insulin is secreted into the portal venous system where its concentration is 3 to 10 times that found in the peripheral circulation. Approximately half of the insulin delivered to the liver is extracted in a single circulatory passage. This suggests a special metabolic role for high concentrations of insulin within the liver and constitutes an important difference in the mode of insulin delivery in the normal and in the insulin treated patient. In the latter, insulin injected subcutaneously is distributed to the peripheral tissues in proportion to blood flow and not preferentially to the liver. It is therefore possible in the insulin treated patient for peripheral tissues to be exposed to excessive amounts of insulin, while the liver has available to it a less than optimum supply.

Regular or crystalline zinc insulin and semilente insulin exhibit rapid onset of effect and short duration of action. In order to prolong the period of insulin action, modifications have been introduced which delay the onset and prolong the duration of effect. Insulins in current use are summarized in Table 1.

TABLE 1.   Insulins in Current Use*

TYPE	ONSET (HR.)	PEAK (HR.)	DURATION (HR.)	INTENSITY OF PEAK
Rapid-acting				
Crystalline zinc (insulin injection, U.S.P.) ("regular" insulin)	½	2 to 4	6 to 8	Marked
Semilente (prompt insulin zinc suspension, U.S.P.)	½	2 to 4	10 to 12	Marked
Intermediate-acting				
Globin (globin zinc insulin injection, U.S.P.)	2	6 to 10	12 to 18	Moderate
NPH (isophane insulin suspension, U.S.P.)	2	8 to 10	18 to 24	Moderate
Lente (insulin zinc suspension, U.S.P.)	2	8 to 12	20 to 26	Moderate
Prolonged-acting				
Ultralente (extended insulin zinc suspension, U.S.P.)	6	18 to 24	36+	Mild
Protamine zinc (PZI) (protamine zinc insulin suspension, U.S.P.)	6	14 to 20	24 to 36	Mild

*From Shirkey, H. C. (ed.): Pediatric Therapy. Edition 4. St. Louis, C. V. Mosby Co., 1972, with permission.

Insulins for routine use are available in several concentrations—U40, U80, U100—that is, 40, 80 or 100 units per ml. U100 insulin contains lower concentrations of impurities and its use is less often associated with lipoatrophy. Its injection into lipoatrophic sites often reverses the process. Insulin lipomata, which are swellings of fat-engorged subcutaneous tissue, are best avoided by rotation of injection sites.

Adjustment of Insulin Dosage. A combination of a rapidly and intermediately acting insulin administered in the same syringe is generally used and may provide the means of controlling the blood glucose concentration for 24 hours. Regular or semilente insulin (rapid-acting insulins) is utilized to limit post-breakfast hyperglycemia and glycosuria and lente or NPH (intermediate acting insulins) for control during the remainder of the day. Peak effects, including hypoglycemic reactions, of the rapidly acting insulins given before breakfast are noted in the mid-morning, and of the intermediate acting insulins in mid-afternoon. To counteract potential hypoglycemia, snacks are given at these times and also before bed-time.

The peak effectiveness characteristics of the insulins indicate how tests for glycosuria at specific times can be utilized as a guide for adjustment of insulin dosage. If the test for urinary glucose before the evening meal is consistently high on two consecutive days, the dosage of NPH* or lente is increased by 2 units.

*This applies to lente as well. NPH and lente are considered to be interchangeable. In order to avoid alterations of the properties of insulin mixtures given in the same syringe, regular and NPH are used together and semilente and lente are employed in combination.

This procedure is repeated at 2 day intervals until the magnitude of glycosuria is reduced below the 4+ level. If, on the other hand, tests for urinary glucose are negative for 2 days in the pre-supper specimen, the dosage of NPH is reduced by this amount. In this way, glycemic control is set at a level designed to avoid excessive hyperglycemia on the one hand and hypoglycemia on the other. The NPH dosage is given priority in adjustments because its longer duration of action has a greater effect on the 24 hour level of blood glucose than a change of an equal number of units of short-acting insulin. A similar method of adjustment of the short-acting insulin, regular or semilente, is made based on the quantity of glycosuria in the urine specimen obtained prior to the noon meal.

A second injection of insulin before the evening meal is indicated when glycosuria is well controlled during the period from breakfast to dinner but becomes excessive later in the day as indicated by the tests done before bed-time and the following morning. Under these circumstances, it is not feasible to attempt to reduce the late evening and early morning hyperglycemia and glycosuria by an increase in the morning dosage of NPH or lente, as the glycosuria at the time of its maximum effectiveness is already satisfactory and a further increase might induce a hypoglycemic reaction in the late afternoon while failing to significantly reduce the excessive glycosuria later in the day. Adding a second injection before dinner of a mixture of regular and NPH insulin is an effective way of dealing with this situation. Here, the guide to the appropriateness of the evening injection of regular insulin is the test before bed-time, and for the evening NPH, the test before breakfast the following day.

When a second daily injection of insulin is indicated a safe starting point is 10 per cent of the morning dose divided equally between regular and NPH insulin. For example, a patient receiving a total of 40 units of insulin should be started on a total of 4 units before supper, 2 units of regular and 2 units of NPH. When introducing an evening dose of insulin according to the above criteria, it is appropriate to make an equal reduction in the quantity of insulin given in the morning. This recommendation is based on the fact that when the pre-lunch and pre-supper tests are already satisfactory, the introduction of an evening dose of insulin will provide a lower baseline of pre-breakfast glycemia on which the insulin given at that time will operate. Reducing the pre-breakfast insulin dose will serve to avoid hypoglycemia before lunch and before dinner.

It is desirable to instruct parents in the foregoing guides so that they may assume, with time, the responsibility of adjusting the insulin dose between visits to the physician on the basis of the urine testing results. This practice increases the potential for securing the most complete and safe control of glycosuria of which the individual patient is capable.

Initial Insulin Treatment.   Most children with newly diagnosed diabetes are in relatively good condition, without significant acidosis, dehydration or vomiting which would necessitate the provision of water, electrolytes and glucose by the parenteral route. For these patients, a normal meal pattern with a bed-time snack is provided. Regular insulin in a dosage of 0.2 units per kg. is administered subcutaneously 15 minutes before the three meals and the bed-time snack. The dosage is adjusted by 25 to 50 per cent depending on the effectiveness of the preceding dose in reducing glycosuria and acetonuria in the urine tests spanning the interval between successive doses. If the next urine test shows no improvement in terms of decreased glycosuria and acetonuria, the dosage is increased as described above. Occurrence of an hypoglycemic reaction or negative tests for glucose and acetone in the urine indicate a comparable reduction in dosage. In this way the individual patient's insulin requirement is titrated.

After 5 to 8 days of this regimen a definite fall in insulin requirement usually occurs, evidenced by continued negative tests for glucosuria on a progressively reduced dose of insulin. This phase is called a "partial remission" and reflects the improved metabolic state accomplished by correction of the insulin deficiency present prior to treatment. With insulin therapy, glucose is converted to glycogen and fat; amino acids are synthesized to protein and excessive lipolysis is stopped. This is in contrast to the excessive glycogenolysis, gluconeogenesis and lipolysis which is manifested in the untreated diabetic patient. It seems reasonable to ascribe the "partial remission" to this metabolic shift from a catabolic to an anabolic state with a consequent reduced insulin requirement to maintain energy balance.

When the stage of minimum insulin requirement is attained, a mixture of regular and NPH insulin given in the same syringe before breakfast is substituted for the four injections of regular insulin previously administered. The dosage of regular insulin is approximately 80 per cent of the pre-breakfast dose of the preceding day. The requirement for NPH is about 80 per cent of the sum of the three injections of regular insulin given before lunch, before supper and at bed-time. Subsequent adjustments are made as described above.

Insulin Adjustments During Special Situations.   INFECTION.   The stress of infection may increase the output of the counter-regulatory hormones which oppose the action of insulin: cortisol, growth hormone, glucagon and epinephrine. When this stimulation is sufficient to cause the appearance of ketones in the urine, supplements of insulin should be given in addition to the basal dosage. Regular insulin equal to 10 per cent of the total daily requirement of the individual patient is administered if acetone is detected in any of the routine urine tests done before meals and at bed-time. By this means symptomatic ketonuria can usually be avoided.

VOMITING EPISODES.   Insulin should not be omitted in spite of the expected reduction in caloric intake in order to avoid uncontrolled lipolysis and ketosis. Insulin is given in 80 per cent of the usual dose, and carbohydrate in the form of fruit juice or carbonated beverage is administered in divided doses of 2 to 4 oz./hr. depending on the size of the child. Insulin resistance accompanying stress makes the development of hypoglycemia unlikely even though caloric intake is reduced. Supplementary insulin is given as needed according to the system described above for infections. Fortunately, most episodes of vomiting terminate spontaneously in 4 to 6 hours and permit ingestion of easily digested carbohydrate-containing foods such as applesauce, gelatin or custards and toast or crackers with jelly. In the few instances in which oral carbohydrate cannot be retained after the 4 to 6 hour trial, intravenous administration of glucose is mandatory to prevent hypoglycemia.

SURGERY.   Operative procedures do not

usually require an increase in insulin dosage. It is our practice to administer half the patient's total dose as intermediate-acting insulin prior to the operation, with the balance of the insulin given at 6 hour intervals as regular insulin. This estimate can be adjusted upward or downward in units of 2 to 4, depending on the urinary findings. Adequate carbohydrate and sodium chloride will be furnished by provision of the child's water requirement as 10 per cent glucose in one-fourth strength physiologic saline.

Insulin Resistance and Allergy.   A small number of patients will require increments in insulin to extremely high levels without achieving control of glycosuria. Daily insulin requirements greater than 40 units in children under 6 years, 60 units in children under 10 years, and 150 units in adolescents warrant the designation of insulin resistance. The resistant state is usually due to excessive formation of antibodies to beef insulin present in commercial insulin made from mixed bovine and porcine sources. The use of pure pork insulin* is usually effective in overcoming resistance and bringing the insulin dose into an average range. A favorable response may be delayed for 3 to 14 days. Patients who fail to benefit from this therapy will usually respond to treatment with corticosteroids. Prednisone, in a dosage of 2 mg./kg./24 hr., is administered with a reduced dosage of insulin. Prednisone is reduced as the insulin requirement declines. A maintenance dosage of 2.5 to 5 mg./24 hr. may be necessary. Fortunately, most episodes of insulin resistance are of limited duration.

Redness and swelling at the site of insulin injection are common in the early states of treatment and usually prove to be transitory. If they persist or evolve into a more generalized urticaria, antihistamines and desensitization should be carried out.

URINE TESTING FOR GLUCOSE

There are several considerations relating to urine testing which warrant some discussion. Clinitest tablets provide a more accurate estimation of the quantity of glycosuria than do the various tape or strip tests, such as Diastix. Using the latter it is difficult to differentiate between small and large amounts of urinary glucose. It should be emphasized that under the usual circumstances of urine testing, glucose concentration rather than quantity is measured. The latter determination requires the additional measurement of urine volume.

*Obtained by special order from Eli Lilly & Co., Indianapolis, Indiana.

Concentration alone may be used as an index of the magnitude of glucosuria, although highly concentrated or dilute urine specimens may yield potentially misleading information.

At times, patients may experience symptoms suggestive of hypoglycemia, while urine voided at the time may be of high glucose concentration. This may occur because the voided specimen is made up of urine formed over a period of time, during the early part of which high concentrations of glucose may have been present, whereas urine formed later may be free of glucose. Urine voided at the time of the hypoglycemic reaction will therefore represent a mixture of glucose-containing and glucose-free urine and test positively for glucose.

"Double-voided" specimens avoid this problem, as the initial urine is discarded and testing is done on a second specimen passed 10 to 15 minutes later. This has obvious advantages but is troublesome to the patient and family and is utilized only when there is a discrepancy between the results of urine testing and the clinical condition of the patient.

SOMOGYI EFFECT

Following an episode of hypoglycemia, urinary excretions of glucose and ketones are frequently elevated. This sequence is the result of activation of the counter-regulatory hormones described above which oppose insulin. If the mechanism of this "rebound effect" is not understood, additional insulin may be prescribed with exaggeration of the phenomenon, the Somogyi effect. Patients so treated may become brittle diabetics, alternating between acidosis and hypoglycemia, depending on whether insulin or its antagonists predominate at the time. This situation may be suspected when a brittle diabetic apparently requires an unusually large dosage of insulin (greater than 0.4 to 0.7 units/lb. in the young child and the adolescent, respectively). Gradual reduction of the insulin dosage will lower the level of insulin antagonists and restore stability.

RECOGNITION AND TREATMENT OF HYPOGLYCEMIA

Hypoglycemia stimulates the secretion of the counter-regulatory hormones in order to elevate the level of blood glucose. The effects of one of these, Adrenalin, produce signs and symptoms that can alert the patient and informed observers to the need for ingestion of carbohydrate. Adrenalin hypersecretion is associated with pallor, a feeling of anxiety, tachycardia, hypertension and less often with sweating and pupillary dilatation. Further progression of hypoglycemia is accompanied by irritability, negativistic behavior and finally by unconsciousness and convulsions. This sequence may be interrupted by the administration of carbohydrate in a rapidly absorbed form such as orange juice or carbonated beverage. In the unconscious patient, unable to swallow, glucagon (0.5 to 1.0 mg.) administered intramuscularly will often raise the blood glucose concentration and terminate the episode, obviating the need for administration of intravenous glucose.

A slow decline in blood glucose concentration is often accompanied by headache or sleepiness at an inappropriate time. It should also be pointed out that hypoglycemia may progress to unconsciousness in a matter of minutes, whereas the coma of diabetic acidosis is the result of a process requiring hours or days for full development.

DIABETIC KEOTACIDOSIS

Diabetic ketoacidosis is the culmination of the metabolic alterations consequent to insulin deficiency. Treatment is designed to reverse these derangements by providing adequate amounts of insulin, water, electrolytes and energy in the form of glucose. General principles of treatment of diabetic ketoacidosis are as follows.

Hyperosmolality. Extracellular glucose is osmotically active and increases extracellular osmolality by 10 mOsm./liter for each increment of glucose concentration of 180 mg./dl. above physiologic levels. Marked hyperglycemia therefore leads to transfer of water from the intracellular to the extracellular compartment and serves to maintain blood volume threatened by renal solute diuresis. With insulin treatment and reduction in blood glucose levels, the flow of water is reversed and cerebral edema may occur. This complication can be avoided by maintaining blood glucose levels at approximately 250 mg./dl. during the first day of treatment. Withholding glucose from the initial infusate avoids further increases in osmolality and intracellular dehydration. Five per cent glucose should be added to the infusate when the blood glucose concentration approaches 250 mg./dl. The initial infusion of physiologic saline solution provides expansion of blood volume as reduction in hyperglycemia induces transfer of water intracellularly.

Correction of Acidosis. pH levels of approximately 6.9 to 7.0 are accompanied by depression of the respiratory center and decreased myocardial contractility, both of which may be lethal and avoided by the administration of alkali. The use of alkali in the treatment of diabetic ketoacidosis should be reserved for those situations in which respiratory and myocardial depression constitute real threats to the patient's survival. This limitation is based on the fact that an abrupt increase in pH reduces the dissociation of oxyhemoglobin and therefore the delivery of oxygen to the tissues and also paradoxically lowers central nervous system pH.

Acidosis is associated with two alterations in the characteristics of the hemoglobin-oxygen dissociation curve which tend to neutralize each other. The first results from decreased glycolysis in the red cell leading to a reduction in 2,3-diphosphoglycerate (2,3-DPG) and impaired release of oxygen from oxyhemoglobin. This change is offset by increased liberation of oxygen as a consequence of lowered pH. Abrupt increase in pH, with the administration of exogenous alkali, deprives the subject of the beneficial effects of the enhanced oxygen delivery associated with acidosis, while the reduced oxygen delivery consequent to 2,3-DPG depletion is still operative and is only corrected as glycolysis is stimulated with restoration of pH toward normal.

The paradoxical lowering of cerebrospinal fluid pH as systemic pH rises is the consequence of differential permeability of the blood-brain barrier to CO_2 and HCO_3. The former is freely diffusible, whereas the latter equilibrates more slowly. Administration of alkali elevates blood pH and reduces the minute volume of ventilation leading to systemic increase in pCO_2 and HCO_3^-. The increased CO_2 equilibrates rapidly with the cerebrospinal fluid, while HCO_3^- movement is delayed with the result that central nervous system pH falls and systemic pH rises. The increased acidosis of the central nervous system may be associated with decreased consciousness. These considerations suggest that patients whose acidosis is moderate (pH > 7.1 or $HCO_3^- > 8$ mEq./liter) are best treated by reliance upon endogenous regeneration of HCO_3^- with ketone body oxidation under the influence of insulin therapy. More severe acidosis with its attendant threat of respiratory and myocardial depression warrants administration of $NaHCO_3$, 2.0 to 2.5 mEq./kg.

Insulin. Continuous intravenous infusion of low doses of insulin has received much attention in the medical literature of the last several years. Proponents of its use have made several valid arguments in its favor. It is inappropriate to rely on prompt absorption of subcutaneous insulin in patients with impaired peripheral circulation. Intravenous bolus administration of insulin is limited in effectiveness by its short half-life (2 to 4 minutes) resulting in concentrations approaching 0 in 30 minutes. The validity of these considerations relating to route and mode of administration cannot be challenged, but the extension to "low dose" treatment leaves some problems unanswered.

Low dose insulin infusion, 0.1 unit/kg./hr., results in peripheral insulin concentrations comparable to those observed after a glucose load 40 to 120 μU/ml. However, there is no proof that the elevated portal vein and hepatic concentrations (5 to 10 times systemic) observed under physiologic conditions are achieved by this regimen. The possibility of inadequate insulinization of the liver with failure to suppress ketogenesis is suggested by a more prolonged duration of acidosis observed in patients treated by this method. There is also evidence that potassium retention is minimal in the "low dose" regimen, unless large amounts of alkali are administered.

Although there is no question that a large number of patients with severe diabetic acidosis have been successfully treated by this regimen, there remains reason for caution regarding its general adoption. It should be emphasized that conventional treatment methods have resulted in 98 per cent survival of ketoacidotic patients in the absence of complicating myocardial infarction or severe infection. There is concern that some patients may be lost who would have survived under more established treatment procedures. For these reasons, continued adherence to conventional, "moderate insulin dose" therapy is advocated.

As a basis for estimating the initial insulin dosage and frequency of injection, it has been useful to classify patients into grades of progressive severity, according to the criteria in Table 2. Improved clinical condition with

treatment results in increased insulin sensitivity and lower insulin requirements. The table provides guidelines which are applicable to a patient with ketoacidotic coma and to the relatively well child with untreated diabetes which has been diagnosed early.

Grading based on clinical observation and examination of urine for glucose and acetone should be supported by measurement of blood glucose, CO_2 content of serum and semiquantitative determination of serum acetone, and in the severely ill child, of sodium, potassium chloride, pH and BUN as well. Serial dilutions of serum are tested with Acetest tablets. The test has limitations as an index of severity of ketoacidosis, as it fails to measure betahydroxybutyrate, the major ketone body in diabetic acidosis, and reacts with acetone which is undissociated and plays no role in acid-base balance. Also, acetone may be released from adipose tissue for many hours after acidosis is corrected.

Administration of Water and Electrolytes. The ketoacidotic patient requires water for maintenance (1500 to 1800 ml./m²/24 hr.) plus approximately 70 ml./kg. for deficit repair. Maintenance requirements for water and electrolytes are given in Table 3 and approximate deficits of water and electrolyte in diabetic ketoacidosis in Table 4. Intracellular and extracellular water deficits are approximately equal. As restoration of the intracellular deficit is dependent upon the limited capacity of cells to take up potassium, only 70 per cent of the estimated water deficit is administered in the first 24 hours. Continued solute diuresis increases the quantity of water necessary for maintenance. The renal component of maintenance water (800 ml./m²/24 hr. or 100 ml./m²/3 hr.) serves as a guide to the additional quantity of water which must be added to ap-

---

TABLE 2.   Initial Insulin Treatment Based on Clinical State*

| | GRADE | | | | |
	IV	III	IIa	IIb	I
↓ Consciousness	+	−	−	−	−
Hyperventilation	+	+	−	−	−
Dehydration	+	+	−	−	−
↓ CO_2 content	+	+	+	+	−
↑ Serum ketones	+	+	+	+	±
4+ glycosuria	+	+	+	+	±
Acetonuria	+	+	+	+	±
Vomiting or nausea	+	+	+	−	−
Route of fluid therapy	IV	IV	IV	O	O
Initial insulin dose (units/kg.)	1 to 2†	1	0.5	0.25	0.2
Subsequent dose (units/kg.)	0.5 to 1	0.5	0.25	0.25 ± 50%	0.2 ± 50%
Frequency of insulin injections (hr)	1 to 2	2 to 4	4	4 to 6	6

*From Shirkey, H. C. (ed.): Pediatric Therapy. Edition 4. St. Louis, C. V. Mosby Co., 1972, with permission.
†Half intravenously and half intramuscularly.

TABLE 3. Maintenance Requirements* by Body Weight and Surface Area†

WT (kg.)	SURFACE AREA (m²)	WATER (ml.) kg.	WATER (ml.) m²	SODIUM (mEq.) kg.	SODIUM (mEq.) m²	POTASSIUM (mEq.) kg.	POTASSIUM (mEq.) m²	GLUCOSE (gm.) kg.	GLUCOSE (gm.) m²
3	0.20	100	1500–1800	3	60	2	50	6–10	150
5	0.27	90	1500–1800	3	60	2	50	6–10	150
10	0.45	75	1500–1800	3	60	2	50	6–10	150
15	0.64	65	1500–1800	—	60	—	50	—	150
30	1.10	55	1500–1800	—	60	—	50	—	150
50	1.50	45	1500–1800	—	60	—	50	—	150
70	1.73	40	1500–1800	—	60	—	50	—	150

*These quantities of water, sodium, and potassium will be approximated by using Butler's solution (concentrations in mEq./liter; Na, 40; K, 35; Cl, 40; HCO_3, 20; and P, 15) in the above specified quantities. Another suitable solution is provided by saline in one fourth of physiologic concentration supplemented by appropriate amounts of a potassium concentrate (1 mEq./ml.).

†From Shirkey, H. C. (ed.): Pediatric Therapy. Edition 4. St. Louis, C. V. Mosby Co., 1972, with permission.

proximate maintenance requirements under these conditions. Intravenous fluids are given at a rate to provide 50 per cent of the estimated 24 hour requirement in the first 8 hours.

Administration of Sodium. Initially, sodium chloride in isotonic solution is administered intravenously in a volume of 20 to 30 ml./kg. in 2 to 3 hours. If pH is in the range of 7.1 to 7.15 or below, $NaHCO_3$ (2.0 to 2.5 mEq./kg.) should be substituted for an equal quantity of sodium chloride (10 mEq. of isotonic sodium chloride contain 1.5 mEq. of sodium). Concentrates of $NaHCO_3$ containing approximately 1.0 mEq./ml. are available. Successive reductions in concentration of sodium chloride from isotonic (150 mEq./liter) to one-half normal saline (75 mEq./liter) to one-fourth normal saline (37.5 mEq./liter) should be administered to achieve the required amount (60 mEq./m² for maintenance and 10 mEq./kg. for repair of deficit).

Potassium Administration. Because of the presence of acidosis, serum potassium concentrations are usually normal or elevated at the outset of treatment. Therefore, the administration of potassium is delayed for 1 to 2 hours and until there is evidence of adequate urine flow. As the rate of cellular uptake is lim-

ited, only 3.5 mEq./kg., which is approximately one-third of the estimated deficit, is administered in the first 24 hours. Serial determinations of serum potassium concentration should be obtained and additional amounts given if hypokalemia threatens. Concentration of potassium in parenteral fluids should usually not exceed 40 mEq./liter.

Administration of PO₄. Hypophosphatemia may occur due to renal losses and intracellular shifts with insulin treatment. Low levels of serum phosphate are associated with depletion of 2,3-DPG and reduced oxygen delivery to the tissues and hemolysis. It is therefore appropriate to administer half of the potassium as K_2HPO_4, which is available as a concentrate. (Potassium phosphate injection, 4.4 mEq of potassium/ml., Abbott Laboratories.)

The first two insulin injections are given in the quantity and at the time intervals specified in Table 2. Following this, the patient's clinical condition and sensitivity to insulin will have improved sufficiently to permit application of the schedule for the next less severely affected grade. Grade IIb is usually reached in about 16 hours, at which time fruit juices and carbonated drinks may be taken orally in small amounts. On the second day, oral fluids may be given to supplement the parenteral fluids in a total quantity approximately 50 per cent above maintenance requirements for water and electrolytes. The potassium concentrations (in mEq./liter) of some useful fluids are:

TABLE 4. Water and Electrolyte Deficits* in Diabetic Coma†

	TOTAL	PER KG. BODY WEIGHT
Water	5 to 11 ml.	100 ml.
Sodium	300 to 700 mEq.	7 to 10 mEq.
Chloride	350 to 500 mEq.	5 to 7 mEq.
Potassium	200 to 700 mEq.	5 to 10 mEq.

*Approximate, based on retention of water and electrolyte during treatment of ketoacidosis.

†Modified from Bradley, R. F., and Rees, S. B.: Water, electrolyte and hydrogen ion abnormalities in diabetes mellitus. In Bland, J. H. (ed.): Clinical Metabolism of Body Water and Electrolytes. Philadelphia, W. B. Saunders Co., 1963.

Apple juice	26
Coca Cola	12
Ginger ale	0.1
Grape juice	30
Orange juice	49
Pepsi Cola	0.8

At the end of the second day a soft diet can usually be started and insulin administered on a four times daily basis, before meals and at bed-time as described above.

GENERAL PRINCIPLES OF MANAGEMENT

Probably the most important factor in the successful management of the diabetic child is adequate instruction of the parents in the rudiments of diabetic pathophysiology. This should include an explanation of the mode of action of insulin, recognition and treatment of hypoglycemia and the steps in progression of insulin deficiency to symptomatic ketoacidosis. The principles of adjustment of insulin dosage in relation to the temporal characteristics of glycosuria and the use of glucagon in the management of severe hypoglycemic episodes should be explained.

It is important to state clearly the objectives of treatment. These should include the major goal of fostering satisfactory physical and emotional development and the provision of sufficient insulin to avoid the reappearance of diabetic symptoms and findings. The inability of currently available treatment regimens to secure adequate control of hypoglycemia and glycosuria is discussed. Nevertheless, the family is assured that a continuous effort will be made to limit glycosuria as far as possible in their child.

Adolescence is often a difficult time for the child who finds the diabetic state particularly odious as he seeks a sense of independence from his parents and identity with peers. In order to minimize this stress, it is important to attempt to transfer most of the responsibility of management to the diabetic teenager and thus remove some of the causes of contention which occur when the parents continue to carry the major responsibility for diabetic care.

Blood glucose determinations at office visits are useful to detect the presence of reduced renal threshold for glycosuria and to validate the reliability of urinary glucose measurements.

Prognosis. The prospects for achievement of healthy growth and development of the diabetic during childhood and the teens are excellent. However, the long-term prognosis remains disappointing. The availability of insulin has increased the life expectancy from the few months that was characteristic of the pre-insulin era. Today a diabetic child aged 10 years may look forward to only 44 more years of life in contrast to the 62 years to be anticipated by his normal peers. The outcome of childhood diabetes has not improved significantly since antibiotics came into general use in the 1950's. The major causes of morbidity and mortality in juvenile diabetes are macroan-

giopathy and microangiopathy. There is an impressive body of information which relates the pathogenesis of these complications to the imperfect metabolic control achieved by current methods of treatment. Efforts to develop safe and effective pancreatic transplantation and to build an artificial pancreas are responses to this situation.

Priscilla White has summarized her experience with 702 juvenile diabetics surviving 20 years or more and has found the following incidence of complications.

Gangrene	3%
Blindness	4%
Cerebral vascular lesions	18%
Retinitis	80%
Retinitis proliferans	33%
Hypertension	43%
Proteinuria	60%

While these figures are a cause for concern, they offer some hope in that a significant number of patients escape severe complications after this duration of illness.

Hypoglycemia

NOEL KEITH MACLAREN, M.D., *and* MARVIN CORNBLATH, M.D.

Clinical hypoglycemia is the association of an abnormally low blood sugar with a variety of signs and symptoms which are improved with glucose administration or food. The clinical state results from decreased glucose availability to the central nervous system and the induced catecholamine response. Weakness, apathy, irritability, hunger, bizarre behavior, mental confusion, apnea, cyanosis, hypothermia, convulsions and coma, together with pallor, sweating, tremulousness, tachycardia and shock may result.

The Dextrostix is a useful screening technique, but a reliable laboratory glucose determination of blood or cerebrospinal fluid must be done in every patient before therapy is initiated. In addition, a further blood sample should be obtained prior to treating the acute episode of hypoglycemia, since a definitive diagnosis determines long-term therapy and thus prognosis. A minimum of 1 or 2 ml. of serum or plasma should be frozen and saved for determination of insulin, growth hormone, cortisol as well as metabolites, such as alanine and lactate. The first urine specimen after the episode should be analyzed for ketones and reducing sugars (Clinitest tablet).

In neonates with persistent or recurrent hypoglycemia, as well as in older infants and children, an abbreviated glucagon (0.05 mg./ kg., not to exceed 1 mg., given intramuscularly or intravenously) tolerance test (0, 10, 20 minutes) may differentiate between hypoglycemia due to hyperinsulinism and that due to other etiologies. A brisk significant hyperglycemic response to glucagon implicates hyperinsulinism.

NEONATAL HYPOGLYCEMIA

Hypoglycemia has been defined in the neonate as replicate whole blood glucose values of less than 20 mg./100 ml. in the infant under 2500 gm., less than 30 mg./100 ml. in full-size infants during the first 72 hours of life, and less than 40 mg./100 ml. thereafter. Plasma or serum glucose values tend to be 15 to 20 per cent higher than those of whole blood, depending upon hematocrit. Most infants with hypoglycemia have clinical manifestations, such as twitching, jitteriness, apathy, cyanotic spells, hypothermia, pallor, sweating or convulsions. Symptomatic infants should be treated if the Dextrostix reads under 30 mg./ 100 ml. while waiting for the diagnostic laboratory blood results.

Give 2 to 4 ml. (0.5 to 1 gm.) per kg. of 25 per cent glucose intravenously at the rate of 1 ml./min., and continue the infusion with glucose in water to provide 8 to 10 mg./kg./min. for at least 24 hours, or at increased rates until the blood sugar is stable in the normal range. The total 24-hour fluid requirement determines the concentration of glucose to be used. If the total requirement is 65 to 85 ml./kg./day, use 15 to 20 per cent glucose; if it is 115 to 145 ml./kg./day, use 10 per cent glucose. After 24 to 48 hours of age, continue the infusion with 10 per cent glucose in 0.22 per cent saline at a rate to maintain a normal glucose level. If parenteral fluid therapy alone is required beyond 48 hours, add potassium (1 to 2 mEq./ kg./day as KCL) and monitor serum potassium levels. Oral feedings should be introduced as soon as clinical manifestations subside. Therapy can be tapered off after blood sugar levels have remained over 30 to 40 mg./100 ml. for 24 to 48 hours by changing to 5 per cent glucose and then stopping.

Never discontinue hypertonic glucose abruptly, for a reactive hypoglycemia may ensue.

If symptoms persist beyond 2 to 4 hours despite a sustained elevation in blood sugar, the hypoglycemia may have been secondary to one of a variety of underlying conditions. Among the latter, CNS, hemorrhage, congenital defects, sepsis, respiratory distress syndrome, hypoplastic left heart syndrome, asphyxia or anoxia, and metabolic aberrations

such as hypocalcemia are the most common. Thus it is necessary to diagnose and treat the underlying disease as well.

If blood sugar levels remain under 30 mg./100 ml. with adequate glucose therapy, start hydrocortisone (Solu-Cortef), 5 mg./kg./ day every 8 hours, by the oral, intramuscular or intravenous route. Hydrocortisone can be tapered when the blood sugar has remained over 30 mg./100 ml. for 48 hours, and stopped after 3 days. During treatment, blood sugar should be monitored at 2 to 6 hour intervals.

Glucagon, 0.5 mg./kg. intramuscularly or intravenously, can be used with effect in asymptomatic infants of diabetic mothers or initially in symptomatic infants while the intravenous infusions are being started. However, glucagon and epinephrine are not recommended for treating any other neonate with hypoglycemia.

Rarely, despite the above therapies, chronic or persistent hypoglycemia may occur, can be life-threatening and may be responsible for permanent CNS damage. Thus an aggressive diagnostic and therapeutic approach is indicated as noted below (see diazoxide and pancreatic surgery for hyperinsulinism).

HYPOGLYCEMIA OF INFANCY

Inborn Errors of Hepatic Carbohydrate Metabolism

Such disorders may result in hypoglycemia episodes from the neonatal period or from early infancy, and tend to ameliorate with age.

Hepatic Glycogen Storage Diseases. *Type I* (glucose-6-phosphatase deficiency). A diet containing 60 to 70 per cent of the caloric requirement as carbohydrate (glucose, maltose or starch), 15 per cent as protein and the remainder as fat, given at 3 to 4 hour intervals, plus a continuous nasogastric drip of Vivonex-HN (glucose, oligiosaccharides, fat 0.8 per cent and protein 18 per cent) during the night is indicated for older children. See page 356.

Type III (amylo-1,6-glucosidase or "debrancher" deficiency). Hypoglycemia is less frequent and usually follows episodes of caloric deprivation, intercurrent infections or gastrointestinal upset. Since gluconeogenesis is intact, a high protein diet with regular meals and a bedtime snack is advised.

Types VI and IX (phosphorylase and phosphorylase-kinase deficiency). Hypoglycemic episodes are mild and infrequent. The measures for type III generally apply.

Synthetase deficiency is probably extremely

rare, and severe hypoglycemia is reported within a few hours of fasting. Frequent feedings, high in any carbohydrate and protein, should be the basic approach.

Galactosemia (galactose-1-phosphate uridyl transferase). Strict avoidance of lactose-containing milk, foods and sweets is essential to prevent the associated postprandial hypoglycemia and other sequelae (see p. 361).

Fructose Intolerance (fructose-1-phosphate aldolase deficiency). Postprandial hypoglycemia episodes date from the introduction of sucrose into the diet. Give a fructose-free diet avoiding table sugars, sweets and fruits, and substitute glucose as the dietary sugar (see p. 358).

Fructose-1,6-Diphosphatase Deficiency. A special diet consisting of 56 per cent utilizable carbohydrate (glucose, maltose or lactose), 12 per cent protein and 32 per cent fat has been reported to be effective; however, intercurrent illness may require alkali and glucose therapy (see p. 358).

Endocrine Disorders Associated with Hypoglycemia

Hypopituitarism. A syndrome of congenital hypopituitarism has been described which may result in profound life-threatening hypoglycemia from the first hours of life. Associated findings include jaundice, hepatomegaly, midline abnormalities, edema and frequently a microphallus in the male. Multiple endocrine deficiencies are usually present, and therapy consists of glucose and steroids, followed by specific replacement therapy. Growth hormone deficiency may result in hypoglycemic episodes from early life; however, such episodes become less frequent during the school years, due perhaps to larger body size. Replacement therapy with human growth hormone at 1 to 2 units thrice weekly is indicated. In combined GH and corticotropin deficiency, a trial of GH therapy alone appears to be justified (only in the absence of mineralocorticoid deficiency), since glucocorticoid therapy retards the growth response from GH treatment. If hypoglycemia persists, cortisone acetate, 0.75 to 1.0 mg./kg./day (25 mg./m²/day) in divided doses (half this dose if intramuscular), is effective.

Adrenal Insufficiency. Congenital hypoplasia of the adrenals, corticotropin unresponsiveness and rarely congenital virilizing hyperplasia may be associated with hypoglycemia. Cortisone replacement therapy as above is indicated. During intercurrent illnesses, the dose should be doubled.

Hyperinsulinism. Inappropriately high insulin secretion may occur in infancy, associated with the "infant giant," Beckwith-Wiedeman syndrome, or without physical stigmata. Histologically the pancreas may show beta cell hyperplasia, nesidioblastosis or beta cell tumor. Surgery is often required in such cases and should not be delayed in infants refractory to adequate glucose, diazoxide, and/or glucocorticoid therapy. If a discrete tumor is not palpated at laparotomy, a subtotal pancreatectomy removing at least 80 to 90 per cent of the pancreas should be carried out. Diazoxide may be used postoperatively, should it be necessary, but considerable salt retention may occur in smaller infants (see below). Infants exhibiting hypoglycemia and elevated insulin values after oral leucine should be managed with low leucine diets. The diet must be adequate in leucine for growth, but divided into three or more meals to provide small amounts of leucine. Offer carbohydrate before sleep. For infants, S-14 (Wyeth) is recommended, but SMA-26, Enfamil, Bremil or Similac can be used. Diazoxide may induce striking improvement in those responding poorly to diet. Partial pancreatectomy may be necessary in leucine-sensitive patients with beta cell hyperplasia or adenoma.

Idiopathic

Occasionally, no specific cause for the hypoglycemia is found. Emergency treatment with intravenous glucose is given as outlined under Neonatal Hypoglycemia. Dietary management with frequent carbohydrate-containing feedings, avoiding prolonged fasts, is basic.

Drug Therapy

For many infants, regular feeding schedules and avoidance of overnight fasting are adequate. For others, attacks become recurrent and further measures are necessary.

Diazoxide. This drug is a thiazide derivative. It has a major action in inhibiting insulin secretion. Its side effects include hypotension, salt retention, hyperuricemia and low IgG levels. In practice, hirsutism (hypertrichiasis lanuginosa) is frequently encountered, and parents should be warned about this prior to its appearance.

Start with 6 mg./kg./day in 8 to 12 hour doses by mouth, and increase as necessary to 20 to 25 mg./kg./day. Doses near 10 mg./kg./day are usually effective. Diazoxide should *not* be discontinued *suddenly* after prolonged use.

Steroids. Oral cortisone acetate (5 mg./kg./day) or prednisone (1 to 2 mg./kg./day) in two to three divided doses, is often effective.

The steroid dosage should be reduced by approximately 20 per cent weekly until the lowest dose compatible with freedom from hypoglycemia is reached. Steroids will retard growth, as well as cause other problems, and should be slowly withdrawn after prolonged use.

Adrenergic Drugs. These compounds offer the theoretical advantages of inhibiting insulin release, mobilizing fat stores and promoting hyperglycemia. Sus-Phrine or epinephrine, 0.3 ml. subcutaneously, may be useful in treating an acute episode and can be given by parents in an emergency. Ephedrine may be used in long-term management, particularly in patients who fail to respond to hypoglycemia with increased catecholamine output.

Glucagon. In infants with hyperinsulinism, glucagon may produce a dramatic response. Give 0.05 mg./kg., not to exceed 1.0 mg. total dose, intravenously or intramuscularly. If the infant responds to glucagon, parents should be shown how to administer it at home in an emergency.

HYPOGLYCEMIA IN LATE INFANCY AND CHILDHOOD

Any of the previously mentioned endocrinopathies may occur at this age. Hypoglycemia may occur in children with psychosocial growth retardation. These patients have a functional hypopituitarism with GH and ACTH deficiency. Removal of the child from his environment to one providing affection and concern produces a dramatic improvement.

The frequency of *islet cell tumor* increases with age, but it remains a rare cause of hypoglycemia at any age. Treatment is surgical. In patients who have persistent hypoglycemia after partial pancreatectomy, diazoxide may be effective. Streptozotocin, which selectively destroys the pancreatic beta cells in animals, has had restricted and limited use in humans with beta cell carcinoma. For adults, 2 to 5 gm. have been given as an intravenous infusion at 1 to 4 week intervals for two to three doses. Nausea and vomiting are usual. This drug is experimental, highly unstable, and difficult to use.

Drug ingestion or the malicious administration of insulin should always be considered as a cause of hypoglycemia. Overdose of insulin or hypoglycemic drugs may respond to glucagon (0.5 to 1 mg. by injection). Alcohol taken during fasting can cause serious hypoglycemia by inhibiting hepatic gluconeogenesis. In all cases of *alcohol ingestion,* the child should have his stomach washed out and be admitted to the hospital for monitoring blood sugar levels. If the child is drowsy, intravenous glucose is given at a rate of 6 to 8 mg./kg./min. Hypoglycemia may complicate severe aspirin overdose. Glucose therapy as outlined previously is given for hypoglycemia occurring in Reye's syndrome, hypothermia, malnutrition states and diarrheal disorders.

Idiopathic Hypoglycemia of Childhood

Ketotic hypoglycemia is the most common syndrome of hypoglycemia in childhood. It rarely occurs before 1 year of age, and attacks seldom persist into puberty. Hypoglycemic episodes are widely spaced and can be largely prevented with frequent low fat, high protein, high carbohydrate meals coupled with the routine testing for ketonuria at bed time, on rising and at times of illness. If ketonuria is found, attacks may be prevented with sugar in the form of candy, carbonated drinks or sweetened juices. This must be continued until the ketonuria clears. If vomiting, coma or convulsions occur, give Instant Glucose* or 0.5 to 1 gm. of intravenous glucose per kilogram by push, followed by 0.5 gm./kg./hour until food can be taken. Glucagon is characteristically ineffective and the poor response is often diagnostic. Treatment with glucose is essential. Steroids have been shown to prevent attacks, but are seldom required since most children respond to dietary measures.

Hypoglycemia often constitutes a medical emergency and glucose administration is required, although some patients will respond to glucagon or epinephrine. Rational therapy subsequently depends on identification of the cause.

Diabetes Insipidus

ZVI LARON, M.D., *and* RIVKA KAULI, M.D.

When polyuria or polydipsia develops, whether suddenly or gradually, the differential diagnosis must be made among several conditions:

1. Diabetes insipidus
   a. neurohypophyseal (ADH-sensitive)
   b. nephrogenic (ADH-insensitive)
2. Diabetes mellitus
3. Renal tubular failure
4. Compulsive (psychogenic) water drinking.

Diabetes mellitus is the most frequent cause of the above symptoms and should be considered

---

*Tubes of Instant Glucose and absorbable gel are available from the Diabetes Association of Greater Cleveland, 10205 Carnegie Avenue, Cleveland, Ohio 44106.

first. It is diagnosed by the finding of glycosuria and fasting hyperglycemia, and hypertonic urine in the presence of polyuria is characteristic. The rare association between diabetes mellitus and ADH-sensitive diabetes insipidus has been described, however. Renal tubular failure is generally preceded by the signs and symptoms of chronic renal disease and can be confirmed by pathological urinary findings and elevated levels of urea nitrogen and creatinine in the blood. Compulsive water drinking, which is rare in childhood, is differentiated from true diabetes insipidus by the ability of the patient to diminish his urinary output and to concentrate the urine when water intake is restricted. When no diminution of urinary volume and no urine concentration is achieved during the water deprivation test, the differential diagnosis between ADH-sensitive and ADH-insensitive diabetes insipidus is made by the administration of a test dose of ADH.

ADH-SENSITIVE DIABETES INSIPIDUS

Adequate treatment of diabetes insipidus is especially important in children since in addition to the interference with normal school attendance, social activities and night rest, normal growth is disturbed by the imbalance of water and electrolyte metabolism.

Most of the drugs used until recently, such as lysine-vasopressin nasal spray, nasal pitressin powder and vasopressin tannate in oil, have proved unsatisfactory. Recently, a synthetic analogue of the natural human antidiuretic hormone, 1-deamino-8-D-arginine (DDAVP, Minirin, Desmopressin), has been found to be the drug of choice. DDAVP has been used in Europe and elsewhere, and at the time of this writing the Food and Drug Administration is considering its release in the United States. It is dispensed in vials of 2.5 ml. (1 ml. = 0.1 mg. of DDAVP) with a small marked tube which makes possible the aspiration of as little as 0.05 ml. (= 0.005 mg.) and its nasal insufflation. Older children easily learn how to administer the drug to themselves. The dose for small children is 0.05 ml. applied twice daily and for adolescents usually 0.1 ml. In rare cases, a double dose is required. The range of effectiveness is 10 to 14 hours.

No local or general allergic reactions have been ascribed to this drug. On the same day therapy is instituted, there is a restoration of normal hydration, volume of urine and drinking habits. In infants the dose can be further diminished by diluting the drug with sodium chloride 0.9 gm. chlorobutanol 0.5 gm. and water to make 100 ml. (pH adjusted to a range of 4.0 to 4.5 using 0.1 per cent normal hydrochloride).

The drug is taken in the morning and in the evening before retiring. On this regimen the polyuria and polydipsia are satisfactorily controlled for periods of 10 to 14 hours, granting the patient a feeling of comfort and security during the day. The antidiuretic effect of DDAVP is most pronounced during the morning hours, assuring uninterrupted work at school. The evening dose permits the patient an uninterrupted night's sleep without bed wetting. When using DDAVP it is unnecessary to carry along an antidiuretic drug when leaving home for several hours. This drug also enables children and adolescents with diabetes insipidus to participate in social activities, which they previously avoided. Even in the presence of upper respiratory infections, sufficient absorption of DDAVP is achieved when the nose is properly cleaned prior to the application of the drug. It is therefore beyond doubt that at present DDAVP is the drug of choice for the treatment of ADH-sensitive diabetes insipidus.

Other drugs still employed are vasopressin tannate in oil dispensed in vials containing 5 I.U./ml. An intramuscular injection in a dose of 0.5 to 1.0 ml. usually is effective for 36 to 48 hours. The effectiveness decreases gradually and often irregularly, usually leaving the patient uncomfortable and wetting during the second night. An inadequate effect often is registered on the second morning. Because of its long-lasting effect, injection made more frequently than every 48 hours can lead to water intoxication. The Pitressin does not always dissolve in the oily vehicle; therefore before injection the vial should be heated in warm water to reduce viscosity, and the vial is shaken or turned until the Pitressin, seen as a dark spot, has properly dispersed. To ensure adequate absorption the intramuscular injection has to be made with a long needle.

In patients undergoing surgical removal of a craniopharyngioma, it is advisable to give an injection of Pitressin tannate (2.5 to 5 I.U.) before and perhaps one day after operation. The administration of Pitressin tannate is also advisable in patients unconscious after operation or trauma.

Pitressin powder, an unpurified preparation used either as nasal snuff or by insufflation (with a bulb inflator), has been used for many years. The dosage ranges between 20 and 40 mg. twice daily, having to be adjusted individually. The effectiveness of a dose is between 6 and 10 hours. This preparation cannot be used during rhinitis. Some patients develop an allergy to this powder and its use has to be discontinued.

Lysine-vasopressin nasal spray is an aqueous solution of 20 I.U./ml. which is effective for only 3 to 4 hours and has to be used 3 or 4 times a day, not covering the night. It also cannot be used during upper respiratory infections, and if too large doses are used may cause vasospasm and contraction of the gastrointestinal muscles. Vasopressin linguettes have been tried but the duration of effectiveness is short.

Other nonhormonal drugs have been found to be partially effective in ADH-sensitive diabetes insipidus but their use is hazardous and not recommended. Among them are thiazides, carbamazepine, clofibrate and chlorpropamide.

Chlorpropamide (Diabinese), an oral hypoglycemic agent, acts either by sensitizing the renal tubules to the effect of circulating ADH (thus is only effective if there is some endogenous ADH production still present) or by exerting an ADH-like action. It reduces the polyuria when used in doses of 200 to 250 mg./m²/day in 2 or 3 divided doses, but its hypoglycemic effect is a major and dangerous disadvantage. It should never be used when antidiuretic hormone as a drug is available.

ADH-sensitive diabetes insipidus can be an isolated hormone deficiency of transitory or permanent duration or may be combined with other hypothalamic pituitary hormone deficiency states. It can be caused by a cranial tumor such as craniopharyngioma, pinealoma or diencephalic glioma or may appear as a sequela to the surgical removal of the tumor. It can be associated with histiocytosis, leukemia, or encephalitis or can occur after meningitis, vaccination and cranial trauma. It has also been described in association with the Laurence-Moon-Biedl syndrome and diabetes mellitus.

In case of multiple hypothalamic pituitary hormone deficiency including ADH, it is necessary to institute ADH replacement therapy prior to assessment of the reserve of other hormones. When there is suboptimal hydration, false negative results may be obtained.

ADH-INSENSITIVE DIABETES INSIPIDUS

Treatment of this disease has posed great problems to pediatricians. If untreated in early childhood, there may be growth retardation and cerebral damage in addition to the discomfort it causes. Ideally the treatment is based on a low-solute diet to reduce the osmolar load to the kidney, and drugs are aimed to affect water reabsorption. Chlorothiazide, 1 gm./m²/day divided in 3 doses, reduces water requirement by 20 to 40% by paradoxically decreasing free water clearance. The judicious use of this drug provides the patient with sufficient sodium for

growth and a moderate state of discomfort. Other diuretics such as hydrochlorothiazide, spironolactone, furosemide (1 to 2 mg./kg.) and ethacrynic acid have also been used.

Psychological counseling of the family and gradual restriction of the water intake are usually helpful.

Rickets

LAURENCE FINBERG, M.D.

PREVENTION

Dietary deficiency rickets may be prevented by oral intake of 400 to 1000 I.U. of vitamin D per day exclusive of sunlight exposure. Most cow milk sold in the United States is fortified with 400 I.U. of vitamin D per quart or reconstituted quart. Breast-fed infants and prematurely born infants on less than a quart of milk per day require supplementation. Older infants on a general diet and receiving some sunlight exposure will not require supplementation. Those infants and children with fat malabsorption may need fivefold to tenfold the usual amount of vitamin D to have a sufficient amount absorbed. Patients on anticonvulsant drugs may also need a threefold to fourfold increase because of the overly rapid metabolism and subsequent excretion of the cholecalciferol molecule induced by such drugs.

An alternate preventive regimen may be 600,000 units of vitamin D given orally or intramuscularly every 6 to 9 months. Used in some parts of Europe, this technique is not common in the United States except in some centers using long-term, total parenteral nutrition for a small number of infants.

TREATMENT

Deficiency Rickets. At virtually any stage of this disturbance, treatment will be effective in every way unless severe deformities have already occurred. Therapy may be accomplished in a single day by oral intake of approximately 600,000 I.U. of vitamin D either as a single dose or divided over six doses during 24 hours. Care should be taken not to use a preparation suspended in propylene glycol because the dilution is usually such that the vehicle would be toxic at this dose level given at one time. Alternatively, 5,000 to 10,000 I.U. of vitamin D per day for eight weeks will also be effective. When single day therapy is employed, the phosphorus level in serum rises to normal within five days or less providing differential diagnostic discrimination from some of the varieties of metabolic rickets.

Malabsorptive States. Rickets of the deficiency type may occur when there is malabsorption of fat for any reason. Usually, simply increasing the daily intake to 10,000 to 20,000 I.U. of vitamin D daily followed by individualized increased intake after healing will suffice. The propylene glycol preparations are useful in these circumstances. Parenteral therapy, preferably 600,000 I.U. of vitamin D in a single injection, may also be utilized.

Liver Disease. Ideally, 25-hydroxy vitamin D is preferable for patients with hepatic impairment. Since this compound is still experimental, the technique described above for use in malabsorption will be effective in reversible hepatic disease such as acute hepatitis. Presumably, the effect is by mass action kinetics.

Primary Hypophosphatemic Rickets (Vitamin D-Resistant Rickets). Whether the familial X-linked, the sporadic, or autosomal dominant form, therapy may be the same. All of these patients require an increased intake of some form of vitamin D active substance. We prefer dihydrotachysterol (DHT) because it is rapidly excreted and inadvertent overdosage will not persist in body stores as it does with vitamin D. The usual dosage is 0.5 to 1.4 mg./day after a priming period of 1.5 to 2.0 mg./day for 7 to 10 days. When DHT is used alone the phosphorus level in the serum should not ever be expected to rise to normal levels. A sensitive biochemical marker for early toxicity is the calcium:creatinine ratio in urine over a 24 hour period. When both are measured in milligrams, the ratio is usually 0.25 or less and when over 0.4, toxic damage is imminent.

Most of our patients have been managed successfully with DHT alone, monitored at three month intervals after close initial observation and achieving a stable dose. Other workers have successfully recommended a lower dose of vitamin D or DHT coupled with a high phosphate intake. This method raises phosphorus levels to the normal range but requires large daily dosage of phosphate salts (1.5 to 2.0 gm.) which must be divided into four or five doses to avoid bowel symptoms. A preparation such as Neutraphos may be used with 150 ml. (0.5 gm. of phosphorus) given four times daily. The DHT dose may then be reduced to 0.2 to 1.0 mg. per day, but some such compound will still be required because the phosphate intake will otherwise overly suppress calcium absorption.

Fanconi Syndrome (Cystinosis or Tyrosinemia). With either of these generalized aminoacidopathies, the rachitic component may be managed by DHT, 0.2 to 1.0 mg. daily.

Vitamin D-Dependent Rickets. The optimal treatment of this disorder is the daily use of the hormone 1,25-dihydroxy-D since the disorder results from inadequate synthesis of this compound. Until the substance is commercially available, however, 5,000 to 40,000 I.U. of vitamin D per day is effective in treating these patients. The precise dosage must be ascertained by following serum levels of phosphorus and alkaline phosphatase, and by use of the calcium:creatinine excretion ratio as discussed above.

Renal Tubular Acidosis. When unaccompanied by aminoaciduria, rickets in acidemic patients will heal following correction of the acidemia by alkali.

Tetany

LAURENCE FINBERG, M.D.

Tetany results from reduced levels in the extracellular fluid of ionized calcium (Ca^{++}), magnesium ions, or hydrogen ions singly or in combination. As used here, the term will apply to reduced levels (< 3 mg./dl. = 1.5 mEq./liter = 0.75 mM/liter) of Ca^{++}. When hypocalcemia is secondary to rickets or chronic hypoparathyroidism, the long-term management is that of the underlying condition. Refer to the appropriate section. For emergency management of any hypocalcemic state, extracellular fluid levels may be raised by the continuous infusion of calcium gluconate which is available as a 10 per cent solution. A trial dose of 2 ml./kg. up to 10 ml. given at a rate that does not induce bradycardia may be used for a diagnostic test. Subsequently, 0.5 ml./kg./day (50 mg./kg./day) may be given by continuous infusion either diluted in glucose water with other electrolytes (no bicarbonate!) or by slow pump. Bolus intravenous therapy will not be effective because of rapid uptake by the skeleton and the pathophysiologic conditions which obtain. Once the symptomatic period is past, other more conservative measures will succeed while the underlying condition is corrected.

Tetany of the Newborn. The hypocalcemia of the early hours following birth in stressed infants probably has multifactorial etiology, and possibly more than one pathophysiologic process may be operative. It tends to be short-lived, and when symptomatic may be managed intravenously as above. Calcium salts should not be given intramuscularly for any condition because of local tissue damage.

The entity of hypocalcemic tetany seen after a few days of life, which presumably results from a "physiologic" relative deficiency of parathormone in the face of a high phosphate feeding, should be managed over a period of several weeks. Such infants are usually receiving cow milk feeds. The aim of management is to reduce phosphate absorption from the gut. This may be done by selecting a low phosphate feeding or more simply by adding excess calcium salts to milk feedings. A suitable excess is a mg.:mg., calcium:phosphorus ratio of 4:1. Calcium chloride is very irritating to gastric mucosa and in addition will produce an acidosis and acidemia by enhancing H^+ absorption. While this will correct tetany, acidemia has its own undesirable risks, so that it is wiser to choose an alkaline calcium salt such as the lactate or gluconate. Calcium lactate is 13 per cent calcium, and calcium gluconate is 9 per cent calcium. In the newborn given an adjusted feeding, Ca^{++} and phosphate levels may be watched every week, and after several weeks the "relative hypoparathyroidism" will spontaneously abate. A special case of this entity is the infant of the hypercalcemic (during pregnancy) mother.

Hypomagnesemic Tetany. This uncommon entity may be treated by the intramuscular injection of 0.2 ml./kg. of a 50 per cent solution of $MgSO_4 \cdot 12 H_2O$. The dose may be repeated at four to six hour intervals if needed. Levels of magnesium should be followed if more than a few doses are required. Long-term management is discussed in the section on hypomagnesemic states.

Alkalotic Tetany. The usual cause of this type of tetany is a lowered Pco_2 secondary to hyperventilation. Restoration of Pco_2 by slowing ventilation or breathing CO_2 will be quickly effective. Metabolic alkalosis which rarely causes tetany may be corrected by any appropriate acidifying regimen and replacement of K^+ and Cl^- ions.

Idiopathic Hypercalcemia

LAURENCE FINBERG, M.D.

This is a rare disorder in the United States and it resembles (and in fact may be) an excess of vitamin D. There is great sensitivity to any administered vitamin D so that all substances with vitamin D activity must be withheld. In addition, a diet very low in calcium should be arranged, which means elimination of milk and substitution of a low calcium infant formula. If the calcium level in serum is very high ($Ca^{++} > 6$ mg./dl. or total $Ca > 13$ mg./dl.), a 10

day course of steroid, e.g., prednisone, 2 mg./kg./day, should be started.

If the hypercalcemia is symptomatic, a rapid reduction in extracellular fluid calcium may be achieved by several doses of furosemide, 2 mg./kg. every six to eight hours, for a day or two. The water, sodium, potassium and magnesium salts of the urine should be replaced as they are lost.

Long-term management seldom goes beyond a few months. Close observation of serum levels and of the skeleton should be maintained to adjust therapy.

Magnesium Deficiency

LAURENCE FINBERG, M.D.

Symptomatic magnesium deficiency occurs uncommonly. Most often when it does occur, it is a late manifestation of a chronic problem. Chronic diarrheal disease whether from regional enteritis, ulcerative colitis, laxative abuse, or other causes may produce severe magnesium depletion. Other conditions include chronic malnutrition and hypoparathyroid states. The recent increased use of total parenteral nutrition for quick "hyperalimentation" of the chronically undernourished may precipitate low extracellular fluid levels of magnesium through the rapid production of new intracellular fluid, magnesium, like potassium, being primarily an intracellular ion. Symptomatic magnesium deficiency invariably means low (below 1.2 mg./dl. or 1 mEq./liter) levels in the extracellular fluid.

Quick correction for any of these situations may be achieved by the intramuscular administration of a 50 per cent solution of $MgSO_4 \cdot 12 H_2O$ in a dosage of up to 0.2 ml./kg. every four to six hours until symptoms are controlled or serum levels are normal.

For continued therapy the oral route may be used when the bowel permits. Many magnesium salts are laxative owing to poor absorption. Magnesium gluconate, 2 to 3 mEq./kg. per day, is a suitable preparation and dosage. Aside from diarrhea, side effects are unimportant. On the other hand, parenteral administration of magnesium may produce cardiac arrhythmia when given intravenously, and severe neurologic depression when given intramuscularly. Intravenous use should not ordinarily be employed and intramuscular usage should be closely monitored by serum levels. The presence of elicitable deep tendon reflexes generally indicates an absence of significant magnesium toxicity.

Hepatolenticular Degeneration

(Wilson's Disease)

NORMAN B. JAVITT, M.D., Ph.D.

The awareness of liver disease in children together with the increasing availability of specific diagnostic tests such as serum ceruloplasmin, serum α-1-antitrypsin, and serum hepatitis BsAg has improved early diagnosis. Absent or markedly reduced serum ceruloplasmin establishes the diagnosis of Wilson's disease. However, the previous view that excessive copper retention with chronic toxicity manifested by liver and/or central nervous system disease be classified as Wilson's disease, regardless of serum ceruloplasmin levels, is no longer tenable. Cholestasis occurring at birth and persisting through childhood can also be associated with excessive copper accumulation. In addition to the difference in serum ceruloplasmin levels, children with cholestasis have symptoms of pruritus earlier in life and have markedly elevated serum bile acids and 5-nucleotidase at the earliest stages of the disease. Treatment of the cholestasis as well as the copper retention is indicated.

TREATMENT

Diet. Although by the time the diagnosis is usually made, excessive amounts of copper have already accumulated, reduction of copper in the diet facilitates depletion of body stores with therapeutic agents. Foods rich in copper are nuts, chocolate including cocoa, shellfish, liver, mushrooms, and dried fruit.

Penicillamine ($\beta\beta$-Dimethylcysteine). Hydrolysis of penicillin gives rise to penicillamine which possesses a free amino group and free sulfhydryl group on adjacent carbons. The α amino carbon is asymmetric so that two isomers, d and l, are possible. The d isomer (d-penicillamine, Cuprimine) has less of an inhibitory effect on pyridoxal-dependent enzyme systems.

Via the free SH group penicillamine chelates with copper, lead, mercury, and gold. It will react with cysteine to form a mixed disulfide. The reactivity of the sulfhydryl group may also account for other biological activities such as interference with collagen and elastin maturation causing diminished tensile strength. Prior to therapy, liver function, renal function, and hematologic parameters should be evaluated. For these purposes urinary excretion of copper, ceruloplasmin, SGOT and SGPT, bilirubin, prothrombin time, albumin, BUN, and creatinine, and hemoglobin, white blood count, and differential with either a platelet count or smear should be done. Immunoglobulin levels, particularly IgA, may also require monitoring since selective IgA deficiency has been reported.

A wide range of doses has been used and it is possible to achieve amounts of 40 mg./kg./day. It is probably best to begin with a 250 mg. capsule three times daily (approximately 20 mg./kg.) one hour before meals. At this dose, nausea, vomiting, and anorexia are not likely to occur and the dose can be doubled in several weeks if there have been no hypersensitivity reactions as manifested by fever, rash, lymphadenopathy, neutropenia, or thrombocytopenia. In this event, the dose can be reduced or stopped and steroids (prednisone, 20 mg./day) instituted for several weeks. Recurrence of hypersensitivity phenomena, particularly if there is evidence for a developing nephrotic syndrome or agranulocytosis, indicates that d-penicillamine should be discontinued, and an alternate but less efficacious form of therapy will be necessary.

At 1500 mg./day a marked increase in copper excretion should occur and be documented. After a year of continuous therapy, urinary copper excretion may fall and a reduction in hepatic copper should have occurred. At this time, particularly when evidence for improvement in liver function has been obtained, lowering of the dose can be attempted. It may be found that a reduction in d-penicillamine dose does not greatly affect cupruresis. In principle the lowest dose that maintains high urinary copper excretion is least likely to result in the long-term side effects on skin and mucous membranes. Since d-penicillamine will be needed throughout life, establishing the lowest effective dose has merit. Pyridoxine, 50 mg./day, is often prescribed in the hope of reducing the possibility of adverse reactions.

Potassium Sulfide. Thirty to 40 mg./day with meals can reduce copper absorption from the diet. Although toxicity is unlikely, body odor can become offensive.

Triethylene Tetramine (TETA). This chelating agent in the amount of 400 mg. three times daily can bring about a cupruresis of 3 mg./day. Compared with d-penicillamine on a molar basis, it is less efficient at chelating copper. However, it is a reasonable alternative when d-penicillamine is contraindicated because of severe untoward reactions such as thrombocytopenia, agranulocytosis, or nephrotic syndrome.

Sufficient experience has not been obtained to define its toxic effects so that extra precautions should be taken in monitoring for toxicity when the drug is used. Clearly, some form of chelation therapy must be instituted to prevent progression of the disease and hopefully to reverse established deficiencies.

Dimercaprol (BAL). This compound, designed for the treatment of arsine poisoning, will bind other metals including copper. It is given by intramuscular injection and doses of 3 to 5 mg./kg. are frequently associated with nausea, headaches, and transient hypertension. Although cupruresis is obtained, the need for continual parenteral administration is a serious hindrance to long-term use.

Anion-Exchange Resins. There is no need for these agents in the treatment of Wilson's disease. Occasionally marked elevations of bile acids in serum is found in children with liver disease, excessive copper retention, and normal or reduced ceruloplasmin. Administration of cholestyramine in amounts of 8 to 12 gm./day reduces serum bile acid levels and improves liver function. Concomitant use of copper chelating agents is probably also beneficial. The exact nature of their disease is not defined.

Phenylketonuria

HELEN K. BERRY, M.A.

Screening programs carried out for detection of phenylketonuria (PKU) have revealed a spectrum of biochemical disorders in which phenylalanine concentrations range from only slightly above normal to over 30 mg./100 ml., the concentration usually associated with classic phenylketonuria. The need to provide a diet low in phenylalanine for children with classic phenylketonuria is no longer questioned. Less certain is whether children with variant forms of phenylketonuria or hyperphenylalaninemia should have restricted phenylalanine intake. It is not easy to distinguish the various forms of phenylketonuria early in infancy. Only about two-thirds of individuals with persistent elevations of phenylalanine in blood prove to have a form of phenylketonuria requiring treatment with a low-phenylalanine diet.

The dietary treatment of phenylketonuria consists of providing a nutritionally balanced diet containing enough phenylalanine to meet the needs of a growing child without exceeding his limited capacity to utilize it. The outcome of treatment of phenylketonuria is dependent on the quality of treatment, which includes avoidance of nutritional deficiencies, as well as avoidance of excess phenylalanine in the diet.

Decision for Treatment. The decision to treat or not to treat a child with elevated serum phenylalanine concentration should be based on the considered judgment of whether the elevation is sufficient to constitute a risk to the child's future development. The conservative measures described below ensure that a child without phenylketonuria will not be subjected unnecessarily to a phenylalanine restricted diet, but a child with PKU will be protected against excess phenylalanine. If serum phenylalanine concentrations are consistently below 15 mg./100 ml., a low-phenylalanine diet is not recommended. If serum phenylalanine concentrations are above 20 mg./100 ml., the prudent course is to place the infant on a low-phenylalanine formula while adding enough phenylalanine to the diet to maintain serum phenylalanine concentrations between 3 and 10 mg./100 ml. If serum phenylalanine concentrations are between 15 and 20 mg./100 ml., decrease in protein in the diet may be sufficient to lower the level. If phenylalanine concentrations persist above 15 mg./100 ml. on a protein intake of 2.0 to 2.2 gm./kg./day, a low-phenylalanine formula may be needed to reduce phenylalanine in the diet. If the amount of phenylalanine needed to maintain serum levels at 3 mg./100 ml. is over 100 mg./kg./day, at any time, the low-phenylalanine formula should be stopped and the diagnosis of a form of phenylketonuria should be reconsidered. In some infants the categorization as classic or variant may not be apparent until several years later. The reason for maintaining serum phenylalanine concentrations above 3 mg./100 ml. is to prevent the harm that comes from exaggerated stringency in the treatment, which, in the past, led to chronic phenylalanine deficiency and impairment of cognitive and behavioral development.

Low-Phenylalanine Diet. Compared with diets of most children, the low-phenylalanine diet is severely restricted. Foods that are rich in protein such as milk, meat, cheese, fish, eggs, and beans must be limited rigidly. The phenylalanine intake is reduced to one-fourth to one-seventh that furnished by a normal infant diet. Proteins of both plant and animal origin contain approximately 4 to 5 per cent phenylalanine. Thus it is impossible to obtain enough protein from ordinary foods without obtaining excess phenylalanine. Special products from which most or all the phenylalanine has been removed are used as the major protein source. The formulas available in the United States are Lofenalac, a casein hydrolysate low in phenylalanine, and PKU-aid, a beef serum protein hydrolysate virtually free of phenylalanine. Compositions of

TABLE 1.　Composition of Low-Phenylalanine Products

	LOFENALAC*	PKU-AID†
Calories/100 gm.	454	240
Protein (gm./100 gm.)	15	60
Fat (gm./100 gm.)	18	0
Carbohydrate (gm./100 gm.)	60	0
Phenylalanine (gm./100 gm.)	.08	<.07

*Lofenalac is a product of the Mead Johnson Co., Evansville, Indiana.

†PKU-aid is a product of the Milner Scientific and Medical Research Co., Ltd., Liverpool, England.

these two products are compared in Table 1. The important differences are the higher caloric content of Lofenalac and the higher protein content of PKU-aid. Because of its higher protein content, the amount of phenylalanine contributed by PKU-aid to the daily diet is negligible. Formulas based on PKU-aid must be supplemented with fat and carbohydrate. The products may be used interchangeably or in combination. Both products contain a good balance of essential amino acids other than phenylalanine. Both contain minerals and vitamins in amounts to meet the recommended daily allowance when fed in the quantity to meet the protein requirement.

Treatment in Specialized Centers. Facilities for the frequent testing of blood and urine and the nutritional training and skills necessary to evaluate and monitor the phenylalanine content of the diet are not generally available except in large medical centers. Because of difficulties inherent in administration of this highly restrictive diet, affected children should be referred for treatment to centers where there is a team consisting of pediatrician, pediatric nutritionist, biochemist, and psychologist. The staff in such centers have experience in caring for children with phenylketonuria; laboratory facilities are available immediately; proper dietary supervision can be supplied; and the effect of treatment can be assessed. Inclusion in the treatment team of a nurse and social worker facilitates the long-term management necessary for this chronic disease. It is important that pediatricians involved in other aspects of care of phenylketonuric children understand the goals and principles of the therapy being used, enabling them to work closely with families to reinforce recommendations of specialists responsible for the child's treatment. The more thoroughly parents understand details of the treatment program, the more easily can effective long-term control be achieved.

Initiation of Dietary Treatment. Once the decision has been made to treat the child, the infant is taken off the regular formula and the low-phenylalanine formula is begun. The low-phenylalanine diet may be initiated on an outpatient or inpatient basis. For an individual infant dietary prescriptions initially are based on recommendations shown in Table 2. The protein and caloric recommendations are based on those of the National Research Council. The protein recommendation is calculated to be met entirely from the low-phenylalanine source. A small amount of additional protein is provided by the natural food supplement needed to furnish the phenylalanine requirement, but this is not considered in the calculation shown in Table 2, providing a desirable small excess.

Young babies ordinarily accept the low-phenylalanine formula well. The formula may be given alone for one to two days to bring about a rapid decline in serum phenylalanine levels. A source of phenylalanine should be supplied by the third day. It is convenient to use cow's milk initially. If one of the low-protein milks is used, correction should be made in calculating the amount needed to supply the daily phenylalanine requirement. Serum phenylalanine concentrations should be measured frequently during the initial period of dietary treatment. The amount of phenylalanine in the form of milk may be raised or lowered according to the rate of serum phenylalanine decline. Dietary prescriptions are altered according to individual needs, determined by growth progress, appetite and biochemical changes. Phenylalanine intake is adjusted so that the greatest tolerated intake that maintains the approporiate serum phenylalanine level is ingested. The dietary

TABLE 2.　Recommended Daily Intakes of Nutrients for Children with Classic Phenylketonuria

AGE	PHENYLALANINE (mg./kg.)	PROTEIN (gm./kg.)	CALORIES (cal./kg.)
0–3 mos.	50–60	2.2–2.5	110–120
6 mos.	40–50	2.0–2.5	110–120
1 yr.	30–35	1.8–2.5	100
2 yr.	25–30	1.8–2.0	95
3 yr.	20–30	1.8–2.0	90
4 yr.	20–25	1.8–2.0	90
5 yr.	18–25	1.6–1.8	85
6–7 yr.	15–25	1.6–1.8	80
8–9 yr.	15–25	1.4–1.6	75
10–12 yr.	10–25	1.4–1.6	60–70
13–15 yr.	5–15	1.0–1.5	50–60
16–20 yr.	5–10	1.0–1.3	40–50
During pregnancy	10	1.3	50

regimen is constructed by the nutritionist to fit within the family pattern of eating and within the stages of development of eating habits.

MANAGING THE DIET. During the first month of treatment, determination of the amount of milk required to stabilize serum phenylalanine levels between 3 and 10 mg./100 ml. aids in establishment of the amount of phenylalanine which can be allowed from natural foods. Following the newborn period, cereals and low-protein fruits and vegetables gradually replace milk as a source of dietary phenylalanine. Infant foods are introduced in the same fashion and at the same times for phenylketonuric infants as for normal infants. Iron and vitamin supplements are given in usual doses. Small amounts of high-protein foods may be included so the child can become accustomed to their tastes. Table foods are introduced at the same time as they would be for children without phenylketonuria. For optimal growth, strict attention must be paid to appropriate increases in the prescription for protein from the low-phenylalanine formula. With the introduction of cup feedings, the demand for formula may become less. To avert a decrease in protein intake, a prescribed amount of low-phenylalanine diet may be made up in a small volume or prepared in a paste form. It is important to maintain an adequate intake of energy. Nonprotein sources such as Dextri-Maltose, corn syrup, sugar or margarine may be used to maintain caloric intakes.

The adequacy of dietary treatment is assessed by frequent measurements of height and weight, psychological and neurological evaluations, together with frequent monitoring of serum phenylalanine concentrations in relation to dietary intakes. During the first year, daily diet records are usually kept. Parents are given lists of phenylalanine contents of a wide variety of foods to aid them in selection of the kinds and amounts of food needed to meet a specific prescription. After the first year usually seven days of diet records per month are sufficiently representative to permit calculations of nutrient intakes. Serum phenylalanine determinations are usually carried out once or twice a week during the first three months of treatment and weekly until six months of age. After a year of age, as the growth rate slows, monthly monitoring of serum phenylalanine levels is usually satisfactory.

The first two years of treatment are probably the most critical in preventing mental retardation from phenylketonuria. During this time the child makes the transition from bottle to cup feedings, from strained to chopped foods to table foods, and to self-feeding practices. The major burden of treatment falls on the parents. They need assurance that the formula and other foods will nourish the child. They should understand that the total amount prescribed may not always be taken each day and there is no need to force feed or coax the child to eat. They must learn to manage the prescription for a limited amount of phenylalanine in the diet, while at the same time ensuring adequate intake of the protein substitute and of calories. In most programs parents collect the frequent blood specimens needed for biochemical monitoring.

As the child grows older, he must be taught that his food is special and that he may eat only what is given him by parents. Siblings, relatives, neighbors and teachers must be instructed not to offer food without consulting the parents. When the child reaches kindergarten or first grade, planning of low-phenylalanine school lunches is needed.

By six to eight years of age some relaxation of the stringency of the diet is usually permitted, and serum phenylalanine values may range from 5 to 12 mg./100 ml. Occasional temporary lapses in the rigidity of the diet for holidays or other special occasions do not appear to be harmful. It is important that the child begin early to accept some responsibility for the diet and be allowed some freedom in selecting foods. The diet should follow that of the family as closely as possible, though some foods will necessarily have to be restricted.

Illnesses and infections may have a temporary effect on phenylalanine balance, and elevated serum phenylalanine levels often accompany declining appetites. Therapy appropriate to the illness is given. The low-phenylalanine formula should be continued and supplemented with low-phenylalanine fluids and sources of calories. Children hospitalized for surgical procedures such as tonsillectomy, requiring only an overnight stay, may have the diet ordinarily prescribed for such procedures. If hospitalization is prolonged, the low-phenylalanine diet should be continued in the hospital.

Results of Treatment. Many reports confirm intellectual development in the normal range for children in whom treatment began early in life. Nevertheless, a small but significant deficit in intellectual ability, compared with that predicted from unaffected family members, has been found in many phenylketonuric children in spite of early treatment. Prolonged malnutrition from phenylalanine deficiency has been associated with mild to moderate mental retardation in spite of early treatment. Fortunately over-treatment rarely occurs now. Long periods of elevation of serum phenylalanine over 10 mg./100 ml. during the first two years of life may also be related to intellectual impairment.

Variant Types of Phenylketonuria. Phenylalanine hydroxylase is usually absent in liver of patients with classic phenylketonuria. Patients with atypical or variant forms have liver phenylalanine hydroxylase activity ranging from 5 to 20 per cent of normal. A number of patients with a new form of phenylketonuria have been described recently in which phenylalanine hydroxylase activity was normal or only slightly reduced. Patients showed progressive neurological deterioration and death, in some instances, even when serum phenylalanine levels were controlled. Levels of dihydropteridine reductase, another component of the phenylalanine hydroxylase system, were reduced in liver, brain and fibroblasts. The recognition of forms which do not respond to low-phenylalanine diet suggests restraint in offering a good prognosis following dietary treatment. The neurological symptoms probably result from impairment of neurotransmitter synthesis in brain. Intravenous administration of tetrahydrobiopterin was effective in reducing serum phenylalanine levels, but caused no clinical improvement. High doses of this substance would be required to support hydroxylation of aromatic amino acids. Tetrahydrobiopterin does not readily enter the brain where it would be needed for synthesis of dopamine and serotonin. Promising results have been attained from administration of the neurotransmitter precursors, L-dopa and 5-hydroxytryptophan, to a child who was not responsive to the low-phenylalanine diet.

Termination of Dietary Treatment. For many years it has been assumed that the low-phenylalanine diet could be terminated when major phases of brain growth were completed. This conclusion is now less certain. Concerns about discontinuation of diet therapy for early treated children center around possible adverse behavioral changes, decreases in functional intellectual capacity, abnormal changes in electroencephalograms, lessening in general well-being and subsequent pregnancies of phenylketonuric women. Visual-perceptual deficits, overactivity, distractability and short attention span often interfere with school performance and acquisition of academic skills by phenylketonuric children after dietary treatment is stopped, although no consistent decrease in intellectual performance has been shown. There have been very few long-term follow-up studies. The electroencephalogram may become abnormal, and other symptoms of untreated phenylketonuria such as eczema and the unpleasant odor may appear. Reports of psychotic behavior associated with phenylketonuria in individuals with normal intelligence are particularly disturbing. It seems likely that phenylketonuria has two effects: irreversible structural damage to the developing central nervous system and reversible interference with function of the central nervous system related to serum phenylalanine levels, possibly associated with deficiency of catecholamines and serotonin. Present evidence suggests that phenylalanine accumulation can interfere with the chemical basis of learning. Caution is called for and it may be safer to continue the low-phenylalanine diet indefinitely.

Alternate Approaches to Treatment. As phenylketonuric children grow older it becomes increasingly difficult to maintain serum phenylalanine levels within the range of 3 to 12 mg./100 ml. Phenylalanine requirements steadily decrease while the desire for a normal life, particularly regarding food, becomes urgent as the treatment is successful in producing normal physical and intellectual development. Alternate methods of treatment need study so that either control of blood phenylalanine levels can be continued into the adult years or some form of treatment can be developed which might inhibit the deleterious effect of phenylalanine on the central nervous system.

The most promising adjunct of dietary treatment of phenylketonuria at present is the administration of excess quantities of the branched-chain amino acids, valine, isoleucine, and leucine, together with the low-phenylalanine diet. Since these amino acids share a common transport system with phenylalanine, their inclusion in the diet in increased amounts inhibits the transport of phenylalanine into the brain. Higher concentrations of phenylalanine in the blood might be permitted, provided access of phenylalanine to the brain could be inhibited. Other avenues for exploration include absorption of dietary phenylalanine from the gastrointestinal tract by some inert substance prior to absorption. Activated charcoal is used to prepare the low-phenylalanine protein hydrolysates. This substance has a long history of medicinal use in removing toxic substances from the gastrointestinal tract. Current experimentation centers around the use of activated charcoal in binding excess phenylalanine and thus preventing its absorption by phenylketonuric children.

Amino Acid Disorders

MARY G. AMPOLA, M.D.
See tables on following pages.

DISEASE (AND APPROXIMATE INCIDENCE)*	CLINICAL FEATURES	ABNORMAL ENZYME	AMINO ACIDS INCREASED IN BLOOD	AMINO ACIDS INCREASED IN URINE	COMMENTS	TREATMENT
Phenylketonuria						
Phenylketonuria, classic. (1:15,000)	Mental retardation; also seizures, eczema and fair skin, eyes, and hair in some patients.	Phenylalanine hydroxylase (virtually total absence).	Phenylalanine—levels usually over 30 mg./100 ml.	Phenylalanine; phenyl-pyruvic, -lactic acids, ortho-hydroxyphenylacetic acid also increased.	Increasing evidence treatment cannot be stopped at age 4 to 6 without intellectual deterioration.	Low phenylalanine diet.
Phenylketonuria, atypical. (1:90,000)	Mental retardation; often less severe than in classic form.	Phenylalanine hydroxylase (partial defect).	Phenylalanine—levels not as high as in classic form, about 20 mg./100 ml.	Same as in the classic form but often in smaller amounts.	May not need treatment to maintain normal blood phenylalanine after early childhood.	Low phenylalanine diet to tolerance.
Hyperphenylalaninemia, persistent mild. (1:20,000)	Normal in all respects.	Phenylalanine hydroxylase (partial defect—more enzyme remains).	Phenylalanine—levels in range of 6-8 mg./100 ml.	None.	Mental and physical development normal.	None necessary.
Disorders of Ammonia Metabolism			NOTE: Glutamine elevated in blood and urine in all hyperammonemia situations, but often difficult to detect on screening.			
Urea Cycle Diseases						
Carbamyl phosphate synthetase deficiency. (rare)	Episodic vomiting, acidosis, cyclic neutropenia.	Carbamyl phosphate synthetase.	Glycine.	Glycine.	Postprandial hyperammonemia.	Low protein diet (1 gm./kg./day), also alpha-keto acids.
Ornithine transcarbamylase deficiency. (rare)	Episodic vomiting, and stupor, failure to thrive, hepatomegaly, seizures; mental retardation usually.	Ornithine transcarbamylase (also some decrease in carbamyl phosphate synthetase).	—	—	Postprandial hyperammonemia.	Low protein diet (1 gm./kg./day), also alpha-keto acids.
Citrullinemia. (rare)	Vomiting, seizures, failure to thrive, mental retardation; may die in neonatal period.	Argininosuccinic acid synthetase.	Citrulline.	Citrulline.	Postprandial hyperammonemia.	Low protein diet (1–1.5 gm./kg./day).
Argininosuccinic Aciduria. (1:70,000)	Ataxia, seizures, mental retardation, friable hair, hepatomegaly; may die in neonatal period.	Argininosuccinase.	Argininosuccinic acid.	Argininosuccinic acid.	Postprandial hyperammonemia.	Low protein diet (1–1.5 gm./kg./day).

Disorder	Clinical features	Enzyme defect			Laboratory findings	Treatment
Hyperargininemia. (rare)	Seizures, spasticity, mental retardation.	Arginase.	Arginine.	Arginine; lysine, ornithine, and cystine also present at times.	Postprandial hyperammonemia may be present.	Low protein diet (1.5 gm./kg./day).
Other Hyperammonemias						
"Hyperglycinemia, ketotic form." (1:300,000)	Periodic vomiting, lethargy, ketosis, myoclonic jerks, osteoporosis, neutropenia and thrombocytopenia.	Not specific; deficiencies of the following are known: (1) carbamyl PO_4 synthetase, (2) methylmalonyl CoA carbonylmutase and (3) proprionyl CoA carboxylase.	Glycine, occasionally lysine.	Glycine, occasionally lysine.	Hyperammonemia may be present.	Low protein diet (1–1.5 gm./kg./day).
Ornithinemia (type I) (with homocitrullinuria). (rare)	Irritability, ataxia, myoclonic seizures, aversion to protein, mental retardation.	Unknown	Ornithine.	Homocitrulline; ornithine may be normal.	Hyperammonemia.	Low protein diet (1.5 gm./kg./day).
Familial protein intolerance with hyperdibasic aminoaciduria. (rare)	Vomiting and diarrhea, failure to thrive, neutropenia, aversion to protein, hepatomegaly.	Defective transport of dibasic amino acids in kidney; also in intestine in some.	—	Arginine, lysine.	Usually normal intelligence. Ammonia intoxication after high protein intake.	Low protein diet (1 gm./kg./day): arginine supplement (2 gm./day) to improve urea formation from ammonia.
OTHER AMINO ACID DISORDERS						
Cystathioninuria. (1:100,000)	Probably benign.	Cystathionase.	Trace of cystathionine.	Cystathionine.	—	None necessary (although pyridoxine, 25 to 100 mg. daily, will clear cystathionine).
Cystinosis, nephropathic. (rare)	Fanconi syndrome in urine, failure to thrive, vitamin D-resistant rickets.	Unknown.	Essentially normal, including cystine and cysteine.	Generalized aminoaciduria.	Phosphaturia, glycosuria; cystine deposits in many tissues.	Symptomatic; vitamin D (10,000 to 15,000 U/day): limited success with low-cystine diets and D-penicillamine. Renal transplantation.

DISEASE (AND APPROXIMATE INCIDENCE)*	CLINICAL FEATURES	ABNORMAL ENZYME	AMINO ACIDS INCREASED IN BLOOD	AMINO ACIDS INCREASED IN URINE	COMMENTS	TREATMENT
Cystinuria. (1:15,000)	Renal calculi; ? mental retardation in some.	Defective transport of cystine and the dibasic amino acids in kidney and intestine.	—	Cystine and dibasic amino acids.	—	High fluid intake; add D-penicillamine if calculi appear. Alkalization of urine and low methionine diet effective but difficult to maintain.
Hyperglycinemia, nonketotic form. (1:150,000)	Lethargy, seizures, spasticity, mental retardation.	Defect in an enzyme catalyzing conversion of glycine to CO_2, NH_3 and a one-carbon tetrahydrofolate derivative.	Glycine.	Glycine; occasionally not elevated.	—	No effective therapy. Low-glycine, low-serine diet; supplemental methionine of possible value.
Hartnup disease. (1:18,000)	May be benign; lightsensitive rash, ataxia, psychosis, mental retardation in some.	Defective transport of neutral amino acids in kidney and intestine.	None: indeed, neutral amino acids about 30 per cent less than normal.	Neutral amino acids.	Indoles produced by intestinal bacteria from tryptophan are absorbed and excreted into the urine.	None necessary in some; nicotinamide for rash (up to 400 mg./day); high protein diet for general nutrition.
Histidinemia. (1:20,000)	Probably benign.	Histidase.	Histidine.	Histidine.	Urocanic acid absent in skin homogenates and sweat; low serotonin in serum.	None necessary.
Homocystinuria. (1:200,000)	Dislocated lenses (downward), malar flush, intravascular thromboses, long, thin extremities, osteoporosis; mental retardation in some.	Cystathionine synthetase.	Methionine; small amount of homocystine.	Homocystine.	Two variants: pyridoxine-responsive and nonresponsive.	Up to 500 mg. daily of pyridoxine for responders; otherwise, low-methionine diet with cystine supplement.
Hyperlysinemia. (rare)	May be benign in some; mental retardation and other minor features in others.	Lysine - ketoglutarate reductase in some patients; saccharopine dehydrogenase in others.	Lysine.	Lysine; some also have increased saccharopine.	—	Therapy may not be necessary; low-protein diet (1.5 gm./kg/day).

Disorder (incidence)	Clinical features	Enzyme defect	Amino acid	Laboratory findings	Comments	Treatment
Maple syrup urine disease (severe infantile form). (1:450,000)	Vomiting, progressive hypertonicity, acidosis, coma, early death.	Branched-chain keto acid decarboxylase (absence virtually complete).	Leucine, isoleucine, valine.	Leucine, isoleucine, valine (with their three corresponding keto acids).	Urine has odor of maple syrup.	Partially synthetic diet low in leucine, isoleucine, and valine; peritoneal dialysis during crises.
Maple syrup urine disease (intermittent form). (rare)	Episodic vomiting, lethargy and coma, often with infection; normal between episodes including I.Q.	Branched-chain keto acid decarboxylase (activity 12 to 18 per cent of normal).	Leucine, isoleucine, valine only during acute attacks.	Leucine, isoleucine, valine (with their three corresponding keto acids only during acute attacks).	Odor of maple syrup when ill; disease may be fatal during crises.	Low protein diet during exacerbations (0 to 1 gm./kg./day).
Ornithinemia (type II). (rare)	Prolonged neonatal jaundice, failure to thrive, liver cirrhosis, mental retardation.	Ornithine keto-acid transaminase.	Ornithine.	Ornithine may be normal; generalized aminoaciduria, glycosuria.	Normal serum ammonia even after protein loading.	Low protein diet (1 gm./kg./day).
Hyperprolinemia (type I). (rare)	May have seizures, mental retardation, hereditary nephritis and deafness; others completely normal.	Proline oxidase.	Proline.	Proline; hydroxyproline and glycine may also be elevated.	—	? necessary; low-proline, low-protein diet tried with some success.
Hyperprolinemia (type II). (rare)	Seizures, mental retardation in some; others completely normal.	Δ^1-pyrroline-5-carboxylate dehydrogenase.	Proline.	Proline, Δ^1-pyrroline-5-carboxylate, hydroxyproline and glycine.	—	? necessary; low-proline, low-protein diet tried with some success.
Sarcosinemia. (rare)	? mild mental retardation; variable clinical picture in patients reported.	? Sarcosine dehydrogenase.	Sarcosine.	Sarcosine.	—	? necessary; no special diet tried.
Tyrosinemia, hereditary. (rare)	Failure to thrive, vomiting, diarrhea, liver cirrhosis, renal tubular defects, vitamin D–resistant rickets.	Unknown.	Tyrosine, methionine.	Generalized aminoaciduria with especially large amounts of tyrosine.	Glycosuria, phosphaturia, hypoglycemia, hypophosphatemia.	Low-phenylalanine, low-tyrosine diet.

*Incidence figures are from the State of Massachusetts Metabolic Screening Program as of November 1974 (courtesy of Dr. Harvey Levy) and from review of the literature. The figures presented are approximations; in many cases the disease is not detectable on routine screening and true incidence is unknown.

Inborn Errors of Carbohydrate Metabolism

NOEL KEITH MACLAREN, M.D., *and*
MARVIN CORNBLATH, M.D.

There are a rich variety of enzymatic deficiencies in carbohydrate metabolism important to the practice of pediatrics. Most patients with such disorders can be greatly helped clinically, provided that the underlying disease has been recognized and characterized. Galactosemia is discussed elsewhere.

THE GLYCOGENOSES

Disorders involving pathological storage of glycogen within the body can be subdivided into two groups, those involving principally the liver (kidney)—types I, III, VI and IX, and those with skeletal muscle involvement—types II (heart) and V (limb musculature).

Hepato (Renal) Syndromes

Type I (Von Gierke's). The disease results from a deficiency of glucose-6-phosphatase. Since hydrolysis of glucose-6-phosphate to glucose is the common end event for gluconeogenesis and glycogenolysis, hypoglycemia is severe. Further, new glucose-6-phosphate is diverted into glycogen deposition, to lactic acid formation and indirectly to triglyceride synthesis following generation of diphosphopyridine nucleotide from pentose shunt activity.

HYPOGLYCEMIA. In the severely affected infant, blood glucose levels regularly fall to the hypoglycemic range within a few hours of eating. Curiously, symptoms such as associated CNS disturbance may be blunted, presumably because of some cerebral capacity to utilize substrates other than glucose for its energy needs. However, symptoms of the associated sympathetic response (pallor, sweating, and so on) are more common.

Recent evidence suggests that many of the features of the disease (such as hepatomegaly, lipemia, hyperuric acidemia, lactic acidosis, growth retardation, bruising) may improve markedly if hypoglycemia is minimized. To this end, infants must be fed every 3 hours night and day. We use Cho-Free with 10 gm./100 ml. (10 per cent) glucose added and avoid sucrose (cane sugar) and lactose (milk sugar), since the contained fructose and galactose cannot form new glucose but rather tend to be stored as glycogen or be directed to lactic acid formation. Glucose water (10 per cent) may be offered between feedings as needed. The diet should provide 60 to 70 per cent carbohydrate (glucose, maltose starches), 12 to 15 per cent protein and 10 to 25 per cent fat.

Burr, Greene and colleagues have shown the benefits of long-term continuous intragastric feeding during night time periods in the older child. Such feedings consist of Vivonex* delivered via a small nasogastric tube from a continuous infusion pump (see below) over a 12 hour period to provide one-third of the total daily calories. The remaining two thirds of the caloric requirement are best given as 2 to 3 hour feedings for the 12 hour period of the daytime regimen. Although there appears to be a tendency for clinical improvement with increasing age, perhaps due in part to cerebral adaptive processes, prevention of hypoglycemia, whether clinically apparent or not, remains the goal in therapy.

There is probably no place in therapy for drugs such as diazoxide, ephedrine or glucagon. Portacaval shunting procedures have been reported to induce increased blood glucose levels, reduction of hyperlipemia, diminution of liver glycogen and lipid content, and improvement in growth. However, the procedure should be considered experimental at this time since encephalopathic changes may result, the shunts may close spontaneously with time, and simpler methods involving dietary manipulations, as outlined above, may achieve the same end.

ACIDOSIS. Episodes of lactic acidosis are not uncommon during infancy and are often associated with infections. Acidosis is worsened in the presence of dehydration. For acute acidosis (pH <7.2), give 2 mEq./kg. of intravenous bicarbonate suitably diluted with 5 per cent dextrose (such as 1 part to 5), and monitor the subsequent response. This dose should be sufficient to raise the serum bicarbonate level by approximately 5 mEq./liter. Buffering with sodium lactate is contraindicated. Parenteral glucose should also be given as indicated by the blood glucose level. For chronic acidosis, we use sodium bicarbonate, 2 to 4 mEq./kg./day in divided doses; that is, ½ teaspoon per feed for infants, and 0.5 to 1.0 gm. tablets 3 to 6 times daily for older infants and children.

HEMORRHAGIC DIATHESIS. A tendency to increased bleeding or bruising is common, with epistaxis being the most frequent manifestation. Studies have suggested that the origin of these problems lies in disordered platelet func-

---

* Vivonex—89 per cent of calories as glucose and glucose oligosaccharides, 1.8 per cent as safflower oil and 9.2 per cent as crystalline amino acids.

tioning. Application of cold compresses to the nose and face, together with rest, is all that is usually required. For severe epistaxis, nasal packing and transfusions of whole fresh blood or platelets are appropriate management. Major surgical procedures should be carefully planned and monitored.

HYPERURICEMIA. Raised blood levels of uric acid occur frequently, yet may be reduced by careful frequent feeding (as above). Transient joint pain may occur in young patients; however, gouty arthritis occurs mainly in older patients. If dietary management is insufficient to control uric acid levels, then allopurinol,* a methyl xanthine inhibitor, at a dose of from 5 to 10 mg./kg./day (maximum 300 mg.), is the drug of choice. Uric acid nephropathy should be prevented by maintaining as normal blood uric acid levels as possible and by avoiding chronic acidosis with frequent feeding regimens or alkalis.

HYPERLIPIDEMIA. In type I disease, triglyceride levels may be greatly raised with more modest elevations of blood cholesterol. Again, avoidance of hypoglycemia with accompanying elevations of glucagon, growth hormone and catecholamines, is associated with an improvement of lipid levels. However, should hyperlipidemia persist, clofibrate (Atromid-S)† can be used with effect at a dose of 50 mg./kg./day in 2 divided daily doses, although long-term trials with the drug still need to be carried out.

Type III. This disease results from a deficiency of amylo-1,6-glucosidase (debrancher enzyme). The patients have an illness similar to but milder than that with type I disease. Hypoglycemia on fasting accompanied by hepatomegaly of moderate severity are the usual clinical findings. Lactic acidosis, abnormal bleeding, hyperuricemia and hyperlipemia are not usual problems clinically. Treatment consists of avoiding prolonged fasting. A late night snack consisting of protein with carbohydrate is important. During intercurrent illnesses associated with poor food intake, carbonated drinks are useful to prevent hypoglycemia. The parents should be taught to test for ketonuria (Ketostix), as presence of ketones provides a warning that hypoglycemia is imminent. Glucagon is of no value for treatment of hypoglycemia, however Instant Glucose (see p. 342) may be administered at home

with effect. Diet restrictions as for type I do not apply; however, the diet should be high in protein.

Type VI and Type IX. These disorders result from deficiencies of hepatic phosphorylase and phosphorylase activating enzymes. The latter disease is sex-linked and is associated with a defect in phosphorylase kinase. These disorders resemble *type III disease* clinically and are much milder clinical disorders than type I. The therapy for these types has been outlined under type III.

Type IV. The disease results from a deficiency of alpha-1, 4 glucan: 1,4 glucan 6-glycosly transferase or brancher enzyme. Affected infants have progressive hepatomegaly with increasing signs of portal hypertension and congestive failure resulting in death within 2 years of life. Therapy is supportive. Attempts at specific therapy utilizing purified alpha glucosidase from *Aspergillus niger* have been encouraging but have not altered prognosis appreciably.

Muscle Glycogen Storage Syndromes

Type II (Pompe's disease). The disease results from a deficiency of the lysosomal hydrolase, acid maltase. Lack of this enzyme results in a massive accumulation of glycogen within cardiac muscle and neuromuscular tissue. Hypoglycemia is not a characteristic clinical finding. Cardiac hypertrophy with attendant cardiac failure is usually unremitting, and affected infants can seldom be supported beyond one year of age despite the use of antibiotics, digitalis, nasogastric feedings and the like. Specific therapy is unavailable although alpha glucosidase purified from a fungal source has been used with limited success.

Type V (McArdle's disease). The disease has been characterized as a deficiency of muscle phosphorylase. During the second decade, patients may suffer muscle fatigue on exercise. However, noncustomary exercise during adulthood precipitates the characteristic muscle pains, often in the calves, associated with red myoglobinuria. Fructose ingestion (30 gm.) prior to exercise may improve the capacity for exercise. However, recognition of the inability of the patient to withstand much muscular exercise will allow for avoidance of attacks. No specific therapies appear effective; however, apart from the rare occurrence of acute renal failure following an episode, longevity appears to be unaffected.

DISORDERS OF FRUCTOSE METABOLISM

The principal disorder involving fructose metabolism is that of hereditary fructose intolerance, and this condition needs to be dis-

---

*Manufacturer's precaution: Allopurinol is contraindicated in children with the exception of those with hyperuricemia secondary to malignancy.

†Clofibrate is not recommended by the manufacturer for use in children, and should be given with caution in all cases with apparent renal disease of hypoprothrombinemia. Serial hepatic enzymes should be monitored.

tinguished from the gluconeogenic defect, fructose-1, 6-diphosphatase deficiency and benign fructosuria.

Hereditary Fructose Intolerance

Severely affected infants may suffer hypoglycemia with vomiting, apnea and/or convulsions following sucrose-containing feedings. Continued sucrose feedings may lead to hepatomegaly with hepatic dysfunction (ascites, bleeding diathesis, jaundice and so on), Fanconi-like syndrome following renal damage, and recurrent hypoglycemia which may be accompanied by acidosis. Older infants and children have abdominal symptoms and hypoglycemia. The defect is one of deficiency of the enzyme fructose aldolase in liver, kidney and intestinal mucosa. Acute hypoglycemic episodes should be treated with intravenous glucose.

Sucrose should be strictly avoided in the diet. Besides sucrose-containing sweets, drinks and cookies, the following should be avoided completely: ham, bacon, lunch meats, sweet potatoes, all fruits and fruit juices, bread, sugar-containing cereals, salad dressings, most desserts, catsup, pickles, jam, preserves and honey. Allowable foods include beef, veal, lamb, pork, fish, poultry, cheese, cabbage, cauliflower, celery, green beans, lettuce, spinach, peppers, wax beans, white potatoes, macaroni, noodles, spaghetti, rice, crackers, nonsugared cereals, dietetic gelatin and ice cream, and vegetable juices (not tomato) and soups made from allowable meats and vegetables. All processed packaged foods should be viewed with suspicion and the list of contents carefully examined.

Friends and school teachers should be given a list of allowable foods and warned of the dangers of sucrose-containing food or drinks. Some potatoes, especially if fresh, certain vegetables such as broccoli, cucumber, and gourds, and some varieties of peas and rhubarb may contain small amounts of sucrose or fructose and should be viewed with caution and/or avoided. Invert sugar, sorbitol or levulose must never be administered intravenously. Whereas some tolerance to fructose develops over time, the above dieting principles should be lifelong.

Fructose-1, 6-Diphosphatase Deficiency

This disease manifests with hypoglycemic attacks which may be precipitated by fasting or by the ingestion of fructose or glycerol. Lactic acidosis usually accompanies hypoglycemia. The disease is often present within the first months of life and hepatomegaly may be ap-

parent. Feedings should be frequent and fasting avoided. Sucrose, fructose and sorbitol should be eliminated from the diet. A diet consisting of 56 per cent carbohydrate, 32 per cent fat and 12 per cent protein has resulted in normal growth and development. Acute hypoglycemic attacks must be treated promptly with intravenous glucose and sodium bicarbonate as required (see above), since fatalities have resulted from such episodes. Specific therapy is unavailable.

Essential Fructosuria. This is a rare and benign inborn error of carbohydrate metabolism. Fructose is a reducing sugar and reacts positively with Clinitest tablets or Benedict's solution, but not to the glucose oxidase system which is specific for glucose (Testape, Clinistix, Dextrostix). No treatment is required.

OTHER MELITURIAS

Sucrosuria may occur after sucrose ingestion in association with various gastrointestinal disorders, such as gastroenteritis. Sucrose is not a reducing sugar and may be detected by testing the urine with Clinitest tablets after hydrolysis of the urine with glacial acetic acid and boiling. In itself, sucrosuria is benign.

Benign pentosuria is another rare disorder which results in urinary excretion of L-xylulose but has no associated medical problems. The urine shows a constant small quantity of reducing sugar, which can be shown to be other than glucose by specific glucose oxidase (as above). Provided the patient is not mistakenly treated for diabetes, the condition is of little consequence.

Inborn Errors of Serum Lipoproteins

JUNE K. LLOYD, M.D., F.R.C.P.

PRIMARY HYPERLIPOPROTEINEMIAS

Familial Hyperchylomicronemia (Type I Hyperlipoproteinemia). The basis of therapy for this rare disorder is restriction of dietary fat. This will reduce, but usually not abolish, the hyperchylomicronemia and will alleviate the clinical features of eruptive xanthomata, abdominal pain and hepatosplenomegaly.

If the patient presents with an acute abdominal crisis, all fat should be withdrawn from the diet, and intravenous fluids may be required until the symptoms subside. If the presenting symptoms are less severe, reduction of dietary fat to between 2 and 5 gm./day will usually result in clearing of the grossly turbid serum and a fall in serum triglyceride toward normal values in about 7 to 10 days. Thereafter dietary fat may be increased to around 15 to 20 gm./day, provided that the child remains symptom-free. Tolerance of fat does not increase with age and a low-fat diet will have to be maintained on a life-long basis.

In order to improve the palatability of a low-fat diet, medium-chain triglycerides (MCT), whose fatty acids are largely absorbed into the portal vein and do not enter into chylomicron formation, may be used as an adjunct to therapy. MCT oil is useful for frying and baking, and filled dried milk preparations containing MCT can be used if energy requirements are not met by skim milk alone. MCT should never be used undiluted and by itself has no specific therapeutic effect. All children receiving low-fat diets require supplementary vitamins, and these should be given regularly in amounts corresponding to normal daily requirements.

Follow-up by a pediatrician is advisable throughout childhood in order that growth progress can be monitored, the serum lipoproteins periodically checked, and dietary problems discussed. Transfer of care to a physician knowledgeable about the disorder should occur at an appropriate age.

Familial Hyperbetalipoproteinemia (Type II Hyperlipoproteinemia, Familial Hypercholesterolemia). HETEROZYGOUS FORM. Most children with this disorder have the heterozygous form, with serum cholesterol concentraions ranging from 270 to 400 mg./100 ml. (6.9 to 10.2 mM/liter). Treatment designed to lower the serum cholesterol is instituted in the hope that the development of atheroma will be prevented or at least delayed. As treatment must be life-long, it is especially important that the diagnosis is correctly established and, although this is usually relatively easy, difficulties may be encountered when serum cholesterol levels are in the "borderline normal" area. Wherever possible, evidence of the same disorder in a first degree relative should be obtained, and the presence of tendinous xanthomata or premature coronary heart disease in an adult relative is helpful in this respect.

Treatment of children over the age of 1 year should be started as soon as the diagnosis is established. Boys and girls are usually treated equally even though the risk of subsequent coronary heart disease is less for the girls. Current therapy relies on diet or drugs or a combination of both.

Diet involves a reduction in ordinary fat intake (largely saturated fat) to about 15 to 20 gm./day. Such a diet is likely to be boring and can be made more palatable by the use of oils and margarines rich in polyunsaturated fat. Polyunsaturated fat itself, however, has no specific hypocholesterolemic effect in familial hypercholesterolemia. Limitation of dietary cholesterol to below 300 mg./day is stressed by some investigators, but as most dietary cholesterol consumed by children is in the form of eggs or other foods rich in saturated fat, a strict low-fat diet effectively limits cholesterol intake, and formal instructions regarding this component seem unnecessary. The description of the diet as a low-cholesterol diet should be discouraged, as this fails to emphasize that the most important aspect of the diet is the reduction in saturated fat.

Dietary treatment alone may be expected to achieve a reduction in serum cholesterol of about 20 per cent of the pretreatment value. If the aim of treatment is to achieve cholesterol levels below 250 mg./100 ml. (6.4 mM/liter), diet by itself is unlikely to be adequate therapy for children whose initial values are over 350 mg./100 ml. (8.9 mM/liter).

Dietary treatment, even when initially effective, is likely to prove difficult to maintain on a long-term basis; as many as 80 per cent of children may no longer have adequate control of serum cholesterol after the first 1½ to 2 years of dietary treatment. However, for the minority of children who achieve good long-term compliance and have a satisfactory response, diet alone can be expected to maintain reasonable levels of serum cholesterol over the years.

Drugs are likely to be needed for the control of hypercholesterolemia in the majority of children either because diet produces inadequate lowering of serum cholesterol, or because it is not adhered to over the years. Clofibrate has only a weak hypocholesterolemic effect in familial hypercholesterolemia; furthermore, it has to be given in conjunction with diet and for these reasons it probably has no place in the management of children with this disorder. Nicotinic acid and d-thryoxine have potential side effects which limit their use in pediatric practice.

Cholestyramine,* a nonabsorbable ion exchange resin which binds bile acids in the intes-

---

*Manufacturer's precaution: As experience in infants and children is limited, a practical dosage schedule has not been established. The effects of long term administration, as well as its effect in maintaining lowered cholesterol levels in pediatric patients, are unknown.

tine, is currently the drug of choice. It has been shown to be effective without the need for dietary restriction, and can be given in twice daily dosage. The amount of cholesterol lowering is proportional to the size of the dose, and reduction of about 35 per cent in serum cholesterol can be achieved with a mean daily dose of about 0.6 gm./kg. Compliance with this treatment is better than for any regimen involving a strict diet, but even so about 40 per cent fail to be satisfactorily controlled after 3 to 4 years. The major reason for nonadherence is unpalatability of the resin, and studies with more palatable and less bulky preparations are clearly indicated.

Side effects are limited to those caused by discomfort due to the bulk of the resin (rare in childhood), or due to interference with absorption. Folate deficiency occurs due to binding of folic acid to the resin, and can be corrected by additional oral folate (5 mg./day), which should always be given to children on long-term therapy. Steatorrhea and progressive lowering of serum concentrations of vitamins A and E and inorganic phosphate may occur, and, although no adverse clinical effects have been reported, long-term follow-up with investigations for possible adverse consequences need to be continued on all children receiving resin therapy.

The advisability of instituting treatment under the age of 1 year is still debatable. The diagnosis may be made at birth if one parent is known to be heterozygous for the disorder. Serum cholesterol concentrations in early infancy are lower in babies fed milk formulas with a high polyunsaturated fat content than in those who are breast fed or fed on cow's milk preparations containing butter fat. Breast feeding has so many advantages that it should certainly not be discouraged for such infants. Once bottle feeding is started, however, a formula with high polyunsaturated fat may be used, and foods with high saturated fat content can be avoided at weaning. Drugs are not indicated at this age.

Control of other risk factors for coronary heart disease is important in overall management. A combination of risk factors is known to greatly enhance the risk for coronary heart disease in adults, and investigations of children with familial hypercholesterolemia should include assessment of fatness and measurement of blood pressure, as well as inquiry about family smoking and exercise patterns. Obesity and hypertension should be treated and the risks of cigarette smoking explained. Parents should be told that the likelihood of children smoking becomes much greater if their parents smoke.

A parent who has the disorder, with or without clinical coronary heart disease, should stop smoking. Parents may be prepared to give up smoking for the sake of their children's health, even when they would not do it for their own.

Follow-up should be strictly maintained with regular estimations of serum cholesterol, the intervals between estimations depending upon individual response. Because overall compliance with current forms of treatment is poor, and new types of therapy need to be evaluated, children are probably best treated in clinics with special interest in and expertise with the disorder. Until more acceptable therapy is available and reasonable long-term compliance can be expected, it would seem appropriate to confine treatment to those children from families in which coronary heart disease has already occurred and motivation can be expected to be high. The psychological effects of treating outwardly healthy and symptom-free children with a restricted diet or unpleasant drugs have not been critically evaluated. Experience with high risk families who have themselves requested help suggests that, in this highly selected group, the need for treatment is well accepted and general family anxiety may be allayed, at least in the short term.

HOMOZYGOUS FORM. The homozygous form of familial hypercholesterolemia is rare, and serum cholesterol levels are usually over 800 mg./100 ml. (20.5 mM/liter). Because tendinous xanthomata and coronary heart disease occur during childhood, treatment is essential but unfortunately seldom satisfactory. Combined use of diet, cholestyramine (0.6 gm./kg./day, or as large a dose as can be tolerated in 2 or more doses per day), and nicotinic acid (100 mg./kg./day, or as large a dose as can be tolerated in 2 or more doses per day) appears to be the most effective medical regimen for lowering serum cholesterol, although levels below 500 mg./100 ml. (12.8 mM/liter) are seldom achieved. Such a regimen requires supplementation with folic acid, fat soluble vitamins, and possibly iron. Other procedures such as plasmapheresis, ileal bypass and portacaval shunt require further evaluation.

Broad-Beta Disease (Familial Type III Hyperlipoproteinemia). This form of hyperlipoproteinemia is rare during childhood. If the child is obese, weight reduction by means of diet in which calories and saturated fat are reduced is the initial treatment, and serum lipids may fall to normal. If hyperlipoproteinemia is not controlled by diet, clofibrate is the drug of choice and should be given twice daily in a dose of 20 to 30 mg./kg./day.

Primary Prebetalipoproteinemia (Famil-

ial Type IV Hyperlipoproteinemia). This is also a rare disorder in children. Reduction in dietary carbohydrate to 25 to 30 per cent of total calories may result in a fall in serum triglyceride concentrations to normal. Clofibrate, 20 to 30 mg./day, is likely to be the most effective drug.

PRIMARY HYPOLIPOPROTEINEMIAS

Abetalipoproteinemia. Replacement therapy with beta-apoprotein is not practicable; furthermore results of investigations in which plasma infusions have been used to keep circulating betalipoprotein at normal concentrations for as long as six days suggest that restoration of plasma levels alone may be ineffective. No improvement in fat absorption or in red cell morphology has been observed during such periods.

Treatment is therefore symptomatic. Steatorrhea can be controlled by reducing the intake of dietary fat, and this measure alone can result in marked clinical improvement and growth acceleration. The degree of fat restriction varies; some patients only tolerate 5 gm. of fat daily, whereas others can take up to 20 to 25 gm. Some polyunsaturated fat (for example, corn oil) may be included in the daily allowance of fat and will increase the linoleic acid content of plasma and tissue lipids; it is not known whether this is of clinical benefit. Medium-chain triglycerides, whose fatty acids are absorbed into the portal vein, may provide a useful additional source of calories for some patients and also improve the palatability of the low-fat diet. Large amounts of medium-chain triglycerides should be avoided, as competition for binding sites in the portal blood stream may exacerbate the malabsorption of long-chain triglycerides.

Additional fat soluble vitamins should be given orally. Normal quantities of vitamin D appear sufficient to prevent rickets, but large doses of vitamin A (up to 20,000 I.U./day) are required to maintain normal plasma levels. Vitamin K is important and enough should be given to maintain a normal prothrombin time. Vitamin E, 100/mg./kg./day divided in 3 or 4 doses, will usually result in correction of red cell peroxide hemolysis and may enable small amounts of the vitamin to be detected in the plasma.

Such a treatment regimen, started early in life as soon as the diagnosis is made, will not only maintain normal growth but will also probably delay the onset of the neurological and ophthalmological manifestations of the disorder.

Familial Hypobetalipoproteinemia. If steatorrhea is present, treatment with a low-fat diet as described for abetalipoproteinemia is indicated. In such cases additional fat soluble vitamins should be given, but very large doses of vitamins A and E are not required.

Tangier Disease (Familial High-Density Lipoprotein Deficiency). No treatment is known for this disorder.

Galactosemia

M. MICHAEL THALER, M.D.

The outstanding manifestations of untreated galactosemia are rapidly progressive liver disease, cataracts and the gradual appearance of mental retardation. Galactosemia can be fatal in early infancy, the mortality being due largely to cirrhosis and its complications (ascites, edema and bleeding). The most serious abnormalities in galactosemic children who survive past infancy are low intelligence and various poorly defined psychological problems.

A galactose-free diet is the only treatment available. Such a diet is dramatically effective in some respects: all signs of liver involvement disappear, and the development of cataracts is arrested or reversed. The effectiveness of strict dietary measures as protection against the deterioration of intellectual and psychological functions is less obvious, possibly because brain damage may have already occurred in utero in certain cases. Whether significant recovery from mental retardation is possible in galactosemia continues to be debated.

A galactose-free diet should be instituted as soon as galactosemia is suspected and before definitive proof can be obtained. Several galactose-free formulas are readily available, such as Nutramigen, soy protein, Cho-Free and meat base preparations. As the infant responds to treatment, his appetite rapidly increases, vomiting and diarrhea subside, jaundice disappears and weight gain is notable even after only a few days. In older children, any food containing milk or milk products should be omitted from the diet. Labels on canned and processed foods should be examined for the presence of lactose or galactose. Among meats, hot dogs and sausages should be avoided, as well as organ meats rich in galactose, such as liver, pancreas and brain. Most vegetables are safe, except those that have been buttered or creamed and those processed with lactose. Breads, rolls or biscuits made with milk should be excluded, as well as commercial cookies, cakes and custard puddings. Chocolate, milk-containing ice cream, and fruits processed with lactose complete the list of common forbidden foods. It is still unclear whether greater tolerance for galactose is acquired with age, but a strict diet should be maintained at least through the period of active growth and probably beyond.

The thoroughness with which galactose intake has been eliminated can be monitored with periodic determinations of galactose-1-phosphate in red cells.

Complications of galactosemia in young infants include dehydration and electrolyte losses due to vomiting and diarrhea, ascites due to portal hypertension and hypoalbuminemia, bleeding due to prothrombin deficiency and frequent infections. These problems should be treated according to standard measures described elsewhere in this text. Detailed growth and development records, supplemented with yearly intelligence tests, are useful indices of progress after infancy. The completeness with which galactose is excluded from the diet should be reevaluated when physical or intellectual growth shows signs of slowing down.

Cataracts which are refractory to dietary management may require surgical excision.

Disorders of Porphyrin, Hemoglobin, and Purine Metabolism

RICHARD D. LEVERE, M.D., *and* STANLEY L. WALLACE, M.D.

THE PORPHYRIAS

Congenital Erythropoietic Porphyria. This rare type of porphyria usually first makes its clinical appearance shortly after birth. Severe photosensitivity is the most disabling manifestation of this disorder of erythrocyte porphyrin metabolism, and avoidance of direct sunlight is mandatory. Also helpful is the use of protective clothing and barrier creams to shield out incident ultraviolet light. When cutaneous bullae and vesicles occur, they frequently become infected and should be treated with local and systemic antibiotics as indicated by the appropriate cultures.

Congenital erythropoietic porphyria is frequently complicated by hemolytic anemia, and the resulting anemia often requires blood transfusion. The transfusion requirement may be alleviated by splenectomy, but this procedure should be postponed until as late in childhood as possible because of the repeated exposure to skin infections and the possibility of resultant sepsis.

Erythrodontia (pinkish-brown discoloration of the teeth due to porphyrin deposition) is another cardinal manifestation of this disease. If cosmetically disturbing it may be treated with jacket crowns, but this treatment may prove difficult because of the frequently associated gingivitis which may lead to loss of the crowns.

Congenital Erythropoietic Protoporphyria. This disorder of erythroid porphyrin metabolism is less rare than erythropoietic porphyria, but the symptomatology is much milder in intensity. Photosensitivity is the most disturbing manifestation, and protection from sunlight, coupled with protective clothing and barrier creams, is essential. The production of carotenemia with the oral administration of 30 mg. of beta-carotene beadlets once a day has been reported useful in the management of the photosensitivity. Hemolytic anemia is a rare complication of this disease, but when it does occur it may be ameliorated by splenectomy.

Acute Intermittent Porphyria. Development of clinical symptomatology in this form of hepatic porphyria is frequently precipitated by exposure to various exogenous agents. Barbiturates, sulfonamides, ethyl sulfones, griseofulvin and sulfonylureas have been known to produce acute exacerbations of acute porphyria and are, therefore, contraindicated in anyone with a personal or family history of the disease. During periods of remission strict attention should be directed toward the maintenance of good nutrition, since a diet deficient in carbohydrate can predispose the patient to an acute attack.

Large quantities of carbohydrate, in the form of glucose in water, should be used to treat the acute attack. This requires the placement of a catheter into one of the great veins so as to permit infusion of 10 to 15 per cent glucose solutions in order to reach a goal of 450 to 600 gm. of glucose administered in each 24 hour period. Pain and distress are best treated with chlorpromazine; opiates should be discouraged because of the fear of addiction. Inappropriate secretion of antidiuretic hormone is a not infrequently associated feature of the acute attack. The resultant hyponatremia should be managed with fluid restriction, and if refractory, by the cautious intravenous administration of hypertonic NaCl solution. Severe hypertension may occasionally accompany the acute attack and this should be managed in the same manner as primary malignant hypertension. Propranolol,* 40 to 240 mg. daily, has

---

*Manufacturer's precaution: Data on dosages of propranol in children are too limited to permit adequate directions for use.

also been successfully used to treat the hypertension and tachycardia accompanying acute attacks.

Paralysis of the muscles of respiration with resultant respiratory insufficiency is a common mode of death. Since paresis is often reversible in acute porphyria, this manifestation should be treated vigorously with the hope of maintaining life until remission occurs. The patient is best treated in a respiratory care unit with a tracheostomy and a mechanical respirator while blood gases are constantly monitored.

Recently, intravenous hematin has been used experimentally during acute attacks with dramatically beneficial effects in the few patients so treated.

Congenital Cutaneous Hepatic Porphyria (Porphyria Variegata).   This disorder of porphyrin metabolism is often exacerbated by the same drugs which adversely affect acute intermittent porphyria, and therefore they are contraindicated in these patients as well. Photosensitivity is a cardinal manifestation and should be managed by protection from sunlight and barrier creams. Oral administration of cholestyramine in a dose of 12 gm. per day* may prove helpful in the management of the cutaneous lesions because of its ability to bind porphyrins in the intestinal tract and prevent their reabsorption. Caution must be exercised when using cholestyramine to make sure that the patient does not become depleted of fat-soluble vitamins. When acute neurological symptoms develop in this form of porphyria they are managed as described under acute intermittent porphyria.

Acquired Hepatic Porphyria (Porphyria Cutanea Tarda Symptomatica).   This type of porphyria may be seen in patients with alcoholic cirrhosis or with chronic exposure to certain chemicals such as hexachlorobenzene, ethyl sulfone, stilbestrol, griseofulvin and sulfonylureas. The majority of these patients have associated chronic liver disease which requires dietary management. The photosensitivity should be managed as outlined for the congenital porphyrias. In addition, iron-unloading by repeated phlebotomies has proven helpful in those patients who have demonstrated evidence of hepatic hemosiderosis. The goal of this venesection therapy is to remove a total of 3 to 3.5 gm. of iron.

METHEMOGLOBINEMIA AND SULFHEMOGLOBINEMIA

Hereditary Methemoglobinemia with Normal Hemoglobin Structure. *Congenital*

methemoglobin reductase (diaphorase) deficiency is usually due to a deficiency of NADH-methemoglobin reductase (diaphorase I). Hereditary deficiency of NADPH-methemoglobin reductase (diaphorase II) is not associated with methemoglobinemia unless the patient is exposed to oxidant drugs. A transient deficiency of NADH-methemoglobin reductase may occasionally be seen in newborn infants of mothers who receive prilocaine during caudal anesthesia.

Patients with methemoglobin reductase deficiency usually do not require treatment except for cosmetic reasons (to decrease the associated cyanosis). Chronic oral administration of either ascorbic acid or methylene blue will decrease the cyanosis and can be useful in alleviating any associated symptoms such as headache. Ascorbic acid is given in a dose of 300 to 600 mg. per day and methylene blue at a dose of 60 mg. four times a day. Care should be taken when administering methylene blue, since excessive doses may be toxic and cause an increase in methemoglobinemia.

Towne's variant of hereditary methemoglobinemia is associated with normal levels of methemoglobin reductase but a decrease in total erythrocyte glutathione content. These patients also respond to orally administered ascorbic acid.

Hereditary methemoglobinemia with abnormal hemoglobin structure is seen in association with hemoglobin M and the unstable hemoglobins (Zürich, Köln, etc.). Patients with unstable hemoglobins are particularly sensitive to oxidant drugs, and these should be avoided. Ascorbic acid and methylene blue are of no value. Transfusion may be necessary if hemolysis and the associated anemia are severe.

Congenital sulfhemoglobinemia is extremely rare and relatively benign and requires no therapy.

Acquired Methemoglobinemia. A number of drugs are capable of activating the oxidation of ferrous hemoglobin to ferric hemoglobin, leading to methemoglobinemia. Nitrites, sulfonamides and aniline derivatives have been the most frequently incriminated. Other compounds include acetanilid, phenacetin, chlorates, quinones, sulfones, and nitrobenzene. Infants and children may acquire methemoglobinemia from aniline dyes used in marking inks on diapers or other clothing. Aniline dyes may also be absorbed from recently dyed blankets or shoes. Benzocaine ointments have also been implicated in the production of methemoglobinemia in children. Children may also be affected by drinking well water with a high nitrite content.

Acute and severe drug-induced methe-

*Manufacturer's precaution: Dosage of cholestyramine resin for infants and children has not been established.

moglobinemia requires treatment with intravenous methylene blue. The recommended dosage for infants is 2 mg./kg., for older children 1.5 mg/kg., given as a 1 per cent aqueous solution. If cyanosis persists the dose may be repeated in 1 to 2 hours. In extremely severe cases transfusion may be indicated. Milder cases may require only discontinuance of exposure to the offending agent. If mild symptoms are present oral ascorbic acid or methylene blue should be administered as described in the section dealing with hereditary methemoglobinemia.

Acquired Sulfhemoglobinemia. The same drugs which cause methemoglobinemia may also lead to sulfhemoglobinemia; however, sulfhemoglobin cannot be reduced. Treatment consists of removal of any causative agent and correction of constipation when present. If anoxia occurs transfusion is indicated.

MYOGLOBINURIA

Familial Myoglobinuria (Meyer-Betz Disease). Infection or severe exertion may precipitate acute episodes of this disease, and strenuous activity is therefore contraindicated in susceptible individuals. Acute attacks may be associated with severe muscle weakness and respiratory paralysis, which should be treated with a mechanical respirator. The degree of associated renal insufficiency usually determines the ultimate prognosis, and this complication should be treated in the usual manner.

Secondary Myoglobinuria. Myoglobinuria may be seen in association with crush injuries, high-voltage electric shock, extensive infarction as in the main artery of a limb, alcoholic polymyopathy and polymyositis. If respiratory failure occurs, respiration must be supported. Among the predisposing factors, crush injury is the most common cause of associated renal failure, which should be treated in the usual manner.

Myoglobinuria in McArdle's Syndrome. Severe exertion may cause myoglobinuria in McArdle's syndrome (myophosphorylase deficiency glycogenosis). Patients should be instructed to limit activities, avoid tight garments and increase carbohydrate intake before attempting increased physical exertion.

GOUT

Traditionally, the treatment of gout is divided into three parts: (1) control of the acute episode, (2) prevention of subsequent attacks, and (3) dissolution of tophaceous deposits or stones by reducing the serum urate level to normal. Juvenile and adolescent gout is almost always associated with significant urate overproduction. For this reason, the prevention of recurrences and the treatment of deposited urate can be considered together.

The four most effective agents in the treatment of acute attacks of gout are colchicine, phenylbutazone,* indomethacin* and adrenocorticotropic hormone. The earlier in the course of the acute attack any of these are used, the more effective the drug is in eradicating the episode.

Colchicine has both diagnostic and therapeutic value in acute gout. A dramatic, objective response in an inflamed joint strongly suggests that the patient has had acute gout. The drug is given by mouth as a single 0.5 mg. or 0.6 mg. tablet once hourly, until one of three eventualities occurs: objective improvement, gastrointestinal side effects, or, if neither of the preceding occurs first, an arbitrary maximum dose. For the adolescent, the oral colchicine dose should not exceed 6 mg. as total therapy for an attack; the size of the total dose should be roughly proportional to body size and weight. However, about 80 per cent of patients so treated develop major gastrointestinal side effects, including abdominal cramping, diarrhea, nausea and vomiting. For this reason, colchicine should be given intravenously if possible rather than by mouth. The effective dose is 1 to 3 mg. as a single total dose with the dose again selected according to body size and weight. Gastrointestinal side effects occur very rarely after intravenous colchicine. Colchicine solutions are strong chemical irritants, so that it is vital to be certain that the material is being given well into the vein, and slowly.

Phenylbutazone* is effective in 90 per cent of patients with acute gout. Once the diagnosis is made, phenylbutazone is the orally administered drug of choice. Doses vary with body size, ranging from 200 to 500 mg. per day for 3 days, in divided doses. Indomethacin is about as effective as phenylbutazone, in divided doses of 75 to 200 mg. per day for 5 days.* However, with these doses, frequent gastrointestinal and central nervous system side effects occur. Several of the newer nonsteroidal anti-inflammatory drugs (ibuprofen, fenoprofen) have been shown to be moderately effective in adult gout; experience with these agents in adolescents is limited. Adrenocorticotropic hormone, in doses of 100 mg. of the

---

*Manufacturer's note: Phenylbutazone and indomethacin are contraindicated in children under 14 years of age.

gel intramuscularly daily for 5 days, is effective in the treatment of acute gout. However, as many as one third of patients so treated rebound after therapy with an acute gouty recurrence. Adrenocorticotropic hormone therefore must be given with and followed by colchicine therapy, 0.6 mg./day for 14 days, to prevent the flareup.

Treatment to prevent recurrences and to dissolve tophi and stones involves the return of the miscible pool of urate to normal. The miscible pool can be considered normal 6 or more months after the last recognized tophus has disappeared, or in the patient without visible tophi, after about 1 year of a normal serum urate level.

Drugs capable of lowering serum urate levels include a xanthine oxidase inhibitor and several uricosuric drugs. Allopurinol,* the xanthine oxidase inhibitor, lowers both serum and urinary urate levels. Doses must be titrated to accomplish the urate level reduction needed. Such doses range from 100 to 500 mg. per day. Toxic effects are infrequent. Severe disseminated vasculitis has been reported. Mild cutaneous vasculitides, hepatocellular chemical changes, and nausea and diarrhea may occur. Allopurinol has also been shown to alter enzyme function in liver microsomes, prolonging the half-life of bishydroxycoumarin and antipyrine by inhibiting their biotransformation.

When allopurinol has reduced the serum level to normal, but deposited urate still persists, there is an increased potential for new attacks of acute gout. Colchicine is necessary, in doses of 0.6 mg. once daily, to prevent these, and must be given with allopurinol until the urate miscible pool is normal (see above).

For those rare patients with juvenile or adolescent gout unable to tolerate allopurinol, the uricosuric drugs probenecid, sulfinpyrazone and aspirin are available. These reduce serum levels but increase urinary urate content. Probenecid† doses range from 0.5 to 2 gm. per day, while sulfinpyrazone doses range from 100 to 400 mg. per day. Aspirin doses need to be large enough to produce serum levels of at least 20 mg./100 ml., and gastrointestinal distress may follow. The major risk in the use of any of these agents is the precipitation of renal calculus. Large fluid intake and urinary output is imperative in conjunction with their use. Triggering of fresh attacks of gout is also possible with these agents; colchicine, 0.6 mg. per day, should be given along with them.

Dietary restrictions can be mild, with the elimination only of foods high in purine content, such as organ meats (kidneys, sweetbreads, brain and liver), anchovies, sardines, meat extracts and wild game.

HYPERURICEMIA DUE TO HEMATOLOGIC NEOPLASMS AND THEIR TREATMENT

Hyperuricemia occurs frequently in association with leukemia and lymphoma; the treatment of these disorders with cytolytic agents leads to major overproduction of uric acid due to the rapid breakdown of cellular nucleic acids. This in turn may result in the precipitation of uric acid in the upper and lower urinary tract, and sometimes in total urinary obstruction.

Treatment of choice in the prevention of such precipitation is the use of allopurinol. Since it takes about 72 hours for allopurinol to reach its maximal inhibition of xanthine oxidase, with the consequent maximal lowering of serum and urinary urate concentrations, allopurinol therapy in these disorders should precede cytotoxic therapy by at least 3 days, and preferably 5 to 7 days, if possible. In situations where pretreatment is not feasible, allopurinol should be used concurrently with cytotoxic agents. Optimal doses range from 100 to 500 mg. per day, roughly according to body weight. However, individual measurement of serum urate is necessary to accomplish the appropriate reduction.

Mercaptopurine is also degraded by xanthine oxidase. For this reason, when the cytotoxic agents mercaptopurine and azathioprine are used in conjunction with allopurinol, doses of the former must be reduced sharply. Potential toxic manifestations of allopurinol are described above. Since allopurinol interferes with xanthine oxidase function, patients receiving this agent excrete increased amounts of xanthine and hypoxanthine. Xanthine stones have been reported during such therapy in one patient with lymphosarcoma and two children with Lesch-Nyhan syndrome (see below).

Other therapeutic approaches to minimizing uric acid lithiasis during treatment of hematologic neoplasms include (1) cautious initiation of cytolytic therapy; (2) vigorous administration of fluids; and (3) administration of alkali or acetazolamide in an attempt to alkalinize the urine, thus increasing solubility of uric acid.

Once uric acid is already precipitated, al-

---

*Manufacturer's note: Pending further investigation, allopurinol is contraindicated for use in children with the exception of those with hyperuricemia secondary to malignancy.

†Manufacturer's note: Probenecid is contraindicated in children under 2 years of age.

lopurinol, fluid and alkali therapy may not be adequate, and peritoneal dialysis or hemodialysis may be required.

LESCH-NYHAN SYNDROME

The profound uric acid overproduction in the Lesch-Nyhan syndrome (hyperuricemia associated with choreoathetosis, mental retardation, and self-mutilation), caused by severe deficiency of hypoxanthine-guanine phosphoribosyl transferase, is characteristically associated with hyperuricosuria and with urate gravel or stone. Optimal therapy must include allopurinol in doses sufficient to return the serum urate level and urinary excretion of urate to normal. Customary doses range from 100 to 300 mg. of allopurinol per day in divided amounts, but must be individually titrated to accomplish the desired reduction in serum and urinary urate levels. Increasing the fluid intake and urinary output (diluting the excreted uric acid and the increased xanthinuria associated with allopurinol therapy) also is of value in preventing uric acid or xanthine stones.

There is no evidence that allopurinol, even if therapy is initiated at birth, can prevent the neurologic manifestations of the syndrome.

OROTIC ACIDURIA

Uridine* in divided doses totaling 150 mg./kg./day has resulted in hematologic remission in orotic aciduria, with decreased urinary excretion of orotic acid. A uridine-resistant patient has been reported to respond partially to folic and folinic acid (2.5 mg. per day), with a bone marrow remission and a rise in hemoglobin. Glucocorticoid therapy can produce a partial hematologic remission without reversal of the megaloblastic marrow. Prednisone in doses of 10 to 20 mg. per day by mouth will accomplish this result. A large fluid intake will dilute urinary orotic acid and minimize the likelihood of precipitation. Uracil has been shown to be ineffective as therapy.

XANTHINURIA

The purpose of treatment in xanthinuria is to inhibit the formation of xanthine stones. Reducing the concentration of xanthine in the urine in patients with xanthinuria can be accomplished either by restricting the content of purine in the diet, or by increasing the fluid intake, or preferably both. Foods high in purine content include the organ meats, meat

---

*Uridine is investigational.

extracts and concentrates (gravies, etc.), anchovies, sardines and wild game.

Xanthine has limited solubility in acid urine, so that alkalinization of the urine may be necessary in selected cases. However, the hazards of continuous alkalinization of the urine (calcium stones, infection with certain alkaline-preferring organisms) must be considered. Once xanthine stones are present, surgical removal may be necessary.

Lipid Storage Diseases

LARRY J. SHAPIRO, M.D., and
MICHAEL M. KABACK, M.D.

The genetic lipidoses are a group of inherited disorders with highly variable modes of onset, organ system involvement, and clinical courses. In spite of this diversity, major advances have been made in the past decade which bring this seemingly disparate group of disorders together. The first description of a disease state in man due to deficient activity of a lysosomal enzyme occured in 1963. Since that time, approximately 40 distinct clinical entities have been identified which share a common pathogenetic mechanism: massive intralysosomal accumulation of a naturally occurring biopolymer which takes place because of a genetically determined reduction in activity of a specific acid hydrolase.

The lipid storage diseases as well as the mucopolysaccharidoses and mucolipidoses are examples of these disorders. It is thought that the varied manifestations of these conditions are a function of the type of macromolecules which accumulate, the rate at which the accretion of polymer occurs, and the specific tissues in which the storage is found. It is outside the scope of this section to describe in detail the clinical features or biochemical findings of these disorders. However, those conditions in which lipid accumulation predominates are listed in Table 1 along with the relevant enzyme deficiency and stored molecule.

At the present time, no effective, specific therapy exists for these diseases. Evaluation of a number of treatment modalities has been attempted but has been hampered by several innate features of most of these conditions. First, they are relatively rare disorders and so it is difficult for a single center to accumulate enough experience with therapy to get meaningful results. Second, these disorders have an insidious and progressive clinical course. There is evidence that pathologic lipid storage commences in fetal life and often precedes

TABLE 1. Lipid Storage Diseases

CLINICAL DISORDER	AGE OF ONSET	INITIAL SIGNS OR SYMPTOMS	PROGNOSIS	MATERIAL STORED	ENZYME DEFECT	MANAGEMENT*
GM₁ Gangliosidoses Generalized	Neonatal	Bone deformities, organomegaly, course facies, cherry red spot	Death by age 2	GM_1 ganglioside	Acid β-galactosidase	HD,† PD†
Juvenile	6 to 18 mos.	Weakness, seizures, ataxia	Death by 5 to 10 yrs.	GM_1 ganglioside $\pm$ Mucopolysaccharide $\pm$ Glycoprotein	Acid β-galactosidase	HD, PD
GM₂ Gangliosidoses Type I—Tay-Sachs disease	4 to 8 mos.	No organomegaly, hyperacousis, weakness, slow development, cherry red spot, Ashkenazi Jews (predominantly)	Death by age 5	GM_2 ganglioside	Hexosaminidase A	HD,† PD† population screening
Type II—Sandhoff's disease	4 to 8 mos.	Organomegaly, cherry red spot, developmental delay	Death by age 5	GM_2 ganglioside	Hexosaminidase A and B	HD,† PD†
Type III—Juvenile	1 to 2 yrs.	Spasticity and weakness	Death by 5 to 15 yrs.	GM_2 ganglioside	Hexosaminidase A (partial)	HD, PD
Gaucher's Disease Infantile	Neonatal	Strabismus, opisthotonus, CNS impairment, organomegaly	Death by age 2	Glucocerebroside	Glucocerebrosidase (Acid) (β-glucosidase)	HD,† PD†
Juvenile	4 to 8 yrs.	Visceromegaly, retardation, Swedish (predominantly)	Death by 10 to 15 yrs.	Glucocerebroside	Glucocerebrosidase	HD, PD
Adult	Any	Massive splenomegaly, bone disease, Ashkenazi Jews (predominantly)	Variable	Glucocerebroside	Glucocerebrosidase	HD,† PD†
Niemann-Pick Disease Type I—Infantile	Infancy	Retardation, visceromegaly, cherry red spot, Ashkenazi Jews (predominantly)	Death by age 3	Sphingomyelin	Sphingomyelinase	HD,† PD†
Type II—Adult	Any (adolescence most common)	Visceromegaly, CNS spared	Variable	Sphingomyelin	Sphingomyelinase	HD, PD
Type III—Late infantile	Early to mid-childhood	Mild visceromegaly, progressive retardation	Death by adolescence	Sphingomyelin	Unknown	
Type IV—Nova Scotia	Early to mid-childhood	Visceromegaly, retardation, Nova Scotian	Death by adolescence	Sphingomyelin	Unknown	
Metachromatic Leukodystrophy Type I—Late infantile	12 to 14 mos.	Motor dysfunction, ataxia, spasticity, progressive deterioration	Death by 5 to 6 yrs.	Cerebroside Sulfatide	Cerebroside Sulfatidase (Arylsulfatase A)	HD,† PD†

Continued

TABLE 1. Lipid Storage Diseases (continued)

CLINICAL DISORDER	AGE OF ONSET	INITIAL SIGNS OR SYMPTOMS	PROGNOSIS	MATERIAL STORED	ENZYME DEFECT	MANAGEMENT*
Type II—Juvenile	4 to 8 yrs.	Ataxia, spasticity, progressive deterioration	Death by 10 to 15 yrs.	Cerebroside Sulfatide	Cerebroside Sulfatidase (Arylsulfatase A)	HD,† PD†
Type III—Adult	15 yrs. or greater	Dementia, depression, motor signs	Prolonged survival	Cerebroside Sulfatide	Cerebroside Sulfatidase (Arylsulfatase A)	HD,† PD†
Type IV—Multiple sulfatase deficiency	1 to 2 yrs.	Similar to late infantile MLD, visceromegaly	Death by age 10	Cerebroside Sulfatide Mucopolysaccharide ? Steroid sulfates	Arylsulfatase A, B, C Iduronate sulfatase Heparan sulfamidase	HD, PD
Krabbe's Disease	Early infancy	Blindness, seizures, spasticity	Death by age 2	Galactocerebroside	Galactocerebrosidase	HD,† PD†
Fabry's Disease	15 yrs. or greater	Angiokeratoma, corneal opacities, renal failure, pain crises, X-linked inheritance	Dependent upon renal and cardiovascular diseases	Cerebroside trihexoside	Cerebroside trihexosidase Acid α-Galactosidase	HD,† PD† Renal dialysis Renal transplantation
Fucosidosis	1st few yrs.	Skeletal abnormalities, neurologic deterioration, frequent infections, hepatomegaly, skeletal involvement, ± rash, ± increased sweat electrolytes	Death usual 5 to 10 yrs.	Fucose-containing lipids, glycoproteins, and polysaccharides	α-L-fucosidase	HD,† PD†
Batten's Ceroid Lipofuscinoses						
Type I—Jansky-Bielschowsky	2 to 4 yrs.	Seizures, late blindness, dementia	Death by age 8	Lipofuscin	Unknown	
Type II—Spielmeyer-Vogt	6 to 10 yrs.	Blindness, late seizures, dementia	Death in 2nd decade	Lipofuscin	Unknown	
Type III—Kufs' disease	15 yrs. or greater	Psychosis, progressive dementia, late blindness	Death in 3rd decade	Lipofuscin	Unknown	
Farber's Disease	Infancy (usually)	Hoarse cry, restriction of joint mobility, subcutaneous lipogranulomas	Death usually in 1st or 2nd yr.	Ceramide	Ceramidase	HD, PD
Wolman's Disease	Infancy	GI symptoms, failure to thrive, hepatosplenomegaly, adrenal calcifications	Death in 15+ yr.	Neutral lipids, particularly cholesterol esters	Acid lipase	HD, PD
Cholesterol Ester Storage Disease	Infancy 0 to 20 yrs.	Hepatomegaly with marked lipid accumulation, failure to thrive, hyperlipidemia, increased plasma low-density lipoprotein	Prolonged survival	Triglycerides Cholesteryl esters	Acid lipase	HD, PD

*HD = heterozygote detection potentially possible; PD = prenatal diagnosis potentially possible.

physical signs and symptoms. It is uncertain in most of the lipidoses how much tissue damage is irreversible and how much could be remedied by postnatal removal of excessively accumulated lipid. Therefore, therapeutic experiments performed at different stages in the evolution of the natural history of these diseases might give different results.

The third factor hampering therapeutic progress is the increasing appreciation of heterogeneity of the clinical features in these disorders. New, biochemically indistinguishable variants are being described at a rapid rate, making the direct comparison of different treatment modalities quite difficult. A fourth source of problems comes from the relative lack of meaningful physiologic or chemical parameters which can be objectively quantitated during the evaluation of potential therapies.

In spite of all of these problems, much has been learned regarding the clinical management of these patients. Through the use of appropriate supportive symptomatic therapy such as orthopedic procedures, physical therapy, antibiotics, anticonvulsant medication and the like, it has been possible to extend the length and hopefully the quantity of life of these patients. Careful attention to diet, including the use of blendarized tube feedings and adequate hydration, can improve the often compromised nutritional status of the patient. Bowel care and judicious use of stool softeners can obviate the frequent problems of fecal impaction in the terminal stages of these diseases. More specific therapies such as splenectomy in adult patients with Gaucher's disease with sequestration of formed blood elements, and kidney transplantation and/or dialysis in patients with Fabry's disease with end-stage renal disease are clearly of benefit.

Since the causal association of specific hydrolase deficiencies with lipid storage diseases has been appreciated, consideration has been given to enzyme replacement therapy. Many potential sources and routes of delivery of enzyme have been considered including bacterial, plant, or other heterologous enzymes (with predictable immunologic complications), crude human enzymes in the form of plasma, purified human enzymes (usually from placenta), and transplantation of leukocytes, spleen, liver, kidney, and skin fibroblasts in attempts to restore lysosomal function. To date no sustained objective clinical improvement has been documented where such efforts have been made, although there is some encouraging preliminary data. Most investigators now feel that the proper preparation, "packaging," modification, and routes of administration will be crucial to any future successes in this area. One substantive issue in those diseases with a substantial cerebral component of lipid storage is whether or not sufficient quantities of enzyme placed in the vascular compartment by any means can effectively negotiate the blood brain barrier.

Although enzyme replacement therapy appears at least several years off, and direct manipulation of the genome even further in the future, a number of positive alternatives in the management and treatment of *families* in which lipid storage diseases occur have developed within the past several years. Adequate genetic and reproductive counseling can be of great value in alleviating the serious burden of genetic disease on a family. The inheritance patterns of these diseases are now well understood and accurate recurrence risks can be given. They are all inherited as autosomal recessive traits except for Fabry's disease which is X-linked. Carrier detection is possible for most of these conditions, and large scale population screening for heterozygotes for Tay-Sachs disease has been accomplished.

Finally, accurate mid-trimester prenatal diagnosis has either been achieved or is possible for the remaining disorders. This capability offers a positive alternative to many "at risk" families, enabling them to have normal children without fear of recurrence of the disease in question. The physician treating a child with a lipid storage disease as with any other heritable malady must remind himself that his interest and influence can and must extend to the family at large.

11

Connective Tissue

The Rheumatic Diseases

JOHN J. MILLER, III, M.D., PH.D.

Although the causes of the "rheumatic" or "collagen" diseases of children remain unknown, they are all assumed to be manifestations of altered immune responses. Deposition of antigen-antibody complexes is probably triggering the complement system in some of these diseases. In others, abnormal reactivity of thymus-derived cells (T-cells) may be more important. In all, both mechanisms may play some part. All these diseases are treated by attempting to reduce the effects of inflammation or to stop the abnormal immunologic reactivity. Similar manifestations of the different diseases are treated similarly, and some important general principles apply to all.

Patience and a good relationship with the family are essential. All of the diseases are chronic and none has a medical cure. The courses are unpredictable and relapses may occur after prolonged remissions. Nevertheless, the prognosis for all has improved in the last two decades. Active parental and patient cooperation is necessary for optimal treatment. These require time for education by physicians and by other therapists. The chronicity creates frustration in child, parent, and physician and exacerbates whatever social problems the family already has. A large amount of misinformation is fed to parents about these diseases. Overly bleak expectations may be based on older family members' experiences or older medical literature. Outright quackery is heavily sold to the arthritic patient. Often the most appropriate treatment appears trivial to the parents. All these problems must be handled realistically and patiently. Explanations and trust must be adequate to gain compliance.

The drugs used to treat these diseases are dangerous. Mortality in all the rheumatic diseases of children is now more commonly due to the treatment than to a manifestation of the disease. This applies most specifically to the adrenocorticosteroids and immunolytic drugs. In addition to the increased danger of infection and hypertension, steroids are now known to increase blood lipids and probably produce precocious arteriosclerosis. Chronic use of the immunolytic drugs appears to increase the risk of lymphoreticular neoplasms and opportunistic infections.

Treat the manifestations, not the diagnosis. The particular diagnosis defines the long-term prognosis and potential complications; however, most of these diseases share manifestations which can be treated effectively by the same methods. For instance, splints and salicylates are useful in treating the arthritis of juvenile rheumatoid arthritis (JRA), systemic lupus erythematosus (SLE), or dermatomyositis. Life-threatening manifestations of any of the diseases are treated vigorously with adrenocorticosteroids in essentially similar ways. However, when considering treatment it is important to be sure that all active manifestations of the particular disease are being covered; these will vary with the diagnosis. Thus, if arthritis flares in a patient with SLE, a search must be made for asymptomatic nephritis, which would require strenuous therapy, whereas this would not be a consideration if the diagnosis were JRA.

Do not "cold turkey" anti-inflammatory drugs. Suddenly stopping aspirin, adrenocorticosteroids, and even the immunolytic drugs will often result in a severe flare of disease. This is true whether a disease is mildly active or in apparent remission. The need for slow tapering of adrenocorticosteroids is generally understood but even aspirin should be withdrawn over at least a two week period. Occasionally this phenomenon is a helpful diagnostic aid in a child who is referred with an equivocal history and who is already under treatment, but a sudden withdrawal for diagnostic purposes should be done in a hospital.

Use allied health professionals fully. Very often the physical therapist or occupational therapist, who sees the child more frequently and who is less threatening to the child than the physician, will know more about the psychosocial and medical status. On occasion a nurse or teacher may have this role. These therapists are sources of information for the physician, and serve as important channels of education for child and family.

JUVENILE RHEUMATOID ARTHRITIS

Physical therapy and drug therapy are the two essential components of the treatment of JRA. Surgery is sometimes required and orthopedic surgeons or physiatrists should be consulted to help in long-range planning for the severely involved children.

Physical Therapy. Balanced programs of rest and exercise are essential to maintain joint function and position. An important paradox must be appreciated in planning physical therapy: resting a joint reduces the inflammation but rapidly causes loss of strength and of range of motion. Do not completely immobilize a joint in a cylindrical cast. Inflamed joints can be splinted or kept in a bivalved cast if they are moved for brief periods once or twice a day, but they must be moved. Less active joints should be moved more vigorously and for longer periods. During remissions, exercises to increase and maintain strength are needed.

The prescription for therapy must also be adjusted for the personalities and experiences of both child and therapist. A therapist experienced with rheumatoid children can safely perform gentle passive exercises for range of motion. If the therapist is more accustomed to spastic children, passive exercises may be performed too vigorously (a particular hazard for fingers). Thus active exercises which allow the child to control the degree of motion are usually better. Few children will perform so vigorously as to harm themselves. However, occasional problems with motivating children to do enough will be found if only active exercises are prescribed.

The application of heat before a therapy session reduces pain and aids muscle relaxation, which allows greater motion and more productive exercise. Since water is buoyant and protects joints from the stress of weight bearing, exercise in warm water is ideal.

Contractures or subluxations of wrists or knees can be prevented by the use of night splints. Splints for knees should be made in the maximal possible degree of extension. Wrist splints should be in a slightly dorsiflexed, neutral position and should include the fingers at night. A wrist splint allowing finger flexion may be used during the day to provide both wrist stability and hand function. A number of materials are available for making splints. The older heat-labile plastics such as Orthoplast or Prenyl tend to lose shape. Newer plastics such as Polyform are more stable and lighter. Cheap and easily replaceable splints can be made by molding four or five layers of a resin-containing plaster (Zoroc) to the joint. A thin plaster splint may be strengthened and made permanent by applying a soluble plastic to the back of the plaster (Aircast, if available). When hard, this makes a cheap, light, durable, and nonirritating splint.

Appropriate placement of pillows or towels around a patient in bed may be used for short or long periods to maintain the position of joints which cannot be splinted. Lying in prone position helps to prevent hip and knee flexion contractures. It is important to remember that most contractures appear because of the tendency to flex joints to decrease pain, and that extension is easier to maintain than it is to regain.

Medical Therapy. Aspirin is still the mainstay in the treatment of arthritis. Starting doses should be 100 mg./kg./day, but this usually needs adjustment. The dosage should be split evenly and given four times per day, with meals and a bedtime snack. The enzymes that detoxify aspirin have complex kinetics, and a consistent serum level is not reached for two weeks. Parents should be warned about the signs or symptoms of hypersalicylism: hyperventilation in small children and tinnitus in older ones. Check serum salicylate levels in two weeks and at intervals thereafter. When hypersalicylism is suspected, obtain a serum level, stop the aspirin for two or three doses and restart at a lower level. By the end of two weeks of constant dosage, the serum salicylate level should be close to 25 mg./dl.

Gastric irritation is reduced by administering aspirin with meals or milk. Occasional postprandial pain can be treated with an antacid as needed. Constant use of antacids decreases gastric absorption, increases renal excretion and requires an increased total dose of salicylate. Giving dissolved aspirin may reduce gastritis. Enteric-coated aspirin or sodium salicylate has unpredictable and often inadequate absorption. Choline salicylate (Arthropan) may be substituted but has poor acceptance because of its bad taste. Aminopyrine and acetophenetidin are not effective in treating arthritis and cannot be used as substitutes for aspirin. They may be used as adjuncts to control fever.

A great deal of attention has recently been paid to the elevated serum transaminase levels associated with aspirin therapy. These usually appear at the start of therapy but may occur sporadically in children on constant dosage. The transaminase levels are related to salicylate concentrations, but not predictably so from child to child, nor from time to time in an individual child. There have been no reports of chronic liver damage from aspirin. It is a good practice to follow transaminase levels and to treat elevations over 100 I.U./liter in the same way as an episode of acute symptomatic hypersalicylism (see above). Elevated transaminases *per se* are not reasons for stopping salicylate therapy.

Aspirin should be given for at least six months (some pediatric rheumatologists advise two years) after the last sign or symptom of arthritis has disappeared. The dose should then be tapered over several weeks to avoid a severe relapse.

If a child is getting worse during the first six months of salicylate treatment, or if significant active rheumatoid disease persists at six months, "gold" should be considered. Sodium aurothiomalate (Myochrysine)* is given by intramuscular injection at weekly intervals with an initial injection of 0.25 mg./kg. Some children will react with fever, rash and malaise for one to two days. No further injections are given if this occurs; otherwise, the full dose of 1 mg./kg. may be given a week later. Toxicity of gold includes stomatitis, eczematoid rash, bone marrow depression, and liver or renal disease. The child, the serum, and the urine must be examined weekly. A response takes at least eight weeks. When a good response occurs, reduce the dose of gold by increasing the time between injections to two weeks, then three weeks, and eventually four weeks. If no improvement is seen within 20 weeks, stop the injections.

Hydroxychloroquine (Plaquenil) has proven anti-inflammatory activity in arthritis and may be considered if aspirin and gold have failed. It has a high risk of causing retinitis which may progress to blindness even after the drug is stopped. Its use should be limited in JRA. The dose should not exceed 4 mg./kg./day and, since the toxic effects on the eye are believed to be cumulative, it should not be used for indefinite periods.

The role of the new, nonsteroid anti-inflammatory drugs—naproxen (Naprosyn), ibuprofen (Motrin), fenoprofen (Nalfon), and tolmetin (Tolectin)—is not yet certain in children. Although naproxen and ibuprofen have been used in children fairly extensively in Europe, only tolmetin has been systematically studied in children in this country. In general, these drugs are slightly less active than aspirin as anti-inflammatory agents. However, they cause less gastritis and are therefore preferred by some patients. Optimal doses and long-term toxicities are not adequately known for children. The older nonsteroid anti-inflammatory agents indomethacin and phenylbutazone are considered too toxic for children under 14 years of age.

Daily adrenocorticosteroids should only be used to save lives or eyesight. The specific indications are pericarditis with threatening tamponade, myocarditis with congestive heart failure, or iridocyclitis not controllable by local therapy. Daily steroids provide relief of symptoms, but joints continue to deteriorate, and destruction may become worse and more crippling than need be. Osteoporosis and vertebral collapse are common in children treated with steroids for JRA, and definitely add to the disease's own deleterious effect on bone and cartilage. Moreover, eventual steroid withdrawal is often followed by a flare of disease as bad as or worse than when the drugs are started.

To avoid the ill effects of daily steroids, the experimental use of an alternate morning schedule of short-acting steroids has been tried. The day on which steroids are not given is usually very difficult for the patient during initial stages of such treatment, but eventually general improvement may occur. It is not yet clear which side effects can be avoided by this method. Cataracts and glaucoma do appear with alternate day steroids.

The intra-articular injection of steroids may be useful in the rare situation in which a single joint is severely involved and interfering significantly with function. Most typically this will be a knee. Although rapid relief is possible, intra-articular steroids will themselves destroy cartilage. Injections can be repeated only once or twice into a single joint. A number of steroid

---

*Manufacturer's precaution: Do not give more than 25 mg. of sodium aurothiomalate in a single dose to children under 12 years of age.

preparations are used. Doses vary with the particular steroid and with the size of the joint. Crystalline forms are used to prolong the effect, but may be more destructive than soluble preparations.

Surgery. Surgical consultation is useful early to help plan long-term management of difficult cases. The greatest recent surgical advance pertinent to children with JRA is the early success of total hip replacement. Proof of the value of this operation in the long run is still lacking. No other joint replacement operation is as successful, but improvements are likely during the life span of children now being treated. It is essential that joint position and surrounding soft tissues be maintained for replacement surgery. When contractures which resist physical and medical therapy are seen, surgical soft tissue releases should be considered before nerve and vascular shortness develops. This complication prevents the establishment of normal joint extension, and precludes replacement surgery.

Iridocyclitis. Optimal treatment of this frequently recurrent problem requires an awareness of its incidence and of the lack of early symptoms. It may occur with any form of JRA, but is most common in young girls with relatively few inflamed joints and with positive antinuclear antibody tests. It does not cause pain in the younger child and unless slit-lamp examinations are done, its presence will be missed until late changes are present. Treatment with local mydriatics and steroids is usually successful, but some children have progressive disease requiring systemic steroids and surgery.

ANKYLOSING SPONDYLITIS AND REITER'S SYNDROME

Ankylosing spondylitis may start in childhood as a peripheral arthritis. Most often it will present in the 10 to 14 year old boy as a pauciarticular arthritis involving hips, knees, or ankles. Reiter's syndrome may occur in this same age and sex group. In general, treatment is similar to that for JRA. The first drug to try is aspirin. However, the importance in making these diagnoses as early as possible is that there is often a better response to indomethacin (Indocin), either alone or when added to aspirin. The presence of the HLA-B27 antigen on the child's lymphocytes may help in making these diagnoses when doubt exists. Indomethacin should be started at 50 mg./day and increased in 25 mg./day increments to a maximum of 150 mg./day; this is the adult dosage. Phenylbutazone (Butazolidin) may be more effective than indomethacin. It is used in doses from 100 to 400 mg./day for short periods. Both these drugs are toxic and their use must be limited to postpubertal patients. They are specifically useful only for these two diseases.

SYSTEMIC LUPUS ERYTHEMATOSUS

The prognosis for SLE has improved remarkably in the last 10 to 20 years. Some children even appear to reach permanent remissions. A large number of factors appear to be involved: recognition of milder disease, better methods of detection of relapses, more precise indications for the use of steroids and immunolytic agents, and improved antimicrobial treatment. It is hard to generalize about therapy because patients vary a great deal. For this reason, the major requirement is that consultation with experienced and comprehensive sources be established. At different times an individual child may present problems for the rheumatologist, nephrologist, neurologist, cardiologist, pulmonary disease specialist or infectious disease specialist. Obviously, there must also be a single person in charge to whom the patient and family can relate, presumably the pediatrician.

Early treatment improves the short-term prognosis. Therefore, identification of the insidious or atypical presentation of SLE is important; so too is the early recognition of a relapse. Certain laboratory abnormalities should be treated before clinical evidence of relapses appears. The two most valuable laboratory predictors of impending active disease are rising titers of antibody to native DNA and falling levels of serum complement. Either change should be considered evidence of potentially severe activity. Less specific laboratory abnormalities—high sedimentation rate, anemia, low white blood cell or platelet counts, and changes in any of the other unusual antibodies present in SLE—may give warning, but do not carry as grave import as changes in complement and anti-DNA concentrations.

The mainstay of therapy remains adrenocorticosteroids. Prednisone or prednisolone are most used. Initial therapy of renal involvement or slowly progressing diseases of other vital organs should be with a dose of 60 mg./m²/day of prednisone or its equivalent. This can usually be given once a day in the morning. This high dose should be maintained for four to six weeks even if the response is rapid. Immediately life-threatening central nervous system disease, myocarditis or pulmonary vasculitis should be treated with intravenous steroids. One or two gm. of hydrocortisone (Solu-Cortef) every four to six hours are used in these emergencies. This should be reduced when possible, but an oral dose of 60 mg./m²/day of prednisone or its equivalent should be maintained for at least four to six weeks after such an episode.

Since there is high morbidity and mortality associated with this level of steroid therapy, reduction in dosage consistent with activity of the disease must be a constant aim. The usual method is to decrease the daily dose at two to four week intervals. Initial reductions may be large, but below 30 mg./m²/day individual reductions should be no greater than 5 mg./day. Sometimes as little as 1 mg./day appears to make a difference. Recently success has been reported in switching from high dosage daily doses to alternate morning prednisone without a long withdrawal period on daily doses. The alternate day dosage should be at least 2½ times the daily dose at the time of the switch. Not all of the side effects of steroids can be reduced by alternate morning dosage, but there does appear to be less change in appearance and less suppression of growth. To realize the adrenal-saving effect of alternate day dosage, it is important to use a steroid with a short in vivo life, such as prednisone, and to give the dose in the morning.

If the disease remains uncontrolled after six weeks of treatment with high doses of steroids, one of the immunolytic drugs should be added. The choice is difficult. Azathioprine (Imuran),* 1 to 2 mg./kg./day, is used most often, but its effectiveness in SLE is still controversial and, at best, slow in onset. It appears to be less toxic than other immunolytic drugs, but it may increase the incidence of neoplasia. Alkylating agents such as cyclophosphamide (Cytoxan) and chlorambucil (Leukeran) are more rapidly and more convincingly effective, but only when added to steroid therapy.† In effective doses they are almost universally associated with significant side effects. An intravenous alkylating agent should be used if a life-threatening episode is not responding to intravenous steroids.

When there is no evidence of active disease in a vital organ, the relatively minor manifestations, particularly the rash, arthritis and serositis can be treated with salicylates and hydroxychloroquine.‡ Hydroxychloroquine has long been used for discoid skin lesions, but recently has been shown to have a real role in treating the arthritis and minor subjective

symptoms. It does not reduce the incidence of serious relapses. The doses of salicylates and hydroxychloroquine should be those used in JRA.

Occult infection and gastrointestinal ulcers remain serious and frequent causes of morbidity and mortality during periods of steroid and immunolytic therapy. Constant vigilance is required. Specific bacterial, protozoal and virological diasgnoses are essential to take advantage of the improved choice and specificity of current antibiotics. Prophylactic use of antacids is used by some but is associated with its own complications. Maintaining a high level of suspicion is probably adequate, particularly since it is now thought that steroids hide rather than cause ulcers. It is vital to remember that these side effects of therapy are more likely to be the immediate cause of death in SLE than is the disease itself. The best protection is to be certain that an indication exists for each drug being used at any specific phase of the disease.

DRUG-INDUCED SLE

The drugs most commonly implicated in inducing lupus-like syndromes in children are anticonvulsants, specifically trimethadione (Tridione), ethosuximide (Zarontin), mephenytoin (Mesantoin), and phenytoin (Dilantin). The syndrome associated with these drugs includes rash, arthritis, serositis and the abnormal serology of spontaneous SLE. However, renal disease appears rarely, if ever. For most patients a cure can be obtained by simply stopping the offending drug and providing symptomatic treatment as the syndrome subsides. A few patients will have significant pericarditis, anemia, or leukopenia requiring high doses of adrenocorticosteroids (prednisone, 60 mg./m²/day). The length of treatment will generally be short and the tapering of steroid dosage can be more rapid than when treating spontaneous SLE.

DERMATOMYOSITIS

Dermatomyositis is another disease in which the prognosis has markedly improved in the last 15 years. In contrast to the previously expected 30 per cent mortality in the first two years, very few deaths are now expected.

The principal medication again is prednisone in doses of 60 mg./m²/day during the initial episode and during relapses. This is given as long as the muscle-derived enzymes, creatinine phosphokinase (CPK), serum glutamic oxaloacetic transaminase (SGOT), or aldolase are elevated. Even in those cases in which the serum concentrations of these enzymes fall rapidly, high dose therapy with

---

*This use of Imuran is not indicated by the manufacturer.

†This use of cyclophosphamide and chlorambucil is not indicated by the manufacturers.

‡Aspirin has been reported to cause a reversible decrease in creatinine clearance and increase in serum creatinine when given to patients with systemic lupus erythematosus. The significance of this change is unknown, but it can confuse approaches to therapy.

prednisone should be continued for four to six weeks before starting reduction. If remission has been established but the enzymes begin to rise, or if weakness increases, high doses should be reinstituted. Occasionally the skin manifestations will become worse without evidence of active muscle disease. It is not possible to generalize about the use of prednisone in that situation, since cosmetic problems are perceived differently by each patient.

Prednisone may be effective if given once a day, and the dose may be reduced slowly every two weeks. Relapses occur if the alternate morning method is introduced too early during withdrawal. Relapses usually have a subtle onset, and sometimes respond to a small increment in dosage if discovered early. However, a return to a dose of 60 mg./m²/day may be required. An alternate day schedule should be tried only when the patient is in remission while taking 10 mg./day or less of prednisone. Some pediatric rheumatologists recommend maintaining prednisone therapy for at least two years in all patients. I have tried to stop the drug after six to eight months but then watch carefully for relapses, which may occur many years after the initial episode.

A few patients will not respond to prednisone, or will become so toxic as to require withdrawal. Immunolytic drugs may be used in these patients, but there are no good choices. Greatest experience has been with A-methopterin (methotrexate) given 1 mg./kg. intravenously at weekly or biweekly intervals. This is rarely necessary and is an experimental use of this severely toxic drug.

During the acute phases of the disease, aspiration pneumonia, infections and occult gastrointestinal ulcers are hazards. Adequate treatment requires alertness and early diagnosis. Patients with dermatomyositis may have arthritis as a prodromal or chronically persisting symptom. In the absence of muscle disease, arthritis may be treated with aspirin.

Physical therapy is vital for these children. Since this disease is thought to be primarily a vasculitis which occludes small vessels and damages muscle by producing microinfarcts, initial therapy should not increase the oxygen demand of the muscle. Exercises should be passive and aimed at maintenance of range of motion. Contractures develop during the healing stages, and vigorous stretching may become necessary later. Once the muscle-derived enzyme concentrations in the serum are normal, active strengthening exercises may be started and pursued vigorously. Children in remission should continue to be examined at intervals because weakness and contractures can persist and even progress slightly for many years. A physical therapy program may be needed indefinitely, although the intensity required will decrease.

There is no proven medical therapy for the subcutaneous and perimysial calcinosis that develops in many of these children. The calcium will resorb slowly in most, but new deposits may appear for many years. Surgical removal may be necessary when calcium deposits interfere with function. Experimental use of probenecid (Benemid) has been reported from England, but has not been evaluated by rigorous study. All other attempts to alter calcium deposition have been discarded.

SCLERODERMA

Scleroderma in children is still usually classified as "morphea" or as "progressive systemic sclerosis." A recently added classification is "eosinophilic fasciitis." There is controversy about the concept of morphea as a benign and self-limited disease. Some believe it may become progressive and that systemic sclerosis is more common in children than is usually thought.

Medical therapy is usually unsuccessful in the long term. However, eosinophilic fasciitis has been reported to respond well to steroid treatment. Occasionally other cases of scleroderma will also respond to steroids, but this is unpredictable. Certainly prednisone should be tried if life or function is threatened. Immunolytic agents may also be tried, particularly when there are high titers of antinuclear antibodies or other immunologic abnormalities, but success is limited and toxicity high. Penicillamine has been used in England. It may prove to have a place in treating mild or early cases, but it is associated with chronic nephritis when used for long periods and is not approved for this use in the United States.

Physical therapy and splinting help prevent the formation of contractures in some cases of scleroderma. The extent and depth of the lesion determine the nature of the program and its success. Surgical release of contractures is often complicated by lack of adequate tissue deep to the skin, as well as by poor healing of skin lesions and grafts. Amputation of a limb is occasionally necessary, and may be preferable to multiple attempts at soft tissue release.

POLYARTERITIS

Polyarteritis may present in children as an acute or rapidly evolving disease with nodular aneurysms as seen in adults or in an infantile form. The adult form of polyarteritis is a multisystem process with a poor prognosis due to renal, CNS, and pulmonary disease. This syndrome responds well to high dose steroid therapy (60 mg./m²/day of prednisone or its equivalent). Cyclophosphamide (Cytoxan) and azathioprine (Imuran) have been added with apparent success when the response to prednisone was too slow.* Treatment should be prolonged but apparently permanent remissions have been reported.

The infantile syndrome kills by coronary artery dilatation and occlusion, and is usually only diagnosed at autopsy. The only reported survivors have been treated with high dose steroids. However, some or all cases may be manifestations of the mucocutaneous lymph node syndrome (see p. 485) which is not clearly responsive to steroids. Until more certain information is available, infants with coronary or disseminated polyarteritis should be treated with high dose steroids.

MCTD

Mixed connective tissue disease (MCTD) is another recently described syndrome which combines features of scleroderma, myositis, and SLE. Originally thought to be benign, it is now known to be associated with a significant mortality due to pulmonary and renal disease. It is distinguished by the presence of high titers of antibody to an easily extractable ribonucleoprotein of calf thymus cell nuclei. Raynaud's phenomenon is frequent. Although rarer in children than is SLE or dermatomyositis, it is probably about as frequent as polyarteritis. This disease, even more than the related ones already discussed, should be treated for the systems involved at any given time. The Raynaud's phenomenon is best managed by avoidance of cold and may be helped by vasodilators. Arthritis is treated by aspirin as in JRA. Major organ involvement requires high doses of steroids and occasionally immunolytic drugs as in SLE.

ANAPHYLACTOID PURPURA (HENOCH-SCHÖNLEIN SYNDROME)

The exact etiology of anaphylactoid purpura is unknown and may vary. The pathogenesis includes deposition of antigen-antibody complexes, but the duration of activity is self-limited, lasting weeks or at most a few months. Therapy depends on the severity and the particular manifestations of each case.

Mild cases with principally rash and arthritis may be treated symptomatically for pain and need not be hospitalized. Hematuria and melena should be anticipated and careful follow-up for several weeks is necessary. Aminopyrine and acetophenetidin are less likely to cause the appearance of occult blood in feces than aspirin, and are preferable only for that reason; however, aspirin may be used, particularly if the arthritis is severe.

Children with abdominal pain should be admitted to the hospital and observed for intussusception or significant bleeding. If either of these complications occurs, or if abdominal pain becomes severe, intravenous hydrocortisone (Solu-Cortef) should be used, 100 to 500 mg. every four to six hours. The duration of treatment is as short as possible.

The treatment of the renal disease remains controversial. Traditionally steroids have been considered of no benefit. However, the studies usually cited predate modern usage. Another problem is that the natural history of the renal disease is variable and not entirely predictable. Onset of hematuria in the first week may indicate a worse prognosis for acute nephritic complications, for chronic nephritis, or for the nephrotic syndrome. However, initially mild disease may progress to chronicity. The older idea that chronic nephritis could appear de novo after long intervals is no longer accepted. The child with onset of mild hematuria in the second or third week of illness may not need treatment. Until rigorously tested data become available, it is probably wiser to treat the child with early onset, severe, or persisting hematuria with high doses of steroids (prednisone, 60 mg./m²/day or its equivalent) until it is clear that renal failure or the nephrotic syndrome is not appearing. Very severe cases have been treated with azathioprine (Imuran) or cyclophosphamide (Cytoxan) as well as steroids, but the effectiveness of these drugs is also assumed rather than proven. In the rare case which progresses to systemic vasculitis or polyarteritis, steroids and immunolytics are used as described for SLE.

---

*This use of cyclophosphamide and azathioprine is not indicated by the manufacturers.

12

Genitourinary Tract

Renal Hypoplasia and Dysplasia

LARRY E. FLEISCHMANN, M.D.

The term renal hypoplasia includes a number of conditions characterized by a decreased number of nephrons. The patient's kidneys are small but initially anatomically no aberrant tissue is present. Patients with renal dysplasia, probably a consequence of intrauterine urinary obstruction in the vast majority of cases, show both reduction of functional mass and the presence of aberrant tissue—metaplastic cartilage, primitive ducts, and so forth. These kidneys vary in size from small nubbins, capping an atretic ureter, to large multicystic organs presenting as flank masses. These two groups of congenital renal disturbances, though disparate in their pathogenesis and anatomic features, are alike in that their victims often share features of deranged renal physiology—those of decreased numbers of functioning nephrons and abnormal function of remaining nephrons. The former defect leads to complications of decreased excretion, the latter to those of decreased conservation. Therapy for the accumulation of unexcreted products is directed toward minimization of effects; treatment of increased losses involves supplementation therapy. In addition, infection and hypertension can complicate both groups of conditions; surgical therapy is often of value in children with renal dysplasia secondary to obstruction.

Since obstruction of the urinary tract is usually the inciting event leading to the development of renal dysplasia, a thorough evaluation of the state of urinary drainage is imperative in these children. Cystourethrography, in-cluding voiding studies, is mandatory to assess the need for surgical procedures on the lower tracts. Intravenous urography usually is the best guide to the drainage status of the calyces and renal pelves. Cystourethroscopy may be necessary to determine insertion sites of ectopic ureters, often associated with dysplastic, duplicated renal segments, and regularly requiring surgical revision or resection.

Surgical therapy of the dysplastic renal mass is directed toward the preservation of a maximal number of functioning nephrons. Segments of kidneys or whole organs are *not* removed unless there is essentially no chance of repair and later function, or unless continued infection of the area or organ severely threatens the patient's well being. Today's pediatric urologists regularly accomplish feats of repair with conservation of renal mass that would have been considered foolish to attempt within the recent past. The surgical correction of residual obstruction will usually prevent further hydronephrotic damage, but dysplastic tissue will not become normal. One cannot expect cartilage to redifferentiate to collecting duct.

Further damage in both types of renal abnormality may occur from infection. There appears to be a higher incidence of infection in dysplastic and hypoplastic organs. Urine is cultured regularly and antibiotics are chosen with three principles in mind: (1) effectiveness against the bacterium as determined by sensitivity tests, (2) possible systemic *side effects,* especially nephrotoxicity, and (3) effect of decreased renal function on the above. The aminoglycosides, for example, may prove effective against the infecting organisms in most cases, but should be reserved for serious infections because of their nephrotoxicity. When they must be used, serum levels are monitored and the dosage schedule modified if the disposal rate (half-life) is increased. Failure to modify the dosage schedule will lead to the accumulation of toxic levels of drugs when the patient's glomerular filtration rate is decreased.

Typically, children with renal hypoplasia or dysplasia present with severe problems in infancy. Most often these are related to renal tubular dysfunction, out of proportion to glomerular insufficiency.

Patients may excrete a high volume of dilute urine, with salt wasting and acidosis. The inability to conserve water, sodium, potassium and bicarbonate may exist in combination or separately in these patients; close monitoring of clinical status in the initial period of stabilization is necessary to guide therapy. Provision of an adequate volume of water to compensate for the inability to elaborate a concentrated urine may often be accomplished by adding supplements of glucose water to the diet. Cow's milk and high protein formulas impose an added solute load and require a greater volume of water for their excretion, and should be avoided in severe cases. Low solute formulas such as Similac PM 60/40 and SMA S26 may be of value. Additional calories, when required, may be provided in the form of high carbohydrate supplements: they impose no added solute load.

Bicarbonate wasting may be a prominent feature in these children; acidosis to a degree requiring supplementation with bicarbonate or citrate salts (citrate is ususally better tolerated) is often found. The dose of base required often ranges up to 3 to 5 mEq./kg./day; it can be determined only by close monitoring of the patient's acid-base status. In the acidotic patient the bicarbonate or citrate supplements, usually furnished as sodium salts, generally provide sufficient sodium to overcome the inability of the renal tubules to conserve that ion. Occasionally potassium and chloride may be wasted in excess, so provision for adequate replacement of these electrolytes must be made. Renal tubular phosphate loss is less common in this group of conditions than it is in the congenital renal tubular abnormalities included in the broad category of the Fanconi syndrome; however, it may occur and may be treated with supplementation with mixtures of monobasic and dibasic sodium phosphate such as Nutra-Phos or Phospho-Soda. When phosphate salts are administered, the end-point for effective therapy is often the degree of gastrointestinal irritation that these products produce.

When scarring progresses, or when growth of the dysplastic or hypoplastic organ fails to keep up with the patient's growth and maturation, signs of glomerular insufficiency may supervene. Typically, the patient who has been stabilized as a newborn or in early infancy progresses well for a matter of years and then, with the approach of the puberal growth spurt, begins to exhibit signs of glomerular insufficiency.

Concomitant with this event, bone disease, which may not have been a prominent feature of the condition early on, may increase in severity and require appropriate treatment. The principles underlying the prevention and cure of renal osteodystrophy include close monitoring of the patient's serum calcium balance and provision of adequate calcium supplementation, usually in the form of calcium carbonate. This salt, together with judicious use of aluminum hydroxide, may also be used to bind phosphorus in the gut and prevent its absorption; as glomerular insufficiency progresses, the amount of phosphate filtered falls and phosphorus tends to accumulate in the blood. This hyperphosphatemia interferes with the normal course of bone formation by stimulating the parathyroid glands and producing secondary hyperparathyroidism. In addition to adequate calcium and phosphorus regulation, the patients often will require supplemental doses of vitamin D analogue. Recently the kidneys have been found to play an important role in the activation of both exogenous and endogenous vitamin D; by the process of 1-hydroxylation they convert it to the active hormone which fosters calcium absorption. The analogue we have found most useful in treating children is dihydrotachysterol (DHT). This preparation appears to be of greater physiologic activity on a milligram for milligram basis than do the other commercially available products. One mg. of DHT equals approximately 40,000 units of vitamin D. Dosage requirements of DHT vary widely; patients may require as little as 0.1 mg. or as much as 1 mg. DHT has the additional advantage of a rapid onset of action and rapid metabolism so that if hypercalcemia occurs, discontinuation of the drug is followed by rapid fall in the serum calcium.

The most important limitation placed on these children as glomerular insufficiency occurs is that of the toxic side effects of the accumulation of protein metabolic products. Severe protein restriction must be avoided, for sufficient protein must be supplied to foster continued growth; approximately 1.5 to 2 gm. of protein/kg./day should be sufficient. The intake should consist primarily of complete proteins, usually of animal origin; proteins lacking in one or more essential amino acids are ineffective as anabolic agents and are metabolized as an energy source, adding further to the solute disposal problem. Occasionally, supplementation with carbohydrate and amino acid mixtures (Amin-aid) may be of value in these children whose appetites often fall as glomerular insufficiency advances.

It must be remembered that the clinical status of these children is often a dynamic one, constantly changing with the progression of time and the state of growth and development. Therapy which is appropriate at one point in the progression of disease may be entirely inappropriate in another; the patient who required supplements of water and electrolyte at one period of time may later, when glomerular insufficiency develops, require restriction of those same products.

Hypertension may be a complicating factor in either form of these two groups of congenital anomalies. It tends to present earlier in patients with renal dysplasia than in patients with hypoplasia, but may be a prominent feature in both groups later in the course of the disease. We consider hydralazine to be the best antihypertensive agent in this group of patients because of its wide range of dosage and efficacy (0.75 to 4.0 mg./kg./day). Moderately severe cases of hypertension may require the addition of other agents such as propranolol in a dose of 1.0 to 4.0 mg./kg./day.* This agent, however, since its primary mode of action is probably a decrease in cardiac output, should be avoided in patients with compromised cardiovascular status. It tends to induce bradycardia; this effect may serve as a useful feature in counteracting the tachycardiac side effect of hydralazine. Guanethidine and other autonomic blocking agents have generally been replaced by the above combinations in our practice; however, some cases may be of such severity that they require the addition of this potent agent. Its side effects often are almost incapacitating, however. Hypertensive emergencies may occur, usually associated with episodes of acute volume overload. We have found the most effective drug in the treatment of hypertensive emergencies to be diazoxide,†

administered intravenously in a bolus of from 3 to 5 mg./kg. over a 20 second period. Hypotension rarely supervenes in these patients unless they have also been receiving hydralazine, another vasodilator. We have not found hyperglycemia to be a limiting side effect in the use of this agent if it is reserved for the acute emergent patient.

Every effort should be made to establish a definitive diagnosis in each of these patients, for while most occurrences of renal hypoplasia and dysplasia represent congenital, nongenetically determined conditions, some of the more rare varieties may be familial, and genetic counseling may prove advisable.

Hydronephrosis and Ureteral Disorders

FRANK HINMAN, Jr., M.D.

Hydronephrosis. *Unilateral* hydronephrosis, usually induced by congenital obstruction of the ureteropelvic junction, is treated by observation, repair, or nephrectomy.

Observation—with intravenous urograms obtained at regular intervals—is indicated if the obstruction is mild, with minimal or no dilatation of the calices. This form of therapy is especially applicable to the teenager. In infants, progression of the hydronephrosis is more frequent, often requiring operation.

Repair by ureteropelvioplasty, often without the need for nephrostomy drainage or stents, is advisable for most childhood obstructions, since the damage found at the age when the young patient is seen can be expected to increase at an accelerated rate.

Nephrectomy is done when the parenchyma is so thinned and destroyed that, even after repair and recovery, the kidney alone could not support life with its less than one-fifth of total function revealed by renal scanning. The younger the child, the greater the ability for recovery; thus nephrectomy should be reserved for cases of extreme unilateral damage in infancy.

If the obstruction is *bilateral,* repair of both sides is advisable despite severe damage, since the child needs every nephron for survival, and since stimulus for recovery is greater when neither kidney is normal (renal counterbalance).

Ureteral Disorders. Vesicoureteral reflux, the most common abnormality, occurs because the ureterovesical junction does not close as the bladder fills and empties; either it is congenitally deficient, or deranged by persistently

---

*The use of propranolol in pediatric practice for the treatment of hypertension has not yet been recognized by the Food and Drug Administration. Pediatric experience in the use of this agent indicates that it is an effective antihypertensive agent in the dose quoted which is not outside the body size adjusted dose range recommended for adult patients for this purpose.

†Manufacturer's note: Safety of intravenous diazoxide in children has not been established.

abnormal voiding, or distorted by inflammation caused by infection.

The congenitally abnormal ureterovesical junction appears grossly impaired on cystoscopy, often with a golf hole configuration. Treatment by reimplantation (ureterovesicoplasty) is to be delayed until the physician is certain that competency cannot be regained even though infection is suppressed and voiding patterns are normal.

The ureterovesical junction deranged by persistently abnormal voiding—a consequence of incoordination, either neurogenic (usually from meningomyelocele) or psychogenic (the so-called dysfunctional bladder)—cannot be repaired with any assurance of cure until bladder function is restored to normal. With the neurogenic bladder, intermittent catheterization may lead to restoration of normal valve function. In cases of the dysfunctional bladder, coordination can be improved by myoneural drugs such as propantheline bromide (Pro-Banthine) at a dosage of 7.5 mg. four times daily and phenoxybenzamine hydrochloride (Dibenzyline), 5 mg. daily, or by retraining techniques, sometimes including suggestion and hypnosis.*

Infection itself deranges the ureterovesical junction. Eradication of bacteriuria and prevention of reinfection by suppressive medication may allow the ureteral orifice to return to normal and operation to be avoided.

Obstruction of the terminal ureter from local congenital malformation is treated by ureteral reimplantation when it is severe or progressive; otherwise it requires no operation.

Ureterocele, associated with ureteral duplication, generally obstructs itself and often blocks the accompanying ureter. Reimplantation is required.

Malignant Tumors of the Kidney

RICHARD M. EHRLICH, M.D.

Nephroblastoma, or Wilms' tumor, has been reported to compose from 6 to 30 per cent of malignant solid abdominal tumors in children, and is second only to neuroblastoma in overall frequency. It is the most common malignant renal tumor of childhood (approximately 1 in every 13,500 live births) and has an incidence of about 2 new cases per year per million population. Approximately 500 new cases per year are discovered in the United States; thus an indepth study of this fascinating neoplasm is difficult.

The necessity for treatment by an interdisciplinary team, consisting of skilled surgeon, pediatric oncologist, and radiotherapist, is undisputed. The rise from a dismal cure rate of 14.9 per cent and 16 per cent in those patients treated by surgery alone in 1914 to 1930 and 1943 respectively to the present 2 year survival rate of between 60 and 80 per cent in localized disease utilizing the combined therapeutic modalities of surgery, radiotherapy, and chemotherapy attests to this triumph of cooperation.

It has been unequivocally demonstrated that with all stages of disease, the results of nephrectomy alone are not as good as those obtained when nephrectomy is combined with these other modalities.

Early diagnosis, improved surgical technique, advances in pre- and postoperative care, and the growth of experience of those who are particularly interested in treatment of this tumor have added greatly to more favorable results.

Surgical excision, however, remains the cornerstone of therapy for all children with Wilms' tumor. In one large series it has been shown that without nephrectomy, no patient survives.

Thorough preoperative evaluation is mandatory. As opposed to the "emergency surgery" advocated 20 years ago, special attention to the metabolic status of the child is crucial. Often there is hemorrhage within the tumor (which may be the event leading to diagnosis), and preoperative transfusions become necessary. Roentgenograms and tomography of the chest are important. With the use of femoral venography to visualize the vena cava and excretory urography to visualize the kidneys, retrograde pyelograms are rarely necessary. Arteriography is usually not employed nor necessary, yet it may provide useful information in differentiating large or questionable lesions from neuroblastoma. The above studies can usually be completed within a 48-hour period and surgery accomplished soon thereafter.

A generous transverse transperitoneal incision is most desirable. It may be curved in any direction depending upon the size of the tumor and may be extended into the thorax if the tumor is large and arises from the upper pole. In addition, this latter approach may be helpful in the excision of an ipsilateral solitary pulmonary metastasis. A formal thoracoabdominal approach is particularly suited to a large upper pole lesion.

Thorough inspection of the intraabdominal

---

*This use of propantheline bromide and phenoxybenzamine hydrochloride is not mentioned in the manufacturers' instructions.

contents is next performed, with particular attention to the liver and paraaortic areas. The tumor, often large and friable, must be handled with minimum manipulation to prevent tumor spillage. Tumor spillage at surgery worsens prognosis, but postoperative radiotherapy and cyclical chemotherapy have improved survival markedly, even in these difficult circumstances.

Since between 2 and 10 per cent of Wilms' tumors are bilateral, formal mobilization of the contralateral kidney from its perirenal fat is mandatory to ascertain if a second lesion is present. It should be emphasized that manual palpation through the peritoneum is inadequate in making this judgment.

Both the anterior and posterior surfaces of the contralateral kidney must be visually inspected and palpated. Any suspicious nodule must be totally excised if possible, or the site marked with metallic clips for the radiotherapist if only biopsy is possible.

The entire mass, including perirenal fascia and fat, should be removed. Occasionally, contiguous structures, such as the tail of the pancreas, spleen, diaphragm or colon, must be removed en bloc with the specimen. Psoas fascia and/or muscle may have to be removed as well if direct extension is present. The margins of any tumor not amenable to resection should be identified with metallic clips. The primary tumor should not be biopsied prior to removal to prevent tumor spillage. The adrenal gland should be removed in continuity with the specimen in cases of upper pole lesions.

With an adequate incision it is rare that the tumor cannot be removed despite direct extension to adjacent viscera. Every effort should be expended to remove as much tumor bulk as possible, even if distant metastases are present, to afford greater success with postoperative radiotherapy and chemotherapy.

Preoperative inferior vena cavography via a femoral vein, which also permits excretory urography at the time of initial diagnosis, may be helpful in establishing the presence of vena caval involvement. Renal vein tumor thrombus must be carefully sought for and removed if found, after first gaining proximal and distal control of the vena cava. The vena cava may be ligated and resected below the level of the renal veins if absolutely necessary.

Metastases occur via retroperitoneal lymphatics as well as hematogenous routes primarily to the lungs, and less commonly to the liver, brain, and skeleton. Nodal metastases are more common than once thought. Thus thorough and complete lymph node dissection from the level of the diaphragm to the aortic bifurcation is mandatory for both staging of the disease and removal of any residual tumor. The importance of staging cannot be overemphasized, and the performance of simultaneous lymphadenectomy with nephrectomy has gained considerable support.

In order to refine therapy to include only those modalities (radiation therapy and chemotherapy) which are absolutely essential, the National Wilms' Tumor Study I conceived staging categories which dictated treatment regimens. Begun in 1969 and reported in 1976, this crucial study answered multiple questions regarding refinement of treatment. The reader is encouraged to seek out this important reference before embarking on any treatment regimen in the child with Wilms' tumor (Cancer, *38*:633–646, 1976).

Certain facts deserve emphasis. Prolonged, cyclical treatment with actinomycin D and vincristine sulfate is more effective than either agent alone. Actinomycin D (Cosmegen)* is administered intravenously in a dose of 15 μg./kg. for 5 days for a total dose of 75 μg./kg. per course. No single injection should exceed 500 μg., and less than 15 μg./kg./day may be given if the above is poorly tolerated. If less is given (such as 10 μg.), the therapy should be continued for 7 days. If there is no question in diagnosis prior to surgery, it is suggested that the first dose be given in the operating room prior to making the incision to help kill circulating tumor cells coincident with tumor handling. If the diagnosis is questionable, actinomycin D can be started in the immediate postoperative period once the diagnosis is confirmed. The five day courses are then given at 6 weeks and every 3 months to a total of 7 courses over 15 months. Toxicity includes nausea, vomiting, bone marrow suppression with anemia, leukopenia, thrombocytopenia, and alopecia, dermatitis and stomatitis.

Vincristine sulfate (Oncovin) is administered intravenously weekly for 6 weeks in a dose of 1.5 mg./m²/week. No single injection should exceed 2 mg. The neurologic effects include hyporeflexia, wrist or foot drop, and paresthesias. Gastrointestinal symptoms may also result. Alopecia may occur and anemia and leukopenia occur more frequently than does thrombocytopenia. The notable lack of bone marrow toxicity, however, allows this agent to be administered safely with actinomycin D. The side effects of both drugs are reversible, although neurologic consequences of vincristine are slow to resolve. It is particularly important that a good intravenous line be established prior to the administration of these drugs, as subcutaneous infiltration results in severe tissue necrosis. It should further be emphasized that due to severe toxicity of these agents, particular care in dosage calculations must be assured and the regimen supervised by a skilled pediatric chemotherapist.

---

*Manufacturer's precaution: Actinomycin D should not be given to infants under the age of 6 to 12 months because of the greater frequency of toxic effects.

Recent data from the National Wilms' Tumor Study II suggest that all drugs administered to children 11 months of age at time of therapy be reduced to one-half the standard dosage to avoid toxicity in this young age group: that is, a total of 37.5 μg./kg. of actinomycin D per course; 0.75 mg./m² of vincristine sulfate per dose; and if Adriamycin is used, 30 mg./m² per course be employed. Potentiation of toxicity with the use of chemotherapy must also be borne in mind, and the state of nutrition and hydration in young infants is crucial.

Adriamycin is presently under investigation in the National Wilms' Tumor Study II and does appear to have important adjunctive use. In the first study it was shown that patients who relapsed after adequate therapy with actinomycin D and vincristine were not benefited by further treatment with these same drugs. It is possible that Adriamycin may well have a place in this setting in the future. The toxicity of Adriamycin is mostly gastrointestinal and hematologic but cardiac toxicity may occur.

Radiation therapy is the third modality which has been shown to be mandatory except in very special circumstances. It is begun shortly after surgery (within 24 to 72 hours) with the aim to render nonviable cells that may have spilled during surgery. The size of the field depends on the findings at surgery, but in all cases the liver, spleen and opposite kidney are carefully shielded. To prevent scoliosis, the entire width of the vertebral epiphyseal plates are radiated. Routine preoperative therapy is not advocated unless the tumor is massive and deemed possibly unresectable. In this setting, preoperative therapy may well reduce tumor bulk, making surgery easier. There are several reports as well that preoperative vincristine sulfate helps in reducing tumor bulk, but there is as of yet no evidence that the prognosis is positively affected.

Data from National Wilms' Tumor Study I indicate that postoperative radiotherapy need not be given to children under age 2 with unequivocal group I lesions with the tumor sharply confined within the kidney capsule and totally removed at the time of surgery. In older children over age 2 and those instances in which the question of assigning the lesion to group I is not certain, it is then recommended that postoperative irradiation therapy be given.

Therapy for children with bilateral Wilms' tumor is difficult and requires aggressive management, close surveillance and long-term follow-up. When possible, bilateral partial nephrectomy followed by radiotherapy and chemotherapy is the treatment of choice. If one tumor is large and not amenable to partial nephrectomy, the entire kidney should be removed. Partial nephrectomy on the opposite side should then be done if possible and adjunctive radiotherapy and chemotherapy given. If at the time of initial exploration diffuse involvement of both kidneys is found, bilateral biopsy followed by radiotherapy and chemotherapy is suggested. Depending on the response to therapy, arteriography followed by a second look exploration is warranted in the hope that partial nephrectomy on one or both sides may be feasible. It may be that workbench surgery with newer methods of renal preservation will provide increased success with this approach.

Despite the complications of immunosuppression, renal transplantation may have a bona fide place in the therapy of bilateral Wilms' tumors but should be reserved for patients whose neoplasms cannot be controlled with aggressive surgery and adjuvant chemotherapy and radiotherapy. Transplantation should be offered only to those patients whose diseases are not controllable with the usual modalities and not as an initial undertaking.

Routine physical examination should be undertaken at least every three months during the first several years and then every six months for the following five years. It is important that blood counts be determined on the first day and on four days during the five day course of actinomycin therapy. With vincristine sulfate, this should be accomplished weekly at three times a week during radiotherapy.

Chest x-rays should be taken at six weeks, three months and every three months thereafter for the first 24 months.

Intavenous pyelography should be obtained each year until the third year and liver and bone scans done as necessary. Liver and renal functions should be carried out every six months for two years and then yearly through the fifth year.

Other primary malignant tumors of the kidney are rare and are treated with radical nephrectomy and lymphadenectomy. Both postoperative radiation therapy and chemotherapy may be given if metastases are present, but the response rate is not nearly as good as with Wilms' tumor.

Glomerulonephritis

JOHN E. LEWY, M.D.

The management of a child with glomerulonephritis differs depending on the etiology of the process and whether it is acute or chronic. This section deals primarily with the treatment of acute glomerulonephritis since the treatment of chronic glomerulonephritis is covered under the broader topic of chronic renal insufficiency. The therapy of acute poststreptococcal glomerulonephritis is directed toward correcting the physiologic abnormalities associated with this disease since the process itself is generally self-limited. In conditions such as systemic lupus erythematosus, treatment must be directed not only toward correcting the physiologic abnormalities but also toward specific depression of the disease process. The more severe complications of acute glomerulonephritis such as hypertensive encephalopathy, acute renal failure with hyperkalemia, pulmonary edema, hypocalcemia or uremia require intensive and experienced care.

Hospitalization. The main considerations in determining whether hospitalization is required are the severity of clinical abnormalities and the family and physician's ability to provide close observation and care at home. The children with moderate to severe reductions in renal function (creatinine clearance less than 60 ml./min./1.73 m^2, BUN greater than 50 mg./dl.) should be hospitalized as should any child with uremic symptoms or signs. Patients with marked oliguria (urinary output less than 20 ml./kg./day), significant edema or pulmonary congestion should be promptly hospitalized, as should children with hypertension, vomiting or lethargy. If renal function is normal or only mildly depressed, and edema, oliguria, vomiting and hypertension are absent, hospitalization can often be avoided. Children treated for acute glomerulonephritis at home must have the same care and observation as the hospitalized child.

Bed Rest. It is recommended that children who have gross hematuria, hypertension, edema, evidence of circulatory congestion or moderate to severe depression of renal function be kept as quiet as practicable. Bed rest is ideal but difficult to achieve in the young child. Encouraging quiet activities that can be carried out in bed or on a chair or sofa is often adequate. The child should be kept reasonably inactive during the period when clinical signs are raidly changing. Once edema, hypertension, azotemia, oliguria and gross hematuria have abated and the creatinine clearance is rising, children can be returned to activities as tolerated. Microscopic hematuria and proteinuria may remain for months or years despite ultimate complete recovery and therefore are not indications for restricting activity. I generally allow the child to return to school within one week after ambulation but continue to restrict competitive activities until the urinary sediment has normalized.

Dietary Management. I do not usually limit dietary protein if the BUN is less than 75 mg./dl. If azotemia is more severe, I generally restrict protein intake initially to 0.5 gm./kg./day. Provision of adequate calories is particularly important to reduce catabolism. We encourage the child to ingest at least 50 per cent of the minimum daily requirement of calories for age and size. Numerous dietary supplements are available to provide calories with a minimum of protein and electrolyte. These are available in both liquid and solid form. Sodium restriction is indicated in the presence of hypertension and edema. I generally limit sodium intake to 1 gm. (2 gm. sodium chloride) per m^2/day. Severe sodium restriction leads to poor caloric intake, whereas moderate degrees of sodium restriction sufficient to assist in blood pressure or edema control do not severely restrict the diet.

Fluids should be restricted in the presence of edema or oliguria. Patients should be provided with fluids amounting to their insensible water loss plus measured urinary output. Insensible water loss amounts to approximately 20 ml./kg./24 hours in young children and about 15 ml./kg./24 hours in older children. These replacement calculations should be accomplished by measuring spontaneously voided urine and should *not* require catheterization. The best check on fluid therapy is to monitor the child's weight. The child's intake minus output will be equal to the change in body weight. Fluids should be adjusted to maintain body weight if the patient is not edematous or restricted sufficiently to gradually reduce weight in the edematous child.

Oliguria may be caused by other factors including underhydration. If the patient is not obviously edematous or appears dehydrated or has lost weight, it is often useful to give full maintenance or slightly increased amounts of fluids for the first 6 to 12 hours to ensure that dehydration is not contributing to the oliguria. Mannitol or furosemide can also be given to test renal responsiveness. A single intravenous infusion of mannitol* (0.5 gm./kg. as a 12.5 per cent solution = 2 ml.-kg. of 25 per cent mannitol diluted with an equal volume of 5 per cent dextrose and water) may be given as a test dose. A satisfactory response is a urinary output in the next two to three hours of about three times the volume of injected solution (10 to 12 ml./kg.). Furosemide, 1 mg./kg., may be given intravenously or 2 mg./kg. orally, in which case a similar output should occur within two to four hours. If the urinary output remains reduced despite appropriate hydration and a test with mannitol or furosemide, oliguria is most likely related to intrarenal causes and is not promptly reversible. Fluids should then be restricted to insensible water loss plus urinary output.

Hyperkalemia. Hyperkalemia is a serious and potentialy life-threatening complication in the patient with acute renal failure. Consultation by a physician experienced in the therapy of renal failure and electrolyte imbalance should be sought. Dietary modification should avoid all foods with substantial amounts of potassium. Sodium polystyrene sulfonate (Kayexalate) can be given by rectal enema, 1 gm./kg., and will decrease the serum potassium by approximately 1 mEq./liter. A Kayexalate enema takes approximately two hours to be effective and therefore cannot be given as the only therapy for the immediate treatment of severe hyperkalemia. Kayexalate enemas can be repeated at four to six hour intervals until the serum potassium is below 5 mEq./liter.

Severe hyperkalemia is treated by the intravenous administration of sodium bicarbonate. Two to three mEq. of sodium bicarbonate/kg. can be infused intravenously. This is often effective in reducing serum potassium by increasing potassium movement into cells. Bicarbonate infusion leads to decreased hydrogen ion concentration in the extracellular fluid. Hydrogen ion then moves out of cells and potassium into cells. Since this is merely a shift of potassium into cells rather than the removal of potassium from the body, Kayexalate enemas are still needed. Calcium infusion may be required if the electrocardiogram shows evidence of severe hyperkalemic changes (4 mg. of elemental calcium/kg. usually given as calcium gluconate). Severe hyperkalemia that does not respond promptly to the above measures is an indication for dialysis.

---

*Manufacturer's precaution: Dosage requirements of mannitol for patients 12 years and under have not been established.

Hypocalcemia. Hypocalcemia may manifest itself as tetany as acidosis is corrected. The child with severe or symptomatic hypocalcemia can be treated with intravenous calcium gluconate calculated to deliver an infusion of 4 mg. of elemental calcium/kg./hour for each of four hours. This has been shown to raise the serum calcium by approximately 2 mg./dl. Such an infusion should be given slowly and in an intravenous bottle that contains no sodium bicarbonate. Sodium bicarbonate in the same intravenous solution with calcium gluconate will form calcium carbonate precipitate in the intravenous bottle or tubing. Calcium should only be given intravenously when the patient's electrocardiogram and pulse rate can be closely monitored. Subsequently, oral calcium (calcium gluconate or calcium carbonate) can be provided to assure that the total oral calcium intake is at least 1 gm. of elemental calcium per day.

Hyperphosphatemia is generally present in the child with acute or chronic renal failure. Hyperphosphatemia must be reduced to minimize secondary hyperparathyroidism and to assist in normalization of serum calcium. This is accomplished gradually by dietary restriction of phosphate rich foods and by the oral administration of aluminum hydroxide gels to bind phosphorus in the intestine. It is important that phosphate-binding gels containing only aluminum hydroxide be used. Many phosphate-binding agents contain magnesium hydroxide and are contraindicated in the presence of renal failure.

Hypertension. Hypertension often resolves with bed rest alone. A child should be placed at bed rest and his blood pressure response observed. If the diastolic blood pressure is less than 100 mm. Hg and falls toward normal levels on bed rest, sodium restriction and bed rest are sufficient therapy. If the blood pressure does not decline with this management or if there are symptoms of encephalopathy (headaches, vomiting, nausea, seizures), treatent should be instituted promptly. Hydralazine, 0.15 mg./kg. intramuscularly, is usually quite effective in reducing blood pressure in acute glomerlonephritis. This dosage may be repeated every six hours as needed. Reserpine, 0.07 mg./kg. intramuscularly (maximum dose 2 mg.), may also be effective and may be repeated in 12 hours. A reserpine and hydralazine combination appears to be synergistic. If hypertension responds but only transiently, hydralazine may then be given orally with a starting dose of 0.7 mg./kg./day in four divided doses. This may be gradually increased as needed to a maximum of 200 mg./day. When blood pressure is normal for 24 to 48 hours the medication may be gradually tapered and discontinued. Sustained hypertension may require sustained therapy with hydralazine or therapy with agents such as alpha methyldopa, guanethidine or propranolol. Diazoxide, 5 mg./kg. by rapid intravenous infusion, is extremely effective in treating severe hypertension with encephalopathy.*

Diuretics. Diuretics are indicated to reduce edema, as a test of renal responsiveness, and as an adjunct to the therapy of hypertension. The use of mannitol and furosemide to test renal responsiveness has been discussed. Persistent edema can be treated with furosemide, 2 mg./kg./dose orally, which may be given once or twice daily. Hydrochlorothiazide, 2 mg./kg./day, is effective when renal function is normal or slightly reduced but not when there is marked depression of glomerular filtration rate. Vascular congestion can generally be treated effectively by limiting fluid and sodium in the diet, and by the use of furosemide given orally twice a day until signs of vascular congestion have abated. Digitalis is infrequently indicated and usually ineffective in the treatment of the vascular congestion associated with acute glomerulonephritis, since myocardial failure is usually not present.

Anemia. The anemia associated with acute poststreptococcal glomerulonephritis usually does not require therapy. The hematocrit is generally not reduced to less than 25 per cent in this disease. If the hematocrit is more severely reduced, the physician should look for evidence of concomitant iron deficiency or other causes of anemia (such as a hemolytic process). Transfusion is rarely necessary and should be reserved for those children with symptomatic anemia. If transfusion is required, it should be carried out with washed buffy coat poor cells since these have less free potassium and decreased antigenicity.

Antibiotics. We generally treat all children with acute poststreptococcal glomerulonephritis with a 10 day course of penicillin or an appropriate substitute. Throat cultures should be obtained from immediate family members and those with positive cultures should also receive treatment. I do not give antibiotics beyond the 10 day course except for specific clinical indications. During the conva-

lescent phase of acute glomerulonephritis, hematuria may increase with any infectious process and is generally transient. I therefore do not favor the use of prophylactic antibiotics during the convalescent period or subsequently.

Renal Biopsy. Renal biopsy is not essential in most children with acute poststreptococcal glomerulonephritis. Renal biopsy is important in those with acute nephritis in whom this diagnosis cannot be clearly made or in the more severe forms of this disease and particularly if specific therapeutic agents are being considered. Renal biopsy is most useful when performed early in the course of the disease when a good correlation has been found between the severity of the clinical disease and severity of the morphologic lesion. If a poststreptococcal etiology cannot be established, renal biopsy may be diagnostically helpful. If improvement in renal function does not occur in two or three weeks, or if the serum complement has not returned to normal within six weeks, renal biopsy is indicated for diagnostic purposes.

Corticosteroid and Immunosuppressive Therapy. I do not employ corticosteroids or other immunosuppressive drugs in the treatment of acute poststreptococcal glomerulonephritis. The use of immunosuppressive drugs in the diffuse proliferative glomerulonephritis of systemic lupus erythematosus has been shown to be effective but should be conducted in consultation with a nephrologist experienced in the therapy of this disease. The use of steroids or immunosuppressive drugs in other proliferative glomerulonephritides such as Henoch-Schönlein purpura with nephritis and rapidly progressive glomerulonephritis remains controversial; thus this therapy is also best carried out in consultation with an experienced pediatric nephrologist.

Follow-up. Serum creatinine, BUN and urinalysis should be re-checked after activity has been resumed to be sure that recovery is progressing. Serum B_1C complement should return to normal in acute poststreptococcal glomerulonephritis within six weeks of onset. We would repeat the urinalysis and serum creatinine and creatinine clearance in one week and one, three and six months after ambulation, and at six month intervals until all findings have returned to normal. The creatinine clearance generally normalizes within the first month but microscopic hematuria may persist for months to years despite ultimate recovery.

---

*Manufacturer's warning: Safety of diazoxide injection in children has not been established.

The Nephrotic Syndrome

JEAN E. ROBILLARD, M.D., *and*
FRED G. SMITH, JR., M.D.

Nephrotic syndrome is a clinical entity which is characterized by proteinuria, hypoalbuminemia, hypercholesterolemia, and may be the result of intrinsic renal disease or occur secondary to systemic diseases which damage the glomeruli (i.e., systemic lupus erythematosus, Henoch-Schönlein purpura, nephritis, acute poststreptococcal glomerulonephritis, syphilis, etc.). In children, the nephrotic syndrome is due to intrinsic renal abnormality in 90 per cent of the cases, and the incidence of nephrotic syndrome in children has been reported to be between 2.3 and 2.8 new cases per 100,000 white children under 19 years of age, with a peak incidence at onset between two and three years of age. Renal biopsy findings in children with the nephrotic syndrome indicate that only minimal pathological changes are present in 70 to 80 per cent of the patients.

Generally the physician has two goals in the treatment of the nephrotic syndrome. The first is to eliminate the disease completely by inducing permanent remission; if that cannot be achieved, one should attempt to improve the quality of life by bringing about a partial remission.

Diet. In order to minimize edema before steroids take effect, dietary sodium should be limited. A diet containing 1 to 2 gm./day of sodium chloride is usually tolerable. There is no need for rigid water restriction. In fact, this may be dangerous since it may aggravate the commonly associated hypovolemia. A generous intake of protein is beneficial and is especially important in the growing child. The presence of azotemia and renal failure is, of course, a contraindication to a high-protein diet.

Antibiotics. One of the major advances in the treatment of nephrotic syndrome has been the introduction of antibacterial agents. Before antibiotics, the mortality at five years from onset of the disease was 70 per cent. This has been decreased to 20 per cent after antibiotic therapy was introduced.

Presently, antibiotics are not used prophylactically because their long-term use may predispose the patient to infection with unusual and resistant organisms. However, the life-threatening nature of infection in the nephrotic patient and the large risk of bacterial peritonitis must always be recognized. Prompt intensive antibiotic therapy is then mandatory.

Actually, gram-negative bacillary infections and staphylococcal infections are more frequent than pneumococcal infections in children with nephrotic syndrome under steroid therapy.

Antiserum against herpes zoster and herpes varicellae virus should be used when the danger for these infections occurs in a patient being treated with prednisone and immunosuppressive drugs. Also, during these diseases prednisone dosage should be reduced to physiologic levels (6 mg./m²/day) and immunosuppressive drugs discontinued.

Immunization. No live virus vaccine should be administered when the child is on steroid and immunosuppressive therapy. However, the nephrotic syndrome per se is not a contraindication for routine immunization during the period of remission, although recurrence of nephrotic syndrome has been associated with immunization against influenza viral infections.

Activity. Normal activity can be permitted unless the physical location of the edema prevents normal mobility. In this case careful attention is needed to protect the edematous skin from injury and subsequent infection. After the child becomes free of edema, full activity is permitted and a rapid return to school is encouraged.

Diuretic Therapy. Standard diuretic therapy, while not curative, can give prompt relief to the edematous nephrotic child while waiting for steroids to take effect; however diuretics should be given cautiously.

In the patient with edema secondary to low plasma proteins, the intravascular space is depleted and plasma water and salt shift to the extravascular space. Therefore any therapy which will decrease further the intravascular volume must be monitored carefully. When an edematous nephrotic child needs diuretic therapy, he should be under observation in the hospital during the initial diuresis. Also, his blood pressure and peripheral circulation should be regularly assessed.

Generally, hydrochlorothiazide, 2 to 4 mg./kg./day, given in three or four doses orally, will produce effective diuresis. In less responsive children, more potent diuretics such as furosemide may be required. Initially, 1 mg./kg./day of furosemide is usually effective, but up to 250 mg. or more may be required, especially in the face of renal impairment. Frequent determination of the serum sodium and potassium concentrations should be done during the period of diuretic therapy and especially during the diuresis phase. Supplemental intake of potassium may be necessary.

Patients may be resistant even to potent diuretics because of an important contracted vascular volume that stimulates sodium retention. In these cases, 10 to 25 gm. of salt-poor albumin (1 gm./kg.) may be given intravenously followed by intravenously administered furosemide (1 mg./kg./dose). This may be repeated on three to four successive days as necessary. We reserve this therapy only for patients with serious side effects from their edematous state. We will not institute such therapy in mild states of edema even if refractory to diuretics.

Also, we never recommend paracentesis in the edematous nephrotic child because of the danger of acute shift of water and electrolytes from the vascular space to the peritoneal cavity, which may precipitate a state of severe hypovolemia and shock. Second, children with nephrotic syndrome are more susceptible to infection, and penetrating the peritoneal membrane increases the possibility of peritonitis.

Steroid Therapy. The initial treatment with steroids is usually started as soon as the diagnosis of idiopathic nephrotic syndrome is established. Patients are started on prednisone orally, 60 mg./m²/day (maximum 60 mg./day). It is given daily in three divided doses until the urine becomes free of protein for two or three days or for a total of 28 days if the child does not respond early. Almost all children who will respond to steroid therapy will have responded within four weeks of full therapy. The failure to respond during the first four weeks of therapy may result from the presence of infection, as we have witnessed on several occasions. Thereafter, the same amount (60 mg./m²/day) is given every other day for a two-month period and then withdrawn slowly over the next month.

After this initial therapy, approximately 90 per cent of children with idiopathic nephrotic syndrome will be free of protein. When there is a relapse, the patient again receives prednisone, 60 mg./m²/day, until the urine is free of protein for two or three days or for a total of 28 days, then 60 mg./m² on alternate days for one month, and then tapered over another month. However, respiratory infections are frequently associated with recurrences of proteinuria lasting two to three days. Also, steroid therapy is reintroduced only if the proteinuria persists more than three days in these cases. Those patients who experience frequent relapses but remain responsive to prednisone are retreated for short courses of alternate day prednisone (two or three

months). After two relapses, we believe that a renal biopsy should be performed in order to rule out significant parenchymal renal damage.

If the patient fails to respond to daily steroids for 28 days, he or she is classified as "resistant." We think renal biopsies should be performed in all patients who are "resistant." We prefer to treat "steroid resistant" patients with an alternate day regimen; approximately 30 to 40 per cent will become "protein-free" after six months of treatment.

Side Effects of Steroid Therapy. Complications of steroid therapy are multiple. We must be particularly concerned in the steroid-resistant and steroid-dependent patients who require large doses of prednisone over long periods of time.

Growth failure, hypertension, and disfiguring Cushing's syndrome are the most frequent and the most physically and psychologically damaging side effects. Other complications have included diabetes, osteoporosis, aseptic necrosis, posterior subcapsular cataracts, decreased resistance to infection, myopathy, psychiatric disorders, and increased tendency toward intravascular coagulation.

Immunosuppressive Agents. Immunosuppressive agents such as azathioprine, cyclophosphamide, chlorambucil,* and so forth have been used alone or in combination with prednisone in the management of nephrotic children who are resistant to steroids or who are frequent relapsers. We believe cyclophosphamide is useful in the management of the child who is having frequent relapses and is experiencing significant side effects from steroid therapy. In this latter group, we have used cyclophosphamide, 2 to 3 mg./kg./day, for no more than 42 days in combination with prednisone, 60 mg./m²/day, on alternate days. The parent and child must be informed of the potential hazards of cyclophosphamide which include leukopenia, alopecia, cystitis, nausea, increased susceptibility to severe viral infections, and permanent gonadal damage which may result in sterility.

We do not recommend the use of immunosuppressive agents in the treatment of the child who is resistant to steroids except on rare occasions. Carefully designed studies are needed before the usefulness of cyclophosphamide can be determined in steroid-resistant children.

---

*This use of azathioprine, cyclophosphamide, and chlorambucil is not indicated by their manufacturers.

Chronic Renal Insufficiency

JOSÉ STRAUSS, M.D.

Chronic renal insufficiency or chronic renal failure is the chronic state in which the kidney is unable to perform its function, usually diagnosed when glomerular filtration rate decreases permanently or progressively at least 20 per cent. The various derangements which may be found usually appear gradually but become more prominent as glomerular filtration rate falls below 8 ml./min./1.73 m². These derangements and treatment recommendations are summarized in alphabetical order.

Acidosis. Initially, the metabolic increase in H+ concentration in arterial blood is not clinically detectable; it is mainly compensated by respiratory means and what is left of the renal ability to eliminate H+. Since even mild acidosis may decrease a person's sense of well being, it should be treated with an alkalinizing agent. Doses can only be given as rough guides since the amount required by each patient will depend upon individual ability to correct acidosis and the degree of decompensation. Usually periods with a higher catabolic rate or with respiratory problems will require an increase in the amount of alkalinizer administered.

Initially, when CO_2 of arterial blood is 12 mM/liter, an increase in caloric intake and a decrease in protein intake may suffice. Subsequently, 1 to 3 mEq./kg./day of sodium bicarbonate or calcium carbonate should be administered as needed in divided doses throughout the day. Control of hyperphosphatemia will help in the control of acidosis. Severe acidosis unresponsive to alkali administration or in a patient with fluid overload may benefit from hemodialysis or peritoneal dialysis. The use of Tris-THAM is contraindicated in patients with renal disease but may be helpful in correcting severe acidosis while the patient is being transported or while the dialysis procedure is being set up. Overcorrection should be avoided since alkalosis will decrease ionized calcium and may lead to seizures and cardiac arrhythmias.

Anemia. The typical anemia of the patient with renal disease is normochromic and normocytic. It is an important component of sickle cell nephritis and hereditary nephronophthisis even before appearance of markedly elevated BUN and serum creatinine. Levels of hemoglobin around 8 gm./100 ml. usually are asymptomatic and require no treatment. Hemoglobin of 5 to 8 gm./100 ml. should be treated with iron supplement (sulfate or fumarate, 2 to 5 mg./kg./day of elemental iron in three divided doses), folic acid (1 mg./day), and in older adolescent and young adult males, testosterone enanthate (50 mg. intramuscularly once monthly) or fluoxymesterone (10 to 30 mg./day orally).

Levels of hemoglobin below 5 gm./100 ml. or of hematocrit below 12 per cent require a transfusion of packed and washed or frozen red blood cells (10 to 20 ml./kg.). If the above are not available, whole blood should be transfused, taking care to discard the "buffy coat" or top layer. These measures help reduce the degree of antibody production which will interfere if the patient later receives a kidney transplant.

Special precautions in the treatment of anemia pertain to: testosterone—early epiphyseal fusion in growing children; and transfusions—fluid overload and a poorly understood pulmonary edema for which chlorpromazine (1 mg./kg. intramuscularly prophylactically) is recommended.

Azotemia. The accumulation of various metabolic products and resulting derangements constitute the basis of the complex picture called azotemia. The indispensable component, a continuous and progressively elevated BUN, is taken mainly as a reflection of the accumulation of other toxic products. Initially, adequate hydration (to maintain stable weight) and dietary modification consisting of decreased protein (0.75 gm./kg. preferably of high quality—egg, milk and meat) and increased carbohydrate and fat intake (to supply 50 to 75 cal./kg.) may suffice. Subsequently, only the addition of dialytic procedures and renal transplantation will correct the problem. Care should be taken to avoid excessive decrease of protein intake.

Bone Disease. Osteodystrophy (demineralization, cysts and so on) and rachitism are the manifestations of bone disease related to chronic renal failure in children. Since the bone disturbance is at least related to and may be produced or aggravated by the calcium-phosphorus imbalance, treatment of the accompanying hypocalcemia and hyperphosphatemia should help in controlling its progression. Iatrogenic hypophosphatemia also seems to worsen the osteomalacia.

The bone disease of chronic renal failure, especially when rachitism is present, seems mainly to be caused by the lack of vitamin D or decreased renal conversion of this vitamin to its active metabolite 1, 25-(OH) 2-cholecalciferol. Administration of this product should be the ultimate goal, but it is not yet available commercially. The products available for this purpose are dihydrotachysterol (0.125 mg. orally three times a day) or calciferol (vitamin D_2, usually 500 to 1000 I.U./kg./day and up to 200,000 I.U./day orally). Monitoring serum calcium, phosphorus, and alkaline phosphatase and PTH levels is imperative.

Bleeding and Hematological Aspects. The accumulation of toxic products present in chronic renal failure seems to cause the bleeding tendency observed in these patients. Some type of vasculitis together with liver and bone marrow disturbances forms the basis for this tendency. There is a hemorrhagic tendency (gastrointestinal or genitourinary bleeding, epistaxis) apparently due to a platelet defect. Thrombocytopenia is not common but may occur, especially in systemic disorders; most commonly there is a qualitative platelet defect.

Other hematological changes that may occur are: moderate reticulocytosis, reticulocytopenia, morphological distortion of red blood cells, shortened red blood cell survival, increased autohemolysis, decreased iron incorporation into red blood cells with normal serum iron and iron-binding capacity, and increased adenosine triphosphate and 2,3 diphosphoglycerate of red blood cells. Bone marrow may be normal, hypoplastic or hyperplastic; leukocytes may be normal or increased, but leukopenia may develop in the chronic renal failure of systemic disorders.

General measures directed at minimizing azotemia and improving nutrition should help this problem. Administration of steroids and antimetabolites, if successful in controlling the systemic disorder, also should improve the hematologic components.

Dehydration. Indiscriminate reduction in the amount of water ingested or allowed in patients with poor renal ability to conserve water will lead to dehydration. This problem is magnified in warm climates or when the patient is febrile. Patients should be allowed free access to water unless they require restriction due to fluid overloading and hypertension. In correcting the dehydration of a polyuric patient, the large urinary output disproportionate to intake should be entered in the calculations.

To establish the patient's water needs, 24 hour intake and output should be carefully measured. Approximately 50 per cent of the intake should be voided. The water requirements can be calculated as 500 ml./m^2/day (or 45 ml./100 cal./day) for insensible water loss, to which the measurable losses (urine, vomit, bleeding, and suctioned fluids) should be added. A correct estimate should allow the patient to remain at his normal "dry" weight without undue losses or gains. Overcorrection will lead to problems characteristic of overhydration.

Edema. In the patient with chronic renal failure, edema usually is due to overhydration; only rarely is it due to the nephrotic syndrome. In the newborn, edema is found together with renal agenesis; in infancy and preschool age, with severe congenital anomalies of the genitourinary tract; and later, with any type of chronic renal failure.

Control of salt and fluid intake or addition of a diuretic agent to the therapeutic regimen should control most cases of edema. In the more advanced cases when other factors determine a change in therapeutic modality, hemodialysis will help to remove retained fluids. When the nephrotic syndrome is present, rapid (30 min.) administration of volume expanders (albumin, mannitol* or dextran, 1 gm./kg.) followed by a diuretic (furosemide or ethacrynic acid,† 1 to 5 mg./kg. by intravenous push) should produce diuresis if glomerular filtration rate is not decreased to the point of interference with this therapeutic modality.

Growth Retardation. Failure to thrive or some degree of growth impairment is present in infants with congenital uropathy and renal tubular acidosis; in preschool children with Fanconi syndrome, nephronophthisis, hydronephrosis, obstructive uropathy and sickle cell disease; and in school-age children with segmental renal hypoplasia.

The problem of stunted growth lacks definition, though it is unquestionably present in patients with longstanding impairment in renal functions. The patient's growth curve may have been normal up to the time the renal disease developed. The interference with growth varies with each patient, type of renal disease, treatment used, and degree, type and duration of renal disturbance.

Use of steroids may, to some degree, worsen the existing growth problem; their role in retarding growth is not clear. Chronic malnutrition, whether present prior to the onset of chronic renal failure or secondary to the dietary manipulations, may play a role in the patient's growth. Prolonged dialysis stunts growth for unknown reasons. Institution of good dietary habits (ingestion of high quality

---

*Manufacturer's precaution: Dosage requirements of mannitol for patients 12 years and under have not been established.

†Manufacturer's note: Insufficient pediatric experience precludes recommendation for this age group of intravenous dosage of ethacrynic acid.

proteins and high caloric diet), correction of osteodystrophy, and renal transplantation should help in restoring the growth pattern toward normal. Use of anabolic steroids is of questionable value.

Heart Failure. Fluid overload, arterial hypertension, chronic malnutrition and coexistence of systemic disease (diabetes, atherosclerosis, systemic lupus erythematosus, and so on) are among the causes of this disturbance. Placement of an arteriovenous bypass (external shunt or internal fistula or bovine graft) for chronic hemodialysis creates extra work for the heart. The degree to which this procedure is tolerated depends largely on the size and location of the bypass—the larger and closer to the heart, the greater the extra cardiac load and the possibility of cardiac decompensation.

Treatment should aim at restoring a good state of nutrition, proper vitamin intake, elimination of fluid overload, control of hypertension and the systemic disease if present, placement of the smallest bypass possible as distally as possible, and administration of digitalis. The latter should be undertaken as a last resort and discontinued as soon as possible.

Hyperkalemia. Hyperkalemia, the usual cause of concern in a newly diagnosed patient or in a patient known to have poor dietary control, can be fatal. Its clinical definition is elusive since a blood level by itself is not sufficient; it is a dynamic state where rate of increase, pH, and ratio of intracellular to extracellular potassium levels, among others, play a role. Most laboratories accept a normal range of 3.5 to 5.6 mEq./liter; accordingly, a laboratory diagnosis of hyperkalemia is made with a serum level of potassium greater than 6 mEq./liter. A clinically useful diagnosis requires electrocardiographic changes; they may appear at levels of 7 mEq./liter or higher, depending upon blood pH and serum calcium, among other factors.

Treatment of hyperkalemia in a patient with chronic renal failure must include dietary control with reduction of protein intake and increase in calories. Administration of Kayexalate (resin which exchanges potassium for hydrogen and sodium ions) orally or by retention enema at daily doses of 0.5 gm./kg. two or three times daily, is extremely helpful. Oral intake is facilitated by preparing capsules with the necessary amount rather than having to ingest the resin in a suspension.

For acute exacerbations or when a patient arrives with marked electrocardiographic changes, rapid but transient correction can be achieved by administration of glucose in water together with insulin, both intravenously. Since this treatment displaces potassium from the extracellular to the intracellular spaces, a normal pH is essential. Accordingly, if the patient is acidotic, an alkalinizing agent also should be administered. Since this is only a transient maneuver and allows potassium to remain in the body, exchange resins should be instituted at the same time and continued indefinitely.

Once the patient's glomerular filtration rate has decreased below a level of 8 ml./min./1.73 m^2, either one of the dialytic procedures (hemodialysis or peritoneal dialysis) must be considered. Avoidance of hypokalemia is important since it will induce neuromuscular derangements which also can be fatal; for this reason, potassium chloride supplements should be provided to all patients on chronic diuretic therapy, and potassium should be added as soon as possible to the solution used in any dialysis procedure.

Hyperphosphatemia. Most likely this derangement starts with phosphorus retention secondary to a decreased glomerular filtration rate in most cases of chronic renal failure; it may appear for unexplained reasons in renal tubular acidosis. It is characteristically present in the newborn with renal agenesis and in the older infant or child with renal tubular acidosis and renal hypoplasia. Before therapeutic modifications, it is accompanied by hypocalcemia.

Treatment must be directed at decreasing phosphorus intake (similar to protein intake), increasing caloric intake, reducing phosphorus absorption (Amphojel or Basaljel, 1200 to 2700 mg. daily), calcium supplementation and vitamin D or analogs. An unresolved question is how early to start treatment. Avoidance of hypophosphatemia is essential since it will aggravate the bone disease and may affect cellular metabolism.

Hypertension. Elevations in arterial blood pressure can be present early in the neonate with congenital uropathy and in the older infant and child with polyarteritis nodosa, systemic lupus erythematosus, and segmental hypoplasia. Eventually, it will appear in most cases of chronic renal failure, especially when overhydration is present. Accordingly, treatment should be directed at the cause, to correct overhydration and to administer the necessary drugs. Chronically, orally administered drugs such as diuretics, peripheral vasodilators (hydralazine, 1 to 10 mg./kg./day; minoxidil,* 0.1 to 1.5 mg./kg./day),

---

*Minoxidil is an investigational drug.

and sympathetic inhibitors (methyldopa, 10 to 50 mg./kg./day; clonidine,* 0.2 to 2.4 mg./day; propranolol hydrochloride,† 1 to 5 mg./kg./day), alone or combined, usually will suffice to control hypertension. Under acute conditions, overhydration will produce hypertension which may be severe and require dialytic procedures for rapid correction; intravenous medication can be life-saving (sodium nitroprusside, 0.5 to 8 µg./kg./min. infused continuously; diazoxide,‡ 3 to 5 mg./kg. by intravenous push). As of this writing, sodium nitroprusside has not been approved by the Food and Drug Administration for use in children.

It is imperative to monitor patients frequently to avoid overcorrection of hypertension. This is particularly true of acute episodes in which an emergency develops and powerful drugs are administered intravenously or hemodialysis is performed to remove fluids rapidly.

Hyperuricemia. Uric acid serum levels increase with various renal diseases at different rates for reasons not well understood. Administration of diuretics or of urine acidifiers favors hyperuricemia; decreasing urine pH also decreases uric acid solubility and excretion.

Treatment consists of dietary control (decrease in alcohol and protein ingestion, increase in caloric intake), reduction in diuretic administration, use of urine alkalinizers, induction of water diuresis, and administration of uricosuric agents (probenecid, 25 to 40 mg./kg./day) or of agents limiting the production of uric acid (allopurinol, 50 to 100 mg./day).§

Possible complications of treatment include precipitation of uric acid crystals with formation of calculi when an uricosuric agent is administered in the presence of scant and acid urine; allergic reaction to allopurinol consists of an itchy rash on the legs which disappears upon discontinuation of the drug.

Hypoalbuminemia. The nephrotic syndrome accompanying chronic renal failure has a decreased albumin serum level secondary to albuminuria and probably worsened by chronic malnutrition and liver impairment. Edema is a more constant accompaniment of chronic renal failure in these cases; a mild degree of overhydration may lead to formation of edema. However, the relationship between edema formation and hypoalbuminemia is not constant since edema may be present without hypoalbuminemia or overhydration and no edema may be detected with very low levels of serum albumin (<1.5 to 2 gm./100 ml.). Obviously, factors other than serum albumin are at play in the formation of edema; hypersensitivity to environmental antigens or allergens and hormonal changes may be at least partially responsible.

Treatment of hypoalbuminemia can await severe accumulation of edema. Otherwise, attempts to increase the albumin levels in serum are doomed to failure as the infused albumin is promptly lost in the urine. Acute administration of plasma expanders and diuretics should help in the symptomatic correction of the edema. Cautious supervision should be exercised to avoid hypertension as fluid is brought into the intravascular compartment; dehydration could ensue as diuresis is established. Prolonged use of diuretics may perpetuate the edema and increase the possibility of venous thrombosis described in nephrotic patients.

Hypocalcemia. A constant accompaniment of chronic renal failure, hypocalcemia is closely related to bone disease, hyperphosphatemia and hypercalciuria. In most cases the initiating problem may be a reduction in glomerular filtration rate which leads to hyperphosphatemia and in turn induces hypocalcemia to maintain the needed Ca/P ratio. The stimulus to the parathyroid gland produces hypersecretion of parathyroid hormone and bone disease. Some patients have a primary hypercalciuria.

Besides controlling the hyperphosphatemia as described above, hypocalcemia should be treated by oral administration of 10 to 20 mg./kg./day of calcium as calcium gluconate, lactate or carbonate in three or four doses, and by administration of vitamin or analogs. Acute episodes of hypocalcemia with convulsions and muscular contractions should be treated with slow intravenous infusions of 10 per cent calcium lactate or gluconate at a rate of 0.1 ml./kg./min., provided that the heart rate does not decrease by >10 beats/minute.

Hyponatremia. Since patients with chronic renal failure have a tendency to lose salt excessively in the urine, indiscriminate salt

---

*Manufacturer's precaution: No clinical experience is available with the use of clonidine in children. The maximum effective daily dose is 2.4 mg., but doses as high as this have rarely been employed.

†Manufacturer's note: Data on the use of propranolol in the pediatric age group are too limited to permit adequate directions for use.

‡Manufacturer's precaution. The safety of intravenous diazoxide in children has not yet been established.

§Allopurinol has not been approved for use in children, except in those with hyperuricemia secondary to malignancy.

restriction will lead to body sodium depletion and decrease in sodium serum level. The only manner in which salt-losing patients can be identified and the actual sodium needs determined is by measurement of intake and output. In patients with excessive salt losses in the urine, a normal salt intake can be allowed if the patient is not hypertensive or retaining fluids excessively.

It is useful to remember that hypoproteinemic diets contain 10 to 20 mEq. of sodium without the addition of sodium chloride (each gram of which equals about 400 mg. or 17 mEq. of sodium). All additional forms of sodium ingested should be taken into account in attempting to establish total sodium intake; sodium exchanged for other ions (Kayexalate, 1 gm. leads to retention of 3 mEq. of sodium); sodium in alkalinizing agents (sodium bicarbonate, 1 gm. is equal to about 12 mEq. of sodium); and various other drugs administered as sodium salt.

Treatment of hyponatremia consists of oral replacement of the lost salt or restriction of fluids in the amount needed to restore balance. Subsequently, prophylaxis consists of supplements of salt in the amounts lost in the urine.

Hypovitaminosis. Patients with chronic renal failure have such distorted food intake (by prescription, poor dietary advice, or lack of appetite) that often they do not receive the minimum daily requirement of vitamins. Added to this is the drain caused by dialysis. It has become routine to administer multivitamins, iron and folic acid.

Immunologic Disorders. Many diseases leading to chronic renal failure have immunologic bases. Unfortunately, no clear-cut assessment can be made at this time regarding specific factors leading to progression of the renal disease; the therapeutic implications of what is known or suspected have not been well documented.

The only exception to the above may be renal transplantation which involves survival of a homograft kidney; it is readily and universally accepted that failure to administer prednisone and antimetabolites leads to graft rejection. Even so, the mechanism of action of these agents is not clear.

Prednisone, antimetabolites and anticoagulants, individually or combined, are being used in renal disorders with serum total complement decrease, glomerular or tubular basement membrane changes, glomerular epithelial cell proliferation, microangiopathy, angiopathy or coagulopathies. No fixed recommendations can be made for all these patients. One rule generally applied is that at onset, observation, symptomatic treatment and diagnostic procedures should be instituted. General measures of protection should be enforced. Avoidance of exposure to toxins or allergens is desirable; increasing numbers of patients are being reported as evidencing allergic manifestations to various environmental factors (including foodstuffs) at the time of clinical onset of the disease or of exacerbations. If the allergen (antigen) is known, it should be promptly eliminated from the patient's environment or diet. If close to 100 per cent of glomeruli are severely affected (epithelial crescents present) and the glomerular filtration rate follows a downgrade course, a trial with antimetabolites and some of the other agents may be warranted on an empirical, unproven regimen. Since such treatment does not have the approval of the Food and Drug Administration, a special informed consent for use of experimental drugs must be secured from parents and older children.

Infection, Inflammation, and Fever. This subject may be closely related to immunologic disorders. Some of the above statements may be pertinent here, especially in relationship to systemic diseases such as systemic lupus erythematosus (SLE), Henoch-Schönlein purpura, and so on.

No definitive data are available yet on the types of renal involvement (diffuse versus focal) which, if untreated, will progress to chronic renal failure and, if treated, will disappear, progress more slowly or stop progressing. SLE (not an uncommon disease in children) may produce severe decrease in glomerular filtration rate to the point that hemodialysis is required. Institution of prednisone and antimetabolite therapy or increase in prednisone dose can restore the glomerular filtration rate to its previous level. What effect such a reduction in glomerular function has on the final outcome or how much the steroid-antimetabolite combination affects the progression of the disease is not known. Currently, there are controlled efforts to quantitate these variables in the most severe group of patients (those with diffuse glomerular involvement).

Patients with chronic renal failure may evidence inflammatory processes which are related to the basic illness or unrelated to any specific factors. It is important to keep in mind that patients may not be able to respond normally to bacterial invasion and that an otherwise controllable situation may overwhelm some of them. The nephrotic syndrome present in some, the functional asplenia described in the SS hemoglobinopathy, and the use of steroids and antimetabolites create special situations regarding infections. An active search for infective pathogens in urine, skin, throat, blood and CNS fluid (as indicated), even with paucity of signs or symptoms in a suspected patient, is the only way to diagnose an infection.

Treatment with antibiotics should be aggressive and as specific as possible with antibiotic sensitivities obtained from any positive culture. The inflammatory episode of systemic diseases such as SLE usually will respond to larger doses of steroids or antimetabolites.

Neurologic Disorders. The systemic disease leading to chronic renal failure also may affect the central nervous system as in the case of SLE and acute or chronic endogenous or exogenous poisonings. Chronic renal failure, with the disturbances induced by restrictions in intake, administration of steroids, accumulation of various products, or by removal of various substances from the bloodstream, may lead to neurological changes. These may range from minor sensory disturbances to gross cerebral and peripheral nerve dysfunction: metabolic encephalopathy (generalized myoclonic convulsions, Wernicke encephalopathy, akinetic mutism, and Balint syndrome); neuromuscular irritability (asterixis or metabolic flap, myoclonus, and muscular wasting or degeneration); cranial nerve (sixth nerve weakness, deafness and vertigo and amaurosis) or peripheral nerve changes (asymmetry, hyperreflexia and hyporeflexia); and CSF alterations (elevated pressure, protein content and cell count).

When the glomerular filtration rate falls below 8 ml./min./1.73 m², dialysis and transplantation must be regarded as likely therapeutic procedures. They are discussed separately in this text.

Chronic renal insufficiency or failure is a complex state with a multiplicity of factors involved and a large armamentarium of therapeutic tools available. It is essential that diagnosis be made early so that management can be instituted at the proper time. The relatively slow course of renal deterioration induced by some disorders (especially congenital urological anomalies) makes it ideal for thorough medical, emotional and financial reviews as soon as the suspicion of a progressive disorder is entertained. The readily available dialysis and transplantation measures for the care of patients in end stage renal disease should not lead to a sense of complacency. Rather, the large number of these patients should be a stimulus to find the causes and

implement the prophylactic measures to prevent the development of congenital anomalies of the genitourinary tract and of the various progressive nephropathies.

Peritoneal Dialysis

JOSÉ STRAUSS, M.D.

Any situation in which there is accumulation of waste products (acute or chronic renal failure) or of drugs (acute or chronic intoxication or poisoning) should benefit from peritoneal dialysis. The only limitation is that the substances to be removed must diffuse through semipermeable membranes.

Materials ready-made for this purpose are: solutions (two concentrations); special infusion-drainage set; trocar with special set (adult and pediatric sizes); and balance sheet. Materials available for general use and adapted for this purpose in place of above are: glucose solutions, potassium chloride solution; electrolyte solutions; feeding tubes; intravenous sets; Buretrol; blood warmer; intracath; intake and output sheet; vital signs sheet; and bed scale.

Technique. In the abdominal midline between the umbilicus and the symphysis pubis (about one-third the distance below the umbilicus), a point is marked. A local anesthetic (1 to 2 per cent Xylocaine) is injected intradermally and then subcutaneously. After proper surgical preparation (three cleansings with Betadine or similar solution and formation of a surgical field with sterile paper or cloth towels), a hole is punctured with a No. 12-14 Intracath needle. The needle is advanced for about ¼" or until the peritoneum is pierced, at which time the metal part is removed and the plastic cannula is advanced all the way up to the adapter. A solution of 2.5 per cent dextrose in water in 0.45 per cent sodium chloride is instilled through the cannula until the abdominal wall is distended without interfering with respiration. The Intracath is removed and in the same spot a larger hole is made with a No. 11 pointed scalpel blade thrust in until the peritoneum is pierced. The special dialysis catheter (pediatric size), with its trocar inside to maintain a straight form, is pushed through the hole until the "pop" sound is heard, characteristic of the peritoneum being pierced. Gently, the catheter is pushed toward one of the iliac fossae with the trocar inside initially but not subsequently or at any time is pressure applied. If not done before, the trocar is removed when the tip of the catheter reaches its final location. The special catheter is taped to the skin by using wide adhesive tape with a hole in the center. A suture holding the catheter to the skin or the tape may be useful.

The catheter is cut down to about one inch from the abdominal surface and then connected to the special dialysis tubing. This tubing is connected sequentially as follows: "In": warmer, short (about 2 feet) single tubing, Buretrol, bottle and "Out" from catheter to measuring bag for discarded fluid.

The volume of fluid used will depend upon the specific patient. A general rule is 20 to 40 ml./kg. with a maximum of 1200 ml./m² surface area. Some authors with extensive experience use up to 70 ml./kg. in infants. The absolute rule is to observe the degree of abdominal distention and to fill the abdomen only up to a point which does not interfere with cardiorespiratory function. This volume usually is in the range of 150 to 300 ml. for infants, 300 to 500 ml. for preschoolers and 500 to 1500 ml. for older children and adolescents. Initially, heparin is added to the solutions (1000 units/liter); if there are no specific indications for its use, heparin is discontinued.

Each volume is kept in for 30 to 45 minutes; the remainder of the hour is used to retrieve the instilled dialysis fluid plus any extra fluid. It is essential that accurate records be kept with clear labels as to time and amount of fluid "in" and "out."

The type of fluid used is modified to meet the specific patient's needs. The general approach consists in instilling a solution which contains less than normal solute concentration, or none of that which is in excess in the patient. For hyperkalemia, no potassium chloride is added to the dialysis solution (which has no potassium) or only 2 mEq./liter of potassium are added to the initial dialysis washings. Once a trend has been established and the serum potassium is decreasing, the potassium in the dialysis solution is increased to 3 to 4 mEq./L.

Mild deviations from normal in serum calcium, phosphorus, uric acid and sodium should improve by dialyzing the patient with a solution containing the normal concentration of those solutes. Severe deviations from normal require use of solutions with addition or subtraction of the solute in low or high concentration, respectively; for uric acid, increase in the solution's pH is highly desirable. When excess fluid needs to be removed, the concentration of solutes in the afferent fluid is increased. The solution may have the following compositions: 1.5 per cent and 4.5 per cent dextrose in water; fortunately, a higher glucose concentration solution has been discontinued because of the frequency of complication and lack of indication.

Moderate water removal is to be expected under most circumstances by using the dialysis solution with the lowest glucose concentration (1.5 per cent). Large water removal requires use of the higher concentration of glucose. It is important that the concentration of glucose be as close to 1.5 per cent as soon as possible to avoid excessive correction of fluid overload and the development of severe hyperglycemia.

The levels of blood glucose must be monitored frequently to be sure that safe limits are not exceeded, especially when using the dialysis solution with high glucose concentration and when diazoxide is administered concomitantly for the control of hypertension.

For the removal of drugs from the circulation, the general measures outlined above should suffice. Specific instructions from each pharmaceutical company should be followed to enhance removal of a certain agent; simple changes such as an increase in the pH of the solution or addition of albumin to the dialysate will greatly modify the solubility and removal of a given compound. (Emerg. Med., 1972, pp. 48–52.)

Complications. HEMORRHAGES.   Piercing the abdominal wall too close to the umbilicus may damage the vessels of that area. Rough edges of a freshly cut catheter tip may produce abrasions. Jerking and thrusting the catheter back and forth may lead to small vessel damage at the interface of tissues. In all the above cases, a faint pink color indicates mild bleeding which usually requires no corrective measures. A darker color or clearly red fluid requires the continuous addition of heparin (1000 units/liter) in the dialysis solution or temporary discontinuation of the procedure; if dialysis needs to be continued, the problem may be solved by the use of another abdominal site for the tip of the catheter or of another point of penetrance in the abdominal wall.

INFECTION.   This complication may develop despite all precautions and any length of time the dialysis continues. Some basic steps will greatly reduce the chances of infection: (1) any sign of peritonitis is a contraindication for peritoneal dialysis or should lead to treatment of peritonitis prior to the start of peritoneal dialysis; (2) all standard precautions are taken to ensure that only sterile equipment and supplies are used; (3) the skin is prepared as for surgery in the area and at least five inches around where the catheter will be introduced; (4) the catheter is firmly secured to avoid in-and-out movements which will introduce contaminated segments of the catheter inside the abdominal wall or peritoneum, and (5) the catheter is removed as soon as it is not needed. It should be properly covered during and between procedures. Infections seem to be less frequent when the catheter is withdrawn and re-implanted for peritoneal dialysis with intervals greater than 24 hours between procedures.

The routine prophylactic use of antibiotics either in the dialysis solution or parenterally is not recommended. Awareness of the possibility of infection should lead to an early diagnosis of this complication; specific treatment for the organism involved should be effective, especially if administered both intraperitoneally and systemically.

LEAKAGE. This problem may be decreased or eliminated by making a tight fitting around the catheter. In addition, no side holes should be outside of the peritoneum. In small children, a special pediatric catheter should be used; for newborns and infants, an Intracath sleeve can be used provided side holes are burnt near the tip with a needle.

PERFORATION. A hollow organ (urinary bladder, intestinal loop, and so on) can be penetrated by the Intracath needle, the scalpel blade, or the trocar. The best precaution against perforation is to remain as superficial as possible with these sharp instruments. The operator should handle the tool with the index finger and the thumb while supporting the hand by means of the small finger pressing on the abdominal wall; preferably, both hands should be used at the same time for greater force and control.

Perforation by catheter is unlikely but it can occur under extreme conditions. A distended and fixed organ will be easier to perforate than a deflated movable organ (normal state). A catheter which has been shortened at the penetrating (proximal) end may have sharp edges or a bevel tip; this can mimic a needle or scalpel and facilitate perforation of a viscus. Therefore shortening of catheters should be avoided if at all possible; if not, the following precautions are mandatory: cut the catheter at its distal end; if the proximal end *must* be cut, file out or burn the sharp edges prior to use.

PLUGGING. The dialysis catheter has a large hole at the tip and multiple small holes to facilitate movement of fluid in and out of the abdominal cavity. One single large hole at the end of the catheter in line with its longest measurement is undesirable because of less efficient drainage, greater likelihood of occlusion by the omenta, and greater risk of trauma to internal organs.

The small holes are located in the sides of the dialysis catheter near its tip. These holes can be plugged by precipitated proteins, omenta, or blood; their usefulness can be greatly decreased by contact with the abdominal wall and the surface of relatively fixed intestinal loops.

HYPOKALEMIA. Institution of peritoneal dialysis because of hyperkalemia can lead to overcorrection and the development of hypokalemia. To avoid this and sudden changes in the total body content and blood levels of potassium, the dialysate should always contain some potassium. The amount to be added must be decided by the individual physician and tailored to each patient's needs. The intake and output of potassium must be carefully recorded. Care should be exercised to avoid worsening a depletion of total body potassium with normal or elevated serum potassium due to acidosis.

DEHYDRATION. Peritoneal dialysis performed with any available solution for that purpose is hyperosmotic and therefore will produce movement of water into the peritoneal cavity. If this water is removed and not replaced in a carefully planned manner, eventually dehydration will ensue. This is particularly true of situations in which there is overhydration and fluid removal is one of the therapeutic aims. In such case a solution with a higher concentration of glucose, and consequently with a higher osmolality, is used and the fluid removal magnified; therefore, the danger of dehydration is greater than with the standard solution. To minimize the danger of dehydration, only the standatd solution should be used in situations in which there is poor control of intake and output and only infrequent weighing of the patient.

HYPERGLYCEMIA. All solutions used for peritoneal dialysis have a glucose concentration greater than that of blood and therefore will lead to hyperglycemia. This is especially true when using the solution with higher glucose concentration (to remove water) and even more so if diazoxide is used concomitantly in order to control severe hypertension. Only extremely careful monitoring of blood sugar will avoid catastrophic consequences under those conditions.

Treatment of such a complication should be as conservative as possible and mainly oriented at decreasing the supply of glucose. Too aggressive treatment with insulin will only lead to unavoidable hypoglycemia. Whenever possible, insulin should be withheld or only administered cautiously in several small doses as indicated.

Patient Control. Peritoneal dialysis is relatively safe and simple, provided the personnel are familiar with the procedure, exercise proper caution and have access to the necessary monitoring equipment.

The receptacle for the fluid withdrawn from the peritoneal cavity should be readily accessible, well sealed, transparent and graduated. Its position should be at a level below that of the patient to make drainage by gravity possible. To minimize infection it should be connected to the dialysis catheter through a sealed system and emptied without breaking the continuity of this system.

The sheet on which the balance of fluid and the various laboratory results are entered should be clearly labeled and easily read at a glance. The concept of "positive" and "negative" balance should be clearly stated so that reporting is not misinterpreted and decisions are not made contrary to the patient's needs.

Repeat Procedures. Usually peritoneal dialysis is performed for periods of 6 to 48 hours, after which another dialysis may be needed 24 to 72 hours later. The need for repeat dialysis will be decreased if the catabolism is reduced to a minimum by administration of high calorie-low protein diets, and if complications such as infection are treated promptly.

The approach to follow regarding removal of the catheter is a subject of controversy. In general, the catheter should be maintained in place during intervals of 24 to 48 hours; for longer intervals the catheter should be removed and re-implanted when needed again.

For temporary renal failure, this procedure may be repeated as often as needed. For chronic renal failure (in the absence of hemodialysis) a "button" is inserted in the abdominal wall to provide ready access to the peritoneal cavity.

It can be stated categorically that peritoneal dialysis is a relatively simple procedure which is extremely useful in the treatment of renal failure and of intoxications. Though proper training, personnel, equipment and facilities are essential, even the smallest hospital may render this valuable and rewarding therapy.

Hemodialysis

JOSÉ STRAUSS, M.D.

Hemodialysis is indicated for removal of accumulated waste products in acute or chronic renal failure, removal of excess fluid, and removal of dialyzable poisons and drugs. This mode of therapy should be used whenever the serum creatinine is above 8 mg./dl. or the creatinine clearance is below 8 ml./min./1.73m^2, when the patient shows severe, life-threatening changes, or when the patient has intractable pulmonary edema or cardiac failure.

Facilities and Personnel. Approximately 100 square feet per patient are indispensable to accommodate equipment around the patient. Any good dialysis machine should be adequate if the personnel are familiar with the machine and the procedure. The ratio of nurses to patients varies with the severity of the problem, ranging from one nurse to four patients in the chronic, old, stable or adolescent setting to one nurse per patient or even one nurse and one technician per patient in the acute pediatric emergency situation and in the dialysis of a young unstable child.

Equipment and Solutions. Numerous options in this area make a choice more difficult.

DIALYZING MACHINES. A variety of dialysis machines are available. Basically, they are comparable; differences are minor when looked at from the point of view of performance of the desired treatment. One recycles the dialysate but final trials have not been performed; thus its reliability remains somewhat uncertain. Other machines are also portable but bulkier than the nonportable.

DIALYZING SOLUTIONS. In areas with water substantially rich in minerals, it may be necessary to establish special procedures. Otherwise, the simple de-ionizing system is sufficient in most situations.

DELIVERY SYSTEMS. New systems for central delivery of dialyzing solutions have simplified and at the same time complicated this aspect. The simplification consists of the use of only one reservoir with no need to use modifications in the water entering each machine. The complication is the accumulation of pools of water in various areas leading to growth of water-related germs (Pseudomonas, and so on). For small clinical units, time-tested individual delivery systems seem to be most highly desirable and are preferred.

SINGLE NEEDLE ADMINISTRATION. Without question, the machines which make possible the application of dialysis into an especially prepared vessel through a single needle is to be preferred over the system which requires two needles. Patient acceptance is greater and procedure performance quality seems to be equal.

DIALYZERS. These are the main components to consider for the most efficient dialysis tailored to the needs of each patient. By mass transfer, solutes are removed; by changes in the pressures within the system, fluid is removed. The above characteristics plus the ease and completeness of blood recovery (especially in small children) should be guides in the choice of dialyzer.

There are three main types: (1) parallel flow dialyzer, made of dialyzing membrane alternating with supporting layers; the dialysate flows between support and membrane while blood flows between the two membrane layers; (2) coil dialyzer, made of membrane wrapped around a cylinder; the dialysate flows through the membrane support while the blood flows between two membrane layers; and (3) hollow fiber capillary kidney, made of many capillaries laying side by side; the dialysate flows among the capillaries while the blood flows through them.

Desirable and undesirable aspects of each dialyzer are as follows: (1) the parallel flow does not require a blood pump, small priming volume, unlikely to induce hypotension, relatively inefficient with low mass transfer rate; (2) the coil is efficient, easy-to-use, needs small amounts of heparin, a blood pump is essential, leaks more frequent than with other dialyzers, difficult to predict needed priming and ultrafiltration volumes; and (3) hollow fiber capillary is extremely efficient, easy-to-predict priming and ultrafiltration volumes, may be used without a blood pump, requires larger amounts of heparin. It seems safe to state that for newborns and infants the parallel flow dialyzer should be preferred, for young children the hollow fiber capillary does a good job, and for older children and adolescents the coil is the easiest to use.

Vascular Access. For emergency situations we use an external shunt with one Teflon tubing inserted into a vein and another into an artery of an upper or lower extremity, depending upon patient size and vessel size. Once an acute or emergency situation has subsided, if the need for dialysis persists, the patient then will have a permanent subcutaneous fistula or a bovine graft inserted. Our results seem to be equally good with the fistula or the graft, though in patients with small vessels, the graft seems to be preferred.

General recommendations suggest the following placement for vascular access: for children who weigh more than 8 kg., peripheral radial artery and cephalic or basilic vein; for those who weigh 4 to 8 kg., brachial artery and cephalic or basilic vein; for those who weigh less than 4 kg., profunda or superficial femoral artery and saphenous vein; and for newborns, the umbilical vessels. The above recommendations should be modified to suit an individual patient; for instance, a child with a weight greater than 8 kg. but who has small vessels may need to have a vascular access usually recommended for patients who weigh less than 8 kg.

Monitoring. In patients who are overweight and need to lose fluid, continuous monitoring of weight can be best accomplished with an electronic scale. This useful tool requires the staff's thorough familiarization with details. Often, even though available, this scale is not used because its operation has not been adequately explained. If an electronic scale is not available, weighing the patient at the beginning and end of each procedure is mandatory. The aim of each dialysis should be to end as close as possible to the patient's "dry" or "true" weight.

Blood pressure should be checked frequently in order to avoid hypotension while attempting to remove fluids; hypertension may be due to fluid overload even in a patient who seems to be dry (mistaken "true" or "dry" weight?) but who could benefit from further removal of fluids. In acute situations, continuous monitoring of heart rate and electrocardiogram is desirable in order to avoid marked changes in cardiac function. Monitoring of pulse rate should be frequently performed and a cardiac monitor installed if there is any indication of arrhythmia. Body temperature should be checked frequently in order to avoid excessive temperature change induced by the machine. Blood chemistries should be checked before and after each procedure until the patient stabilizes, and in chronic patients until a routine mode of management is established.

Subsequently, monitoring of electrolytes and complete blood count should be done less frequently. The complete evaluation of total protein, uric acid, albumin, phosphorus, Australia antigen, serum iron, serum iron-binding capacity, and so on, should be done at least once monthly. Bone appearance and serum parathyroid hormone should be monitored every three months and bone age once annually in a patient with chronic renal disease. Other monitoring such as bone marrow, chest x-ray, electroencephalogram and electrocardiogram should be performed in all patients but timed according to the patient's individual problems.

Reason for Treatment. If the purpose of the hemodialysis is to remove fluids, increased venous resistance is applied. The speed at which the machine is set to circulate the blood and the dialysate will depend upon the efficiency desired to remove solutes. Initially, short dialysis at a slower rate is desirable; both time and rate can be increased with repeated dialysis performed daily until the patient stabilizes or the blood chemistries are within tolerable ranges.

Dialysis Prior to Transplantation. This

question must be solved on an individual basis. In the past some have believed that patients with anti-kidney antibodies should be dialyzed for several months prior to transplantation; this practice has not been supported by experience, nor have solid data been accumulated to prove this point. If a patient is not a good surgical risk, hemodialysis may be used prior to transplantation to reduce the level of accumulated substances or to remove excess fluids and correct hypertension; otherwise, hemodialysis is not necessary.

Prophylactic Dialysis. In patients who have deteriorated but are ready to have a transplant performed, some advise the installation of external shunts and performance of dialysis prior to transplantation. An external shunt would facilitate performance of the dialysis if the transplanted kidney were to be rejected acutely. An acceptable alternative is to place the external shunt at the specific time needed, thus avoiding unnecessary surgery.

Complications. If dialysis is initiated in a patient with extremely high levels of BUN (> 100 mg./dl.), serum creatinine (> 10 mg./dl.), or serum osmolality (> 310 mOsm./kg.); or if too aggressive a dialysis is performed, often the patient will have convulsions. To minimize this, mannitol (20 per cent solution) or plasma proteins (5 per cent solution) (0.5 to 1 gm./kg.) should be administered throughout the procedure, and the dialysis should be performed slowly and for a short period of time.* When too aggressive dialysis to remove fluid is performed, especially in patients on antihypertensive medication, hypotension may complicate the procedure; this can be corrected by administration of 0.9 per cent sodium chloride (200 ml./m^2/hr.), mannitol (20 per cent) or plasma proteins (5 per cent). Antihypertensives should be discontinued at least six hours before dialysis and short-acting drugs (hydralazine, sodium nitroprusside) should be used preferentially.†

Infections may develop, usually due to poor sterilization of the equipment, or contamination of the vascular access when the patient is connected to or disconnected from the machine (especially with an external shunt). Australia antigen positive hepatitis may be acquired from other patients or personnel. Clotting of the dialysis system can occur for unknown reasons, especially when using the capillary flow systems. In this case, an added amount of heparin should be used; subsequently, this problem may disappear without a clearly explainable reason.

Vomiting is a frequent occurrence during dialysis and seems to affect children more often than adults; treatment may be unnecessary except when associated with hypotension. Cardiac arrhythmia should be well documented and treated along with correction of the electrolyte imbalance which may be present at the same time. Acid base imbalances are infrequent and usually do not require special treatment.

When there is a break in the line, immediate clamping of the various parts of the system will prevent exsanguination. Electrical shocks can occur if the machine is improperly grounded or if the common grounding system is not used for the various electrical tools. When this happens, a defibrillator may need to be used to restart a heart which has gone into ventricular fibrillation or arrest. Failure of various alarms to detect foam, air, or changes in various pressures may lead to serious complications. These can be prevented by continuous maintenance to ensure excellent function of the equipment.

Osteodystrophy. This may be present prior to the onset of hemodialysis or develop during a chronic maintenance period. Both preventive and therapeutic administration of vitamin D or its metabolites have their supporters. Maintenance of a normal level of serum phosphorus by phosphate binders (Amphojel, Basaljel); administration of supplemental calcium (as gluconate, lactate or carbonate); and vitamin D (10,000 to 50,000 I.U.) should at least delay bone deterioration. In a patient with osteodystrophy, hyperphosphatemia and hypocalcemia, a higher than normal (6 mg./dl.) calcium level in the dialysate solution may be beneficial.

Diet. An acceptable state of nutrition may be attained by providing 50 to 75 cal./kg./day and 1 to 3 gm. of protein/kg./day. Recommendations vary on dietary restriction and the desirable or tolerable level of fluid and urea accumulation. In general, normotensive patients should be on a nonrestricted fluid, sodium and protein intake, provided they come to dialysis three times per week for up to six hours or as long as needed. In patients who do not come three times a week, or cannot be dialyzed for as long as needed, or are hypertensive, dietary restrictions are mandatory: 1.0 to 1.5 gm. of sodium, 0.75 to 1.0 gm. of protein/kg./day and only enough fluid to maintain a stable body weight. In addition, cation

---

*Manufacturer's precaution: Dosage requirements of mannitol for patients 12 years of age and under have not been established.

†Sodium nitroprusside has not been approved for use in children.

exchange resins, phosphate binders, supplemental calcium, and low potassium intake may be necessary. Supplemental vitamins, folic acid (1 mg./day) and iron must be provided.

Hematological Aspects. Transfusions of frozen blood, packed and washed red blood cells, or whole blood without supernatant should be administered when hemoglobin and hematocrit decrease markedly. For practical purposes, a blood hematocrit of 12 per cent is the lowest tolerated without a transfusion. Iron should be administered either orally or parenterally; the intravenous route can be used readily in patients on chronic hemodialysis (50 mg. every six months). Because of masculinization and early epiphyseal closure, androgens should not be used in children; in older adolescents and young adults they may help in reducing the rate of transfusions. Nephrectomy should be postponed for as long as possible in order to maintain erythropoietin production.

Psychosocial Aspects. Patients with chronic renal disease, especially those requiring transplant and hemodialysis, are under great stress and require careful psychosocial evaluation and guidance. Early involvement of the family is essential, and needs to be encouraged in a careful and professional manner. The relatively long period of time between onset of chronic renal failure and end stage renal disease in patients with congenital anomalies of the genitourinary tract should make this easier.

Familiarization of the patient and relatives with the machines and the operation of the hemodialysis unit is valuable. Subsequently, frequent meetings to discuss and work out difficulties seem to prevent major problems. Meetings of the staff without the patients or families, and subsequently with all parties involved, are highly desirable. Because of the severely stressful conditions which exist, time should be allowed to discuss emotions created in patients and in staff.

General Measures and Regulations. Food should not be allowed in the dialysis area for other than the patients. Personnel should wear gloves not only to protect themselves but also to keep the lines sterile. Handwashing should be mandatory after connecting a patient to the machine. Monthly checkups for liver function tests and Australia antigen should be performed on all personnel involved regularly in dialysis. Emergency systems should be available immediately as needed. Alarm systems easily reached to call for assistance should be installed throughout the unit. A laboratory should be adjacent to the patient area; centrifugation of blood should be able to be performed within an adjacent and closed area to avoid dissemination of Australia antigen viruses should they be present. Regular meetings should be held to work out difficulties, evaluate the condition of the patients, and introduce needed changes.

Conclusion. Hemodialysis has proved to be a highly effective tool for the rapid correction of biochemical and cardiovascular derangements in patients with acute and chronic renal failure, and for the removal of some drugs and poisons. Performance of this procedure should be reserved for secondary or tertiary (referral) medical centers since complex equipment and specially trained personnel are essential. The high efficiency of this procedure may readily induce complications; its dramatic impact in the life of patients and their families and the demands imposed upon the medical and paramedical personnel require that careful attention be given to psychosocial aspects.

Hemolytic-Uremic Syndrome

R. R. MONTGOMERY, M.D., D. DURANTE, M.D., *and* R. M. McINTOSH, M.D.

Hematologic and renal problems are of greatest concern to the physician confronted with a patient with the hemolytic-uremic syndrome. This disease is most frequent in younger children and usually follows a prodrome characterized by bloody diarrhea. The child usually presents with pallor, bleeding problems and renal insufficiency and its complications.

HEMATOLOGIC COMPLICATIONS

The hematologic complications associated with the hemolytic-uremic syndrome include acute hemolytic anemia, thrombocytopenia, and a variable coagulopathy.

Anemia. The hemolytic anemia present in hemolytic-uremic syndrome is associated with a negative Coombs' test, and the peripheral blood smear shows numerous distorted and fragmented red cells. Since hypervolemia is usually a problem, red cell transfusions should be given only for severe symptomatic anemia (hemoglobin <6 gm./dl.). If transfusions are given, they should be given slowly and as packed red blood cells. Frequent small transfusions are preferable to total correction of the anemia with one transfusion.

Thrombocytopenia. The thrombocytopenia is due to platelet consumption and is usually severe (<50,000/mm^3). Transfused platelets undergo rapid destruction and are therefore not used except for major life-threatening hemorrhage or when used in conjunction with some form of anticoagulation (see below).

Coagulopathy. The coagulation abnormalities have been extensively reviewed and include a spectrum of cases from classic disseminated intravascular coagulation (DIC) with thrombocytopenia, low clotting factors, and elevated fibrin degradation products (FDP) to what appears to be isolated platelet consumption with thrombocytopenia, normal clotting factors, and normal fibrinogen turnover. Therapy of these coagulation abnormalities ranges from no therapy to combined therapy with heparin, fibrinolytic agents, and platelet function inhibitors. The following approach used in Denver directs the therapy to one of these two processes, depending upon the coagulation findings.

Once the diagnosis of hemolytic-uremic syndrome is suspected, baseline coagulation studies are obtained including platelet count, partial thromboplastin time (PTT), prothrombin time (PT), thrombin time (TT), fibrinogen, and FDP. Specific coagulation factor assays are often helpful in substantiating these tests.

When the diagnosis is made and if it appears that the major abnormality is platelet consumption, i.e., normal PTT, PT, TT, and fibrinogen with elevated FDP and thrombocytopenia, the patient is begun on antiplatelet therapy. Dipyridamole, 2.5 mg./kg. orally twice daily, and aspirin, 60 to 75 mg./year of age once daily, are begun and the coagulation studies followed daily. The platelet count usually increases to greater than 100,000/mm³ over the next 48 to 72 hours on this therapy. Once the platelet count is stabilized for 3 to 5 days, therapy is discontinued and the patient followed closely. If during therapy evidence of DIC develops, the aspirin and dipyridamole are discontinued and the patient managed as below.

If at the time of initial diagnosis there is evidence of DIC (prolonged PTT, PT, and TT, a low fibrinogen, factor V, factor VIII, and platelet count as well as elevated FDP), the patient is given an intravenous push of heparin (100 units/kg.) along with fresh platelets (if the platelet count is <30,000/mm³) or fresh frozen plasma to replace the deficient coagulation factors. Fluid balance must be followed closely with these transfusions. Subsequent doses of heparin are given in the same dose every 4 to 6 hours. Coagulation studies are obtained just prior to the next dose of heparin and the dose adjusted if necessary. When appropriate clotting factors are replaced, this dose of heparin has not been associated with hemorrhagic

complications. Additional fresh frozen plasma and platelets are given as needed.

The experience with this approach has been favorable with a more prompt termination of the thrombocytopenia. Most patients fall into the first group and are treated just with antiplatelet agents. The long-term effect on the renal pathology is as yet unknown.

Other forms of therapy have been used. Steroids have not proved useful and fibrinolytic therapy, although theoretically well based, has been associated with excessive hemorrhagic complications and is not recommended.

RENAL DISEASE

Despite the almost universal occurrence in hemolytic-uremic syndrome of frequently severe hematologic abnormalities, acute renal failure and its complications are by far the most common cause of early mortality and chronic morbidity. Proper management has greatly reduced the incidence of mortality in the acute period. However, whether the frequency of chronic sequelae is altered by any therapeutic regimen must still be established. The principles of management of acute renal insufficiency have been covered elsewhere in this book; we will review them briefly with special reference to the problems which occur most frequently in this syndrome.

Initial Patient Assessment. It should be kept in mind that bloody diarrhea, oliguria, and azotemia, common features of hemolytic-uremic syndrome, may be seen as well in cases of severe infectious gastroenteritis. In these cases the azotemia is caused by prerenal factors, that is, digestion of blood in the gastrointestinal tract and diminished effective renal blood flow secondary to hydration. Even when the diagnosis of hemolytic-uremic syndrome is established by the appropriate hematologic evaluation, azotemia may still be partly related to similar prerenal factors. A prerenal component to azotemia is suggested by evidence of hypovolemia on physical examination and by a disproportionate elevation of the blood urea nitrogen to serum creatinine level (beyond a 10:1 ratio). Confirmatory studies include a urine sodium concentration less than 10 mEq./liter, a urine to serum creatinine concentration ratio greater than 14:1, and a urine osmolality which exceeds the serum osmolality by 50 mOsm./liter (Table 1).

In addition, placement via an antecubital vein of a line for measuring the central venous pressure is often necessary for accurate determination of the patient's volume status at initial evaluation and during subsequent manage-

TABLE 1.   Prerenal Versus Renal Failure

LABORATORY TEST	PRERENAL	ACUTE RENAL FAILURE
Urine versus plasma osmolality	50 mOsm./kg. greater than plasma osmolality	Equal to or less than plasma osmolality
Urine sodium concentration	Less than 10 mEq./liter	Greater than 20 mEq./liter
Urine creatinine concentration to plasma creatinine concentration	Greater than 14 to 1	Less than 14 to 1
Urine specific gravity	Greater than or equal to 1020	1010 to 1018

ment. If the central venous pressure and other studies indicate the presence of hypovolemia, cautious fluid replacement is indicated, and diuretic therapy (furosemide, 1 mg./kg. intravenously) may help initiate urine flow. Even in cases of associated intrinsic renal disease such as hemolytic-uremic syndrome, detection and correction of prerenal factors may reduce the severity of oliguria as well as azotemia. However, the great majority of patients will remain in oliguric acute renal failure and many will be hypervolemic at presentation. Management of these patients involves attention to the following critical areas.

Fluid Management.   The oliguric patient (urine output less than 250 cc./m^2/day) should be restricted to 20 per cent of the usual maintenance fluid requirements, with appropriate adjustments for fever, ongoing diarrheal losses, mist therapy and so on. If the patient is not hypervolemic, any urine losses should also be replaced. Fluid status is monitored and recorded on a flow sheet showing daily weights, frequent vital signs, cardiopulmonary evaluations and, in difficult cases, central venous pressure determinations. A daily weight loss of approximately 1 per cent is to be expected during the oliguric period. Catheterization of the urinary bladder is usually not necessary for fluid management, and often results in superimposed urinary tract infection.

Fluid should be given as glucose in water in the highest concentration that can be tolerated by peripheral veins (usually 15 per cent dextrose in water) with monitoring of the blood glucose level. Provision of the highest possible caloric intake, by minimizing tissue catabolism, will help limit the rate of development of azotemia, hyperkalemia and acidosis.

Vitamins B and C should be added if intravenous therapy is prolonged. If oral feedings can be tolerated, glucose and water may be given. Increasing concentrations of glucose may be given as feeding progresses and the blood sugar remains stable. If the BUN stabilizes (either in the natural course of the disease or by dialysis), high quality protein, as in the common infant milk-based formulas, may be given. High fat foods provide a good caloric source.

Electrolytes and Minerals.   If there is a significant urine output, the urinary sodium concentration is measured and replaced by addition of sodium with chloride or bicarbonate to the maintenance fluid. There is usually no indication for potassium replacement.

Hyponatremia is a frequent problem on presentation in hemolytic-uremic syndrome, resulting from fluid retention and some diarrheal losses of sodium. If the serum sodium concentration is less than 120 mEq./liter, or there has been a rapid fall in the serum sodium concentration with symptoms referable to hyponatremia (stupor, convulsions), rapid improvement in the sodium level is attempted. Unless the patient is in severe fluid overload (impending pulmonary edema or severe hypertension), a small amount of 3 per cent sodium chloride may be given, calculated to raise the serum sodium concentration to 125 mEq./liter.* Further gradual correction may be attained by more stringent fluid restriction and additional sodium if necessary. If the patient is severely oliguric, or if he is markedly overloaded with fluids at the onset, correction of the hyponatremia usually requires immediate dialysis.

Hyperkalemia is another frequent complication in these patients. Management is outlined elsewhere in this text. Persistent hyperkalemia or rapidly rebounding hyperkalemia following conservative therapy, often in a patient whose fluid status prohibits further therapy with sodium bicarbonate or glucose, is a common indication for immediate dialysis.

Serum calcium and phosphate derangements are other frequently encountered problems. Hypocalcemia may persist beyond the duration of hyperphosphatemia. If the serum calcium is below the lower limit of normal for that particular laboratory and the patient dis-

---

*mEq. of sodium required = 0.6 × body weight in kg. × (desired sodium concentration − actual sodium concentration). Three per cent sodium chloride contains approximately 510 mEq. of sodium/liter.

plays clinical evidence of hypocalcemia (tetany, seizures, electrocardiographic changes), then calcium may be given as 10 per cent calcium gluconate, 0.5 cc./kg. by slow intravenous push with electrocardiographic monitoring. However, if the patient is asymptomatic, the pathological effects of hypocalcemia may be mitigated by an associated acidosis or, occasionally, hypoproteinemia. In such cases, rapid correction of the serum calcium level is not indicated; rather, supplementation may be given orally (0.5 to 2.0 gm. of calcium gluconate in 4 doses daily) or by intravenous maintenance (120 cc./m²/day of 10 per cent calcium gluconate) as the acidosis is repaired.

Hyperphosphatemia may be treated by nonmagnesium-containing oral phosphate binders (Amphogel, Basaljel, or Titralac) in dosages equivalent to 50 to 150 mg./kg. of aluminum hydroxide, provided the patient is on significant oral feedings.

Acidosis. The metabolic acidosis of acute renal failure may be managed by sodium bicarbonate administration, 2 to 3 mEq./kg. of bicarbonate by slow intravenous push if the serum bicarbonate is less than 10 mEq./liter, or similar amounts by more gradual oral or intravenous daily replacement if the acidosis is not as severe. The amount of sodium administered should, of course, be included in calculations of the patient's sodium intake. However, frequently a volume-expanded oliguric patient will not be able to tolerate the sodium load which such therapy involves; often dialysis is required for correction of the acidosis.

Hypertension. The management of acute hypertension is described elsewhere in this text. The same principles apply to patients with hemolytic-uremic syndrome. If the patient is symptomatic (agitation, depressed consciousness, retinopathy, or seizures) or the diastolic pressure is above 100 mm. Hg, then diazoxide, 3 to 5 mg./kg. by intravenous push, is given.* The normotensive effect usually lasts 12 to 24 hours. Other antihypertensive medications commonly employed include hydralazine, 0.3 to 0.5 mg./kg. intramuscularly, or 0.3 mg./kg. intravenously. The intravenous dose is doubled every 20 minutes until an effect is obtained (maximum is three doses). Alpha methyldopa, 5 to 10 mg./kg. intravenously over 10 minutes, is also used. Each antihypertensive may be repeated every six hours. As with the metabolic problems, dialysis may be necessary to correct hypervolemia-related hypertension.

Seizures. Seizures and other neurological disturbances are more common in hemolytic-uremic syndrome than in other forms of acute renal failure. Several pathogenic factors may play a role in any individual patient. As described above, metabolic derangements include hyponatremia, hypocalcemia and uremia. Hypertensive encephalopathy may also occur. Occasional patients probably have microangiopathic changes in organ systems other than the kidney, including the central nervous system. Central nervous system hemorrhage secondary to thrombocytopenia may also occur. Finally, some patients seem to have seizures not readily explicable by any one of these mechanisms.

Diazepam (Valium) may be given during a seizure in a dose of 0.1 mg./kg. by slow intravenous push with attention to respiration.* This dose may be repeated in 15 minutes if seizures recur. The physician should be aware that intermediate metabolic products of diazepam with central nervous system depressant effects may accumulate in renal failure. Phenobarbital and phenytoin may be used for maintenance anticonvulsant therapy. The dosage interval for phenobarbital should be doubled for the patient in renal failure who is not on dialysis. Decreased protein binding of phenytoin in renal failure shortens the half-life, although toxicity may occur at lower serum levels. Of course, therapy aimed toward correction of any underlying etiology should be instituted whenever possible.

Dialysis. By far the most significant contribution to the improved survival rates of patients with hemolytic-uremic syndrome has been the recognition of the importance of early institution of dialysis. In the foregoing discussion, we have alluded to several critical indications for dialysis—intractable hyperkalemia, intractable acidosis, severe volume overload with pulmonary edema, hyponatremia, or severe hypertension, and uremic complications such as encephalopathy or aggravated bleeding tendency. However, as in other forms of acute renal failure in children, dialysis is most effective in altering mortality and morbidity if it is performed early. As a prophylactic procedure, dialysis avoids life-threatening uremic complications. We institute dialysis at a BUN of 80 mg./100 ml. or serum creatinine of 7 mg./100 ml., if none of the above complications has intervened to require earlier dialysis. Others institute dialysis after 48 hours of severe

---

*Manufacturer's precaution: The safety of intravenous diazoxide in children has not yet been established.

---

*Manufacturer's precaution: The safety and efficacy of injectable diazepam have not been established in the neonate.

oliguria. Although the equipment and technical knowledge are now available for hemodialysis in even the youngest infant, most of these patients can be well managed by peritoneal dialysis in a pediatric intensive care unit (see p. 393). Patients who need rapid correction of life-threatening metabolic derangements, such as hyperkalemia with serious arrhythmias, or severe pulmonary edema, may require hemodialysis in a specialized setting.

Prognosis. The prognosis of the acute situations relies most heavily on early recognition of the syndrome and early application of the basic principles of management. Many cases of early fatality and some of the most severe nonrenal chronic morbidity problems are related to potentially avoidable complications such as repetitive seizures from prolonged hyponatremia.

The long-term outcome of most patients is still difficult to predict. Although there is some correlation between the severity of the acute episode and the long-term renal status, it should be remembered that patients with mild initial involvement and those with apparent complete recovery shortly after the acute disease may eventually develop hypertension and other evidence of declining renal function. On the other hand, some patients may show slow but progressive improvement from the initial episode over the course of several years. It is obvious that all patients must be examined periodically, with urine collections for renal function and careful measurement of blood pressure to detect and manage any complications. There are no recognized chronic hematologic sequelae.

Renal biopsy, while not necessary for diagnosis, may provide some prognostic information by revealing the presence of either sclerosing or proliferative lesions. We do not as yet routinely perform either early or late biopsies in this disease, and rely for the most part on close clinical and laboratory long-term follow-up in these patients, although other groups have found early renal biopsy to be an important and accurate prognostic tool.

Renal Vein Thrombosis

RICHARD A. COHN, M.D., *and*
S. MICHAEL MAUER, M.D.

IN INFANCY

The diagnosis of renal vein thrombosis (RVT) must be suspected in an infant with hematuria or flank mass, particularly if associated with dehydration, thrombopenia, sepsis, birth trauma, or maternal diabetes. Management of these babies requires radiologic confirmation and precise delineation of the extent of the thrombotic process while excluding other causes of renal masses in infants.

Basic principles of pediatric therapy must be applied. Babies with dehydration and hyperosmolality should have appropriate fluids with correction of electrolyte imbalances. Infectious processes are often etiologic in RVT. Urine, blood, and cerebrospinal fluid cultures should be obtained and, if appropriate, antibacterial treatment begun with doses adjusted for the infant's renal and hepatic function. It is important to withhold potassium administration until the adequacy of renal function has been established. Similarly, hypertonic sodium bicarbonate for correction of acidosis should be given cautiously, especially if evidence of fluid overload is present. Pulmonary edema from fluid overload may require positive pressure ventilation, phlebotomy (approximately 10 ml. blood per kg), oxygen, and sorbitol administration. The latter rapidly promotes osmotic diarrhea and can be used at 2 to 4 hour intervals in doses of 2 ml./kg. of the 70 per cent solution by mouth, or 10 ml./kg. of the 20 per cent solution by enema. Diuretics are generally ineffective in the presence of little or no renal function. Hemodialysis with vigorous ultrafiltration or peritoneal dialysis with 4.25 per cent Dianeal rapidly removes excess extracellular fluid, if necessary.

When significant impairment of renal function, fluid overload and hyperelectrolytemia are present, dialytic therapy can effect immediate clinical improvement and successfully prevent the complications of extreme hyperosmolality—intracranial bleeding, convulsions and coma—and thus permit subsequent contrast radiographic studies to be undertaken with safety. The intravenous pyelogram or isotopic renogram will define whether functional impairment is unilateral or bilateral. Arteriography or alternatively cavography with renal vein phlebography will determine the extent of the thrombosis. The diagnosis of renal vein thrombosis cannot be certain unless confirmed by these vascular studies. One pitfall of cavography is the false appearance of caval obstruction with collateral drainage from the Valsalva effect of crying or straining of the infant. We have performed successful cavography in infants and small children by rapid infusion of contrast material into a foot vein while a tourniquet is tightly applied to the contralateral leg to reduce dilution of the contrast agent. Bilateral renal vein thrombosis in infancy is almost always associated with caval thrombosis.

Unilateral RVT, unassociated with infection or uremia, generally resolves with medical management, including anticoagulation. Contralateral extension of the thrombus and recurrence after cessation of anticoagulation tend not to occur in infants. Intravenous heparin is given as an initial 20 units/kg., followed by a constant infusion of 20 units/kg./hr. The effect of heparin is noted both by the thrombin time (TT), which is very sensitive to low heparin concentrations, and by the activated partial thromboplastin time (PTT), which has a linear relationship to heparin levels. Adequate heparin effect is present when the PTT is 1½ times baseline values, and the TT is between 20 and 80 seconds at a 1:4 dilution. With significant thrombopenia a TT of 20 to 80 seconds at a 1:2 dilution is adequate. An advantage of a continuous infusion is that samples for anticoagulation testing may be drawn at any time, as the plasma heparin levels remain constant. Heparin therapy is continued for 10 to 14 days. Long-term oral anticoagulation is generally unnecessary. Fibrinolytic therapy (streptokinase or urokinase) has been used in RVT; the therapy is too risky and experience too limited for general usage. Surgery is mandatory if sepsis is present since the infected thrombosed kidney must be removed.

Surgery is still the treatment of choice for acute bilateral RVT; thrombosis of the inferior vena cava commonly occurs, preventing establishment of collateral renal venous drainage, inviting bilateral renal infarction and death. Successful nonoperative management of bilateral RVT proven angiographically, with convincing resolution on follow-up, has not been documented. The infant with bilateral RVT should be prepared for surgery by the rapid correction of fluid electrolyte and uremic abnormalities as outlined above. With incision of the inferior vena cava, thrombus can be removed from this vessel and from the renal veins. Following removal of renal vein clots, particularly if brisk bleeding from the renal vein does not occur, the kidney should be flushed via its artery with 25 to 50 ml. of 0.9 per cent saline containing 100 units of heparin; this will dislodge many tiny thrombi from the intrarenal venous radicals. If oliguria is present the infant should receive furosemide, 1 mg./kg., and mannitol, 1 gm./kg. intravenously, immediately after thrombectomy to help establish good urine flow.* Anticoagulation with heparin should be started at surgery to prevent recurrence of thrombosis. The an-

ticoagulation is maintained for 10 to 14 days as described above. Unilateral renal infarction found at surgery for bilateral RVT is best treated by nephrectomy along with thrombectomy. However, if diagnosed and treated rapidly, the majority of patients can be managed without nephrectomy.

The involved kidney(s) require careful attention in follow-up. Hypertension may result from either segmental renal infarction or atrophy of an entire kidney and may necessitate nephrectomy months to years after the acute thrombotic event. If bilateral renal cortical scarring results, medical therapy of the hypertension is the only course available. Renal tubular dysfunction, including defective concentrating ability, renal tubular acidosis, and Fanconi's syndrome, may be a permanent sequela despite adequate excretory function.

IN OLDER CHILDREN

Beyond infancy, RVT is generally associated with the nephrotic syndrome. Predisposing factors include a hypercoagulable state, hypovolemia with hemoconcentration, and corticosteroid therapy. RVT can be associated with any pathologic variety of idiopathic nephrotic syndrome but is most commonly seen with membranous glomerulopathy. It has also been described in association with systemic diseases such as lupus erythematosus, diabetes mellitus, and anaphylactoid purpura. Additional etiologic factors include trauma, invasive tumors, cardiac catheterization, renal transplantation, and other surgical procedures. Therapy must be directed, if possible, at both the underlying cause as well as the thrombotic process per se.

RVT may develop acutely with symptoms of flank pain, hematuria, leg edema and thromboembolic signs or may develop gradually and asymptomatically. The gradual onset allows time for collateral drainage to develop, minimizing infarction and renal insufficiency. In such cases fluid and anticoagulation therapy as outlined above, after radiologic documentation, are generally adequate and allow reestablishment of renal vein patency while reducing the chance of potentially fatal pulmonary emboli. Many cases of acute RVT have been managed successfully with anticoagulation as long as renal function remains intact. With acute bilateral RVT associated with impaired renal function, thrombectomy and anticoagulation have been employed. If the underlying cause of RVT cannot be eliminated (e.g., nephrotic syndrome which is resistant to therapy), long-term treatment with oral anticoagulants is indicated.

---

*Manufacturer's precaution: Dosage requirements of mannitol for patients 12 years and under have not been established.

Perinephritis and Perirenal Abscess

C. W. DAESCHNER, M.D.

Bacterial infection of the perirenal tissue is characterized by the acute onset of high septic fever, chills, malaise and *intense* local pain. The pain is unilateral, but localization to the flank, hip, psoas or abdominal area depends upon the site and distribution of the primary process. The infection may originate from rupture of a septic renal cortical abscess, primary cellulitis of the perirenal tissue or penetrating trauma. Although etiologic bacteria may vary widely, the Staphylococcus is the most common offender. Broad antibiotic coverage is indicated unless the specific etiologic agent is known. Frequently surgical drainage will be necessary to release loculated pus before signs and symptoms are relieved. In recent years perinephritic infections have been uncommon.

Urinary Tract Infections

HUGO F. CARVAJAL, M.D.

Though the management of patients with urinary tract infections remains controversial and localization of the infection site to either the kidneys or the urinary bladder has not gained widespread use, it has become increasingly evident that therapeutic generalizations made to include both types of infections lack effectiveness. The need for greater diagnostic specificity is obvious: pyelonephritis represents an infection to a vital organ, cystitis does not; pyelonephritis once established may well be self-perpetuating, a fact that does not apply to bladder infections. Finally, and perhaps most important, the potential morbidity of kidney infections is far greater than even the most severe bladder infection. Judging from recent reports, lower urinary tract infections, whether symptomatic or asymptomatic, are probably self-limiting, innocuous, and in the absence of reflux or obstruction appear to impose no significant threat to the kidneys. Renal parenchymal infections, on the other hand, are difficult to eradicate and frequently result in anatomic and functional derangement. During pregnancy, pyelonephritis carries a significant risk of toxemia, premature delivery and perinatal death. Once chronic disease is allowed to develop, cure may not be possible despite a host of therapeutic agents and techniques. If the goals of therapy are to be attained, namely elimination of chronic pyelonephritis and its complications, parenchymal infections must be prevented or completely eradicated soon after their inception. Early differentiation between the two conditions is therefore essential for proper selection of effective treatment programs.

The successful management of patients with urinary tract infections evolves from fulfillment of five major therapeutic principles: (1) diagnosis of infection; (2) localization of the infection site; (3) selection of proper antimicrobial agents and therapeutic regimens; (4) early surgical correction of predisposing anatomical defects; and (5) adequate follow-up.

Diagnosis of Infection.   One of the most common therapeutic errors is initiation of antibiotic therapy without documentation of infection. This does not imply that antibiotics need to be withheld until the responsible organism has been identified; it means that the institution of specific therapy should be preceded by careful examination of the urinary sediment for bacteria and that a "properly collected" urine specimen is obtained for culture and antibiotic sensitivity testing before treatment is started. Whenever possible, one should await the bacteriological report and obtain additional cultures for confirmation.

Bacteria are not filtered by the glomerulus; hence the urine formed by the kidneys under normal circumstances is sterile. If the normal architecture of the urinary tract is maintained, bladder urine should likewise be sterile. During the act of voiding, however, the urine is frequently contaminated with bacteria from the urethra, glans, labia, vagina, skin, and so forth. Careful washing of the external genitalia and surrounding structures minimizes the likelihood of contamination but does not ensure sterility.

To establish the diagnosis, one must demonstrate that the pathogenic organism is present in quantities not likely to be the result of contamination. Colony counts of 100,000 per ml. of urine or greater are generally accepted as evidence of infection. Colony counts below this level, however, need to be interpreted according to the method and technique used for urine collection. If the sample was obtained by spontaneous voiding, a colony count less than 10,000 can be regarded as being the result of contamination. Colony counts in the 10,000 to 100,000 range, however, should be viewed with concern, as they may represent either infection or contamination (faulty technique).

When the urine is obtained by catheterization or suprapubic aspiration of the bladder, the possibility of contamination at the time of collection is practically eliminated and counts below 10,000 can be indicative of significant infection.

Regardless of methodology, falsely low counts may be the result of prior antimicrobial therapy, polyuria or an obstructed ureter. The examination and culture of at least two urine samples is therefore needed before a high level of reliability is assumed.

When facilities for quantitative cultures are not convenient, a relatively reliable evaluation can be accompanied by microscopic examination of the urinary sediment after Gram or methylene blue staining. The presence of clearly defined bacteria in each field is highly suggestive of a significant colony count but failure to identify bacteria by this means does not exclude infection. Semiquantitative culture methods for office use are now available as inexpensive and relatively reliable disposable units (Testuria or slide culture methods).

Localization of the Infection Site. The determination of the infection site represents a further step in the diagnostic evaluation of patients with infections of the urinary tract. Physicians must be cognizant of the fact that such accuracy in diagnosis cannot be attained on the basis of clinical symptomatology, bacteriologic or even radiologic data, and that specific diagnostic procedures must be used to establish the site of infection. The most popular direct methods (require isolation of the infecting organism) are culture of kidney tissue (autopsy or biopsy), culture of ureteric urine (Stamey's test), and culture of urine from the bladder after sterilization (bladder washout test). Indirect methods useful in localization of the site of infection are assessment of maximal urine concentrating capacity, determination of specific serum antibodies to the infecting organism, leukocyte excretion rate, antibody-coated bacteria test, quantitative measurement of C-reactive protein, and urinary LDH isoenzyme assay. A detailed description of each one of these is beyond the scope of this communication but the reader must recognize their importance and is urged to review the appropriate literature. The direct methods are based on isolation of the infecting organism from kidney biopsy material, ureteral urine, or bladder washout specimens. The indirect methods rely on the demonstration, in either blood or urine, of functional, hematologic, or biochemical alterations resulting from bacterial invasion of kidney parenchyma. The direct methods while reliable are invasive, time-consuming, expensive and potentially hazardous; therefore they are applicable to only a small segment of the patient population. With the exception of the LDH isoenyzme assay and possibly the antibody-coated bacteria test, the indirect methods, although usually easier to perform, are generally less specific.

The urinary LDH isoenzyme assay has the advantage over other equally reliable diagnostic procedures (bilateral ureteral catheterization, bladder washout test and antibody-coated bacteria test) in that it is simple, inexpensive and can be performed on a routine basis by most clinical laboratories; hence it affords greater applicability to the patient population.

Selection of Antimicrobial Agent. Antibiotic treatment is indicated in all patients and must be initiated as soon as the diagnosis is well established. The selection of the antibiotic to be used must be based on recent and reliable epidemiological data.

Since *E. coli* continues to be responsible for most initial urinary tract infections the antibiotic of choice should be one that will eradicate this organism. Nitrofurantoin* is particularly useful in *E. coli* urinary tract infections and is effective against most other urinary pathogens. At the usual recommended dose of 5 to 7 mg./kg./day, disproportionately high concentrations of the drug develop in the kidney. This is apparently related to the recycling of the drug by the renal tubule, a fact that also explains the greater effectiveness of the drug in urinary as contrasted to systemic bacterial infections. It is our habit to begin treatment with this drug in patients with symptomatic and even systemic evidence of infection, but in the latter case we recommend the addition of a parenteral bactericidal antibiotic. Except for mild gastrointestinal irritation which usually disappears when the dose is reduced, the drug is well tolerated. The fact that it does not modify stool or periurethral flora makes it suitable for prolonged suppressive therapy as well.

Judging from recent reports, *E. coli* sensitivity to the sulfonamides is changing and today a significant percentage of common urinary pathogens may be resistant to this agent. Treatment of urinary tract infections with sulfonamides, best represented by sulfisoxazole (Gantrisin), however, continues to offer certain advantages. These include the good tissue and urine levels, the relative freedom from toxic side effects, and the low cost to the patient. In the case of sulfisoxazole,† an initial loading dose of 0.1 gm./kg., followed by .05 gm./kg.

---

*Manufacturer's precaution: Nitrofurantoin should not be administered to infants under one month of age.

†Manufacturer's precaution: Sulfisoxazole (Gantrisin) is contraindicated in infants under two months of age.

every 8 hours for a total of 2 weeks, is usually sufficient to eradicate most sensitive urinary pathogens.

For several years, ampicillin enjoyed an excellent reputation in urinary tract infections and was considered by many to be the antibiotic of choice. However, in recent years, the reports of *E. coli* strains resistant to this agent have increased and it is estimated that 30 to 50 per cent of urinary *E. coli* strains are now highly resistant. Although no longer considered a drug of primary choice, ampicillin is well tolerated, gives excellent blood and tissue levels, and is still useful in the management of selected patients with urinary tract infections. The drug is bactericidal and when given orally in doses of 100 mg./kg. day (four divided doses), adequate urinary levels are achieved.

In patients requiring parenteral antibiotics, gentamicin and kanamycin are certainly the leaders. The former, having replaced polymyxin B, currently enjoys the greater popularity.

Length of Therapy. Although length of therapy continues to be a controversial subject and there is a lack of necessary data to propose ideal therapeutic programs, it is the author's current belief that kidney parenchymal infections require a minimum of six weeks of continuous antibiotic therapy for eradication. The standard two week course should be reserved for patients with infections limited to the lower urinary tract. What to do with patients in whom the site of infection has not been determined remains a therapeutic dilemma. To propose that they be treated for only two weeks may be inadequate as there will be some whose infections have invaded the kidneys; to recommend that they be subjected to six weeks of therapy would represent gross overtreatment for those with infections confined to the urinary bladder. Since either may prove to be erroneous, every attempt should be made to localize the site of infection.

Correction of Predisposing Anatomical Defects. The radiologic and urologic workup of patients with urinary tract infections is aimed at detection of surgically correctable anatomic defects which predispose to recurrent infections and particularly invasion of kidney parenchyma. While early detection of urinary tract anomalies may allow the institution of preventive surgical procedures, in most cases acute or chronic pyelonephritis develops before the anatomic defects are uncovered. Therefore, an intravenous pyelogram and a voiding cystourethrogram are indicated, if not in all children with urinary tract infections, certainly in all of those with proven kidney infections.

This initial evaluation may be misleading if done while the inflammatory process is active, as the effects of the latter may be difficult to differentiate from true anatomic defects. The evaluation of the urinary tract, whether radiologic or urologic, then should be postponed until two to three weeks after treatment has begun. Obstruction, whether functional or anatomic, must be promptly corrected if recurrent infection and progressive deterioration of kidney function are to be prevented.

Follow-up. Proper management does not end with a course of antibiotic therapy or surgical correction of anatomic defects. Judging from various prospective studies, 25 to 75 per cent of female patients with initial urinary tract infections will have a recurrence within two to three years from onset. The physician's responsibility is to promptly detect and eradicate these infections. This can best be accomplished through well organized follow-up programs in which cultures are obtained routinely at fixed intervals.

It is appropriate to begin therapy with an antibiotic likely to be effective, but soon thereafter one must demonstrate its in vivo efficacy or recognize its failure. If the antimicrobial agent selected is an effective one, the patient's urine should be sterile in 48 to 72 hours. It is therefore good practice to obtain a culture two or three days after the initiation of treatment either to confirm the suitability of the therapeutic choice or as a basis for making a new selection. The patient should not be dismissed until post-treatment cultures obtained within a week of stopping therapy are negative. Subsequent cultures at 1, 2, 3, 6, 9, 15, 24 and 36 months after the last infection are in order if the at-risk patient is to be identified early and the number of chronic infections reduced.

Recurrent Infections. These patients present quite a different problem. Not infrequently they have multiple acute episodes, and some require years of intermittent or continuous therapy. It is essential that the etiologic organism be identified and tested for antibiotic sensitivity. Use of the specific antibiotic in full therapeutic doses for two weeks should be followed by suppressive therapy (reduced dose) for several weeks, months or even years as necessary.

A detailed discussion of all the antibiotics is unnecessary here; however, some characteristics of certain less commonly required agents should be mentioned. The tetracyclines have a broad antibacterial spectrum, which includes most of the common urinary pathogens with the exception of Proteus and Pseudomonas. The latter are rare in uncomplicated urinary tract infections. Since the tetracyclines are well absorbed following oral administration and produce good tissue and urine concentrations of active drug, they might be expected to be desirable agents for the management of urinary tract infections. However, experience indicates that during therapy, resistant strains emerge rapidly and that when prolonged or repeated administration is necessary there is a tendency for the original sensitive organisms to be replaced by more resistant strains or species (e.g., Proteus or Pseudomonas). Their marked tendency, when given to small children, to cause permanent dental staining further detracts from their usefulness in pediatrics.

The cephalosporins now available (cephaloridine and cephalothin) are quite effective against all coliform bacteria except Aerobacter and Pseudomonas. They are excreted in the urine in an unmodified, active form. Their renal toxicity limits their use to patients with good renal function and good hydration. Oral forms, particularly cephalexin, show promise in long-term management of urinary tract infection.

Carbenicillin is a broad-spectrum penicillin which has been shown to be effective in Pseudomonas and Proteus infections of the urinary tract. Carbenicillin offers the advantage of producing excellent urinary levels and low toxicity and should be considered in treatment of acute or chronic infections.

Gentamicin is a parenteral antibiotic which has played a significant role in the management of Pseudomonas urinary tract infections. A propensity of this agent to both ototoxicity and nephrotoxicity (particularly in the presence of impaired renal function) requires that it be used with caution and only when the infecting organisms are not amenable to other antimicrobial agents. The patient must be observed carefully to maintain good hydration and to detect early signs of drug toxicity.

Finally, it should be remembered that in vitro sensitivity testing generally may be misleading and in vivo trial of an agent is often indicated when its therapeutic spectrum includes the etiologic organism.

Chronic Infection. Chronic infection of the urinary tract is frequently silent and is most often associated with significant anatomic or functional abnormalities. When the functional abnormalities can be eradicated, the hope for cure is reasonable; when they cannot, cure is infrequent. Culture and sensitivity testing is particularly important, because the etiologic organism is less predictable, and not infrequently mixed infection exists. Initial treatment in these patients should be similar to that for acute recurrent infections, and good

symptomatic relief can be expected; however, the frequent recurrence of symptoms or persisting silent bacteriuria following cessation of therapy may encourage the physician to give prolonged periods of antimicrobial therapy.

As renal insufficiency develops, supportive therapy to combat hypertension and hypoplastic anemia should be added as appropriate clinical indications appear. Unilateral pyelonephritis with renal atrophy and hypertension may indicate nephrectomy, but only when the other kidney is uninvolved and function in the infected kidney is negligible.

Renal Tuberculosis. This is an infrequent but serious form of urinary tract infection both because it usually implies significant involvement of the kidney, and because if untreated it is quite contagious. The diagnosis is usually suspected by the presence of a positive tuberculin test or chest radiogram in a patient with painless gross hematuria or "sterile" pyuria. It can be confirmed by urine culture and requires prolonged therapy.

Hemorrhagic Cystitis. This occurs infrequently in children and may represent chemical, mechanical or infectious inflammation of the urinary bladder. There is usually fever, acute suprapubic pain, dysuria, urgency and frequency, together with grossly hematuric urine—sometimes containing clots, but never erythrocyte or hemoglobin casts. The bacterial etiology is most often *E. coli*, and treatment with a sulfonamide, nitrofurantoin or ampicillin, as for acute urinary tract infection, is effective. In many of these patients the illness is self-limited and no bacterial agent is found; therefore a viral etiology is assumed.

Foreign bodies, calculi and tumors may also present the clinical syndrome of hemorrhagic cystitis. Cyclophosphamide therapy may produce an acute hemorrhagic cystitis and in some cases lead to permanent vascular changes (telangiectasia) in the bladder mucosa. When possible, removal of the offending agent is the obvious treatment for these patients.

Urolithiasis

A. BARRY BELMAN, M.D., M.S.

Patients with urinary calculi present most frequently with hematuria or symptoms of urinary tract infection. Abdominal pain may also be the primary complaint, particularly in the presence of obstruction. The diagnosis of urinary tract calculi is made secondarily, i.e., when patients with hematuria, urinary tract infections or abdominal discomfort undergo urography in an effort to ascertain the cause of their presenting complaints. The necessity for complete evaluation of patients with hematuria or urinary tract infection is underscored by the high incidence of anatomic abnormalities noted when such screening is carried out.

Approximately half the patients with stones who are seen by the physician will have anatomic abnormality, usually of an obstructive type, as the underlying cause. Most of these present with infection and calcium ammonium phosphate stones. Obstruction resulting in renal calculi may occur at the ureteropelvic junction, along the course of the ureter (most often at the ureterovesical junction), at the bladder outlet, or intraurethrally. Stones may be lodged at any point proximal to the obstruction. Patients with stone disease in association with obstruction frequently have severe damage to the involved renal unit, particularly if the obstruction has been present for a long time.

Identifiable metabolic disorders are the underlying cause of stones in 10 to 20 per cent of children. Idiopathic hypercalciuria or hypercalciuria secondary to hyperparathyroidism or hypercortisonism produces radiopaque calcium stones. Familial forms of oxaluria, cystinuria or other forms of aminoaciduria may result in calculi, the composition of which is related to the metabolic disorder.

Iatrogenic calculi may result from the milk alkali syndrome or excessive vitamin D ingestion. Foreign bodies in the urinary tract produce stones and are usually seen in the bladders of little girls, though boys are not immune. Immobilization occurring with prolonged orthopedic manipulations also may be associated with stone disease in children, but is nowhere nearly as frequent as in immoblized adults. Urinary calculi have not been associated with metabolic bone disease in children in any of the recent reviews. Nephrocalcinosis has been noted with renal tubular acidosis, with oxalosis, and in patients on long-term exogenous steroids.

Stones associated with infection and obstruction are best treated by finding the underlying cause of the obstruction and correcting it. Calculi are removed simultaneously, such as removal of a renal pelvic stone in conjunction with repair of a ureteropelvic junction obstruction. It is imperative that all of the calculus be removed at the time of operation, since any residual fragments serve as a nidus for recurrence. In the absence of a known underlying cause which can be treated, maintenance of a dilute urine may be the only therapeutic device possible. This usually requires that the patient awaken during the night to drink additional water in an effort to avoid nocturnal urinary concentration. Additionally, aluminum gels have been used in the treatment of phosphatic calculi.

Patients with cystine stones are treated with alkalinization of the urine or with penicillamine under careful supervision, since the side effects are multiple. Alkalinization is attained with an oral citrate mixture (Polycitra) and is verified by frequent monitoring of the urinary pH. It has been suggested that the urine need not be continuously alkaline in these patients. Since cystine is highly soluble, intermittent alkalinity during each 24-hour period prevents stone formation. Stone formation secondary to hyperoxaluria has been successfully controlled with oral magnesium oxide.

Vesicoureteral Reflux

ALAN B. RETIK, M.D.

Vesicoureteral reflux is an abnormal condition which has been detected in 30 to 70 per cent of children undergoing urologic investigation for recurrent urinary tract infections. The treatment of reflux depends to a large extent upon the etiologic factors involved. A systematic evaluation of the child with urinary tract infection is essential for accurate diagnosis, prognosis and therapy. The diagnostic tools employed are the excretory urogram, voiding cystourethrogram and cystoscopy.

It is well documented that urinary infection may be a cause as well as a result of reflux. Radiologic evaluation of a child with a urinary tract infection should be delayed until the urine has been sterile for 3 to 4 weeks. This will usually eliminate the group of children with reflux secondary to inflammatory changes. However, if there is difficulty sterilizing the urine or if the child remains symptomatic, these investigations should be performed sooner because a serious disorder may be present.

Anatomic lesions of the ureterovesical junction associated with reflux include absence or partial absence of the intravesical ureter, a paraureteral diverticulum in which the intravesical ureter lacks muscular support, and a markedly underdeveloped trigone with laterally placed patulous ureteral orifices. Reflux is often seen in children with autonomous neurogenic bladders and is associated with loss of tone in the bladder detrusor. A small percentage of children may have reflux secondary to obstruction at or distal to the bladder neck.

Children with bladder exstrophy and those born with the syndrome of absence of abdominal musculature, cryptorchidism and urinary tract abnormalities often exhibit reflux associated with one of the previously mentioned primary abnormalities at the ureterovesical junction.

Treatment must be individualized; such factors as length of history, age at onset, number of infections and the ease with which they are controlled should be considered in deciding whether surgery should be performed.

Operative Repair. The indications for antireflux surgery are (1) recurrent urinary infection despite continuous chemotherapy, (2) severe reflux with chronic pyelonephritis, or (3) persistent reflux associated with a basic anatomic abnormality at the ureterovesical junction. Obstructions at or distal to the bladder neck associated with reflux should be corrected. Surgical correction of the reflux should be performed as well if the ureterovesical junction is anatomically abnormal. Antireflux surgery in children with neurogenic bladder dysfunction has been employed in specific instances when it is ascertained that the bladder is able to empty completely.

The type of antireflux surgery most often employed is the Politano-Leadbetter operation with the creation of an adequate submucosal tunnel. The surgical success rate following such a procedure is almost 99 per cent. About one quarter of children following surgery continue to have recurrent urinary tract infections, but these are invariably confined to the bladder. Acute pyelonephritis is uncommon following successful corrective surgery.

Nonoperative Treatment. It is generally agreed that reflux in the absence of infection does not cause renal damage. Therefore, if it is decided to pursue a nonoperative program, it is imperative that continuous chemotherapy be employed as long as reflux persists. The drugs most often used for this purpose are sulfisoxazole, nitrofurantoin and methenamine mandelate. Urinalysis and culture with colony count should be obtained at 4 to 8 week intervals. Excretory urograms and voiding cystourethrograms are repeated every 6 to 12 months. In the infant and young child with severe vesicoureteral reflux, pyelonephritis may progress rapidly, and x-ray studies should be performed at more frequent intervals. Other measures designed to reduce the incidence of urinary stasis and infection should be encouraged. These include adequate hydration, attention to proper perineal hygiene, a frequent voiding schedule and double voiding in the older cooperative child. Measures designed to reduce outlet resistance, such as urethral dilatation, meatotomy or internal urethrotomy, may be helpful in eliminating minor degrees of reflux or in reducing the severity of reflux.

The ultimate goal of nonoperative management is the cessation of reflux. This has been reported to occur by maturation of the trigone or by healing of a chronically inflamed ureterovesical junction. When reflux is still present at puberty, it is likely to persist and surgical intervention should be recommended.

Neurogenic Vesical Dysfunction

ALAN B. RETIK, M.D.

Neurogenic vesical dysfunction in childhood is most often due to spina bifida with myelomeningocele or sacral deformities. It is but one aspect of the difficult problem confronting the pediatrician, neurosurgeon, orthopedic surgeon, urologist and psychiatrist. However, the ultimate prognosis in those children who have survived the early hazards of meningitis and hydrocephalus depends upon the severity of their renal disease. Progressive renal dilatation and deterioration may occur over a period of years in urinary tracts which initially appear to be anatomically and functionally normal. Not only does renal failure cause serious morbidity, but urinary incontinence plays an important role in the social acceptability of the child. In general, the bladder disturbance is of the lower neuron type, although it is difficult to correlate bladder behavior with the level of the spinal lesion and the degree of paralysis of other functions.

The goals of therapy in the neurogenic bladder are preservation of renal function and urinary continence. Infants and children are managed by conservative means, providing that chemical and radiological evidence of renal deterioration is not present, urinary infection is controlled, and Credé and other maneuvers produce reasonably dry intervals. The bladder must be evacuated by manual expression at regular intervals to ensure a low residual urine and reduce dribbling incontinence. Older children readily learn to Credé themselves. Fecal impaction must be avoided to aid bladder expression. This is most readily achieved by the use of stool softeners, but often enemas two or three times a week or even digital assistance may be necessary.

An excretory urogram should be performed during the first month of life and repeated at regular intervals. Urinalysis and urine culture with colony counts must be obtained every 2 to 4 months. Severe vesicoureteral reflux demonstrated by voiding cystourethrography occurs frequently and may lead to chronic urinary infection and severe pyelonephritis. Continuous chemotherapy is often necessary in these children.

When the bladder fails to empty properly following conservative measures, operations designed to lower urethral resistance may be undertaken. Transurethral resection of the bladder neck, sphincterotomy, or unilateral pudendal neurectomy may be of occasional benefit in the boy. In the girl, extensive urethral dilatation or internal urethrotomy has been effective in lowering resistance to voiding. Anticholinergic drugs such as propantheline bromide, 7.5 to 15 mg. three times a day, may be of some help in the spastic bladder. Similarly, bethanechol chloride (Urecholine), 0.6 mg./kg./day, may help to evacuate a large atonic bladder.

Many children have some degree of incontinence, requiring either intermittent catheterization, an external collecting apparatus, therapy with imipramine or a combination of the above. In the boy, incontinence can often be managed with a penile urinal, providing that the phallus is large enough. Intermittent catheterization has become increasingly effective in both male and female. Incontinence is rarely the sole indication for urinary diversion.

Indications for urinary diversion are hydronephrosis, progressively decreasing renal function, or repeated attacks of pyelonephritis. The sigmoid conduit has replaced the ileal conduit as the most satisfactory form of urinary diversion. The ureters are anastomosed to an isolated segment of sigmoid colon using an antireflux technique. This prevents reflux and consequently pyelonephritis. Stomal problems may also be less with this method of diversion. In a severely uremic child with dilated, tortuous ureters, ureterostomy should be considered as an alternative and simpler procedure. Stomal problems are not uncommon with all methods of tubeless urinary diversion, and stomal revisions may be necessary.

Exstrophy of the Bladder

ALAN B. RETIK, M.D., *and*
STUART B. BAUER, M.D.

When a child is born with an exstrophy and epispadias, the consequences of this abnormality extend far beyond the anatomic defect. The multitude of problems must be handled in an individualized manner for each child.

The congenital anomaly arises as a result of failure of fusion of the mesodermal component of the lower abdominal wall. The cloacal membrane is overdeveloped and more ventrally placed than normal, thus preventing mesodermal fusion. When the membrane normally splits creating the urogenital opening, the underlying vesical wall and urogenital ridge are exposed and fail to close off. The entire urogenital tract is thus laid open.

After birth an excretory urogram will reveal the status of the upper urinary tract and provide a basis for future comparison. The size of the bladder and condition of the kidneys and ureters will determine the therapeutic management for each individual child. Until that decision is made, however, the exstrophied mucosa and surrounding skin is best managed with Saran Wrap coverings underneath the diaper.

Sometime before the end of the first year, the baby is reevaluated. If the vesical wall is soft and supple and the bladder capacity large enough to permit satisfactory closure, the repair is carried out then with an attempt at a continence procedure after age 3. Only selected infants should be handled in this manner, because continence is achieved in a small number of children. If continence is not obtained after one or possibly two operations on the bladder neck, then the authors feel that urinary diversion by a nonrefluxing colon conduit is warranted and should be performed soon thereafter.

Reflux occurs in 80 per cent of closed bladders because of an abnormal vesical wall and position of ureteral entrance. An antireflux operation may be necessary to prevent ascending infection as well as to allow for a continence procedure on the bladder neck. They can be performed simultaneously. In addition, the bladder wall may not be entirely normal. Detrusor function in these closed bladders is not always present, and may not be effective even when evident. When upper tract damage, either from hydronephrosis or pyelonephritis, and impaired vesical function are seen, urinary diversion is indicated even though continence has been achieved.

When the decision is made not to close the bladder (and this is generally the case) because of small capacity and thick fibrotic walls, then the child is spared the multitude of operations previously discussed. Urinary diversion is preferentially delayed until the time between 12 and 18 months of age when the surgeon can assess the functional status of the anal sphincter. Ureterosigmoidostomy with an antireflux ureteral anastomosis is preferred because this frees the child from any external urinary appliances. If there is any question about the competency of the anal sphincter, then a sigmoid conduit is performed. This can later be turned in and implanted into the rectum if and when the anal sphincter proves to be effective. A mucosal cystectomy is recommended when diverting the urine either primarily or secondarily after attempted bladder closure. The transitional cell epithelial lining frequently undergoes metaplastic change in response to chronic inflammation, and an increased incidence of cancer in corrected exstrophy patients has been cited later in life. The abdominal defect is closed with the bladder wall aiding in the closure.

The penile epispadias commonly associated with exstrophy may be repaired either at the time of exstrophy closure or subsequently. When the child is not a candidate for bladder closure, the epispadias is corrected separately, some time after primary diversion has been accomplished. In both instances however, the repair is completed before puberty. In addition, a penil lengthening procedure will invariably be needed whether or not the bladder is retained. Most males have been able to attain satisfactory sexual relations and some have even fathered children.

In female children, the epispadiac urethra is closed at the time the bladder is repaired, or in conjunction with an anti-incontinence operation. If the urine has been diverted, then the urethra is removed during the mucosal cystectomy. The bifid clitoris and widely separated pubic hair distribution can be made to look more normal with rotation of the skin flaps when the urethra is repaired or removed. A vaginoplasty to enlarge the normally placed yet stenosed vaginal orifice is accomplished sometime after puberty.

Patent Urachus and Urachal Cysts

EDMOND T. GONZALES, Jr., M.D.

The urachus is a normal embryologic structure which connects the bladder dome with the allantois. Normally, it is a fibrous band composed of three discrete layers: an inner layer of transitional epithelium, a connective tissue layer of blood and lymph vessels, and an external layer of involuntary muscle continuous with the normal detrusor. The mucosal lining is normally nonsecreting, but a tiny lumen can often be identified histologically. Urachal abnormalities are rare and include both con-

genital and acquired lesions. The former include patent urachus, external sinus and internal sinus. Acquired lesions include urachal cyst and urachal carcinoma. Urachal carcinoma is almost exclusively a problem in adults, the youngest reported case being in a 15 year old female.

During embryogenesis, the bladder is positioned in the abdomen just beneath the umbilicus. At birth, it has begun to descend into the pelvis, and the urachus averages 2.5 cm. in length. Patent urachus presents most often in the neonatal period. If the bladder has failed to descend, a "vesicoumbilical" fistula will result with no identifiable urachal remnant and profuse flow of urine. In other cases, the long narrow urachus allows only a few drops of urine to be evident at the umbilicus. The diagnosis is generally evident with sloughing of the cord, but may be suspected if the cord is tense or hydropic shortly after birth. Management involves an appropriate diagnosis followed by surgical excision of all of the urachus and a small segment of bladder dome. A curvilinear infraumbilical incision allows adequate exposure in the neonate with cosmetic closure. Cauterization of the tract is not recommended, since recurrence is almost inevitable. An intravenous urogram and voiding cinecystourethrogram should be obtained in all patients with patent urachus, since nearly 10 per cent are associated with infravesical obstruction.

External urachal sinus occurs when the vesical communication of the urachus obliterates, but the umbilical opening remains patent. The tract periodically drains purulent material and desquamated cells, and must be differentiated from chronic granuloma of the umbilicus or persistent vitelline duct. Rarely, the sinus may alternately drain between both the umbilicus and bladder.

Urachal cysts are rare and represent a collection of mucus and cellular debris which accumulates in the lumen of the urachus. At times they ultimately present at the umbilicus as a urachal sinus.

Both of these disorders are best managed by complete extraperitoneal excision, as described for patent urachus.

If the urachus is patent at the bladder but obliterated near the umbilicus, a diverticulum will result at the bladder dome. Generally, these are small and asymptomatic and require no therapy. When large, they are often poorly contractile and contribute to residual urine and urinary infection. In this case, surgical excision of the diverticulum is indicated. Urachal diverticula may also be seen with infravesical obstruction and are especially common in the "prune-belly" syndrome.

Tumors of the Bladder and Prostate

EDMOND T. GONZALES, Jr., M.D.

BENIGN TUMORS

Tumors of the lower urinary tract (bladder, prostate and urethra) are rare in children. Both benign and malignant lesions may occur. Two benign tumors have been described in the urinary bladder of children: neurofibromas and hemangiomas. Neurofibromas usually occur with generalized neurofibromatosis. They cause no harm unless so positioned as to cause ureteral or bladder neck obstruction and are best observed unless such complications occur.

Bladder hemangiomas present with total, gross, painless hematuria. About one-third of patients may have hemangiomas in other organs as well. The lesions are universally benign, but surgical therapy is often necessary to control troublesome hematuria. Very small lesions may be controlled by transurethral resection, but most will require open partial cystectomy.

MALIGNANT TUMORS

Three malignant tumors may occur in the bladders of children: transitional cell carcinoma, urachal carcinoma and embryonal rhabdomyosarcoma. Urachal carcinoma is exceedingly rare, only one case having been reported in a child.

Transitional cell tumors have been reported in only about 12 cases. They present with hematuria and histologically are usually low-grade papillary lesions which have not recurred after transurethral resection. Only one case is known to have metastasized.

Embryonal rhabdomyosarcoma is the most common and most serious tumor which occurs in the lower urinary tract of children. Rhabdomyosarcoma represents 10 to 15 per cent of solid tumors in children, and 15 per cent of these occur in the urogenital tract. Tumors occurring in the bladder and in the prostate differ slightly. Rhabdomyosarcoma of the bladder tends to remain localized with extensive submucosal extension and intraluminal protrusion of large "grape-like" masses of tumor described as sarcoma botryoides. Prostatic rhabdomyosarcomas are more sessile and infiltrative, although a botryoid pattern can occur if the neoplasm extends into the bladder. Prostatic lesions are more likely to have metastasized at the time of diagnosis than those originating in the bladder.

Both types of tumors usually present with urinary obstructive symptoms. Strangury may occur if large masses of tumor fall into the vesical neck with voiding. Hematuria is uncommon but may occur if ulceration of the mucosa occurs. Biopsy to confirm the diagnosis should be obtained transurethrally if at all possible.

Treatment is multimodal, involving surgery, radiotherapy and chemotherapy, and over the past few years dramatic improvement in survival has occurred. Presently, recommendations for therapy include surgical extirpation of all grossly involved tissue, radiotherapy if residual tumor is left behind or regional lymph nodes are positive, and cyclic chemotherapy with actinomycin-D, vincristine and cyclophosphamide. Some centers also include Adriamycin in the chemotherapeutic protocol.

In the male, surgical excision requires total cystoprostatectomy and proximal urethrectomy. In the female, if the lesion has not extended beyond the bladder, only a total cystourethrectomy might be accomplished. If the lesion, though, has invaded into the paravesical tissues, hysterectomy and vaginectomy should be included. In both sexes, the tumors may extend for a considerable distance submucosally, and frozen sections should be obtained to confirm that the margins of the dissection are free of tumor.

Recently, a few reports have shown dramatic regression of pelvic rhabdomyosarcoma with chemotherapy only. It is hoped that confirmation of these observations will allow improved survival with less mutilating procedures than have been accomplished in the past.

Disorders of the Bladder, Prostate and Urethra

EDMOND T. GONZALES, Jr., M.D.

BLADDER

Exstrophic Disorders. The exstrophic disorders include a spectrum of anomalies from simple glanular epispadias to exstrophy of the cloaca. Exstrophy of the bladder (which includes urethral epispadias) is the most common form and occurs in about 1 of 20,000 live births. The disorder is twice as common in males. Subsymphyseal epispadias is the next most common variant.

Treatment of bladder exstrophy is controversial. Until recently procedures designed to preserve the bladder resulted in a high incidence of urinary incontinence and upper tract deterioration. Early, primary urinary diversion became the procedure of choice in most centers and is still the standard by which newer techniques must be compared. Uretero-intestinal-cutaneous anastomoses (which require an external collecting device) or ureterosigmoidostomy (which avoids a device) may be chosen, depending on the age of the patient, appearance of the upper urinary tract and the presence or absence of anal continence. I prefer primary ureterosigmoidostomy for infants under two years of age who have normal kidneys and ureters. The ability to hold "liquid feces" can be judged preoperatively by giving the child an oatmeal enema of a consistency similar to a mixture of urine and feces.

Recently, interest has increased again in trying to accomplish functional bladder closure. A better understanding of the urethral sphincteric mechanism, current antibiotics and staged surgical reconstruction has improved results compared with past years. Careful patient selection is important in determining the proper procedure.

Subsymphyseal epispadias is a variant of bladder exstrophy and is associated with urinary incontinence. Here, though, there is usually a near normal bladder to work with, and surgical procedures on the bladder neck can achieve satisfactory continence in at least 50 per cent of these children.

Bladder Diverticula. Bladder diverticula are seen occasionally in children. In the presence of infravesical obstruction, marked trabeculations and cellule formation occur. These diverticula are usually small, and if the infravesical obstruction is relieved, they are of no clinical concern. Many diverticula, though, are congenital in origin and are not related to obstruction. They are usually present near the edge of the trigone, may be quite large, empty poorly and contribute to persisting or recurring urinary infection. On occasion they may obstruct the ipsilateral ureter, or if they dissect behind the bladder neck, they can cause bladder outlet obstruction. Surgical excision is required only for complications of infection or obstruction. Diverticula associated with the ureteral orifice are common and usually are associated with vesicoureteral reflux. They are excised if ureteroneocystostomy is performed.

Bladder Septa. Various partial or complete septa can occur in the bladder. They are thought to be due to development of accessory urorectal septa or to adherence of redundant mucosal folds. When small, they are often of no clinical concern, but large septa are commonly associated with infection and hydronephrosis. Appropriate excision of the septum and reconstruction of dilated upper tracts are definitive.

PROSTATE

Posterior Urethral Valves. Disorders of the prostate are rare and consist of posterior urethral valves and cysts of the utricle. Posterior urethral valves are obstructive lesions in the male which may result in severe renal insufficiency. Neonates with severe obstruction may present with palpable masses or with marked dehydration, acidosis and azotemia. Older infants are more likely to have associated urinary infection also.

When renal function is near normal, the procedure of choice is transurethral destruction of the valves by electrocautery. When the obstruction is relieved, even massive ureteral dilation will gradually improve. Infants with significant decreases in renal function or with persisting infection require some sort of temporary tubeless diversion, such as vesicostomy or loop ureterostomy. Occasionally, a primary total upper tract reconstruction may be accomplished in the neonatal period. Many of these infants demonstrate a significant impairment in urinary concentrating ability, and dehydration with acidosis is likely during episodes of acute illness from any cause, especially diarrhea.

Utricular Cysts. Utricular cysts are exceedingly rare and result from disordered regression of the müllerian ducts in the male. Because of their location, they may cause bladder neck obstruction and must be distinguished from posterior urethral valves. Options in management are similar to those described for urethral valves.

URETHRAL ANOMALIES

Hypospadias. Hypospadias is common and occurs in 1 of every 200 live male births. The location of the meatus varies from the most mild subglanular position to a perineal meatus with bifid scrotum. The more severe degrees of hypospadias, especially when associated with cryptorchidism, require evaluation for possible intersex anomalies.

Hypospadias is repaired for cosmetic and functional reasons, and numerous techniques have been described. Repair can be accomplished in a single stage in many cases, but more severe forms require multiple stages. Most significant degrees of hypospadias are also associated with chordee (ventral curvature of the penile shaft) which requires correction at the same time. Chordee may be seen without hypospadias, but similar techniques are utilized for its repair. Timing for repair must take into account the psychosexual development of the child, the psychological effects of genital surgery and technical considerations. If a one-stage reconstruction is chosen, the repair is usually accomplished between the age of three and four years. This allows reconstruction before school age, when separation anxieties and genital maiming fears can be handled. If a multiple-stage repair is required, the initial procedure may have to be done by 18 months to allow adequate time to complete the repair before school age.

Urethral Stricture. Congenital urethral strictures occur just distal to the membranous urethra and appear as concentric filmy diaphragms. They are thought to represent inadequate resolution of the cloacal membrane and can be cured by simple urethral dilation.

Acquired strictures in children are usually due to perineal trauma of instrumentation. They respond less well to dilation and often require open urethroplasty.

Meatal Stenosis. Following circumcision, urethral meatitis is common with secondary formation of a thin membrane across the meatus ventrally. Urethral meatal stenosis in male children is subsequently diagnosed commonly, but accurate calibration of the meatus or urodynamic evaluation to confirm this diagnosis is unusual. In children with minor bladder irritative symptoms (frequency, dysuria, terminal hematuria) but without urinary infection, who have a small urethral meatus visually, it is reasonable to accomplish a meatotomy under local anesthesia in the office. If the symptoms do not resolve, a more complete urologic evaluation may ultimately be required.

Urethral Diverticulum. Anterior urethral diverticula represent defects in fusion of the urethral folds. Some are small and require no treatment, but many are obstructive and must be surgically excised.

Urethral Prolapse. Prolapse of the urethral mucosa is seen principally in black girls. It presents with either irritative symptoms or introital bleeding. Though easy to recognize in most cases, prolapse of the urethra may be confused with prolapsed ureteroceles or rarely sarcoma botryoides. Surgical excision with careful mucosa-to-mucosa anastomosis is the preferred treatment.

Accessory Urethra. Accessory urethra is seen occasionally. If the extra urethra drains from the bladder, incontinence and dorsal chordee are common. If the duplication is partial and distal to the membranous urethra, symptoms are uncommon. Occasionally, obstruction may occur at the junction of the two urethras. When necessary, simple excision is accomplished.

Megalourethra. Megalourethra results from congenital absence of the corpus spongiosum. The large inelastic urethra is unsightly and also may promote urinary infection by poor drainage. Some cases are also accompanied by deficiency or absence of the erectile bodies (corpora cavernosa). Repair must take into consideration not only a functional urethra but a functional sexual organ also. Children with deficient erectile bodies will ultimately require some form of penile impotency device at puberty.

Undescended Testes

EDMOND T. GONZALES, Jr., M.D.

Undescended testes are common and affect nearly 0.5 per cent of males. At birth cryptorchidism is present in 2 per cent of live-born male infants, so that a few undescended testes descend shortly after birth. Spontaneous descent, though, probably does not occur after one year of age.

During childhood the cremasteric reflex is very active and is able to bring the testis well into the groin. An incorrect diagnosis of cryptorchidism in these cases can easily be made. Careful manipulation of the testis in the supine or squatting position will allow most retractile testes to be brought into the scrotum. The parents may note that the testis is down during a warm bath. Rarely, an unsuspected retractile testis will be found in the scrotum when the child is anesthetized for orchidopexy. Retractile testes require no therapy. Children with bilateral cryptorchidism and hypospadias should be evaluated for possible intersex abnormalities.

Treatment of cryptorchidism may be nonsurgical or surgical. The timing of treatment remains somewhat controversial, but recent data support earlier repair than has generally been done in the past. By age five years, differences in the germinal epithelium between undescended and descended testes can be observed by light microscopy. Some observers have extended these observations to age two years with electron microscopy. Since spontaneous descent is rarely, if ever, observed after 12 months of age, it is reasonable to initiate therapy at any time after age two years that the diagnosis is made. It is not clear at this time if early orchidopexy lessens the increased risk of tumorigenesis seen in cryptorchid testes, but preliminary data suggest that this may also be the case. If surgical exploration is required at any age for symptomatic inguinal hernia with cryptorchidism or testicular torsion, simultaneous orchidopexy should be accomplished.

The nonsurgical management of cryptorchidism is based on the observation that spontaneous descent occurs occasionally at puberty, although whether these testes are truly cryptorchid or merely retractile remains controversial. Nonetheless, this observation has stimulated interest in the use of chorionic gonadotropin to effect descent without orchidopexy. Ehrlich and associates noted that testicular descent occurred in one-third of children with bilateral cryptorchidism treated with human chorionic gonadotropin (HCG), and that it did not matter whether the drug was administered in a short course (10,000 units total: 3300 units every other day) or a long course (10,000 units total: 500 units every other day). In children with unilateral cryptorchidism, only 16 per cent responded, primarily those who received a long course of therapy. Androgenic side effects were minimal, but some increased penile growth and development of pubic hair were observed in a few children. In both groups, the response to HCG was better in children two to five years of age than in older children.

Surgical management of cryptorchidism is the standard by which other therapeutic modalities must be compared. Although many techniques have been described to fix the testis in the scrotum, traction or fixation of the testis to the thigh should not be required for adequate placement. If adequate length of the testicular vessel is not obtained with the initial dissection, it is preferable to place the testis where it lies without tension and plan a second stage for completion of orchidopexy.

A short course of HCG is recommended for younger patients (under five years of age) with bilateral cryptorchidism with both testes palpable near the external inguinal ring. A primary surgical approach is recommended for all other patients.

When a testis is not found in the inguinal canal, a complete transperitoneal exploration must be accomplished. Some intraabdominal testes are near normal and should be placed in the scrotum if possible, but many are small and dysgenetic and are best excised. A primary orchiectomy is indicated in most cases of cryptorchidism seen initially after puberty.

Because of the 30 times increased incidence of tumorigenesis associated with cryptorchidism, parents should be advised to encourage these patients to practice self-examination of the testes following puberty.

Disorders of the Penis and Testis

EDMOND T. GONZALES, Jr., M.D.

Phimosis and Paraphimosis. At birth, the space between the foreskin and glans penis is incompletely developed and a physiologic phimosis exists. Often the foreskin can only be retracted sufficient to expose the external urethral meatus. As the child gets older, the preputial space develops normally. If the foreskin is retracted gently but firmly for cleansing, separation of the foreskin and glans will be hastened. It is not necessary to forcibly disrupt these adhesions if the child has had no troubles. In a few cases, development of the preputial space will leave small pockets or crypts which may become infected and packed with desquamated epithelium, resulting in balanoposthitis. In this situation complete retraction of the foreskin will allow drainage of the purulent material and cleansing of the glans penis. An elective circumcision is not required if local hygiene is adequate.

Paraphimosis results when the foreskin becomes trapped behind the coronal sulcus. Initially, manual reduction is possible, but swelling ensues from lymphatic and venous occlusion and may progress until manual reduction is no longer possible. Sloughing of the foreskin and glans penis may result. A longitudinal incision at this time through the restricting band will allow easy reduction of the paraphimosis. An elective circumcision is indicated but is best delayed until all edema and tissue reaction subside.

Webbed Penis. A webbed penis results from attachment of the scrotal skin along the ventral aspect of the penile shaft. Cosmetic reconstruction of the penoscrotal junction is technically easy and should be accomplished before the child is three years of age. There are no other associated anomalies.

Bifid Penis and Diphallus. These anomalies result from inadequate fusion of the two primordial genital tubercles. In the more severe forms, two complete urethras may be present and the bladder may be bilobed or completely duplicated also. Reconstruction involves cosmetic approximation of the erectile bodies and preservation or formation of a functional urethra.

Micropenis. (See Intersex, p. 323.)

Congenital Absence of the Penis. This is an embryogenic catastrophe that is believed due to complete failure of development of the genital tubercles. The scrotum may be normal or bifid. Since no acceptable surgical technique is available to construct a functional penis, these children should be established and reared in a female gender role.

DISORDERS OF THE TESTIS

Testicular Torsion. Testicular torsion may be seen at any age, although it peaks in two separate periods—in the neonate and in the adolescent.

In the neonate, torsion occurs extravaginally and involves not only the testis but also the entire tunica vaginalis. Some argue that this is more accurately called torsion of the spermatic cord. The lesion is usually noted at birth as a firm, nontender, nontransilluminating scrotal mass. Surgical exploration is generally performed, but reported survival of a testis is extremely rare, since the length of time torsion has been present is undetermined. There is no need to electively secure the opposite testis in cases of extravaginal torsion.

In older children, torsion occurs within the tunica vaginalis and results from extension of the tunica along the posterior surface of the testis, allowing the gonad to hang freely within the cavity of the tunica vaginalis. Torsion is usually associated with the sudden onset of severe scrotal pain, nausea and vomiting. The testis rides high in the scrotum, and the skin of the scrotum is tense and reddened. Torsion of the testis must be differentiated from torsion of the testicular or epididymal appendices and from acute epididymitis. Infected urine and elevation of circulating white blood cells suggest epididymitis. Careful physical examination (sometimes under local or general anesthesia), sodium pertechnetate blood flow scans, or auscultation of the testis with the Doppler ultrasound stethoscope may help distinguish appendiceal torsion from testicular torsion.

Surgical exploration is required urgently, although the length of time torsion may be present before permanent damage is done to the testis is unknown (there is no way to determine the degree of vascular compromise preoperatively). Thus, every effort should be made to save the affected testis, and the other testis should be fixed simultaneously. If the diagnosis of torsion of one of the appendices or of epididymitis can be confirmed clinically, surgical exploration is not necessary. It is preferable, though, to err on the side of a negative exploration rather than to miss a testicular torsion.

Ductal Anomalies. Absence of the vas deferens occurs from loss of the wolffian system. If this occurs before four weeks of development, there will be ipsilateral absence of the kidney also. The vas deferens may be atretic for only a short segment or absent throughout its length. There is an increased incidence of absence of the vas deferens in children with cystic fibrosis. There is no therapy for management of this problem and most will not be diagnosed until they present for evaluation of infertility as adults.

Congenital Anorchia. On occasion, exploration for bilateral cryptorchidism in an otherwise normal male fails to identify any gonadal tissue. Since the presence of a testis is required for development of the genital primordia along male lines, it has been assumed that testicles were originally present but later sustained some accident such as intrauterine torsion.

There is no treatment except cosmetic placement of testicular prostheses and the administration of testosterone during adolescence. It has been suggested that failure of a rise in serum testosterone to injection of HCG (20,000 I.U. spread over five days) indicates the presence of anorchia. While this correlation is good in the small series available, surgical exploration is still indicated at present to confirm that no dysplastic gonadal tissue is present.

Hernia and Hydrocele

STEPHEN L. GANS, M.D.

Herniorrhaphy is the most frequently performed operation in infancy and childhood. This procedure has an excellent record and offers reasonable and ample protection from the more serious and hazardous complications of incarceration and strangulation. These may involve omentum, small or large intestine, bladder, testes, ovaries, tubes and even uteri, any of which may be damaged or destroyed as a consequence. Not only is incarceration troublesome and dangerous per se, but it has a way of happening when the infant or child has a severe upper respiratory infection, contagious disease or other conditions, making emergency anesthesia and surgery more of a problem.

Therefore when the diagnosis of inguinal hernia has been made, operation is advised regardless of age or symptoms. An otherwise well newborn tolerates the procedure as well as an older child when managed by experienced anesthesiologists and surgeons. Failure to thrive, acute illness, some temporary household or psychological problems, or exposure to a contagious disease may prompt delay in surgical correction. Under these circumstances yarn and other trusses have been used, but they are troublesome to the mother, are frequently associated with severe underlying skin irritation or furunculosis, and cannot be depended upon to prevent incarceration. I do not recommend them.

If repair is to be postponed, the parents must be informed about the symptoms and signs of an incarcerated hernia, instructed in simple measures to reduce it, and warned to call if complete relief is not obtained within a reasonably short time (see Incarcerated Hernia).

Hospitalization for uncomplicated herniorrhaphy is now a matter of only a few hours ("outpatient surgery") or at the most one day. Smaller infants are fed up to a few hours before anesthesia in order to prevent dehydration, and appropriate preanesthetic medication is ordered by the anesthesiologist.

When hernias are present bilaterally, both sides are repaired at the same operation. However, when a hernia is present on only one side, should the other side be explored? After many years the controversy still rages and the pendulum swings back and forth with reasonable arguments on both sides. I suggest that the situation be resolved in the following manner. If the history reveals an early undescended testicle which "came down," or a transient hydrocele, or if examination demonstrates thickened cord structures or a "rub" sign, exploration of this side should be considered. This judgment should be tempered by consideration of the experience and skill of the operating surgeon and the anesthesiologist, the amount of time involved in repairing the first side, and the patient's response to the procedure thus far.

Postoperatively the patient is discharged from the hospital as soon as he is fully recovered from the anesthesia and has retained food, usually in four to six hours. The following instructions for home care are given:

1. Sponge baths instead of tub baths should be given for one week.

2. Infants still in diapers should be changed more frequently during the day and once or twice during the night.

3. For pain, if present, Tylenol is usually sufficient.

4. There are no physical restrictions for infants and toddlers. Older children need be restricted only from heavy lifting and pushing, wrestling and fighting, bicycle riding and athletics for a total of three weeks.

5. If of school age, the patient may attend classes as soon as he is comfortable, but he is excused from physical education for the same three week period.

Hydrocele. Most hydroceles of the tunica vaginalis, canal of Nuck or the spermatic cord do not require treatment in the first few months of life, and many of them will disappear spontaneously. However, patients with hydroceles which fluctuate significantly in size during the course of a day or from time to time, or increase greatly in size over a period of several weeks, have a patent processus vaginalis and will eventually come to surgery for repair of this associated hernia. Hydroceles which persist or develop after six months to a year are almost invariably associated with hernias and should be treated as a hernia and for the same reasons.

The operative approach is always through the inguinal region and the hernia sac is ligated high and removed along with a portion of the hydrocele sac. Postoperative care is the same as for herniorrhaphy, but the parents should be told that occasionally discoloration and swelling of the scrotum occur and are temporary.

Incarcerated Inguinal Hernia. Reasonable attempts should be made to reduce an incarcerated hernia in an infant. Emergency surgery for this condition is frequently difficult, and the morbidity, complications and recurrence rate are significantly higher than with elective surgery. At home all the usual efforts to comfort and relax the patient should be tried; even a warm bath may help. Often the hernia will reduce during the ride to the hospital because of the relaxation derived from holding and motion.

Usually the physician can reduce the hernia by gentle firm pressure while the baby industriously works on a pacifier reinforced with sugar. If this maneuver fails, sedative or narcotic medication is given and the infant's buttocks are propped up by pillows or leg traction for as long as an hour. Pressure may be tried again when the patient is well relaxed by the medication. More often than not, reduction will be obtained. If not, immediate surgery is indicated. Nasal gastric suction and intravenous fluids are started. At operation, incarcerated bowel should be examined carefully before returning it to the peritoneal cavity. Ovaries or testes may appear badly traumatized or infarcted, but this is not necessarily an indication for resection. Return of the ovary to the abdomen and the testis to the scrotum is the rule. Postoperative care is much the same as for elective herniorrhaphy, except that the patient should not be discharged for at least 24 hours.

Sometimes it is difficult to distinguish a tense hydrocele of the cord or scrotum from an incarcerated hernia. In such instances it is safer to operate for hernia than to attempt differentiation by needle aspiration.

Whenever possible, successful nonoperative reduction should be followed by elective repair in 48 to 72 hours, when reactive edema and inflammation have subsided.

Inguinal Hernia in Females. In general the same principles apply as in the male, but certain special considerations warrant discussion. When the hernia is represented by a small firm mass in the groin or labium, several possibilities exist. Most frequently it is an incarcerated ovary or tube. Occasionally it will be a sliding hernia with ovary, tube, or even a corner of the uterus making up part of the wall of the sac. Rarely the lump represents a hydrocele of the canal of Nuck. Even when the infant or child appears to be a normal female in all other respects, the mass may be a testis (male pseudohermaphroditism).

If the mass is quite tender and the patient is symptomatic, treatment is carried out without delay as in the male with incarcerated hernia. If the mass is not tender and the patient is asymptomatic, elective surgery should be scheduled at the earliest possible date. Meanwhile buccal smears are done and further history obtained, in order to help rule in or out gonadal abnormalities.

When these investigations prove normal, the operative procedure follows the usual description. Simple hernia in the female is repaired in the same way as in the male. Hydrocele of the canal of Nuck is invariably associated with a hernia; it is removed and the hernia similarly repaired. Sliding hernia requires a different technique. In dissecting out the sac, care is exercised to avoid damage to the ovarian and uterine vessels. The sac is then opened and incised to its neck alongside the sliding element. The tongue of sac with the adnexal structures is returned to the peritoneal cavity, and the sac itself is ligated high at its neck and amputated. Postoperative care is the same as in the male.

If investigations have suggested that male gonads may be found in place of female organs, full discussions should be held with the parents, explaining the possibilities and obtaining permission for possible laparoscopy through the hernia sac, possible exploratory laparotomy, and possible orchiectomy. Selection of treatment is determined by the findings when the hernia sac is opened at surgery, the nature of the gonad is determined and the status of internal pelvic genitalia is known.

Femoral Hernia. Femoral hernias are rare in infants and children. The same principles of treatment apply as in inguinal hernia.

Disorders of the Vulva and Vagina

BARBARA LIPPE, M.D.

CONGENITAL OR DEVELOPMENTAL DISORDERS

Treatment of any congenital or developmental disorder involving the external genitalia and excretory system of the child should be designed to (1) establish the sex of rearing of the child in the neonatal nursery, (2) permit appropriate gender identification by the child prior to 18 to 24 months, (3) allow for potentially adequate sexual function, (4) establish an excretory system which will have the fewest ultimately serious medical consequences, and (5) preserve fertility when possible and compatible with the above. Achieving these goals requires early recognition of abnormalities, appropriate diagnosis, and institution of appropriate medical therapy.

Isolated Clitoromegaly. When present at birth, clitoromegaly without labial scrotal fusion may still indicate prenatal exposure to virilizing steroids of either maternal or fetal origin. Congenital adrenal hyperplasia, gonadal intersex, or a maternal virilizing condition or maternal ingestion of a virilizing substance must be ruled out, and treatment directed to the underlying etiology. Plastic repair of the clitoris may or may not be necessary and the decision can be deferred to 18 months of age, at which time the relative size and erectile nature of the organ should be assessed. If prominent with stimulation or micturition, then a surgical procedure should be so designed to retain the organ, its innervation, and the most normal anatomic appearance possible. This can usually be accomplished by clitoral recession. Clitorectomy is rarely, if ever, indicated.

Ambiguous Genitalia. While the multiple etiologies and specific therapies for ambiguous genitalia are dealt with elsewhere (see p. 322), the principles outlined above apply to reconstruction of the vulva and vagina, or to creation of female genitalia in an infant with a testis. Reconstruction must permit appropriate gender identification and allow for adequate sexual function. In the female, these principles are usually accepted without hesitation. In the male, however, many cases of severe anomalies may mean the assignment of the female gender, and this is often more difficult. The timing of the necessary procedures should include clitoral reconstruction prior to 2 years of age and early removal of the testis with preservation of scrotal tissue for use in construction of an artificial vagina. This recommendation is primarily to relieve the parents from abnormal concerns of the potential effects of a gonad of the opposite sex as well as to prevent the possible confusion on the part of the older child who might misinterpret the nature of the later surgery. Medically, the gonad may be safely left in place until just before puberty.

Reconstruction of the introitus should be done in early puberty prior to menses in females in whom a uterus and ovaries are present, with only isolated absence of the vagina; when there is no uterus, construction of an artificial vagina is timed for the age sexual activity is contemplated. This timing depends on the motivation of the adolescent to use a vaginal dilator or wear an obturator until coitus becomes frequent. The decision for surgery therefore requires a good deal of personal physician-patient communication independent of parental mores.

Finally, the assignment and rearing of a male child as a female may no longer be the "secret" of the parents and physician. Medical and genetic sophistication on the part of society as well as increasing awareness of and desire for knowledge about her own body may in the future dictate a different approach on the part of the physician to the "intersex" patient.

Congenital Absence of the Vagina. This is usually associated with some form of uterine abnormality and with variable abnormalities of the skeleton and urinary tract (Rokitansky-Kuster-Hauser syndrome). When recognized, appropriate diagnostic studies of potentially affected systems are indicated. The ovaries are usually intact. The timing and extent of surgical repair depend upon whether the uterus will develop sufficiently to bleed. Often this cannot be assessed until some stimulation occurs at the time of puberty. At that time, establishment of a vaginal access to the cervix may be necessary, and patency maintained with an obturator or dilatation until coitus becomes frequent.

ACQUIRED HORMONAL FINDINGS

Findings of hormonal stimulation of the vulva and vagina, such as precocious development of pubic hair (adrenarche), enlargement of the clitoris, estrogenization of the labia minora, or menstruation, are all signs of a systemic process and should be so investigated and treated. If isolated precocious adrenarche is diagnosed, no systemic therapy is recom-

mended nor is local removal of pubic hair suggested. Acquired clitoromegaly will be self-limiting after treatment of the virilizing process, and 12 to 18 months should intervene between institution of adequate therapy and evaluation of clitoral size for possible surgical reconstruction. If then necessary, a recession procedure with preservation of both glandular tissue and innervation should be performed. Clitorectomy for acquired enlargement is rarely necessary.

Menstruation, as a sign of isosexual precocious puberty, must be distinguished from exogenous sources of estrogen, such as ingestion of birth control pills, estrogen cream, autonomous ovarian or adrenal sources of estrogen, or treatable central lesions causing sexual precocity, or hypothyroidism. When isosexual precocity is diagnosed and no cause is found, treatment is difficult. Medroxyprogesterone acetate (Depo-Provera), 100 to 200 mg. intramuscularly every 2 weeks, has been used successfully to stop menses.* It does so primarily by causing endometrial atrophy, rather than acting centrally, and has been associated with prolonged amenorrhea following cessation of therapy. Additionally, it does not retard the rapid growth or advancement of bone age associated with this condition.

More recently, cyproterone acetate, an anti-estrogen, has been used successfully by European investigators. This drug is centrally active and appears to stop all hormonal secretions. Clinical trials are currently under way and may be available for selected patients. Local therapy such as curettage is not recommended. Use of tampons is not recommended until the child is responsible enough to remember to insert and remove them (the "forgotten" tampon is a common foreign body in the young adolescent). However, when the child is motivated for their use, they may be recommended at any age, as the hymenal ring is rarely occlusive to proper placement even in the virginal child.

INFECTIOUS AND INFLAMMATORY DISORDERS

Gonorrheal Vulvovaginitis. Diagnosed by appropriate cultures, including anorectal and oral swabs, this disorder is being seen with increasing frequency in prepubertal children. When uncomplicated and not associated with bacteremia, arthritis, conjunctivitis, and so on, single dose therapy is effective. Penicillin G procaine, 100,000 units/kg. intramuscularly in two injection sites (maximum 4.8 million units),

---

*The use of Depo-Provera for this disorder is investigational.

administered simultaneously with probenecid, 25 mg./kg. orally (maximum 1 gm.), is effective. Alternate oral single dose therapy of amoxicillin trihydrate, 50 mg./kg. (maximum 3.5 gm.), with probenecid can be used. In the patient with penicillin allergy, tetracycline may be used, but single dose therapy is not sufficient. A course of oral tetracycline* hydrochloride, 25 mg./kg. initially (maximum 1.5 gm.), followed by 10 mg./kg. four times daily for four days (16 doses), is recommended. A new penicillin-resistant strain of gonorrhea is currently emerging which may require modifications in therapy in the future. Currently this strain is known to be sensitive to spectinomycin (Trobicin), and if this resistant strain is isolated, intramuscular spectinomycin is currently used in adults, but the dose for children has not been established.

Syphilitic Chancre.   This may present as a primary painless chancre with vulvar and inguinal adenopathy. A positive dark field examination or later positive specific serologic test for syphilis (FTA-ABS) requires therapy. Benzathine penicillin G, 1.2 to 2.4 million units intramuscularly in a single dose, is usually sufficient. In a child allergic to penicillin, tetracycline may be used as outlined under gonorrhea, but continued for 14 days.

Streptococcal Vulvovaginitis.   Streptococcus is difficult to eradicate from the genital tract and should be treated in the nonpregnant female only when associated with symptoms. Systemic therapy with oral penicillin, 125 to 250 mg. four times daily for 7 days, is preferred to local antibiotics.

Pinworm Vulvovaginitis.   A new anthelminthic agent, mebendazole (Vermox), is recommended for pinworm vulvovaginitis associated with migration from the anus in the child over two years. A single dose of one chewable tablet is used for family members of all ages. Side effects are minimal but the drug is contraindicated in pregnancy.

Candidiasis and Trichomoniasis.   For candidiasis occurring in the child under 1 year of age or following an oral course of antibiotics, oral nystatin, 100,000 to 1,000,000 units orally four times daily for 7 days, can be used combined within local nystatin cream or suppository therapy every day. In the older nondiabetic child where a primary gastrointestinal source is not suspected, local therapy with either nystatin cream or vaginal suppositories or newer topical antifungal drug, miconazole (MicaTin, Monistat), is used twice daily for 5 days. For trichomoniasis, oral therapy with metronidazole (Flagyl), 10 mg./kg./day in four divided doses for 5 days, is preferred to local treatment.

Nonspecific Vulvovaginitis.   This may be associated with a recent upper respiratory infection, poor hygiene, manipulation or masturbation, excessive irritation from bicycle seat, irritants in bath water (so called bubble bath vaginitis), synthetic undergarments, associated urinary tract infection or ectopic urethra. When possible, therapy should be aimed at improved hygiene and removal or correction of the local problem. Washing is best done by bathing with a mild soap, gently blotting the area dry and applying a nonmedicated cream. If vulvitis is acute, moist and edematous, cleansing should be done with a nonmedicated baby oil rather than soap. If there is no response in one to two weeks, then a trial of topical therapy may be necessary. Furacin-E Urethral Inserts may be placed into the vagina nightly for 7 to 10 days. Local application of estrogen cream to the prepubertal genital tract should be reserved for chronic unresponsive irritation or the lysis of occlusive vaginal synechiae. Premarin or dienestrol vaginal cream can be applied to the outside of the vagina nightly for two weeks and then every other night for two weeks.

Condylomata Acuminata.   Although rare in prepubertal children, condylomata acuminata are being seen more frequently, alone or associated with other infectious agents. Twenty per cent podophyllin resin in tincture of benzoin, applied to the vulva with a cotton applicator and removed by washing after 4 to 6 hours, is used once weekly until the lesion is cleared. Surgical removal is rarely necessary. For the vagina, treatment of an associated infection may result in resolution. Podophyllin is not recommended for mucosal surfaces.

Herpes Genitalis.   Herpes infection of the vulva is rare in the precoital child. If herpetic lesions are present, however, treatment is largely symptomatic, with nonmedicated sitz baths followed by an antibiotic ointment such as Neo-Polycin to prevent secondary infections. Phototherapy is no longer recommended, as it was found to have no therapeutic benefit in double blind studies. No currently available antiviral agents are as yet recommended.

---

*Manfacturer's note: The use of tetracyclines during tooth development (last half of pregnancy, infancy and childhood to age 8 years) may cause permanent discoloration of teeth. This adverse reaction is more common during long-term use of the drug but has been observed following repeated short-term courses.

OTHER ACQUIRED MEDICAL OR SURGICAL CONDITIONS

Adhesions of the Labia Minora (Synechia Vulvae). Partial adhesions without interference with micturition may not require treatment. Symptomatic, extensive or occlusive adhesions which interfere with micturition or produce a vaginal mucocele can be divided by application of Premarin or Dienestrol vaginal cream to the line of the adhesion twice daily for 7 to 14 days. Repeated courses of estrogen therapy are, however, not recommended. Should symptomatic occlusion recur, then surgical division, with chromic sutures of the divided labial edge to the vaginal wall, may be indicated.

Urethral Prolapse. Circular urethral prolapse may present with bleeding and a mass in the vaginal introitus simulating a vaginal neoplasm. Bed rest and sitz baths are usually unsuccessful in reducing the prolapse and afford only temporary relief until surgical excision can be performed.

Vaginal Prolapse. In the neonatal and early infant period, redundant estrogenized vaginal mucosa may protrude or prolapse into the introitus, presenting as a tumor mass. No therapy is recommended as long as the condition is appropriately distinguished from a tumor by physical examination. It is usually self-limiting. A lesser lesion, such as hymenal tag, may similarly be present. Surgical excision is recommended if the tissue is significant in size or subject to trauma or irritation.

Vaginal Foreign Body. Although removal should be attempted under local anesthesia with topical Xylocaine jelly for material which is judged not to be sharp or deeply imbedded in tissue, removal under general anesthesia may be necessary.

Lichen Sclerosis et Atrophicus. This is a generalized skin disease which, when it involves the vulva, may result in pruritus and susceptibility to trauma and ecchymoses. Nonantibiotic-containing topical corticosteroid creams such as Cort-Dome, ⅛ per cent, or Kenalog, 0.025 per cent, may be used to control the pruritus. Estrogen creams are not indicated nor is vulvectomy.

TRAUMA

Appropriate surgical measures should be taken to achieve hemostasis, restore anatomy and prevent secondary infection in trauma to the vulva and vagina, as in any other area. Vaginal stenosis or denervation as a consequence of trauma is most unlikely, and concerns about later sexual or reproductive function should be minimized. In evaluating the extent of the injury, examination under anesthesia may be necessary to distinguish and treat damage to the urethra, bladder, or rectum and possible intraperitoneal penetration. When physically inflicted trauma such as child abuse or sexual molestation is suspected, additional measures need to be employed. Vaginal and rectal and urethral cultures should be obtained in appropriate media for detection of gonococcus and therapy instituted if the cultures are positive (see infectious disorders). A specific VDRL (FTA-ABS) should be obtained after 6 weeks and if positive, treatment with penicillin G is the drug of choice (see infectious disorders). If the child is menarcheal, then the so-called "morning after" contraceptive, stilbestrol, 25 mg. orally, is instituted within 48 hours and is given for 5 days. Prior to administration, a pregnancy test and consent form should be obtained. Additional diagnostic and forensic studies such as examination of vaginal washings for sperm should be part of an organized child abuse and molestation program including medicolegal, social service and psychological support.

TUMORS OF THE VULVA AND VAGINA

Hemangiomas. Vulvar hemangiomas, either of the capillary or cavernous type, are rarely neoplastic and their treatment depends on size, rapidity of growth and susceptibility to injury. Cryotherapy has been used for the capillary lesion which either ulcerates or bleeds. This is seldom sufficient for the symptomatic cavernous lesion. If large, symptomatic and associated with thrombocytopenia, a short course of corticosteroids, prednisone, 2 mg./kg./day for 3 weeks, tapered over 3 to 6 weeks, may afford reduction in size. Surgical ligation of the blood vessels with skin grafting, if necessary, may be indicated.

Cysts. These lesions, arising as developmental anomalies of the urogenital tract, are usually not associated with other major lesions. Their excision is recommended only when they are painful or large, or if they interfere with urination.

Vaginal Adenosis and Clear Cell Adenocarcinoma. Since the reported association between in utero exposure to maternally administered diethylstilbestrol (DES), dienestrol, and hexestrol and the development of vaginal adenosis and clear cell adenocarcinoma of the vagina and cervix in young women, these lesions are being recognized with increasing frequency. The risk of adenocarcinoma in the DES-exposed women appears to be about 1.4 per thousand, whereas the incidence of adenosis in exposed women is reported to be as high as 90 per cent.

When clear cell adenocarcinoma is diagnosed, the treatment is aggressive, as the lesion is invasive and malignant and may metastasize. Staging the extent of spread may assist in the decision as to the procedures of choice. However, vaginectomy, hysterectomy, abdominopelvic lymph node dissection, adjunctive chemotherapy and radiotherapy may all be indicated. Local excision or local radiation of even small lesions to preserve reproductive function is viewed with great caution in light of evidence that small superficially invasive tumors have potential for lymph node spread. If vaginectomy is to be performed and local irradiation is not contemplated, then simultaneous vaginal reconstruction with skin grafts should be done. All cases of clear cell adenocarcinoma in DES-exposed women should be reported to Dr. A. L. Herbst, Registry of Clear Cell Adenocarcinoma, Room 303, 5841 Maryland Avenue, Chicago, Ill. 60610.

Vaginal adenosis, the presence of glandular epithelium resembling that of the endocervix and associated with transverse vaginal and cervical ridges, has been found in a large majority of DES-exposed women. As most women are cancer-free at the time adenosis is discovered, no immediate therapy is indicated, but long-term gynecologic follow-up at six month intervals is recommended. There is a suggestion that these women may be at risk for later development of other lesions such as squamous cell carcinoma. While there is no evidence for a deleterious effect of estrogen-containing contraceptives in these women, mechanical means of contraception are judged more prudent. Pregnancy is not contraindicated.

Sarcoma Botryoides. The extent of treatment depends upon local staging and the presence or absence of metastatic disease. Surgical treatment includes exenteration of the vagina, cervix and uterus and possibly excision of the vulva and rectum; the decision to preserve ovarian function by elevating them out of the pelvis at the time of surgery is again dependent on the extent of the pelvic involvement. Aggressive postoperative chemotherapy protocols are being evaluated using combinations of vincristine, cyclophosphamide, actinomycin D and doxorubicin hydrochloride (Adriamycin). Radiation therapy is often incorporated into the postoperative multimodal therapeutic regimen. When extensive metastases are present at the time of diagnosis, chemotherapy and radiation may be employed first, and depending on response, followed by surgery. Vaginal reconstruction should be done when coitus is contemplated.

Disorders of the Uterus, Tubes and Ovaries

BARBARA LIPPE, M.D.

DEVELOPMENTAL DISORDERS

Congenital Absence of the Uterus. This may occur alone or in association with skeletal and genitourinary abnormalities. If noted radiologically or surgically in the prepubertal child, no therapy is recommended except for routine intravenous pyelogram. The ovaries are usually intact, and feminization without menstruation occurs at puberty. There is no therapy as yet for this form of infertility.

Duplication or Bicornuate Uterus. This requires no therapy in premenarcheal child. Post-menarcheal surgical correction to establish fertility may be necessary.

Hydrometrocolpos - Hematosalpinx - Hematometra. Nonsanguineous fluid or blood may distend the vagina, uterus and tubes, appearing as a pelvic or abdominal mass. In the neonate, imperforate hymen or a transverse vaginal septum are the most common causes. Therefore, surgical treatment to correct the obstruction should first be done vaginally, and abdominal exploration is usually not necessary. Associated congenital anomalies should be suspected and evaluated radiologically. In the menarcheal female, obstruction at the level of the hymen, upper vagina, or cervical os will require gynecologic evaluation and surgical repair.

Abnormal Ovarian Descent. The ovary will most often be located in the canal of Nuck and be associated with an inguinal hernia. The ovary should be returned to the peritoneal cavity and the hernia repaired. Attempt should be made to visualize associated müllerian structures such as a fimbriated tube, broad ligament or uterus. Conversely, the cervical os may be visualized at surgery using a pediatric cytoscope. Should there be no demonstration of normal müllerian structures, then postoperative evaluation including blood chromosomal studies and endocrinologic evaluation is in order to ensure that the herniating gonad was indeed an ovary.

Gonadal Dysgenesis (Turner's Syndrome); Mixed Gonadal Dysgenesis: Pure Gonadal Dysgenesis. Chromosomal karyotype on blood leukocytes should be performed on all patients with suspected gonadal dysgenesis to confirm the diagnosis and to look for a Y chromosome. A buccal smear is not sufficient since it does not distinguish the presence or absence of a Y chromosome. The presence of a Y (as in the mosaic karyotype 45XO/46XY) puts the patient at risk for the development of a gonadoblastoma in the streak gonad, and either long-term gynecologic follow-up with peritoneoscopy or pelvic ultrasonography, or prophylactic surgical removal of the streaks is indicated. In typical 45XO gonadal dysgenesis, surgical exploration is not necessary as the streaks may remain in situ. Hormonal replacement therapy is begun after gonadal failure is demonstrated physiologically by elevated plasma FSH and LH concentrations, usually at age 11 to 12. Low-dose estrogen replacement, 0.01 to 0.02 mg. of ethinyl estradiol, is used continuously for 6 months to prime the uterus and breasts, and then cyclic therapy is recommended. A low-dose estrogen contraceptive such as Loestrin 1/20 or Zorane 1/20 may be used. Alternatively, ethinyl estradiol, 0.01 to 0.02 mg., given from day 1 to day 23, and a progestational agent such as medroxyprogesterone, 2.5 to 10 mg., from day 17 to day 23, have been used. Sequential contraceptives are no longer recommended, and so-called mini-dose contraceptives are of no value for substitution therapy, as these are progestational compounds which do not contain estrogen.

ACQUIRED DISORDERS

Infectious and Inflammatory. Gonorrheal salpingitis or tubo-ovarian abscesses have not been reported to be a problem in the premenarcheal child. Cervicitis is rare. Although usually not recommended, the intrauterine device as a form of contraception is being used in nulliparous adolescents and presents an additional source of infection and inflammation. Removal is recommended if infection is suspected.

Torsion of the Adnexa. The diagnosis may be suspected by history, physical examination and noninvasive imaging techniques such as ultrasound. Treatment involves surgical removal of vascularly compromised gangrenous tissue.

Toxic or Traumatic. Ovarian failure is now being seen following irradiation therapy or high dose chemotherapy for a variety of neoplastic or systemic disorders. Prophylactic ovariectomy of the damaged or atrophic ovary is not usually recommended. Replacement therapy with a low-dose estrogen compound (ethinyl estradiol, 0.01 to 0.02 mg.) given in a cyclic fashion with a progestational agent during the third week, or a low-dose estrogen contraceptive, is recommended.

Tumors of the Uterus, Tubes and Ovaries

BARBARA LIPPE, M.D.

UTERINE TUMORS

Benign tumors of the uterine cervix or corpus occur uncommonly in the preadolescent. Cervical polyps or papillomas should be excisionally biopsied to rule out sarcoma, and the patient reexamined yearly to detect recurrence. Similarly, benign uterine tumors (such as myomas) are rare, and hysterectomy is rarely indicated for benign conditions. For squamous cell carcinoma or adenocarcinoma, surgical excision of uterus, cervix and upper vagina, with sparing of the ovaries, may be possible unless spread is extensive. Sarcoma usually requires more extensive exenteration followed by a program of chemotherapy and radiation similar to that for sarcoma botryoides. Reconstruction surgery for the vagina and hormonal substitution for oophorectomy are recommended.

TUMORS OF THE OVIDUCT

Tumors of the oviduct are, if found on laparotomy, usually inflammatory rather than neoplastic in origin. A tubo-ovarian abscess may present with an adnexal mass, and medical management should be attempted prior to surgical therapy. Tubal pregnancy should be treated with salpingectomy without cornual resection.

OVARIAN TUMORS

Simple Cysts. Follicular cysts of the ovary may occur anytime from the newborn period onward. They are usually unilocular and less than 5 cm. in diameter. When found incidentally at the time of exploratory laparotomy, they should not be removed. When greater than 5 cm., persistent for longer than 6 months or symptomatic secondary to leakage, then attempts should be made to remove only the cyst, leaving the remainder of the ovary intact. Corpus luteum cyst may be associated with an early pregnancy, and if possible should be oversewn rather than removed. Oophorectomy is seldom necessary in managing ovarian cysts.

Benign Tumors. These include teratomas, dermoids, fibromas, myomas and cystadenomas. The most common is the benign cystic teratoma. Treatment for all benign tumors is surgical removal. If the lesion is totally encapsulated and can be removed solely by shelling it away from normal ovarian tissue, then this is preferred. In the case of papillary serous or pseudomucinous cystadenomas, total oophorectomy is recommended. Since both cystic teratomas and cystadenomas tend to be bilateral, most gynecologists recommend careful inspection of the contralateral ovary, with bisection and inspection for tumor.

Malignant and Functional Tumors. The principle of staging the extent of the malignancy, including preoperative determination of distant metastasis, underlies the approach to treatment of all ovarian tumors. Staging may involve lymph node biopsies, pelvic washings, lymphangiography and bivalve examination of the contralateral ovary. Widespread metastatic disease, for example, might prompt a trial of systemic chemotherapy and radiation prior to extensive pelvic surgery. Conversely, lack of evidence for metastatic disease supports aggressive initial surgical management to effect total cure. Reconstruction surgery and hormonal substitution therapy are indicated in all pubertal patients who are in remission and require such therapy.

Carcinoma, Sarcoma and Malignant Teratoma. Therapy is surgical salpingo-oophorectomy for the circumscribed lesion with inspection of the contralateral bisected ovary. If disease has spread beyond the ovary, then staging will determine the extent of surgery and the necessity for adjunctive chemotherapy or radiation. While bilateral oophorectomy requires replacement estrogen therapy, even if hysterectomy is performed, cyclic replacement is still indicated since a combination of estrogen and a progestational agent in a cyclic fashion, rather than estrogen alone, is deemed more physiologic.

Dysgerminoma. The treatment of the early stages of this disorder is quite controversial. For the unilateral mobile encapsulated lesion, salpingo-oophorectomy, examination of the bisected opposite ovary, and unilateral postoperative pelvic irradiation with shielding of the opposite ovary is the moderate therapy recommended; some would not use the additional radiation, whereas others feel the risk of contralateral disease necessitates bilateral oophorectomy and hysterectomy in all patients. In more extensive disease, all agree that bilateral oophorectomy and hysterectomy should be performed. Chemotherapy with a combination of agents including vincristine, actinomycin-D, cyclophosphamide and doxorubicin hydrochloride (Adriamycin) is added to the radiotherapy.

Choriocarcinoma. This hormonally active tumor is highly malignant but relatively rare. Again, the extent of surgical therapy depends upon staging. However, since it has been reported that distant metastases may regress following resection of the primary lesion, extensive pelvic surgery is recommended even in the presence of metastatic disease. Postoperative chemotherapy with courses of methotrexate is recommended. As the tumor produces measurable human chorionic gonadotropin (HCG), hormone titers should be determined preoperatively and then followed at 1 to 2 month intervals postoperatively as a marker for therapy and for recurrence.

Embryonal Carcinoma is a highly malignant tumor for which surgical therapy alone is usually largely palliative. Combination chemotherapy, including newer agents such as Adriamycin as well as vincristine, actinomycin-D and cyclophosphamide have induced remission in some patients.

Granulosa Cell Tumors and Mesenchymomas. Both the feminizing tumors of the granulosal-thecal-luteal group and the virilizing mesenchymomas are usually benign. If localized, unilateral salpingo-oophorectomy is sufficient for initial therapy. Should evidence of malignancy be present, then contralateral oophorectomy, hysterectomy and postoperative radiation therapy are indicated.

13

Bones and Joints

Craniostenosis

J. WILLIAM FUTRELL, M.D.,
MILTON T. EDGERTON, M.D., *and*
JOHN A. JANE, M.D.

Virchow, in 1851, introduced the term craniostenosis (or craniosynostosis) to refer to conditions associated with premature closure of the cranial sutures. Various abnormal head shapes have been described to result from premature bony fusion of the cranial vault, and anatomically descriptive Greek names have been applied to the different conditions: oxycephaly—tower skull; scaphocephaly—boat-shaped head; and plagiocephaly—oblique head. Craniostenosis may occur as a primary isolated cranial bone malformation, as an individual component of certain craniofacial syndromes such as Crouzon's or Apert's deformities, or as a secondary manifestation of other clinical conditions such as following thyroid replacement therapy, in association with idiopathic hypercalcemia, or following hydrocephalus decompression.

Any single suture or at times a combination of several or all cranial sutures including the coronal, sagittal, lambdoidal, metopic, or squamosal sutures may be involved. Normally, the metopic suture is closed at birth, although the remaining sutures do not completely fuse until postpuberty. When premature fusion occurs normal head expansion is restricted and, according to Virchow's postulate, bone growth is inhibited in a direction perpendicular to the obliterated suture line. Excess compensatory growth occurs in other directions creating additional deformity. Diagnosis of craniostenosis is made on the basis of clinical observation of the resultant deformity, palpation of a ridge or bony thickness at the suture line, or by radiographic examination. Recently, radionuclide bone scanning with technetium 99 has occasionally been helpful in identifying prematurely fused sutures which radiographically appear open.

Attention must also be given to detection of associated problems such as intracranial hypertension or hydrocephalus, which should be suspected in the presence of papilledema, bulging fontanelles, wide separation of uninvolved suture lines, cracked-pot percussion sound, or a beaten-silver appearance of the skull on x-ray. Other congenital anomalies often found in association with craniostenosis, such as syndactyly of the fingers or toes, orbital proptosis, or recession or hypoplasia of the midfacial bones, should also alert one to the possibility of premature cranial bone fusion. The urgency of early recognition of abnormal cranial bone fusion is suggested by the fact that brain growth is most rapid during the first three months of life and tends to level off by the ninth month. During the first year of life more than 50 per cent of the total increase in skull circumference occurs and the brain weight increases approximately 135 per cent, with the frontal lobes almost quadrupling in size during the period. In addition to the potential neurologic compromise caused by bony restriction of brain expansion, the physician must also consider the detrimental effects in uncorrected patients, leading to severe secondary facial and skull structural abnormalities.

Sagittal suture fusion alone is the most frequently occurring type of craniostenosis and occurs most often in males. Coronal synostosis is more common in females and is second in overall frequency. Combinations of suture line fusion occur with varied frequency. Premature closure of the sagittal suture is generally found in children with normal intelligence, whereas some degree of mental retardation is commonly associated with coronal synostosis, particularly when other systemic anomalies are also present. Multiple suture closure, especially with microcephaly or significantly increased intracranial pressure, is likely to result in intellectual impairment unless the defect is corrected early. When only a single suture line is fused, brain damage does not normally result in that the potential increase in intracranial pressure can be reasonably well compensated for by brain expansion in abnormal directions.

The lack of intellectual impairment in patients with single suture fusion has in the past led to a false sense of security by physicians in view of the fact that significant structural deformity can and does occur in uncorrected patients. Such preventable secondary deformity can often assume grotesque anatomic proportions, is progressive during growth and is socially stigmatizing. Appropriately planned, early surgery can often avert significant secondary deformity as well as correct the initial malformation. These facts and increasing clinical experience have further established the benefits of early surgical treatment during the first to ninth month of life for virtually all forms of craniostenosis, from single to multiple fusions. It is our current opinion, therefore, that even when a single isolated suture is involved, unless specific contraindications to surgery exist, early correction of the stenotic suture or sutures is almost always indicated.

The counter argument that a single fused suture (particularly the sagittal) carries little risk of neurologic compromise in the unoperated state is less significant because of possible long-term structural deformity, and particularly in view of the refinement in operative techniques and the availability of craniofacial centers specializing in such surgery. There is, correspondingly, less argument regarding the need for early surgery in the presence of intracranial hypertension or when multiple sutures are involved. Likewise, operative indications are clear when cranial synostosis is associated with other faciostenoses, creating facial and orbital deformity such as progressive exophthalmos and/or visual or auditory compromise.

The skull itself develops from mesoderm and it is felt that the brain and dura induce development of the surrounding bony vault. Probably too much attention has been paid to the readily accessible calvarial sutures and not enough to the base of skull sutures in controlling head growth and shape. The rationale for surgery during early infancy is that correction of the abnormal bony fusion can prevent potential neurologic compromise and improve the primary deformity. Equally important is that correction can release the constricting forces, allowing for more normal brain growth, thereby helping to prevent secondary skull and facial abnormalities resulting from abnormal compensatory brain growth. Creation and maintenance of artificial suture lines to allow expansion of the cranium and growth of the brain is the principal goal of treatment.

The surgical procedure itself consists of wide craniectomy creating open sutures, and appropriate repositioning of the secondarily deformed bony structures. At surgery the head must be positioned such that wide exposure, usually through a bicoronal incision, can be obtained. Inspection and palpation of all potentially involved suture lines are performed. Appropriately placed burr holes are made and the desired amount of bone resected. Normal cranial bone can be osteotomized and repositioned as free bone grafts when secondary deformity has already occurred. Occasionally, in infants, total calvariectomy is performed, removing the entire exposed cranium and depending on bone regeneration to provide a more normal contour. The "functional matrix" concept, which implies that skeletal growth is programmed from the underlying brain and dura, has suggested the additional technique of dural release and grafting in areas of constriction, and dural plication in areas of secondary brain protrusion. When indicated, dural expansion is achieved by use of periosteal grafts applied in the released areas, and plication with interrupted mattress sutures placed in the areas of compensatory brain expansion.

In our experience extensive craniectomy and bony repositioning performed at an early age (preferably one to nine months), when complete bone regeneration can be anticipated, has entirely supplanted interposing polyethylene film or Zenker's solution over the opposing bone edges to prevent premature refusion. Intraoperative inspection of even sutures which radiologically are open occasionally identifies the additional need for release of clinically fused suture lines. Special attention is given to minimizing bleeding including the use of bone wax, epinephrine skin infiltration, cautery hemostasis, and hypotensive anesthesia. Blood transfusion is given as needed. Accurate repair of any dural incisions or tears is undertaken to prevent postoperative spinal fluid leakage.

In areas of actual bone deficit following extensive removal, favorable regrowth and remodeling of the skull can be expected to take place in infants operated upon at less than six months of age and perhaps up to twelve months of age. Less favorable natural remodeling can be expected in patients operated upon after the first year of life. If early bone refusion occurs, reoperation may be necessary and staged procedures may be required for total correction. Occasionally, even in children, use of alloplastic cranioplasty material such as methyl methacrylate has been employed. Early ventricular shunting may also be required to alleviate hydrocephalus, particularly when craniostenosis is associated with certain deformities such as the clover leaf skull (Kleblattschadel syndrome) and occasionally with other craniostenoses.

Careful follow-up, including clinical and radiologic re-examination, is necessary. Early recognition of developing secondary deformity must be appreciated and appropriately treated.

Crouzon's Disease and Apert's Syndrome

J. WILLIAM FUTRELL, M.D., MILTON T. EDGERTON, M.D., and JOHN A. JANE, M.D.

Apert, in 1906, and Crouzon, in 1912, described the common association of physical findings which have become known by their individual eponyms. Crouzon's disease and Apert's syndrome are complex craniofacial bone and soft tissue anomalies which are characterized by the premature fusion of one or several cranial sutures and also the premature closure of multiple facial bone suture lines. These anomalies are included in the general category "craniofacial dysostoses," having the common clinical characteristics of midfacial retrusion and hypoplasia of the maxillary bones, exophthalmos with shallow orbital cavities, forehead and cranial bone deformities, and often an anterior open bite between the jaws.

The hallmark of Crouzon's disease is coronal synostosis and faciostenosis with extreme orbital proptosis. In Apert's syndrome (acrocephalosyndactyly), in addition to these findings there are often multiple additional congenital anomalies commonly including cleft palate, syndactylism or complete webbing of the fingers and toes, ankylosis of the limbs, and mental retardation.

Tessier has been largely responsible for the development of a rational surgical plan for the treatment of these individuals, and it is now clear that the best and most appropriate therapy is radical and extensive osteotomy of the middle third of the face, separating the facial bones from the cranial base and allowing a complete repositioning of the involved bone segments. Earlier attempts to provide help by multiple, limited soft tissue surgical procedures have been only minimally successful and in most patients are now indicated only when performed in association with major cranial and facial remodeling. Due to the general inexperience of dealing with these anomalies and the radical complex surgery involved, early referral for treatment by a coordinated interdisciplinary craniofacial surgical team is generally indicated.

The degree of deformity in any individual with Crouzon's or Apert's anomaly may vary widely from minimal involvement to extreme incapacitation, including the propensity to close the eyelids behind grossly proptotic globes. Cleft palate and hyperseborrhea occur more often in Apert's syndrome, although apart from the syndactylism always found in patients with Apert's syndrome, there are no specific characteristic differences between the two deformities. Variant and transitional forms occur which include traits common to both conditions.

The initial work-up should be begun in early infancy and directed toward identification of the degree of craniostenosis and the presence or absence of hydrocephalus. Skull x-rays will identify multiple bony abnormalities and occasionally the "beaten-silver" appearance characteristic of increased intracranial pressure. In the presence of extreme deformity of skull shape such as oxycephaly (tower skull) in addition to appropriate release of the involved suture lines, techniques are currently available for radical remodeling and reshaping of the entire cranial vault prior to one year of age. In severe cases the grotesqueness of the deformity dictates a radical attempt at restoring symmetry and appropriate contour to the skull and face as well as providing for suture release.

Other systemic symptoms such as upper airway breathing difficulty, occasionally the development of cor pulmonale (due to retroposition of the maxillary structures against the posterior pharynx), and failure to thrive are likely to be apparent in early infancy and can be improved by appropriate surgery. A dominant potentially correctable and characteristic of both Crouzon's and Apert's deformities is malformation of the bony orbits resulting in extreme exorbitism. This is thought to be due to the invariable presence of coronal synostosis, with the anterior cranial base malformation resulting in extreme shallowness of the orbital cavity dimensions including sloping and forward protrusion of the walls which project the globes anteriorly. In certain situations early tarsorraphy may be necessary in order to protect the corneas from abrasion.

Divergent strabismus or exotropia is often present due to the shallowness and outward thrust of the orbital globes from the central ethmoid area; if uncorrected, this can lead to binocular vision and amblyopia. Primary optic atrophy either due to increased intracranial pressure or to atresia of the optic canal can also cause visual disturbances. Photophobia and squinting in early infancy are often apparent, particularly in patients with Apert's syndrome, due to hypopigmentation of the retinae. Although mandibular prognathism is frequently thought to be present, this is usually relative in that maxillary hypoplasia and recession is the dominant characteristic. The mandibular arch should, therefore, be taken as the appropriate plane of reference for the projected craniofacial profile when planning treatment by midface advancement. Overcorrection of the deformity is usually indicated, particularly in young patients, in whom there is still mandibular growth potential.

The complexities of total management for patients with such anomalies make it essential that physicians in various areas of expertise see and evaluate the patient. Family genetic counseling and support are an active part of total patient therapy. Otologic and ophthalmologic evaluations, in addition to preparation and planning for extensive craniofacial plastic and neurosurgery, make optimal habilitation possible only through a well integrated team approach, usually in a center specializing in such surgery.

Due to the generally progressive nature of the deformity and the development of extreme secondary deformity with continued growth, early surgical intervention is usually indicated. Considerations of surgical timing, goals, and rationale in isolated craniostenosis apply to the patient with more extensive syndromes involving facial as well as cranial bone malformation. Due to rapid brain growth and head development during the first year of life, ideal management usually involves early release of the involved cranial base and vault sutures, together with needed cranial bone remodeling and positioning. Our current experience suggests that this should be performed initially when the patient is between three and twelve months of age, although even earlier surgery is now being performed. Expansion of the orbital cavities by resection of the constricting supraorbital ridges and release of the periorbital fascia can also be performed at this initial procedure to improve the exorbitism.

Osteotomies and bone grafts for midface advancement by separation of the facial bones from the cranial base are now occasionally being performed on young infants during the first year of life. Evaluation of these results in selected individuals will have to be compared with those obtained from surgery performed more frequently at four years of age or beyond. Surgical osteotomies are basically along the lines of a LeFort III fracture, allowing simultaneous correction of the exorbitism and retromaxillism by forward displacement of the facial mask. At this time additional attention is given to the orbital area including complete decompression of the orbital periosteum, allowing for expansion of the periorbital fat into the enlarged orbital cavities and further correction of the exophthalmos. Rib and iliac crest bone grafts are used for stabilization and anterior buttressing of the mobilized facial structures.

Sophisticated surgical monitoring apparatus including arterial, spinal drainage, and urinary catheters, hypotensive anesthesia, a central venous pressure line, and a postoperative intracranial pressure screw is used for each patient. In spite of the complex nature of the surgical procedures the mortality and morbidity have been acceptably low and the functional and psychological benefits highly gratifying.

In addition to the craniofacial procedures, multiple operations may be required to produce maximally functional hands and feet in the patients with acrocephalosyndactyly. Release and grafting of the lateral digits in the first year of life is usually indicated with more extensive correction of syndactyly subsequently. Narrowing the foot is often beneficial in allowing the patients to wear normal shoes. In spite of the often extreme deformity and the considerable time and effort of the physician, such radical operative procedures coordinated as a team approach to the total patient are now capable of providing a more normal and self-sufficient existence for these individuals. Attention to detail at an early age cannot be overemphasized.

Hypertelorism and Hypotelorism

J. WILLIAM FUTRELL, M.D.,
MILTON T. EDGERTON, M.D., *and*
JOHN A. JANE, M.D.

Hypertelorism refers to an increased distance between the eyes. The preferred term is orbital hypertelorism, which is defined as an abnormally wide space between the orbits when measured from radiographically fixed points on the skull at the dacryon (the point of junction of the posterior and anterior lacrimal crests). Pseudohypertelorism refers to the visual appearance of increased interorbital distance but with normal measurements. Hypotelorism is an abnormally narrow distance between the orbits. Both orbital hypertelorism and hypotelorism are conditions which represent a physical finding that is secondary to other cranial or facial malformations and is not an entity unto itself. Various facial clefts and premature synostosis of the cranial and facial sutures are the principal causes of orbital hypertelorism, whereas hypotelorism is usually associated with maldevelopment of the nasofrontal process. Each condition is most often the result of a congenital deformity in that although trauma may produce a widening between the canthi (telecanthus) or lateral displacement or a part or parts of the orbital frame, it rarely produces true orbital hypertelorism.

The diagnosis of hypertelorism or hypotelorism can be suspected by visual observation and clinical measurements of the distance between the medial canthi, although accurate documentation must be made radiographically. Measurements of the interpupillary distance may give a false impression of widening or narrowing due to pull of the extraocular muscles on the globe causing exophoria or esophoria. When such is the case interpupillary measurement can be interpreted as a false increase or decrease in the interorbital distance. Cephalometric x-rays or a standardized two-meter posterior-anterior Caldwell film is the best means for accurate diagnostic measurement and reproducibility. Published studies have defined the interorbial distance as averaging 16 mm. at birth, and rising to 25 mm. by age twelve. In females this growth increase levels off at approximately 13 years, whereas males show a continued increase in interorbital distance until approximately age 21 years. Average adult interorbital measurements are reported to be 25 mm. in women and 28 mm. in men.

Classification of hypertelorism is based on the measured interorbital distance and the shape of the fronto-orbital region. First degree orbital hypertelorism, as defined by Tessier, refers to a measured distance of 30 to 34 mm.; second degree as greater than 34 mm. with normal shape and orientation of the orbits; and third degree as greater than 40 mm. Tessier has further systematically developed a working classification of 15 potential facial clefts which can occur circumferentially around the orbital cavities and can account for true orbital hypertelorism. Detailed clinical study and observation have demonstrated that many deformities previously considered to be primarily soft tissue involvement are frequently associated with underlying facial clefts.

In addition to bony clefts the various craniofacial dysostoses (such as Apert's and Crouzon's deformities) can cause orbital hypertelorism as can other etiologic factors including midline dermoid cysts, glial tumors of the root of the nose, meningoencephaloceles involving the frontal, nasal, or ethmoid areas, and so on. Pesudohypertelorism and telecanthus should not be confused with true orbital hypertelorism in that this only apparent interorbital wideness can occur with a variety of conditions including Waardenburg's syndrome, blepharophimosis, epicanthal folds, canthus inversus, and facial clefts lateral to the central ethmoid region.

Due to the intricate nature of the surgery involved, appropriate treatment of any of the various deformities associated with orbital hypertelorism or hypotelorism requires a coordinated interdisciplinary team approach. Extensive diagnostic evaluation is necessary preoperatively to determine the extent of deformity and the most appropriate treatment approach. The clinical presentation may vary in severity and there often appears to be considerably more intermixture of syndromes accounting for the deformity than is generally described.

In addition to the diagnostic radiologic work-up, particular care must be given to the patient's total needs including psychosocial and environmental aspects. Optimal habilitation requires expert technical execution of well planned, complex surgical procedures and subsequent comprehensive clinical care with detailed follow-up documentation of the alterations achieved. Patients and primary care physicians should be aware that centers undertaking such efforts must be capable of offering emotional support for the child and entire family as well as the scientific and technical expertise necessary for execution of this highly complicated surgery. Although only one major surgical procedure may be required, more often patients can benefit by additional less extensive corrective procedures, and this should be understood preoperatively. The development and current availability of centers performing such radical surgery to totally reorient the facial bony architecture must be considered to be one of the most significant technical advances of the last decade.

HYPERTELORISM

Children with orbital hypertelorism are generally of normal intelligence and usually without systemic disabilities. The principal anatomic abnormality associated with increased interorbital distance is thought to be a horizontal widening of the ethmoid sinuses. This increase in bony dimensions is localized to the anterior ethmoid structures and does not involve the posterior ethmoid cells and the sphenoid sinus. Since the cribriform plate is generally not significantly increased in width, a surgical procedure preserving this area and mobilizing the anterior orbital structures without disturbing the posterior optic chiasm is possible. When the roof of the ethmoid mass is inferiorly prolapsed, the cribiform plate may be depressed to a point considerably below the orbital floor (an average of 10 mm.), making it necessary to expose and retract the frontal lobes through an anterior craniotomy prior to performing orbital osteotomies.

In certain situations definitive surgery is performed around the second year of life, making early referral important. In other patients surgery is delayed until after four years of age to allow for pneumatization of the maxillary sinuses and descent of the permanent tooth buds. In addition to a complete physical examination to look for other abnormalities, preoperative evaluation for the patient with hypertelorism includes routine skull and facial bone x-rays, frontal and lateral cephalometric films, frontal tomograms of the orbital cavities to delineate the relationship of the cribriform plate to the orbits, at times pneumoencephalography and arteriography, and more recently computerized axial tomography scans. Detailed ophthalmologic examination and physical measurements of facial structures, together with standardized medical photographs, are also necessary for operative planning and serial follow-up.

Mild hypertelorism generally requires no specific treatment. In moderate and severe cases, amblyopia and the lack of binocular vision is inevitable in the uncorrected patient.

The operative procedure required for the patient with moderate to severe hypertelorism involves an intracranial-extracranial approach. Access to the cranial cavity is obtained through a bicoronal scalp incision, turning down the entire forehead and exposing the periorbital structures. A frontal bone flap is raised, allowing for retraction and protection of the frontal lobes and dissection of the olfactory nerves from the anterior cribriform plate. Osteotomies are then performed through the maxillae and around the orbits. Accurate intraoperative measurements are made of the exact bony interorbital distance and the desired amount of correction determined. The appropriate amount of midline bone and septum is removed and, after wide bone and soft tissue mobilization, the orbital cavities are translocated medially, leaving a central bone core around the stationary orbital foramen in each posterior orbit. Some overcorrection of the deformity is generally desired and the new orbits are wired into position and fixed laterally with rib and iliac crest bone grafts.

Postoperative improvement can be dramatic. Surgery required for strabismus is usually postponed for at least six months postoperatively in that most eye muscle changes are transient and frequently self-correcting. Continued long-term follow-up and support are mandatory.

HYPOTELORISM

The extreme forms of hypotelorism are most frequently associated with cerebral maldevelopment and may not be compatible with life. The spectrum of facies associated with the holoprosencephaly-arhinencephaly type of abnormalities can range from complete cyclopia to orbital hypotelorism associated with median cleft lip, or orbital hypotelorism in association with hypoplastic maxillae. As is true for orbital hypertelorism, a mild degree of hypotelorism may occur as a normal variant and requires no treatment. In severe brain abnormalities, no effort at surgical correction of the ocular problem is indicated; the experienced clinician can often recognize such conditions at birth.

When the patient's condition is determined to be compatible with life, a careful clinical and radiologic evaluation similar to that for hyperteloric patients is indicated. Attention to associated problems such as correction of craniostenosis and repair of a cleft lip or palate is also warranted. The total habilitation program should be managed by a coordinated interdisciplinary team familiar with such problems. In situations in which improved functional and social interaction is anticipated, surgical correction of ocular hypotelorism can be considered. Procedures for this have recently been undertaken and consist of a craniofacial approach similar to that for hypertelorism. Expansion of the orbital cavities with lateral translocation and bone grafts between the orbits have been successful in providing considerable improvement.

Disorders of the Spine and Shoulder Girdle

R. A. KLASSEN, M.D.

Skeletal disorders of the spine and shoulder girdle basically can be classified as congenital or acquired. Congenital disorders may be classified as embryonal failures of segmentation, migration, ossification or fusion or defective cellular differentiation. Associated somatic and visceral anomalies occur with great frequency but these may remain clinically silent until increasing pathology becomes evident. Embryonal vertebral and genitourinary systems differentiate at about the same time, about 4 to 8 weeks of development, and in the same vicinity. An insult at that stage of development may produce many serious anomalies, such as the Klippel-Feil syndrome associated with genitourinary system, hearing, shoulder girdle and cardiac anomalies. An absent or hypoplastic odontoid or elements of C1-C2 may be associated with Down or Morquio syndromes. Hip dysplasia may be associated with infantile torticollis. All of the above can result in severe functional disabilities.

Clinically, anomalies of the cervical spine and shoulder girdle may have deceptively similar appearances and are frequently mixed. They are characterized by a variably short appearing neck, torticollis and uneven shoulder level. Clinical and radiological evaluation differentiates the defects.

Perinatally acquired disorders may pose problems in diagnosis. Birth palsies and perinatal infections may mimic congenital disorders. Clavicular fractures, dislocated shoulders or slipped proximal humeral epiphyses can all give the appearance of paralysis or a congenital anomaly.

Klippel-Feil Syndrome. Klippel-Feil syndrome is a disorder resulting from failure of segmentation of the cervical vertebrae. It may be a minor defect, simply an incidental radiological finding commonly at C2 or C3, or the malformation may be extensive with marked shortening of the neck, cranial asymmetry, webbing of the neck, scoliosis and shoulder girdle involvement. Bracing or surgical correction is rarely indicated other than to control progressive or severe deformities. Plastic surgical revision of the neck webbing or shoulder girdle deformities may be indicated. All patients with anomalies of the spine, Down and Morquio syndromes, should be evaluated routinely for the associated anomalies of C1

and C2, as instability in this area may result in severe accidental neurological deficits.

Scoliosis and Kyphosis. Eighteen to twenty per cent of the children have clinically demonstrable spinal deformities. Treatment is predicated upon the severity and etiology of the deformity. Idiopathic or genetic scoliosis is the most common deformity, followed by congenital and neuromuscular scoliosis.

Flexible curves of 20 to 45 degrees in the growing child are treated with a Milwaukee brace or a similar brace. Rigid and progressive curves not responding to brace management require surgical stabilization. In severe curves, treatment consists of preliminary skeletal traction, followed by a posterior spinal fusion and Harrington rod instrumentation of all the involved vertebrae. Postoperative care consists of early ambulation and casting or bracing for a 9 to 12 month period.

Anterior interbody spinal fusion and Dwyer cable fixation are occasionally used in association with a posterior fusion and Harrington rod instrumentation for a severe deformity. Scoliosis due to congenital, neuromuscular, neurofibromatosis and Marfan syndromes frequently requires surgical correction because of the severity of the deformity. Kyphosis is managed in a manner similar to treatment of scoliosis. Scheuermann's disease, or juvenile kyphosis, occurs most frequently. Milwaukee bracing for flexible curves in excess of 45 degrees in a growing child has been effective. Congenital, traumatic, severely rigid progressive juvenile and painful kyphoses may require surgical stabilization. Anterior interbody fusion as well as posterior fusion with Harrington rod instrumentation may be necessary to maintain the correction of the spine.

Spondylolysis and Spondylolisthesis. Spondylolysis is an acquired defect, probably a stress type fracture of the pars interarticularis, occurring usually after age six. It is seen most frequently at the L5 level and occurs in about 5 per cent of the population. Anterior displacement of the affected vertebral body may occur, varying in degree from minimal to complete displacement. The lesion with displacement is called spondylolisthesis. Symptoms include back pain, radicular pain, tight hamstrings and paravertebral muscle spasm. Initial treatment is bed rest and corset or brace immobilization. If symptoms persist or increasing deformity occurs, surgical intervention is indicated. A spinal fusion of the affected level is carried out and, depending on the symptoms or pathology, this may or may not be associated with removal of the entire loose posterior lamina and excision of the fibrous and cartilaginous tissue surrounding the nerve root.

Intervertebral Disc Herniation. Intervertebral disc herniation occurs most commonly at L4-L5 and L5-S1 levels in the adolescent age group. Symptomatology is similar to that in adults but there is a much lower incidence in children. Back pain and muscle spasms are the most common features. Conservative management consists of bed rest and analgesics. In the event of neurologic deficit or intractable pain, myelography and disc excision are indicated.

Discitis and Vertebral Osteomyelitis. Discitis is an infection or an inflammatory lesion affecting children usually between the ages of 2 and 7, characterized by moderately severe back pain with some diffuse radiation to the buttocks. The child prefers to remain recumbent. When in an upright position or walking, the child maintains the spine in an extended position and usually walks with an awkward swagger. Neurologic deficit is usually not present. The patient's temperature may be mildly elevated. Erythrocyte sedimentation rate and white blood count are usually elevated initially. X-rays will usually show a disc space narrowing two or three weeks after the onset of symptoms. Treatment should consist of an attempt at isolating an organism by means of blood cultures. If there is any evidence of a septic course, disc aspiration and culture of the material should be performed with an image intensifier to permit precise placement of the needle. Appropriate antibiotic treatment should then be instituted. A body cast or brace should be worn for 3 to 6 months until the lesion heals and the symptoms are resolved. Significant bony erosion or abscess formation should be dealt with surgically.

Vertebral osteomyelitis is uncommon since the control of tuberculosis, brucellosis and typhoid fever. Currently, the most frequent offending organism is *Staphylococcus*. Symptoms are similar to discitis, and x-ray findings usually consist of evidence of bony erosion and collapse of the vertebral bodies or abscess formation. Treatment is directed toward identification of the organism, use of appropriate antibiotics, and debridement and immobilization of the spine. A spinal fusion may also be performed to prevent progressive deformity.

Vertebra Plana or Calvés Disease. This is a compression or fracture of the vertebral body usually secondary to eosinophilic granuloma. Vertebral hemangioma or an aneurysmal bone cyst may give a similar appearance. The diffuse flattening of the vertebral body noted radiologically is fairly characteristic and biopsy is not indicated for a satisfactory diagnosis. Treatment is symptomatic only and bracing is necessary for the levels involved and when deformity occurs.

Spinal Trauma. Trauma to the spine is seen less frequently in children than in adults, presumably because of the greater mobility of the spine in children. In the cervical spine the upper vertebrae are more susceptible to injury than are the lower cervical segments; in adults this situation is reversed. A critical radiological analysis must be made including flexion and extension views and cine radiography if a lesion is not apparent and if the patient complains of neck pain following an accident. Severe fracture of the thoracic and lumbar vertebrae in a growing child may result in progressive deformity, especially in the quadriplegic and paraplegic. A growing child has the ability to reconstitute compressive and other deformities if adequate support is given. Continued observation should therefore be maintained, and appropriate bracing and spinal fusion may be instituted.

Muscular Torticollis. Muscular torticollis is usually present at birth. Fibrosis of the sternocleidomastoid muscle is usually noted in the form of a palpable nodule. Asymmetry of the face is often an associated finding. The torticollis is usually self-resolving. If it persists beyond a six month span, surgical treatment consisting of muscle release may be indicated. Congenital hip dysplasia may also be present and is evaluated routinely.

Clavicular Congenital Pseudoarthrosis. Congenital pseudoarthrosis is rare, is usually right-sided but occasionally may be bilateral, and is associated with cleidocranial dysostosis. Surgical treatment with internal fixation and bone grafting may be indicated in a young child. Functional impairment is rare.

Sprengel's Deformity. Sprengel's deformity is an embryologic failure of descent and imperfect formation of the shoulder girdle, generally unilateral. The scapula remains deformed, elevated and may be attached to the cervical spine by a fibrous, cartilaginous or bony structure. The clavicle is frequently deformed. Degree of deformity varies from a minimally elevated scapula and shoulder with no functional impairment to a severe deformity with only the vestigial remnants of the scapula and marked limitation of shoulder motion. Marked deformity and limitation of motion warrant surgical correction, usually performed between the ages of 2 and 7. This consists of surgically mobilizing the scapula and deforming structures, applying skeletal traction to the scapula distally, and maintaining with a cast until healing has occurred.

Chest Wall Abnormalities

E. S. GOLLADAY, M.D., *and*
J. ALEX HALLER, JR., M.D.

Failure of sternal fusion, absence of pectoralis major and minor muscles with mammary hypoplasia, thoracic dystrophy, pectus excavatum and pectus carinatum are significant chest wall abnormalities which may affect children.

Pectus excavatum, or funnel chest, is a depression deformity of the anterior chest which is usually central, but may be deeper on one side—nearly always the right side. This anomaly has a familial tendency and not infrequently is associated with Marfan's syndrome. It is congenital and often increases in severity through childhood. Many of these patients have an asthenic habitus and nearly all have a characteristic postural deformity with slumping shoulders and protuberant abdomen. No convincing evidence of cardiopulmonary dysfunction has been documented from the possible distortion of the heart and lung in children; however, several studies and anecdotal reports in adults with severe pectus excavatum indicate moderate to severe physiologic abnormalities. These include restricted cardiac output and diminished pulmonary function. All older children and teenagers are bothered by the ugly deformity. The cosmetic impact, the postural changes and possible prevention of cardiopulmonary dysfunction are the reasons for repair of this abnormality.

Radiologic examination shows displacement of the heart to the left and varying degrees of posterior position of the sternum. Soft midsystolic murmurs along the left sternal border over the pulmonary valve area are frequent. The electrocardiogram may show (1) S_1 S_3 or S_1 Q_3, or (2) negative P in V_1 and qr or RSR^1 in V_1. These apparent cardiac abnormalities are due entirely to rotation and displacement of the heart, although through misinterpretation they have been the basis in the past for physician-induced semi-invalidism.

Multiple etiologies have been suggested; none has been proved. The pathogenesis appears to be deformed costal cartilages which hold the sternum backward. Removal of these abnormal cartilages forms the basis for all corrective procedures.

Decision for surgical correction is made with the child and parents if the surgeon feels the cosmetic and postural deformity is severe. We feel that the best time for elective repair is just prior to entering school when sufficient emotional maturity is present and the hospital experience is easier on the patient. The psychological problems from exposure of the abnormality in the school sports are thus eliminated. The best long-term correction of the postural abnormalities occurs when there is still late childhood and teenage growth ahead.

The repair of choice in our experience consists of a transverse skin incision, elevation of skin flaps, reflection of the pectoral muscles from the chest wall, subperichondral resection of abnormal cartilages, sternal osteotomy above the lowest normal rib and oblique transection of the lowest normal cartilage for dynamic internal support. The sternum is thus elevated and the medial part of the transected costal cartilage is sutured to and supported by its lateral partner. This is the so-called tripod support and it obviates the need for any type of metallic splint. The hospital stay is 7 to 10 days, and a restriction from strenuous exercise for six weeks must be imposed to allow regrowth of the costal cartilages. If a late adolescent patient desires correction, Silastic implantation to correct the cosmetic deformity may be advisable.

Pectus carinatum, or pigeon breast, is a protrusion deformity which is one tenth as common as pectus excavatum. Familial occurrence is higher and there is a rare association with Marfan's disease. This defect is frequently off the midline and may be largely unilateral. It tends to occur later than excavatum and reaches a maximum deformity in the teens. The prominent knob is troublesome from the standpoint of an irritative pressure while in a prone position; it is also unattractive and difficult to conceal by clothing; it may be confused with neoplasia. The etiology is obscure, but prevailing opinion ascribes the condition to overgrowth of costal cartilages. We do not believe that cardiopulmonary or postural dysfunction is associated with this defect. The operation is similar in concept to excavatum repair in that the abnormal cartilages must be excised. It is undertaken for cosmetic reasons and should not be carried out until the late teenage years to avoid recurrence from postoperative re-growth.

Thoracic dystrophy is a familial chondrodystrophy which affects the costochondral junction. The majority of patients succumb during infancy due to chest wall constriction. Splitting and wedging of the sternum may be life-saving if respiratory failure persists in spite of mechanical ventilatory support. Prolonged support of ventilation may be necessary because of inadequate stability of the thorax.

Poland's syndrome is the absence of the pectoralis major and pectoralis minor muscles, absence of costal cartilages and ipsilateral syndactyly. Paradoxical respiration may be present in the involved area (75 per cent on the right) and the nipple and areola may be small or absent. If the costal cartilages are present and no paradoxical motion is present, no operative procedure is necessary until maturity and then only in females in the form of augmentation mammoplasty. If a large section of chest wall is missing, operation to prevent secondary progressive deformity and to eliminate paradoxical motion may be indicated. Ravitch used split sections of contralateral rib to bridge the gap between the rib ends and the sternum, and applied a sheet of Teflon felt to complete a stable repair.

Failure of Sternal Fusions. Absence of the xyphoid is fairly common; complete absence of all sternal elements is extremely rare. If there is no integument covering the heart, the condition is usually lethal. The presence of a beating heart outside the thorax is perhaps the most distressing of congenital anomalies. The defect should be closed with early operation if undue cardiorespiratory distress does not occur on replacement of the heart within the mediastinum. A prosthesis may be necessary for immediate repair and the intracardiac defects left for subsequent procedures.

A lower sternal defect is often associated with embryologically related defects. Those include a midline supraumbilical abdominal wall defect (omphalocele), a deficiency of the anterior diaphragm, a defect in the diaphragmatic pericardium, and an intracardiac defect (VSD, tetralogy of Fallot, cor triloculare with single ventricle, or atrial septal defect, often with a left ventricular diverticulum). The omphalocele, sternal cleft and diaphragmatic closure may be handled at the initial stage.

Summary. Deformities of the sternum and chest wall may be categorized into failure of fusion, depression deformities, protrusion deformities and regional deformities of ribs and costal cartilages. The pathogenesis is obscure, but an approach to therapy is well established.

Orthopedic Disorders of the Extremities

ROBERT B. SALTER, M.D., M.S.

In the form and function of the child's musculoskeletal system the borderline between normality and the subtle beginning of an abnormality is not always clearly defined. If, however, the normal variation is *extreme* and is a source of significant concern to the child or his parents, simple therapeutic methods to make the condition closer to the "average," and hence more acceptable, are justifiable provided they are safe and effective. Unnecessary treatment of the child for the sake of "treating the parents" is not justifiable and should be replaced by "treating" the parents through reassurance.

Variations Due to Joint Laxity. Joint laxity, which is extremely common as a normal variation in infancy, is less common in childhood and relatively uncommon in adult life. Thus, the joint laxity tends to improve spontaneously with age as do the two associated common normal variations, flexible flat feet and knock knees.

FLEXIBLE FLAT FEET (HYPERMOBILE PES PLANUS). At the time children begin to stand and walk the majority still have a considerable degree of generalized joint laxity and consequently their feet look "flat," but only on weight bearing. Indeed, if they stood on their hands they would have flat hands.

As the joint laxity improves spontaneously, so also does the appearance of the child's feet. This is why flat feet are so uncommon in adults. The term "flexible feet" avoids the stigma and anxiety associated with the term "congenital flat feet," while expressions such as "weak arches" and "fallen arches" are inaccurate as well as unduly ominous and should be avoided.

The majority of young children with flexible flat feet require no treatment whatsoever. For the more severe degrees of flat feet the aim of treatment is simply to prevent further stretching of the already lax joints pending the spontaneous improvement in the joint laxity.

For *preschool children* this aim is readily accomplished by means of sturdy boots to which have been added a sponge rubber arch support (scaphoid pad) and a ³/₁₆″ inside heel wedge. Even at this stage, however, the child need not be denied the joy of running barefoot, or in "running shoes," at least part of the time.

For *school age children* with persistent flexible feet the same corrections can be added to sturdy low shoes, but excessive corrections in so-called "orthopedic shoes" force the child's heels to the outer side of the shoe, put the shoe out of shape and cause unnecessary discomfort. Since the muscles are not weak, elaborate exercises designed to strengthen them are understandably of no value in the management of flexible flat feet.

Adolescents with persistent flexible flat feet secondary to more severe degrees of generalized joint laxity are generally comfortable in ordinary foot wear and consequently only those with discomfort need have any type of arch support. It is only very rarely in adolescence that shoe corrections fail to relieve discomfort and only under these unusual circumstances is operative treatment in the form of subtalar joint fusion (arthrodesis) indicated.

Flexible flat feet associated with a tight tendo Achillis may be secondary to either mild cerebral palsy or early muscular dystrophy, whereas rigid flat feet, which are a serious abnormality, are usually secondary to congenital tarsal coalition and are discussed in a subsequent section.

KNOCK KNEES (GENU VALGUM). The common type of knock knees in children is secondary to hypermobility of the knee joints, which in turn is simply a manifestation of generalized joint laxity. Thus knock knees, like flexible flat feet with which they are associated, are most noticeable when the child is standing. Furthermore, knock knees are common in young children but become progressively less common with age because of the tendency toward spontaneous improvement.

The majority of young children with knock knees require no treatment. For the more severe degrees of deformity the aim of treatment is to prevent further stretching of the already lax medial ligaments of the knee pending the spontaneous improvement in the joint laxity.

For *preschool children* boots with inside heel and sole wedges are frequently prescribed with the idea of decreasing the strain on the medial ligaments of the knees, but their efficacy is open to question.

In *older children* and *adolescents* with persistent knock knees, secondary bony deformity may become superimposed upon the joint laxity because of unequal epiphyseal plate growth in the region of the knee. Under these circumstances, a specially designed night splint (which holds the extended knees apart and the feet together) may be used to overcome the bony component of the deformity by influencing subsequent growth. Such a splint has proved efficacious even up to and including the prepubertal growth spurt. Long leg day braces are not only unnecessarily cumbersome and restrictive but also ineffectual, and operative treatment is almost never necessary during childhood.

The common so-called "physiological" type of knock knees must be differentiated from the much less common but much more serious "pathological" type of knock knee deformity that is secondary to epiphyseal plate disturbance in congenital abnormalities (such as hypoplasia of the tibia and fibula), metabolic disturbances (such as the various forms of rickets) and damage to the epiphyseal plates in the region of the knee from either infection or injury.

Variations Due to Torsional Deformities. The growing long bones of the fetus, infant and young child respond to repeated twisting or torsional forces through their epiphyseal plates by becoming twisted. Such torsional forces are applied to the lower limbs of the growing fetus in the cramped quarters of the uterus. Such forces are subsequently applied to the lower limbs of infants and young children by certain habitual sleeping and sitting positions. There is a natural tendency for torsional deformities of the long bones to correct spontaneously, but the aforementioned sleeping and sitting positions may either prevent this spontaneous correction or even create new torsional deformities.

The site and nature of torsional deformities is best determined by examining the child lying down (with his hips and knees extended) and assessing the relationship of the foot to the knee for tibial torsion and the knee to the hip for femoral torsion.

TOEING-OUT. The commonest cause of toeing-out in toddlers is *external femoral torsion* which is secondary to the externally rotated position of the hips during intrauterine life. The child stands with both knees and feet turned outward. The prognosis without treatment is excellent and for those few preschool children with persistent external femoral torsion a Denis Browne night splint with the feet turned inward corrects the residual deformity.

TOEING-IN. In *preschool children* the commonest cause of toeing-in is internal tibial torsion, which is evidenced by the observation that when the knees are facing forward the feet are turned inward. This deformity, which is secondary to the cross-legged position in utero, tends to correct spontaneously unless the child habitually sleeps or sits with the knees flexed and the feet turned in. Under these circumstances the internal tibial torsion will not only fail to correct spontaneously but may even become more marked with growth.

The aim of treatment is to prevent the internal torsional forces on the tibia during postnatal life by training the infant or child to avoid harmful positions in sleeping or sitting. In children over the age of 2 or 3 years in whom the internal tibial torsion is sufficiently severe that the child repeatedly trips over his own feet, treatment is justifiable, since it consists of simply holding the feet in the turned out position in a Denis Browne splint at night for a period of approximately 6 months.

Straight last shoes and outflare shoes may mask the deformity but do nothing to correct it, while having the child wear his boots on the opposite feet only results in corrective comments by relatives and friends. Outside wedges in the shoes are of no proven value and cable "twisters" are both cumbersome and restrictive. Rotation osteotomy of the tibia for simple internal tibial torsion in young children is not necessary and could even be considered meddlesome.

Toeing-in may also be due to obvious foot deformities such as metatarsus varus and club feet which are described in a subsequent section.

In *older children* and *adolescents* the commonest cause of toeing-in is internal femoral torsion, which is evidenced by the observation that when the extended lower limbs are rotated inward, the knees turn in about 90 degrees, whereas when they are rotated outward the knees can be brought only slightly beyond the neutral position. The child stands and walks with both the knees and the feet turned inward. Internal femoral torsion is never present at birth but usually develops by the time the child is 5 years of age secondary to the habitual "television position" of sitting on the floor with the femora internally rotated and the feet out to the side.

The aim of treatment is to prevent the internal torsional forces on the femora during childhood by training the child to avoid the "television position" and to replace this with the cross-legged or "tailor" position.

For more severe and persistent torsional deformity in children over the age of 8 years, it may be necessary to use a specially designed night splint in which the knees are flexed and the femora are externally rotated. As with internal tibial torsion, special shoes and outside wedges are of no proven value; cable "twisters" are both cumbersome and restrictive. Rotation osteotomy of the femora for simple internal femoral torsion is seldom justifiable in the growing child.

Toeing-in due to internal rotation contracture of the hip secondary to the muscle imbalance of conditions such as cerebral palsy may mimic internal femoral torsion but is readily differentiated from it.

Bow Legs (Genu Varum). The common type of bow legs in children is not simply the opposite deformity to knock knees but rather is due to a combination of internal tibial torsion and external femoral torsion, a combination that is caused initially by the intrauterine position. There is a natural tendency for both deformities to correct spontaneously but they may be aggravated by habitual positions of sleeping and sitting.

For more severe degrees of persistent bow legs in children over the age of 2 years or 3 years it may be necessary to use a specially designed night splint which holds the extended knees together and the feet apart. Long leg day braces are cumbersome, restrictive and ineffectual; operative treatment for simple bow legs in young children is almost never necessary.

The common, so-called "physiological" type of bow legs must be differentiated from the less common but more serious bow leg deformity associated with the various forms of rickets, tibia vara (Blount's disease) and damage to the epiphyseal plates in the region of the knee from either infection or injury.

CONGENITAL ABNORMALITIES OF THE EXTREMITIES

The responsibility for the early diagnosis of congenital abnormalities is shared by the family physician, obstetrician and pediatrician. Failure to recognize a congenital abnormality at the earliest possible time is an injustice, not only to the unfortunate infant, but also to his devoted parents. Since the localized congenital abnormalities of the extremities are compatible with longevity, their total care demands farsighted planning, skillful orthopedic treatment and prolonged supervision, for the results must last a lifetime.

Metatarsus Varus (Metatarsus Adductus) (Forefoot Adduction). In many infants with metatarsus varus, the adduction deformity of the forefoot is both mild and flexible, in which case the prognosis is good with simple stretching by the parent and avoidance of sleeping face down with the feet curled in.

When the deformity is more marked and relatively rigid, however, orthopedic treatment should be instituted within the first few weeks of life. This involves the careful application of a series of well molded plaster casts which are changed every 2 weeks, the duration of cast treatment varying from 6 to 12 weeks depending on the resistance to correction. A Denis Browne type of boot splint with the feet turned out is then applied nightly to maintain the correction for another few months.

Untreated congenital metatarsus varus in a child over the age of 1 year may require a soft tissue releasing operation and if the child has reached the age of 4 years without correction, it may be necessary to perform an osteotomy at the base of each metatarsal.

Clubfoot (Talipes Equinovarus). The most important congenital abnormality of the foot is clubfoot or talipes equinovarus, a deformity that is easy to diagnose but difficult to correct completely, even in the hands of an experienced orthopedic surgeon. The combined deformities of forefoot adduction, heel varus and ankle equinus vary in severity and are better assessed by the feel of rigidity of the foot rather than its appearance.

The general principles of treatment, which should be applied very early—at least within the first few *days* of life—include gentle passive correction of the combined deformities, maintenance of correction for a very long period and supervision of the child until the end of growth. Even after full correction of a clubfoot, recurrence of the deformities may develop, particularly during periods of rapid skeletal growth.

The following general plan of treatment, which has proven to be very satisfactory, is suggested for the average clubfoot seen within the first month of life:

1. Weekly application of plaster casts (following gentle and progressive correction of the deformities) which requires about 10 weeks.

2. Maintenance of correction by means of a Denis Browne splint which is to be worn day and night (and removed only for bathing) during the ensuing 3 months, after which it is left off for longer and longer periods during the day until the child is walking. The splint should be used at night for another year or longer in order to decrease the chances of recurrence.

3. Straight last or outflare boots for day wear until age 3 years.

Approximately 60 per cent of clubfeet treated early by these nonoperative methods will have responded satisfactorily within the first 3 months of treatment. The remaining 40 per cent, however, are resistant to these methods, in which case it is better judgment to perform a relatively minor soft tissue operation (lengthening of the heel cord and capsulotomy of the posteromedial joints of the foot) at 3 months for *resistance* rather than be forced to perform a major operation at a later date for *recurrence*. Following this type of early surgery, the aforementioned nonoperative plan is resumed to maintain the correction. The relatively recent emphasis on early minor operation for resistant clubfeet at 3 months of age has greatly decreased the number of recurrent clubfeet.

Neglected clubfeet and recurrent clubfeet always require extensive operative treatment, the nature of which depends on the severity of the deformity and the age of the child. In general, soft tissue operations are effective only in the first 5 years of life, after which bony operations usually become necessary.

Talipes Calcaneovalgus. At birth some infants are found to have one or both feet maintained in a position of dorsiflexion and eversion. This mild and transient deformity of an otherwise normal foot is probably the result of intrauterine position and hence is not comparable to a congenital clubfoot. Daily passive stretching of the foot by the mother usually produces excellent and permanent correction of the deformity; indeed many of these deformities improve spontaneously.

Tarsal Coalition (Rigid Valgus Foot) (Peroneal Spastic Flat Foot). Any two of the tarsal bones on the hindfoot may be congenitally joined together by a bridge or bar (coalition) which at birth is still cartilaginous but later becomes ossified. The foot is flat but unlike the flexible flat foot it is rigid. Usually symptomless in the first 10 years of life, the foot subsequently becomes painful and may require operative treatment in the form of triple arthrodesis.

Accessory Tarsal Navicular (Scaphoid). This accessory navicular bone is not rigidly joined to the main part of the tarsal navicular (scaphoid) bone and produces on the medial side of the foot a bony prominence which may become painful and tender in adolescence. If symptoms persist, surgical excision of the accessory bond and part of the underlying navicular bone may be required.

Dislocation and Subluxation of the Hip. The most challenging congenital abnormality of the musculoskeletal system is congenital dislocation of the hip, an abnormality that is almost as common as clubfoot and yet not so obvious at birth. It demands a specific method of examination for its detection in the newborn and regrettably it is still not being recognized sufficiently early in all children. Unless treated early and well, it leads inevitably to painful crippling degenerative arthritis of the hip in adult life. In no other congenital abnormality of the musculoskeletal system is the effort to make an early diagnosis so rewarding, and the failure to make this effort so tragic!

In the early diagnosis of congenital dislocation of the hip, the pediatrician plays the pivotal part. Indeed, the specific examination of the hips—by means of the Barlow test for *dislocability* of the hip and the Ortolani test for *dislocation* of the hip—should be a routine and essential part of the pediatrican's examination of *every* newborn infant. Furthermore, these tests should be repeated on every occasion the pediatrican sees the infant during at least the first 3 months of life. Even the slightest suspicion of abnormality in the hip is an indication for immediate referral of the infant to an orthopedic surgeon.

The general principles of treatment include gentle reduction of the hips followed by maintenance of the reduction with the hip in a stable (but not extreme) position until the various components of the hip have developed well and the hip has become stable even in the position of bearing weight. Treatment is best discussed in relation to the age at the time it is started.

Birth to 3 Months. Treatment during this most favorable period involves gentle reduction of the hip, which is usually not difficult at this stage, followed by the maintenance of the hip in the stable position of flexion and abduction in some type of nonrigid device such as a Frejka pillow splint. Occasionally, even at this early stage, the hip is too unstable to be kept reduced by any type of splint in which case a plaster hip spica is indicated. When treatment is started within the first 3 months of life a period of about 4 months' protection is usually necessary for the capsule to become tighter and for the reduced femoral head to stimulate development of the hip and thereby reverse the secondary changes. The effects of treatment must be assessed both clinically and radiographically.

3 to 18 Months. In this period, contracture and consequent shortening of the muscles around the hip (especially the adductors) have become marked. Hence, treatment involves preliminary lengthening of these muscles by continuous traction for a few weeks followed by a subcutaneous adductor tenotomy and very gentle closed reduction of the hip under anesthesia. The reduction is maintained in the stable position of marked flexion and only moderate abduction (the "human position") in the plaster hip spica cast. The "frog position" of extreme abduction is a causative factor in producing the serious complication of avascular necrosis of the femoral head; consequently the "frog position" should be reserved for frogs only. The hip spica cast is changed every 2 months until radiographs reveal satisfactory development of both the acetabulum and the femoral head. The period of immobilization varies with the age of the child at the time treatment is started, but is usually at least as many months as the number of months the dislocated hip has been untreated.

18 Months to 5 Years. By this time the unfortunate and neglected child is walking and treatment is fraught with difficulties, dangers and disappointments even in the most experienced hands. After several weeks of preliminary traction, open reduction and capsular repair of the dislocated hip is indicated; this operation is combined with innominate (pelvic) osteotomy to redirect the maldirected acetabulum and thereby render the reduced hip stable in the position of bearing weight. For a subluxated hip in this age group only the innominate osteotomy is required.

Over the Age of 5 Years. Fortunately, few children now reach the age of 5 years with previously untreated congenital dislocation of the hip, though the same cannot be said for congenital subluxation. By this time the secondary changes in a complete dislocation are so marked and their reversibility so limited that even extensive operative procedures cannot be expected to meet with success. Indeed, beyond the age of 6 or 7 years it is unwise to even attempt reduction. Residual subluxation, however, can be improved by innominate osteotomy, at least up to the end of the growing period.

For those unfortunate older children with irreducible congenital dislocation of the hip, palliative and salvage types of operative procedures are frequently required in early adult life for the relief of pain.

Hemihypertrophy. In congenital hemihypertrophy with enlargement of a lower limb and an upper limb as well as half the face and trunk on the same side (relative to the opposite side) the structure of each half of the body and their functions are normal but the two halves are asymmetrical. The only clinical problem that may arise is significant longitudinal overgrowth of the lower limb on the larger side. The resultant leg length discrepancy may be dealt with either by surgical epiphyseal arrest at the appropriate age, or by surgical shortening of the femur at the end of growth.

Congenital Amputations. Treatment of children with significant congenital amputations of either the upper or the lower limb involves early fitting with prosthetic limbs of special design even before the child has started to crawl. The fact that frequent changes will be necessary during the child's growing years is no excuse for either delay or makeshift prostheses. In recent years major improvements in prosthetic design and function have been developed as a result of the establishment of juvenile amputee clinics in which orthopedic surgeons, engineers and limb makers (prosthetists) combine their knowledge and skill.

Clubhand (Hypoplasia of the Radius). In this relatively uncommon but serious abnormality manifest by marked radial deviation of the hand, shortening of the forearm and frequently absence of the thumb, the principles of treatment include very early surgical correction of the radial deviation, maintenance of this correction during growth and, finally, improvement of hand function. Permanent correction of the radial deviation may necessitate bony operations. If the condition is bilateral and both thumbs are absent, the index finger of the dominant hand can be surgically repositioned to function as, and resemble, a thumb (pollicization).

LATE MANIFESTATIONS OF CONGENITAL ABNORMALITIES

Adolescent Hallux Valgus (Bunion). A relatively inconspicuous congenital abnormality of the first (prime) metatarsal consisting of varus, or adduction (metatarsus primus varus) is frequently overlooked for several years. During this time, especially in girls, the pressure of shoes gradually pushes the first toe (hallux) laterally, thereby producing the late secondary deformity of adolescent hallux valgus, with an overlying enlarged bursa (bunion). When hallux valgus develops during adolescence it is usually progressive. If repeated examinations reveal progression of the deformity, the prognosis is bad and the deformity should be corrected by a soft tissue operation around the metatarsophalangeal joint combined with a corrective osteotomy at the base of the medially deviated first metatarsal.

Recurrent Dislocation of the Patella. Congenital generalized joint laxity predisposes the affected adolescent to traumatic lateral dislocation of the patella, particularly in girls. Despite reduction of the dislocation and subsequent immobilization of the knee in extension, a troublesome complication is *recurrent* dislocation of the patella. Moreover, with each dislocation, the articular cartilage of the patella is injured and this leads to chondromalacia of the patella which, in turn, leads to degenerative arthritis. Consequently, recurrent dislocation of the patella is an indication for a reconstructive operation which involves release of tight structures on the lateral side of the joint, repair of the fibrous capsule on the medial side and redirection of the line of pull of the patellar tendon by means of a tenodesis.

DISORDERS OF THE EPIPHYSES

During the growing years the epiphyses are relatively resistant to the disorders seen in other parts of the skeleton. Hematogenous osteomyelitis, for example, never begins in an epiphysis and rarely spreads into it through the epiphyseal plate. Furthermore, during childhood nearly all bone neoplasms, both benign and malignant, avoid the epiphysis. By contrast, however, the epiphyses are particularly vulnerable to an idiopathic type of avascular necrosis (osteochondrosis).

Specific Osteochondroses of Epiphyses. For all of the various osteochondroses the aim of treatment is the same—namely, prevention of deformity of the involved epiphysis by keeping abnormal forces from it during its vulnerable phases of revascularization and healing. However, the time-honored practice of prolonged relief of weight bearing over many years, either by means of bed rest or by weight relieving braces, is neither necessary nor desirable.

FEMORAL HEAD (LEGG-CALVÉ-PERTHES SYNDROME) (COXA PLANA). The most important of the osteochondroses is Legg-Calvé-Perthes syndrome, not only because it is more common than the others but also because potential deformity of the femoral head and resultant incongruity is more serious in the hip joint than it would be in other sites. Indeed, severe incongruity leads eventually to degenerative arthritis of the hip in late adult life.

Treatment must be based on a knowledge of the prognosis for a given child. The age of onset is an important factor; in general, the prognosis is good in children whose onset is under the age of 5 years, fair in children with an onset from 5 to 7 years of age and poor in children with an onset over the age of 7 years. The prognosis is definitely worse when the whole head (as opposed to only part of the head) is involved. Furthermore, radiographic evidence of subluxation is a bad prognostic sign since it is associated with abnormal forces, or stress concentrations, that tend to gradually deform the vulnerable femoral head. Likewise, persistent loss of motion in a hip is a bad prognostic sign and for the same reasons.

In recent years, weight relieving methods of treatment (that vary from continuous confinement of the child to bed in an institution for several years, through various types of weight relieving braces to the use of a sling and crutches) have to a large extent been replaced by weight bearing methods of treatment that are designed to allow weight bearing with the femoral head well contained within the acetabulum. The latter methods overcome any tendency toward subluxation and thereby prevent abnormal forces from deforming the femoral head.

Very young children (ages 4 and under) with only partial resorption of the femoral head have an excellent prognosis and hence do not require treatment, provided subluxation of the involved hip does not supervene.

All children who have resorption of the entire head and also those over the age of 4 years who have resorption of only part of the head merit treatment during the active phases of the disease. An effective nonoperative method of treatment for most children is weight bearing in abduction casts or some types of abduction brace (such as the Toronto brace), both of which prevent subluxation and enable the acetabulum to mold the healing head in such a way that it does not become deformed.

For children 7 years of age or older who have a bad prognosis and a prolonged period of healing, but in whom the femoral head is not yet deformed and there is a good range of motion, an alternative method of weight bearing treatment is pelvic (innominate) osteotomy which redirects the acetabulum and thereby provides better containment of the femoral head in the weight bearing position. Six weeks later, by which time the osteotomy has united, the child may be allowed to walk, run and play unhampered by braces or crutches. The indications and contraindications for surgical treatment, however, are strict. Some orthopedic surgeons employ a femoral osteotomy to achieve the same goal.

In the late stages of the disease, if marked deformity of the femoral head has already developed, the salvage operation of partial excision of the head may improve motion.

METATARSAL HEAD (FREIBERG'S DISEASE). Osteochondrosis of either the second or third metatarsal heads usually develops in adolescence and is more common in girls. Nonoperative treatment by means of low heeled shoes and a transverse metatarsal bar across the sole, proximal to the metatarsal heads, may relieve the symptoms. Frequently, however, in later life excision arthroplasty of the metatarsophalangeal joint is necessary for relief of pain from the complication of degenerative arthritis.

VERTEBRAE (SCHEUERMANN'S DISEASE). Osteochondrosis involving the anterior portion of the ring epiphyses of several adjacent vertebral bodies in the thoracic region leads to the gradual development of exaggerated dorsal kyphosis or round back in adolescents. The aim of treatment is the prevention of progressive kyphosis. In milder forms of the condition, spinal extension exercises are beneficial. During the painful stage, a plaster body cast applied with the spine in as straight a position as possible brings relief of the pain and prevents progression of the kyphosis. More effective for the long-term treatment of the more severe forms of the condition, however, is the Milwaukee brace (which is normally used for scoliosis but which can be modified for the treatment of kyphosis).

DISORDERS OF TRACTION APOPHYSES. *Tibial Tubercle (Osgood-Schlatter's Disease).* The aim of treatment in uncomplicated osteochondrosis of the tibial tubercle is prevention of further irritation during the healing phase. This is accomplished by the avoidance of kneeling and jumping; it is not necessary to immobilize the knee nor to restrain the child from running. Residual nonunion of a proximal fragment after the remainder of the tibial tubercle has healed will continue to cause symptoms; under these circumstances, surgical excision of the ununited fragment is indicated.

Calcaneal Apophysis (Sever's Disease). This self-limiting disorder, which is seen most frequently in active young boys, improves spontaneously in about a year. During this time, however, the pain at the site of attachment of the Achilles tendon can be relieved by decreasing the pull on the tendon; this can be accomplished by a 2 cm. raise in the heels of the shoes.

Chondrodystrophies and Achondroplasia. There is no treatment available for these disorders at the present time.

DISORDERS OF EPIPHYSEAL GROWTH

Slipped Upper Femoral Epiphysis (Adolescent Coxa Vara). In this disorder the femoral head, or upper femoral epiphysis, slips (either gradually or suddenly) downward and backward in relation to the femoral neck, the site of the slip being through a weakened epiphyseal plate. The underlying cause of weakness in the epiphyseal plate is usually an endocrine disturbance as evidenced by the very high incidence in the overweight Fröhlich type of adolescent and also in the very tall, thin, rapidly growing adolescent. Although the slip first becomes apparent in one hip, there is approximately a 30 per cent chance of the second hip becoming involved during the remaining years of growth.

The aim of treatment in the early stages of the gradual or chronic type is to prevent further slip through the weakened epiphyseal plate. Since the precarious blood supply to the femoral head has already been threatened by the slip, forceful manipulation should be avoided. For a minimal slip (less than 1 cm. in the lateral radiographic projection) the femoral head should be stabilized to the neck in situ by means of three threaded pins, following which weight bearing may be resumed.

A sudden or acute slip with complete separation of the epiphysis can usually be reduced to a satisfactory position by means of preliminary traction and a gentle manipulation (provided that it had not been slipping gradually prior to the acute slip). The reduced head is then stabilized by threaded pins, but since there has obviously been complete disruption of the epiphyseal plate, weight bearing must be avoided until the epiphysis has healed to the neck, and this may require several months.

Treatment of the gradual or chronic slip that has already progressed beyond 1 cm. in the lateral radiographic projection is more difficult. Under these circumstances, surgical correction of the deformity (and the associated abnormal relationship between the femoral head and the acetabulum) is most safely accomplished by a compensatory subtrochanteric osteotomy of the femur. Although operative correction in the region of the epiphyseal plate, or even in the femoral neck, would seem more logical, the risk of producing the dreaded complication of iatrogenic avascular necrosis is considerable. Indeed, such an operation might be considered a form of "orthopedic roulette" because the surgeon never knows which time the operation is going to kill the femoral head.

A particularly serious but poorly understood complication of slipped upper femoral epiphysis is acute cartilage necrosis (chondrolysis), which is manifest by painful stiffness of the hip and marked diminution of the radiographic cartilage space. Management of this complication involves prolonged traction followed by the use of crutches for many months.

During the remaining period of skeletal growth, frequent follow-up examinations should include assessment of the opposite hip because of the aforementioned 30 per cent chance of the second hip becoming involved.

Tibia Vara (Blount's Disease). A localized form of epiphyseal dysplasia involving the medial portion of the proximal tibial epiphysis, Blount's disease becomes manifest in early childhood by a progressive growth disturbance. The combination of diminished growth in the medial portion of the underlying epiphyseal plate and continued growth in the lateral portion leads to a progressive bow leg or varus deformity at the knee (tibia vara).

Nonoperative treatment with day braces and night splints is ineffectual. Correction of the progressive deformity must be achieved by means of a tibial osteotomy, which may even have to be repeated on one or more occasions during the remaining period of growth.

COMMON ACUTE DISORDERS OF JOINTS

Acute septic arthritis, rheumatic fever and juvenile rheumatoid arthritis are discussed in other sections of this book. Three common but less serious disorders merit discussion in this section.

Transient Synovitis of the Hip (Idiopathic Monarticular Synovitis). A nonbacterial inflammatory disorder of the hip, transient synovitis—also known as "observation hip"—occurs most commonly in young boys. In essence it is a diagnosis that can be made only after exclusion of more serious local disorders of the hip. Aspiration of the joint is of value when the diagnosis is in doubt.

Treatment consists of bed rest with the hip maintained in the most comfortable position of flexion, abduction and external rotation (the position in which the capsule of the hip joint can accommodate the most fluid) until a full range of painless motion of the joint has returned; this usually requires 1 week. Such treatment is definitely more comfortable and more effective than continuous traction in extension. Relief of weight bearing on the involved hip by means of crutches is advisable for an additional few weeks in an attempt to prevent recurrence.

Since approximately 5 per cent of children who have had transient synovitis of the hip develop radiographic evidence of Legg-Perthes' disease at some time between the ensuing 6 and 18 months, all children with transient synovitis should be examined and their hips radiographed at 6-month intervals for at least 18 months in order to detect the earliest evidence of this complication.

"Sprains" of Joints in Children. Since the major ligaments around joints in children are stronger than the epiphyseal plates in the region of that joint, it is understandable that major tears of ligaments are unusual. The type of joint injury that would cause either a "sprained" or a completely torn ligament in an adult is more likely to cause a separation of the epiphysis through the epiphyseal plate in a child. Indeed, many so-called "sprains" of the ankle and knee in children represent epiphyseal separations with immediately spontaneous reduction. The radiographic examination is therefore normal, but "stress films" of the joint reveal the true nature of the injury. Furthermore, radiographic examination 2 to 3 weeks after the injury reveals evidence of periosteal new bone formation in the region of the epiphyseal plate and metaphysis.

When epiphyseal separation can be recognized as the significant component of an apparent "sprain" of the ligaments around a joint, it is better treated by means of a plaster cast for 3 weeks than by simple strapping.

"Pulled Elbow" ("Nursemaid's Elbow"). Children of preschool age are particularly vulnerable to a sudden pull or jerk on their arms and frequently sustain the very common minor injury known simply as "pulled elbow." A parent, nursemaid or older sibling, while lifting the small child up a step or curb by the hand or pulling him away from potential danger, exerts a sudden strong pull on the extended elbow and thereby produces the injury.

A detachment of a portion of the annular ligament at the moment of the sudden pull allows the radial head to move distally momentarily. The proximal part of the annular ligament and synovial membrane become entrapped between the radial head and the capitellum as the radial head immediately moves upward again. The crying or fretting child holds his injured arm protectively with the elbow flexed and the forearm pronated. Radiographic examination is consistently negative.

Treatment consists simply of encouraging the child to relax and then deftly and quickly supinating the forearm. A slight "click" can usually be felt over the lateral aspect of the elbow as the entrapped portion of the annular ligament is freed from the joint. If the child has been sent to the radiology department prior to treatment, the radiographic technician frequently and unwittingly "treats" the pulled elbow as she supinates the forearm to obtain the anteroposterior projection.

After-treatment consists of a sling for 2 weeks to allow the minor tear in the attachment of the annular ligament to heal. In addition, the parents are advised about the harmful effects of pulling or lifting their small child by the hand.

Infantile Cortical Hyperostosis
(Caffey's Disease)
RICHARD B. GOLDBLOOM, F.R.C.P.(C)

Since the cause of infantile cortical hyperostosis is unknown, no specific treatment is available. Curiously, many pediatricians and pediatric radiologists have noted a striking decline in the prevalence of this condition in recent years.

In most patients, symptoms appear before the age of 6 months. Occasionally prenatal diagnosis by x-ray examination has been reported. In the initial acute phase of the illness, problems requiring management may include fever, irritability, soft tissue swelling and tenderness over affected bones, salivation and refusal of food. Less common complications are proptosis and pleural effusion. Because progressive spontaneous recovery occurs in most patients, a conservative initial approach to treatment is usually advisable. Often within the first week or so of observation, gradual diminution of local and systemic signs and symptoms is evident. If fever is a problem, acetaminophen, 60 mg. every 4 to 6 hours by mouth, may be given for a few days at most. Acetylsalicylic acid should be used with great caution in young infants. If necessary it can be given for a day or two, 30 to 60 mg./kg./day orally in divided doses, but preferably not to infants under 6 months of age.

Although steroids have been observed to relieve the systemic manifestations of the disease, they do not seem to alter the evolution of the subperiosteal hyperostosis. Thus their use should probably be restricted to those rare infants whose disease is unusually severe, and in whom a reasonable period of observation and antipyretic-analgesic therapy has failed to yield signs of spontaneous improvement.

Cortisone can be given in a dose of 5 to 10 mg./kg./day in divided doses, or prednisone in a dose of 1 to 2 mg./kg./day. If steroid therapy is used, it should be continued only until the child has been afebrile for a few days (usually not more than a week or 10 days), and then gradually discontinued.

The child should be handled gently while affected bones and overlying soft tissues are tender. The use of a cross-cut nipple may facilitate feeding since the mandible is regularly involved. Parents should be advised that different bones may be involved at various stages in the evolution of the disease. Late exacerbations, though uncommon, may occur—sometimes several years after the infantile episode has subsided. Several instances of familial occurrence in siblings, cousins and/or successive generations have been reported. Whether this represents genetic disease or "pseudo-heredity" (i.e., susceptibility or exposure to a common environmental agent) is unknown. From a practical viewpoint, familial occurrence and late exacerbation are sufficiently uncommon that parents should not be caused undue anxiety over either possibility. Similarly, although sequelae such as cortical thickening, bowing and dilation of the medullary cavity have been reported, these changes are usually more apparent radiographically than clinically. Thus parents should be advised that clinical recovery is likely to be complete, even though the period required for recovery is variable—weeks or months.

Septic Arthritis and Osteomyelitis

THOMAS R. TETZLAFF, M.D., and
JOHN D. NELSON, M.D.

Acute osteomyelitis and septic arthritis of childhood usually result from the hematogenous seeding of bacteria into the bone or joint space. Less commonly, infection can spread from a contiguously infected area or result from a penetrating wound.

Initial signs and symptoms are those of an acute inflammatory process, with localized tenderness, swelling, and fever being most prominent. In some patients, especially newborn infants, nonspecific constitutional signs are most prominent. In osteomyelitis the metaphyses of the long bones such as the femur, tibia, and humerus are most commonly involved. Septic arthritis usually affects the large joints such as the hip, knee, shoulder, and ankle. In one-third of patients a history of recent infection or trauma can be elicited.

When septic arthritis or osteomyelitis is suspected, every effort should be made to identify the etiologic agent because the choice of antimicrobial agent, the duration and mode of treatment, and the prognosis depend to a large extent on the infecting microorganism and the joint or bone involved.

MANAGEMENT OF SEPTIC ARTHRITIS

Whenever the diagnosis of septic arthritis is entertained on the basis of clinical or radiographic signs or gallium-67 citrate scanning, synovial fluid aspiration with a large bore (18 to 20 gauge) needle should be performed. An orthopedic surgical consultant usually performs this procedure, but it can be done by any physician. A heparinized syringe is used for aspiration to prevent clotting of the specimen. The fluid should be diluted in normal saline for white blood cell count rather than the white cell diluting fluid.

Gram and methylene blue stains of the exudate may give useful hints as to the infecting bacteria, but definitive identification depends upon bacteriological cultures or other techniques such as immunofluorescence or counterimmunoelectrophoresis (CIE). To ensure maximal bacteriological yield, the purulent material should be inoculated into a blood culture bottle which contains antiphagocytic and anticomplementary substances as well as onto routine culture media. Aliquots of joint fluid are also sent for total white blood count with differential morphology, total protein, and glucose content.

Blood cultures provide a bacteriological diagnosis in approximately 20 per cent of cases of septic arthritis when no bacteria are isolated from the joint fluid. Antimicrobial susceptibilities of organisms isolated from blood or from synovial aspirate are usually determined; however, in the case of group A beta-hemolytic streptococci, pneumococci or meningococci, which are uniformly susceptible to penicillin, this is usually not done.

Antimicrobial Therapy. Treatment consists of a combination of medical and orthopedic procedures. Presumptive identification of the etiologic bacteria can often be made from the Gram or methylene blue stains or CIE determination, and appropriate antibiotic therapy instituted. The age group of the patient is also important in selecting initial therapy.

Septic arthritis is rare during the neonatal period. When it occurs it is usually due to group B streptococci, gonococci, coliforms or *Staphylococcus aureus.* If gram-positive cocci are seen in the stained specimen, therapy with a penicillinase-resistant penicillin such as methicillin is started. For gram-negative bacilli an aminoglycoside antibiotic such as kanamycin or gentamicin can be used. (For convenience, methicillin will be used as a generic term to represent the penicillinase-resistant penicillins. Nafcillin or oxacillin would be equally suitable.) Penicillin is given when gram-negative intracellular diplococci are present.

From 1 to 24 months of age *Hemophilus influenzae* and *Streptococcus pneumoniae* are the most common etiologic agents, but *Staphylococcus aureus* is occasionally encountered. If no bacteria are identified in the Gram-stained specimen of synovial fluid, chloramphenicol and methicillin can be used until the etiologic agent is identified and antibiotic sensitivity testing is completed.

Beyond two years of age septic arthritis is most often due to staphylococci or other gram-positive organisms. Thus unless gram-negative rods are seen in the joint fluid stains, treatment can be started with methicillin.

Infection with *Pseudomonas aeruginosa* or anaerobic organisms is rare, but should be suspected in arthritis secondary to penetrating wounds.

In all cases, once bacteriological test results are available, treatment should be changed to the safest effective drug based on susceptibility testing. See Table 1 for preferred antibiotics and recommended dosages for specific etiologic agents.

Adequate synovial fluid antibiotic concentrations are achieved using the intravenous or intramuscular route for antibiotic administration. There is no indication for intra-articular instillation of antibiotics. In special circumstances orally administered antibiotics may be employed, but in this event monitoring the blood and synovial fluid antibiotic concentrations and the bacteriostatic and bactericidal titers of the joint fluid against the infecting bacteria is mandatory. A bactericidal titer of at least 1:8 should be achieved in the serum.

A difficult therapeutic problem is encountered when no microorganisms are seen on Gram-stained specimens, and cultures of syno-

TABLE 1.   Recommended Antibiotics and Dosages for Treatment of Arthritis and Osteomyelitis

BACTERIA	PREFERRED	ALTERNATIVE
Hemophilus influenzae, ampicillin-susceptible	Ampicillin, 150 mg./kg./day in four doses IV or IM	Chloramphenicol sodium succinate, 50 to 70 mg./kg./day in four doses IV or orally
Hemophilus influenzae, ampicillin-resistant	Chloramphenicol sodium succinate (as above)	—
Staphylococcus aureus, penicillin-susceptible	Penicillin G, 100,000 units/ kg./day in six doses IV	—
Staphylococcus aureus, penicillin-resistant	Methicillin* or oxacillin, 200 mg./kg./day, or nafcillin, 150 mg./kg./day in four doses, IV or IM	Cefazolin, 60 mg./kg./ day in three doses IV or IM *or* Lincomycin, 20 mg./kg./ day in three doses IV or IM
Enterococcus	Ampicillin (as above)	Penicillin or ampicillin (as above) *plus* Kanamycin, 15 to 20 mg./kg./day in three doses IM
Neisseria meningitidis, Streptococcus pneumoniae, or other streptococci	Penicillin (as above)	—
Neisseria gonorrheae, penicillin-susceptible	Penicillin G, 100,000 units/ kg./day in six doses IV	Tetracycline, 50 mg./ kg./day in four doses orally†
Neisseria gonorrheae, penicillin-resistant	? A cephalosporin (inadequate clinical efficacy data)	? Erythromycin
Pseudomonas aeruginosa	Carbenicillin, 400 to 600 mg./kg./day in four to six doses IV (max. daily dosage 30 to 40 gm.)	Carbenicillin *plus* gentamicin, 6 to 7.5 mg./kg./day in three doses IM
Coliform bacilli	Gentamicin (as above)	Kanamycin (as above)
Salmonella sp.	Ampicillin (as above)	Chloramphenicol sodium succinate (as above)

Reduce dosage of penicillins and cephalosporins for neonatal infants.

*This dosage of methicillin is higher than that recommended by the manufacturer but has been found safe and effective. The manufacturer gives no specific recommendation for intravenous use of methicillin in infants and children.

†Manufacturer's note: Use of tetracycline during tooth development years may cause permanent discoloration of the teeth.

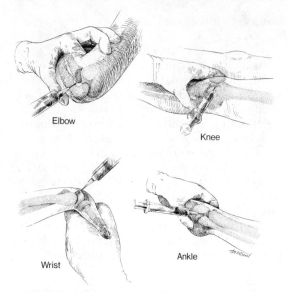

Technique for aspiration of joint fluid. Note particularly the positions of the extremities and of the restraining hands. Sedation may be required. The area is prepared with povidone-iodine or a similar antiseptic. A No. 20 needle is suitable for any age patient and for any joint. (A needle with a stylet is preferred but not essential.) The syringe contains a small amount of heparin to prevent clotting of the specimen.

vial fluid aspirate and blood are sterile. On the basis of the most common etiologic agent involved according to the child's age and the current antibiotic susceptibility of these bacteria, an educated guess should be made and treatment initiated. Other causes of synovitis should be investigated in such children. It should be remembered that leukocyte counts in synovial fluid as high as 100,000/cu. mm. may occur in collagen diseases. In traumatic synovitis the synovial fluid usually has fewer than 2000 cells/cu. mm., but we have seen counts as high as 50,000/cu. mm. develop with continued weight-bearing and repeated trauma to the joint. Granulomatous disease is usually characterized by a predominance of mononuclear cells and low cell counts.

The optimal duration of treatment has never been precisely determined by controlled studies. Based upon general clinical experience the following periods are recommended. For septic arthritis caused by *Staphylococcus aureus* or coliform bacteria, three weeks is considered a minimum period. When disease is due to *H. influenzae,* streptococci or *N. meningitidis,* 10 to 14 days usually suffices. Three days' therapy has been shown to be adequate for gonococcal arthritis in adults and presumably would be in children also. The adequacy of the initial choice of antibiotics and length of therapy will be dictated by the child's clinical response in

each case. When there is persistent fever, localized signs and symptoms, positive joint culture or elevation of the erythrocyte sedimentation rate, one of the following possibilities would merit investigation: there may be an associated area of purulent material (an osteomyelitis or deep tissue abscess); the needle aspiration is inadequately draining the joint; the etiologic agent is resistant to the administered antibiotic; or the antibiotic is being administered in an inadequate dose.

Surgical Management.   The orthopedic management is determined largely by the joint involved. Because the synovial membranes of the hip and shoulder joints extend over the proximal portions of the femoral and humeral bones, pus within the joint space is likely to cause damage to the bones either directly or by compression of their vascular supplies. Surgical incision and drainage are recommended immediately after the diagnosis is made. In septic arthritis of joints other than the hip or shoulder, one or two percutaneous synovial aspirations performed on the days following initiation of therapy will usually suffice to evacuate the purulent material. If, after several days of daily percutaneous aspirations, the amount of synovial fluid does not decrease, open surgical incision and drainage is done. Open drainage is also indicated in arthritis secondary to penetrating wound or foreign body. During open surgical incision and drainage the joint space is copiously irrigated with saline solution.

In the acute inflammatory period, if joints are held in a flexion-contraction position, mild Buck's traction or a splint is indicated. Immobilization is required to maintain functional position of the joint until pain has subsided and passive and active range of motion exercises are instituted.

FOLLOW-UP.   The need for long-term follow-up of infants and children with septic arthritis cannot be overemphasized. Major sequelae occur in up to 30 per cent of episodes and many of these may not be suspected at the time of hospital discharge. This is particularly true of arthritis in infancy when functional disability may not become apparent until many months later when the child begins walking. If shortening of an extremity, impaired joint mobility, flexion-contracture or other deformities are noted, further physical therapy or corrective surgical procedures may be needed.

MANAGEMENT OF OSTEOMYELITIS

When acute osteomyelitis is suspected from the presence of fever and localized erythema, induration, and tenderness, the diagnosis can be confirmed in several ways. The roentgenogram is frequently helpful, showing deep soft tissue swelling, but generally requires 7 to 14 days before the classical changes of periosteal elevation, cortical mottling, and new bone formation appear. Radionucleotide scanning using ^{99m}Tc-phosphate compounds is more helpful and may be positive as early as 24 hours after the onset of symptoms. The most important procedure for establishing the diagnosis of osteomyelitis, however, is needle aspiration of the involved area at the point of maximum tenderness. If pus is not obtained in the subperiosteal space, the needle is forced through the cortex to aspirate metaphyseal material. Any specimen obtained with this method (even those that look like blood rather than pus) should be appropriately stained and cultured for microorganisms.

Blood cultures are positive in approximately 50 per cent of cases of acute hematogenous osteomyelitis. If the joint adjacent to the area involved contains purulent material, this should also be aspirated and the joint infection managed as outlined above.

Antimicrobial Therapy. At any age *Staphylococcus aureus* is the most common agent, so initial treatment consists of a penicillinase-resistant penicillin such as methicillin unless Gram stains of pus suggest another etiology. A cephalosporin or lincomycin may be substituted for methicillin for patients allergic to penicillin.

Antibiotic treatment is later changed to the most appropriate drug based on susceptibility testing of organisms isolated from blood or pus. If the staphylococcus is penicillin-susceptible, penicillin G given intravenously is the drug of choice. In general a drug with a bactericidal mode of action is preferred over one that is bacteriostatic.

Osteomyelitis due to gram-negative enteric organisms occurs occasionally. For these patients gentamicin (7.5 mg./kg./day intramuscularly in three divided doses for infants or 6 mg./kg./day for older children) or another aminoglycosidic antibiotic is used. Infection due to group B streptococci is best treated with intravenous penicillin G.

Anaerobic bacteria rarely cause acute osteomyelitis but may complicate chronic, draining bone infection. Most anaerobes are penicillin-responsive, but *Bacteroides fragilis* requires treatment with chloramphenicol or clindamycin. Carbenicillin or trimethoprim-sulfamethoxazole is also effective.

Osteomyelitis of the maxillary sinus in infancy is characterized by periorbital edema and swelling of the face and nose. *Staphylococcus aureus* has been the etiologic agent in the majority of cases described, so treatment with methicillin should be instituted.

Osteomyelitis of the tarsal bones following a penetrating injury is commonly due to *Pseudomonas aeruginosa*. For these cases carbenicillin is the treatment of choice.

Patients with sickle cell anemia have a proclivity to infection with coliform bacteria or pneumococci. The possibility of *Salmonella* osteomyelitis should always be considered. Ampicillin or trimethoprim-sulfamethoxazole is the treatment of choice in these patients. Chloramphenicol should be avoided in the sicklemic patient because it may cause a precipitous fall in hemoglobin by suppression of reticulocytosis.

Parenteral treatment with antibiotics should be continued for a minimum of three weeks. Four to six weeks is preferable for patients with advanced disease or for any patient who has not had infected bones surgically drained. If treatment is changed to the oral route of administration, the same precautions and controls should be employed as mentioned above for treatment of suppurative arthritis.

A good index of response of the acute inflammatory process is a return to normal of an initially elevated erythrocyte sedimentation rate (ESR). If there is persistent elevation of the ESR after 3 weeks of treatment, treatment is best continued for a longer period of time. The patient should be evaluated for the possibility of infected sequestrum.

Surgical Treatment. If pus is obtained by diagnostic needle aspiration of the affected bone, it is recommended that the patient be taken to surgery and an oval bone window created for drainage. If only a small amount of bloody fluid is obtained but bacteria are seen on the Gram stain of the specimen, antibiotic treatment is started and the patient is reevaluated after 24 to 48 hours. If there has been no improvement, needle aspiration is repeated and, if pus is then obtained, surgical drainage is carried out.

Supportive Therapy. Medication for fever and pain and intravenous fluid and electrolyte therapy are used as indicated by the clinical status of the child. The affected extremity is placed in an appropriately functional and comfortable position with sandbags or splints. After surgery the extremity is often placed in a plaster cast. Previously it was thought that prolonged immobilization was necessary. It is now believed that early moderate exercise and even weight-bearing once the local pain has disappeared may be beneficial in diminishing the sequelae of prolonged immobilization and in hastening recovery.

Management of Relapse or Chronic Osteomyelitis. With adequate surgery and antimicrobial therapy it is now possible to cure subacute and chronic osteomyelitis. Children with these forms of disease require adequate surgical drainage and/or removal of sequestrum and several months, or in many cases, up to a year of oral antimicrobial therapy. This necessitates complete parental compliance and frequent clinic visits. The antibiotic dosage is regulated to attain a bactericidal titer against the offending pathogen of at least 1:8 by the twofold inhibition test with serum taken one hour after a dose.

In spite of prolonged antibiotic therapy and surgical treatment, chronic osteomyelitis may still recur, sometimes after asymptomatic intervals of months or years.

Malignant Bone Tumors

PHILIP R. EXELBY, M.D., *and*
GERALD ROSEN, M.D.

The proper treatment of bone tumors in children begins with an adequate biopsy and accurate diagnosis by the surgeon, radiologist and pathologist. The biopsy should be generous and include a sample of any soft tissue extension of the tumor.

If the tumor is benign the most conservative surgical resection is carried out. This includes excision of exostoses, if symptomatic, and curettage and packing with bone chips for cystic lesions. Hemorrhagic lesions, such as aneurysmal bone cysts, or tumors with a high recurrence rate, such as giant cell tumors, may require cryosurgery in addition to curettage.

If the tumor is malignant the child will require complex multidisciplinary treatment which is most effectively carried out in a center specializing in these diseases. Effective chemotherapy is now available for malignant bone tumors but the treatment is potentially hazardous and requires intensive supportive treatment. Specific treatment varies with the histological type of tumor and will be described for the three commonest malignant bone tumors: osteogenic sarcoma, non-Hodgkin's lymphoma and Ewing's sarcoma.

OSTEOGENIC SARCOMA

This is the most common tumor in the group of malignant spindle cell sarcomas of the bone. Pure chondrosarcoma and fibrosarcoma are rare in children and are usually seen as components of the osteoid-producing osteogenic sarcoma. These tumors in children are all managed as osteogenic sarcoma.

Management of the Primary Tumor. Surgical ablation of the entire involved bone with surrounding soft tissue is the established treatment of osteogenic sarcoma. This means amputation at a level above the involved bone. For distal femur lesions hip disarticulation is recommended, for proximal tibia mid-thigh amputation, and for proximal humerus forequarter amputation. Surgeons at major treatment centers are currently investigating a variety of limb-saving procedures. Total femur resection with prosthetic replacement, bloc excisions with total knee replacemnt, and the Tickhoff-Linberg procedure are examples of such operations. Evaluation of limb function and therapeutic efficacy of these procedures appear promising but must await longer follow-up.

Adjuvant Chemotherapy. Following surgery of the primary tumor all patients should be placed on adjuvant chemotherapy. The most effective regimen used at present is high dose methotrexate with citrovorum factor rescue. Methotrexate, 8 gm./m^2, is given intravenously with citrovorum factor, 10 to 20 mg. orally or intramuscularly, given two hours following methotrexate infusion, and then every six hours for a total of 72 hours. Other agents, such as Adriamycin and cyclophosphamide, have also proved to be of value in treatment of osteogenic sarcoma. Adriamycin is given as a course of 90 mg./m^2/ over two or three days. Cyclophosphamide is given in single pulse doses up to 1200 mg./m^2 intravenously with adequate hydration to prevent hemorrhagic cystitis. Chemotherapeutic agents are given at intervals of two weeks to allow bone marrow recovery. Adjuvant therapy is continued for approximately 12 months. The total cumulative dose of Adriamycin should not exceed 500 mg./m^2 because of the danger of cardiomyopathy. Chest x-rays once a month and bone scans every three months are carried out for the year of adjuvant therapy and for an additional two years after treatment is stopped. Following this regimen approximately 60 per cent of patients with osteogenic sarcoma can be expected to be alive and free of disease two years following definitive surgery for their primary tumor.

Treatment of Pulmonary Metastases in Osteogenic Sarcoma. If pulmonary metastases occur during adjuvant treatment, the patient may still be salvaged by thoracotomy and wedge excisions of the tumor nodules followed by continued chemotherapy. This treatment is most successful where the nodules are solitary or few in number, peripherally located and can be totally excised. Where a few peripheral pulmonary metastases are present at initial presentation, thoracotomy resection of these nodules may be carried out after resection of the primary tumor prior to commencing chemotherapy. Chemotherapy should be delayed for two weeks after surgery to allow adequate wound healing, and skin sutures are left in place for three to four weeks. Patients presenting with diffuse pulmonary metastases present a more difficult management problem since it is doubtful that initial thoracotomy would be able to clear the patient's lungs of all disease. Such patients can be managed with initial aggressive chemotherapy. If the primary tumor is still present, hopefully it will also be controlled by the chemotherapy until definitive surgery can be planned. If the pulmonary metastases and/or the primary tumor do not appear to grow over a period of three to four months while on chemotherapy, and if previously elevated serum alkaline phosphatase levels return to normal, this may indicate that temporary control has been achieved. Such patients can then undergo surgical removal of their primary tumor and then thoracotomies to remove residual disease that may be present in the chest.

It has been our experience that chemotherapy can sometimes control multiple pulmonary metastases; however, they may recur if not surgically removed. Frequently pulmonary metastases that do not change in size after a period of chemotherapy may have no active tumor cells but only tumor osteoid when resected. Again, however, permanent control requires surgical excision. Following the apparent surgical excision of all pulmonary metastases the patient should continue on adjuvant chemotherapy for a period of one year. Utilizing this approach even the patient with pulmonary metastases can be offered a chance for prolonged disease free survival. In our hands, 75 per cent of patients presenting with operable pulmonary metastases and 30 per cent of patients presenting with diffuse pulmonary metastases are alive, well, and free of disease two to three years following the commencement of treatment.

Patients presenting with inoperable primary tumor or bone metastases have a very poor prognosis. The addition of radiation therapy to aggressive chemotherapy may be of some value in controlling disease. Although malignant spindle cell sarcomas are classically resistant to radiation therapy, high dose irradiation has been shown to be synergistic with agents such as high dose methotrexate, and

this approach may provide prolonged control of disease and palliation in this situation. Chemotherapy remains the most effective treatment and radiation must not be allowed to depress bone marrow to an extent that will compromise the patient's ability to tolerate high doses of drugs. At this time the role of immunotherapy in the treatment of osteogenic sarcoma is being evaluated. Although at present the results seem disappointing, trials of immunotherapy in combination with chemotherapy may offer advances in the future treatment of osteogenic sarcoma.

EWING'S SARCOMA

Management of the Primary Tumor. James Ewing described a small round cell sarcoma of bone in 1921 and noted that the tumor was radiosensitive. Historically the treatment of Ewing's sarcoma with high doses of megavoltage radiation (5000 to 7000 rads) to the entire involved bone provided local control of primary tumor in the majority of patients. However approximately 90 per cent of these patients died of metastatic disease within one to two years following diagnosis. The early use of adjuvant chemotherapy begun immediately with high dose irradiation for the primary tumor has improved the survival rate to a reported 50 to 75 per cent at some centers. This improved prolonged survival of patients with Ewing's sarcoma observed after the use of systemic adjuvant chemotherapy has made it evident that local recurrence of the primary tumor occurs in 20 to 30 per cent of patients following irradiation therapy. It is also now understood that patients surviving to adulthood may have limited function of a previously heavily radiated limb, particularly the weight bearing lower extremities.

The suggested therapy for Ewing's sarcoma at this time is high dose radiation therapy (5000 to 6000 rads delivered in 5 to 6 weeks) to the entire bone in upper extremity lesions. For lesions of the weight bearing lower extremities in patients who have attained or nearly attained their adult height, radiation therapy alone may be utilized for treating the primary tumor. However, in young patients in whom radiation therapy to the growing ends of bone would cause excessive leg length discrepancy, surgery should be considered as the primary treatment. This would obviate the problem of local recurrence of primary tumor and the patient would eventually have a better function with a prosthesis than with a very short irradiated limb. The argument that amputation could be carried out after failure of radiation therapy is not entirely tenable because once local recurrence is evident the disease usually becomes widely disseminated with little hope for ultimate cure. Also in proximal femur and humerus lesions amputation may be technically unfeasible because of radiation changes in the skin and soft tissues. Patients who have primary tumors of surgically expendable bones, such as the fibula, scapula, ribs and the bones of the foot, should be treated by surgical excision of the tumorous bone followed by moderate dose radiation therapy. Combinations of moderate doses of irradiation to shrink soft tissue masses followed by en bloc excision of the tumor bearing bone may also be successful in selected cases.

Adjuvant Chemotherapy in Ewing's Sarcoma. Concomitant with the start of management of the primary tumor, the child should be placed on aggressive adjuvant chemotherapy. This treatment utilizes multiple agents that are effectie in the management of Ewing's sarcoma, such as dactinomycin given in dosages of 450 μg./m^2/day intravenously for five days; Adriamycin, 20 mg./m^2/day intravenously for three days; and cyclophosphamide, 1200 mg./m^2 as a single intravenous infusion. Drug treatment should be separated by approximately two weeks to allow time for hematological recovery from the previous drug. Vincristine, 1.5 mg./m^2 intravenously, has also been shown to be of value in the treatment of Ewing's sarcoma. Chemotherapy should be continued for approximately two years, limiting the total dose of Adriamycin to under 500 mg./m^2 to avoid the occurrence of cardiomyopathy.

Throughout the course of treatment and for two years following the cessation of chemotherapy, chest x-rays are taken at monthly intervals and bone scans (technetium diphosphonate or fluorine 18) at three month intervals. Early detection of local recurrence is better appreciated on the bone scan since heavily irradiated primary tumor may not show healing on x-ray. Bone scan will usually detect metastatic bone disease three to four months before it becomes evident on x-ray. Prophylactic pulmonary irradiation in Ewing's sarcoma is of doubtful value since this disease metastasizes to other bones almost as frequently as it does to the lungs. Once pulmonary metastases become evident, however, the use of bilateral pulmonary irradiation may be of value in controlling metastatic disease. Radiation therapy, particularly in combination with chemotherapy, can cause lethal pulmonary fibrosis, and irradiation to the lungs should be limited to 1400 rads delivered in 100 rad fractions. Patients presenting with metastatic Ewing's sarcoma are at a particularly high risk. Some of these children may be salvaged by an aggressive approach to the primary tumor, chemotherapy and in addition local radiation therapy to the various metastatic sites. Again, however, irradiation of large volumes of bone marrow should be avoided because this may compromise the use of systemic chemotherapy.

NON-HODGKIN'S LYMPHOMA OF BONE (RETICULUM CELL SARCOMA)

Non-Hodgkins's lymphoma of bone in children presents the same therapeutic problems as non-Hodgkin's lymphoma of lymph nodes or other organs in children. Although local control can be achieved by radiation or surgery, this disease almost universally recurs, usually presenting a picture of leukemic infiltration of the bone marrow and late central nervous system disease similar to that seen in acute lymphoblastic leukemia. This disease therefore is best managed by achievement of local control of disease followed by the use of adjuvant chemotherapy similar to that used in the treatment of acute lymphoblastic leukemia. Local control can be achieved by surgery or radiation therapy or combinations of the two.

Usually radiation therapy delivered to the primary tumor-bearing bone at the dose of 4000 rads achieves good local control. This tumor is very sensitive to alkylating agents and in our experience a large pulse of cyclophosphamide, 1200 mg./m^2 intravenously, can greatly reduce the size of the primary tumor. It is used therefore as an adjuvant to radiation therapy in the treatment of primary disease. Because in children this disease metastasizes rapidly to the bone marrow and other node-bearing areas, systemic chemotherapy should be started as soon as possible. In addition to a large dose of an alkylating agent such as cyclophosphamide, systemic chemotherapy similar to that used for acute lymphoblastic leukemia is given. This includes central nervous system prophylactic treatment, usually intrathecal methotrexate, which may be combined with cranial radiation. Patients presenting with primary tumor should have adjuvant chemotherapy continued for two years, and where bone marrow involvement is present at diagnosis, chemotherapy is continued for three years. Previously, therapy directed at the primary bone tumor alone resulted in the majority of children relapsing with a "leukemic" bone marrow or meningeal disease. The addition of systemic antileukemic chemotherapy has resulted in prolonged disease free survival in the majority of children with non-Hodgkin's lymphoma at all sites including bone.

REHABILITATION OF CHILDREN WITH MALIGNANT BONE TUMORS

Physical and emotional rehabilitation is part of the initial treatment. The seriousness of the disease must be explained to the patient and family at the outset so that they fully understand the need for aggressive chemotherapy and are prepared for the severe side effects of treatment. Physical rehabilitation is directed toward early ambulation, crutch walking and the early use of prosthesis so as to minimize disability. The child is encouraged to lead as near normal a life as possible by continuing to attend school and by participating in peer group activities. The adolescent is given as much responsibility as possible in managing his own treatment and is encouraged to discuss his problems freely with the physicians. Rehabilitation requires a large effort from the patient, family and staff. The aims are to have the child survive the disease and to have a quality of physical and emotional life as near normal as possible.

Fractures of the Extremities

HENRY H. BANKS, M.D.

In many respects fractures in children differ from those in adults. At the end of each long bone there is a growth plate which if injured may result in shortening of the extremity or distortion of growth. The periosteum is thicker over the shaft of the long bone of a child and allows for more rapid healing and dramatic remodeling than in the adult. A fracture through the shaft of the long bone even with perfect contact and alignment may stimulate longitudinal growth. The patient may then end up with a longer limb on the fractured side. Some patients, especially if young, with fragments overriding 1 to 2 cm. may end up with extremities of equal length.

More severe trauma is necessary to produce a complete fracture in a child than in an adult. The child's skeleton can tolerate a greater degree of deformation than that of an adult. Compression failure of the bone produces a buckle fracture or a ripple in the cortex of a bone. This is far more common in the child and is unusual in the adult. In a child, when a bone is angulated beyond its limit of bending, a green stick fracture results. Nonunion of fractures is unusual in children.

Those caring for children must be aware that whether the child has an injury of the upper or lower extremity, there is usually pain, swelling, and deformity with a fracture. Even

without deformity, the fracture may be so uncomfortable that the child may prefer not to move. It will appear as if the child has a "paralysis," so-called "pseudoparalysis." Careful examination will show that there is no neurologic deficit. The child who has a buckle fracture in the vicinity of the wrist will prefer not to use the hand on this side but will seem normal otherwise. Careful examination and palpation may establish the diagnosis before an x-ray is obtained. In the lower extremity it is not unusual for the child to have an undisplaced crack of the tibia and either walk with a limp protecting the tibia or prefer not to walk at all.

When one first sees a child with what appears to be a fracture of a long bone, splinting until an x-ray has been obtained is essential. If there is mobility at the fracture site, then general alignment should be restored with traction prior immobilization. The neurovascular status of the extremity must be assessed beforehand. If there is an apparent injury of the spinal column, then the child must be carefully moved "as if a log" onto a stretcher until a more definitive diagnosis can be made by examination and x-rays. The child may lose a significant amount of blood into the soft tissues from a fracture of the femur of the pelvis as the adult does. Hence, immobilization and rapid transfer to a hospital are in order, to begin intravenous fluids, monitor blood loss and ensure replacement.

If one sees a child with a clinical fracture of the upper extremity, the simplest type of immobilization until an accurate diagnosis can be made is a sling. Additional immobilization, particularly of the forearm, with a commercial splint, cardboard or a newspaper with an ace bandage will be helpful. In the lower extremity if no traction device or pillow splint is available, simple immobilization to the neighboring extremity may provide comfort. Furthermore, it will prevent further destruction of soft tissues. In the lower extremity a long bone fracture with overriding may be maintained with manual traction if no device is available during transportation to the hospital.

In epiphyseal fracture separations, the separation of the growth plate invariably occurs through the zone of cartilage transformation preserving the zone of growth. Informing a family that the injury involved the growth of an extremity may terribly concern them and requires the understanding and support of the pediatrician.

A clear and complete epiphyseal separation if restored is compatible with normal subsequent growth. If there is a partial separation with a fracture of the epiphysis itself, then anatomic restoration by open reduction may be necessary to preserve growth and to prevent distortion. If there is a compression injury of the growth plate, then distortions of growth may not be avoidable and may require future surgical correction. Epiphyseal injuries require adequate follow-up throughout the growing period to be sure that there is no discrepancy in length or distortion of growth. If there is significant leg length discrepancy, it may be necessary to do an epiphyseal arrest at an appropriate time. Angular distortions of growth may require an osteotomy of the affected bone to correct alignment.

The most common epiphyseal injury of the elbow is to the capitellum. Distortions of growth here classically cause a varus deformity of the elbow with tardy ulnar nerve paralysis. In follow-up the child must be observed with this in mind.

In any injury of the elbow, the possibility of a neurovascular complication, particularly Volkmann's contracture, should be considered. Hence, early immobilization, transportation to the hospital and x-rays are indicated. It is important to do this before undue swelling has occurred. Any fracture of the shaft of the long bone of the lower extremity may also cause a similar neurovascular injury. An anterior compartment syndrome below the knee is the equivalent of the Volkmann's contracture of the upper extremity. Here again, rapid immobilization and transportation to the hospital are indicated.

Accidental injuries are considered the most common single cause of death in children. Automobile accidents and falls are the most common causes of skeletal injuries. Children may have multiple fractures if the trauma is severe enough. While they occur less commonly than in the adult, they demand the same principles of management. Childhood fractures, particularly in the presence of severe trauma, may be associated with injuries of other structures such as the skull, the spinal column, the chest and the abdomen. Do not just treat the fracture but look for injuries of other structures as well.

A fracture of the pelvis is likely in any child who has been hit by a car. Pelvic injuries may be accompanied by vascular or neurologic injuries. Look for blood at the various organ exits. Abdominal and rectal examinations are performed. Pulses are checked as are active movements of the lower extremities.

The initial care of severe injuries requires the assumption that all victims of major accidents have multiple injuries. In the initial examination one seeks to determine the presence of respiratory difficulty, major hemorrhage, depression of the state of consciousness, shock, internal injuries, fractures, and superficial soft tissue injuries.

Initially it is vital to maintain the airway, prevent further blood loss, immobilize the patient and transport him to the hospital as soon as possible. In the hospital further life-saving measures are begun while the extent and nature of the injuries are determined by physical examination and x-rays.

The "Six B's"—breathing, bleeding, brain, bowel, bladder and bone—indicate the order in which attention must be paid to multiple system injuries. Airway exchange must be established and inhalation assisted if necessary; transportation is in a semi-prone position; visible hemorrhage is controlled; if available, intravenous replacement of fluid is begun; the level of consciousness is assessed and pupils are checked for inequality. Changing vital signs may indicate a head injury.

14

Muscles

Congenital Muscular Defects

MICHAEL J. GOLDBERG, M.D.

Congenital absence of muscles is usually asymmetrical and can be diagnosed by careful examination at birth. Although any of the voluntary muscles may be absent, the pectoralis, trapezius, seratus anterior and quadratus femoris are absent most frequently. Absence of these muscles is not accompanied by contracture and no treatment is indicated other than observation to assure that scoliosis does not develop in patients in whom the shoulder girdle muscles are absent.

Absence of the pectoralis major muscle is most common and is not associated with any shoulder weakness. It is, however, associated with a high incidence of abnormalities of the hands, such as syndactyly and hypoplasia. Cosmetic surgery for correcting the chest deformity has generally been unsatisfactory. Since function is normal, the approach to the child should be one of de-emphasizing the condition and preserving the child's confidence and self-image.

Congenital absence of a muscle may result in contractures if the function of the absent muscle is not fulfilled by other muscles controlling the part. This is the situation in congenital absence of forearm and hand muscles. Bracing and exercises to carry the part through a full range of motion may be indicated until the function of the absent muscle can be substituted for by tendon transfers. Congenital absence of the thenar muscles, the extensor muscles to the thumb or the finger extensors requires reconstructive surgery because of impaired hand function, and the patient should be referred to an orthopedic surgeon for

therapy, bracing and muscle-tendon transfers. Congenital absence of the palmaris longus requires no treatment.

Congenital absence of the abdominal muscles, prune belly syndrome or triad syndrome is a rare but disabling disease and is associated with high infant mortality. Early urologic surgery is often needed because of obstructive uropathy with megaureter and advanced hydronephrosis. Extensive urologic reconstructive surgery is the rule. Aggressive medical management of the frequent urinary tract infections is required to prevent further parenchymal loss from the kidneys. Associated malformation of the gastrointestinal tract, usually atresia and loss of intestinal continuity, requires appropriate pediatric surgical consultation and treatment. The high incidence of associated orthopedic malformations includes congenital dislocated hips, bilateral club feet, as well as congenital amputations, and necessitates treatment as soon as the child's condition is stabilized. A significant number of these children have cardiovascular abnormalities requiring either surgical or medical management.

In this syndrome the abdomen is wrinkled and shapeless and hangs down in folds. Upright positioning of the child assists respiration. An abdominal corset or binding improves respiration and the ability to defecate. A corset in the older child is important for cosmesis.

Bilateral paralysis of the face, or Mobius syndrome, is due to congenital absence of the facial nerve or nucleus. It often results in impaired nursing; squeezing the cheeks during feeding is required. The lack of facial expression may result in an erroneous diagnosis of mental retardation. No treatment is effective in this condition. There is a high incidence of associated orthopedic defects.

Arthrogryposis multiplex congenita is a disorder characterized by congenital immobility of multiple joints, fixed in extension or flexion, with decreased active and passive range of motion and marked hypoplasia of the skeletal muscles. A few patients may have involvement of one limb, but usually all four extremities are involved to varying degrees. Early accurate diagnosis and immediate treatment in the nursery yield the best functional results since soft tissue deformities are least rigid soon after birth. Nonoperative treatment in the nursery consists of exercises and range of motion to *every* joint performed many times a day, and in addition light plaster or plastic holding splints to maintain the limb in the corrected position. Flexion and extension splints are used to maintain the range of motion between exercise sessions. Manipulation and application of corrective plaster casts within the first days of life are needed for control of the frequently associated club foot. Congenital dislocated hip and clubfoot, common with arthrogryposis, are notoriously hard to treat and usually require surgery during the first year of life. Scoliosis almost invariably develops during the first decade. The overall goals are to maintain the function and mobility of the hand and upper extremity for feeding and self-care and to maintain the alignment and stability of the lower extremities for weight bearing and ambulation. Recurrence of deformities is the rule, and a meticulous program of braces, night bivalved casts, physical therapy, surgical releases of contracted joint capsules and tendon transfers is continued throughout growth and development of these children.

Torticollis

MICHAEL J. GOLDBERG, M.D.

Torticollis should be considered as a physical sign and not as a diagnosis. Only after determining whether the onset is congenital or acquired, acute or insidious, and after careful physical examination and cervical spine x-rays, can an accurate diagnosis be made and appropriate treatment instituted.

CONGENITAL TORTICOLLIS

In congenital muscular torticollis (infantile muscular torticollis) the head is tilted to the affected side and the face is rotated to the opposite side. It appears at birth or shortly thereafter and is due to a tightening and shortening of one sternocleidomastoid muscle. Asymmetry of the face, eyes, ears and skull is often present in addition to other frequently associated anomalies such as clubfoot and dislocated hip. Treatment consists of stretching exercises to the affected sternocleidomastoid muscle and are performed by the mother only after careful instruction by the physician or therapist. There are two exercises: (1) tilting the head away from the affected side so that the ear is brought in contact with the opposite shoulder and (2) rotating the chin toward the affected side, toward the tight sternocleidomastoid muscle. The head should be held in the stretched position for 10 seconds and each maneuver is performed 20 times at each exercise session. There should be four to six exercise sessions a day, scheduled at feeding or diaper changes.

In addition, the child should be positioned in the crib so that he must actively rotate his head toward the affected side in response to sound or light stimuli. Positioning the head in a neutral position when the baby is sleeping using either a blanket roll or small sand bag can be helpful.

The sternocleidomastoid tumor is present in 50 per cent of cases, appears approximately 10 days after birth and is located in the lower one-half of the muscle. It spontaneously regresses in three to six months and operation for its excision is not indicated. Occasionally a child may have marked tenderness about the sternocleidomastoid tumor when it initially appears, and spasm, thus making it difficult to perform stretching exercises. In these cases, exercises may be postponed a few days, but in the interim, the use of a soft cervical collar to maintain the head in a partially corrected position is recommended.

Various devices for traction have been designed but are difficult to manage and not usually required.

With conservative management, a cure rate approaching 90 per cent can be expected. Operative intervention is considered if there is a failure of conservative treatment after a minimum of six to nine months. It is rare to perform surgery before one year of age. Surgery is indicated in the older child of age two or three who has not been treated. The surgery consists of careful lengthening of the sternocleidomastoid muscle at either the mastoid or clavicular end according to the preference of the orthopedic surgeon, although it is cosmetically preferable if the surgical release can be performed at the mastoid attachment of the muscle behind the ear.

Postoperative management includes head halter traction and bed rest for 7 to 10 days, and then use of a brace for three to six months combined with a detailed physical therapy program to restore muscle strength and balance as well as to improve range of motion of the neck.

Torticollis present at birth can be due to congenital segmentation and fusion anomalies of the cervical spine with cervical scoliosis. Accurate roentgenograms are essential for diagnosis. Occasionally, stretching or flexibility exercises may be beneficial, but more often are disappointing in controlling the curves. Splinting the head with a cervical collar may help, but the essential treatment consists of carefully following any progression of this scoliotic curve, and if it does increase, then the use of a Milwaukee brace and/or surgical fusion is indicated. Because of the associated spinal cord anomalies and the high incidence of genitourinary malformations, patients with congenital scoliosis should undergo both a myelogram and an intravenous pyelogram.

ACQUIRED TORTICOLLIS

Torticollis may be acquired either acutely or insidiously. Acute torticollis is frequently seen in children following trauma and is due to a rotatory subluxation of cervical 1 (atlas) on cervical 2 (axis). Subluxation is also seen in children who have instability of the atlantoaxial junction, a common finding in several syndromes including bone dysplasias and Down syndrome. Treatment for rotatory subluxation due to trauma includes bed rest, head halter traction, heat and aspirin. Once there is reduction, the child is maintained in a cervical collar for four to six weeks. Those with instability due to malformations of the atlantoaxial junction require surgical stabilization.

Acute torticollis is seen occasionally with pharyngeal infection and resolves after appropriate antibiotic treatment.

Acquired torticollis of gradual onset occurs with ocular muscle abnormalities when head positioning by the patient minimizes nystagmus or prevents diplopia. Acquired torticollis is also seen with inner ear conditions, disturbances of vestibular function, inflammatory processes of the neck such as tuberculosis or rheumatoid arthritis, and may be the presenting complaint with intraspinal or posterior fossa tumors.

SPASMODIC TORTICOLLIS

Spasmodic torticollis is not seen during infancy and only rarely during childhood but does occur occasionally during adolescence. It is an intermittent rather than continuous malpositioning of the head and may be either rapid jerky movements or a prolonged dystonic spasm. Treatment is unsatisfactory. Physical therapy is usually of no value. Cervical traction and rigid mechanical supports may offer temporary relief. Medical management including muscle relaxants, diazepam, haloperidol, amantadine, lithium and levodopa have been reported to be successful only infrequently. Cervical rhizotomies and sternocleidomastoid release are rarely recommended. A combined approach utilizing psychotherapy techniques and neurosurgical creation of stereotactic lesions seems to offer most success.

Congenital Hypotonia

N. PAUL ROSMAN, M.D.

The term *congenital hypotonia* implies a reduction in body tone that is present at birth or very early in infancy. It can be caused by a diverse array of nonneurological and neurological disorders. Muscle tone, or the resistance of muscle to stretch, depends on the viscoelastic properties of muscle, joints and tendons, and is influenced by activity of the gamma motor system of the spinal cord. Muscle tone can be phasic or postural. Phasic tone is that accompanying the brief contractions of muscle that occur in response to high intensity stretch, seen when one elicits deep tendon reflexes. Postural tone is that manifested by prolonged contraction in response to low intensity stretch, and is seen in antigravity muscles.

The hypotonic infant shows a reduction in postural tone, with or without associated alteration in phasic tone. Such children tend to assume abnormal postures, such as the "frog-leg" position in the lower limbs, their joints show decreased resistance to passive movement and an increased range of movement, and their spontaneous movements are usually reduced. Muscle weakness may be associated with congenital hypotonia, particularly with diseases of the lower motor neuron (spinal cord, spinal nerve root, peripheral nerve, neuromuscular junction, skeletal muscle). More frequently, however, hypotonia is due to medical illness or disease of the upper motor neuron (brain, spinal cord) and is unaccompanied by muscle paralysis. If hypotonia first appears in early intrauterine life, the child may be born with limb contractures.

Assessment of tone is best achieved in the young infant by ventral suspension or by the traction response. In ventral suspension, the child is supported in a prone position by the examiner's hand placed under the chest. The normal full-term newborn will hold his head somewhat above the horizontal, his back will be straight or only slightly flexed, his arms will be flexed at the elbows and partially extended at the shoulders and his knees will be partially flexed. The hypotonic infant, by contrast, will show floppiness of the head, trunk and limbs. The traction response is elicited by pulling a child from a supine to sitting position by exerting gentle traction on both forearms. The normal newborn will flex his elbows and his neck, whereas the hypotonic infant fails to flex his upper limbs and his head lags behind, tending to remain in contact with the bed. An additional means of assessing tone is by vertical suspension, during which the child is supported in an upright position by the examiner's hands placed beneath the axillae. The normal infant will maintain some scapular fixation during that maneuver, whereas the hypotonic infant tends to "slip through" the examiner's fingers.

Clinical Signs. A detailed gestational, perinatal, and postnatal history must be obtained. Inquiry should be made about the vigor of fetal movements and about the presence of intercurrent illness, trauma, hemorrhage, excessive weight gain, drug ingestion and other potentially noxious events during the mother's pregnancy. Since a number of the diseases causing congenital hypotonia are genetically determined, a detailed family history should be obtained. The clinical signs of congenital hypotonia in upper and lower motor neuron diseases are summarized in Table 1.

Children with upper motor neuron (brain) disease usually lack normal social and adaptive responses. Not uncommonly, such children show abnormalities in head size, shape or transillumination. Associated ocular, facial, or other somatic abnormalities may be found, as illustrated by Down's syndrome, a disorder in which hypotonia of cerebral origin is a characteristic feature. The deep tendon reflexes are usually normal when hypotonia is due to upper motor neuron disease.

Children whose hypotonia is caused by lower motor neuron disease tend to have a "bright" appearance and normal social and adaptive responses. They frequently show muscle weakness or paralysis that is usually proximal in distribution. Deep tendon reflexes are characteristically reduced or absent. A minority of such children have a discrete spinal malformation, which may be indicated by an overlying collection of hair, fat pad, hemangioma or sinus tract; occasionally, a discrete sensory level is found. Fasciculations of the tongue are highly suggestive of Werdnig-Hoffmann disease.

Laboratory Signs. The laboratory signs of congenital hypotonia in upper and lower motor neuron diseases are outlined in Table 2. Electromyography (EMG) and measurement of nerve conduction velocities (NCV) are particularly valuable in diagnosis of the causes of hypotonia due to lower motor neuron disease. In primary diseases of muscle, such as polymyositis or congenital myopathies, the resting muscle usually shows little or no electrical activity, though fibrillations may be seen in polymyositis. During volitional contraction in primary muscle disease, the motor unit action potentials are of decreased amplitude, polyphasic, and of shortened duration. In diseases of spinal cord anterior horn cells, spinal nerve roots or peripheral nerves, the resting EMG shows fibrillations; when the denervation is due to anterior horn cell disease, fasciculations also can be seen. During voluntary contraction in denervating diseases, the numbers of motor unit action potentials are greatly reduced and high voltage polyphasic potentials are seen. When this denervation pattern is caused by spinal cord disease, NCV (which average about 30 meters/second in newborns) are usually normal. By contrast, when the denervation is due to peripheral nerve disease, NCV are reduced.

Muscle biopsy is particularly valuable in the evaluation of congenital hypotonia due to lower motor neuron diseases. With combined histological and histochemical staining, three patterns of abnormality can be seen: (1) necrobiosis, or acute necrosis of muscle fibers, can occur in the presence of inflammation, as in

TABLE 1.   Clinical Signs in Congenital Hypotonia

	BRAIN	SPINAL CORD	PERIPHERAL NERVE	MUSCLE
Proximal muscle weakness	±	+	±	+
Hyporeflexia or areflexia	−	±	+	+
Atrophy	±	+	+	+
Sensory loss	±	±	+	−
Fasciculations	−	+	−	−
Direct muscle excitability on percussion	+	+	+	−

Table 2.   Laboratory Signs in Congenital Hypotonia

	BRAIN	SPINAL CORD	PERIPHERAL NERVE	MUSCLE
Abnormal radiographs	±	±	—	—
Abnormal electroencephalogram	+	—	—	—
Elevated CSF protein	±	±	±	—
Elevated serum creatine phosphokinase	—	±	—	±
Abnormal electromyogram	—	+ (neuronopathic)	+ (neuropathic)	+ (myopathic)
Prolonged nerve conduction velocities	—	±	+	—
Abnormal muscle biopsy	±	+	+	+
Abnormal myelogram	—	±	—	—

polymyositis, or in its absence, as in the muscular dystrophies; (2) disfiguration is due to an alteration of muscle organelles or accumulation of material within muscle, and characterizes the congenital and metabolic myopathies; and (3) denervation is seen in myelopathies and radiculoneuropathies. In brain disease and in certain disorders of the lower motor neuron (for example, myasthenia gravis), no obvious or consistent alterations in muscle are found.

A variety of other laboratory tests may be useful in the diagnosis of neurologic, muscular and nonneuromuscular causes of congenital hypotonia. Abnormalities in blood or urine electrolytes, amino acids, "muscle enzymes," or hormones may be found. Elevations in CSF protein may be seen, especially in radiculoneuropathies. Chromosomal abnormalities may be found in hypotonic infants who also have somatic abnormalities. Radiographs of soft tissues may disclose muscle atrophy, not

Table 3.   Treatable Causes of Congenital Hypotonia

DISORDER	TREATMENT
Medical Illness	
Systemic infection	Antimicrobials
Nutritional deficiency (single or multiple)	Replacement
Electrolyte abnormality ($\uparrow$ Ca, $\downarrow$ K, $\uparrow$ or $\downarrow$ Mg)	Correction
Hyperbilirubinemia	Exchange transfusion; phototherapy
Endocrine abnormality ($\downarrow$ thyroid function, $\uparrow$ or $\downarrow$ adrenal function $\downarrow$ pituitary function)	Correction
Aminoacidopathy	Dietary restriction; vitamin therapy
Excessive maternal medication	Respiratory support
Maternal barbiturate addiction	Respiratory support
Brain	
Seizures (from variety of causes)	Anticonvulsants or more specific measures
Tumor	Surgical removal; radiotherapy
Subdural hematoma	Aspiration; surgical removal
Spinal Cord	
Myelomeningocele	Surgical removal; CSF shunt for associated hydrocephalus
Spinal Root and/or Peripheral Nerve	
Chronic radiculoneuropathy	Corticosteroids (?)
Neuromuscular Junction	
Myasthenia gravis (transient neonatal or congenital)	Anticholinesterases
Skeletal Muscle	
Polymyositis	Corticosteroids

easily appreciated on clinical examination because of prominent subcutaneous tissue. Skull and spine x-rays may disclose a variety of abnormalities. In congenital hypothyroidism, wrist films characteristically show a retarded bone age. Computerized axial tomography (CT scan) can delineate a diverse array of intracranial and spinal disease processes. Some of the treatable causes of congenital hypotonia are outlined in Table 3.

Myasthenia Gravis. When the presence of either transient neonatal or congenital myasthenia is suspected, the diagnosis can be confirmed by the administration of anticholinesterases. These agents will result in an improvement in hypotonia, and a reversal of swallowing and respiratory difficulties and, indeed, may be life-saving. Neostigmine methylsulfate, given intramuscularly or subcutaneously in a dosage of 0.125 mg., will result in improvement within 10 to 30 minutes. Alternatively, edrophonium chloride (Tensilon) can be given intravenously in a dosage of 1 mg. in children under 3 months of age, 2 mg. for those between 3 and 12 months of age and 0.15 mg./kg. in older infants. One tenth of the total dose of Tensilon is given first, and if no adverse reaction occurs, the remainder is administered 1 to 2 minutes later. Improvement occurs within a few minutes. On occasion, adverse effects may occur, but these can be overcome by the subcutaneous administration of atropine in a dosage of 0.01 mg./kg., every 2 hours if necessary. Treatment for the myasthenia can be maintained by intramuscular or oral anticholinesterases given 10 to 15 minutes before each four-hourly feeding.

Prognosis. The prognosis in congenital hypotonia is highly variable and ranges from reversal of the underlying disorder with full recovery to rapid progression and death. Clearly, the major determinant is the nature of the underlying illness and its potential for treatment. The success of such treatment depends on accurate diagnosis and prompt institution of appropriate therapy.

Muscular Dystrophy and Related Myopathies

E. G. MURPHY, M.D., F.R.C.P.

The muscular dystrophies compose a group of genetically determined diseases of muscle, by far the most common of which in childhood is the Duchenne type. This disorder usually presents in the first three or four years of life and runs a remorseless downhill course in which the patient rarely survives the second decade.

It is important to emphasize that many disorders of the neuromuscular systems in childhood are superficially similar. Some of these conditions are relatively benign with a relatively good prognosis. In addition these disorders may be inherited in different fashions. Sophisticated testing may be required to differentiate particularly the rare myopathies. Patients with neuromuscular disorders should be investigated at centers interested in such problems. Special investigations include serum enzyme studies, electromyography, and muscle biopsy with full histochemical and electron microscopic evaluation.

As these disorders are genetically determined, it is of prime importance to have a full genetic assessment. It is now well known that female carriers of the sex-linked recessive Duchenne type of dystrophy and the milder Becker type of dystrophy can be detected by creatine kinase studies.

Once the diagnosis of neuromuscular disorder is made, one faces the unfortunate fact that there is no specific remedy for most of them, although the progress of polymyositis, polyneuritis and myasthenia gravis and periodic paralysis can certainly be modified by specific therapy discussed elsewhere. However, a multidisciplinary approach can be highly supportive and can improve the quality of life for these seriously handicapped children and their parents.

The main goal in muscular dystrophy is to keep the patient as mobile and independent as possible at all stages of the disease. It is desirable to keep the patient walking as long as possible. In the Duchenne type of dystrophy long leg bracing has been found to keep the patient ambulatory for 1 or 2 years longer, which could represent about 10 per cent of the life span. In order to fit the patient into braces, Achilles tendon lengthening and transfer of the posterior tibial tendon to the dorsum are usually required as well as tendon releases in the thighs. In the stage of nonambulation, which represents 30 to 50 per cent of the patient's life span, the problem is to prevent progressive spinal deformities.

During the wheelchair-bound stage of the disease, treatment should be aimed at the prevention of early scoliotic deformities by extension of the spine and maintenance of pelvis-based back bracing. Special seating devices have been developed to prevent such deformities. At times, however, it has been necessary to prevent progressive spinal deformities by operative measures. It must be observed that electric wheelchairs have enriched the lives of the wheelchair-bound patients enormously.

Physiotherapy in the ambulatory stages of the disease should be aimed at keeping patients active and modifying the development of contractures. In the nonambulatory phase, attention has to be given to maintenance of respiratory function. Late in the lives of patients with Duchenne type dystrophy and sometimes in those with myotonia dystrophica and the facioscapulohumeral type, cardiomyopathy may develop and has to be treated with small doses of digoxin.

Unfortunately medication has little place in the management of the hereditary myopathies. No medication has been found so far that affects the progression of the various disorders significantly. Myotonia is almost the only exception. Procainamide hydrochloride, 250 mg. to 2 gm./day may be helpful.* More recently phenytoin (Dilantin), 100 mg. 2 to 3 times daily, has been found to be helpful. In addition small doses of prednisone, such as 10 mg. every other day, seem to help some patients. In patients with myotonia dystrophica, weakness is usually more of a problem than myotonia, but if myotonia proves to be troublesome, the drugs outlined above can be used. Muscle cramps occasionally are troublesome in the ambulatory early stages of Duchenne type dystrophy, and if usual home remedies are ineffective small doses of prednisone, 10 to 15 mg. every other day, may prove helpful. The use of prednisone for the management of the Duchenne and other types of dystrophy has been advocated as having an ameliorating effect, but there is no clear-cut evidence of sustained effectiveness.

Penicillamine has shown some beneficial effects in chickens affected by hereditary types of dystrophy. Its action is on inhibition of cross-linkage in the subunits of collagen in the formation of fibrous tissue which is such a feature of most types of muscular dystrophy. Clinical trials are under way in several countries, and it should be clear within a year or two whether this therapy has a beneficial effect in the Duchenne type dystrophy.

Myasthenia Gravis

J. GORDON MILLICHAP, M.D.

NEONATAL MYASTHENIA

The diagnosis of neonatal myasthenia is established by the intravenous injection of edrophonium chloride (Tensilon) in a dose of 1 mg. Symptoms should be relieved almost immediately. In moderate and severe cases and especially those with bulbar symptoms, a positive Tensilon test should be followed by therapy with anticholinesterase drugs. In the milder forms of the disorder the infant may recover spontaneously but respiratory difficulty, choking, dysphagia, or inability to suck are indications for specific therapy.

Pyridostigmine bromide (Mestinon) and neostigmine bromide (Prostigmin) have a less rapid but more prolonged effect than Tensilon and may be effectively used in treatment. Mestinon is preferred because it is less toxic, having fewer muscarinic side effects. The required dosage differs in each patient and must be adjusted according to the individual response. The following have been found satisfactory as initial doses, to be given every four hours at the time of each feeding: oral doses, Mestinon bromide, 5 mg. (5 drops of syrup of Mestinon, containing 60 mg. per 4 ml.), Prostigmin bromide, 1 mg. Parenteral preparations are approximately 30 times as potent as the oral; the intramuscular dose of Prostigmin methylsulfate is 0.05 to 0.1 mg. When a dose level sufficient to relieve bulbar symptoms has been determined, further increments in dosage are unnecessary and may be hazardous.

Overdosage with anticholinesterase medication (cholinergic crisis) is manifested by the following signs: increase in muscle weakness, worsening of respiratory difficulty and dysphagia after each dose of drug, muscular fasciculations, and prominent muscarinic side effects, which include excessive salivation, vomiting, diarrhea, pallor, sweating, and bradycardia. Tensilon, 0.05 ml. (0.5 mg.) given intravenously, will cause a mild and transient exacerbation of cholinergic weakness and may be used to differentiate the crisis due to excessive medication and that associated with a worsening of myasthenia. Atropine may be administered for anticholinesterase overdosage. The oronasopharyngeal secretions should be suctioned repeatedly and oxygen administered when indicated.

After the first week of treatment the gradual withdrawal of medication may be attempted. If symptoms increase, the original dosage is reinstituted, and the effects of withdrawal are observed again after two or three days. The duration of the illness is short, and the natural course is from a few hours to seven weeks. With efficient therapy recovery is complete.

JUVENILE MYASTHENIA GRAVIS

Diagnosis is confirmed by the intravenous injection of Tensilon, which relieves the presenting symptoms within a few minutes. In children weighing up to 34 kg., the dose is 0.2

---

*This use of procainamide is not mentioned in the manufacturer's instructions.

ml. (2 mg.); in those over 34 kg., 0.5 ml. (5 mg.) may be given. If Prostigmin is employed, the intramuscular dose is 0.25 to 1.0 mg. of Prostigmin methylsulfate, dependent on the weight or surface area of the child; the patient is examined for signs of improvement at 5- or 10-minute intervals for a period of 45 minutes, and atropine may be required for the relief of muscarinic side effects.

Treatment with anticholinesterase drugs is instituted and controlled as outlined for neonatal myasthenia. Mestinon is given orally in initial trial doses of 5 to 10 mg. at intervals of two to four hours, or Prostigmin in doses of 1 to 5 mg. orally. Mytelase (ambenonium chloride) is prescribed occasionally; it causes less bronchial secretion than do other anticholinesterase drugs, and its use may be indicated in patients with respiratory paralysis. Five mg. of Mytelase chloride is equivalent to 15 mg. of Prostigmin bromide or 60 mg. of Mestinon bromide.

Other treatments of value in refractory cases include adrenocorticotropic hormone and, in some patients, ephedrine and potassium chloride. A mechanical respirator and tracheostomy may be necessary in advanced cases.

Thymectomy may be followed by improvement and sometimes by complete remission. It is considered of particular value in young female patients who have had the disease for less than five years, and is indicated especially in patients with generalized muscle weakness and bulbar symptoms resistant to therapy.

The prognosis in children is variable but relatively good compared with adults. The case fatality rate is approximately 5 per cent. The course is generally prolonged, and complete remission following drug therapy or thymectomy may be expected in less than 25 per cent of cases up to six years from the onset; complete remission after this time is rare. Ptosis and ocular palsies are often refractory to treatment, and relapse and failure of response to medication are frequently related to systemic or upper respiratory infection and to menstruation.

Familial Periodic Paralysis

PETER R. HUTTENLOCHER, M.D.

Two major types of familial periodic paralysis are described. In the classic form, serum potassium is decreased during attacks (hypokalemic periodic paralysis), and attacks are often precipitated by large carbohydrate meals or during rest following strong exertion. The second type is characterized by elevated serum potassium levels during attacks (hyperkalemic periodic paralysis, adynamia episodica hereditaria, paramyotonia). Heavy exercise, starvation, and high potassium intake appear to be precipitating factors. In this form of periodic paralysis there often is myotonia, which persists between attacks. Both forms of familial periodic paralysis are transmitted as dominant traits, with more severe expression in the male. The therapy of these disorders differs and will be discussed separately.

Treatment of *hypokalemic periodic paralysis* is conveniently divided into acute therapy for attacks of weakness and prophylactic therapy for prevention of future attacks. Adult drug dosages are provided. These have to be adjusted downward for the occasional patient in whom periodic paralysis develops prior to late childhood or adolescence.

Acute therapy includes rapid assessment of the patient's respiratory status and institution of assisted ventilation if there is respiratory failure. Potassium administration will shorten attacks and will abort incipient attacks. If possible, potassium should be given by mouth, since this route of administration is safer. Liquid preparations of potassium should be employed, rather than potassium tablets, since the latter produce gastric irritation. Enteric coated tablets are to be strictly avoided, in view of the risk of ulceration, perforation, or stricture of the small intestine.

Liquid preparations of both potassium chloride and potassium gluconate are available at a concentration of 20 mEq./tablespoon (15 ml.); 60 to 100 mEq. of the elixir are usually needed to ameliorate an attack. This dosage should be given slowly over a period of about one hour, preferably diluted in water. Potassium chloride is given intravenously in severely ill patients who are unable to swallow. Potassium chloride for injection (2 mEq./ml.) is diluted 1:10 with distilled water so as to make a solution of 20 mEq./100 ml.; 20 mEq./hr. is a safe rate of administration in a patient with adequate renal function. Monitoring the electrocardiogram is advisable during intravenous infusion. Electrocardiographic evidence of potassium toxicity includes atrioventricular block and prolongation of P-waves and of the QRS complex.

Prophylactic therapy for hypokalemic periodic paralysis includes education of the patient regarding factors that may precipitate attacks, such as large carbohydrate meals and rest after heavy exercise. Mild exercise, such as walking about, may abort incipient attacks. Patients frequently develop paralysis during overnight sleep, and this may be prevented by administration of potassium chloride or potassium gluconate prior to retiring in the evening, at a dosage of about 60 mEq. (3 tablespoons of the elixir). When taken on a daily basis, acetazolamide is effective in preventing attacks in some patients. The dosage has to be adjusted individually, and varies from 125 mg. twice daily to 250 mg. three times daily. Spironolactone also may prevent recurrent attacks. The amount is 50 to 100 mg./day in two to three divided doses.

Hyperkalemic periodic paralysis usually requires no specific therapy for acute attacks, since these are generally brief, lasting for a few hours only, with weakness largely confined to the lower extremities. Intravenous calcium gluconate, (10 to 20 ml. of a 10 per cent solution) and intravenous glucose infusion have been reported to produce more rapid return in strength. Prophylactic therapy includes avoidance of conditions which may lead to a rise in serum potassium, such as heavy exercise, starvation and excessive intake of high potassium foods. Frequent, small, high-carbohydrate meals may be effective. Drug therapy is directed at maintaining serum potassium in a low normal range. Both chlorothiazide and acetazolamide are effective. The dosage of chlorothiazide varies from 125 mg./day to 500 mg./day; that of acetazolamide varies from 250 to 750 mg./day in two or three divided doses. Serum potassium should be monitored periodically while patients are on chlorothiazide or acetazolamide therapy.

Myositis Ossificans

FREDERICK J. SAMAHA, M.D., *and* YAKUB INATI, M.D.

Two types of myositis ossificans are recognized; one follows trauma to muscle and the other is a rare genetically determined progressive disease. In the former condition, an injury usually involves crushing or shredding of muscle fibers in association with hemorrhage; connective tissue proliferates with metaplasia and subsequent osteoid formation. Calcification of this osteoid concludes the formation of heterotopic bone. The patient will usually relate the occurrence of a crushing injury, as might occur from a high fall or of repeated minor trauma such as pitching a baseball. Following the injury a tender, firm mass gradually appears over several weeks. As bone formation occurs the mass hardens. The x-ray study of the mass will show the typical feathery calcification. Avoidance of further trauma and physical therapy are all that is needed in mild cases. The persistence of pain or discomfort and the breaking down of overlying skin may require surgical removal of the mass.

The clinical features of progressive myositis ossificans are characteristic. Most of the cases begin in the first decade, and more than 90 per cent have their onset in the first 20 years of life. There appears to be no sex predilection, and in less than 5 per cent of cases a family history of myositis ossificans may be obtained. The latter observation, along with a 90 per cent incidence of digital abnormalities in these patients and the occurrence of digital abnormalities alone in the family history, provides the basis for the belief that progressive myositis ossificans may be genetically determined. The most common anomaly is microdactyly or adactyly.

The initial complaints are those of a painful, swollen, tender area, probably following minor trauma, which may be associated with erythematous skin. The pain subsides over several weeks and a firm lump gradually becomes ossified. The heterotopic bone formation occurs in the connective tissue of skeletal muscles, tendons, ligaments and capsules of joints. As in the case of traumatic myositis ossificans, the basic lesion is one of proliferating connective tissue followed by metaplasia, osteoid formation and calcification. The lack of classic inflammatory changes and the lack of direct involvement of muscle cells have moved some clinicians to note that "myositis ossificans" is a misnomer. It is more characteristically a fibrodysplasia. In this regard a case of myositis ossificans has been reported in association with polyostotic fibrous dysplasia.

The prominent areas of involvement are the muscles in the neck, paravertebral area, shoulders and arms, head, face, jaw, hips and legs, in decreasing order of frequency. The episodes of painful swelling and heterotopic bone formation recur over three to four decades until the patient becomes totally immobilized as a "stone man." When intercostal and masseter muscle involvement occurs, death may occur because of respiratory failure and inanition.

Over the last 10 years treatment attempts with ethylenediamine tetra-acetic acid (EDTA), parathyroid extract, triiodothyronine, propylthiouracil, corticosteroids, vitamins and low dietary calcium have failed. On the other hand, physical therapy which attempts to maintain full range of joint motion has been of significant value.

Since 1969, a number of patients with progressive myositis ossificans have been treated with sodium etridonate (EDHP).* The statistics available up to 1973 in a report by W. B. Geho and J. A. Whiteside show that in a total of 52 patients treated for more than six months, 24 were better, 20 were stabilized, and 8 were worse. Our knowledge of individual cases that progressed on EDHP suggests these results are too optimistic; none of the studies published were conclusive. The dosage generally used was 10 mg./kg./day by mouth. More recently, investigators have realized that the drug is poorly absorbed in amounts varying from 1 to 10 per cent of administered dosage.

---

*EDHP is an experimental drug and is available only on this basis.

Because serum level measurements are not available, recent therapeutic regimens have utilized an empirical dosage of 20 mg./kg./day. Serum phosphate levels become elevated on administration of this dosage. EDHP therapy along with surgical removal of some ectopic bone has the therapeutic aim of preventing formation of ectopic bone causing joint fixation and of increasing mobilization of crippled patients. The only probable side effects of EDHP noted have been gastrointestinal in nature and these can be controlled by dividing the total daily medication into two dosages.

Since this experimental drug represents the only possible therapeutic approach, and since its toxicity is apparently low, patients with documented progressive myositis ossificans might benefit by being referred to centers using EDHP.

15

Skin

Topical Therapy: A Formulary for Pediatric Skin Disease

ROBERT M. ADAMS, M.D.

GENERAL CONSIDERATIONS

Choice of Active Ingredient. When writing a prescription which requires the pharmacist to compound medication, the fewer active ingredients you order the better; one usually is enough. Exceptions to the one active ingredient rule are corticosteroids compounded with other active substances such as tars, nystatin and other antibiotics, sulfur with salicylic acid, and others. When compounding with fluorinated steroids, one must consider whether the steroid is released into the skin by the vehicle. Homemade preparations using crushed tablets are probably totally inactive.

The pH of the final preparation is very important. Erythromycin in solution is inactivated in pH concentrations less than 4, and even at an optimum pH the preparation is not stable for long periods. When you are in doubt about the efficacy of any compounded medication, it is advisable to consult a knowledgeable pharmacist for advice.

The concentration of the active ingredient is very important. Choose the smallest concentration which is effective. Hydrocortisone in 0.25 per cent concentration possesses little anti-inflammatory effect. A better choice is a 0.5 or 1 per cent concentration.

Choice of Vehicle. The vehicle is often as important as the active ingredient. Although pharmacologically inert, vehicles possess therapeutic properties based on their physical properties. Ointments, creams and pastes protect the skin and relieve dryness, while lotions and baths clean by removal of crusts, scales and exudate.

Greater penetration occurs with ointments than with creams, pastes and lotions, in decreasing order. Shake lotions, such as calamine, may "cake" on the skin, especially when used on acute, oozing dermatitides, and may thus lead to secondary bacterial or monilial infection.

Cosmetic Effect. The effect of treatment on the patient's appearance is always an important consideration. Iodochlorhydroxyquin may stain the skin yellow and must be used cautiously on the face and other visible areas. Other staining medications are potassium permanganate, gentian violet, silver nitrate, tars and anthralin.

Cost. Prescribe only the amount necessary to treat the disease. By demonstrating how to apply a topical medication during the patient's visit, and supplying written instructions, you will help reduce the cost by decreasing the amount of medication wasted, since most patients apply more topical medication than necessary.

BASIC PRINCIPLES OF TOPICAL THERAPY

Do Not Overtreat. Therapeutic aggressiveness should be inversely proportional to the acuteness of the disease. When treating acutely inflamed skin, use bland medications such as wet dressings and simple, almost inert lotions; creams should be used sparingly, and ointment must never be employed on an acute oozing dermatitis. The irritant properties of the active ingredient(s) and the possibility of allergic sensitization must be considered. Overtreatment may induce a widespread or gen-

463

eralized dermatitis. Systemic absorption may occur from potent medications employed under plastic wrap occlusion, or when intertriginous areas such as the axilla and groin are treated. Avoid prescribing potent fluorinated steroids for use on the face for long periods of time, since atrophy and telangiectasia may result. Also avoid these agents for prolonged use in intertriginous areas because of the possibility of development of striae, in addition to the above.

Remove the Contributing Factors. Success or failure of topical therapy may hinge on the physician's recognition of the influence of environmental factors. In pediatric practice the most important of these are soaps, bubble baths and bath salts, rough or tight clothing, wool blankets, rugs, toys, dirt, sand, heat, cold, moisture and wind. Irritating or sensitizing home remedies used as self-medications are common causes of aggravation.

Decrease Itching. The most effective method of alleviating pruritus is by prompt and adequate treatment of the disease. Topical "caine" anesthetics may produce allergic sensitization. Systemic antihistamines and aspirin are the medications of choice. Menthol and phenol which are frequently found incorporated into topical medications as antipruritic agents may be systemically absorbed when applied to large areas of skin.

Recognize and Promptly Treat Secondary Infection. The appearance of secondary bacterial infection of dermatitic skin may be subtle and thus easily overlooked. Increased pruritus and pain, accompanied by yellow crusting, may signal its development. Children with atopic dermatitis are particularly likely to develop secondary pyogenic infection. Treatment of choice is the use of systemic antibiotics, such as erythromycin, often continued for 10 to 14 days. Topical antibiotics are less effective, and probably should not be employed without concomitant systemic antibiotics.

Individualize Treatment. In pediatrics, tailor the treatment carefully, not only to the patient and disease but also to the parents. Parental concerns which are most frequent are (1) contagiousness, (2) disfigurement, (3) malignancy and (4) inheritance. Reassurance in such matters may play an important role in the successful outcome of the therapeutic program.

FORMULARY

Open Wet Dressings

Open wet dressings, the mildest form of topical therapy, cool the skin by evaporation, relieve itching and clean the surface by loosening and removing crusts and debris. Used on acute blistered dermatitides, open wet dressings may often be the only treatment possible. The principle is based on cooling by evaporation.

Kerlix gauze, plain gauze without absorbent cotton, thin white handkerchiefs or strips of bed linen are most commonly used. Moisten the dressings in the solution and apply them, wet but not runny, to the affected area. One layer is usually sufficient. Wrap fingers separately; wrap arms and legs so that the elbows and knees can bend. The patient must be comfortable during treatment and must be prepared so that he can still look at pictures, play with toys and so forth.

Apply the dressings flat and smooth against the skin and leave them uncovered. When evaporation begins to dry the cloth after 5 to 10 minutes, remove the entire dressing, resoak it in the solution and reapply it to the inflamed area. Never pour or syringe the solution directly over the dressings. The treatment ordinarily has a duration of 30 minutes to 1 hour, three to four times daily. Ordinary tap water is used and it is not necessary to sterilize the water or the dressings. Keep the solutions at room temperature and mix them immediately before each treatment. Do not keep the solutions overnight, since they may become unstable and more concentrated on standing.

Wet dressings are usually discontinued after 36 to 48 hours; if they are continued longer than this, drying of the skin can result. Do not cover more than one-third of the body at any one time, and avoid chilling the patient. After treatment, dry the skin by patting with a towel or washcloth. At this time a lotion or other medication may be applied.

Compresses are preferred to soaks because of the cooling which occurs from evaporation, but soaks may be required when a hand or foot is affected. The duration of treatment should not exceed about 15 minutes to avoid maceration.

Burow's Solution (Domeboro powder packets, tablets) (Dome Laboratories). Composition: aluminum sulfate and calcium acetate, which has an acid pH in solution. Prepare a 1:40 solution by mixing one packet of powder or one tablet in one pint of tap water. The more concentrated 1:20 solutions indicated on the package directions may be somewhat irritating. Burow's solution is mildly astringent and antiseptic and leaves a fresh, dry feeling. It is supplied as tablets in boxes of 12 to 1000, and as powder in packets from 12 to 100.

Potassium Permanganate. Potassium permanganate is available in 300-mg. tablets. A 1:15,000 solution may be prepared by pulverizing one 300-mg. tablet between spoons; add the powder to 4½ quarts of water. Be certain the entire tablet dissolves, since skin contact with particles of tablet may cause a chemical burn. Solutions of potassium permanganate are mildly antiseptic and drying, and are useful for vesicular, oozing dermatitides. Potassium permanganate stains clothing and skin and should never be used on the face.

Silver Nitrate. Silver nitrate is a very effective antiseptic, coagulant, germicidal agent for bacteria, fungi and viruses, especially Pseudomonas organisms. Prepare a 0.5 per cent solution by adding two teaspoonfuls of a 50 per cent aqueous solution to one quart of cool tap water. The concentrated solution must be dispensed in a brown or other opaque bottle. Silver nitrate is expensive and stains the skin dark brown after exposure to light, and will also stain everything else with which it comes in contact, such as teaspoon, containers and floors. In 0.5 per cent concentration, silver nitrate does not irritate normal skin or inhibit epidermal proliferation; it is not antigenic. The chief disadvantages are its staining properties and its costliness.

Bluboro Powder (Derm-Arts Laboratories). Composition: aluminum sulfate, calcium acetate, boric acid and FD&C blue dye number 1. The boric acid is present in each packet at 0.056 gram for its buffering action and in this concentration probably presents no hazard of absorption. Directions for use are similar to Burow's solution.

Boric Acid. Because of the possibility of systemic poisoning, boric acid compresses should never be used.

Soaks and Paints

Formaldehyde Solution. For the treatment of hyperhidrosis of the feet and recurrent multiple plantar verrucae, 3 per cent aqueous formaldehyde solution has been advocated by some. The feet are soaked once or twice daily for 15 to 20 minutes. Formaldehyde solution must be freshly prepared prior to each use and may be sensitizing.

Glutaraldehyde. Glutaraldehyde in a 10 per cent solution may be painted on plantar skin with a cotton swab three times weekly for treatment of hyperhidrosis. Glutaraldehyde is an allergic sensitizer, and cross-reactions with formaldehyde may occur. Remember that the skin will stain yellow following its use. (Note: glutaraldehyde is investigational, not yet having been approved by the Food and Drug Ad-

ministration. It is manufactured by Mathison, Coleman and Bell, Norwood, Ohio.)

Lotions and Solutions

Lotions are suspensions of a powder in liquid and are used most commonly immediately following wet dressings. They are preferable to creams and ointments when the dermatitis is still oozing and showing vesiculation. As the liquid evaporates, a coating of powder remains on the skin surface. Evaporation cools the surface and the powder soothes, protects and dries the skin. Lotions are useful in the treatment of acute dermatitis but must be avoided on oozing surfaces and in hairy or intertriginous areas.

They are most often applied with the fingers or gauze, or with a small paint brush, in which case they should be dispensed in a wide-mouthed bottle. Cotton will soak up most of the preparation, releasing only about half into the skin. Apply evenly; remove by soaking in a portion of the compress solution, not by peeling the dried material from the skin. If used for more than 3 or 4 days, shake lotions may cause chapping. Addition of an oil and a dispersant forms an emulsion.

A BASIC SHAKE LOTION		TO WHICH ONE MAY ADD	
zinc oxide	20%	olive oil	10%
talc	20%	menthol	⅛-¼%
glycerin	15%	ichthammol	2-3%
sufficient water		liquor carbonis detergens	5-10%
to make	120%	Vioform	1-3%
		hydrocortisone	½-1%

Do not add "caine-type" anesthetics or antihistamines.

Calamine Lotion U.S.P. Composition: zinc oxide, ferric oxide and yellow ferric oxide, with glycerine and bentonite magma and calcium hydroxide solution. Calamine solution is inexpensive and has a wide and well deserved reputation. Its disadvantages are that it tends to dry and cake, especially in the presence of oozing.

Caladryl (Parke, Davis) contains Benadryl which may be an occasional contact sensitizer.

Aveeno Lotion (Cooper Laboratories). Composition: 10 per cent Aveeno colloidal oatmeal in an aqueous base consisting of propylene glycol, isopropyl myristate and liquid petrolatum. In acute and subacute dermatoses, Aveeno Lotion forms a flexible adherent coating which does not crack or flake off. It is supplied in 6-ounce plastic bottles.

Cetaphil Lotion (Texas Pharmacal). Cetaphil Lotion is a lipid-free lotion and skin cleanser containing propylene glycol, cetyl alcohol, stearyl alcohol, sodium lauryl sulfate, butyl, methyl and propyl parabens and water. It may be used as a waterless cleaner, especially for atopic dermatitis, and also as a vehicle for various active ingredients, especially hydrocortisone, in the treatment of other forms of dermatitis. Apply by rubbing in two layers to produce a lather. The excess may be permitted to remain on the skin or gently removed with a soft cloth. It is dispensed in one-pint containers.

Steroid-Containing Lotions and Solutions. SYNALAR SOLUTION, 0.01 PER CENT (fluocinolone acetonide) (Syntex Laboratories). The vehicle is propylene glycol with citric acid added as a preservative. It is especially useful in hairy and intertriginous areas, and can be used on the scalp overnight under a plastic bag or a shower cap. It is available in 20- and 60-ml. plastic squeeze bottles.

CORDRAN LOTION (Dista Products). Composition: 0.05 per cent flurandrenolone in glycerine, stearic acid, cetyl alcohol, glycerile monostearate, mineral oil, polyoxyl 40 stearate, menthol, methyl and propyl parabens and water. Cordran Lotion is easy to apply and useful in acute and subacute dermatoses. Available in 15- and 60-ml. plastic squeeze bottles, but rather expensive.

KENALOG LOTION (Squibb). Composition: 0.1 and 0.025 per cent triamcinolone acetonide. The base includes propylene glycol, cetyl and stearyl alcohols and methyl and propyl parabens. It is dispensed in 15- and 60-ml. plastic squeeze bottles. Kenalog Lotion is very effective for seborrheic dermatitis on the face and in intertriginous areas.

Special-Purpose Lotions. ANTIFUNGAL. *Dermatophytes: Halotex Solution* (Westwood). Halotex is haloprogin 3-iodo-2-propynyl 2,4,5-trichlorophenyl ether. It is available also as a cream. Halotex is useful for the topical treatment of trichophyton infections, as well as infections with Microsporum and Epidermophyton infections. It is effective treatment for tinea versicolor, but because large areas are involved, somewhat expensive. It is ineffective treatment for Candida infections. One per cent solution is available in 10- and 30-ml. squeeze bottles with a controlled drop tip and the cream in 15- and 30-gm. tubes.

Tinactin Solution. Composition: 1 per cent tolnaftate solution with butylated hydroxytoluene in a vehicle of polyethylene glycol. It is effective against Trichophyton, Microsporum and Epidermophyton species of fungi, as well as for the latter because of the large amount required. Remember that Tinactin is ineffective against Candida. It is dispensed as a 10-ml. plastic squeeze bottle and is also available as a cream or powder. Recently, Tinactin preparations have become available "over the counter."

Lotrimin Solution (Delbay Pharmaceuticals, Inc.). Lotrimin solution is clotrimazole 1 per cent in polyethylene glycol. Lotrimin is active against Trichophyton, Microsporum and Epidermophyton as well as *Candida albicans*. It is supplied in 10-ml. and 30-ml. plastic bottles, and is available also as a 1 per cent cream.

Candida. Fungizone Lotion (Amphotericin B) (Squibb). Composition: 3 per cent amphotericin B in a vehicle containing thimerosal, titanium dioxide, guar gum, propylene glycol, cetyl alcohol, stearyl alcohol and other ingredients including methyl and propyl parabens. Apply two to four times daily. It is effective against *Candida albicans* infections. It is available in 30-ml. plastic squeeze bottles. Fungizone Lotion discolors fabrics, but the stain may be removed by applying a standard cleaning fluid. It is available also as Fungizone cream 3 per cent and ointment 3 per cent.

Using a fine brush, Fungizone Lotion may be applied under the cuticle two to three times daily as effective treatment for chronic Candida paronychia.

Tinea Versicolor. Tinver Solution (Barnes-Hind). Composition: 25 per cent sodium thiosulfate, 1 per cent salicylic acid, 10 per cent isopropyl alcohol, propylene glycol, menthol, disodium edetate, colloidal alumina and water. Apply after showering, twice daily, for tinea versicolor only. However, it is less effective than Selsun in the treatment of tinea versicolor. It is dispensed in 5-ounce plastic squeeze bottles.

ANTIPARASITIC. Apply gamma benzene hexachloride lotion after showering and leave on 24 hours, then wash thoroughly. Second and third applications may be made at weekly intervals. All clothing and bed linen must be laundered.

Eurax Cream (Geigy). Contains 10 per cent N-ethyl-o-crotonotoluide in a cream base. It is used for treatment of scabies and is also an excellent antipruritic, but it should never be applied to acutely inflamed skin.

Baths

For treatment of a widespread dermatitis, baths are antipruritic and mildly anti-inflammatory. Fill the tub half full of lukewarm water and bathe the patient for 15 to 30 minutes. The bathroom must be well ventilated when volatile tars are used.

Aveeno Colloidal Oatmeal (Cooper Laboratories). This preparation is a concentrated colloid fraction of oatmeal which is useful in the treatment of widespread poison ivy or oak dermatitis, diaper rash, atopic dermatitis and contact dermatitis. Add one cup to a tub of warm water once or twice daily. For infants, add one or two tablespoonfuls to the bathinette. It is available in 1-pound and 4-pound boxes, plain and "oilated." Do not use the oilated type for treatment of acute oozing dermatitis. Individual dose packets are also supplied.

Soyaloid Colloidal Bath (Dome Laboratories). This is a colloidal soya protein complex with 2 per cent polyvinyl pyrrolidone. It is very valuable for the treatment of diaper dermatitis, poison ivy or poison oak and sunburn. Dissolve one packet in a tub of warm water, or two to three tablespoonfuls to each gallon of warm water for an infant's bath.

Potassium Permanganate Baths. These are used for generalized weeping dermatoses; they have some deodorizing properties. Crush 12 300-mg. tablets between two spoons and dissolve the powder by shaking into one quart of lukewarm water. Pour the mixture into a tub of tepid water; this will produce a concentration of about 1:20,000. The particles of potassium permanganate must completely dissolve, since tiny crystals may burn the skin if sat upon; they will also stain any cracks in the porcelain.

Lubricating Baths. These include *Alpha-Keri* (Westwood), *Domol* (Dome Laboratories), *Aveenol* (Cooper Laboratories), *Lubath* (Texas Pharmacal) and *Nutraspa* (Owen Laboratories). Baths are very useful for treatment of dry and pruritic skin, such as from ichthyosis, psoriasis, and atopic dermatitis. They can also be used after showering or sponge bathing, and for general cleansing of dry skin.

Tars. Tar baths may be used for the treatment of widespread dermatoses such as psoriasis, atopic dermatitis, seborrheic dermatitis, and other such diseases in older children and adolescents. The room must be kept well ventilated during treatment. Avoid excessive exposure of treated skin to direct sunlight for three to four days.

Liquor Carbonis Detergens (N.F.). This preparation contains crude coal tar with quillaja, a foaming agent also known as soap bark. Add ½ to 1 ounce to a tub full of water.

Zetar Emulsion (Dermik Laboratories). Zetar emulsion contains 50 per cent colloidal crude coal tar. Three to five capfuls placed directly under the open water tap usually suffice. Available in 6 ounce bottles.

Polytar Bath (Stiefel Laboratories). Polytar Bath is a combination of 25 per cent polytar, which is a blend of juniper tar, pine tar, coal tar solution, polyunsaturated vegetable oil and water-dispersible solubilized crude coal tar, with 25 per cent butyl stearate in a water-miscible emulsion base. It may be used for psoriasis and chronic atopic dermatitis, lichen planus and other dermatoses. It does not discolor the hair, skin or tub. Add two to three capfuls to an 8-inch tub of water.

Creams and Ointments

The most important characteristic of creams and ointments is their ability to be spread evenly over the skin. The fatty component may be composed of (1) animal fat, such as lard or wool fat; (2) mineral substances, such as petrolatum; or (3) vegetable oils. With the addition of emulsifiers, it is possible to incorporate large amounts of water. When rubbed onto the skin, the water evaporates slowly, producing a cooling effect. The cholesterolization of yellow petrolatum produces artificial lanolin-like materials. Aquaphor and Eucerin are the most frequently employed preparations of this type, and they have justifiably found wide acceptance as effective emollients.

Creams are cosmetically more attractive than ointments because they tend to "vanish" when rubbed into the skin. They are less occlusive than ointments, and also cannot be used in intertriginous or hairy areas or for treatment of acute weeping dermatitis.

The useful ointments and creams include the following: *Lubriderm Cream* (Texas Pharmacal), *Unibase* (Parke, Davis), *Aquaphor* (Duke Laboratories), *Nivea Cream* (Duke Laboratories), *Keri Cream* (Westwood Pharmaceuticals), *Nutraderm* (Owen Laboratories).

A useful tar-containing ointment is *Pragmatar* (Smith Kline & French), which contains a coal tar distillate, cetyl alcohol, 3 per cent precipitated sulfur and 3 per cent salicylic acid in an oil and water emulsion base. Pragmatar is particularly useful in the treatment of dandruff and "cradle cap." For treatment of infants' scalps, it should be diluted by mixing in equal parts with either Aristocort Topical Cream 0.1 per cent, or a water-miscible vehicle.

The addition of 10 per cent urea as in *Aquacare HP* (Herbert Laboratories) and *Carmol Cream* (Ingram) provides considerable increase in emolliency and is useful for long-term treatment of keratosis pilaris.

The addition of 5 per cent lactic acid to a water-miscible base such as Unibase or Aquaphor is useful for treatment of very dry skin and ichthyosis.

Pastes

Pastes consist of semisolid mixtures of a powder and ointment base. In pediatrics the one most frequently prescribed is *Lassar's paste* U.S.P., also known as "zinc oxide ointment," which contains 25 gm. each of zinc oxide and starch or talc, with 50 per cent white petrolatum.

Pastes absorb moisture and have a drying effect. They are best applied on gauze or to the skin with a spatula or tongue depressor.

Medications are released much more slowly from pastes than from creams and ointments. They are useful in the treatment of chronic dermatitis and have been extensively employed for diaper dermatitis.

Anthralin, 0.1 to 0.4 per cent, in plain zinc oxide paste "hardened" with the addition of 5 per cent hard paraffin and 0.2 to 0.4 per cent salicylic acid, has been found useful in treating individual lesions of psoriasis. Since anthralin stains the skin and can never be used around the eyes, it is impractical for infants and young children. When used over wide areas of skin, anthralin may be absorbed and produce renal damage.

Powders

Powders are soothing, absorb moisture and protect the skin by reducing friction. They are chemically inert and are used chiefly for prophylaxis, as in intertriginous areas to prevent miliaria. Apply as a fine film which will not cake or form lumps when wet. Frequent application is advisable.

Kaolin and Talc.   Kaolin and talc in equal parts, with the addition of 0.5 per cent spermaceti for added greasiness, is a valuable "general-use" powder.

ZeaSORB (Stiefel Laboratories).   This is a medicated powder containing 45 per cent microporous cellulose, 0.5 per cent hexachlorophene, 0.5 per cent parchlorometaxyallantoinate. ZeaSORB is useful for its water-absorbing capacity and also because it is mildly antibacterial and antifungal.

Neosporin Powder (Burroughs Wellcome).   This preparation contains polymyxin B, neomycin sulfate and zinc bacitracin in a powder base of lactose. It should not be used in intertriginous areas because of the likelihood of sensitization to neomycin. It is available in 10-gm. shaker-top containers.

Mycostatin Topical Powder (Squibb). Mycostatin Topical Powder contains nystatin, a specific antibiotic for moniliasis. Particularly useful in intertriginous areas for treatment of *Candida albicans,* it may also be used as a prophylactic measure. It is available in plastic squeeze bottles of 15 gm.

Tinactin Powder (Schering).   Tinactin Powder contains 1 per cent tolnaftate in cornstarch and talc. It may be used for the daytime treatment of tinea pedis but probably is most effective as a mild prophylactic against recurrence.

Corn Starch.   Corn starch is useless as a therapeutic agent and tends to cake and irritate the skin, providing an excellent medium for growth of bacteria and fungi, especially *Candida albicans.* It should never be recommended and its use should be discouraged whenever possible.

Topical Steroids

Probably the most overused class of medications today are topical steroids. Nevertheless, they are of undisputed value as anti-inflammatory and antipruritic agents.

Triamcinolone Acetonide (Aristocort, Lederle) (Kenalog, Squibb).   This is available in 0.1 and 0.025 per cent cream, lotion or ointment. Aristocort is now available as a 0.5 per cent cream which is very useful for short-term treatment of small, stubborn lesions, especially lichen simplex chronicus and psoriasis. Aristocort A cream and ointment 0.1 and 0.5 per cent are compounded in a hydrophilic base somewhat more "ointment-like" than creams. These preparations are very useful where there is dryness and fissuring. Aristogel and Aristoderm Foam are also supplied.

Kenalog topical preparations include cream (0.025 per cent, 0.1 per cent, and 0.5 per cent), lotion (0.025 and 0.1 per cent), ointment (0.025, 0.1 and 0.5 per cent) and spray. The indications for Kenalog are the same as for Aristocort; Kenalog spray is especially useful for treatment of sunburn, insect bites and poison oak dermatitis.

Fluocinolone Acetonide.   Synalar (Syntex) is available as a cream (0.01 or 0.025 per cent, the latter also with neomycin), ointment (0.025 per cent) or solution (0.01 per cent). Synalar-HP cream contains 0.2 per cent fluocinolone acetonide.

Flurandrenolone Acetonide.   Cordran (Lilly) is available as cream, ointment and lotion and also with neomycin. Cordran tape in two lengths is also available.

Betamethasone.   Valisone (Schering), available as a cream, ointment or spray, is very effective as is Diprosone cream and ointment (0.05 per cent) (betamethasone dipropionate), which is reported to possess a rapid onset of action and is useful in contact dermatitis, atopic dermatitis and psoriasis. It is available in 15- and 45-gm. tubes. *Lidex* (Syntex) and *Synemol* (Syntex) are also effective and widely used.

Nonfluorinated corticosteroids include *Tridesilon Creme* and *Ointment* (both 0.05 per cent), containing prednisolone acetonide. This preparation may be safer for long-term use than the potent fluorinated corticosteroids. Available in 15- and 60-gm. tubes and in 5-lb.

jars. Another preparation *Nutracort Gel,* containing 1 per cent hydrocortisone gel, is especially good because it does not contain parabens as preservatives, but citric acid, which is practically nonsensitizing. *Halog* cream, Halcinonide cream 0.1 per cent, is supplied in 15- and 60-gm. tubes and 240-gm. jars.

Occlusive Dressings. Topical steroids are covered with a thin plastic film followed by a covering of stockinette, cotton glove, stocking, T-shirt, pair of shorts or Ace bandage. Occlusive dressings are very effective in the treatment of chronic dermatitis, such as psoriasis, lichen planus, lichen simplex chronicus (localized neurodermatitis), atopic dermatitis and other conditions. Treatment usually is overnight for a period of 8 to 12 hours. No more than 10 per cent of the body should be treated at any one time, since significant systemic absorption may occur, especially with the fluorinated corticosteroids. Complications include an objectionable odor, folliculitis, sweat retention, secondary irritation and infection. Late sequelae may include atrophy and striae.

For treatment of small and medium-sized lesions of psoriasis, lichen planus and other chronic dermatoses, Cordran Tape (Dista Products) is useful. Before application the area must be cleansed gently to remove scales, crusts, and dried exudate and any traces of medications. Dry the skin thoroughly and apply the tape smoothly against the skin, usually leaving it in place for about 12 hours. The adhesive consists of a synthetic copolymer of an acrylic ester.

Another very useful method of occlusive therapy is a plastic suit, which retains body heat and causes slight maceration of the skin and thus greater penetration of medication. The suit material is a washable vinyl with elastic at the waist, ankles, neck and wrist. This form of treatment must be employed very cautiously in children, since significant systemic absorption of corticosteroid may occur. It is usually better to treat the upper half of the body one night and the lower half the next. Plastic suits are available from the Slim-Ez Company, Box 648, Carrabelle, Florida 32322, and are sold in many sporting goods stores.

Topical Antibiotics

While the efficacy of topical antibiotics has been questioned recently, the most used are those which are rarely employed systemically, such as neomycin, bacitracin, polymyxin and gramicidin. Other therapeutic agents often classed with antibiotics are Vioform and Furacin.

Neosporin-G Cream (Burroughs Wellcome). Neosporin-G Cream contains polymyxin B, neomycin sulfate and gramicidin in a water-miscible vanishing-cream base. Neosporin ointment contains polymyxin B, zinc bacitracin and neomycin sulfate in white petrolatum. Both the cream and ointment are employed for bacterial infections such as impetigo, ecthyma, and secondarily infected dermatoses. The ointment is more effective in the treatment of impetigo than is the cream. Neomycin is a fairly common skin sensitizer. It is available in tubes of 15 gm.

Erythromycin Ointment (Ilotycin ointment) (Dista). This is a better choice for topical treatment of pyoderma than neomycin, and concomitant systemic antibiotics are indicated in most cases because of the possibility of renal complications from B-hemolytic streptococci. Erythromycin topically is almost nonsensitizing.

Garamycin (Schering). Garamycin contains 0.1 per cent gentamicin sulfate as cream or ointment. It is fairly effective for topical treatment in primary and secondary bacterial infections of the skin. It is available in 15-gm. tubes.

Chloromycetin Cream (Parke-Davis). Chloromycetin cream contains chloramphenicol in a water-miscible ointment base with 0.1 per cent propyl paraben. It is useful in superficial skin infections, but can be sensitizing, especially when used over long periods of time. It is supplied in 1-gm. tubes.

Mycolog (Squibb). Mycolog contains nystatin, neomycin sulfate, gramicidin and triamcinolone acetonide. It is one of the most overused preparations in dermatology today, and is often employed without clear-cut indications for its use. The cream contains several possible allergic sensitizers: neomycin and nystatin, ethylenediamine and parabens. The manufacturer does not sufficiently emphasize the importance of sensitization to ethylenediamine in its advertising, in my opinion. Formerly it also contained thimerosal. Striae may result after prolonged use in intertriginous areas. Mycolog should be restricted to short-term use in treatment of conditions where it is clearly indicated, such as in *Candida albicans* infections (moniliasis). Because the ointment does not contain ethylenediamine, it is safer to use although its occlusiveness makes it less desirable for hairy, intertriginous areas.

Sunscreens

Sunscreens are topical preparations to protect the skin from the effects of ultraviolet light. They are either (1) "barriers," which generally impede the passage of ultraviolet light or (2) screens which absorb the light at a particular wavelength. They are extremely valuable for sun-sensitive persons and those with sunlight aggravated disease, such as porphyria, xeroderma pigmentosum, lupus erythematosus and polymorphous light eruptions.

A-Fil (Texas Pharmacal). A-Fil contains 5 per cent titanium dioxide with 5 per cent menthyl anthranilate in a vanishing cream base tinted to blend with the skin color. The titanium dioxide physically screens out wavelengths of light up to 3900 Å, while menthyl anthranilate absorbs the sunburning wavelengths between 2950 and 3200 Å.

Pabafilm (Owen Laboratories). This contains an amino benzoate in an ethyl alcohol base. It effectively blocks out ultraviolet radiation in the 2900 to 3250 Å range. The base is greaseless, dries quickly and will provide protection up to 2 to 3 hours after swimming and 8 to 12 hours in the absence of excessive moisture.

Uval (Dorsey) contains 10 per cent sulisobenzone, a benzophenone in an alcohol-free base.

PreSun (Westwood Pharmaceuticals). PreSun contains 5 per cent paraaminobenzoic acid in an alcohol base with moisturizers. As with Pabafilm, the patient will tan but not burn. PreSun may stain clothing.

Eclipse (Herbert Laboratories) contains 3 per cent glyceryl PABA, 3 per cent octyl-dimethyl PABA in a slightly moisturizing base. Patients sensitive to benzocaine may develop cross reactions to Eclipse, so pre-testing for two days prior to use is advisable.

Sundown (Johnson & Johnson) contains 3.3 per cent octyldimethyl PABA in a non-greasy, water barrier vehicle.

RVP (Paul B. Elder). RVP contains red petrolatum improved with 5 per cent surfactants for easy application. RVP absorbs the sunburn spectrum and additional ultraviolet light to 3400 Å. It resists perspiration and water and can be used around the eyes and lips. It is, however, very greasy. RVPaque is skin tinted and contains zinc oxide, a physical barrier to sunlight. RVPlus contains titanium dioxide, also a physical barrier.

Solbar (Person & Convey). This contains 3 per cent oxybenzone, a benzophene. Solbar is a broad-spectrum ultraviolet sun protective lotion which, after application, dries to a transparent film which has high skin retention, but a "tight" feel which is objectionable to many patients.

Masking Preparations

Covermark (Lydia O'Leary). Covermark is a neutral, opaque, greaseless cream which is a most effective agent for concealing birth-marks, many types of scars and skin discolorations. It is particularly useful for covering lesions of vitiligo, port wine stains and nevi. Ten shades are available and the company provides professional help in selecting the proper shade for the skin and instructing patients in its application. A Lydia O'Leary finishing powder is also available. When applied with skill, Covermark can be a very effective masking agent.

Soaps

Germicidal soaps provide adjunctive therapy for skin infections, especially in prophylaxis for recurrent furunculosis. They are also effective deodorants. Incorporated bactericidal agents include halogenated salicylanilides and carbanilides. The halogenated salicylanilides have occasionally caused allergic contact photodermatitis. Soaps containing one or more of these substances include Dial (Armour), Lifebuoy (Lever Brothers), Safeguard (Procter and Gamble), Zest (Procter & Gamble) and Irish Spring (Colgate-Palmolive).

pHisoHex (Winthrop) contains 3 per cent hexachlorophene in an emulsion. It is an effective surgical scrub and bacteriostatic skin cleanser. It should not be used on burned or denuded skin or over wide body areas. It is now available only on prescription.

Betadine (Purdue Frederick Company). Betadine is a topical microbiocide containing a detergent with iodine and polyvinyl pyrrolidine. It is also available as an aerosol spray, surgical scrub, douche, vaginal gel, mouthwash, gargle and skin cleanser. In pyodermas, Betadine Skin Cleanser is a useful topical adjunct to systemic antimicrobial therapy.

Super-Fatted Soaps. Addition of extra fat, such as lanolin, cold cream or mineral oil, to soap during manufacture makes a soap "super-fatted." The superfat is said to produce a soap somewhat less alkaline than ordinary soap, which hopefully will be less irritating to the skin.

In pediatric practice, super-fatted soaps are used most commonly in the treatment of children with atopic dermatitis and ichthyosis. The effectiveness of these soaps has been overemphasized, but when used in place of ordinary soap they may play a minor therapeutic role. Preparations include Basis (Texas Pharmacal), Oilatum (Stiefel), Emulave (Cooper Laboratories) and Lowila (Westwood).

Shampoos

Regular. Sebulex (Westwood), Ionil (Owen), Head & Shoulders (Procter & Gamble) and Fostex Cream (Westwood) are safe for use in children. Selenium-, cadmium- and zinc-containing shampoos are not indicated for use in pediatric patients.

Tar Shampoos. Tar shampoos are useful for treatment of scalp seborrhea and psoriasis. The most frequently used tar shampoos are Ionil T (Owen), Sebutone (Westwood), Polytar Shampoo (Stiefel) and Zetar Shampoo (Dermik). Remember that tar shampoos may stain the hair a yellowish color.

Antiparasitic Shampoos. Gamma benzene hexachloride shampoo is valuable for treatment of pediculosis capitis pubis. Shampoo the hair for a full 4 minutes, rinse and then dry with a towel. Repeat after 24 hours and once in one week if necessary. Do not use more than two times within one week.

Topical Acne Preparations

Liquid and bar skin cleansers (Fostex and Pernox, Westwood; Komex, Barnes-Hind Laboratories; Acne-Aid, Stiefel; Acnaveen, Cooper Laboratories; and others) contribute to cleansing and degreasing the skin. They should be used on an average of one to two times daily, otherwise excessive dryness can result, which itself may aggravate acne. Many acne patients overuse soaps and abrasive cleansers in the mistaken belief that lack of cleanliness is a major cause of their problem.

Retin-A (Johnson & Johnson) is a tretinoin and it is very useful in the treatment of comedone and mild and moderate papulopustular acne, especially in patients with "oily" skin. It is ineffective in severe papulopustular acne and conglobate acne. Some patients, especially fair-skinned patients with dry skin, cannot tolerate the irritation produced by tretinoin; allergic sensitization is rare. Apply once daily at bedtime. It may be used every other night, alternating with a preparation containing benzoyl peroxide. Retin-A is available as a gel 0.025 per cent in 15-gm. tubes, as a cream 0.05 per cent and 0.1 per cent in 20-gm. tubes, and as a liquid 0.05 per cent and as swabs packaged in aluminum foil, 0.05 per cent.

Benzoyl Peroxide. In concentrations of 5 or 10 per cent (Desquam-X 5 or -X 10 gels, Westwood; Persa-Gel 5 per cent and 10 per cent, Texas Pharmacal; 5 Benzagel and 10 Benzagel, Dermik) benzoyl peroxide produces peeling and drying and may possibly decrease the number of comedones after several months of use. Apply once daily with fingertips after first testing in a small area, because occasionally benzoyl peroxide is a contact sensitizer.

Chemical Cautery

Cauterizing chemicals such as salicylic acid, bichloroacetic acid, silver nitrate, and cantharidin should be used with caution in children, but they are safe if the directions are carefully followed. Caustic agents such as phenol, fuming nitric acid and monochloroacetic acid should never be used in the treatment of children. Phenol especially is rapidly absorbed through intact skin and, following treatment of large areas, severe renal damage may result. Monochloroacetic acid is a highly reactive substance which is rapidly destructive to tissue.

Because chemical cautery may be relatively painless at the time of application, it can be preferable to other destructive methods of treatment, such as liquid nitrogen and electrodesiccation.

Salicylic Acid. Salicylic acid, 40 per cent, in an elastic adhesive plaster has been used in the treatment of plantar warts for a very long time. The plaster must be cut to the exact size of the wart, applied firmly and covered with a strip of adhesive tape. This should be allowed to remain against the skin for 4 days, after which the dressing is removed and the white keratotic tissue is pared using a number 15 blade. A new plaster may be applied at the time and the process repeated until the verruca disappears, usually after four to six treatments. Recurrences are common, however.

Silver Nitrate Sticks. Silver nitrate sticks (available from Arzol) are 75 per cent silver nitrate with 25 per cent potassium nitrate. Moisten the tip with tap water before use and apply to fissures and ulcers to remove excess granulation tissue.

Cantharone (Cantharidin collodion) (Ingram). This preparation consists of 0.7 per cent cantharidin in an acetone and flexible collodion vehicle. Cantharidin is a colorless, crystalline scale obtained from cantharides or dried Spanish flies. It is used chiefly for removal of periungual and plantar warts and molluscum contagiosum. The method is relatively painless during application, but marked discomfort may be experienced after 24 hours. The method leaves no scar.

For periungual warts, apply the substance directly to the wart after paring down excessive keratin with a number 15 blade. If pinpoint bleeding should occur, this can be quickly controlled by touching the bleeding points with a drop of bichloracetic acid. After the film of cantharone has begun to dry and a white membrane appears, cover the wart with a nonporous, waterproof adhesive. Keep the area dry and the bandage in place for 24 to 72 hours, after which the patient replaces the tape with a Band-Aid. In 14 to 21 days, pare off the dead tissue, first obtaining a cleavage line which should be easily found at this time.

Cantharone may be reapplied to any remaining wart tissue. Often one or two treatments suffice.

For plantar warts, pare away the keratotic dead tissue on the surface first, then apply Cantharone generously to the entire lesion. A cut-out cushion bandage made from moleskin is then applied and the whole dressing covered with nonporous tape. The patient should remove the dressing in 2 to 3 days, reapplying the cushion bandage for comfort. The patient returns to the physician in 14 to 21 days for paring of dead tissue and re-treatment if necessary. Two to three treatments often are sufficient.

For molluscum contagiosum, coat each lesion with Cantharone, using a small wooden stick, and cover with a small piece of tape. The patient should return in 1 week and any new lesions are treated in the same manner. The patient should remove the tape after about 6 hours, however.

Podophyllin. Although not a caustic, podophyllin is commonly used in the treatment of venereal warts or condylomata acuminata. Podophyllum resin is derived from dried rhizomes and roots of *Podophyllum peltatum* or May apple. A specific treatment for condylomata, podophyllin is ineffective in the treatment of other types of warts.

Apply a 20 to 25 per cent solution in tincture of benzoin directly to the lesions with a wooden applicator stick. Take special care not to permit the liquid to extend to any extent over normal skin. Instruct the patient to wash the area thoroughly with soap and water using a washcloth in about 12 hours, and to return for re-treatment in 4 to 5 days. Usually three to four treatments suffice.

Podophyllin is an antimitotic agent, and if transferred to eyes by the fingers, can cause severe keratitis. For this reason, perhaps one should use it only in adolescents and older children.

Cryosurgery

Liquid nitrogen is available from the suppliers of liquid gas and can be stored in loosely stoppered thermos bottles. One pint is sufficient to treat 30 to 40 patients and will last for a day or two. With long cotton applicator sticks the liquid is applied with *intermittent,* firm pressure for 10 to 30 seconds, until the lesion blanches and an areola of frozen tissue appears around the lesion. Within a few hours a blister will form which will carry the verrucous tissue into its roof. As sloughing occurs during the next 2 to 3 weeks the wart comes off, leaving no scar. Frequently a small "core" of verrucous tissue remains behind, which can be re-treated with liquid nitrogen in 3 to 4 weeks.

Skin Diseases of the Newborn

GUINTER KAHN, M.D.

SKIN CARE OF THE NEWBORN

Do not assault the skin of the newborn infant with chemical and mechanical cleansers. A soft cloth soaked with tepid tap water may be used to remove blood and meconium from the skin following delivery. Vernix caseosa should be removed only from the face because the material is not as aesthetic as it is physiologic in mitigating the effect of harmful environmental substances. The remaining substance will come off by itself during the hospital stay. Tap water soaks with or without soap may be used to remove urine and stool from the diaper area. Seventy per cent isopropyl alcohol is applied onto and around the cord for two minutes twice daily to limit colonization about the cord. Isolate infants with infected cords and apply antibiotic ointment to the nose and cord, and 3 per cent hexachlorophene to the rest of the skin once or twice. Culture the infected areas and the suspected areas of the nursery. Hexachlorophene should be rinsed off thoroughly and should be used only on full term infants. Because of the recent controversy regarding this use of hexachlorophene, the manufacturer's instructions should be read carefully. Enforce meticulous hygiene and hand washing of nursery personnel. Use iodophors and appropriate epidemiological surveillance. Skin care of the premature infant is similar to that of the mature infant.

TRANSIENT LESIONS OF THE SKIN

Judicious neglect and masterly inactivity combined with appropriate counseling to parents is the treatment of choice for many of the skin lesions seen during the neonatal period.

Birth Injuries. Contusions, erosions, and hematomas rarely cause difficulties other than contributing to anemia or hyperbilirubinemia. Even though resorption may take several weeks, no treatment is indicated. Phototherapy and exchange transfusions for hyperbilirubinemia are discussed elsewhere. Neurosurgical consultation should be obtained for any infant with a depressed skull fracture secondary to a cephalhematoma. Erosions secondary to pressure necrosis of difficult deliveries should be kept dry and clean. When secondary infection occurs, identification of the organism determines the choice of antibiotic after moist gentle debridement.

Aplasia Cutis Congenita. Differentiate this congenital absence of skin from pressure necrosis. Most frequently it occurs as solitary or multiple lesions on the vertex of the scalp involving any layer of the skin and even underlying bone. Familial cases are reported, but mode of inheritance is not known. Therapy is indicated later when the atrophic scar may require cosmetic surgery.

Milia. Milia are superficial epidermal inclusion cysts which are eliminated by normal desquamation of skin. Assure the family that no scarring results. Their counterpart in the mucosa of the mouth is called Epstein's pearls.

Miliaria. The crystalline form of sweat retention is common to infants who are overheated and overclothed in the nursery. Control temperature and humidity, and avoid occlusive clothing or emollients. Allow free evaporation from the surface of the skin and the lesions disappear spontaneously without sequelae.

Transient Neonatal Pustular Melanosis. This recently described condition presents at birth with vesicles which become pustules and disappear within 72 hours leaving dark spots. Lesions are sterile and contain neutrophils. Pigment leaves in three weeks to three months.

Toxic Erythema of the Newborn. This erythema is followed by papulovesicles or pustules which must be differentiated from transient neonatal pustular melanosis. The lesions usually occur about two days after birth and are filled with eosinophils rather than neutrophils. No therapy is indicated for either condition even when pustules are present. However, both conditions must be differentiated from the rare congenital form of cutaneous candidiasis in which the direct (potassium hydroxide or Giemsa) smear shows mycelia and spores.

Sebaceous Gland Hyperplasia. Infants with multiple nonpalpable, yellow, tiny spots on and around the nose have enlarged sebaceous glands, made more prominent by translucent neonatal epidermis. Maternal androgens stimulate the glands so their enlargement is temporary.

Acne Neonatorum. Sebaceous gland hyperplasia plus inflammation may result in the formation of comedones, nodules and cysts in infants. Hormone levels are normal but the gland is overresponsive to androgen. The condition may be temporary. Treatment is difficult and conservative. Do not apply irritating acne salves because infants may rub them into their eyes. For severe acne, 50 mg. of erythomycin daily or 15 mg./lb./day for three weeks may help.

Mottling. Lace-like cutis marmorata is a physiologic vascular pattern developed by neonates exposed to lowered room temperature. Rewarming relieves it.

Harlequin Color Change. This bizarre vascular color change occurs in neonates who are turned onto their sides and develop a sharply demarcated erythematous flush of the upper half of the body. The episodes occur in low birth weight infants during the first week of life. The flush lasts seconds to minutes.

Sucking Blisters. Small blisters on the radial surface of the forearm, dorsum of the fingers and central portion of the upper lip are presumed to occur in utero from sucking by the infant. The lesions rapidly dissolve without therapy.

DISORDERS DUE TO TRANSPLACENTAL PASSAGE

Drugs. The fetus exposed to drugs may present with a nonspecific dermatitis that will leave when the drug leaves the tissue.

Antibody Transfer. Immunoglobulin G readily passes through the placenta from the mother to the fetus and may result in neonatal lupus erythematosus. In the newborn, lupus erythematosus may be polymorphous or typical. Lesions usually fade spontaneously during infancy but may leave atrophic scars.

SUBCUTANEOUS DISEASES

Sclerema Neonatorum. Premature infants subject to life-threatening conditions (metabolic acidosis, hypoglycemia, hypothermia) are susceptible to diffuse hardening of the skin. Severe cold injury and malnutrition play a role in causing the diffuse hardening that causes the skin to become shiny and tight. All attempts must be made to maintain normal body temperature while treating the underlying disease.

Subcutaneous Fat Necrosis. In otherwise healthy newborn infants with sharply demarcated blue nodules or plaques on their backs, lesions spontaneously resolve over a period of weeks without scarring. Fluctuant lesions are carefully drained by needle aspiration. Rarely infants with associated hypercalcemia and visceral complications require low calcium intake, low vitamin D and systemic corticosteroid therapy.

BLISTERING DISEASES

Blistering diseases that occur in the newborn period are discussed in the section on transient diseases (transient neonatal pustular melanosis, toxic erythema neonatorum and sucking blisters), in the section on infectious diseases (impetigo, herpes simplex, syphilis), and in the section on inherited diseases (epidermolysis bullosa and bullous ichthyosis). Other blistering diseases of unknown etiology are discussed throughout the chapter and include acrodermatitis enteropathica, incontinentia pigmenti, mastocytosis, and toxic epidermal necrolysis. Biopsy and Giemsa stain of blister material are valuable aids that guide therapy.

INFECTIOUS DISEASES

The occurrence and treatment of venereal diseases, herpes simplex, varicella, congenital rubella, and listeriosis are discussed elsewhere.

NEVI

Vascular and pigmentary nevi are also discussed elsewhere, but the author emphasizes that black or malignant-appearing nevi should be biopsied before the newborn leaves the hospital. The only vascular nevi that should be treated with prednisone (approximately 1 mg./kg./day for 3 to 6 weeks) are those that meet one of the following criteria: (1) encroach on a vital structure, (2) trap platelets and induce thrombocytopenia, (3) induce high output cardiac failure, and (4) cause severe parental psychological difficulties.

INHERITED SKIN DISEASES

Many inherited diseases present at the time of birth and are discussed throughout this chapter. The therapy is to recognize the disease, utilize existing genetic data, and advise or refer parents to a genetic counselor for information about the risk of recurrence and other precautions. Examples would be neurofibromatosis and adenoma sebaceum (tuberous sclerosis). Both are dominantly inherited and both become worse during pregnancy, puberty, or with the use of hormones (birth control pills).

Eruptions in the Diaper Area

GUINTER KAHN, M.D.

The primary cause of diaper area eruptions is the combination of wetness and Candida organisms. More than any other organism, Candida initiates primary irritancy dermatitis in the diaper area. Evidence substantiates that other organisms and chemicals play a lesser role than previously thought in the production of irritation that is known as diaper dermatitis. Previous discourses and admonitions about ammonia production, ammonia-producing bacteria, and ammonia-neutralizing agents are relatively unimportant. Predisposing factors which are more important

include inheritance of reactive skin that is easily irritated, tendency toward seborrheic diathesis of the anal and genitocrural folds and atopic diathesis. When diaper dermatitis becomes refractory to therapy, rule out systemic diseases such as syphilis, acrodermatitis enteropathica, and Letterer-Siwe disease.

Secondary factors are those which maintain wetness, such as continuous contact with a wet diaper, intensified by the moist heat produced by an impervious rubber or plastic cover. Sweat blockade and retention is secondary to continuous wetness. Other secondary factors include the numerous chemicals and medicaments that act as contact allergens and irritants to already wet or macerated skin. The diaper area also may fall prey to overly assiduous cleansing and treatment. An example is granuloma gluteale infantum, which is the formation of plumb-like nodules secondary to the application of strong steroid salves over a prolonged period of time. Similar lesions may appear from the application of talc (talc granuloma).

Prevent diaper dermatitis by promptly changing wet diapers and gently cleansing and drying the skin with each change. Note that Ivory, Zest and Lowila soaps are drying and irritating, whereas Dove, Oilatum, Neutrogena and Keri are neither drying nor irritating. After using the latter, carefully hold a hair dryer blowing cold air over the area for two minutes. If the eruption is mild, further therapy may not be necessary other than the time-honored application of zinc oxide paste and talcum powder to prevent recurrences. Zinc oxide paste protects the area from irritating chemicals, and talcum powder absorbs moisture and reduces friction. There is microscopic evidence that powder rubbed against opposing skin surfaces is somewhat irritating, therefore the value of powder in acute eruptions of the groin is not substantiated.

Because only 10 Candida organisms per square centimeter on wet gluteal surfaces can initiate diaper dermatitis, application of anticandidal agents is vital. Apply nystatin, amphotericin or miconazole cream or lotion after each diaper change on the first day of therapy. Thereafter, alternate anticandidal therapy with 1 per cent hydrocortisone cream applications. When redness persists and the eruption has the appearance of seborrheic dermatitis, contact dermatitis or refractory diaper dermatitis, use a stronger steroid cream or lotion such as triamcinolone, betamethasone valerate, or fluocinolone. Use stronger agents such as fluocinonide or halcinonide creams only in refractory cases, and for less than one month in order to avoid striae, granuloma gluteale infantum, and systemic side effects of corticosteroid absorption.

There are almost no indications for the use of topical antibiotics in the diaper area. Infections in this area such as impetigo, furunculosis, or ecthyma call for cultures and systemic antibiotics. Do not use local heat on the skin of an infant.

A general statement about the use of disposable diapers is that their added expense plus individual techniques of manufacture must be weighed against their convenience, and that the benefits of appropriately boiled and double rinsed diapers should be considered.

The essence of treatment of diaper dermatitis is prophylaxis: prevent excess heat, change diapers often, remove primary irritants, avoid contact allergens, apply the medications discussed above, and in refractory cases, rule out systemic diseases.

Contact Dermatitis

GEORGE F. WILGRAM, M.D.

Contact dermatitis is encountered much less frequently today than it was in the past, as the cosmetic, garment and jewelry industries have made great strides to prevent hypersensitivity reactions. Although contact dermatitis caused by metal, such as the nickel and chromium found in wrist watches, metal chains and buckles is still seen, the two most common types of contact dermatitis in America are contact dermatitis due to plants (poison ivy, poison oak, poison sumac) and shoe dermatitis.

Plant Dermatitis. Plant dermatitis can be readily diagnosed by a linear or arcuate arrangement of eczematous vesicles produced by the sweeping exposure to the plant oil. If exposure to poison ivy has been extensive, or if the patient has been "sensitized" by previous exposures, extensive involvement of the entire skin may occur. In such cases, eczematous lesions are found in areas of the skin where no actual contact took place. Such severe involvement usually requires the oral administration of steroids, anywhere between 20 and 80 mg. of prednisone per day for one or two weeks. After cessation of prednisone therapy, exacerbation of the sensitization process may take place because plant dermatitis due to poison ivy exposure may last up to six weeks. Milder and more simple cases are readily treated by cool compresses and the application of topical steroid creams.

Although the telephone companies have made great efforts to develop a method of de-

sensitization, none has proved to be successful as yet. The key is prevention of poison ivy rashes by avoiding exposure. Once fixed to the skin, the plant oil cannot be transferred to other areas of the skin of the patient or to the skin of other members in the surroundings. Clothes worn on the day of exposure should be washed thoroughly so that re-exposure to the plant oil in the clothes will not occur.

Shoe Dermatitis. Shoe dermatitis is still found, particularly as a result of athletic footwear, such as sneakers with plasticized rubber, and moccasins. Tannic acid and chromic salt preparations are the offending antigens. Shoe dermatitis is an eczematous eruption, usually well demarcated; it is usually located on the dorsum of the arches rather than on the soles, and it is bilateral and symmetrical. The most important feature in treatment is to identify the offending pair of shoes and to dispose of them; otherwise, the problem will persist. Additionally, cool compresses and the application of topical steroid preparations expedite the clearing of shoe dermatitis.

Rare Contact Dermatitis. Contact dermatitides due to toothpaste, lipstick, cosmetics, rubberized materials in garments, or air-borne contact dermatitis due to pollen, such as on occasion is found in the ragweed season, are rare. Applications of medications to the skin (antibiotic creams, lidocaine, antihistamine creams) may cause contact dermatitis. Treatment consists of avoiding the offending antigen and applying topical steroid preparations.

A special form of contact dermatitis is photo-contact dermatitis caused by the application of a sensitizing antigen to the skin, in combination with sun exposure. This form of contact dermatitis can occur after the application of perfumes, either as such or in soaps, or after the use of antibiotic creams. Photo-contact dermatitides occur exclusively in sun-exposed areas. By and large, photo-contact dermatitis is more common than it was in the past, but its recognition requires expert diagnostic acumen and usually a dermatologic consultation.

Patch Testing. With the exception of plant dermatitis, which is usually diagnosed by the linear or arcuate arrangement of spongiotic vesicles on the areas of exposure, contact dermatitis in many instances can be diagnosed definitively only after patch testing. The suspected antigen, if it is available in powder or in liquid form, should be sufficiently diluted so that there is no primary irritating effect. It should be applied in a 1:10 solution to the skin and covered with a Band-Aid, with provisions being made for air entry. Metals can be tested as such by taping them to the skin. A reading should be taken after 24 and 48 hours respectively. Sensitivity to a contact antigen manifests itself by a typical eczematous reaction, whereas an irritant reaction would present itself by edema, erythema and desquamation.

In supplementation of commonly suspected antigens which might be contacted in everyday living, there are specialized patch test kits available which are used mostly by dermatologists. A pediatrician will rarely find it necessary to perform a patch test himself and should rely on the consultation service of his dermatologic colleagues.

Patch testing should never be performed while contact dermatitis is active, as this may lead to severe exacerbation of the original contact dermatitis and also to generalized "sensitization." Patch testing is performed after all symptoms of the original contact dermatitis have subsided.

Atopic Dermatitis

NANCY B. ESTERLY, M.D., *and*
LAWRENCE M. SOLOMON, M.D.

Atopic dermatitis is characterized in the acute stage by erythema, papulovesicular lesions, oozing and crusting. When the dermatitis becomes chronic the skin is thickened, has increased markings (lichenification) and may be hypopigmented or hyperpigmented. Pruritus is the most distressing and universal symptom. Scaly dryness often compounds the problem and must be alleviated as well if therapy is to be effective. The approach to therapy will depend on the stage of the disease, extent of the involvement and the age of the child.

Cool compresses with tap water will alleviate a moist, oozing dermatitis and are indicated if the eczema is acute or secondarily infected. Compresses should be applied at least four times a day for 20 minutes.

Baths are beneficial at any stage of atopic dermatitis; the water should always be tepid, since extremes in temperature will exacerbate pruritus. The use of a bath oil such as Alpha Keri, Domol, NeutraSpa, Lubath or Aveenol will provide needed lubrication. Mild soaps (e.g., Dove, Lowila, Basis, Oilatum) used very sparingly and rinsed away thoroughly are acceptable. Colloids, such as Aveeno and Aveeno-oilated, may be added to the bath. Patients with dry skin should use a lubricant such as hydrophilic ointment, petrolatum or cold cream immediately after bathing.

Topical corticosteroids have become a mainstay in the treatment of atopic dermatitis.

The most effective preparations are the fluorinated steroids such as Synalar, Cordran, Aristocort, Kenalog, Valisone and Lidex. These agents should be applied 3 or 4 times a day, but the course of treatment should be limited in duration, particularly in infants and small children, because of the hazards of absorption, systemic side effects and unwanted local skin changes. One per cent hydrocortisone may be substituted as the dermatitis improves, and the frequency of application also may be decreased. The type of base (ointment or cream) selected will depend on the degree of dryness and on what the patient will tolerate. Creams are better for moist areas and ointments for dry plaques. Systemically administered corticosteroids are rarely, if ever, indicated in the treatment of atopic dermatitis.

The dry, thickened, lichenified stage of atopic dermatitis may also respond to the applications of a tar preparation. Crude coal tar in petrolatum (1 to 3 per cent) is fine, but a more cosmetically acceptable preparation is liquor carbonis detergens (LCD), a tar distillate, which can be incorporated into a cream or ointment base. Generally a 5 per cent concentration is efficacious when used three times a day, but the concentration may have to be adjusted depending on the response. LCD may also be combined with a corticosteroid in the base of choice.

If the scalp is scaly and itchy an antiseborrheic shampoo (Zetar, Sebulex, Fostex, Ionil, Zincon) may be prescribed. The patient should be instructed to leave the lathered shampoo on the scalp for 5 to 10 minutes prior to rinsing. For marked scalp involvement a steroid lotion (such as Synalar solution) or a gel (Fluorobate or Benisone) may be applied three times daily for a few days.

When pyoderma complicates atopic dermatitis, a systemic antibiotic may be indicated. If a streptococcal infection is suspected and organisms are cultured from the lesion, the patient should receive a 10-day course of penicillin. If there is known allergy to penicillin, erythromycin is the drug of choice. Staphylococcal pyoderma will respond to either systemic or topical therapy, depending on the extent and severity of the infection. Penicillin or erythromycin may be adequate, or, if a penicillin-resistant organism is present, a synthetic penicillin may be required. Polysporin ointment is an appropriate topical antibiotic.

Patients should avoid exposure to excessive heat and cold, windy weather, or rapidly changing ambient temperatures, since they have a deficient cutaneous vascular ability to adapt to these changes. The use of air conditioners during the summer and humidifiers during the winter may be helpful to modify extremes in temperature and humidity. Soft, lightweight cotton fabrics should be substituted for rough, scratchy materials such as wool and certain synthetic fabrics. Strenuous athletic activities should also be avoided. Swimming need not be prohibited providing the child applies a lubricant and/or other topical medications after coming out of the water. Soaps, perfumes, detergents, irritating chemicals or skin preparations may cause a superimposed primary irritant reaction. Atopic dermatitis may flare in times of stress, and efforts should be made to alleviate such situations without becoming totally permissive in disciplining the child. Skin testing is not advised because, although positive skin tests may be elicited, avoidance of these substances is unlikely to alter the course of the disease. Implicit in any treatment regimen is an honest and thorough discussion of the disorder with both parents and patient (when appropriate) concerning the nature of the eruption, the chronicity of its course, possible etiologic mechanisms, exacerbating factors, and the rational basis for use of the various types of medication.

Nummular Eczema. Nummular eczema will, in general, respond to the same therapeutic measures suggested for atopic dermatitis; however these lesions are often more refractory to therapy. For selected recalcitrant plaques it may be helpful to apply a fluorinated corticosteroid under polyethylene wrap for 8 to 12 hours on several consecutive days. For toddlers and small children it is advisable to carry out this procedure during the daytime hours, since wraps may be hazardous if applied at night.

Dyshidrotic Eczema. This type of eczema affects the hands and feet and is characterized by small deep-seated vesicles which are usually pruritic. Hyperhidrosis may be associated, and secondary infection is a common complication.

Compresses with cool tap water are helpful during the tense blister or weeping phase. Larger blisters should be drained, with blister tops left intact for protection of the underlying skin. Corticosteroid creams without occlusive wraps are the treatment of choice. Sedatives may also be helpful.

The hands should be adequately protected by cotton-lined rubber gloves from irritating substances. The feet should be kept dry by use of an unscented talcum powder, frequent changes of socks, and nonocclusive footwear.

Urticaria

GEORGE F. WILGRAM, M.D.

The pathogenesis of acute and chronic urticaria is entirely different and they have little in common except the final clinical manifestation, the urticarial wheal.

Acute Urticaria. In most instances, acute urticaria is due to an antigen that passes through the alimentary canal. This includes drugs, foods and fruits. The onset of the eruption is sudden and rather widespread. A thorough history usually reveals that there has been an intake of medication or consumption of specific foods, such as seafood, spicy meats, strawberries and sometimes eggs. It is important to elicit the offending antigen in order to avoid repeated episodes of urticaria which on occasion, due to laryngeal edema, can be serious. Mild urticaria requires little medication other than an antihistamine, such as oral diphenhydramine, 25 mg. 3 or 4 times daily. In acute urticaria, antihistamines have a direct effect on the pathogenesis. They block histamine released during the antigen-antibody combination at the receptor site and thereby interfere with the actions of histamine on the capillaries. This blocking effect on the action of histamine is clinically gradual. In the more serious and acute cases of urticaria, diphenhydramine is injected intramuscularly or intravenously. In still more acute cases, Adrenalin in oil 1:500 is given by intramuscular injection or Adrenalin solution 1:1000 is administered through oral absorption. In life-threatening laryngeal edema, Adrenalin 1:1000 is injected intramuscularly or even intravenously, with great care taken to observe the side effects of acute Adrenalin administration.

In cases of longer lasting subacute urticaria, such as is encountered with a drug eruption, medium doses of oral steroids (15 to 30 mg./day of prednisone) may have to be resorted to for 7 to 10 days.

Acute urticarial lesions can also be seen as dermatologic manifestations of systemic lupus erythematosus, acute rheumatic fever and acute rheumatoid arthritis. Severe prostration, fever and malaise make it possible to differentiate these complex cases of urticaria from urticaria induced by dietary factors or by drugs.

Chronic Urticaria. In chronic urticaria, urticarial lesions recurring for more than three or four weeks, a careful history has to be taken regarding intake of drugs and foods. Sometimes physical factors such as friction, heat or cold can produce chronic urticaria. Among drugs, aspirin is frequently overlooked and is one of the most common offenders, either alone or in combination with other preparations. Lymphomas, systemic lupus erythematosus, rheumatic fever and rheumatoid arthritis can produce urticarial changes. Parasitic infestation can readily be ruled out by a highly elevated eosinophil count. This also holds true for the urticaria seen with trichinosis or that due to chronic insect bites.

In the vast majority of cases of chronic urticaria, no underlying cause is found and anxiety is assumed to be the etiologic factor, but this is not proven by any means. In chronic urticaria, the parents as well as the child need to be advised that the lesions are harmless, but that they may last in a recurrent fashion for several months and sometimes years. In selected cases, hospital admissions need to be arranged in order to rule out the rarer entities mentioned above and in order to give reassurance. Both the child and parents should be forewarned that the chances for finding the cause of the chronically recurrent hives are not too great.

The treatment of chronic urticaria offers little satisfaction to physicians or patients. Antihistamines have no direct pathogenic effect on chronic urticaria and really do not work, unless given in high dosages, at which level their sedative side effect is frequently more cumbersome than the presence of hives. In case of acute laryngeal edema, Adrenalin may have to be resorted to (in oil 1:500, given by intramuscular injection or in aqueous suspension 1:1000 for oral absorption). The administration of oral steroids is warranted only for short periods, as in the long run the side effects of steroids are more serious than the chronic urticaria. In children with definite emotional problems, which indeed might cause chronic urticaria, psychiatric support is indicated.

Drug Eruptions

GEORGE F. WILGRAM, M.D.

Drug eruptions in children and adults alike may present in all clinical symptoms from plain macular eruptions to severe bullous disease. It is important to stop the administration of the offending antigen immediately as continued intake of the offending drug may lead to life-threatening situations, particularly if the eruption has a bullous component. The erythema multiforme–like bullous drug eruption in children can present a serious threat to survival and needs to be treated with aggressive steroid therapy, between 40 and 120 mg. of prednisone per day. The decision to ad-

minister steroids is sometimes complicated by the fact that the drug eruption initially can mimic a viral exanthem, in which case steroids would not be indicated. As soon as the diagnosis of a drug eruption becomes reasonably established, large doses of steroids are given. In case of an infectious component, antibiotic therapy is given, with great care taken that the antibiotic chosen is not the one that is antigenically related to, or identical to, the one that caused the drug eruption in the first place (e.g., penicillin or ampicillin).

Although bullous drug eruptions frequently require hospitalization and expert dermatologic and pediatric care, milder drug eruptions, particularly the macular or urticarial variety, can be treated more easily. Topical cortisone preparations are rarely justified as they do not provide much relief. Chronic, fixed or solitary drug eruptions are rarely found in children and require dermatologic expertise for diagnosis. Since they are not a major threat to the patient's survival, their recognition is less important than, for instance, swift action in bullous drug eruptions.

Papulosquamous Disorders

ALVIN H. JACOBS, M.D.

PSORIASIS

Psoriasis is a chronic constitutional disorder with a tendency to familial occurrence. No age is exempt; in fact, the onset is usually in childhood or adolescence, and it is even seen occasionally in infancy. Before embarking on treatment, it is of great importance that the patient and the parents understand that the child has a lifelong problem, although remissions are common; that general health is usually unaffected; and that with a persistent and concentrated treatment program much can be accomplished to minimize the problem.

General Therapeutic Measures. Assessment of the emotional status of the patient is important, since tensions and anxiety can exacerbate psoriasis. Attention to family difficulties and school problems may be important. The use of sedatives and tranquilizers should be considered. For daytime use, hydroxyzine hydrochloride (Atarax) is a satisfactory tranquilizer for children; it is given in doses of 5 to 20 mg. three times daily.

It is important that the parents of the patient completely understand the treatment and its rationale. It should also be brought to their attention that injury to the skin may result in more psoriasis (Koebner response). This means that bruises, abrasions, scratches, poorly fitting clothing or shoes may cause skin injury sufficient to generate a reaction.

Most psoriatics are benefited by exposure to sunlight and thus frequently are better in the summer. Advantage should be taken of this in planning the summer activities of the psoriatic child, although caution must be exercised, since sudden overexposure to sunlight can result in enough skin injury to cause an exacerbation.

Since acute guttate (drop-like) psoriasis frequently follows a streptococcal respiratory infection, it is especially important that psoriatic children receive adequate therapy for streptococcal disease. Children with guttate psoriasis should routinely have throat cultures taken, and if beta-hemolytic streptococci are found, a course of penicillin therapy should be instituted before more active therapy for the psoriasis is instituted. In many instances, the psoriasis will improve markedly with treatment only of the streptococcal disease.

Proper general hygiene should be emphasized, especially frequent removal of scales by means of warm tub baths with ordinary soaps or tar soap. A tar bath, made by the addition of 1 ounce of Zetar emulsion, Balnetar or liquor carbonis detergens to a tub of water, may be used.

Systemic Therapy. No systemic drugs currently available are safe for administration to children. Systemic corticosteroids clear psoriasis temporarily but should never be used for this purpose, since cessation of therapy is usually followed by a serious flare-up of the eruption.

Cytotoxic antimetabolite drugs, such as methotrexate, are used in the treatment of severe adult psoriasis. These are very toxic drugs, and although they suppress growth of hyperplastic epidermal cells, they are capable of producing the same effects on other rapidly growing cells. The use of such toxic agents for a nonmalignant disease in childhood is not indicated.

A recent development in the management of severe psoriasis is the use of psoralen and high intensity long wave ultraviolet light (PUVA). Many light boxes are now being manufactured to supply the high intensity UVA. Although this method of treatment has received wide publicity, it is still investigational and should not be used on children, since the long-term effects of this therapy are not yet known.

Topical Therapy. Since psoriasis is a chronic disorder with remissions and exacerbations, and since responsiveness to treatment may vary, it is necessary to have a variety of regimens available and to start with the simplest. The usual effective remedies include salicylic acid, tars, anthralin, and topical corticosteroids. Many times in mild psoriasis it is sufficient to recommend frequent sunbaths (with proper caution) and the use of an emollient to supply adequate moisture to the skin. Eucerin cream is an excellent choice for this purpose, since it is composed of equal parts water and Aquaphor.

Localized Psoriasis

Crude coal tar is very effective in the treatment of psoriatic plaques, but is too messy for home use. A more acceptable tar derivative is liquor carbonis detergens (LCD), which may be prescribed as 5 per cent LCD in hydrophilic ointment (U.S.P.). This should be applied to the plaques three times daily.

A new, more pleasant and effective tar preparation in a gel form has recently been introduced by Westwood Pharmaceuticals as Estar Gel. This may be rubbed into the lesions and the excess wiped off so that there is a minimum of mess and staining of clothing.

Fluorinated steroids, such as 0.1 per cent triamcinolone (Kenalog), 0.025 per cent fluocinolone (Synalar), 0.05 per cent flurandrenolid (Cordran), and 0.1 per cent betamethasone (Valisone) have proved to be the most effective of the topically applied corticosteroids. These preparations in a cream or ointment form should be rubbed into each lesion four or five times daily. These steroids should be used only for short periods, shifting to one of the above tar preparations or emollients after initial improvement is evident.

Generalized Psoriasis

Removal of scales by daily tar baths is often a necessary preliminary to adequate treatment.

Massage 5 per cent liquor carbonis detergens (LCD) in hydrophilic emulsion base (HEB) into all lesions at bedtime; according to the results, the concentration of LCD may be increased to as much as 10 per cent. Estar gel (vide supra) is somewhat more effective although more expensive than the LCD.

Remove the ointment in the morning with mineral oil followed by a cleansing bath or shower.

Ultraviolet light may be used in suberythema doses in the office once or twice weekly, or the patient may purchase a lamp for home use. Natural sunlight, when available, is superior to either. Great care must be exercised in any case, since exacerbation of the lesions can result if the skin is allowed to burn.

If prompt results are not evident, it is best to hospitalize the patient for two or three weeks during which the Goeckerman regimen can be carried out. This treatment consists of applying 5 per cent crude coal tar to the entire body every 2 or 3 hours. Each morning the ointment is removed with mineral oil and the patient is then given a tar bath. After the bath, ultraviolet light is used in suberythema doses and the crude coal tar is reapplied. A very satisfactory remission usually follows this type of therapy.

The length of hospital stay can be reduced by the use of anthralin paste in place of the crude coal tar. This treatment, however, is difficult to carry out and should be supervised by an experienced dermatologist.

Psoriasis of the Scalp

Removal of thick scales may be accomplished by daily warm oil applications. This is carried out by saturating the scalp with mineral oil and then applying hot towels in turban fashion every 10 minutes for half an hour before shampooing.

After several days, if the scales have been adequately removed, one can then use daily tar shampoos. Polytar shampoo is an effective and nonmessy preparation for this purpose.

Following the shampoo, anthralin pomade (Lasan pomade) is rubbed into the affected areas in the scalp. Instead of the pomade one may use a liquid corticosteroid preparation such as 0.1 per cent triamcinolone lotion or Synalar solution.

SEBORRHEIC DERMATITIS

Seborrheic dermatitis is an inflammatory, scaly, crusting eruption involving the body areas containing the greatest concentration of sebaceous glands, namely, the scalp, face, postauricular areas, presternal area and the intertriginous zones. It appears in infancy between 2 and 12 weeks of age and usually clears spontaneously by 8 to 12 months of age. It is not seen again until puberty, after which it remains as a chronic condition.

In infancy, seborrheic dermatitis involves primarily the scalp as well as flexural and intertriginous areas and is very frequently secondarily infected with *Candida albicans*.

Seborrheic Dermatitis of the Scalp

Treatment of cradle cap is best carried out by the use of one of the commercially available antiseborrheic shampoos, such as Sebulex or Ionil. The scalp should be washed thoroughly with the shampoo daily at first and later two or three times each week. If the scale has become too thick and adherent for easy removal by shampooing, it can be loosened first by massaging warm mineral oil into the scalp and allowing it to remain for 15 to 20 minutes followed by the therapeutic shampoo. Mother should be reassured that rubbing the infant's scalp vigorously will not injure the baby's fragile-feeling skull.

Adolescents with seborrheic dermatitis of the scalp may use the same type of shampoo and then rub a corticosteroid lotion, such as Synalar solution, into involved scalp areas after the shampoo.

Seborrheic Dermatitis of the Face

The use of corticosteroid creams will clear the facial and postauricular involvement in a very short time. Since it is advisable to avoid fluorinated steroids on the face, 1.0 per cent hydrocortisone cream should be used for this purpose. Involvement of the eyelids with seborrheic blepharitis can be managed by first removing the marginal crusts with warm water twice daily followed by application of an ophthalmic corticosteroid ointment.

Seborrheic Dermatitis of the Diaper Area

In most instances, *Candida albicans* superinfection must be cleared first. This can be done by application of a nongreasy anticandidal agent, such as Mycostatin dusting powder or Fungizone Lotion. As the candidiasis subsides, one can change to one of the corticosteroid creams mentioned above, or the anticandidal and steroid creams may be used alternately during the day.

PARAPSORIASIS

The term parapsoriasis embraces a poorly defined group of rare maculopapular squamous eruptions of unknown origin. None of these disorders has any relationship to psoriasis. Three conditions which come under this heading can occur in childhood. Pityriasis lichenoides et varioliformis acuta (Mucha-Habermann disease) occurs most commonly in childhood or early adult life. The course of the disease is usually a few weeks to several months and recovery is the rule.

Guttate parapsoriasis occurs mostly in young adults and has a long course, usually from 3 months to 7 years. The ultimate prognosis is good.

Treatment for the above two conditions is purely symptomatic. While awaiting recovery, antipruritic medication such as diphenhydramine (Benadryl), 25 to 50 mg. three times a day orally, may be administered, and emollients, such as Lubriderm or Keri Lotion, applied. Ultraviolet light exposure gives relief from symptoms and seems to shorten the course of the condition.

Parapsoriasis en plaques, which may occur at any age, is regarded as an expression of a lymphoreticular disease. Approximately 25 per cent of these eventually progress to mycosis fungoides. Although treatment of parapsoriasis en plaques is symptomatic, careful long-term follow-up is essential.

PITYRIASIS ROSEA

Pityriasis rosea is a common, mild inflammatory skin disorder characterized by round or oval, discrete or confluent salmon-tinted, slightly scaly macules or rings. The disease is self-limited, lasting about 4 to 6 weeks. Treatment is directed toward allaying anxiety, speeding recovery and relieving pruritus.

Exposure to ultraviolet light to the point of producing erythema and exfoliation may hasten recovery.

Since soap is irritating in this condition, cleansing may be accomplished by colloidal starch baths (one cup of Linit starch to a tub of warm water) or by oatmeal baths, such as Aveeno.

Systemic antipruritic drugs are useful if itching is a problem. Temaril is given in divided doses three or four times daily, following the manufacturer's recommended schedule. If necessary, one or two teaspoonfuls of elixir of Benadryl may be given at bedtime.

PITYRIASIS RUBRA PILARIS

Pityriasis rubra pilaris is a rare disorder characterized by fine, acuminate, horny follicular papules. The hereditary form of the disorder may be present at birth or may develop during infancy. The acquired type may occur at any age. The disease tends to be lifelong.

Some patients have been reported to respond to large doses of vitamin A (150,000 to 200,000 units per day), but this is a toxic and dangerous therapy for use in childhood. More recently, it has been suggested that vitamin A acid (Retin-A) applied locally may be of help. Keratolytic ointments, such as 3 per cent salicylic acid, will result in some improvement.

LICHEN STRIATUS

Lichen striatus is a rare condition of unknown cause occurring in children as a linear band of scaling papules usually appearing suddenly on the extremities. Spontaneous resolution usually occurs in several months. Treatment is usually not necessary, but if desired, local application of topical corticosteroids will relieve pruritus and possibly hasten recovery.

LICHEN NITIDUS

This is an asymptomatic, rare, chronic eruption which consists of small, sharply defined, flesh-colored papules localized on the penis, arms and abdomen. The disease is chronic, although spontaneous resolution after many years may occur. No method of treatment has been found to be effective.

Vesiculobullous Disorders

Dermatitis Herpetiformis, Drug-Induced Toxic Epidermal Necrolysis, Pemphigus Vulgaris and Bullous Pemphigoid

GUINTER KAHN, M.D.

Although the skin of children blisters more easily than that of adults, the chronic blistering diseases occur rarely in young people. Pemphigus vulgaris and bullous pemphigoid are almost unheard of before the teenage years. Drug-induced toxic epidermal necrolysis (TEN) is much less common than staphylococcal toxin-induced TEN in children, especially in infants. Dermatitis herpetiformis (DH) is very uncommon in children, but it does occur throughout the pediatric age group. It appears more often as a bullous eruption and more often in the groin among children than among adults. In the past DH has been called juvenile bullous pemphigoid, a misnomer rectified by the recent advent of diagnostic immunofluorescent tests in these diseases.

DERMATITIS HERPETIFORMIS

The sulfone, diaminophenyl sulfone (dapsone), and the sulfapyridines are the agents of choice for this affliction. Neither the cause of the disease nor the reason why these agents help is known. The dramatic relief of symptoms and signs by either of these drugs is almost therapeutically diagnostic of DH; however, it must be pointed out that the identification of IgA in uninvolved basement membrane and evidence of enteropathy are unequivocal evidence of DH. The agent chosen as first therapy varies with the practitioner's experiences with each drug.

Sulfones

Dapsone (Avlosulfone)* is available as 25 and 100 mg. tablets. It is better tolerated and more economical than sulfapyridine; however, its side effects can be serious.

Dose. Initially, 50 to 200 mg. per day should be given, increasing or decreasing about 50 mg. per day depending on response or side effects of therapy.

Cautions. (1) A glucose-6-phosphate dehydrogenase (G6PD) screening test should be done prior to giving this drug to Negroes or Caucasians of Mediterranean descent because of the increased incidence of severe hemolytic anemia in some of these people following the use of dapsone. (2) Order a urinalysis and complete blood count every month during the first year of therapy, then about every three months.

Side Effects. Methemoglobinemia is common and causes headaches and an ashy gray color. It is not an indication to stop medication if the G6PD test is normal. In weeks, these symptoms diminish while the drug's therapeutic activity continues. Less frequent side effects include febrile reactions, hepatitis, peripheral neuropathy, psychoses, exfoliative erythroderma, and agranulocytosis.

Pediatric Formulation. A liquid suspension can be tailored for children unable to swallow pills (5 to 10 mg./teaspoon). Since its stability is unknown, it should be kept in a refrigerator and used within two weeks after formulation.

Maintenance. A dose which reduces signs and symptoms to a minimum is determined for each patient. About every three to six months, slow withdrawal should be attempted, since the disease may remit spontaneously after years.

Sulfapyridine

Sulfapyridine is available as 500-mg. enteric- or nonenteric-coated tablets. Some clinicians claim that it is more effective than dapsone. Proof is lacking.

Dose. Initially, 250 to 1000 mg./day should be given, depending on the size of the patient. Increase the medication by doubling the dose about every other day until symptoms or signs abate or nausea occurs. Thereafter, tailor dosage weekly according to symptoms, signs and side effects.

Cautions. (1) The patient should be encouraged to consume large quantities of fluids to avoid renal crystalline aggregates. (2) The

enteric-coated tablet causes much less nausea because often it is not absorbed. The patient should closely examine his stools for tablets. (3) When using nonenteric-coated tablets, the dose must be kept extremely low initially and must be given with meals; otherwise, severe nausea often occurs. (4) Order a urinalysis and complete blood count monthly.

Side Effects. Nausea and vomiting are usually the first and most common side effects. Others include fever, headaches, leukopenia, agranulocytosis, hepatitis and renal damage (from sulfa crystal aggregates).

Maintenance and Pediatric Formulation. See dapsone.

Discussion

Some patients respond to one of these agents in preference to the other. Occasionally, patients need the combination of both medicines. Rarely, patients will be refractory to both drugs, and such patients are given large doses (4 to 6 mg./kg./day) of prednisone to effect a remission.

DRUG-INDUCED TOXIC EPIDERMAL NECROLYSIS (TEN), THE SCALDED SKIN SYNDROME (LYELL'S DISEASE)

The extent of involvement varies from a few small, flaccid bullae to widespread denudation of skin and mucous membranes. Accordingly, therapy varies from cautious neglect and observation to that of a total body burn regimen. But basic to any therapy for this condition is to avoid the provoking medication and substances with which it may cross-react.

Caution. Children with recurrent TEN should make the physician suspicious of recurrent burns. The physician should look for any other signs or symptoms of neglect or cruelty (battered child syndrome).

Therapy. Death occurs in about 25 per cent of all patients, but much less often in children. Therapeutic measures will be described for the severest, generalized form, and the practitioner can scale down therapy in proportion to the clinical presentation.

Death follows a pattern similar to that in burns, that is, secondary infection, dehydration, decreased electrolytes and serum proteins. Therefore, when available, these patients should be transferred to a burn unit and be under the surveillance of a physician experienced with burn therapy and of a dermatologist.

TEN patients, however, differ from burn patients in that the remaining "normal" epidermis readily shears away from the underlying dermis (Nikolsky's sign) with the slightest

---

*This use of Avlosulfone is not mentioned by the manufacturer.

trauma. Personnel must be warned to minimize trauma or handling of the patient's skin. A vibrating, flannel-covered mattress should be used to avoid creating local pressure zones. The patient's skin and mucosa must be observed daily, since the course of blistering can change suddenly and spread rampantly.

Blistered areas should be treated aseptically. Isolation techniques are advisable; blisters should be punctured with the covering left on. However, infected and necrotic tissue should be removed, the base cultured, and systemic antibiotics chosen as needed on the basis of sensitivity studies. Silver nitrate wet dressings (0.5 per cent) should be applied to involved skin daily or more often in the presence of purulence. Fluids and electrolytes must be monitored, especially since silver ion application can rapidly deplete serum sodium. Silver sulfadiazine cream (Silvadene) may be used as is done for the management of thermal burns. Silver sulfadiazine should *not* be used in newborns during the first month of life. Similar precautions to those noted for the use of dapsone in DH relative to G6PD must be followed.

An alternate proven form of topical therapy is the application of warm, dry air 40° C. and 20 per cent humidity through a quietly vibrating porous mattress. An air conditioner giving 2000 liters per minute of air quickly dries the moist wound surfaces. The 40° C. ambient temperature relieves the body's metabolic need to produce heat as fluid is evaporated from the skin's surface.

The value of steroids here is not proved, but considering the severe possible prognosis, they commonly are used. Prednisone should be given in adequate doses (4 to 6 mg./kg.) and the dose doubled daily if the course of the disease is not abated. Appropriate intravenous corticosteroids such as hydrocortisone sodium succinate (Solu-Cortef) or sodium succinate methyl prednisolone (Solu-Medrol) should be used for those patients incapable of swallowing oral doses. One must always weigh the necessity for using large doses of corticosteroids against the possibility of producing iatrogenic disease.

Mucosal Care. Topical steroid ointment may be helpful and if used should be applied four times daily. The involved eyes and vulvar surfaces should be separated widely after each application to avoid synechiae. Eye care sould be supervised by an ophthalmologist. The patient with oral-pharyngeal problems should rinse the mouth with 4 per cent viscous lidocaine to encourage eating. Meals should be liquid or soft but not hot.

The family should be warned of possible sequelae even with successful treatment: permanent scars, keloids, corneal scarring and, less often, ectropion and nail loss.

PEMPHIGUS

The vulgaris form is extremely rare in children, whereas the more superficial foliaceous form is more common and less severe. It is endemic to parts of Brazil. The youngest case reported was that of an 18 month old girl who responded to 0.5 per cent triamcinolone cream applied four times a day. Nevertheless, we recommend systemic prednisone, 3 to 6 mg./kg./day, depending on the severity of the process. These figures may be revised upward if the process is inadequately suppressed. When the progression of the disease has been checked and no new lesions appear for two weeks, the dosage may be reduced by about 20 per cent every two weeks. As one approaches maintenance dosage (2 to 5 months after onset of therapy for severe cases), alternate-morning prednisone becomes the preferred therapy because steroid side effects are reduced. Alternate-morning prednisone is the initial therapy of choice for those mild to moderate forms of pemphigus that would require less than 100 mg./day to control. The second choice would be to control the patient on a daily early morning (6 to 8 A.M.) prednisone regimen. Side effects are less than with the daily divided dose regimen, which is needed only in the acute stage of the severest form of the disease.

Uncommonly, severe cases do not respond to large doses of steroids, so that the dose must be doubled about every week until the disorder is stabilized. For unknown reasons, in these rare instances, patients may respond to nominal ACTH dosage, about 80 units per day initially, while they appear refractory to systemically administered corticosteroids.

Once a maintenance dose is established for such difficult patients, immunosuppressives may be added to the regimen, since they allow for the further reduction of steroid dosage. Methotrexate, Imuran and Cytoxan have been used successfully in doses varying with the severity of the process. The physician should be cautious in the use of these drugs, which presently are experimental for the treatment of pemphigus and could be potential mutagens in a child. A basic dictum is: the younger the patient, the shorter the course of drug; and contraceptive measures are used when indicated. Hepatic, renal and hematologic systems are monitored by the laboratory when antimetabolites become part of the regimen. The use of intramuscular gold has recently been advocated for the treatment of adult pemphigus patients, and the author is aware of its successful use in juvenile pemphigus.

PEMPHIGOID

Because the course is similar but less severe than that for pemphigus, treatment is similar and response is usually quicker than for pemphigus. Only one preteen patient with this disease is known to the author.

Discoid Lupus Erythematosus

WALTER F. LEVER, M.D.

Although in childhood chronic discoid lupus erythematosus (DLE) is rarer than systemic lupus erythematosus (SLE), it is estimated that 3 per cent of the cases of DLE have their onset under 15 years of age. Occasionally it requires detailed examination to arrive at a decision as to whether a child has DLE or SLE. It also must be kept in mind that DLE may change into SLE. Characteristically, the cutaneous lesions of DLE consist of well defined, erythematous, "discoid" patches that often show adherent scales and follicular plugging. Older lesions often show atrophic scarring, although involution of the lesions without scarring can occur. Sun-exposed areas are involved most commonly.

DLE in many instances responds to applications of corticosteroid creams either with or without occlusive dressings; in other cases it responds to intralesional or sublesional injections of a corticosteroid suspension. For application, either fluocinolone acetonide cream (Synalar), 0.01 or 0.025 per cent, or betamethasone valerate cream (Valisone), 0.1 per cent, is massaged into the lesions, preferably six times daily at least in the beginning. Although using the corticosteroid cream for 10 to 16 hours overnight with an occlusive dressing applied over it greatly enhances the penetration of the cream into the skin, it is a cumbersome procedure except on the extremities and the scalp. Thus on the hands one may use disposable plastic gloves, on the feet plastic baggies, and on the arms and legs a thin plastic film. The gloves or baggies must be made airtight above the ankles or wrists with tape, and the plastic film can be held in place with an elastic bandage. For the scalp a plastic shower cap with an elastic band may be used for occlusion. For lesions on the face and trunk but also for small lesions elsewhere on the skin, Cordran tape containing flurandrenolide in the adhesive layer is recommended. Cutting it to the size of each lesion, it is left in place for 23 hours daily or for 11 hours twice daily, allowing the skin to dry for one hour before applying new tape. Allowing the skin to dry between applications usually prevents the development of miliaria or folliculitis.

Intralesional injections of a corticosteroid suspension often give better results than topical applications of corticosteroids. Triamcinolone (Aristocort), 25 mg./ml., or betamethasone (Celestone), 6 mg./ml., may be used for this purpose. The suspension is injected (preferably intradermally, but subcutaneously into larger areas) using a syringe with a 26-gauge needle. A 4 sq. cm. area may be injected with 0.4 ml. of the suspension. Several areas may be injected through a single puncture by withdrawing the needle partially and then extending it in other directions. If multiple needle punctures are required because of the large size of a lesion, for purpose of anesthesia the corticosteroid suspension may be diluted with one part of a 2 per cent solution of lidocaine for two parts of the corticosteroid suspension. The injections may be carried out at intervals of two to three weeks. Intralesional injections of corticosteroids may produce temporary atrophy of subcutaneous fat.

Systemic treatment of discoid lupus erythematosus with antimalarial drugs is merited in patients in whom the lesions are spreading, numerous or not amenable to the topical or intralesional administration of corticosteroids. It is no longer necessary to avoid the antimalarial drugs completely since reasonably safe dosage levels have been established and ophthalmologic examinations prior to and during treatment have become standard practice. The recommended rules are to avoid the use of chloroquine since it is the most likely antimalarial drug to produce retinopathy, to give hydroxychloroquine (Plaquenil)* intermittently and no longer than 6 months at a time, and to give preference to quinacrine (Atabrine) which is not known ever to have caused retinal damage. At doses of 200 mg. daily, Atabrine causes yellowing of the skin and sclerae within a few months in adults, and at lower doses in children, but this gradually subsides after discontinuance of the drug.†

The dosage of the antimalarial drugs is dependent on age. Larger initial doses are

---

*Manufacturer does not list children's dosage of hydroxychloroquine for treatment of discord lupus erythematosus.

†This use of quinacrine is not mentioned in the manufacturer's instructions.

used, followed by smaller maintenance doses after improvement has become evident (usually in one to two months). For adolescents over age 15 the starting dose of hydroxychloroquine is 600 mg./day. In children under 20 kg. the starting dose is 100 mg. daily, and for children over 20 kg. the starting dose is 200 mg. daily (250 mg./m²/24 hours). If improvement is inadequate in two months, quinacrine is added to hydroxychloroquine. The initial dose for adolescents over age 15 is 200 mg./day. In children under 20 kg. the starting dose is 50 mg. daily, and for children over 20 kg. the starting dose is 100 mg. daily (125 mg./m²/24 hours). Quinacrine may be the first drug to be given if either parents or the family physician are overly concerned about the possibility of retinopathy with hydroxychloroquine. Because the antimalarial medications have a bitter taste, it is advised that the tablets of medication be crushed and mixed with applesauce and be swallowed rather than be chewed. Gastric irritation from antimalarial drugs is lessened by giving the medication with meals.

Even though the chance that retinal damage may develop is extremely low when using the above mentioned dosages of hydroxychloroquine, all patients taking hydroxychloroquine should have an ophthalmologic evaluation before hydroxychloroquine is started and at four month intervals thereafter. This evaluation should include slit lamp, visual field and funduscopic examinations. A more common ocular complication than retinopathy is blurring of vision as the result of depositions of hydroxychloroquine particles in the cornea. This complication may set in within a few weeks after starting the medication, but it is a rare occurrence at the recommended doses. The blurring of vision is reversible when the medication is stopped and thus is harmless. Temporary hypopigmentation of the hair may occur with hydroxychloroquine. Lichenoid eruptions and exfoliative dermatitis are rare complications of therapy with both hydroxychloroquine and quinacrine. In rare instances quinacrine may cause depression of bone marrow function that may result in aplastic anemia. A complete blood count every two months is therefore advisable.

In many patients with DLE the lesions exacerbate or disseminate on exposure to ultraviolet light. In addition to avoiding exposure to sunlight in the middle of the day, the application first of PreSun, a short ultraviolet sunscreen, and then of Uval, a long ultraviolet sunscreen, is recommended. For application to the lips, A-Fil Sun Stick is acceptable.

Mucocutaneous Lymph Node Syndrome

MARIAN E. MELISH, M.D.

Mucocutaneous lymph node syndrome (MCLS, MLNS, Kawasaki disease) is a recently recognized symptom complex consisting of: (1) fever persisting for more than seven days unresponsive to antibiotics or antipyretics; (2) discrete vascular engorgement of ocular conjunctivae without ulceration or exudate; (3) changes in the mouth consisting of (a) erythema, dryness and fissuring of the lips, (b) prominence of papillae of the tongue creating a "strawberry" appearance, and (c) diffuse erythema of the oral and pharyngeal mucosa; (4) changes in the extremities consisting of (a) striking erythema of the palms and soles in the initial phase of the illness, (b) firm indurative swelling of the palms and soles initially, and (c) desquamation from fingertips in convalescence; (5) an erythematous rash, variously scarlatiniform, morbilliform, or multiform without vesicles, bullae or crusts; and (6) acute nonpurulent enlargement of lymph node of greater then 1.5 cm. diameter (usually unilateral and cervical). The majority of patients have all these manifestations. At least five should be present to consider this diagnosis.

Associated features include sterile pyuria, aseptic meningitis with mild CSF pleocytosis, arthritis, diarrhea and liver function abnormalities. Laboratory abnormalities include significant leukocytosis (>18,000) with a polymorphonuclear predominance and immature granulocyte forms, elevated sedimentation rate and elevated C' reactive protein and thrombocytosis in the second and third weeks of the illness.

Males are affected more often than females. The syndrome occurs most commonly in children under 18 months of age but cases are seen up to puberty. No etiologic agent has been found and no pathognomonic clinical or laboratory features have emerged.

The differential diagnosis includes streptococcal scarlet fever, Stevens-Johnson syndrome, acute exanthematous viral syndrome, collagen vascular disease, and especially acute rheumatoid arthritis. Rocky Mountain spotted fever and Henoch-Schönlein purpura may also be considered.

Although patients with mucocutaneous lymph node syndrome may appear seriously ill and have evidence of multisystem involvement, the illness is generally self-limited, with fever and acute manifestations lasting 2 to 3 weeks. Originally called benign mucocutaneous lymph node syndrome, the large experience in Japan has led to the recognition that there is a measurable fatality rate. Surveys taken by the Japanese Research Committee of MCLS have indicated that nearly 2 per cent of children affected with this syndrome experience sudden death in the third to sixth week after onset.

Pathologic evaluation reveals the cause of death to be secondary to coronary artery thromboarteritis leading to myocardial infarction or ischemia. Involvement of medium-sized muscular arteries in other areas of the body is seen to a greater or lesser degree. The pathologic findings of fatal MCLS are identical with those of infantile periarteritis nodosa, which had been essentially a postmortem diagnosis.

Coronary artery aneurysms and various degrees of cardiac dysfunction have been documented in surviving children with clinical MCLS, but the frequency with which nonfatal cardiac involvement occurs in unselected patients is unknown.

Rational therapy for MCLS awaits an understanding of its etiology. Until that time there are three important aspects of patient management: (1) The patient should have a careful clinical and laboratory workup to exclude another etiology for fever and associated symptoms. (2) Supportive care should be provided throughout the acute phase. (3) The child will need careful follow-up designed to detect possible complications.

MCLS remains a diagnosis of exclusion. A minimal workup includes complete blood count, platelet count, urinalysis, urine culture, sedimentation rate, ASO titer, multiple cultures to rule out bacterial infection, viral cultures, antinuclear antibody, IgE determination, chest x-ray and EKG. If antibiotics have been started they should be discontinued when bacterial infection has been ruled out. Lymph node aspirates and lymph node biopsy may be helpful in excluding a bacterial cause for the lymphadenopathy but are not helpful in diagnosis. Pathologic evaluation in MCLS reveals only lymphoid hyperplasia. Biopsies of skin and muscle are unlikely to yield specific information.

During the acute phase of the illness most children are highly febrile and quite lethargic. Some are semicomatose. We have treated children with high fever or overt arthritis with suppressive anti-inflammatory doses of aspirin. Aspirin is given in a dose designed to keep the serum salicylate level at approximately 25 mg./100 ml. This can usually be achieved with a dose of 100 mg./kg./day in four divided doses. Aspirin is continued until all acute manifestations of the disease have disappeared, until the sedimentation rate is near normal and until thrombocytosis has resolved. Aspirin may prove to be of benefit for its antipyretic and anti-inflammatory effects and for its action on platelet function.

Certain patients have significant diarrhea which may lead to dehydration or lethargy causing poor oral intake; these patients should receive intravenous hydration. We have observed one case of increased intracranial pressure (pseudotumor cerebri) of short duration. This problem may require evaluation and treatment as detailed elsewhere in this volume. The problems of urethritis, conjunctival engorgement, and hand and foot induration do not require specific attention.

Patients who have the symptom complex compatible with MCLS must be followed carefully through the convalescent phase for at least 6 weeks. This period, from 3 to 6 weeks after the onset of the acute syndrome, is the time when the likelihood of cardiac complications is the greatest. Coronary artery complications are more common in males, infants less than 1 year, those with fever persisting for two weeks or more, those with recrudescent fever or rash, and those with white blood cell counts over 30,000 and sedimentation rates over 60 mm./hour. Thrombocytosis, when present, is also likely to be at its peak by the third week of the illness.

Patients should be followed for evidence of arrhythmias, EKG abnormalities and cardiomegaly. If cardiac decompensation or evidence of myocardial infarction occurs, an aortogram should be done to evaluate coronary pathology. Aneurysms and narrowing of the coronaries have both been described. Once coronary pathology has been demonstrated, the patient will require the sort of care provided in an intensive care unit, with continuous cardiac and blood pressure monitoring, and measurement of cardiac enzymes.

No comparative studies have been done on the effects of anti-inflammatory therapy in the coronary artery disease of MCLS. At present, either aspirin in doses of 100 mg./kg./day or corticosteroids (2 mg./kg./day of prednisone or the equivalent) seem to be indicated on the basis of pathologic studies which show a necrotizing vasculitis. If corticosteroids are used, anticoagulation with heparin should also be employed to combat the thrombotic tendency.

Patients who have developed evidence of coronary artery disease months to years after acute MCLS have been described as having chronic myocardial disease. Careful coronary artery evaluation is indicated in these children. Regression of coronary aneurysms has occurred, and apparently complete healing is possible. Successful coronary bypass grafting has been performed in one child with persistent obstruction.

Although still not commonly recognized outside Japan, reports of cases in children of various ethnic groups have been reported from North America, Europe and the Far East. The epidemiology of the syndrome in the United States is almost completely unknown. In order to learn more about the epidemiology and hopefully the etiology of this puzzling syndrome, the Center for Disease Control has established a registry. Reports of suspected cases should be sent to the Viral Disease Branch, Bureau of Epidemiology, Center for Disease Control, Atlanta, Georgia 30333.

Fungous Infections

ROBERT F. TILLEY, M.D.

Griseofulvin is the medication of choice for the treatment of tinea capitis and some of the chronic fungal infections of the nails and skin. Miconazole (MicaTin), clotrimazole (Lotrimin) and haloprogin (Halotex) have demonstrated their value in treating fungal infections of the skin including those produced by the dermatophytes (Trichophyta, Microspora, Epidermophyton), the common yeast pathogen *(Candida albicans)*. Tinea versicolor also responds to these agents. Tolnaftate (Tinactin) is effective against dermatophytes. Other older agents of value are the halogenated quinolones (Vioform) for secondarily bacterial infected dermatophytosis, and sodium thiosulfate, selenium sulfide and acrisorcin (Akrinol) for tinea versicolor and nystatin for candidiasis.

DERMATOPHYTOSIS

Tinea capitis caused by several different species of fungi responds to adequate amounts of griseofulvin. The oral dose of microcrystalline griseofulvin is 125 to 250 mg./day for those weighing 30 to 50 lbs. and 250 to 500 mg./day for those weighing over 50 lbs. This amount given after a meal containing fats or midday is continued for at least four weeks and usually for eight weeks. A new form of griseofulvin—"ultra microsize" dispersed in polyethylene glycol—is available as Gris-PEG. The recommended dose of this form is one half of that used with the microcrystalline form. Thus children weighing over 25 kg. should receive 125 to 250 mg./day of Gris-PEG* daily, and those weighing 15 to 25 kg. should receive 62.5 to 125 mg./day. Each form of griseofulvin should be continued for four to eight weeks in managing tinea capitis. Medication should be continued until all clinical and laboratory examinations confirm the absence of the fungus. Griseofulvin is contraindicated if there is a history of porphyria, hepatic disease or prior allergic reactions to griseofulvin.

Local measures utilized to lessen the possible spread of the infection include (1) clipping or shaving of the involved areas twice a week, (2) twice daily application of antifungal cream (MicaTin, Halotex, Lotrimin, or Tinactin), (3) frequent shampoos, and (4) head covering when associating with other children at home, school or at play.

Post treatment observations include (1) inspection of the scalp, (2) Wood's light examination, (3) direct examination of scalp hairs, and (4) cultures. These studies should be done every two weeks for a total of eight weeks before discharging patient as cured.

TINEA CORPORIS AND TINEA CRURIS

The newer local agents miconazole, clotrimazole, haloprogin and tolnaftate are effective in managing the localized ringworm infections of the body. Occasionally systemic griseofulvin is also necessary in combination with local agents. Therapy usually is continued for three to four weeks, even though clinical complete clearing is seen 7 to 10 days after initial treatment.

TINEA PEDIS

Acute vesicobullous dermatophytic infections of the feet require (1) systemic griseofulvin therapy, (2) bed rest, (3) drainage of the bullous lesions; (4) Burow's solution soaks; (5) topical applications of antifungal agents such as miconazole, haloprogin, clotrimazole and tolnaftate. The course of griseofulvin should be continued for at least two weeks. Local measures should be done three to four times each day during that period. Subsequent management should be directed to prevention of re-infection. These include (1) proper cleansing and drying of the feet twice a day, (2) light-weight cotton socks, (3) perforated shoes, and (4) foot powder during the day (ZeaSORB or Tinactin) and antifungal cream at bedtime.

Chronic tinea pedia manifested by scaling and erythema with no vesicles is most recalcitrant. Griseofulvin orally, sometimes for 6 to 12 months, is required. Daily application of the antifungal creams is also helpful.

ONYCHOMYCOSIS

Nail infection in children is fortunately rarely seen. If it occurs it is usually associated with other fungal involvement of the skin. It may be seen as a manifestation of other serious systemic illness or with the use of therapeutic

---

*Manufacturer's precaution: Dosage of griseolfulvin ultramicrosize (Gris-PEG) has not been established for children 2 years of age and younger.

agents that suppress the child's defense against infections. If due to one of the dermatophytes, griseofulvin orally may be necessary for a period of 6 to 12 months. If the organism isolated is *Candida albicans,* local use of nystatin, miconazole, clotrimazole or haloprogin is indicated. Again, these later agents may be needed for months.

CANDIDIASIS (MONILIASIS OR YEAST INFECTION)

Localized yeast infections of the skin may be found in any of the moist areas of the body, especially the body folds (axillary, crural, perineal, perianal, interdigital, vulvar and scrotal). These are generally acute moist erythematous eruptions. Management includes (1) gentle cleaning with either Betadine or Burow's solution, (2) gentle drying, and (3) application of antifungal creams. Occasionally Mycolog (a combination of antibacterial and anti-yeast agents and corticosteroid) is helpful. Powders containing nystatin may also be employed.

TINEA VERSICOLOR

This disease is rarely seen in children. It can, however, be chronic and recurrent once it is acquired. Therapy must be thorough and prolonged. Recurrences are usual and should be treated immediately to prevent extensive involvement. Sulfur, either as sodium thiosulfate or as selinium sulfide, is the old standby. The newer agents miconazole, clotrimazole and haloprogin are very effective. Scalp involvement, difficult to identify, may serve as a source of re-infection. Scalp involvement (real or potential) can be treated by the use of a shampoo containing sulfur (Selsun, Fostex, or Meted).

Warts and Molluscum Contagiosum

SIDNEY KIBRICK, M.D.

WARTS (VERRUCAE)

Warts are benign, viral-induced, epithelial tumors characterized by epidermal and papillary hypertrophy. In pediatrics, the following wart types commonly are seen: verruca vulgaris (the common wart), most frequent on the hands; verruca plana juvenilis (the flat wart), often occurring in large numbers especially on the face; and verruca plantaris (the plantar wart), which resembles a callus and generally occurs on the plantar surface of the foot, occasionally on the palm. Clustered plantar warts are known as mosaic warts. Occasionally

filiform verrucae, small stalk-like growths resembling skin tabs, are seen. When warts are present in a moist intertriginous area, such as the anogenital region, they usually assume a fleshy exuberant form, the so-called condylomata acuminata or moist warts.

The multiplicity of treatments for warts indicates that no one method is satisfactory. The fact that these lesions may disappear spontaneously, reappear after their removal or spread after prolonged quiescence makes it difficult to evaluate treatment. About two-thirds of untreated warts in children disappear within two years. It is important therefore that the treatment not produce changes worse than the presence of the wart. Since warts are limited to the epidermis, therapeutic procedures should be confined to this level to avoid scarring.

Warts in some children present a special problem since painful office procedures may induce apprehension, resistance and psychic trauma. Accordingly, where a choice is available, those treatments associated with immediate pain should be avoided in favor of those with a delayed response. Since several approaches may be required before the lesions disappear, a variety of treatments is described. Whenever practical, warts should be carefully pared both before and during the course of treatment.

The most benign approach to therapy is the use of suggestion, which has been estimated to be effective against common warts in as high as 50 per cent of children. Suggestion involves repeated reassurance that the warts will disappear, reinforced by daily or more frequent applications of placebos. This procedure appears to be especially effective against flat warts. Innocuous solutions such as dyed castor oil or, more commonly, exfoliative lotions of the type used for acne are employed, such as topical retinoic acid (Retin-A, 0.05 per cent cream, Johnson & Johnson),* 5 to 10 per cent benzoyl peroxide, and double strength Whitfield's ointment. These latter preparations are generally used until an exfoliative reaction ensues.

Small numbers of common and filiform warts generally can be treated effectively by cryotherapy, preferably with liquid nitrogen. To minimize discomfort, local anesthesia is used for all but the smallest lesions. After procaine infiltration beneath the lesion base, an applicator with a loose cotton tip is dipped into liquid nitrogen, then applied to the wart until it turns white (30 seconds to several minutes). A

---

*This use of retinoic acid is not mentioned in the manufacturer's instructions.

1 mm. border of normal tissue should be included. Hours to a day later, a blister develops. If hemorrhagic or painful it may be drained, but the roof, which contains the wart, should be left intact to dry up and separate. When cryotherapy is used on the hands, care should be taken to avoid freezing the peripheral nerves which run along the lateral aspects of the fingers.

Common and filiform warts can also be removed under local anesthesia by curette or by electrodesiccation and curetting of the burnt tissue. Care should be taken to avoid damage to the dermis.

Common warts may be treated with chemical agents (escharotics, keratolytics). Such treatment is simple, generally less painful, often effective and rarely causes scarring. It does, however, require more time and patient cooperation. A few chemical regimens which have been found to be useful are described below.

Small Warts. The bare end of an applicator stick is dipped into liquid phenol and applied with pressure for several seconds to the base of the trimmed lesion. This is immediately followed by a similar application of concentrated nitric acid which inhibits further phenol action and is escharotic. The treatment is repeated once weekly on the trimmed wart until it disappears. Other escharotic or keratolytic agents also give good results, such as weekly applications of trichloroacetic acid, either alone or followed by rubbing the moist lesion with a silver nitrate stick, or daily applications of Duofilm (16.7 per cent salicylic and 16.7 per cent lactic acid in flexible collodion) followed by Band-Aid occlusion.

Large Warts. An ointment consisting of 40 per cent salicylic acid in petrolatum or a piece of 40 per cent salicylic acid plaster cut to wart size is applied to the lesion, which is then covered with Blenderm or adhesive tape to increase maceration and prevent spread of the medication. The area should be kept dry or the medication and dressing reapplied after washing. At weekly intervals, the tape is removed, the wart is trimmed and the treatment is repeated. Alternately, Duofilm may be used as previously described. Several weeks or longer may be required for a satisfactory response. Such salicylic acid dressings are generally used in conjunction with the phenol, nitric acid or trichloroacetic acid, or silver nitrate treatments described above.

Cantharidin, 0.7 per cent, in equal parts of acetone and flexible collodion (commercially available as Cantharone), is also effective. This drug is a vesicant and induces a blister, the roof of which contains most of the wart. The solution may be applied with a toothpick, using only enough medication to cover the lesion. When the area has dried it is covered with a wart-size piece of plastic adhesive, which in turn is protected by a Band-Aid. The adhesive is removed after one to two days, or earlier if pain is noted, and the lesion is washed. If a painful blister forms, it may be nicked for relief. At one week, the top of the blister is removed and the treatment is repeated for any remaining warty tissue. From one to six weekly treatments may be required. If inflammation occurs, water or saline soaks may be used and treatments should be deferred until it subsides. This preparation should be checked before use to ensure that excessive evaporation of the vehicle has not occurred.

The chemical treatment of periungual warts is similar to that of large warts. They present a special problem, however, since they tend to extend and are difficult to eradicate. When treating the base of the nail, care must be taken to avoid injury to the nail matrix.

Plantar Warts. These may be exquisitely painful if located on points of pressure. Most treatments are relatively unsatisfactory. Neither excision nor any other treatment that could lead to scarring should be used since the resulting scars may be more painful than the wart. The risks associated with x-ray therapy (radiodermatitis, ulceration, scarring, epiphyseal arrest) are not generally justified, especially in children. Plantar warts preferably are treated conservatively with doughnut dressings or "corn pads" to relieve pressure, pending their spontaneous resolution. At least 25 per cent of such lesions disappear spontaneously within one year.

If the wart is associated with disability in walking, however, the following regimens may be tried: (1) any of the treatments described above under large warts, with the exception of cantharidin (not recommended for plantar lesions), or (2) applications, after paring, of 20 per cent podophyllum solutions in compound tincture of benzoin. This is applied at two to three day intervals, with the lesion kept covered by adhesive tape after each application. Repeated applications for several weeks or longer may be necessary. Mosaic plantar warts are treated by the same regimens. For plantar warts under treatment, doughnut dressings may be used for relief of pain from pressure.

Moist Warts. Although these warts are uncommon in children, a simple and effective treatment is available. The growth, surrounded by a protective layer of petrolatum or zinc oxide paste, is treated with a single application of 20 per cent podophyllum in compound tincture of benzoin. The site is washed off thoroughly after four to six hours. There is no immediate reaction but after a few hours pain may occur, and several days later the lesion sloughs off. Sitz baths help to relieve discomfort. The treatment is repeated as needed at intervals of one to two weeks, depending upon the time required for the reaction in the adjacent tissues to subside. If the lesions are numerous, only a few should be treated at a time. The patient should also be checked for the presence of rectal lesions since these may act as a source of reinfection and must be removed (by electrocautery) before cure can be achieved. Electrocautery may also be used for the occasional patient who fails to respond or who develops a hypersensitivity to podophyllum.

MOLLUSCUM CONTAGIOSUM

This viral disease of the skin is characterized by one or more small globular yellow to pinkish tumors with umbilicated centers. The lesions are most simply treated by curettage (local anesthesia with ethyl chloride may be helpful). Bleeding from the base may be controlled by simple pressure. An alternative treatment consists of making a superficial incision through the roof of each lesion, expressing the cheese-like contents or core with forceps or a comedo extractor and applying phenol to the central cavity with a toothpick. Healing occurs within a week with no scarring. All lesions should be removed since the disease, although of low infectivity, is transmissible by autoinoculation.

The above procedures are associated with some discomfort and may present a problem in young children, especially if extensive lesions are present. In such cases the lesions may be treated with trichloroacetic acid applied daily with a toothpick, by the mother, with careful instructions to avoid adjacent normal skin. If numerous lesions persist, it may be desirable to remove them at one session under anesthesia.

The presence of such nodules on the lid margins may be associated with chronic conjunctivitis and keratitis due apparently to the toxic effect on the eye of desquamated material from the lesions. Cure may be effected by excision of these nodules.

Arthropod Bites and Stings

RICHARD S. BERGER, M.D.

Arthropods make up the largest phylum in the animal kingdom with over one million species. They are constant members of man's environment. The two classes, Insecta and Arachnida, contain hundreds of species known to cause cutaneous and systemic problems by their bites and stings.

ARACHNIDS

Spiders

Brown Recluse (and other Loxosceles spiders). The bite of this arachnid produces a toxic reaction due to an enzymatic venomous substance. If a small amount of venom is injected by the spider or if the patient is immune due to previous bites, only erythema and edema occur. In the more severe cases, the venom damages dermal blood vessels and produces hemorrhage, blanching within 24 to 72 hours and finally necrosis. Systemic symptoms, seen mainly in severe reactions, begin as early as 36 hours and include morbilliform rash, urticaria, fever, nausea and vomiting, and occasionally hemolysis or diffuse intravascular coagulation. Presently, no satisfactory treatment is available to prevent the cutaneous necrosis, although systemic and intralesional steroids are used by many physicians.

For minor reactions, antihistamines will control the symptoms. In more severe cases with toxic systemic symptoms, systemic steroids (60 to 80 mg. of prednisone daily) are required. Heparin therapy is recommended if signs of diffuse intravascular coagulation are present. Excision and repair of the area of necrosis should be delayed until the area of necrosis is well delineated and healing has begun.

Black Widow. The neurotoxic effects of the spider's venom produces severe cramps, waves of pain, and a board-like abdomen—symptoms which mimic those of an acute abdomen. Systemic treatment with muscle relaxants and intravenous calcium gluconate helps relieve the muscle spasm. Narcotics may be required for pain. A specific antivenin, Lyovac, is available for high risk patients, i.e., small children and the aged. It is administered intramuscularly after appropriate skin tests for allergy to normal horse serum are found to be negative.

Scorpions

In most areas of the United States, the sting from the scorpion only causes a painful local reaction similar to a bee sting. In the Southwest, however, envenomation by a small scorpion, Centruroides sculpturatus, produces neurotoxic symptoms similar to the black widow spider and is potentially lethal. Specific antivenin is available in the poison centers in the region. Atropine and phenobarbital are given for symptomatic relief.

Ticks

Most people are unaware of the bite with which the tick attaches himself. If the tick is not removed, a painful inflammatory reaction develops. Tick saliva activates a component of complement producing local tissue destruction and chemotaxis. Additionally, if mouth parts remain after removing the tick, secondary infection and ulceration or a foreign body granuloma may develop. The latter may be treated by simple excision or intralesional steroids. While various home remedies for tick removal are rife, simple slow traction using forceps is safe and adequate.

If the tick is not removed within a few hours, it is a potential vector of serious diseases, including rickettsial infections and tick paralysis. The exact mechanism of tick paralysis is disputed. It starts with ataxia and areflexia and progresses to a motor weakness such as that seen in the Landry-Guillain-Barre syndrome. Removal of the tick cures the paralysis. Tetracycline is the treatment of choice for rickettsial infections. Insect repellents and washing the hair with tar shampoos will discourage the initial attachment of the tick.

MITES

Scabies. The scabies mite burrows under the upper layer of the skin inducing an inflammatory response which produces tremendous itching. The diagnostic signs on the skin are multiple papules, minute vesicles and occasional linear tracts located in the fingerwebs, around the wrists, axillae, nipples, waist, umbilicus, buttocks, and genitalia. The upper part of the back, the palms and soles, and the head and neck are usually spared. Often secondary excoriation, eczematization, and infection are present.

Diagnosis is confirmed by placing a drop of immersion oil on a No.15 blade and scraping a burrow and examining it under low power (4 × objective). In the majority of cases (but not all), a mite, an ovum, or fecal pellets can be seen. Lesions other than burrows are much less likely to be "positive."

Treatment consists of applying 1 per cent gamma benzene hexachloride cream or lotion from the chin to the toes after bathing. This is allowed to remain on the skin for 24 hours. A repeat application in one week may be required. More frequent applications may be dangerous due to absorption of the chemicals. In instances of treatment failure, 10 per cent N-ethyl-o-crotonotoluide (Eurax) applied for two successive nights and a cleansing bath taken 48 hours after the last application, or 25 per cent benzyl benzoate emulsion applied for three successive nights, may be used. For infants, 6 per cent sulfur in petrolatum applied twice daily for two or three days is considered safer than 1 per cent gamma benzene.

Chiggers. The tiny orange larva of this mite attaches to the base of the hair follicle usually in areas of constrictive clothing. Introduction of enzymes which liquify the surrounding tissue causes an intense pruritus and erythematous macules, papules, or wheals within 12 to 24 hours. Scratching often results in secondary eczematization and infection. Topical steroids provide symptomatic relief. Insect repellents and toxicants such as Off, Deet, Eurax and benzyl benzoate provide protection from chiggers. Secondary infection should be treated with systemic antibiotics.

INSECTS

Lice

Man is host to three varieties of lice which are named by the area of the body they attack. While obtaining their blood meal, the lice secrete an irritating substance which causes a great deal of itching and subsequent scratching.

Pediculosis pubis usually occurs in the hair of the genital region but may spread to other hairy regions of the body such as the axillae and even the eyelashes. *Pediculosis capitis* affects the scalp hair. In *Pediculosis corporis* the organism is more readily found in the clothes rather than on the body. In addition to bites, a nonspecific papular urticaria sometimes results.

Gamma benzene hexachloride lotion is the therapy of choice for pediculosis pubis. It is left on for 24 hours and then washed off thoroughly. A second application may be repeated in one week if viable eggs persist. For pediculosis capitis gamma benzene hexachloride shampoo is used. After lathering for at least four minutes, rinse hair thoroughly and rub with a dry towel. If necessary, repeat treatment in 24 hours but no more than twice within one week. For pediculosis of the eyelashes, coating the lashes with petrolatum (twice daily for eight days) will eliminate lice.

Flies and Mosquitoes

Usually these bites do not create serious problems and are usually not seen by physicians unless secondarily infected or unless the patient has an extreme sensitivity to the bite. In the sensitive individual, local cool compresses and systemic antihistamines provide relief.

Fleas

Fleas often bite two or three times in a line and usually attack the lower leg because they are coming from the ground or carpet. The bites are not perceptible for the first day or two, then erythematous, pruritic papules develop. A central punctum or vesicle is often present. Not all individuals react to the bites and often only one or two of the people in a household will complain of problems. Treatment is aimed at reducing the pruritus. This is best accomplished with soothing lotions or steroid cream or sprays. Eradication of the fleas from the household pet and the home by use of insecticides is essential to prevent recurrences.

Blister Beetles

This insect causes no problem unless you apply pressure to it. Even slight pressure causes a fluid containing cantharidin to exude from the knee joints, prothorax and genitalia. A stinging sensation develops in 10 minutes, followed in 8 to 12 hours by bulla formation. The blisters usually occur on exposed areas, often in a linear fashion. The beetle should be removed without crushing it and the area should be cleaned with a solvent and then soap and water.

Caterpillars

The nettling hair of the caterpillar produces both a toxic and mechanical injury to the skin. The signs and symptoms range from erythema, edema and pruritus to epidermal necrosis. Often the whole extremity is swollen. Treatment is nonspecific, such as elevation of the extremity and cool compresses. Toxic systemic symptoms may develop including muscle cramps, severe headaches, and tachycardia. Intravenous calcium gluconate and narcotics will alleviate these systemic symptoms.

Hymenoptera

Fire Ants. The fire ant venom causes a painful sensation which accounts for their name. It gives rise to a characteristic pustular reaction. Multiple stings and allergic reactions can be life-threatening. Necrosis may lead to secondary infection. Local treatment, such as soaks, is usually sufficient unless systemic infection or allergic type reactions develop. Allergic reactions require systemic antihistamines and possibly epinephrine.

Bees, Wasps, Hornets. Of all the venomous arthropods, the sting of the bee, wasp and hornet account for the greatest number of deaths owing to hypersensitivity reactions. The treatment for this type of reaction is systemic antihistamines and epinephrine. A patient known to be very allergic to the Hymenoptera venom should receive desensitization. Presently, whole body extracts are used; however, work is progressing on purified venom extract. For local reactions, cold compresses will help relieve the discomfort.

Melanin Pigmentary Disorders

ALVIN H. JACOBS, M.D.

HYPERPIGMENTATION

Café au lait spots are light tan spots of various sizes and with regular borders. They are usually of no significance and need no treatment. However, it is said that a patient with six or more such spots greater than 1.5 cm. in diameter may be assumed to have neurofibromatosis. Café au lait spots also occur commonly with Albright's disease and tuberous sclerosis.

Freckles are small, light-brown circumscribed macules which occur in response to exposure to sun. Depigmentation treatment as described below is inadvisable in the case of freckles. One may wish to provide the patient with a good sunscreen preparation such as PreSun or Eclipse to lessen the number of freckles that occur with sun exposure during the summer months.

Lentigines are small dark-brown macules which are not related to sun exposures and, in fact, are more common on unexposed parts of the body. Generalized lentigines in association with cardiac, ocular, and auditory abnormalities have been described as the generalized lentigines (leopard) syndrome.

Melasma is a patchy, tan-to-brown pigmentation located predominantly on the cheeks and forehead of girls or women who are pregnant or who are taking oral contraceptives. In dark-skinned persons with much exposure to sun, melasma can be a serious cosmetic problem, and one may wish to consider depigmentation treatment (described below). It is advisable to provide a good sunscreen preparation such as PreSun or Eclipse to pregnant girls or those on contraceptive pills during the summer months.

Postinflammatory hyperpigmentation may occur following subsidence of erythema due to any type of inflammation. This fades slowly over a period of months, but in dark-skinned individuals the fading is slower and depigmentation treatment as described below may be necessary.

Moles (nevus-cell nevi) are discussed under Nevi and Nevoid Tumors (page 496).

Agents to Decrease Pigmentation. Hydroquinone is an inhibitor of melanin formation and may be used to "bleach" areas of hyperpigmentation. Since treated areas must be protected from ultraviolet light, a convenient preparation to use is Eldopaque Forte (Elder Co.) in which 4 per cent hydroquinone is incorporated in an opaque base which occludes all light.* This should be applied 2 or 3 times daily for weeks to months. The hyperpigmented areas fade more rapidly and completely than surrounding normal skin.

Hydroquinone treatment should not be used for management of freckles, but is quite useful for melasma and for larger areas of postinflammatory hyperpigmentation.

HYPOPIGMENTATION

Albinism is a rare congenital disturbance (failure of the skin to form melanin pigment) which results from an enzymatic defect in the melanocyte. The most significant result of this absence of melanin is a strong hypersensitivity to light. There is no therapy other than prophylactic measures aimed at the light hypersensitivity. These patients must learn to avoid sunlight exposure and to use sunscreen preparations on exposed surfaces. PreSun, Eclipse, and Solbar are among the better sunscreen agents.

Vitiligo is an acquired cutaneous achromia characterized by variously sized and shaped single or multiple patches of milk-white color, usually with hyperpigmented borders and a tendency to enlarge peripherally. The skin presents no textural changes and is normal in every way except for a sensitivity to solar radiation. Some patients report some repigmentation from the border and in small perifollicular patches on exposure to sunlight in the summer, but disappearance of the repigmented areas in the winter.

Repigmentation in patients with vitiligo can be accomplished by administration of the psoralen compounds followed by gradually increasing exposure to sunlight or long wave ultraviolet (UVA). This therapy is most effective in patients with a relatively short history of vitiligo. The newest and safest of these drugs is Trimethylpsoralen (Trisoralen). The daily dosage recommended by the package insert is 10 mg. However, all leading dermatology cen-

ters are now using doses of 30 mg., increasing to as much as 50 mg. if necessary. There have been no reports of adverse effects from this drug and studies have now been reported in the literature of its safe administration to children of all ages. The manufacturer's application to increase the dosage is now under consideration by the Food and Drug Administration.

Successful treatment of vitiligo requires careful attention to the details of the regimen. The full daily dose of Trisoralen is given at one time, followed in 2 hours by measured exposure to sunlight or an artificial source of long wave ultraviolet light (UVA). The ordinary commercial sun lamps are deficient in this wave length of UV and are ineffective for this purpose. The duration of exposure should be sufficient to produce an erythema but no blistering, and should be increased as indicated. During the remainder of the day, involved areas not covered by clothing should be protected from additional sunburn by application of a washable sunscreen such as Uval. On days where sun exposure cannot be carried out, the dosage of Trisoralen is omitted.

Repigmentation may begin after a few weeks; however, significant results may take as long as 6 months. Once repigmentation has occurred it is usually permanent, although retreatment is occasionally necessary.

White macules exist in more than 90 per cent of patients with tuberous sclerosis when no other visible lesions typical of the disorder are evident. These hypopigmented macules are present at birth but may not be very obvious in fair-skinned infants and so must be looked for with a Wood's lamp. No treatment of the macule is necessary, but this clue should alert one to the possible future development of other manifestations of tuberous sclerosis.

Leukoderma is a patchy depigmentation usually occurring as a result of many inflammatory dermatoses and skin injuries and is frequently preceded by hyperpigmentation. These postinflammatory leukodermas are generally transient and decrease with time. Treatment should be directed only to the primary dermatosis.

An interesting type of leukoderma is the "halo nevus," or leukoderma acquisitum centrifugum. Here, a brown mole becomes surrounded by a depigmented halo that has all the earmarks of vitiligo and may be associated with vitiliginous patches in the same patient. Usually the central nevus also becomes depigmented and disappears completely. The halo nevus should not be treated, since it clears spontaneously in time.

*Manufacturer's precaution: Hydroquinone should not be used in children under 12 years of age.

Photodermatoses

M. T. FLIEGELMAN, M.D., *and*
L. G. OWEN, M.D.

Photosensitizers may induce an abnormal reaction in skin exposed to sun, or the reaction can be caused by artificial light sources such as an ultraviolet light lamp, a welding arc or fluorescent lights.

A list of photosensitizers adapted from Fitzpatrick's *Dermatology in General Practice* is given in Table 1.

Drugs may induce photosensitivity by either phototoxic or photoallergic means. In phototoxic reactions the clinical picture is that of an exaggerated sunburn and develops within hours of exposure to ultraviolet light. A mild phototoxic reaction will usually subside within a few days, but in a few cases, an unexpected new eruption flares up a week or 10 days after the original eruption and in the same areas on the skin. This latter eruption is spontaneous and not related to additional UVL exposure. The clinical picture is also quite different in that it can resemble eczema or dermatitis venenata—vesicles, urticaria or even purpura. This delayed eruption is a true allergic reaction of the cell-mediated type.

An abnormal reaction of the skin to light characterizes these dermatoses, and the distribution of the eruption (face, neck, "V" of the chest, backs of the hands, forearms and lower parts of the legs in children) are of more significance than its morphology.

Sunburn is the most common of these disorders. Cool compresses or baths (plain or colloidal) followed by topical corticosteroids are soothing and healing. Systemic symptoms are treated, if indicated.

Solar urticaria is rare in children and localized hives immediately follow minimal exposure to sunlight and heat. Antihistamines in appropriate doses are often helpful. Erythropoietic protoporphyria and systemic lupus erythematosus must be ruled out.

Polymorphous light eruptions usually appear 1 to 4 days after sun exposure, tending to recur annually. The various eruptions (vesicles, papules, papular plaques) on exposed areas apparently have no other cause except sensitivity to sunlight. Treatment is symptomatic: antihistamines, topical corticosteroids and occasionally doses of parenteral steroids.

Antimalarials are frequently effective, but their toxicity must be borne in mind. Sunscreens are helpful.

Contact photosensitivity is limited to areas involving both the chemical and sunlight. Contact allergens with which children might be affected included antibacterial soaps, fruits, perfumes, plants and coal tar derivatives.

Systemic photosensitivity is caused by many drugs (see Table 1). Treatment consists of removal of the patient from the contact or systemic sensitizers and then symptomatic treatment with compresses or colloidal baths, topical or systemic steroids if indicated.

Furthermore, certain known diseases are aggravated by light. Genetic disorders with this characteristic include porphyria, albinism, xeroderma pigmentosa and hydroa aestivale (a rare familial disorder exhibiting blistered crusts on the nose, cheeks, ears and back of the hands, which sometimes leads to scarring; it appears in early childhood and frequently subsides with puberty). Herpes simplex infections, porphyrias, pellagra and systemic lupus erythematosus are other examples of diseases aggravated by exposure to light.

In making the diagnosis look for the distribution of the eruption. Are the face, extensor surfaces of the forearms or the "V" of the neck involved? Are eyelids and creases of the neck spared? Rule out common etiologies such as certain soaps or drug-related photodermatitis before searching for rarer systemic diseases. Have the patient avoid sunlight, even through window glass or by reflection (from water or sand). Use protective clothing, such as wide-brimmed hats, stockings and long-sleeved shirts.

Sunscreens such as PreSun Lotion, Pabafilm or Solbar are good for sunburn radiation; 5 per cent PABA (para-aminobenzoic acid), 2 per cent titanium dioxide or 1 to 2 per cent neutracolor in hydrophilic ointment will block out all harmful radiation but is less acceptable cosmetically.

Faced with an eruption various forms of topical treatment are most helpful; antihistamines are frequently not very helpful. Topical and systemic steroids may be used if the reaction is severe, tapering off over 1 to 3 weeks.

Being a good detective is of paramount importance!

TABLE 1.   Classification of Abnormal Reactions to Light in Man

TYPE	LIGHT ALONE	LIGHT PLUS EXOGENOUS AGENT	LIGHT PLUS METABOLITE	LIGHT PLUS ABNORMAL SKIN OR DISEASE
Genetic	Ephelides (freckles)		Porphyria Erythropoietic porphyria	Xeroderma pigmentosum Hartnup syndrome Oculocutaneous albinism Cockayne's syndrome Rothmund-Thomas syndrome Hailey-Hailey disease Vitiligo Darier-White disease Bloom's syndrome
Chemical, phototoxic		*Topical and oral drugs* Sulfonamide Eosin and erythrosine Furocoumarins *Oral drugs* Dyes, eosin, trypaflavin, etc. Barbiturates Arsphenamine Gold Quinine Chlorothiazide Griseofulvin Sulfonylurea Demethylchlortetracycline Aminolevulinic acid Hematoporphyrin *Topical drugs:* Coal tar p-Aminobenzoic acid	Porphyria from hexachlorobenzene Griseofulvin Alcohol	
Photoallergic	Solar urticaria Polymorphic photodermatitis	Halogenated salicylanilides Hexachlorophene Sulfanilamide Jadit (4-chloro-2-hydroxybenzoic acid-N-n-butylamide)		
Nutritional				Kwashiorkor Pellagra
Infectious				Lymphogranuloma venereum Herpes simplex
Miscellaneous	Connective tissue degeneration Telangiectasia Polymorphic photodermatitis Solar urticaria Hydroa aestivale and hydroa vacciniforme Disseminated superficial actinic porokeratosis	Phytophotodermatitis	Porphyria Porphyria cutanea tarda	Lupus erythematosus (cutaneous and systemic) Malignant carcinoid Pemphigus foliaceous and pemphigus erythematodes

Nevi and Nevoid Tumors

MICHAEL B. LEWIS, M.D., *and*
MURRAY FEINGOLD, M.D.

MELANOCYTIC TUMORS

Although the term nevus is defined as a circumscribed new growth of the skin of congenital origin (either vascular or nonvascular), it is commonly used in reference to the pigmented variety (either congenital or acquired). A mole is a pigmented nevus and the two words (mole, nevus) are often used interchangeably.

The critical therapeutic decision in dealing with pigmented lesions is to determine which is malignant, which is premalignant or potentially malignant, and which is benign and likely to remain so. It is estimated that about 50 per cent of all malignant melanomas develop in preexisting pigmented lesions but this usually does not happen until after puberty (except for the giant pigmented nevus). The incidence of melanoma in the adult population is approximately 3 per 100,000 and since the average adult has 15 to 20 pigmented lesions, the chance of malignant degeneration occurring in a single pigmented lesion is extremely small. The excision of every pigmented lesion to exclude the possibility of melanoma developing would be impossible and is not indicated. Judgment is required in deciding which lesion to excise and which one not to. Certain characteristics of pigmented lesions should alert the physician to the possibility of melanoma or its chance of developing. Examination of the pigmented lesion under 2 to 4 X magnification is useful in discerning these characteristics. It should be stated from the outset, however, that if doubt exists, the lesion should be excised for biopsy or an incisional biopsy performed. Additionally, it is sometimes advisable to excise nevi because their location exposes them to constant irritation and breakdown or makes them esthetically undesirable.

Moles. The common mole can be found anywhere on the body and presents in a variety of ways. The location of the melanocytes within the skin determines the clinical appearance. Junctional, compound, and dermal pigmented nevi are probably progressive stages of the same lesion. The junctional nevus is a smooth, flat, pigmented lesion in which melanocytes are concentrated just above the basement membrane. They usually appear in early childhood. With the passage of time some of the melanocytes migrate into the dermis creating a compound nevus which is slightly elevated. When all the melanocytes have moved into the dermis a dome-shaped dermal (intradermal) nevus is formed. The majority of moles require no treatment. Only when sudden changes occur which make one suspicious of malignancy should excision be undertaken for pathological examination. Changes in size or color, bleeding, tenderness, itching and ulceration are early warning signs of melanoma.

Halo Nevus. The halo nevus is another presentation of the compound or dermal nevus in which peripheral depigmentation has occurred resulting in a white "halo." Although the sudden recognition of this change might be disconcerting, no treatment is required. Usually the depigmentation process continues to involve the entire mole.

Blue Nevus. The ordinary blue nevus is another form of the dermal nevus in which the melanocytes are located extremely deep in the dermis. Because of their deep location a blue or grayish-blue color is imparted to the lesion. Blue nevi are benign lesions and require no treatment. If there is any difficulty in differentiating a blue nevus from a malignant melanoma, excision is required for histological diagnosis.

Mongolian Spot. Another form of blue nevus is the mongolian spot, which is usually located in the lumbosacral region. It occurs in up to 90 per cent of Negro, Oriental and American Indian infants and in approximately 5 per cent of Caucasian infants. It is macular with irregular borders and varies in size up to 10 cm. in diameter. Mongolian spots usually fade within the first year or two of life, but a small number may persist into late childhood. No treatment is required.

Nevus of Ota. This is another congenital form of blue nevus involving the orbital and zygomatic regions unilaterally, occurring in natives of Japan and Samoa, American Indians, and Negroes. Its occurrence is rare. Indications for treatment are esthetic only. Occlusive, covering makeup is probably the best means of dealing with this lesion.

Spitz Nevus. The lesion is also called benign juvenile melanoma and is typically a dome-shaped, pink-tan lesion which appears rather suddenly on the face, upper limbs, or trunk of children or young adults. It is a highly vascular lesion and diascopy is useful in diagnosis. This maneuver involves pressing a clean glass slide firmly against the lesion, emptying the many capillaries and venules permitting visualization of the brown melanin pigmentation. Simple excision is curative.

Giant Pigmented Nevus. This nevus is present at birth, tends to occur in the distribution of dermatomes, or in a bathing trunk, vest, sleeve, or stocking pattern. It is most common in the head and pelvic regions. Occasionally in giant pigmented nevi overlying the neural canal, leptomeningeal melanocytosis occurs producing focal neurological signs. The giant pigmented nevus is truly a premalignant lesion. The exact incidence of malignant melanoma in these lesions is unknown but reported series vary between 2 and 42 per cent. Forty per cent of all melanomas in children develop in the giant pigmented nevus. Sixty per cent of these melanomas will develop in the first decade, so early aggressive prophylactic excision is indicated. Complete staged excision to include skin and subcutaneous tissue with free skin graft and flap reconstruction is the method of choice.

Data involving smaller congenital nevi are less clear. Melanomas arising in these lesions may occur but the exact incidence of melanoma is unknown. Therefore either a course of careful and frequent observation with excision at the first sign of change or early excision is reasonable.

Malignant Melanoma. These are rare in children and aggressive radical surgical management is indicated. Wide local excision down to the overlying muscular fascia with free skin graft or flap reconstruction is required. Regional lymph node dissection is required if nodes are clinically involved or if the lesion invades the dermis beyond level two.

A summary of indications for excision or diagnostic biopsy of pigmented lesion includes the consideration of three variables: history, appearance, and site of the lesion.

The possibility of malignant change should be considered if: the lesion changes in size or color; there is bleeding, itching, or tenderness; a congenital lesion is greater than 1.5 cm. in diameter; and there is a family history of melanoma. Other characteristics of the individual lesion include: a variegated blue, gray-white, and red admixed to a brown and black color; an irregular or notched border; and an irregular surface and ulceration. The anatomical sites of lesions which require careful consideration include the reproductive organ area, mucous membranes and the sites of repeated trauma occurring anywhere on the body including the scalp.

VASCULAR NEVI

Vascular nevi occur frequently in infants and children and are almost always benign. There are, however, a great variety of such lesions.

Salmon Patches (Nevus Simplex). These are pink-colored lesions usually located at the nape of the neck, glabella, forehead, and upper eyelids and occur in approximately 40 per cent of all infants. No treatment is indicated, as they usually involute spontaneously. A slight erythematous discoloration may be present in adult life with temperature and emotional variations.

Capillary and Cavernous Hemangioma and Strawberry Marks. Although these lesions may be present at birth, they frequently are not obvious. They may initially appear as "whitish" flat areas and then have a very rapid growth. At approximately age one they start to involute and the color turns from red to gray and white starting in the center of the hemangioma. By age 7 the majority have spontaneously regressed. However, with temperature and emotional changes these lesions may appear erythematous. Although treatment is usually not indicated, therapy may be necessary for some of the lesions because of their size or location, or for cosmetic reasons. Hemangiomas located in areas where there is frequent irritation may break down and become infected and subsequently scar. This is especially true of hemangiomas located in the corners of the mouth.

When treatment is indicated prednisone, 3 mg./kg., is given either in the morning or in divided doses two or three times a day. Improvement usually occurs within the first two weeks of therapy. If there are no signs of regression, therapy is discontinued. If, however, treatment is successful the medication can be given for a total of three weeks and then tapered. In our experience approximately 20 to 25 per cent of the patients have a very good to good response. Other investigators have reported a higher percentage. Approximately half of the patients who initially respond to therapy have regrowth following the discontinuation of the medication. If regrowth does occur another course of steroid therapy may be initiated, especially if the hemangioma is in a critical area such as in the orbit with occlusion of the eye. Occasionally surgery may be indicated after age 5 for certain cavernous lesions in order to improve either appearance or function.

Port Wine Stains. Although there are a variety of surgical methods used to treat this lesion, including medical tattooing and excision, most of them are not very successful. At the present time, various covering makeups are used to cover the stains. Patients who have port wine stains on the face, especially in the area of the distribution of the facial nerve, should be evaluated for the possibility of the Sturge-Weber syndrome.

Spider Nevi. These lesions are very small, erythematous, and have a generalized distribution with the trunk being least involved. They may go away spontaneously. If cosmetic treatment is indicated a desiccating diathermy needle applied at the center of the nevus will produce a thrombosis and subsequent clearing.

Congenital Phlebectasia. This has also been called cutis marmorata telangiectatica congenita. These lesions are secondary to dilatation of superficial veins and capillaries and appear as mottling of the skin. The course is different from that of a hemangioma in that it does not have rapid growth nor does it involute by age one year. Regression may take place but a certain percentage remain. Generally no treatment is indicated.

Blue Rubber Bleb Nevus. This is a type of cavernous hemangioma which has a bluish-purplish color, is usually very small and has a generalized distribution. The lesions may involute but generally cause a cosmetic problem. Unfortunately there is no specific treatment available for removal of all these lesions. Similar lesions may be present in the gastrointestinal tract, bone and other areas.

Other Skin Tumors

BARBARA GILCHREST, M.D.

Skin tumors are common in childhood. Most are benign and their importance lies in the cosmetic defect they may create, in their occasional association with systemic disease, and in their separation from the much less common malignant tumors which may also occur in children.

TUMORS OF THE EPIDERMIS

Basal Cell Epithelioma (BCE). Reported in over 100 children, the BCE usually occurs on the head or neck in patients with fair complexion and chronic sun exposure. The tumor grows slowly, often requiring many years to attain a diameter of 1 cm. The early lesion is an opalescent or pearly papule with fine telangiectatic vessels on its surface. Larger lesions may ulcerate centrally, but retain a characteristic border. The lesions almost never metastasize, but invade locally.

The cure rate is 90 to 95 per cent with all accepted treatment modalities; the remainder recur locally. The choice of therapy depends on size, site and character of the tumor as well as on age and complexion of the patient. The best treatment in the pediatric age group is plastic excision in an office or hospital setting by either a dermatologist or surgeon. Larger prominently located lesions should be removed by a plastic surgeon. Periorbital lesions are usually referred to an ophthalmologist for excision. An alternative approach is cryotherapy with liquid nitrogen by a dermatologist experienced in the technique. This may leave a hypopigmented circular scar, especially acceptable in fair-skinned persons, but should be avoided on the scalp, in the periorbital area, and on the lower extremities. Electrodesiccation and curettage is an office procedure, routinely performed by most dermatologists, which leaves a small and imperceptible scar in the case of small tumors. Mohs' chemotherapy may be useful for very large or recurrent tumors, but is a lengthy ordeal for the patient and usually requires referral to a large medical center. X-irradiation, often used for the treatment of BCE in the older adult, should always be avoided in children because of late sequelae. Recurrent BCE, those of the morphea type, and those with squamous differentiation should be treated more aggressively because of their relative resistance to therapy. All patients with BCE should be examined by a dermatologist annually to detect new lesions and should be instructed in the daily use of an effective sunscreen, for example, 5 per cent para-aminobenzoic acid (PABA) in alcohol.

Basal cell nevus syndrome, an autosomal dominant disorder associated with bony, cutaneous and neurologic findings, is characterized by numerous BCE which often begin to appear by the second decade. Standard treatments are appropriate; in addition, topical 5-fluorouracil may be justified for areas with many, rapidly appearing tumors.

Squamous Cell Carcinoma. This tumor is exceedingly rare in children. The treatment modalities listed above are acceptable.

Keratoacanthoma. Rapidly growing and usually self-limited, this lesion is considered by some authorities to be a variant of squamous cell carcinoma and should be treated as a malignancy according to the modalities listed above. It is rare in children, but has been reported even in infants.

Clavis (Corn). This chronic painful discrete hyperkeratotic lesion occurs almost exclusively on the feet and not infrequently begins in the second decade. Because the corn is a response to abnormal pressure, treatment should include correctly fitted shoes and in extreme cases corrective orthopedic surgery to alter the underlying bony architecture. Keratolytic agents applied daily quickly soften the corn and eliminate symptoms while their use is continued. One such product is the 40 per cent salicylic acid plaster, cut by the patient from a rectangular sheet to just cover the corn and held in place with a Band-Aid or adhesive tape. Softened keratotic debris may be removed with a pumice stone or by paring.

Calluses.   Treatment is the same as for corns. Avoiding the precipitating mechanical trauma results in gradual resolution.

Dermatosis Papulosa Nigra.   Minute black papules located on the face and neck are very common in black adults and may be quite numerous. Onset may be in the second decade. Lesions may be removed for cosmetic reasons with simple scissors excision, light electrodesiccation and curettage with or without prior local anesthesia, or by liquid nitrogen therapy.

Acrochordon (Skin Tag).   Lesions may appear on the lateral neck and intertriginous areas of obese children or those with a familial predisposition. Cosmetic removal is easily accomplished by cutting at the base with iris scissors while holding the tag perpendicular to the skin surface with forceps. Anesthesia and additional hemostasis are rarely needed. Electrodesiccation and cryotherapy with liquid nitrogen are also effective.

Epidermal Nevus.   This benign hyperpigmented verrucous lesion is usually single, often linear in configuration, and may be "systematized" involving a limb and/or quadrant of the trunk, in which case the term nevus unius lateris may be used. Cosmetic excision may be performed by a dermatologist or plastic surgeon. Liquid nitrogen cryotherapy or electrodesiccation is effective if sufficiently aggressive to produce scarring. Lesser doses of these modalities or dermabrasion may permit regrowth of the lesion. Patients with nevus unius lateris should be observed periodically for the rare appearance of BCE within the lesion and for a possible increased risk of internal malignancy. Extensive epidermal nevi are sometimes associated with developmental defects of the central nervous syndrome.

Acanthosis Nigricans.   This combination of hyperpigmentation and papillomatous thickening of the epidermis results in dark velvety-feeling skin, usually symmetrically involving the lateral neck, axillae, and other body folds. There is no effective therapy except correction of a known precipitant (such as obesity, endocrine disease, or internal malignancy) when present. The above disorders should be carefully excluded in all children with acanthosis nigricans unless it is a documented familial trait.

TUMORS OF THE EPIDERMAL APPENDAGES

Sebaceous Nevus (of Jadassohn).   An orange-tan plaque is present at birth but is inconspicuous until puberty when glandular hypertrophy makes it raised and deeper in color. It is located most commonly on the scalp, face or neck. The lesion should be excised because of the frequent postpubertal development of basal cell carcinomas and other tumors within it. In most cases, the wound can be closed primarily; no margin of normal skin is necessary. Therapy with liquid nitrogen or electrodesiccation usually leaves an unsightly scar. Central nervous system lesions seem to be restricted to patients with extensive developmental abnormalities of the epidermis in addition to a sebaceous nevus and are not a concern in routine cases.

Trichoepithelioma.   These small flesh-colored often telangiectatic papules may appear at puberty, may be single or multiple, and occur principally on the face. A biopsy should be performed to confirm the diagnosis and to exclude basal cell carcinoma, which is similar in appearance. No treatment is necessary because the lesions are benign and rarely exceed a few millimeters in diameter. Multiple lesions may be treated for cosmetic reasons with excision or gentle electrosurgery by an experienced dermatologist. Patients should be advised that lesions will probably continue to appear into adulthood and that the condition is often dominantly inherited.

Syringoma.   Small benign flesh-colored papules resembling trichoepitheliomata and occurring commonly in the periorbital area tend to arise during adolescence. They are multiple and may be excised or eradicated by judicious electrosurgery.

Wen (Pilar or Sebaceous Cyst).   Wens are firm, discrete, slightly compressible nodules which may appear at any time after puberty, most commonly on the face, scalp, back or scrotum. Lesions vary from a few millimeters to several centimeters in size and are asymptomatic. A small incision under local Xylocaine anesthesia confirms the diagnosis and allows expression of the cyst's cheesy contents. Recurrence can be avoided by extracting the cyst wall with a toothed forceps or mosquito clamp. A large cruciate incision often leaves an unsightly scar and is never necessary. An infected wen, which presents as a sudden painful enlargement of a preexisting lesion, should be treated with local compresses and a 10 day course of an antibiotic such as erythromycin or semisynthetic penicillin. Incision should not be attempted until the acute inflammation has resolved.

Other.   A large variety of benign appendage tumors may rarely present in childhood. Diagnosis almost always requires biopsy of the lesion; treatment is required only for cosmetic reasons and usually consists of excision.

TUMORS OF THE DERMIS

Adenoma Sebaceum (Angiofibroma). Flesh-colored papules begin to appear in the nasolabial folds at puberty in patients with tuberous sclerosis, an autosomal dominant disorder, and rarely in patients without other stigmata of that condition. The lesions need not be treated, but electrosurgery or dermabrasion may considerably improve their appearance. Any child with biopsy-proven adenoma sebaceum should be carefully examined under a Wood's lamp for ash-leaf spots, as well as for a shagreen patch, periungual fibromas, and neurologic deficits.

Angiokeratoma. These small, soft, purple papules are composed of dilated venules. Numerous angiokeratomas are scattered on the lower trunk and proximal extremities of patients with Fabry disease and may precede other manifestations of the disease. Biopsy is diagnostic. A clinically indistinguishable but medically insignificant variety of angiokeratomas (Mibelli) may present as a solitary lesion in childhood and can be differentiated histologically. No therapy beyond biopsy is necessary, but lesions may be destroyed by electrosurgery for cosmetic reasons.

Dermatofibroma. One or more of these benign pink to dark brown papules are common in adults and may also occur in children. Diagnosis can be made clinically by use of the "dimpling sign": when compressed laterally between the thumb and forefinger, the surrounding normal skin rides up over the edges of the lesion. If the lesion is painful at times or considered unsightly, it may be removed by elliptical excision.

Hypertrophic Scars and Keloids. These lesions may be considered together for purposes of therapy. They are especially common and troublesome in blacks. The best therapy is prevention. Incisions and other cutaneous insults should be avoided in children known to heal in this manner. If an incision is made or an existing scar is excised, the freshly sutured wound should be injected with a steroid suspension such as triamcinolone acetonide, 40 mg./ml. at 2 week intervals until healed. Increased rate of resolution has been claimed for hypertrophic scars treated with continuous compressive bandages for weeks to months.

Elastosis Perforans Serpiginosa. Benign clusters of flesh-colored to brown hyperkeratotic papules, often in linear array and located on the nape of the neck or on the knees, are important because of their association in about one-third of patients with one of several systemic disorders. Patients should be screened for Ehlers-Danlos, Marfan, and Down syndromes, pseudoxanthoma elasticum, and osteogenesis imperfecta. Lesions may be excised for cosmetic reasons, although this is rarely necessary.

Neurofibroma. Soft flesh-colored neurofibroma nodules may appear as an isolated usually single lesion in a healthy child or may be a marker for the dominantly inherited von Recklinghausen's disease (neurofibromatosis). Biopsy is required to diagnose the lesions in patients not obviously affected with neurofibromatosis. The most disfiguring lesions are often also most difficult to remove, but cosmetic excision may be appropriate in certain patients. Large plexiform neurofibromas have a small but definite incidence of associated fibrosarcoma in later life, and excision should be performed prophylactically when anatomically feasible. All children with one or more neurofibromas should be carefully screened for café-au-lait spots and other stigmata of neurofibromatosis. Parents and siblings should also be thoroughly examined. In unclear cases, if one or more café-au-lait spots are present, electron microscopy can identify the giant melanosomes characteristic of neurofibromatosis. Like all autosomal dominant disorders, the condition often arises de novo and may vary markedly in severity within a kinship. Genetic counseling should be provided.

Connective Tissue Nevus (Shagreen Patch). Flesh-colored to tan pebbly plaques occur most often on the trunk, especially the lower back, as a single lesion present since birth. They may be an isolated lesion or a marker for tuberous sclerosis. All patients should be examined under a Wood's lamp for ash-leaf spots and for other stigmata of this disease. Diagnosis of the nevus can usually be made on clinical grounds. Cosmetic excision is usually difficult and rarely warranted.

Juvenile Xanthogranuloma. Small firm yellow-tan nodules may be present at birth and usually appear before the end of the first year. Often several lesions appear over a period of months. They tend to resolve spontaneously, are benign, and require no therapy.

Urticaria Pigmentosum. Benign aggregates of mast cells appear as one or, more often, several orange-tan papules, usually in early childhood. Urtication after trauma such as rubbing the lesion (Darier's sign) is diagnostic, whereas a biopsy may be incorrectly interpreted as normal skin if the specimen is "degranulated" during excision or not fixed in absolute alcohol. A large single lesion may be excised if necessary to prevent the symptoms of histamine release (bulla formation, pruritus and flushing). Multiple lesions may be considered unsightly, but therapy should be withheld, as virtually all involute spontaneously by adolescence. Parents should be advised that symptoms associated with lesions usually abate after one or two years, even before the lesions disappear. Children with numerous lesions should avoid morphine and related narcotics, aspirin, alcohol, and polymyxin, as these agents cause mast cell degranulation. Rarely physical trauma such as diving into cold water may also do this. Children with numerous lesions and those with onset after age five years should be screened for the infrequent involvement of other organs with a bone scan, peripheral blood smear and, if indicated by the history, a gastrointestinal survey.

Lipoma. This common benign tumor is actually in the subcutaneous, not dermal, compartment. The lesions are flesh-colored, soft and pseudoencapsulated. Those larger than 10 cm. in diameter may undergo malignant transformation and should be excised if possible; surgical exploration is required if such a lesion changes clinically. Smaller lesions require no therapy. Cosmetic excision may result in a depressed area.

The Genodermatoses

SIDNEY HURWITZ, M.D.

The genodermatoses represent a group of cutaneous disorders dependent upon genetic mutation or the transmission of abnormal genes. Because of the inherited nature of these diseases, genetic counseling should be provided to patients and their families, with frank discussion of all available facts concerning the etiology, clinical course, mode of transmission, and possible complications associated with the disorder in question. Although genetically determined cutaneous diseases are not curable, recent advances in pathophysiology offer helpful therapeutic approaches which may assist in the management of these disorders by patients and their families.

ICHTHYOSIS

The term ichthyosis refers to a group of genodermatoses characterized by dryness and scaling. The recent introduction of reliable measurements of cellular kinetics has provided clearer understanding and organization of this disorder and allows a division into four major classifications: (1) ichthyosis vulgaris (autosomal dominant), (2) sex-linked ichthyosis (X-linked recessive), (3) lamellar ichthyosis (autosomal recessive), and (4) epidermolytic hyperkeratosis (autosomal dominant). In the past, lamellar ichthyosis and epidermolytic hyperkeratosis were designated as nonbullous and bullous congenital ichthyosiform erythrodermas.

The management of all types of dry skin consists of retardation of water loss, rehydration and softening of the stratum corneum, and alleviation of scaliness and associated pruritus. Ichthyosis vulgaris and X-linked ichthyosis can be managed quite well by topical application of emollients and the use of keratolytic agents to facilitate removal of scale from the skin surface. Limited baths with a mild soap and hydration of dry skin by frequent use of lubricating creams or lotions over moisture is helpful. Urea, in concentrations of 10 to 20 per cent, in a cream, lotion, or ointment base has a softening and moisturing effect on the stratum corneum and is helpful in the control of dry skin and pruritus. Propylene glycol (40 to 60 per cent in water), applied overnight under plastic occlusion, hydrates the skin and causes desquamation of scales. Salicylic acid is an effective keratolytic agent and at concentrations between three and six per cent promotes shedding of scales and softening of the stratum corneum. When used to cover large surface areas for prolonged periods, however, care should be taken to ensure that salicylate toxicity does not occur. Keralyt gel, a proprietary preparation containing six per cent salicylic acid in propylene glycol, is often helpful following hydration of the involved area. This preparation, when used properly either alone or under occlusive polyethylene wrapping, has been most successful in patients with ichthyosis vulgaris and X-linked ichthyosis. Recent studies suggest that alpha hydroxy preparations, lactic or pyruvic acids, are beneficial in the treatment of ichthyosiform dermatoses. Lactic acid is available as a proprietary preparation (LactiCare lotion, Stiefel) or may be added to lubricating lotions or emollient creams in a five or ten per cent concentration.

The treatment of lamellar ichthyosis by frequent lubrication or the addition of urea, salicylic acid, or lactic acid to lubricating creams or lotions, although encouraging, is not as effective as in the treatment of ichthyosis vulgaris and X-linked ichthyosis. Although oral vitamin A has been used in the treatment of lamellar ichthyosis it appears to be ineffective except in large dosages. The hazards of toxicity, therefore, preclude its use in infants and small children. Topical vitamin A acid, although potentially irritating, is beneficial in the treatment of lamellar ichthyosis. This preparation should be used cautiously, on a daily or alternate day routine, as tolerated. The therapy of epidermolytic hyperkeratosis is similar to that of lamellar ichthyosis, with the exception that antibiotics are frequently required to control the secondary infection of bullous lesions.

DARIER'S DISEASE (KERATOSIS FOLLICULARIS)

Darier's disease is an autosomal dominant defect characterized by greasy, crusted papules on the scalp, face, neck, seborrheic areas of the trunk, and flexures of the extremities. At present there is no satisfactory specific therapy for this disorder. Patients should be instructed to avoid excessive sun exposure, heat, and humidity, since this disorder characteristically is more severe during summer and is aggravated by sunlight or ultraviolet exposure, perspiration, heat, and humidity. Large doses of oral vitamin A (200,000 to 300,000 units per day for a period of months) have been used with variable results. This treatment, however, is not generally recommended in children because of possible toxicity to such dosages. Topical vitamin A acid, although potentially irritating, has been helpful (the irritation can be minimized by use of adequate yet threshold concentrations, or by the conjoint use of topical steroids).

FAMILIAL BENIGN CHRONIC PEMPHIGUS (HAILEY-HAILEY DISEASE)

Familial benign chronic pemphigus (Hailey-Hailey disease) is an autosomal dominant disorder with incomplete penetrance characterized by recurrent episodes of flaccid vesicles on erythematous skin on the nape or sides of the neck and in the axillae and groin. Less frequently other intertriginous areas of the body may be involved. The disease is characterized by recurrent periods of involvement alternating with periods of complete remission. There is as yet no treatment that will correct the basic defect or prevent exacerbations. An attempt should be made to have the patient avoid the precipitating factors of heat, high humidity, and excessive perspiration. Proper dress and the avoidance of contact irritants and sunburn are helpful prophylactic measures. The topical and systemic use of antibiotics has been of benefit to some patients. The systemic administration of corticosteroids, also effective in suppressing the manifestations of familial benign chronic pemphigus, is not advisable since the disease can show a severe rebound phenomenon when the dosage of the corticosteroid is reduced below the effective level.

EPIDERMOLYSIS BULLOSA

Epidermolysis bullosa refers to a group of inherited disorders characterized by blisters and erosions which develop spontaneously at sites of minor trauma. Modes of inheritance, clinical patterns, and the absence or presence of permanent scarring allow epidermolysis bullosa to be divided into two major classifications with several varieties of each type. Epidermolysis bullosa simplex, recurrent bullous dermatosis of the hands and feet (Weber-Cockayne disease), and some cases of epidermolysis bullosa dystrophica are transmitted as autosomal dominant traits. An autosomal recessive mode of inheritance has been demonstrated in other cases of epidermolysis bullosa dystrophica and epidermolysis bullosa letalis.

The treatment of epidermolysis bullosa is, in general, palliative with avoidance of trauma and control of secondary infection. Since blisters result from mechanical injury, measures should be taken to relieve pressure and prevent unnecessary trauma. When blisters occur, extension may be prevented by aseptic aspiration of blister fluid. Large denuded areas should be treated by the open method (as in treatment of burns) with intravenous replacement fluids and appropriate systemic antibiotics when indicated. Systemic steroids in high concentrations may be life-saving for severe dystrophic forms during the neonatal period, although they appear to have little or no effect on blister formation. The value of systemic corticosteroids in the reduction of esophageal strictures is debatable, although an attempt to correct esophageal strictures may be made by cautious dilatation. Plastic surgical techniques may be helpful, in selected cases, for fusion and flexion deformities of the hands and feet, and in cases of esophageal dysphagia. The value of systemic steroids in the long-term management of severe forms of epidermolysis bullosa remains controversial.

CONGENITAL ECTODERMAL DEFECTS

Ectodermal dysplasia is a descriptive term for an inherited group of defects which involve the skin and its appendageal structures. Although these defects share involvement of similar structures, they are distinct nosologic entities, genetically unrelated, with individual clinical and histologic manifestations.

Aplasia cutis congenita is an anomaly characterized by absence of localized areas of the integument (epidermis, dermis, and at times the subcutaneous tissue). The most common type of aplasia cutis is an oval, or circular, sharply outlined ulcer 1 to 3 cm. in diameter, on the vertex of the scalp at or about the level of the posterior fontanel. Treatment during the newborn period consists of control of secondary infection. As the child matures, most scars become inconspicuous and require no correction. Obvious scars may be treated by multiple punch-graft hair transplants or surgical excision with plastic repair.

Anhidrotic ectodermal dysplasia is an inherited disorder characterized by partial to complete absence of eccrine sweat glands, hair and dental abnormalities, and associated congenital defects. More than 90 per cent of affected patients have been males, with a sex-linked recessive pattern as the most common mode of transmission. Most affected individuals have a distinctive pathognomonic facies with a square forehead with frontal bossing, saddle nose, wide cheekbones, thick everted lips, and a prominent chin. Therapy of anhidrotic ectodermal dysplasia is difficult and should be directed toward temperature regulation, restriction of excessive physical exertion, and the avoidance of warm climates. Cool baths, air conditioning, light clothing, and reducing the causes of normal perspiration are beneficial. Regular dental supervision may help preserve teeth and reduce cosmetic disfigurement.

Hidrotic ectodermal dysplasia is an autosomal dominant disorder of keratinization characterized by hyperkeratosis of the palms and soles and nail dystrophy, with normal facies and no abnormality of the eccrine sweat glands. Body hair may be sparse, eyebrows and eyelashes may be thinned or absent, and scalp hair, generally normal during infancy and childhood, may become thin, fragile, and sparse to absent following puberty. Extreme hyperkeratosis of the palms and soles may be controlled to a degree by topical keratolytic agents (three to six per cent salicylic acid, or 10 to 20 per cent urea, in an emollient cream).

EHLERS-DANLOS SYNDROME

Ehlers-Danlos syndrome (cutis hyperelastica) is a dominantly inherited disorder of connective tissue characterized by hyperextensible, fragile, easily scarred skin, loose-jointedness, subcutaneous hemorrhages, and hemangioma-like pseudotumors around large joints and pressure points. Treatment is directed toward avoidance of or protection against trauma to the skin and joints, and includes the use of compression bandages over hematomas to help prevent pseudotumor formation. Since tissues are friable and difficult to suture, cuts and wounds should have their edges approximated with appropriate sutures and adhesive closure to facilitate healing and minimize the potentially large gaping scars characteristically seen in this disorder.

PSEUDOXANTHOMA ELASTICUM

Pseudoxanthoma elasticum is a recessively inherited disorder of the elastic tissue which involves the skin, eyes, and cardiovascular system. Cutaneous lesions consist of soft yellowish papules and polygonal plaques which resemble plucked chicken skin on the neck, below the clavicles, and in the axillae, antecubital fossae, periumbilical areas, perineum and thighs. Elastic tissue defects may be detected in the eyes (angioid streaks), in the gastrointestinal tract (hemorrhage), and in the vascular system (occlusion and claudication). Although there is no specific therapy for this disorder, plastic surgery may improve the cosmetic appearance. Gastrointestinal hemorrhage can usually be treated by a conservative medical approach, although surgical intervention may be necessary. Since a disabling aspect of this disease is a slow but progressive loss of vision, regular examinations by an ophthalmologist are important.

CUTIS LAXA

Generalized elastolysis (cutis laxa) is a rare disorder of elastic tissue characterized by inelastic, loose, pendulous skin resulting in an aged, bloodhound-like appearance. Patients with this disorder may develop diverticula in the gastrointestinal tract or urinary bladder, rectal prolapse, and ventral or inguinal hernias. The disease is gradually progressive and death from pulmonary complications related to emphysema may occur in the second to fourth decade. There is no specific treatment for this disorder. Surgery can correct diverticula, rectal prolapse, or hernias. Plastic surgery may help the cosmetic appearance, and pulmonary function studies may aid in the early detection of emphysema.

INCONTINENTIA PIGMENTI

Incontinentia pigmenti is a hereditary disorder which affects the skin, skeletal system, heart, eyes, and central nervous system. The syndrome develops almost exclusively in female infants and, although the genetics are not entirely clarified, it has been suggested that transmission is either autosomal dominant (with expression mainly in females) or sex-linked and lethal to males. The disease usually appears at birth with vesicles or bullae which may persist for several months, followed by verrucous lesions on the backs of the hands and feet, and eventually by a highly characteristic blue-gray to slate-brown whorled or splattered Chinese figure–like pigmentation.

No specific therapy is required for the skin lesions. Genetic counseling is advisable, however, since at least 50 per cent of affected children have associated congenital defects (cataracts, microcephaly, spastic paralysis, strabismus, alopecia, delayed or impaired dentition, epilepsy, or mental retardation).

ACRODERMATITIS ENTEROPATHICA

Acrodermatitis enteropathica is an autosomal recessive disorder which appears in early infancy and is characterized by vesiculobullous eruptions on an erythematous base which involve the periorificial areas of the mouth, nose, eyes, ears, buttocks, and perineum, and the extensor surfaces of the major joints, the fingers, and toes, with nail dystrophy, alopecia, personality disorders, diarrhea, and a failure to thrive.

Although the pathogenesis of this disorder is unclear, its course and prognosis were greatly improved since the introduction of treatment by diiodohydroxyquinoline in 1963. Until recently diiodohydroxyquinoline with or without breast milk was the mainstay of therapy. Although it has been successful in dosages of 200 to 2000 mg. per day, serious side effects, especially optic atrophy and/or a neurological syndrome of subacute myeloptic neuropathy, have been seen.

In 1973 studies suggested the basic defect in acrodermatitis enteropathica to be a gastrointestinal malabsorption of zinc. Although many questions concerning the pathogenesis remain unanswered, zinc therapy (in dosages of 10 to 15 mg. three times a day) provides a safe and inexpensive form of treatment for this formerly severe disease.

Diseases of the Hair and Scalp

L. G. OWEN, M.D. *and*
M. T. FLIEGELMAN, M.D.

BACTERIAL INFECTIONS

Folliculitis is a staphylococcal infection of the hair follicle. It is seen more commonly in individuals with poor hygiene or in those who pick and scratch the scalp frequently. Impetigo is a superficial bacterial infection of the skin, developing just beneath the stratum corneum. Impetigo may be due to either a streptococcal or staphylococcal infection. It is frequently associated with impetigo in other areas of the body. Both of these conditions may develop in the summer secondary to insect bites. In both conditions, the skin shows redness, pustular formation and crusting. The condition is treated by using an antibacterial shampoo containing hexachlorophene and the use of either penicillin or erythromycin orally.

FUNGAL INFECTIONS

Tinea capitis has both inflammatory and noninflammatory types. The inflammatory types are due to Microsporon organisms, *Microsporon canis* being most inflammatory and very common. It is frequently contracted from dogs and cats. The involved areas of the scalp show redness with oozing and crusting. Irregular areas of hair loss may be present. Circumscribed red, scaly to oozing plaques may be found on other exposed areas of the body. The diagnosis can be confirmed by doing a KOH mount of both scales and hairs from the involved sites. Long hyphae are noted in the scales and numerous small uniform spores surround the hair shafts. Wood's light examination reveals a yellowish to green fluorescence.

The noninflammatory type of tinea capitis is due to *Trichophyton tonsurans*. This is the so-called "black dot" type of tinea capitis. It produces a penny to quarter size area of hair loss. The involved areas may show some short hairs protruding from the surface of the scalp producing the so-called "black dots." Minimal scaling may be present. Spores and hyphal elements can be seen with a KOH preparation. It is most important to remember that this type of tinea capitis does *not* fluoresce with Wood's light. If the diagnosis is in doubt, a fungal culture should be done, placing scales and involved hair on Sabouraud's agar.

Treatment consists of griseofulvin orally. If the condition is severe it may be necessary to cut the hair short and shampoo daily with hexachlorophene. If the adjacent scalp becomes edematous, red and tender, it usually indicates the formation of a kerion, which is the rupture of hair follicles involved with fungus into the adjacent dermis, producing an intense inflammatory response. It may be necessary to treat a kerion with a short-term course of steroids to prevent permanent scarring and hair loss.

INFLAMMATORY ECZEMA (DERMATITIS)

Eczemas (dermatitis) are inflammatory conditions of the skin manifested in the acute stage by erythema, vesiculation and in the chronic stage by lichenification and scaliness. Eczemas may be of known etiology, such as contact eczema due to poison ivy, in which lymphocytes become sensitized to the Rhus antigen, or of unknown etiology, as is the case with seborrheic eczema (dermatitis). Seborrheic eczema is by far the most common inflammatory dermatitis of the scalp and is commonly referred to as cradle cap in infants. It is manifest by erythema and scaliness of the scalp, nasolabial folds, eyebrows and ears. Treatment consists of using a tar shampoo such as Xseb-T each day plus a steroid preparation topically, such as Synalar Solution.

The scalp is often involved in atopic dermatitis, which occurs in individuals with a family background of hay fever or asthma. The eczema itself is not due to any contactant and recent evidence has shown that atopics have a relative T-cell deficiency, so that they are less likely to develop contact dermatitis even when exposed to multiple antigens. Atopics often perpetuate their dermatitis by rubbing and scratching; therefore antihistamines such as hydroxyzine (Atarax), promethazine (Phenergan) or diphenhydramine (Benadryl) are recommended along with Xseb-T shampoo and Synalar Solution to the scalp at night time. Bath oils such as Alpha-Keri and lubricating lotions such as Ultraderm Lotion are useful for treating the dry skin which is frequently a component of the atopic picture.

Contact dermatitis only occasionally develops on the scalp and is manifested by intense itching and vesiculation. It is usually associated with involvement of the face or neck. Treatment consists of compresses of saline or Burow's solution, topical steroids and oral antihistamines. Parenteral steroids may be necessary for a few days when the involvement is extensive.

COLLAGEN DISEASES

Lupus erythematosus often involves the scalp and produces a scarring type of alopecia. There is erythema, scaliness, "carpet tack" plugging and atrophy of the skin along with hair loss. Similar lesions are frequently present in other exposed areas such as the face, hands and the V of the neck. A collagen disease workup is necessary to rule out internal involvement. The skin lesions respond readily to fluorinated steroids such as betamethasone valerate (Valisone Cream). A benign type of scleroderma (morphea) occurs on the scalp and is known as coup de sabre. This is manifested by a linear area of hair loss with atrophy and hardening of the underlying skin.

PSYCHOGENIC CAUSES

Alopecia areata occurs commonly in children and is manifest by noninflammatory alopecia. The individual lesions are frequently the size of a nickel, smooth and completely without hair. This condition frequently develops a few weeks after an emotional insult. Treatment consists of intralesional triamcinolone in a concentration of 3 to 4 mg./ml. diluted in saline. A 25 or 30 gauge needle should be used for injection and only a very small amount injected in any one site. Trichotillomania is a condition in which the patient pulls out the hair. It is manifested by the lack of inflammation plus numerous broken hairs of varying size. Treatment consists mainly of psychotherapy.

DIFFUSE HAIR LOSS

Anagen hair loss occurs when the growing hair drops out. This hair has a tapered root and has no bulb attached to the end, the bulb being the hallmark of the resting (telogen) hair. Anagen hair loss develops after the ingestion of poisons such as thallium or antimetabolites such as methotrexate. It develops between 19 and 21 days after the insult.

Telogen hair loss develops after the hair passes from the growing phase to the resting phase. It develops approximately 3 months after the initial insult, which may be a high fever or severe debilitating systemic disease. Often no treatment is indicated for the hair loss unless the condition is extremely severe, in which case topical fluorinated steroids such as Synalar Solution may be applied to the scalp at night time.

CONGENITAL ALOPECIAS

Structural abnormalities are diagnosed by looking at several hairs under the low-power objective lens of the microscope. Trichorrhexis nodosa is the most common of all hair shaft abnormalities. It may simply indicate excessive, harsh hair grooming or may signal serious metabolic disorders in which the hair is an important diagnostic clue. A typical defect or "node" appears in the light microscope as a hair shaft fracture in which the individual cells of the hair splay out, resembling the ends of two brushes pushed into one another. Trichorrhexis nodosa may occur in infants with mental retardation and argininosuccinic aciduria. Severe mental retardation is evident in the first year of life and large amounts of argininosuccinic acid are found in the urine, blood and cerebrospinal fluid. An acquired form may develop in individuals who overbrush their hair, in which case the patient should cut off the affected ends and use a comb or brush very gently.

Bamboo hair (trichorrhexis invaginata) is a defect in which the hair is very fragile due to abnormal invagination along the shafts which resemble the ball and cup joints of bamboo. It occurs with a rare genodermatosis known as Netherton's disease. Other features include a dry scaly erythroderma and atopic diathesis. The mode of inheritance appears to be autosomal recessive with greater penetrance in females.

Diseases of Sweat and Sebaceous Glands

SIDNEY HURWITZ, M.D.

ACNE

Although the basic cause of acne vulgaris is as yet unknown, considerable data on its pathogenesis accumulated in recent years allow a much more rational and successful therapeutic approach to this perplexing skin disorder of the adolescent. To date there is no single treatment for acne. The choice of therapy must be individualized to each patient with appropriate modifications as the activity of the disease fluctuates. The success of therapy depends upon the cooperation of the patient and the interest, enthusiasm, and careful selection of medications on the part of the physician.

A clear understanding of the pathogenesis of acne vulgaris can simplify one's therapeutic approach to this disorder. Acne usually begins at puberty due to androgenic stimulation of the sebaceous glands and a faulty keratinization process which results in retention of keratinocytes, obstruction of the pilosebaceous unit, and impaction of horny cells and sebum within the lumen of the sebaceous follicle. This impaction results in the formation of comedones: the open comedo or "blackhead" and the closed comedo or "whitehead." The inflammatory response that occurs in acne results principally from sebum, which escapes into the dermis through ruptures in the follicular walls of closed comedones.

Sebum is made up of a mixture of triglycerides, wax esters, squalene, and sterol esters. Free fatty acids are released by hydrolysis of triglycerides by bacterial lipases within the pilosebaceous follicles, principally those of the anaerobic diphtheroid *Propionibacterium* (previously termed *Corynebacterium*) *acnes*. They are the most irritating component of sebum and appear to be the primary cause of the inflammatory reaction seen in acne vulgaris.

The goal of successful acne therapy is to arrest the natural evolution of its lesions. Effective acne therapy, therefore, depends upon the ability to prevent follicular hyperkeratosis, to lower the level of *Propionibacterium acnes* and

free fatty acids, and to arrest the formation of comedones, and the resulting papules, pustules, cysts, and nodules.

Appropriate topical therapy is essential to the successful management of acne. For years therapy consisted of various cleansing agents, abrasives, astringents, and exfoliants designed to remove blackheads and lipids on the skin surface. Contrary to previously held concepts, there is little evidence to support the reputed beneficial effect of such preparations. Not only are they ineffective, but, due to their tendency to cause dryness and chapping, they often inhibit the effective use of potent topical agents.

Relative to diet, carefully controlled studies refute the value of dietary restrictions imposed upon acne patients. Although some patients still attest to flares of their disease after ingestion of certain foods, there is no evidence to support the value of dietary restrictions in the management of this disorder. For those few who insist that certain foods tend to aggravate their condition, it is judicious to eliminate the suspected agents until their true influence can be appropriately and individually assessed.

Preparations currently available for acne therapy include irritants, keratolytics, antibacterial agents, and hormones. Of the available topical agents, those which have had the greatest popularity include sulfur, resorcin, salicyic acid, benzoyl peroxide, and vitamin A acid (tretinoin). The mode of action of sulfur, resorcin, and salicylic acid is uncertain. Their efficacy is limited and appears to be related to their capacity to produce erythema and desquamation. Although they tend to help dry and peel existing comedones, papules, and pustules, they fail to limit the formation of closed comedones (whiteheads) and the lesions that arise from these comedones.

Benzoyl peroxide and vitamin A acid, conversely, are highly effective preparations for the topical therapy of acne vulgaris. Benzoyl peroxide is currently available in lotion form (Benoxyl, Oxy-5, Persadox, Vanoxide, Loroxide) or in the more potent and penetrating gel formulations available on prescription only (Benzagel, Desquam-X, PanOxyl, Persa-Gel). These preparations offer more than a form of epidermal irritation. They cause a fine desquamation, help reduce the level of the free fatty acids, and appear to be bacteriostatic for *Proprionibacterium acnes*. A relatively low incidence of allergic contact dermatitis to benzoyl peroxide (1 to 2.5 per cent), however, suggest a certain degree of caution in their use.

Oral vitamin A, long used in acne therapy for its theoretical inhibition of keratinization, has been found ineffective (except in potentially toxic levels) and therefore has no place in the management of acne today. Topical vitamin A acid (tretinoin, retinoic acid), however, when used properly, is particularly valuable in the topical therapy of acne vulgaris. Available as Aberel or Retin-A, in swabs or liquid (0.05 per cent), or as Retin-A creams (0.05 or 0.1 per cent) and Retin-A gel (0.025 per cent), tretinoin seems to have several beneficial effects on the skin of patients with acne vulgaris. Included among these benefits are dehiscence of horny cells with resulting thinning of the horny layer, decreased comedo formation, sloughing and expulsion of existing comedones from their sebaceous follicles, and reduction in the number of inflammatory lesions which arise from these comedones.

Because of its known capacity to cause irritation and peeling, topical vitamin A acid therapy should be initiated conservatively, on an alternate-day or, occasionally, an every-third-day regimen, preferably with the less irritating cream or gel preparations. Irritation can be minimized to a great extent if certain precautions are followed. Patients should avoid astringents, abrasives, and all other local medications; only noncomedogenic oil-free cosmetics should be used, and excessive sun exposure should be limited. Patients should be instructed to wash with a mild soap no more than two or three times a day, and to wait at least 20 to 30 minutes after washing (to ensure that the skin is completely dry) before application of vitamin A acid. If prolonged sun exposure is anticipated, patients must be cautioned to use a protective sun screen.

Although success in the management of acne vulgaris can be achieved by the topical vitamin A acid or benzoyl peroxide alone, it now appears that the therapeutic effect can be substantially increased by the use of the two agents in combination. Although vitamin A acid, when used alone, can be irritating to the skin, benzoyl peroxide appears to toughen the epidermis against this cutaneous reaction. Therefore, when the two agents are used in combination (one in the morning and one at night), there appears to be less irritation than when vitamin A acid is used alone. By this combination dramatic therapeutic effects can be achieved in a relatively short time in a high percentage of patients, even those with severe pustulocystic forms of this disorder.

Systemic antibiotics suppress *P. acnes* and inhibit bacterial lipases, causing a reduction in the concentration of free fatty acids (the primary irritant of sebum). For years, broad-spectrum antibiotics have been invaluable in the treatment of inflammatory pustules, nodules, and cystic lesions. Today, however, the use of systemic antibiotics can be decreased and often eliminated with the growth of experience and sophistication in the use of effective topical agents. Since little or no improvement can be expected with noninflammatory lesions (comedones), antibiotics are unnecessary in patients in whom these lesions appear as the sole manifestation of their acne problem.

When antibiotics are considered necessary, tetracycline, the antibiotic most frequently prescribed, is effective, inexpensive, and relatively free of side effects. Erythromycin, clindamycin, and minocycline also are beneficial when inflammatory and pustular lesions fail to respond to oral doses of tetracycline. Of these, erythromycin is the least expensive and has the fewest complications. Clindamycin, although effective, has a tendency to cause pancytopenia and pseudomembranous colitis, which precludes its routine use in the treatment of acne. Minocycline appears to have merit in patients unresponsive to tetracycline or erythromycin therapy, although caution must be exercised, since this tetracycline derivative appears to have an affinity for the central nervous system, with a resulting high incidence of headaches and dizziness. The use of sulfone (diaminodiphenylsulfone) has been suggested for the management of very severe, resistant, nodulocystic, and conglobate acne. This preparation should be used only with extreme caution, with full awareness of the risk of hemolytic anemia, cyanosis, and methemoglobinemia. Penicillin appears to be of no value in the treatment of acne. Sulfa drugs have been used but their clinical results are not as favorable as those of broad-spectrum antibiotics.

Tetracycline therapy generally begins with a dosage of 1000 mg./day, which is gradually decreased to the lowest optimal level and usually maintained at a dosage of 250 mg./day or every other day until clinical improvement allows its discontinuation. Long-term low dosage may be continued for many months with relatively few side effects. The possibility of tetracycline staining of teeth precludes its use for children under 12 years of age and for pregnant women after the first trimester of pregnancy. Monilial vaginitis, an occasional complication in adolescents, is more common in females who are receiving both oral contraceptives and tetracycline.

The incidence of photoreactivity to oral tetracycline is unknown but appears to be extremely low, except in the case of demethylchlortetracycline (Declomycin), in which photosensitivity appears to develop in about 20 per cent of cases. Recent reports also describe unusual porphyria-like photosensitivity with bullae on the hands of patients on tetracycline therapy. Occasionally, patients on long-term tetracycline therapy may develop a gram-negative folliculitis due to *Klebsiella* or *Proteus* overgrowth. This complication is manifested by a pustular folliculitis along the ala nasi or by deep nodulocystic lesions of the face. The ingestion of outdated tetracycline may cause severe toxicity. It is particularly dangerous in children who use "leftover" medication and who start and stop therapy on their own without proper medical guidance.

It is desirable to avoid oral or systemic therapy in the treatment of skin diseases if an equally potent topical agent can be used. Recent investigations have shown that topical tetracycline, topical erythromycin, and topical clindamycin, when used in appropriate vehicles, can inhibit the growth of *P. acnes* and produce a decrease in comedones, papules, and pustules in acne patients. Although studies are incomplete and these products are not yet available commercially, it appears that topical antibiotics may to a great degree replace oral antibiotic therapy in the near future.

Anovulatory drugs suppress the androgenic stimulation of sebum production and are beneficial in 50 to 70 per cent of females with severe, recalcitrant, pustulocystic acne. If estrogen is used, it must contain a minimum of 0.1 mg. of ethinyl estradiol or its 3-methyl ether derivative (mestranol). Side effects to be considered include nausea, weight gain, monilial vaginitis, chloasma and thromboembolic phenomena. Estrogens should never be prescribed in males, since the dose required for sebum suppression will produce feminizing side effects. These drugs should not be administered to patients under the age of 16, when possible bone growth inhibition is a consideration. Even though acne is not listed among the manufacturers' indications for use of anovulatory drugs, these preparations have been used for many years to treat acne, producing good results and a minimum of ill effects.

The value of artificial ultraviolet light is debatable. Its major effect is to give the patient a feeling of well-being, mild erythema, desquamation, and a resultant tan, which helps to conceal acne lesions. The risk of overexposure and conjunctival inflammation from failure to shield the eyes suggests the use of caution and the limitations of this as a method of home therapy.

X-ray, once widely used in the treatment of acne, has generally been abandoned as more effective forms of therapy have developed. Superficial x-ray has been shown to reduce the size of sebaceous glands; however, problems often recur when the glands regenerate after three to four months.

Acne scars may improve to a surprising degree over a period of two to three years, but often the patient's final appearance is less than desirable. Topical chemotherapy by trichloroacetic acid and cryosurgery with liquid nitrogen have been beneficial for patients with unsightly pitting and keloidal scars. Dermabrasion, popular in the past, still offers hope for improvement in a small group of patients with residual cystic scarring and nodular lesions. It is important to note that following dermabrasion, people who pigment easily occasionally develop hyperpigmentation which appears more unattractive than the original scars. Dermabrasion therefore should be executed only in carefully selected cases by a dermatologist or plastic surgeon familiar with its techniques and potential consequences.

HYPERHIDROSIS

Hyperhidrosis is a disorder characterized by an excessive production of perspiration in response to heat or emotional stimuli. Topical and systemic therapy can be temporarily suppressive but are basically unsatisfactory. Treatment with systemic anticholinergic agents (atropine, 0.01 mg./kg. every 4 to 6 hours, or Pro-Banthine, 1.5 mg./kg./day), effective to variable degrees, is limited by side effects such as mucous membrane dryness, blurred vision and mydriasis. Sedative or tranquilizing drugs appear to be beneficial for axillary or palmar hyperhidrosis, as are aluminum salts applied locally (10 to 25 per cent aluminum chloride in distilled water).

In palmar hyperhidrosis, local astringents of value are those which inhibit the production of perspiration (Burow's soaks 1:40 or potassium permanganate 1:4000). Dusting powders, such as ZeaSORB, may be helpful. Plantar hyperhidrosis may be suppressed with a solution of 10 per cent glutaraldehyde (investigational) buffered with sodium bicarbonate to a pH of 7.5 (1.65 gm. $NaHCO_3$ per ml.) applied topically daily or every other day. This solution causes staining and therefore is not a useful modality for treatment of the palms.

DYSHIDROSIS

Dyshidrosis (pompholyx) is a term applied to a condition of recurring vesiculation of the palms and soles in which hyperhidrosis and retention of sweat precede the eruption. Although this condition may not be a disorder of the glands per se, hyperhidrosis is an important accessory factor; treatment directed toward the hyperhidrosis may prove beneficial. Topical steroid creams (Aristocort 0.1 per cent, Valisone 0.1 per cent or their equivalents) and efforts to minimize excessive perspiration are helpful in controlling this disorder.

BROMIDROSIS

Bromidrosis is an embarrassing malodorous condition caused by decomposition of apocrine sweat and keratin which has been softened by excessive secretion of the feet and intertriginous areas. This disorder can be controlled by scrupulous hygiene, repeated cleansing, preferably with antibacterial soaps, frequent changes of clothing and the use of topical bacteriostatic agents and commercial deodorants. Topical aluminum salts (10 to 25 per cent aluminum chloride in distilled water) and oral anticholinergic drugs (Pro-Banthine, 1.5 mg./kg./day) may help axillary eccrine hyperhidrosis, but there is little evidence to their effect upon apocrine gland secretion. Dusting powders (ZeaSORB) may absorb excessive perspiration; disagreeable odors may be reduced by soaks with Burow's solution (1:40) or potassium permanganate (1:4000).

MILIARIA

Miliaria, a common dermatosis caused by sweat retention, is characterized by a vesicular eruption secondary to prolonged exposure to perspiration, with subsequent maceration and obstruction of the eccrine ducts. There are three forms of this disorder: miliaria crystallina (sudamina), miliaria rubra (prickly heat) and miliaria profunda (a more severe form of miliaria rubra commonly seen in the tropics). Therapy is directed toward avoidance of excessive heat and humidity. Light clothing, cool baths and air conditioning are invaluable. Calamine lotion, with or without 0.25 per cent menthol and 0.5 per cent phenol, is effective yet has a tendency to cause excessive dryness; emollient creams such as Eucerin may be helpful. Resorcinol, 3 per cent in alcohol or in Cetaphil Lotion, is therapeutically beneficial in this disorder.

ANHIDROSIS

Anhidrosis is an abnormal absence of perspiration from the surface of the skin in the presence of appropriate stimuli, often resulting in hyperthermia. This condition may be caused by a deficiency or abnormality of the sweat gland (as in anhidrotic ectodermal dysplasia) or of the nervous pathways from the peripheral or central nervous system leading to the sweat gland (as in syringomyelia, leprosy, anticholinergic drug therapy or sympathectomy). Cool baths, air conditioning, light clothing and reducing the causes of normal perspiration help to relieve symptoms.

Miscellaneous Dermatoses

ALVIN H. JACOBS, M.D.

GRANULOMA ANNULARE

The typical lesions are smooth, skin-colored, firm nodules grouped in an arciform or annular arrangement. They occur most commonly on the backs of the hands and fingers, although they often also appear about the feet and ankles.

Granuloma annulare resolves completely in 2 to 4 years. Response to treatment is erratic but the best results are from intralesional injections of triamcinolone. The solution for injection is prepared by mixing in the syringe one part of triamcinolone acetonide (Kenalog—10 injection, 10 mg. per ml.) with three parts physiologic saline solution. Depending on the size of the area to be treated, 0.2 to 2 ml. of the mixture may be injected from one or several points so that the entire lesion is infiltrated. Injections may be given at 4 week intervals, but should be terminated if no resolution of the lesion has appeared after four treatments. Warning must be given that a temporary skin atrophy may supervene.

LICHEN SPINULOSUS

This is an uncommon disorder of unknown etiology. Spiny keratinous, follicular projections grouped in large patches may appear on any part of the body. They are asymptomatic. Treatment is usually unnecessary but, if desired, mild keratolytics may be helpful. For this purpose one may use 5 per cent salicylic acid in Aquaphor or Carmol Cream, which contains 20 per cent urea.

GIANOTTI-CROSTI SYNDROME

Gianotti-Crosti syndrome (papular acrodermatitis of childhood) is a slightly infectious, nonrelapsing disease of childhood characterized by (1) papular eruption on the face and limbs lasting 20 days or more, (2) reactive reticulohistiocytic lymphadenitis, and (3) acute hepatitis, usually anicteric. Australia antigen is always present; it is detectable 10 or more days after the onset of the skin eruption. Liver status should be investigated, but topical treatment of the rash is not necessary.

16

The Eye

The Eye

JULES L. BAUM, M.D.

GENERAL REMARKS ON DRUG THERAPY

Drug therapy by the ophthalmologist is largely restricted to three types of pharmaceuticals: antimicrobial agents, corticosteroids and those drugs which constrict (miotics) and dilate (mydriatrics and cycloplegics) the pupil. Two of these three groups, the corticosteroids and the drugs affecting the pupil size, should not in my opinion be used by the pediatrician to initiate therapy in the treatment of ocular disease.

The use of corticosteroids may induce glaucoma and cataract formation in susceptible individuals and exacerbate infections of the cornea. More drug enters the eye when given topically than when given systemically, and the development of steroid-induced glaucoma and cataract is dose-dependent. While steroid-induced glaucoma usually begins within weeks after starting topical steroid treatment, cataracts of the posterior subcapsular type usually become evident some months after corticosteroids are initiated. While the ophthalmologist may use corticosteroids to reduce inflammation and control allergic processes, he or she monitors intraocular pressure and examines the lens with a slit lamp. Without this ability to monitor the patient, the pediatrician should avoid the use of corticosteroids in the treatment of ocular disease. Corticosteroids have also been shown to exacerbate viral (herpes simplex), fungal and bacterial infections of the cornea.

The ophthalmologist often uses cycloplegic drugs such as atropine, scopolamine, cyclopentolate (Cyclogyl) or tropicamide (Mydriacyl) to dilate the pupil and put the ciliary body at rest in treating intraocular inflammation. These drugs should not be used therapeutically by the pediatrician unless the ophthalmologist has initiated such therapy and advised its continuation.

The following points may prove helpful in treating pediatric cases.

1. Always remember to press on the lacrimal sac (on the side of the nose medial to the medial canthus) for 30 to 60 seconds after a parasympatholytic drug in drop form has been instilled in the eye to avoid systemic parasympatholytic effects. Pressure on the lacrimal sac reduces the chance of the drug's entering the nose and being absorbed systemically through the nasal mucosa.

2. In many instances it is easier to instill eye drops or ointments while a child is asleep.

3. Never use topical anesthetics to relieve chronic eye pain or discomfort.

4. Topical therapy in ointment form is probably more effective than eye drops when given to a child who is crying and struggling. Squeezing of eyelids and tearing dilute the medication, forcing it out of the eye and down the cheek.

OPHTHALMIC HISTORY

As in general pediatrics, the taking of a history is dependent on the age of the child and the astuteness of child and parent. A parent may recognize bilateral, decreased visual acuity by noting the inability of the infant or child to fixate on an object. The eyes appear to wander in wide swings called searching movements, similar to those of an infant 4 months old or younger who cannot fixate on an object. Parents may also recognize decreased visual acuity in both eyes by failure of the infant or child to pick up or recognize small objects, or the necessity of holding objects very close to the eyes.

An older child, or for that matter an adult, may fail to appreciate the loss of vision in one eye. A clue to the onset of decreased vision in one eye may be gained by determining when an eye first turned either in (esotropia) or out (exotropia). When an eye turns early in life, suppression and decreased visual acuity of the turned eye may result. When an eye turns later in childhood, usually after 7 years of age, diplopia results, as the child cannot suppress the double image. When an esotropia or exotropia is seen, the parents should be questioned about relatives with a similar condition, as heterotropia has a tendency to run in families.

If a younger child has an irritative ocular condition, parents will report such symptoms as rubbing of the eyes, blinking, squeezing of the eyes (blepharospasm), tearing, injection of the conjunctiva, and photophobia. A simple conjunctivitis usually causes only a gritty sensation, while involvement of the cornea and inflammation of the iris or ciliary body usually induce the triad of true pain, photophobia and lacrimation.

Ask the parents if the child's lids stick together in the morning. Tearing may result either from an increased output of the tear gland (lacrimation) or from a decreased outflow through the lacrimal canaliculi-lacrimal sac-lacrimal duct system (epiphora). If a parent asserts that a difference in pupil size has become evident, ask for old photographs with which to compare the condition. Anisocoria without any other associated abnormality occurs in approximately 7 per cent of the population. Obtain a family history of ocular disease or blindness.

I have left headache and "failure to do well at school" for last, as these are two of the most frequent ocular problems which pediatricians encounter. Certainly, children with headache should have an eye examination. However, headaches caused by refractive errors or extraocular muscle imbalance (heterophorias) account for only a small percentage of headaches. Relief of such symptoms cannot be expected where there is no significant ocular problem.

The chance of the ophthalmologist's finding ocular pathology in a child said to have dyslexia is approximately the same as for a normal population of a similar age group. Dyslexia, in almost every instance, is not a disease of the eyes and cannot be effectively treated by the ophthalmologist or the optometrist.

EXAMINATION

The initial procedure of every ocular examination involves the determination of visual acuity. In an infant younger than 4 months of age, a familiar object (his mother's face is the best) is placed within the infant's visual field. The eyes turn toward the familiar object, but cannot hold fixation. The object should be moved to another place and the process repeated several times. Each eye should be tested independently by covering the other eye. Since fixation develops at approximately 4 months, an older infant can follow an object as it passes through the field of vision. Remember that eyes turn in the direction of a noise. Objects like keys should not be used, as auditory stimuli confuse interpretation of visual stimuli.

Vision in preschool children may be determined using Allen cards (familiar objects) or a letter "E" chart. Preschool children are learning their numbers much earlier these days due to television programs such as "Sesame Street"; hence number and letter charts may be used for bright preschool children.

Children 4 years and under may not read better than 20/25 to 20/40, even with perfect eyes. Although some believe this decreased visual acuity may be a function of undeveloped vision, others feel it represents failure to concentrate on small objects.

Beyond infancy, a child's cooperation is a prerequisite for a thorough eye examination. Some time should be spent gaining a child's confidence before the actual examination begins. Usually, children relate better to their pediatrician than to an ophthalmologist who is seen infrequently. An infant's eyes open more easily when the infant is sitting up and sucking on a bottle. Another approach is to stand behind the mother as she holds the child with the infant's head resting on her shoulder. Older children respond to a handheld animal figure or a moving object at the far end of the room.

It may be necessary to restrain an uncooperative child, in which case forcible opening of the lids may become necessary. Lid retractors may be employed after a drop of proparacaine, 0.5 per cent. If no lid retractors are available, sterilized paper clips may be bent into the shape of a lid retractor and used in their place.

The symmetry of the corneal reflexes in a younger child and the alternate cover test (covering one eye and then the other while watching for movement of the eyes) for the older child are the most appropriate tests when a pediatrician wishes to diagnose an esotropia or exotropia.

Phenylephrine (Neo-Synephrine), 2.5 per cent, tropicamide (Mydriacyl), 0.5 to 1.0 per cent, or cyclopentolate (Cyclogyl), 0.5 to 1.0 per cent, may be used to dilate a child's eyes for visualization of the lens, vitreous and fundus. Several drops of one or two of these agents may be required to dilate the pupil. Of the three, tropicamide acts most rapidly, and effects of cycloplegia dissipate most rapidly. Cyclopentolate and phenylephrine are more powerful dilators, but their effect lasts for many more hours. Phenylephrine is a mydriatic and dilates the pupil without paralyzing accommodation, whereas cyclopentolate, a cycloplegic, dilates the pupil and paralyzes accommodation. Always remember to press on the lacrimal sac area for 30 to 60 seconds following instillation of these drops to decrease systemic absorption of the drugs. It is more difficult to dilate pupils in brown-eyed children than in blue-eyed children; it may be necessary to give several drops several minutes apart to achieve dilation.

When attempting to evert the upper lid, have the child look down. It is impossible to evert an upper lid when a child is looking up. Flip the upper lid by pulling it up while applying counter pressure to the upper border of the tarsus with a match, Q-tip or finger.

It is often helpful to employ a magnifying glass or loupe when examining the lids, conjunctiva or globe itself.

INJURIES

It is often difficult for a pediatrician to assess the full extent of ocular trauma following injury to the eyes; even an ophthalmologist may have difficulty determining whether a globe has been ruptured. Cases of ocular trauma should be referred to the ophthalmologist, and the examination should start with an assessment of visual acuity. If the possibility of a ruptured globe exists, no pressure should be applied to the globe. In examining an uncooperative child, always open the eyelids with your fingers resting on the orbital bones. In this way pressure is never exerted on the globe itself. If the history or cursory physical examination before even touching the patient suggests the possibility of a ruptured globe, the child should be sent to an ophthalmologist immediately, as children, while fighting an ocular examination and squeezing their lids shut, may cause herniation of uveal tissue through a lacerated globe.

Conjunctival and Corneal Foreign Bodies. A history is most important. If children have been watching their father work with a high-speed drill, an x-ray should be taken to rule out an intraocular foreign body—even if one finds another foreign body on the cornea or conjunctiva. The fornices should be inspected using a good light and loupe. The upper lids should be everted.

If a foreign body is located on the conjunctiva, it can be removed with a moist cotton swab. A topical anesthetic such as proparacaine, 0.5 per cent, may be helpful. If the foreign body is seen on the cornea, first try to irrigate it off without touching the cornea. Use an ocular irrigating solution such as Dacriose, which comes in a 0.9 ounce plastic squeeze-type bottle that emits the irrigating solution in a fine jet stream. If a superficial corneal foreign body cannot be removed with the jet stream, a sterile wet cotton-tipped applicator may be used. If both of these procedures fail to dislodge the foreign body, it is best removed by an ophthalmologist.

Following removal of the foreign body, fluorescein should be instilled by applying a moist fluorescein-impregnated paper strip to the lower fornix while pulling down the lower lid and having the patient look up. An assessment is thus made of the extent of the accompanying corneal abrasion. The abraded area stains green.

An appropriate antibiotic ointment such as bacitracin-polymyxin B is applied and the eye is patched for 24 hours. A tight patch can best be applied by fluffing out one or two sterile 4 × 4 gauze pads, depending on the depth of the socket, stuffing them over the closed eye and taping the eye shut using multiple strips of tape. Keep the eye closed tightly by applying pressure to the gauze with a finger until the pressure from the tape strips is sufficient to keep the eye firmly closed. A loose patch is worse than no patch at all, because if the eye opens, the gauze can rub against the cornea, further injuring it.

The child should be examined 24 hours later. In most cases, there is no staining with fluorescein, the eye is quiet and the child asymptomatic. The eye may be repatched for another 24 hours with antibiotic ointment if significant staining persists. If it appears to be getting worse or there is not complete healing within 48 hours, an ophthalmologist should be consulted immediately.

A corneal foreign body made of iron may leave residual iron in the cornea, which is called a rust ring. It may have to be removed by an ophthalmologist, most often 24 to 48 hours following removal of the foreign body itself.

Following trauma associated with shattering of glass, instill proparacaine and irrigate copiously. Inspect the conjunctiva and cornea for small pieces of glass. Then dry the conjunctiva and fornices with sterile cotton applicators and inspect again, as tears may cover small glass particles.

Corneal Abrasion. In suspected cases of corneal trauma, the corneal epithelium, its most superficial layer, may be damaged, in which case fluorescein application as described above may be used to diagnose the corneal abrasion. Damaged or absent corneal epithelium increases the susceptibility of the cornea to infection. Since a bacterial or fungal corneal ulcer may result in blindness, every corneal abrasion must be treated as a potential catastrophe, even though the typical abrasion heals within 24 hours without sequelae.

After examining for the possibility of a foreign body, antibiotic ointment and a pressure patch are applied (see above). The eye should be examined in approximately 24 hours. An abrasion per se does not decrease the crystal clear appearance of a cornea. If a haze or whitening is seen, it may be indicative of an incipient corneal infection, and the patient should be seen immediately by an ophthalmologist. If an incipient bacterial or fungal corneal ulcer is suspected, do not patch the eye, as patching favors the growth of microorganisms.

Lacerations. Any injury resulting in an eyelid laceration should be referred to an ophthalmologist for a complete ocular examination. If one were certain that there was no injury to the globe and that the lid laceration did not involve the lid margin or lacrimal outflow system, any physician trained in surgery could suture the lid. In practice any laceration of the globe should be treated as a potentially ruptured globe. Once the ophthalmologist confirms a ruptured globe, systemic antibiotics and possibly a tetanus toxoid booster may be required. The ophthalmologist would be grateful if a tetanus toxoid history and any history of antibiotic allergy accompanied the patient. Parents should be advised to withhold oral intake if immediate surgery is contemplated.

Contusions. All except the most innocuous of contusions should be referred to the ophthalmologist, as pediatricians may fail to recognize fractures of the orbital bones including blowout fractures, lacerations of the globe, ruptured globe, corneal edema, hyphema, traumatic iridocyclitis, iridoplegia, secondary glaucoma, traumatic subluxation of the lens, retinal detachment, vitreous hemorrhage, extraocular muscle injury, iridodialysis, traumatic recession of the anterior chamber angle, retinal hemorrhages and edema, central retinal artery occlusion, papilledema and avulsion of the optic nerve.

Chemical Burns. The only true emergency in cases of ocular trauma involves chemical burns to the cornea. These must be treated immediately; minutes, even seconds, count in alkali and acid injuries. Irrigation should be immediate and profuse, lasting 30 minutes. Following application of topical proparacaine, either squeeze-type irrigating solutions or an intravenous bottle of isotonic saline mounted on a pole and connected to intravenous tubing should be employed. Solutions of weak acids or bases as neutralizing solutions are no more effective than isotonic saline.

The fornices should be inspected carefully for evidence of particulate matter such as pieces of mortar or plaster (calcium hydroxide) which may serve as a reservoir for continued alkalization of the cornea. Ethylenediamine tetraacetic acid (EDTA), the disodium salt without calcium, 0.05 M, pH 7.0 to 7.5 used as an irrigating solution, aids in the removal of small pieces of plaster.

Following lavage, the patient should be referred immediately to the ophthalmologist. Burns with strong acid precipitate tissue proteins instantly and the full extent of the ocular damage can be assessed immediately. In cases of burns with strong alkali, however, deterioration of tissue continues over a period of time. What may seem an innocuous alkali burn when first seen, may progress to a perforated globe within one to two weeks.

Thermal Burns. Rapid reflex lid closure usually prevents serious damage to the globe. Serious thermal injury to the eyelids necessitates immediate referral. However, if only minimal eyelid injury is seen, and the cornea stains only minimally with fluorescein, or if there is no corneal stain, an antibiotic ointment should be applied and the patient re-examined the next day.

Ultraviolet Burns. Ultraviolet radiation injury usually occurs following exposure to "suntan" lamps without adequate shielding for the eyes. These rays do not penetrate the eye and cause only surface damage. There is usually a lag of 6 to 10 hours before symptoms become apparent. Unless topical anesthesia is applied, the intense pain, photophobia and blepharospasm preclude a good examination. Usually the history alone makes the diagnosis obvious.

I have previously cautioned against the use of topical anesthesia as treatment, but in these cases, the pain is usually intolerable, and a few drops of proparacaine, 0.5 per cent, immediately relieves almost all pain. Cycloplegic drops such as cyclopentolate, 0.5 to 1.0 per cent, or scopolamine, 0.2 to 0.3 per cent, should be instilled, and both eyes patched if possible. Sometimes it is possible to patch only the worse eye, as the child may not permit total closure of both eyes. An ophthalmologist should be consulted for further treatment. Even severe ultraviolet burns usually heal without residua in 24 to 48 hours.

DISEASES OF THE EYE

Treatable by the Pediatrician

Diseases of the Eyelids. BLEPHARITIS. The two most common types of blepharitis, probably accounting for over 90 per cent of cases of chronic blepharitis in the United States, are staphylococcal and seborrheic. These two types may often occur together.

The lid margins of most children with chronic *staphylococcal blepharitis* are constantly red, and often there is crusting at the base of the cilia. In long-standing cases, there may be loss of eyelashes and recurrent chalazia. The longer the condition is present, the harder it is to eradicate. It is important to culture the eyelid margins by rubbing a wet swab back and forth on the skin side of the eyelid margin. Even when a clinical diagnosis of staphylococcal blepharitis is most likely, it may be difficult to culture the organisms, as they often lie below the surface within the meibomian glands.

Treatment consists of a combination of local hygienic care and specific local anti-staphylococcal therapy. The crusts are removed with sterile moistened cotton applicators, followed by bacitracin ophthalmic ointment, 500 units/gm., placed on a sterile cotton applicator and rubbed into the base of the cilia. When treatment is started it is necessary to apply the ointment approximately four times daily. A response should be evident within 1 to 2 weeks. If, after several weeks, the condition improves, antibiotic application may be reduced to twice daily. Once the eyelids appear normal, nightly application of a bacitracin ointment should be continued for a month. In my experience, if treatment is stopped too soon, the condition recurs.

If bacitracin ointment therapy proves ineffective, sensitivity studies should suggest an appropriate topical antibiotic. Erythromycin ophthalmic ointment, 5 mg./gm., may be appropriate. Staphylococcal exotoxin may add to eyelid margin erythema; the judicious use of topical corticosteroids by the ophthalmologist may reduce this erythema. I know of no evidence substantiating the use of systemic an-

tibiotic therapy in the treatment of chronic staphylococcal blepharitis. The use of staphylococcal toxoid is debatable. Many authorities state that its use is without scientific justification. However, I have observed some cases of chronic staphylococcal blepharitis respond dramatically to staphylococcal toxoid when all other measures have failed, and have heard of other instances of similar results.

Seborrheic blepharitis is manifested by the appearance of greasy scales at the lid margins at the base of the cilia. This may be accompanied by minimal erythema in cases which are not secondarily infected with staphylococcus. In almost all instances seborrhea of the scalp or eyebrows accompanies seborrheic blepharitis. This condition of the eyelids is hard to treat unless the seborrheic conditions of the scalp and eyebrows are cleared first. Antiseborrheic preparations such as selenium sulfide (Selsun)* shampoo may be used on the scalp and eyebrows. In most instances its irritative properties preclude its use around the eyes. Cotton applicators may be used periodically to keep the eyelids clean.

Angular blepharitis. Several decades ago the most common cause of blepharitis affecting the lateral canthal area was moraxella, a bacteria rarely encountered in systemic disease but well known to the ophthalmologist. In recent years, however, angular blepharitis is caused more often by the staphylococcus. Moraxella is sensitive to neomycin. An antibiotic ointment containing neomycin is applied to the involved lid margin four times daily. However, there is a high incidence of sensitivity of the skin, conjunctiva and cornea associated with neomycin therapy. Chloromycetin ophthalmic ointment, 1 per cent, may prove effective. Zinc sulfate solution, 0.25 to 0.5 per cent 4 times daily, is a useful addition to antibiotic therapy in moraxella infections. It does not eradicate the organism, but in some way neutralizes its noxious products, perhaps enzymes, and is clinically effective in reducing the inflammation induced by the bacteria.

HORDEOLUM (STY), MEIBOMITIS AND CHALAZION. A hordeolum is an acute pyogenic infection of the glands of Zeis, while an acute meibomitis is a similar infection of the meibomian glands. Acute infections of these sebaceous glands of the eyelid are almost invariably caused by staphylococcus. A chalazion is a granulomatous process involving the meibomian glands following an acute meibomitis.

---

*Manufacturer's precaution: Safety for the use of selenium sulfide on infants has not been established.

Since the glands of Zeis are located superficially along the lid margin, hordeola present as small painful indurated erythematous infections which quickly localize as small abscesses and usually point within 24 to 48 hours. Because the meibomian glands are located deeper within the lids, staphylococcal infections of these glands do not point, rupture and drain externally. A granuloma usually ensues, leading to the formation of a chalazion.

Cases of single nonrecurrent hordeola or acute meibomitis should be treated with hot compresses only. Resolution of hordeola may be hastened by incising a hordeolum when it is fluctuant and pointing. Antibiotic therapy, in my experience, is ineffective. Cases of recurrent hordeola and meibomitis should be treated as outlined above under chronic staphylococcal blepharitis.

Approximately 50 per cent of chalazia disappear spontaneously within a month. Those that remain can be either left alone or excised by an ophthalmologist. Excising a chalazion is a simple office procedure in the adult, but requires general anesthesia for children. The pediatrician and ophthalmologist should therefore weigh the balance of risks accordingly. Except for cosmetic reasons, there is no contraindication to leaving a small chalazion alone until the child is old enough to have it removed under local anesthesia.

Diseases of the Conjunctiva. Conjunctivitis. Previous sections have outlined signs and symptoms of conjunctivitis which set it apart from more serious inflammations of the eye. Conjunctivitis is known by the laity as "pink eye." Once a diagnosis of *bacterial conjunctivitis* has been made, an antibiotic drop such as gentamicin 0.3 per cent, neomycin, gramacidin-polymyxin B, chloromycetin 0.5 per cent or an antibiotic ointment such as bacitracin-polymyxin B, gentamicin 0.3 per cent or chloromycetin 1 per cent, is usually applied 5 or 6 times daily. In addition the eyelids should be kept clean with sterile cotton applicators moistened with boiled water or a commercial sterile irrigating solution. Since ointments tend to blur vision, drops are usually used during the day and ointments at bedtime. If the child cries during drug administration, ointments should be used.

Bacterial conjunctivitis caused by streptococci, pneumococci, *Hemophilus aegypticus* (Koch-Weeks bacillus), and *Hemophilus influenzae* respond well to this regimen. Two other bacteria, moraxella and staphylococcus, may also respond to this therapy; however, infections by these two bacteria also involve the skin of the eyelid and tend to become chronic

unless quickly eradicated. If a chronic blepharoconjunctivitis ensues, the patient should be referred to an ophthalmologist. Since bacterial conjunctivitis can lead to a bacterial corneal ulcer, a patient with any sign of corneal involvement such as staining with fluorescein or even the smallest infiltrate should be referred immediately to the ophthalmologist.

Neomycin induces a high frequency of punctate staining of the cornea and might best be avoided in treating mild cases of bacterial conjunctivitis. Zinc sulfate drops, 0.25 to 0.5 per cent, are effective in reducing the signs and symptoms of moraxella conjunctivitis, but should be used in combination with antibiotic therapy. Systemic antibiotics and topical or systemic corticosteroids should not be used in the treatment of bacterial conjunctivitis.

Staphylococcal conjunctivitis is best treated with bacitracin ophthalmic ointment, 500 units/gm., 5 or 6 times daily initially, the frequency decreasing as the condition improves. Since staphylococcal conjunctivitis tends to become chronic, it is advisable to instill bacitracin ointment at bedtime for 1 month after all signs of the conjunctivitis have disappeared. As 30 to 50 per cent of all inflamed conjunctiva may have *S. epidermidis* cultured out because it is part of the normal flora, commitment to long antibiotic therapy in cases of staphylococcal conjunctivitis should probably be restricted to isolation of *S. aureus*, coagulase positive.

True membranous conjunctivitis is rare and usually associated with diphtheria. In such cases a gray-yellow membrane is seen on the conjunctiva, and its removal results in multiple areas of bleeding. Treatment of the primary disease usually effects an ocular cure. *Pseudomembranous conjunctivitis* may be caused by many bacteria and some viruses.

Viral conjunctivitis is almost always accompanied by the appearance of follicles on the palpebral conjunctiva, and is often seen with preauricular lymphadenopathy. The most common form of adenoviral conjunctivitis in children is pharyngoconjunctival fever. Adenovirus type 3 is the most frequent pathogen, although other types have been implicated. No specific therapy is available. The disease is self-limited, resolving in 2 or 3 weeks. In cases of corneal involvement, however, ophthalmic consultation is advisable.

Epidemic keratoconjunctivitis (EKC), caused by type 8 adenovirus, begins as a typical viral conjunctivitis. Approximately 7 to 10 days later a keratitis appears, consisting of multiple subepithelial corneal infiltrates. These are often difficult to see without magnification. The conjunctivitis usually disappears in several weeks, but the corneal infiltrates may persist for months. As in all cases of conjunctivitis, ophthalmic consultation should be obtained if there is any corneal involvement. The ophthalmic consultation is necessary not so much for instituting therapy, which in most cases is nonspecific, but rather for verifying a diagnosis when so important a tissue as the cornea is involved.

As stated above, follicle formation of the palpebral conjunctiva is almost always seen with viral conjunctivitis. Young children, with a tendency toward lymphoid hyperplasia, frequently exhibit conjunctival folliculosis, follicle formation of the palpebral conjunctiva without any sign of inflammation. In children, a red eye may combine with conjunctival folliculosis to suggest a spurious diagnosis of viral conjunctivitis.

Following vaccination for smallpox, accidental transfer of the virus from the site of inoculation to the eye may result in *vaccinial* conjunctivitis or keratitis. Vaccine-immune globulin (VIG) may be used in cases of lid or conjunctival involvement, but may exacerbate a keratitis induced by this virus.

The four most common types of *conjunctivitis in the newborn* are chemical, gonococcal, staphylococcal and inclusion conjunctivitis. The time of onset may provide a good clue to diagnosis. Chemical conjunctivitis usually begins on the first or second day of life, soon after silver nitrate is instilled. Gonococcal conjunctivitis usually begins on day 3 or 4, inclusion conjunctivitis on day 7 to 10. Staphylococcal conjunctivitis may begin at any time.

A severe purulent reaction is seen with both gonococcal and inclusion conjunctivitis. Since untreated gonococcal conjunctivitis may rapidly progress to a fulminating corneal ulcer, a Gram stain should be performed immediately on conjunctival exudate to rule out gonococcal conjunctivitis. If the smear is negative the infant should be seen several times during the next 24 to 48 hours to guard against corneal involvement while the culture is incubating.

Treatment of chemical conjunctivitis in the newborn is nonspecific. Therapy for the staphylococcal variety is similar to that described above under staphylococcal conjunctivitis. In gonococcal conjunctivitis, the uninvolved eye must be kept free of contamination. The involved eye should be opened frequently to let the pus drain, as large quantities of it may build up under the tightly closed swollen lids. The pressure from the entrapped pus may induce corneal damage with a resulting gonoccocal corneal ulcer. Be careful to protect yourself from any squirting of the purulent material when the infant's eye is opened. Specific therapy consists of intramuscular or intravenous penicillin G, 50,000 units/kg. daily for 7 days, and penicillin G eye drops. The eye drops are not available commercially but can be prepared with sterile water from the parenteral preparation to a concentration of 10,000 units/ml. and given every 30 to 60 minutes for several days and then tapered to 4 times daily for 7 more days. If the child is older than 8 years and is allergic to penicillin, tetracycline should be administered intramuscularly or intravenously, 125 to 150 mg./kg./day in 4 divided doses for 7 to 10 days. Topical tetracycline 1 per cent drops in oil should also be administered every hour for the first few days and then reduced to 4 to 6 times daily for the remainder of the 7 to 10 day treatment period.

Chlamydial inclusion conjunctivitis invariably responds well to frequent topical applications of tetracycline ointment 1 per cent 4 to 6 times daily over a 3 week period.

Prophylaxis in the newborn: In 1881, Crede demonstrated that a 1:40 solution of silver nitrate reduced the incidence of newborn ophthalmia from over 10 per cent of births to under 0.5 per cent. Until the introduction of antibiotics, instillation of 1 per cent silver nitrate into newborn eyes was standard procedure. Over the last 30 years, topical applications of various antibiotics have been used as a substitute for silver nitrate therapy. Advocates of antibiotic prophylaxis state, and rightly so, that the chemical conjunctivitis following silver nitrate therapy is avoided. They also point out that long-standing solutions of 1 per cent silver nitrate may evaporate, thus increasing the concentration to a level which may cause ocular damage. Modern single dose packaging eliminates this potential hazard for all practical purposes. Some authorities have suggested that prophylaxis be eliminated in the newborn because gonococcal conjunctivitis can be treated effectively once it appears. After reviewing all available material, I have concluded that silver nitrate is the simplest, most effective type of prophylaxis and should be employed. The chemical conjunctivitis associated with its use is acceptable compared to the risk involved when no prophylactic therapy has been instituted.

Having just dealt with inclusion conjunctivitis in the newborn, there remain two other types of *ocular chlamydial disease* to discuss. *Trachoma* is probably the leading cause of blindness in the world today. It is rarely seen in the United States except in the Southwest, where it is endemic in the Indian population. Although topical tetracycline and sulfonamides have been used with success in treating the more virulent form of the disease in the Middle East, their use in the typically mild form found in the southwestern United States has been largely ineffective. The disease in the United States runs a usually mild course over a period of many years. Local hygiene decreases the incidence of secondary bacterial infection and the spread of the disease. Systemic sulfonamide therapy in the form of sulfisoxazole should be given for at least several weeks in combination with topical tetracycline 1 per cent or sulfonamide preparations or both. Systemic tetracycline, 1 gm./day for patients weighing less than 70 kg. and 1.5 gm./day for patients weighing more than 70 kg., may also be used in older children and adults, but should be avoided in children under 8 years and used with caution in children under 12 years.

Inclusion conjunctivitis may occur in older children and adults as well as in the newborn (see above). Whereas inclusion bodies may be found following scraping of the conjunctiva and Giemsa staining in the newborn, it is much harder to find inclusion bodies in older children and adults. Acute follicular conjunctivitis may be chlamydial or viral, but chronic follicular conjunctivitis lasting longer than 2 or 3 weeks should be considered chlamydial until proven otherwise. Treatment is as outlined for trachoma, consisting of systemic and topical tetracycline for a period of 4 weeks. Whereas inclusion conjunctivitis in the newborn invariably responds to topical therapy alone, even a combination of topical and systemic therapy may prove ineffective at times in the older child or adult.

To Be Referred to the Ophthalmologist

Some types of conjunctivitis may, and should, be treated by the pediatrician. Most respond well to either nonspecific or specific therapy and resolve without sequelae. If a diagnosis is in doubt, if the course of the disease is protracted, or if the cornea is involved, ophthalmic consultation should be sought. In addition, all patients with decreased visual acuity, ocular pain, photophobia, lacrimation, or exhibiting ciliary flush, significant anisocoria, decrease in the optical clarity of the media (lens, vitreous) or any abnormality of the fundus or optic nerve, should be referred to an ophthalmologist.

The treatment for *acute staphylococcal blepharokeratoconjunctivitis* is outlined above. When the entity becomes subacute or chronic or when corneal involvement occurs, in the form of punctate epithelial staining with fluorescein, or peripheral corneal infiltrates, ophthalmic consultation is advised.

Chalazion: See above.

Gonococcal conjunctivitis is initially treated by the pediatrician because of the need for immediate specific therapy. Ophthalmic consultation is necessary to help guard against corneal complications.

Bacterial and fungal corneal ulcers may quickly and permanently destroy the optical clarity of the cornea. Whenever a pediatrician sees a painful red eye in combination with a corneal infiltrate, an ophthalmologist should be consulted immediately. Most bacterial and fungal ulcers are treated with subconjunctival injections and multiple topical instillations of antibiotics or antifungal agents, in combination with cycloplegics.

A pediatrician, otolaryngologist and ophthalmologist should cooperate in treating *orbital cellulitis*. The infection usually originates in an infected sinus. Unilateral exophthalmos with lid edema, fever and toxicity combine to make a diagnosis. *H. influenzae* is the prime offender in an infant or young child; grampositive bacteria can account for most infections in the older child. Initial therapy before the age of 6 years consists of oxacillin, 50 to 100 mg./kg./day intramuscularly or intravenously in divided doses every 3 to 4 hours, combined with streptomycin, 30 mg./kg./day intramuscularly or intravenously every 6 hours. After the age of 6 years, oxacillin therapy usually suffices. Parenteral antibiotic therapy should be continued for 7 to 10 days. This therapy may be modified according to patient response and culture reports. A number of ampicillin-resistant strains are beginning to appear. An ophthalmologist should monitor the child to guard against complications such as papilledema, optic atrophy, or exposure keratitis with secondary corneal ulcer. On occasion it may be necessary and perhaps even advisable to drain an orbital abscess.

Acute suppurative *dacryoadenitis* may at times look like orbital cellulitis, except that the greatest swelling is seen in the upper outer quadrant of the anterior orbit under the lid. Treatment of the two conditions is similar. Chronic dacryoadenitis may be seen secondary to mumps, sarcoid, lymphomas, or less often with other systemic disease.

Infection and obstruction of the lacrimal outflow tract. Authorities differ as to whether newborn infants tear. Some do and some do not. The development of the lacrimal duct is usually complete by birth, but in some infants it may not canalize until several months after birth. Epiphora within the first few months of life may be indicative of obstruction of the lacrimal outflow tract or infection of the lacrimal sac. Infection often accompanies stasis. Usually the infection is lowgrade and chronic. It may be diagnosed by a history of pus at the inner corner of the eye or by the appearance of a purulent reflux from the punctum following pressure on the lacrimal sac area.

Since infection usually cannot be cured without establishing the patency of the lacrimal outflow system, irrigation and probing plus specific antibiotic therapy should be instituted soon after diagnosis. I generally wait up to four months following birth before probing the lacrimal duct when there is no sign of infection. In many instances the duct spontaneously becomes patent and epiphora disappears. If epiphora continues beyond the age of 4 months the infant should undergo lacrimal probing and irrigation by the ophthalmologist.

Acute dacryocystitis in children is, in most instances, due to gram-positive bacteria. Before the age of 6 years, *H. influenzae* is a common pathogen and treatment consists of oxacillin, 50 to 100 mg./kg./day, intramuscularly or intravenously in divided doses every 3 to 4 hours combined with streptomycin, 30 mg./kg./day, intramuscularly or intravenously every 6 hours. After the age of 6 years, oxacillin therapy usually suffices. Parenteral antibiotic therapy should be continued for 7 to 10 days.

Chlamydial disease: See previous section.

Herpes simplex infection of the eye in children has been divided into two types, primary and secondary herpes. Unfortunately one type blends into the other and the classification breaks down. In general, however, it may be said that children are more likely to develop herpetic infections of the face, lid and conjunctiva. When there is no involvement of the cornea, as evidenced by a crystal clear cornea without fluorescein staining, and no evidence of iritis, the disease may be managed by the pediatrician. Treatment is nonspecific and consists of local hygienic care.

In two thirds of cases, however, the cornea becomes involved and the patient should be seen immediately by an ophthalmologist. Antiviral therapy in the form of 5-iodo-2'-desoxyuridine (IDU) ointment is usually instituted. By the time this textbook is published adenine arabinoside (Ara-A), a superior antiherpes simplex agent, may be commercially available. Ara-A may also be used to treat severe forms of systemic herpes simplex infection. In older children and adults, herpes simplex keratitis takes the form of a dendritic corneal ulcer without skin or lid lesions, and should be referred immediately to an ophthalmologist for specific therapy. Occasionally a dendritic figure of the cornea is seen in an infant without skin or lid lesions. In cases of suspected herpes simplex keratoconjunctivitis a pediatrician should never use topical corticosteroids, as this exacerbates and prolongs the infection.

Herpes zoster infections of the eye may involve multiple sites such as cornea, iris, ciliary body, retina, optic nerve and extraocular muscles. Combined corticosteroid-cycloplegic therapy is usually employed by the ophthalmologist.

Molluscum contagiosum and *verruca* viruses produce small tumor-like growths on the lid margins and secondarily induce a keratoconjunctivitis. Excision of the lesions is the treatment of choice.

Epidemic keratoconjunctivitis: See previous section.

Oculoglandular syndrome of Parinaud is nonspecific and consists of a conjunctivitis, lid edema and preauricular lymphadenopathy. It may be caused by tuberculosis, cat scratch fever, tularemia, and several other entities.

Symptoms and signs of *allergic conjunctivitis* have been discussed in a previous section. If the symptoms are mild and the signs are few or absent, antihistamines given by mouth or a mild eye drop containing antihistamine or both should be given. Examples are naphazoline hydrochloride (Albalon, Vasocon), naphazoline plus antazoline (Vasocon A), and tetrahydrozoline (Visine). In more severe cases the patient should be referred to an ophthalmologist for topical corticosteroid therapy.

Vernal conjunctivitis is a recurrent bilateral conjunctivitis, probably immunologically induced, consisting of cobblestone papules found on the palpebral conjunctiva of the upper lid. Corticosteroid therapy by the ophthalmologist is the treatment of choice. The disease is often refractory to treatment.

A 1 to 2 mm. mass straddling the limbus, a red eye and extreme photophobia combine to make a diagnosis of *phlyctenule*. There is a higher incidence of phlyctenules in impoverished populations, and phlyctenules have been associated with tuberculosis. It is probably immunologically induced and responds dramatically to topical corticosteroid therapy.

Erythema multiforme and *toxic epidermal necrolysis*. Although severe forms of these diseases may induce a severe conjunctivitis which clears without residua, many cases induce symblepharon formation of the conjunctiva with tragic sequelae of conjunctival scarring, decreased tear formation, decreased integrity of the tear film, a dry eye syndrome with corneal scarring and blindness. I have excellent success in preventing these sequelae using high-dose systemic and topical corticosteroid therapy in combination with reverse sterile precautions and topical antibiotics.

Dry eye syndrome. Entities such as erythema multiforme, toxic epidermal necrolysis, familial dysautonomia, exposure keratitis and neuroparalytic keratitis may result in a dry eye syndrome caused by diminished tear production, diminished production of mucin from diseased conjunctival goblet cells, inadequate blinking or inadequate protection of the cornea by the lids. Drying of the cornea ensues. Once a cornea becomes dry its epithelial layer degenerates and corneal scarring, with or without infection, soon occurs. Tear replacement in the form of artificial tears may help to alleviate the condition. More recently soft contact lenses have been successfully used to protect the compromised cornea.

Episcleritis and *scleritis* are localized areas of inflammation on the white of the eye, usually accompanied by pain. Episcleritis is much more common than scleritis and responds better to topical corticosteroid therapy. Scleritis may be refractory to treatment.

Iritis, iridocyclitis and *posterior uveitis* are caused by multiple immunologic and infectious agents, many of which are still unknown. Iritis and iridocyclitis in the adult is almost always accompanied by pain, lacrimation and photophobia, but they may smolder along asymptomatically in children. This is often the case in iridocyclitis accompanying juvenile rheumatoid arthritis, usually of the pauciarticular type. Periodic referrals to an ophthalmologist are often necessary to guard against asymptomatic iridocyclitis. All cases of iridocyclitis are treated with a combination of topical cycloplegia and corticosteroids.

Usually the only symptom of posterior uveitis is diminished visual acuity. The ophthalmologist generally uses systemic or retrobulbar corticosteroid therapy, since determination of a specific etiologic agent is often difficult. Toxoplastic chorioretinitis is usually treated with pyrimethamine (Daraprim), triple sulfa and corticosteriods systemically when diagnosed in the acute stage. In its chronic stage treatment is ineffective, as the organisms are encysted.

The usual forms of childhood *strabismus* are esotropia and exotropia. Many infants and young children appear to be esotropic because the epicanthal folds create such an appearance. Asymmetry of the corneal reflexes serves as a better guide in diagnosing strabismus. It is often erroneously stated that ocular deviations diagnosed within the first 12 to 18 months of life need not be referred to an ophthalmologist since they are usually outgrown. Although a normal eye may occasionally wander before the age of 18 months to 2 years, it is imperative that all children with strabismus be referred to an ophthalmologist for diagnosis and therapy no matter what age. It is important to remember that any disease which reduces vision may result in strabismus.

Treatment of strabismus may be delayed according to the individual ophthalmologist; however all ophthalmologists agree that suppression amblyopia (decreased vision) in the turned eye should be treated as soon as the diagnosis is made if the child is less than 6 years old. Patching of the good eye is necessary to make the turned eye "work." When patching is instituted before the age of 5 or 6 years, vision will often return to the amblyopic eye. The earlier suppression amblyopia is treated, the more quickly vision returns. A week of patching in a 2 year old may restore vision to approximately the same level as that obtained following a month of patching in a 5 year old. All efforts should be made to induce the child to wear a patch. Substitutes such as atropinization of the eye or the use of frosted lenses are poor seconds to full-time patching. If the strabismus is accommodative in type it may respond either fully or partially to the use of glasses or miotics such as phospholine iodide. Nonaccommodative comitant (nonparalytic) strabismus and the residua of the accommodative type are surgically correctable. Orthoptic therapy (training of the extraocular muscles) may be used to help straighten the eyes.

Torticollis. Certain types of strabismus, usually paresis of the superior oblique muscle, cause a child to keep his head constantly tilted in an effort to compensate for the effects of the paresis. Ophthalmic consultation should be sought when torticollis without an obvious cause has been diagnosed.

Sturge-Weber disease is characterized by a port-wine angioma of the skin on one side of the face and an ipsilateral angioma of the choroid. I have included this entity here, as many children with it have accompanying glaucoma. They should be referred to an ophthalmologist.

Congenital glaucoma usually occurs within the first year of life. Photophobia in an infant should alert the pediatrician to the diagnosis, especially when accompanied by eyes that appear large with corneal diameters greater than 12 mm. The treatment of congenital glaucoma is surgical.

Congenital glaucoma is often associated with *aniridia,* but even more important, it is mandatory to rule out the possibility of an accompanying Wilms' tumor.

"White pupil." Severe congenital cataracts and certain diseases of the vitreous and retina such as retinoblastoma, retinal dysplasia, some types of retinal detachment, inflammatory membranes at the iris level and persistent hyperplastic primary vitreous, create the appearance of a white pupil. Persistent hyperplastic primary vitreous is usually excised. Retinal detachment in the infant is usually secondary to another disease process.

There is no medical treatment for most *congenital cataracts.* However, cataracts secondary to galactosemia, if diagnosed early, may regress following institution of dietary control. A pediatrician usually diagnoses rubella and galactokinase cataracts. The ophthalmologist must decide whether a cataract is severe enough to require surgery. If significant vision is to be restored, surgery should be performed early, if possible within the first 4 months of life. If an infant has had surgery to remove severe bilateral cataracts it is possible to restore vision using cataract glasses. A child will never tolerate glasses following removal of one cataract if the other eye is normal. In such a case a contact lens may be fitted. Some children tolerate contact lenses; others do not.

Retinoblastoma is the most common malignant tumor affecting a child's eye. If a parent has had retinoblastoma the child has approximately a 40 to 50 per cent chance of developing the same tumor. Bilateral involvement occurs in approximately one third of cases. The more involved eye or the only involved eye is usually enucleated, while the less involved eye is treated by chemotherapy or radiation or both.

Until recently there has been no treatment for *retrolental fibroplasia.* Several recent studies indicate that laser therapy to the abnormal blood vessels may help preserve eyesight.

17

The Ear

Foreign Bodies in the Ear

WERNER CHASIN, M.D.

Most foreign bodies in the ear have been inserted by the child itself. They include objects such as beads, peas, matchsticks, and chewing gum. Foreign objects may also consist of insects, maggots, and cotton which has become dislodged from the end of a Q-Tip. Any child with a self-inserted foreign body in the ear should be searched for other such objects in the other orifices of the body. The child with a self-inserted foreign body is often unusually frightened because of a feeling of guilt and is therefore terrified about having the object removed.

In preparing to remove a foreign body from the ear the following principles should be observed:

1. If the child is uncooperative or terrified, the procedure is best performed under general anesthesia.

2. The proper instruments consist of a small suction tube such as a Baron 5 French tube, an ear alligator forceps with serrated jaws, a small or medium Billeau ear loop, and a small blunt hook such as an incus hook.

3. Any child who has had a foreign body removed successfully should have the ear reexamined in one to two weeks after the canal skin has healed to rule out any residual damage to either the ear canal, tympanic membrane, or middle ear.

4. If the foreign object cannot be removed easily the child should be referred to an otologist.

Globular objects such as beads and artificial pearls are large enough to become impacted in the inner half of the external auditory canal. Unsuccessful attempts at removal result at best in a lacerated, bleeding, swollen skin of the external canal. At worst they result in damage to the tympanic membrane with a resulting perforation, dislocation of the ossicles, and even damage to the inner ear from an inadvertent subluxation of the stapes in the oval window.

Maggots in the ear canal cause a necrotizing external otitis and are not easily recognized unless the physician looks carefully for their slow undulating movement usually in the inner half of the ear canal near the drumhead. This must be removed with the suction tube. An antibiotic-steroid otic solution is then prescribed for several days and the ear is reexamined for healing of the skin.

Otologic Infections

RICHARD H. MEADE, III, M.D.

ACUTE OTITIS MEDIA

Suppurative otitis media must be treated for a longer time and often with larger antibiotic doses than are necessary for pharyngitis. Both infections can make the tympanic membrane appear red. Although fever, earache, and regional lymphadenopathy in addition to the presence of a red drum suggest suppurative otitis media, it is wise to look for immobilization of the tympanic membrane by pneumatic otoscopy to confirm it.

Although the cause of middle ear infection can be determined most accurately by needle aspiration through the drum, it is not necessary for all children. It should be considered: (1) if the drum is red, bulging and very painful in association with high fever and signs of generalized severe infection, especially meningitis in which there are no visible bacteria in the spinal fluid; (2) to identify the cause of acute exacerbations of chronic otitis media because the variety of bacteria responsible are such that standard therapy has little chance of being effective; (3) in the child who fails to respond to therapy for an acute infection as in otitis caused by *Staphylococcus aureus*, *Staphylococcus epidermidis* or even *Mycobacterium tuberculosis*; and (4) in the child with compromised host defense as in leukemia or chronic granulomatous disease, or whose otitis media developed after receiving antibiotics for another infection.

not as reliable a guide to the ...is media as aspiration of the middle ...fully done nasopharyngeal swabs are ...lue. A Gram-stained smear showing a ...rge number of polymorphonuclear cells and a predominant bacterial population of one type is good evidence for the presence and etiology of suppurative otitis media. In the absence of polymorphonuclear cells or the presence of a variety of bacteria, the smear helps to rule out bacterial infection. Aspiration or smears of the nasopharynx are not usually needed to diagnose suppurative otitis media or to select therapy. There are, however, an increasing number of children for whom these procedures are an essential part of the diagnostic process.

Most infections are due to *S. pneumoniae* and as such are susceptible to penicillin or to erythromycin. In up to 25 per cent of children under four, *Hemophilus influenzae* is the pathogen. Only 10 per cent of these strains are typable, so that the incidence of ampicillin-resistant infection is low enough at present to permit use of this antibiotic. *Streptococcus pyogenes* types A and B are susceptible to all of these antibiotics and represent no therapeutic problem even if not recognized. A greater problem is posed by the infrequent acute infections due to *Staphylococcus aureus* and *Staphylococcus epidermidis*. The presence of these and other organisms resistant to antibiotics such as ampicillin is announced by the results of aspiration, suggested by Gram-stained smears from the nasopharynx and implied by the lack of response to treatment.

Antimicrobial Agents

Penicillin alone is satisfactory for most children four years or older, although occasionally *Hemophilus influenzae* is the pathogen. Phenoxymethyl penicillin and benzathine penicillin G (in a single intramuscular dose) have also been reported to be effective. Erythromycin can be used for children allergic to penicillin.

Although either penicillin or erythromycin used alone has worked as well as ampicillin in pediatric practices, neither works as well in specific therapy of *Hemophilus influenzae* otitis media. The addition of sulfisoxazole to either of these antibiotics has been effective, as are ampicillin and its analogue, amoxicillin. Allergy to penicillin would make it necessary to use erythromycin and sulfisoxazole. Cephalexin has been proposed as a method of treating all of the common forms of otitis media including infection due to *Hemophilus influenzae* and can be used, with caution, in patients allergic to penicillin.

Uncommonly staphylococci are the cause of acute otitis media. For the child who exhibits no signs of disseminated disease, pneumonia, mastoiditis or meningitis, treatment can be given by mouth. Oxacillin for those not allergic to penicillin is effective against most strains of staphylococci (aureus or epidermidis). Penicillin allergy would require use of erythromycin or of cephalexin. In the particularly sick infant or child, or one not responding to treatment, it is of utmost importance to obtain material from the ear by aspiration both to identify the cause and to determine its sensitivities and to give antibiotic treatment parenterally.

Bullous meningitis has been attributed by some to viral infection. It is also the result of infections with pneumonococci and Group A *S. pyogenes*. Treatment of the febrile child with otitis media when bullae are present should be directed against these bacterial pathogens.

Mycoplasma pneumoniae is an occasional cause of otitis media in children. It is not reliably associated with bullous myringitis. If the diagnosis is suspected because of the course of the disease, lack of response to penicillin or ampicillin, or the presence of sterile fluid in the middle ear, erythromycin should be used.

Antibiotic therapy for acute otitis media should be given for a period of 10 days. Susceptible bacteria are ordinarily killed within 24 to 36 hours and within that period of time evidence of clinical improvement should be discernible. Reexamination of the ear within several days provides assurance that treatment is having the desired effect and that it has prevented extension into the mastoid air cells.

Oral decongestants are usually given to children with the expectation that they will decompress the eustachian tube to allow drainage of middle ear contents and maintain normal pressure. They are not required in all cases and are best used if there is physical evidence of pharyngitis or of rhinitis with visible mucosal edema.

NEONATAL OTITIS MEDIA

Middle ear infections in the infant under 6 weeks of age can be hard to see and to differentiate from irritative changes in the tympanic membranes from contaminated amniotic fluid. Otitis media and such complications as temporal osteitis have been found as the cause of infantile death. Uncomplicated localized middle ear infection has been found in neonates from birth to 6 weeks of age. The most important single finding in making the diagnosis is poor mobility of the drum. Although both pneumococci and *H. influenzae* have been found as causes of infection in this age group, *E. coli, K. pneumoniae,* and *S. aureus* are commoner pathogens and emphasize the necessity of obtaining fluid from the middle ear for cultures. Getting fluid can be difficult. It has been stressed before and is reiterated here that it requires a skilled otolaryngologist to obtain it. Most infants in this age group require parenteral antibiotics using the agent to which the causative organism is susceptible.

For the bacteria listed, and these are not the only ones that have been found, cephalothin is likely to be the most effective agent. For the gram-negative bacilli named above and for others such as *Proteus* or *Pseudomonas*, kanamycin or gentamicin may be required instead. If the causative organism is unknown at the time treatment is started, it is reasonable to combine cephalothin and gentamicin until its identity is known.

CHRONIC OTITIS MEDIA

Recurrent suppurative infections of the middle ear occurs for a number of reasons including anatomic anomalies such as cleft palate, eustachian tube malformation or obstruction, or persistent middle ear effusion with retraction of the drum. They are also due to mastoiditis or to antritis, and in a number of patients are due to no recognizable anatomic defect or chronically infected focus. Persistent otitis media with chronic drainage and wide or multiple perforations of the drum are due to *Mycobacterium tuberculosis*. Treatment with antibiotics is required for acute exacerbations and for tuberculosis, but except for the latter will be ineffective in preventing recurrent attacks. Recurrent episodes have been prevented in some by the continued administration of an oral sulfonamide. Mastoidectomy is indicated if infection is present and deemed unresponsive to antibiotic therapy. Adenoidectomy has been of value in those instances in which compression of the eustachian orifice can be demonstrated. Treatment of the persistent middle ear effusion associated with frequent recurrences of acute otitis media has been accomplished with the installation of plastic tympanostomy tubes. They have also been used to control persistent middle ear effusion even without recurrent infections, and hearing loss associated with retraction of the drums.

OTITIS EXTERNA

Inflammation of the walls of the external canal associated with a mucopurulent exudate that occludes the canal and with pain is a mixed problem. It is associated with hyperkeratosis and plugging of the sweat and sebaceous glands. Secondary invasion by skin bacteria including micrococci, diphtheroids and

Pseudomonas aeruginosa is a complication. Treatment is accomplished with a combination of topical corticosteroid and a mixture of neomycin and polymyxin. The antibiotics inhibit multiplication of surface bacteria and prevent invasion.

Infection can develop in the canal, or of the pinna due to bacteria complicating otitis externa or as the result of trauma (wrestling for example) or of extension from a furuncle, from cellulitis involving adjacent skin, or from erysipelas. While staphylococci or streptococci are the cause of furuncles or cellulitis, *Pseudomonas* is apt to be the cause of the infection following compressive injury of the ear. Treatment of this infection that involves the skin and threatens the cartilage has to be selected carefully. For cellulitis or for furuncles complicated by spreading infection, oxacillin by mouth is sufficient by itself or with surgical drainage. The presence of systemic signs of infection, or of failure of otitis to respond to oral medication requires that the exudate be cultured, the sensitivity of the organism be determined and that treatment be given parenterally. The duration of treatment should be at least 7 days; however, staphylococcal and *Pseudomonas* infection will require from 14 to 28 days to control and eradicate. Extension of infection through the floor of the external canal and into the bone beneath including the temporal bone and the floor of the skull is a rare and dreaded complication. It is to prevent this that long courses of parenteral antibiotic treatment may be needed.

TABLE 1.   Daily Dosage Schedule for Antibiotic Treatment of Otologic Infection

ANTIMICROBIAL AGENT	ROUTE	DOSAGE AND SCHEDULE
Penicillin G	PO	200,000 to 400,000 units 4 times daily
Penicillin G (aqueous)	IM or IV	200,000 to 500,000 units every 3 to 6 hours
Penicillin G (benzathine salt)	IM	600,000 units in one dose
Ampicillin	PO	50 mg./kg./day in 4 doses
Amoxicillin	PO	25 mg./kg./day in 3 doses
Phenoxymethyl-penicillin	PO	50 mg./kg./day in 4 doses
Oxacillin	PO	50 mg./kg./day in 4 doses
	IV	100 mg./kg./day in 4 hour doses
Cephalexin	PO	25 to 50 mg./kg./day in 4 doses
Erythromycin	PO	25 to 50 mg./kg./day in 4 doses
Kanamycin	IM	15 mg./kg./day in 2 doses
Sulfisoxazole*	PO	100 mg./kg./day in 4 doses
Gentamicin	IM or IV	5 mg./kg./day in 3 doses
Cephalothin	IM or IV	100 mg./kg./day in 3 or 4 hour doses

*Systemic sulfonamides are contraindicated in infants under 2 months of age.

Labyrinthitis

PAUL A. SHURIN, M.D.

Vertigo is the prime manifestation of labyrinthine disorders, but the characteristic complaint of a sense of motion of the body or the surroundings may not be elicited in young children. Disease of the labyrinth or its neural pathways may be suggested by dysequilibrium, abnormal gait or head posture, or nystagmus, and can be documented by a diminished response to caloric testing. Determination of the anatomic location of disease of this system requires otologic and neurologic examination, audiometry, and radiologic studies. The association of vertigo with hearing loss or alteration of consciousness suggests that the disorder is not limited to the labyrinth.

Suppurative Labyrinthitis. Bacterial infection of the labyrinth is now unusual. Most cases arise in infection of the middle ear or mastoid. Chronic ear disease, cholesteatoma, certain congenital anomalies of the middle ear, or head trauma may predispose to labyrinthitis. Meningitis, epidural or brain abscess and dural sinus thrombosis are frequently associated with labyrinthitis and may dominate the clinical picture.

The specific bacterial etiology of labyrinthitis has not been studied. In suspected cases of suppurative labyrinthine infection, cultures should be obtained and antimicrobial therapy instituted promptly. When there is associated acute otitis media, *Streptococcus pneumoniae* or *Hemophilus influenzae* are the most likely agents, and therapy is the same as for meningitis caused by these organisms. The presence of chronic otitis or mastoiditis, or of intracranial abscess formation, suggests involvement by anaerobic bacteria. Therapy with penicillin G (250,000 units/kg./day intravenously in 6 divided doses) plus chloramphenicol sodium succinate (100 mg./kg./day intravenously in 4 divided doses) can be used initially in such cases. The results of Gram-stained smears of infected material, cultures, and sensitivity tests may permit modification of this therapy. Adequate cultures of the middle ear cavity, blood, and cerebrospinal fluid must be obtained. Cultures to be processed for anaerobic bacteria must be processed rapidly and without exposure to air. Care is required to avoid contamination by skin flora. This may not be possible in sites such as the external ear canal, and culture of surgically obtained material may be required.

Surgical drainage of the primary infected focus is indicated in most instances. The approach will be determined by the extent of infection and the need for debridement of an infected mastoid or epidural abscess, removal of cholesteatoma, or repair of a perilymphatic fistula. A rapid clinical response to antibiotics may permit surgery to be delayed until the initial toxic course has resolved.

Recovery from labyrinthitis is usually accompanied by loss of hearing in the affected ear. This may be a significant educational or occupational handicap, as directional hearing is lost. Underwater swimming and diving are hazardous when vestibular function is deficient. For most other activities, patients develop effective compensation for labyrinthine destruction.

Nonsuppurative Labyrinthitis. Attacks of vertigo appearing spontaneously and without other manifestations of auditory or neurological disorder are often ascribed to viral infection of the labyrinth or vestibular nerve. This etiology remains unproved. Disease of this sort is uncommon in children. Vertigo may, however, be a manifestation of epilepsy, migraine, cerebrovascular anomaly, late congenital syphilis, or tumors of the cerebellum, brainstem or cranial nerves. In these disorders, altered consciousness, hearing loss, convulsive manifestations, diplopia or headache are indications that involvement is not limited to the labyrinth.

Benign paroxysmal vertigo of childhood is characterized by recurrent, self-limited attacks. Patients exhibit no sign of infection or other systemic disease. Dimenhydrinate, 10 to 20 mg. orally three times daily, has been reported to relieve symptoms in some patients; other children do well without treatment, and the disorder ultimately resolves without sequelae. (Dosages have not been established for use of dimenhydrinate in children less than 6 years of age.)

Injuries to the Middle Ear

WERNER CHASIN, M.D.

The rational management of injuries to the middle ear depends on a careful assessment of the morphological and functional alterations of the ear caused by the injury. Injuries result from fractures of the temporal bone, concussion of the ear, and from sudden pressure changes such as occur during flying and diving, especially when the eustachian tube is occluded by a cold. Injuries may also occur as a result of foreign objects being thrust into the ear (Q-Tips, hair pins, twigs), from thermal and electrical burns, and from slaps on the ear which perforate the tympanic membrane. Whereas the middle ear alone may be injured, the inner ear is often also damaged.

The morphologic changes which can be produced by injuries are perforation of the tympanic membrane, subluxation of part or all of the ossicular chain, hemotympanum (the presence of blood in the middle ear behind an intact drumhead, giving the membrane a strikingly blue or blue-purple color), cerebrospinal fluid otorrhea, facial paralysis, and irregularity or step-abnormality in the usually smooth walls of the external auditory canal caused by a fracture. During the acute phase the skin of the external auditory canal is lacerated over the fracture.

The functional alterations which may be caused by an injury to the middle ear depend on exactly which structures have been damaged. These alterations include some or all of the following: hearing loss (conductive, mixed, or sensorineural), vertigo, ataxia, nystagmus, and loss of sense of taste in the ipsilateral side of the tongue.

The complete evaluation of the child with a possible injury includes otoscopy with adequate magnification; audiologic evaluation including tests of air conduction, bone conduction, speech reception threshold and auditory discrimination; impedance audiometry; and plain mastoid x-rays and polytomograms of the temporal bone. Special tests such as those of facial nerve integrity, taste, and hearing, vestibular tests, and tests for possible spinal fluid leakage are not required unless such abnormalities are suggested by the functional evaluation of the patient.

Fractures of the external auditory canal are left alone. The ear is protected against water by suggesting that the meatus be plugged with lamb's wool or cotton impregnated with Vaseline when the child is being washed.

A hemotympanum is left alone since the blood will be cleaned spontaneously by the eustachian tube within one to two weeks. An attempt might be made to repair a fresh perforation of the tympanic membrane by taking the child to the operating room and under the microscope, laying out the torn flaps of the membrane onto a disc of dry compressed Gelfoam which has been introduced into the middle ear through the perforation. A perforation which fails to heal spontaneously should be protected against entry of dirt and water until a myringoplasty operation can be planned as an elective procedure. Antibiotics and ear drops are not required unless an infection manifested by otorrhea occurs.

The timing of surgical procedures to correct ossicular chain injuries depends on whether inner ear damage has occurred. If the child is found to have vertigo, ataxia, or nystagmus of aural origin then the operation must be performed as an emergency. The concern is that of trying to save the function of the inner ear which may be at risk because of a subluxation of the stapes footplate. If inner ear signs are not present then the repair of the ossicular chain is regarded as an elective operation and can be scheduled at any time in the future without penalty.

A facial paralysis which has its onset immediately after the injury is an indication that the nerve may be severed or that bone spicules have entered the nerve. In such an event an immediate exploratory operation is indicated. Depending upon the site of lesion tests, the operation may involve simply an exploration of the middle ear or may be a more extensive procedure such as a middle cranial fossa craniotomy or a mastoidectomy with facial nerve exploration.

A cerebrospinal fluid leak into the middle ear may be apparent or occult. It is easily diagnosed when clear fluid escapes through a perforated drumhead. It is occult when a tympanic membrane perforation does not exist and the fluid drains into the throat via the eustachian tube. In either case the problem calls for a surgical procedure as soon as the diagnosis has been made and the condition of the child permits surgery. The nature of the operation depends on the location of the communication between subarachnoid space and ear. The procedure may consist of a craniotomy with repair of the leak from the ear or it may involve an otologic operation to repair the leak from below.

Perilymphatic fistulae are suspected when a sensorineural or mixed hearing loss is accompanied by vertigo or ataxia. These leaks require a surgical repair via a tympanotomy under general anesthesia. The leak, which usually occurs through one of the middle ear windows, is sealed with autologous tissue such as ear lobe fat, tragal perichondrium, or temporalis fascia.

Hearing Loss in Children

B. PATRICK COX, Ph.D., *and*
KATHLEEN FOUST BLANE, M.S.

Hearing-impaired* children represent a small percentage of the pediatrician's overall caseload. However, since the pediatrician is

---

*The term hearing-impaired is used here to denote all degrees of hearing loss and is considered synonymous with hard-of-hearing and deaf.

often the primary medical caretaker, it is important for him or her to know about screening, diagnostic, habilitative and educational services appropriate for hearing-impaired youngsters. Indeed, the effectiveness of the audiologic-educational program is dependent on the pediatrician's advocacy on behalf of the hearing-impaired child.

Basic Information Obtained from Routine Hearing Assessment. All hearing test efforts aside from screening attempt to define the degree and type of hearing loss. The degree of hearing loss varies from no loss to a profound loss as determined by air conduction, speech awareness and speech reception threshold audiometry. Results of these measures are often categorized:

Hearing Level dB*	Interpretation
−10 to 20	normal hearing
25 to 45	mild hearing loss
50 to 65	moderate hearing loss
70 to 85	severe hearing loss
90 to 110	profound hearing loss

The type of hearing loss is routinely determined by the relationship of air conduction and bone conduction responses as well as impedance, particularly tympanometry, results. These measures may be categorized as to the expected results for conductive, sensorineural and mixed hearing loss (Table 1.)

Speech discrimination tests are also an important part of the basic battery. These tests indicate how well the child understands speech when it is presented loudly enough. Children with hearing loss or pathologies involving the auditory pathway may have reduced understanding.

Once the audiologist has determined the degree and type of hearing impairment from these routine measures, it may be necessary to perform more specialized procedures to further delineate the type of loss. Although it is beyond the scope of this presentation to elaborate on these procedures, it is important that the pediatrician be aware of such tests. These include Bekesy audiometry, tone decay tests, the Short Increment Sensitivity Index (SISI) test and a variety of altered speech tests. Generally stated these procedures help determine whether a hearing impairment is of cochlear or retrocochlear origin. Because these procedures require a more sophisticated behavior repertoire, they are not used frequently in very young or developmentally delayed children.

---

*Decibel references are A.N.S.I. 1969 standards referenced to audiometric zero.

They are, however, extremely valuable in children suspected of having retrocochlear lesions.

Hearing Screening Recommendations. The foregoing discussion centered on routine audiologic tests which the audiologist uses to define degree and type of hearing loss. However, it is not possible from a logistic or financial standpoint to expect these procedures to be available to all children. Consequently the audiologist is dependent on the pediatrician, school and other professional community members to be hearing advocates for all children. The role of these individuals in the total audiologic program is to provide appropriate hearing screening and referral. For organizational purposes, screening is divided into two categories—newborn-neonate and preschool-school age.

It is recommended that the newborn-neonate hearing screening program be based on three steps: use of a high risk register for hearing loss, parent questionnaire and screening by an audiologist in a sound-treated environment. High risk conditions for hearing loss include many factors but, as a minimum, should include: affected family member (particularly persons with onset before adulthood); bilirubin elevations greater than 20 mg./ml.; congenital maternal rubella or other intrauterine infections such as cytomegalovirus or toxoplasmosis; obvious defects of the ear, nose, throat or eyes; and low birth-weight (below 1500 gm., either premature or small for gestational age).

Parent questionnaires, including items related to auditory behavior and general development, should be given to parents of babies at high risk for hearing loss at regular well baby visits or in intensive care nursery follow-up programs. It is axiomatic in childhood deafness that parents are the first to notice a hearing loss in their child. Unfortunately, it is equally true that these same parents are oftentimes told by health professionals that "he'll grow out of it." The use of parents as hearing screeners is an underestimated resource.

Finally, babies who are at risk by history or parent report should be seen by an audiologist. The audiologist should screen the child's hearing in a sound-treated environment, making use of a combination of sound stimuli such as speech, music and pure tones. The child's abilty to demonstrate response to these stimuli shows a gradual decrement in dB level needed to elicit the response as the child grows older. The skilled audiologist takes this factor into account and thereby adjusts screening criteria. Babies referred to an audiologist should be re-screened at periodic intervals because some

TABLE 1.   Categorization of Results According to Type of Hearing Loss

TYPE OF LOSS	AIR CONDUCTION/ BONE CONDUCTION RELATIONSHIP	TYMPANOMETRY
Conductive	Bone conduction better than air conduction by at least 10 dB	Reduced pressure compliance Greatly increased pressure compliance with no peak value Marked negative middle ear pressure
Sensorineural	Air conduction and bone conduction responses similar	Normal pressure compliance curves
Mixed	At some frequencies there is better bone conduction than air conduction *or* at all frequencies bone conduction responses are better than air conduction responses, but are still not within normal limits	May show conductive-type responses

congenital hearing impairments become apparent only later in the first year of life.

Screening of preschool and school age children should be done routinely through grade three, with periodic rechecks no more than three years apart after that. Children in this category who are at particular risk include those who have frequent otitis media, upper respiratory infections and allergies, as well as those who show general developmental lag, have abrupt behavior changes, exhibit school problems, have protracted or major illnesses, or are teacher- or parent-referred.

The use of pure tone air conduction signals for screening for this age group is the stimuli of choice. The sole use of speech materials for screening is not recommended due to the real possibility of missing significant hearing losses. As speech is a broad-frequency signal, the child with near-normal hearing for even part of the frequency range may pass the screening and still have a major hearing loss for the important communication range.

It is recommended that the child be screened at the frequencies of 1000, 2000 and 4000 Hertz at levels of 20 dB hearing level for 1000 and 2000 Hertz and 25 dB hearing level for 4000 Hertz. If a child fails at any one frequency in either ear, he or she should be rescreened. If the child fails the screening again, referral to an audiologist for a complete assessment is indicated. The use of these recommended frequencies and screening levels assumes a relatively quiet, distraction-free test environment and use of well maintained, calibrated equipment.

Current Pediatric Audiologic Procedures.   In order to obtain reliable results from either hearing screening or diagnostic procedures, it is necessary to make use of the child's developmental strengths. Hence it is important to select a procedure which is within the child's present behavior repertoire. The responses necessitated by any of the procedures in use

today can be divided into those using reflexive behaviors and those using operant (learned) behaviors as shown in the following listing:

Operant (Learned) Procedures	Reflexive Procedures
	Moro
	Startle
	Localization
Behavior observation audiometry	Impedance audiometry
Visually reinforced audiometry	Evoked response audiometry
Play audiometry	Cochleography
Tangible reinforced operant conditioned audiometry (TROCA)	EKG audiometry
Routine audiometry	

In routine practice the majority of reflexive procedures are reserved for children who cannot be tested through more conventional means (that is, operant procedures). The single exception to this is impedance audiometry which is now a routine clinical procedure. Impedance audiometry comprises three subtests: tympanometry, static compliance and acoustic reflex testing. Typanometry attempts to measure the compliance of the middle ear system while undergoing pressure changes. Static compliance, the least used subtest, gives information concerning the compliance of the system based on a volume ratio between the middle ear in its poorest compliance state and in its most compliant state. Acoustic reflex testing measures the resultant compliance change when the stapedius muscle contracts, usually in the presence of a loud sound. All of these impedance measurements can be useful in determining the presence of middle ear pathology and, in many cases, differentiate within the middle ear structures. Impedance audiometry has been used in newborns and infants. It requires the ability to form a proper seal at the beginning of the external auditory canal and reasonable cooperation from the child.

Operant procedures comprise the bulk of the audiologist's tools for audiologic testing. In the newborn and during the first 2 to 3 months of age, the audiologist is dependent on more reflexive behaviors such as the Moro and startle responses. However, as early as 3 months of age the child begins to localize to sound. These localizations, if appropriately reinforced, can be used to test the youngster's hearing.

Behavior observation audiometry involves the presentation of sound stimuli of known intensity and frequency characteristics to the child while observing to see if the stimuli consistently elicit a response. This procedure is used for youngsters from birth and may also be used with older children. Frequently this involves calling the child's name, playing music, giving simple commands, and presenting environmental sounds or warbled pure tones (that is, single frequency sounds which are slightly varied in terms of frequency). Behavior observation audiometry can provide reliable data sufficient to screen out children with normal hearing and to identify the degree of hearing loss in hearing-impaired children. Its use assumes testing in a sound-treated environment with well calibrated equipment. Skill in observing behavioral changes to sound is a prerequisite for the audiologist who uses this procedure.

Visually reinforced audiometry builds on a child's localization abilities. Although there are equipment variations the basic procedure involves reinforcing a child's sound localizations with lighted toys of some kind. This procedure can be used with children as young as 7 to 8 months of age and yields reliable data concerning the degree of hearing loss and, with some children, may yield information concerning the type of loss.

Play audiometry, as the name implies, involves teaching the child to perform a specific motor act only in the presence of the test stimuli. Frequently used activities include putting pegs in a pegboard, rings on a peg, or dropping clothespins in a bottle. This technique is often attempted with children as young as 18 months and yields reliable information concerning the degree and type of hearing loss.

Tangible reinforced operant conditioned audiometry (TROCA) is a procedure in which the child is taught to push a button in the presence of the test stimuli. If his or her response is correct, the response is reinforced with a tangible reinforcer (such as cereal, candy, small building blocks). TROCA has been used with youngsters as young as 7 months, but is probably most used clinically from 24 months. This procedure yields reli-able data concerning the type and degree of loss.

Finally, routine audiometry involves teaching the child to raise his or her hand, push a button or give some other signal when the test stimulus is heard. Routine audiometry may be successful with children as young as 36 months.

MEDICAL AND NONMEDICAL HABILITATION

Medical. The conductive hearing loss, while elusive, often can be dealt with and corrected medically. The pediatrician is usually the first to encounter the young child with frequent episodes of serous otitis media. Naturally, if this is the child's first or second episode in the past year, the chances of existing serous hearing impairment are low. If, however, this is the third or fourth episode in the past 6 months, a referral for audiologic evaluation is indicated. At that point it would also seem appropriate to request consultation with an otolaryngologist to see if more aggressive medical treatment, such as surgery, is indicated. The pediatrician, otolaryngologist and audiologist can work well as a team, assuring thorough medical care as well as prophylactic treatment for the unnecessary handicap imposed by even a slight conductive hearing loss. This is especially pertinent, as educational programs are likely to follow the advice of a family pediatrician in the management of a child. Letters suggesting preferential classroom seating from the pediatrician, in conjunction with the audiologist and otolaryngologist, would reinforce the need for proper educational management.

The child with a sensorineural hearing loss, whose loss is not due primarily to active medical pathology, presents a unique case for the pediatrician. Often this child's middle ear problems are not seen as detrimental to hearing simply because the child already has significant hearing loss. However, the incidence of serous otitis media in children with sensorineural hearing loss is as high as it is in children with normal hearing. Even the slightest presence of middle ear effusion or significant negative middle ear pressure can mean the difference in hearing or not hearing minimal auditory cues which are so vital to the hearing-impaired child's communication development. The pediatrician is the first person to whom the parent will turn and should be prepared to make the appropriate referral as soon as possible in order to maintain the best hearing available for the hearing-impaired child.

Nonmedical. If medical or surgical intervention is not successful or indicated, the next alternative is to provide the hearing-impaired child with aural habilitation services which may include hearing aid selection and orientation, auditory training, speech reading and appropriate educational placement.

The comprehensive habilitation program must start with a thorough diagnostic assessment which includes a complete medical work-up (pediatric and otolaryngologic) as well as audiologic, psychologic, educational and sociologic evaluations. All of these areas are potential problem areas for the hearing-impaired child and will contribute to the success of the habilitative program. Following the complete work-up, an evaluation for the use of a hearing aid should occur.

HEARING AIDS. The hearing aid, in briefest terms, is a miniature device which amplifies sound. Hearing aids are available in many types and styles; those most commonly used by children include the body-worn and ear-level air conduction types. A child may use one hearing aid or binaural hearing aids. All hearing aids consist basically of a microphone which picks up sound (acoustic energy) and converts it into a weak, electrical signal; an amplifier, which makes the weak signal louder; and a receiver, which changes the enlarged electrical signal back to sound (acoustic energy) and presents this louder sound to the ear. The degree of success a child experiences with a hearing aid depends on factors such as the type and degree of hearing loss, age of onset of loss, age of discovery of loss, as well as factors such as educational placement, parental involvement, and the presence of other handicapping conditions (such as blindness, mental retardation, and so on).

Since the hearing aid mainly compensates for loss of loudness, a hearing loss which only causes attenuation of sound, that is, a conductive loss, will be optimally helped. On the other hand, a hearing loss involving loudness and distortion problems, as may occur in sensorineural hearing loss, may not be completely corrected with a hearing aid. This is not to imply that children with sensorineural hearing loss do not benefit from amplification. In fact, coupled with the appropriate comprehensive habilitation program, the hearing aid can be the major key to successful development of communication skills.

It is important to stress here that it is not appropriate to select at random any hearing aid, place it on a child, send him or her off to school and expect the optimal aided performance. Rather, the selection of a hearing aid should be carried out by an audiologist who is trained in audiology as well as in the com-

municative needs of the hearing-impaired. The audiologist can perform a number of tests, depending on the child's age and level of functioning. These tests can provide basic information regarding the child's auditory sensitivity, ability to discriminate speech, and the prognosis for successful hearing aid use. These tests can also provide direction for the habilitation program.

Purchase of the hearing aid may be problematic for the child's family. After the appropriate hearing aid has been identified by the audiologist, the parents may purchase the aid from a hearing aid dealer. For families unable to afford the cost of a hearing aid, assistance may be sought from community agencies such as the Easter Seal or hearing society programs in many communities, or from government-supported crippled children's programs located in most states. The hearing aid should be purchased on a trial basis (2 or 3 weeks) at first, particularly with infants, as it is difficult to know at that age if that particular hearing aid will be best suited for the child's needs. Part of a comprehensive program allows for the useful informal trial of the aid outside the clinic environment.

OTHER HABILITATIVE PROCEDURES. Once the child has been fitted with appropriate amplification, it may be necessary to provide additional habilitative support. Frequently the hearing-impaired child can benefit from: auditory training to help make optimal use of residual hearing; speech reading to help the child to learn to use visual cues in conjunction with auditory information; language stimulation to aid development of language and/or to maintain whatever language skills are already developed; and speech, aimed at developing intelligible speech for communication purposes. The decision to provide such services is dependent on the child's overall needs with particular reference to auditory strengths and weaknesses.

EDUCATIONAL NEEDS. The hearing-impaired child presents a unique problem to general education. Since most academic skills (such as reading, language or math) are learned through auditory and visual channels, sensory deficits in either channel cause major delays in the acquisition of these skills. Educational remediation must be aimed at maximizing the child's use of his strengths.

Although it is apparent that the pediatrician cannot assume the major role in deciding the best educational placement for the child or in the crucial follow-up to determine the child's growth, he or she can strengthen the educational component in several ways. It is helpful for the pediatrician to be aware of the various

TABLE 2.   Methods of Communication and Instruction Used in Programs for Hearing-Impaired Children

AUDITORY	AUDITORY AND VISUAL	VISUAL
Unisensory Use of residual hearing alone. Child is not encouraged to make use of any cues other than auditory ones during habilitation.	*Oral-Aural* Child is encouraged to use residual hearing, speech reading, natural gestures, and contextual cues in all communicative situations. *Cued Speech* In addition to aspects noted in the oral-aural system, child is taught with, and learns to use, 8 hand configurations which add more meaning to the visual configurations of speech reading. *Total Communication* In addition to aspects noted in the oral-aural system, child is taught with, and learns to use, hand signs and fingerspelling which reduce the ambiguity of speechreading and the distortion of listening through a distorted auditory system.	*Manual Communication* Child uses hand signs and fingerspelling without use of residual hearing and, oftentimes, without use of speech reading cues.

programs available for the hearing-impaired child within the community. The pediatrician should also be aware of the relationship between the degree of hearing loss and other auditory and nonauditory characteristics of the child which influence educational progress. In addition, the pediatrician, once informed about appropriate community facilities and programs, should exert influence on school programs on behalf of the hearing-impaired child. Finally the pediatrician can be invaluable in supporting and reinforcing the recommendations of the educational team to the parents.

Programs for the hearing-impaired, regardless of the community in which they exist, can generally be viewed along several continuums. Programs may be organized in terms of the services available to hearing-impaired youngsters with various degrees of integration with normal hearing children: class for normal hearing students (CNH), no special support; CNH with itinerant audiologic-education support; class of hearing impaired with only token interaction with normal hearing (physical education, etc.); class of hearing impaired, no integration. Programs may also be viewed in terms of whether they are day schools or residential programs: day class in school, hearing and speech clinic, hospital clinic, day student at residential program; residential program with weekends spent at home; residential program

with limited stay (holidays, summers) at home. Programs may also be examined according to the method of communication and instruction used (Table 2).

There are many factors which influence the decision of which educational placement is best suited to a given child. Among these are:

Degree of hearing loss
Configuration of hearing loss
Type of hearing loss
Discrimination abilities (does the child understand anything through hearing alone, aided or unaided?)
Age of onset
Progressive nature of hearing loss
Etiology of hearing loss
Family constellation (deaf parents or siblings?)
Use of amplification (performance with hearing aid when first used?)
Intelligence
Academic achievement
General health
Intactness of other sensory channels, particularly vision
Other handicapping conditions, particularly those involving the central nervous system
Speechreading abilities
Community facilities

It should be stressed that no one of these factors is predictive of educational success. Rather, it is important that all of these, as well as others, be considered as a composite when educational decisions are made.

18

Infectious Diseases

Neonatal Septicemia, Meningitis and Pneumonia

GEORGE A. McCRACKEN, JR., M.D.

The principal goals of therapy for neonatal septicemia and meningitis are early diagnosis and prompt institution of antimicrobial therapy. Because objective signs of infection in neonates are often lacking, therapy must be initiated before the diagnosis can be established and before the offending pathogen can be accurately identified. In most areas of the United States *Escherichia coli* and group B beta-hemolytic streptococci account for the majority of septicemia and meningitis during the newborn period. Pseudomonas species cause significant disease in some neonatal units; this is usually on the basis of nosocomial acquisition of the organism from contaminated fomites. Other bacteria which may cause neonatal diseases include *Listeria monocytogenes,* Klebsiella-Enterobacter species and rarely staphylococci, pneumococci, Salmonella and Proteus species. The physician must be aware of the historical and epidemiological experience of the institution in order to intelligently select chemotherapeutic agents. Initial antibiotic therapy is based on knowledge of the etiologic agents encountered in a nursery and on the antimicrobial susceptibilities of these pathogens.

NEONATAL SEPTICEMIA

Once septicemia is suspected, suitable cultures should be obtained and therapy started immediately using ampicillin and either kanamycin or gentamicin. Ampicillin is administered intravenously or intramuscularly in a dose of 50 mg./kg./day for infants under one week of age and 100 to 150 mg./kg./day for infants 1 to 4 weeks of age. Selection of the aminoglycosidic drug is based on the antibiotic susceptibilities of the enteric organisms isolated from infants in each institution.

Kanamycin is the drug of choice for the treatment of infections caused by susceptible gram-negative organisms and may be administered either intramuscularly or by a 20-minute intravenous infusion. The dosage schedule is based on birth weight and postnatal age. Infants with birthweights of 2000 gm. or less are treated with 7.5 mg./kg. doses given every 12 hours (15 mg./kg./day) during the first week of life and with 10 mg./kg. doses every 12 hours (20 mg./kg./day) thereafter. All larger birthweight babies are treated with 10 mg./kg. doses; infants less than 7 days of age should receive the dose every 12 hours (20 mg./kg./day), while those 1 to 4 weeks receive the dose every 8 hours (30 mg./kg./day).

This regimen results in serum concentrations of kanamycin which are consistently within the therapeutic range. Although the ototoxic potential of this revised dosage schedule has not been adequately assessed, the total dosage of kanamycin administered to most infants is less than the 500 mg./kg. amount which is considered ototoxic. The possible exception is the older and larger neonate with meningitis who is treated with 30 mg./kg./day for two to three weeks. The potential risk of adverse effects in such an infant is justified considering the poor prognosis associated with neonatal meningitis caused by gram-negative enteric organisms.

It should be noted that kanamycin-resistant *E. coli* have been encountered in some

531

nurseries in North America. In these nurseries, and when an isolate from an infant is shown to be resistant to kanamycin, gentamicin is used in a dosage of 2.5 mg./kg. every 12 hours for infants under 1 week of age, and 2.5 mg./kg. every 8 hours for infants 1 to 4 weeks of age. The drug may be given intramuscularly or by a 20-minute intravenous infusion. Extensive studies have shown gentamicin to be effective in the treatment of neonatal septicemia, and there has been no evidence of acute renal or hematologic toxicity when these dosages are used during the neonatal period. Significant ototoxicity has not been observed in infants followed for four years after treatment with either gentamicin or kanamycin in the first 4 weeks of life.

When type of skin lesion or historical experience suggests the possibility of Pseudomonas infection, combined therapy with carbenicillin and gentamicin is indicated. Carbenicillin is administered intravenously or intramuscularly in a dosage of 100 mg./kg. every 12 hours (200 mg./kg./day) during the first week of life. Thereafter, the 100 mg./kg. dose is given every 8 hours to low birth weight (≤ 2000 gm.) infants and every 6 hours to the larger babies. Experience has shown carbenicillin to be a safe drug when administered in this dosage for periods of 10 to 14 days. Carbenicillin may occasionally cause hypokalemic, hypochloremic metabolic alkalosis. When gentamicin is to be administered with carbenicillin, the drugs should not be mixed in the same solution prior to intravenous infusion.

Tobramycin (4 to 6 mg./kg./day) and amikacin (15 mg./kg./day) are effective against *Pseudomonas aeruginosa* and other coliforms, but should not be used unless the infant's pathogen is resistant to gentamicin and kanamycin. The long-term toxicity of tobramycin and amikacin has not been assessed. The polymyxins are not first line anti-Pseudomonas drugs. They should be used only when the above mentioned drugs are contraindicated.

When staphylococcal septicemia is suspected, parenteral methicillin is used as initial therapy because many of the staphylococci encountered in neonatal units are resistant to penicillin. The standard dosage of methicillin is 25 mg./kg./dose; only the frequency of administration is altered on the basis of the infant's birth weight and chronologic age. For low birth weight (≤ 2000 gm.) babies, this dose is given every 12 hours (50 mg./kg./day) for the first 2 weeks of life and every 8 hours (75 mg./kg./day) thereafter. For infants weighing greater than 2000 gm. at birth, the 25 mg./kg. dose is repeated every 8 hours during the first

two weeks and every 6 hours from 2 to 4 weeks of age. While kanamycin and gentamicin possess activity against most staphylococci, these drugs do not represent optimal therapy.

Once the pathogen has been identified and its antimicrobial susceptibilities defined, the most appropriate drug or combination of drugs should be selected. In general, kanamycin alone or combined with ampicillin is used for susceptible *E. coli* and Klebsiella-Enterobacter species, while gentamicin alone or combined with ampicillin is indicated for infections caused by kanamycin-resistant enteric organisms. Penicillin is preferred for therapy group B streptococcal infections. Carbenicillin and gentamicin are recommended for diseases caused by *Pseudomonas aeruginosa,* and ampicillin is the drug of choice for *Proteus mirabilis,* enterococcus and *L. monocytogenes.* Methicillin or one of the other penicillin congeners is used for penicillin-resistant staphylococcal disease.

Guidelines for determining duration of therapy in the neonatal period are often lacking because objective evidence of illness may be minimal. Culture of the blood should be repeated 24 to 48 hours after initiation of therapy. If positive, alteration of therapy may be necessary. In the absence of deep tissue involvement or abscess formation, treatment is usually continued 5 to 7 days after clinical improvement. When multiple organs are involved or clinical response is slow, it may be necessary to continue therapy for 2 to 3 weeks.

Supportive Therapy. The case-fatality rate in neonatal septicemia is 20 per cent to 50 per cent depending on the etiologic agent, underlying condition of the infant and the experience of hospital personnel in managing these infants. Improved outcome in many institutions is due to excellent intensive care nursing and attention to assisted ventilation and fluid and electrolyte balance which is essential during the first few days of therapy. The patient must be monitored constantly for evidence of shock, spread of infection or development of adverse reactions to therapy. The value of whole blood or fresh frozen plasma transfusions in neonatal bacterial infections is unknown.

NEONATAL MENINGITIS

Meningitis is caused by the same bacterial pathogens as encountered in septicemia. *E. coli* and group B streptococci account for approximately 70 per cent of all cases of neonatal meningitis. Early diagnosis may be hampered by confusion regarding interpretation of the cerebrospinal fluid examination. Although there is overlap between the findings in normal infants and in those with meningitis, less than 1 per cent of neonates with proved meningitis have completely normal cerebrospinal fluid values on initial examination. Further, the use of counterimmunoelectrophoresis for detection of bacterial antigen and of the limulus lysate assay for measurement of endotoxin in cerebrospinal fluid has provided a rapid, specific and sensitive means of differentiating bacterial from nonbacterial disease.

Systemic antibiotic therapy for meningitis is similar to that described for neonatal septicemia. The main differences are the dosages of the penicillins and the duration of therapy. The dosages of penicillin (100,000 to 250,000 units/kg.) and ampicillin (100 to 200 mg./kg.) are approximately twice those used for septicemia. As a general rule, therapy is continued for at least two weeks after sterilization of cerebrospinal fluid is documented. We recommend a minimum of two weeks for meningitis caused by gram-positive organisms and three weeks for disease caused by gram-negative enteric bacteria.

A major dilemma in treatment of neonatal meningitis is delivery of adequate antimicrobial activity to the site of infection within the central nervous system. The concentrations of penicillin and ampicillin in cerebrospinal fluid are 10- to 50-fold greater than the minimal inhibitory concentrations (MIC) of these drugs for group B streptococci and *Listeria monocytogenes*. As a result, spinal fluid cultures are usually sterile within 24 hours of initiation of therapy in most infants. By contrast, the concentrations of the aminoglycosidic drugs in cerebrospinal fluid usually approximate the MIC values for the gram-negative pathogens, and cultures remain positive for an average of 3.3 days after start of therapy.

The Neonatal Meningitis Cooperative Study Group was created to evaluate intrathecal gentamicin therapy in newborn and young infants with gram-negative meningitis. Patients received on a random basis either systemic therapy alone or systemic therapy plus 1 mg. of gentamicin administered daily into the lumbar intrathecal space for a minimum of 3 days.* The case-fatality rate was approximately 30 per cent and the quality of survival was almost identical for both treatment groups. Approximately 65 per cent of survivors were normal at 2 to 5 years after disease.

The most likely explanation for why intrathecal therapy did not improve survivorship in neonatal meningitis is that the drug which is instilled into the lumbar space does not diffuse away from the area and certainly does not reach the ventricles. Because ventriculitis is diagnosed frequently in babies with persistently positive lumbar cerebrospinal fluid cultures, a more direct approach to this site of infection appears indicated. The Neonatal Meningitis Cooperative Study Group is currently assessing intraventricular therapy in neonatal gram-negative meningitis. Until this study is complete, we recommend that systemic therapy with ampicillin and gentamicin be started in all infants with suspected or proved bacterial meningitis. If the lumbar spinal fluid contains gram-negative rods after 24 to 36 hours of therapy, a ventricular tap by a neurosurgeon should be performed. If ventriculitis (> 50 white blood cells/cu. mm. and/or bacteria are demonstrated on stained smears or culture) is diagnosed, 2 to 2.5 mg. of gentamicin is instilled into the ventricles daily for a minimum of 3 days or until cultures are sterile.

The safest method of administering antibiotics into the ventricles is unknown. Some neurosurgeons favor repeated needling, whereas others prefer placement of a reservoir. Preliminary data from the Cooperative Study indicate that gentamicin delivered directly into the ventricles diffuses rapidly and evenly throughout the cerebrospinal fluid space. Concentrations of gentamicin as high as 30 to 60 μg./ml. (approximately 10- to 50-fold greater than MIC values of most gram-negative pathogens) are observed in the lumbar spinal fluid several hours after intraventricular administration. Although we have not encountered any untoward effects to date, all patients treated with intraventricular antibiotics must be followed closely for evidence of toxicity.

Attention to general supportive therapy is of utmost importance in caring for infants with meningitis. Disturbances of fluid and electrolyte balance are common, particularly in the first several days of illness when inappropriate antidiuretic hormone secretion may lead to fluid retention and hyponatremia. Ventilatory assistance may be necessary.

Convulsions frequently occur with meningitis and are treated by the use of intravenous diazepam (Valium),* up to 10 mg. administered slowly, or with phenobarbital sodium, 4 mg./kg. given intramuscularly. If phenobarbital does not achieve the desired effect, an additional 2 mg./kg. can be injected every 45

---

*The intrathecal use of gentamicin is not mentioned in the manufacturer's instructions.

*Manufacturer's precaution: The safety and efficacy of injectable diazepam in the neonate have not been established.

minutes until the convulsions have ceased or a total of 12 mg./kg. has been administered. If convulsions are not controlled within an hour or two after the start of sedation, phenytoin (Dilantin) in a dosage of 5 to 7 mg./kg./day may be employed, and given in a single dose intravenously or intramuscularly.

NEONATAL PNEUMONIA

Congenital and Intrapartum Pneumonia. Pneumonias acquired at or before delivery usually become clinically apparent during the first two weeks of life, although some may be delayed in onset until 6 to 8 weeks. These infections are usually caused by the same organisms which colonize the maternal genitourinary or gastrointestinal tracts. Group B streptococci and *E. coli* are the most frequent bacterial pathogens, whereas cytomegalovirus leads the list of possible viral agents which cause congenital pneumonia. Chlamydia have been incriminated recently as a cause of interstitial pneumonia associated with eosinophilia in infants 1 to 3 months of age.

Cultures for bacteria and viruses should be obtained from the nasopharynx of the infant and the genitourinary tract of the mother. Material for isolation of chlamydia must be cultured on McCoy cells; this is not available in most hospitals. In addition a blood culture from the infant is taken prior to initiating antimicrobial therapy. A pencillin and an aminoglycosidic drug are usually started in a dosage appropriate for therapy of septicemia. If the cultures are sterile and the clinical course of illness indicates a noninfectious etiology of the pneumonic process, antibiotics are stopped. The role of antibiotics in chlamydial interstitial pneumonia of infancy has not been defined. It should be emphasized that aspiration pneumonia, pulmonary hemorrhage and atelectasis may be indistinguishable clinically from bacterial pneumonia. The former conditions do not require antimicrobial therapy.

Pneumonias During the Later Neonatal Period. Pneumonias acquired after the first week of life may be caused by bacterial or viral agents. The most common bacteria encountered are *S. pneumoniae,* group B streptococcus, and *Staphylococcus aureus,* whereas *Hemophilus influenzae, Klebsiella pneumoniae* and *Pseudomonas aeruginosa* are seen less frequently. The physician should make every effort to establish the etiology because therapy and prognosis are different for each condition. Culture of blood and of material obtained on tracheal aspiration (when indicated) should be obtained. If pleural fluid is present, this should be examined for bacteria and white blood cells and cultured. A percutaneous lung puncture is indicated in a neonate with progressive pneumonia who has failed to respond clinically to conventional antimicrobial therapy.

When staphylococcal pneumonia is suspected on the basis of epidemiological, roentgenographic or bacteriologic findings, an antistaphylococcal penicillin such as methicillin is used as initial therapy. The dosage is identical to that used for septicemia. If the organism is shown to be susceptible to penicillin, this drug is employed for the balance of therapy. Pleural empyema must be drained by the largest caliber tube or tubes and these are kept in place for approximately 5 to 7 days. The identification of a single infant with staphylococcal disease should prompt an epidemiologic investigation of the nursery in which the infant may have acquired the organism.

Pneumonias caused by *D. pneumoniae* or group B streptococci are best treated with 25,000 units/kg. of penicillin given every 6 to 8 hours depending on birthweight and postnatal age. Coliform pneumonias are treated with either kanamycin or gentamicin depending on the susceptibilities of these organisms in the particular institution. Disease caused by *Pseudomonas aeruginosa* is frequently nosocomial in origin and occurs in neonates who require prolonged intubation for assisted ventilation or other invasive procedures. A combination of carbenicillin and gentamicin is preferred for therapy of Pseudomonas pneumonia.

The duration of antibiotic therapy is tailored to the cause and extent of disease in each infant. In general, pneumonia due to *S. aureus,* coliforms and Pseudomonas species should be treated for 3 weeks or longer, whereas those due to streptococci require 10 to 14 days of therapy.

Supportive Therapy. If fluid or air accumulates in the chest, even in relatively small amounts, either open or closed drainage should usually be employed. Since pyopneumothorax as well as tension pneumothorax occurs relatively commonly, these patients are closely observed for manifestations of these events. It is usually not necessary to leave the tubes in the chest for more than 7 days.

Infants with pneumonia should receive oxygen for respiratory distress and for cyanosis. An incubator is used to maintain body temperature. Because of respiratory distress, oral feedings should be discontinued until the infant can tolerate them and replaced with intravenous administration of suitable parenteral fluids. Adequate pulmonary toilet is an important adjunct to therapy. The injection of antibiotics into the pleural cavity, or the use of enzymes to "dissolve" pus is not recommended in infants because they are ineffective and side effects are on occasion quite severe.

Bacterial Meningitis and Septicemia Beyond the Neonatal Period

RALPH D. FEIGIN, M.D.

MENINGITIS

Bacterial meningitis remains a significant problem in the antibiotic era. Although the number of reported fatalities from infectious diseases decreased by 10- to 200-fold between 1935 and 1968, the number of deaths due to bacterial meningitis were only halved during this period of time. Although any bacterial organism may produce meningitis in a susceptible host, *Hemophilus influenzae*, type b, *Streptococcus pneumoniae* and *Neisseria meningitidis* are the microorganisms which are responsible in approximately 95 per cent of children who are over two months of age. *Hemophilus influenzae*, type b accounts for more than 60 per cent of all cases.

The diagnosis of bacterial meningitis is dependent upon careful examination of cerebrospinal fluid (CSF) obtained by lumbar puncture. If a lumbar puncture has been performed because of the suspicion of meningitis, the CSF specimens always should be cultured even when the fluid appears to be crystal clear and acellular or nearly so. Blood, CSF, and urine may be evaluated for the presence of *H. influenzae*, type b, *Streptococcus pneumoniae*, and *Neisseria meningitidis*. The results obtained are not dependent upon the presence of viable organisms. Thus it is a particularly important diagnostic aid in the patient who has received antibiotic therapy prior to the initial lumbar puncture.

The appearance throughout the United States of strains of *Hemophilus influenzae*, type b which are resistant to ampicillin has necessitated a change in the initial antibiotic therapy given to children with bacterial meningitis. Ampicillin may be used in areas where resistant strains have not emerged, but this option can be exercised with decreasing frequency, for strains of *H. influenzae* resistant to ampicillin have been reported from an ever increasing number of geographic areas.

Generally, treatment should be initiated with ampicillin and chloramphenicol. Ampicillin is administered intravenously in a dosage of 200 to 300 mg./kg./day in six divided doses.* Chloramphenicol sodium succinate is administered intravenously in a dose of 100 mg./kg./24 hours in four divided doses. If *N. meningitidis*, *S. pneumoniae*, or *H. influenzae* sensitive to ampicillin are identified, chloramphenicol can be discontinued. Conversely, if an ampicillin-resistant strain of *H. influenzae* is identified, ampicillin is discontinued.

Still another option is the initiation of treatment with chloramphenicol as above and aqueous penicillin G administered intravenously in a dosage of 250,000 to 300,000 units/kg./24 hours in six divided doses. If an *H. influenzae* is recovered, chloramphenicol treatment is continued, whereas penicillin alone is continued if *S. pneumoniae* or *N. meningitidis* are identified as the causative agents.

Strains of *H. influenzae*, type b which are identified as resistant to ampicillin by a standardized disc susceptibility method should be reassessed utilizing tube dilution sensitivity tests. Specific colorimetric assays are presently available which permit the identification of beta-lactamase production (indicates resistance to ampicillin) within 1 to 15 minutes. These methods all should be employed in the evaluation of *H. influenzae*, and strains which are resistant to greater than 1.5 μg./ml. of ampicillin and/or which produce beta-lactamase should be sent to the Center for Disease Control for confirmation and additional study.

If a history of significant allergy to penicillin is documented (anaphylaxis, urticaria, exfoliation, dermatitis), chloramphenicol may be used as a single drug for suspected or proven bacterial meningitis.

An appropriate antibiotic should be continued until the patient is afebrile for 5 days but for at least 7 to 10 days in all cases. If clinical improvement ensues within 24 hours, a repeat lumbar puncture is not necessary during the course of treatment. When clinical improvement is not noted, or is slower than anticipated, a repeat examination of CSF is indicated at any time. In some medical centers, a lumbar puncture is performed 48 hours after treatment is discontinued. This practice was instituted in an attempt to discern at an early date the possibility of relapse following treatment of *H. influenzae* meningitis with ampicillin. We favor this approach since it permits the physician to document bacteriologic sterility

---

*This dosage of ampicillin is higher than that recommended by the manufacturer but it is both safe and effective.

following the conclusion of treatment. It should be noted that at the conclusion of therapy, white blood cell counts within CSF and CSF protein concentration generally have not returned completely to normal and the CSF:blood glucose ratio may remain depressed. In every case, CSF Gram stain, CSF-CIE and CSF cultures should be sterile; retreatment is mandatory if they are not and also may be suggested if more than 10 per cent of the cells are polymorphonuclear leukocytes or if the CSF glucose or the CSF:blood glucose ratio was less than 20 mg./100 ml. or 20 per cent respectively.

Supportive Care. The blood pressure, pulse rate, and respiratory rates of all children with suspected or proven bacterial meningitis should be monitored closely. Generally, vital signs can be measured every 15 minutes until stable and then every hour for the first several days. Temperature should be measured rectally every four hours.

A complete neurologic evaluation should be performed at the time of admission and daily thereafter. A rapid neurologic evaluation to include assessment of cortical findings, pupillary response to light, extraocular motility, the symmetry of movement and deep tendon reflexes should be performed 6 to 12 times a day during the first several days of treatment.

Generally the patient should receive nothing by mouth since vomiting may ensue and aspiration is best avoided. Of equal importance, careful measurement of intake and output can be achieved more readily in the child who is receiving fluids intravenously.

Every child with meningitis should be evaluated carefully and studied in a manner that will permit identification of patients with inappropriate secretion of antidiuretic hormone (ADH), recognition of seizure activity and the development of subdural effusions. In an attempt to monitor the presence and severity of inappropriate secretion of ADH, body weight, serum electrolytes, and serum and urine osmolalities should be measured at the time of admission. These studies may be repeated several times during the first 24 to 36 hours in hospital and daily for several days thereafter. Urine should be obtained sequentially and careful measurements made of volume and specific gravity. Inappropriate secretion of ADH in children with bacterial meningitis is more the rule than the exception and is countered best by fluid restriction. A multiple electrolyte solution containing approximately 40 mEq./liter of sodium and chloride, 35 mEq./liter of potassium and 20 mEq./liter of acetate or lactate should be administered at a rate of 800 to 1000 ml./m²/day. Fluid restriction is continued until it can be documented on the basis of the measurements detailed above that the ADH effect is not a factor or has dissipated. The best indication of fluid retention in excess of solute is the body weight and serum sodium. As serum sodium increases toward normal (140 mEq./liter), fluid administration may be liberalized progressively to normal maintenance levels of 1500 to 1700 ml./m²/day.

Head circumference should be measured and the head should be transilluminated at the time of admission and daily thereafter. These simple techniques permit assessment of the development of subdural effusions or may suggest other causes for an enlarging head. It was documented over a decade ago that transillumination is as useful in the evaluation of subdural effusions as is the presence of seizure activity, full fontanelle, fever, irritability, vomiting, or even isotope scans. Recent experience has documented that transillumination is a more reliable indicator of the presence of a small subdural effusion than is computerized axial tomography.

The treatment of subdural effusions has been a source of considerable debate. Recent studies suggest that treatment should consist of subdural paracentesis only to curtail specific symptoms of increased intracranial pressure or when one suspects that the effusions may be responsible for seizure activity or the presence of focal neurologic signs. In most cases, no subdural taps are required. In those patients subjected to subdural paracentesis, repetitive taps are rarely indicated. In over 1000 patients followed in this manner, persistent subdural effusions (beyond three months) were not found. When vigorously sought, the frequency of subdural effusions in young children with bacterial meningitis is such that it can be viewed as part of the general disease process rather than as a persistent or troublesome complication of the meningeal infection.

Seizures may be reported prior to hospitalization or noted during the first several days of treatment in approximately 30 per cent of children with bacterial meningitis. When seizures are noted, a patent airway must be maintained and appropriate anticonvulsants administered. Sodium phenobarbital, 7 mg./kg. as an initial dose, may be administered parenterally. Seizure control may be sustained with phenytoin, 5 mg./kg./day, provided in two divided doses intramuscularly. Phenytoin generally does not depress the respiratory center to the same extent as phenobarbital; it also may benefit the host by inhibiting the secretion of ADH. Shock and/or disseminated intravascular coagulation may complicate meningitis. When this occurs, additional supportive measures are indicated (see Meningococcal Disease).

Total evaluation of the child with meningitis must include detailed neurologic, psychometric and audiometric evaluation following discharge from the hospital to permit the institution of corrective measures, where possible, as early as possible.

SEPTICEMIA

Septicemia beyond the neonatal period may be caused by any microorganism. In general, a careful history and physical examination will provide clues to a bacteriologic diagnosis. In the infant, the neonatal history may suggest specific infection with Streptococcus agalactiae, (Group B, beta-hemolytic streptococci), Staphylococcus aureus, Pseudomonas or other enteric pathogens. Sepsis in patients with impetiginous lesions or a history of recent surgery may be due to S. aureus or Streptococcus pyogenes. Fever of greater than 103° F. without focal findings in a child between 7 and 21 months of age whose white blood cell count is more than 15,000 per cu. mm. suggests septicemia due to Streptococcus pneumoniae or, less frequently, H. influenzae. Infection with S. pneumoniae is even more likely in patients who have been splenectomized. Infection with S. pneumoniae or Salmonella is more frequent in children with sickle cell disease or other hemoglobinopathies than in the normal population.

Whenever septicemia is suspected, two or three sets of blood cultures should be obtained over a period of several hours and antibiotic treatment should be initiated. A careful search should be made for the focus of infection. When, following a careful physical examination, no source is discernible, a chest radiograph should be obtained and cultures of urine and CSF (if indicated) should be performed.

Until bacteriologic diagnosis is established, ampicillin, 200 mg./kg./day in four divided doses; gentamicin, 5 to 7.5 mg./kg./day in three divided doses; or kanamycin, 20 to 30 mg./kg./day in two or three divided doses, should be provided intramuscularly or intravenously to cover enteric microorganisms.* Alternatively, penicillin G, 100,000 to 200,000 ml./kg./day intravenously in six divided doses, and chloramphenicol sodium succinate, 100 mg./kg./day intravenously in four divided doses, may be utilized.

Shock and bleeding are common concomitants of septicemia, particularly when gram-negative organisms are recovered. In these patients, gentamicin or kanamycin should be given intravenously and administered over a period of 30 minutes to 1 hour. If renal failure ensues, the usual dose of the aminoglycoside may be given on the first day but subsequently dosage must be altered. Subsequent adjustments are managed best by measuring the concentration of aminoglycoside in blood specifically. When this cannot be done, and when renal failure is moderate, subsequent doses of aminoglycosides can be repeated every two or three days. In severe renal failure, one half of the usual dose is given every three or four days.

When the cause of septicemia is due to Streptococcus pneumoniae, Streptococcus pyogenes, Streptococcus agalactiae, Neisseria gonorrhoeae, Neisseria meningitidis or a penicillin-susceptible S. aureus, penicillin (as above) may be utilized alone. Hemophilus influenzae septicemia may be treated with ampicillin (as for meningitis) if the organism proves susceptible or with chloramphenicol. The treatment of Salmonella septicemia must be guided by the sensitivity of the microorganism. In general, ampicillin or chloramphenicol may be utilized; chloramphenicol is preferred if Salmonella typhosa is identified.

Penicillin-resistant staphylococcal infection should be treated with methicillin administered intravenously in a dosage of 200 mg./kg./day in four divided doses.* Oxacillin and nafcillin, 200 mg./kg./day in four divided doses intravenously, are acceptable alternatives. A cephalosporin or clindamycin will provide effective coverage for patients who are sensitive to penicillin. Of the cephalosporins, peak blood levels following cefazolin generally are higher than with other derivatives. This drug can be provided in a dose of 50 mg./kg./day in four divided doses intravenously. Clindamycin can be administered in a dose of 30 mg./kg./day in three divided doses intramuscularly or intravenously.

When Pseudomonas is identified, carbenicillin, 400 to 600 mg./kg./day in four divided doses intravenously, should be used alone or preferably (in my opinion) in combination with gentamicin. The polymyxins are less suitable alternatives. Ticarcillin, an antibiotic recently approved for use, may be used in place of carbenicillin in a dose of 200 mg./kg./day in four divided dosages intravenously.

---

*This dosage of kanamycin is higher than that recommended by the manufacturer.

*Manufacturer's note: The number of instances in which methicillin was administered intravenously to infants and children is not large enough to permit specific dosage recommendations.

When septicemia is accompanied by shock or by disseminated intravascular coagulation, supportive care is indicated (see Meningococcal Disease).

Bacterial Endocarditis

CATHERINE A. NEILL, M.D.

The basic principle of therapy in endocarditis is to establish bactericidal levels of the appropriate antibiotic(s) and to maintain them long enough so that the blood is sterilized and the infecting organism destroyed.

This is a serious, debilitating, tedious, expensive and potentially lethal disease, and the difficulties in treating it show some analogies to the problems of guerrilla warfare-identification of the enemy (clinical and bacterial diagnosis), defense mechanisms (drug resistance) and the limits of human tolerance (a sterile blood stream but a dead patient).

The question of *diagnosis* is of such vital import that it cannot be ignored in an article specifically devoted to therapy. Clinical diagnosis depends on a high index of suspicion in susceptible patients and on proper awareness of the protean manifestations of the disease.

Susceptible subjects include all those with congenital or rheumatic heart disease. There is some evidence that the incidence is higher in cyanotic than in acyanotic patients and in those with functioning systemic pulmonary shunts than in others. An occasional case does occur in children without a known preceding cardiac murmur or other evidence of underlying heart disease. There is some discussion as to whether these children have a bicuspid aortic valve which has not given rise to any murmurs. The age distribution is helpful, this condition being rare in children under 5 years of age.

Predisposing factors include dental or other oropharyngeal or genitourinary manipulations without antibiotic coverage, and occasionally oropharyngeal trauma; careful history taking and examination reveals such predisposing factors in 60 to 70 per cent of cases. A recent major predisposing factor is cardiac surgery, particularly open heart.

The classic *clinical syndrome* of fever, anemia, petechiae and splenomegaly is well known. However, atypical modes of presentation are frequent, including chest pain and pulmonary infiltrates, which may simulate pneumonia. This type of presentation is especially frequent in patients with pulmonary stenosis or functioning systemic pulmonary anastomoses. The disease may also be ushered in with symptoms of meningoencephalitis, and occasionally malaise and weight loss without other signs or symptoms apart from low-grade fever may be the chief complaint. Particularly difficult though rare modes of presentation are cardiac failure with nephrotic-like syndrome and a severe macrocytic anemia.

Iatrogenic modification of the clinical syndrome is unfortunately not infrequent. Such a patient might receive, for example, at the onset of a fever a week's penicillin followed by defervescence; then recurrence and a week of chloramphenicol (defervescence, recurrence); then a week of a new antibiotic (defervescence, recurrence). After 6 to 8 weeks of this the patient may present with severe anemia, malaise and fever, and often significant weight loss. Splenomegaly is often slight and petechiae are absent. In addition to the modification of the clinical syndrome by this period of delay, the infecting organism has also been altered to an atypical form which grows out of the blood very slowly and requires a long period for exact identification.

"Changing cardiac murmurs," although repeatedly emphasized, can be characterized as a legendary rather than a useful sign. In pediatric practice a new cardiac murmur means that the patient either has mitral insufficiency from gross anemia or has developed aortic insufficiency due to the valve perforation; almost certainly therapy should have been started several weeks before. In other words, to wait for changing cardiac murmurs is to wait too long. Petechiae are a special problem in cyanotic patients. A few small, frail cyanotic children get recurrent showers of petechiae on the extremities, rarely on the trunk, apparently due to some disorder of capillary fragility. So far, despite multiple venipunctures and many unhappy investigatory hours, we have not yet seen a young blue child presenting with large showers of petechiae who proved to have endocarditis.

In the postoperative patient, following cardiac surgery, differentiation of bacterial endocarditis from postpericardiotomy syndrome and postperfusion syndrome may present real difficulties. The presence of friction rubs and effusions in the former, and of leukopenia and atypical lymphocytes in the latter are frequently useful clues. Particular difficulty is now being encountered by internists in diagnosing *S. albus* endocarditis on prosthetic valves; as this type of surgery is done more frequently in the young, pediatricians will also encounter it. The only apparent symptoms are low-grade fever and general malaise appearing several months after surgery.

Bacterial diagnosis depends on adequate

blood cultures and a highly competent laboratory. We have had transferred to us several patients with "negative cultures" whose first five or six consecutive cultures all grew out within 48 to 72 hours in our laboratory, and now believe that the clinician attempting to make the diagnosis must be fully and justifiably confident in the skill of the laboratory he is using. The proper laboratory techniques cannot concern us here, except to say that cultures should be both aerobic and anaerobic, and kept for three weeks and then examined with a Gram stain before discarding. The clinician's role is to supply an adequate number of cultures (6 to 10) drawn over a period of 24 to 72 hours, each containing at least 1 ml. of blood for each 10 ml. of culture medium. The culture should of course be drawn with full aseptic precautions, and penicillinase should be added if the patient has recently had either penicillin or one of its analogues. Cultures of arterial blood are thought now by most authorities not to have any particular value, but bone marrow cultures have been useful in a few children who have received antibiotics. The time of day and the degree of fever at the time the cultures are drawn are now thought to be unimportant.

MANAGEMENT

Our present policy is to suspect the diagnosis in any patient with heart disease in whom fever persists for more than 3 to 5 days without an obvious and adequate local cause. Antibiotics are withheld, blood cultures are drawn, and temperature is taken and charted every 4 hours. Persistent fever for 5 to 7 days necessitates hospitalization. The younger the child, the more vital it is that a skilled pediatric house staff be available in the institution.

Following admission and the drawing of an adequate number of blood cultures, a number of decisions must be made. These include when to start therapy, the antibiotic(s) to employ, the use of other medications, the management of complications, the duration of therapy and the role of surgery. Close cooperation with a specialist in infectious disease is helpful at the beginning and throughout the course.

Starting therapy is a major decision and should, except under the very rarest circumstances, be considered an irrevocable one. In other words one should not start intravenous therapy "for a week, until we see how the blood cultures come out." In a patient who is not acutely ill and who has not received prior antibiotics, it is entirely justifiable to withhold therapy for a few days, watching the course of the fever, checking carefully several times daily for petechiae and splinter hemorrhages and awaiting the results of blood cultures, which may be positive after 72 hours. If at the end of that time the majority of the cultures taken in the first 24 hours are positive for the same organism, therapy may be confidently started.

If, after five to seven days of waiting, the clinical picture is clearly that of endocarditis and the cultures remain sterile, a decision may be made to start therapy. It is helpful at this time to make a detailed written note of the exact clinical status and the reasons for starting on this long, somewhat difficult and potentially hazardous course without bacterial diagnosis.

In a few patients therapy may be started within 24 hours of admission, immediately after six or eight blood cultures have been drawn. Indications to do this include (1) a classic clinical picture; (2) a gravely ill patient with enough clinical features to render the diagnosis probable; (3) a probable clinical diagnosis, plus evidence of aortic valve involvement or cerebral or pulmonary embolization; and (4) a prolonged preceding illness of two to three months treated with a multiple short course of antibiotics—under such circumstances the infecting organism, even with very skilled laboratory techniques, may not grow for two to three weeks and may need another week of subculture for complete identification.

Contraindications to starting therapy for endocarditis include the presence of an obvious localized focus of infection (such as pneumonia, tonsillitis), which should be treated appropriately, even though in some cases blood cultures may be drawn. "Positive" blood cultures, particularly with an organism likely to be a contaminant, in a child who is now afebrile should usually not be treated.

Antibiotic Therapy. In all series the clinical course and management have been simpler and more satisfactory if the infecting organism is a penicillin-sensitive *Streptococcus viridans* (alpha strep), as it is in about 60 per cent of all cases, than if cultures reveal another organism or if no organism can be grown. The clinician can have a better and more logical understanding of available therapy if he cooperates with a group specializing in infective disease. He should be prepared for new approaches in the atypical and hazardous types of endocarditis, but in the author's opinion he should not experiment with "short cuts" or new drugs in *S. viridans* infection or in other situations in which ample experience has demonstrated a highly effective mode of therapy.

S. viridans is usually highly sensitive to

penicillin, and intravenous therapy with 10 million units of penicillin G daily is used, usually without any additional antibiotic, for a minimum of 3 weeks. After 3 weeks the decision may be made to use intramuscular or oral therapy in similar doses, and this should be maintained for at least another week. Because intramuscular therapy in such high doses can be painful, we prefer not to use it in children if the veins are still available.

Other organisms include the staphylococcus, the most frequent cause of endocarditis following cardiac surgery, the enterococcus and the penumococcus. Gram-negative infections are rare but highly refractory to treatment, and fungal infections are usually, though not always, preterminal, occurring during therapy for bacterial endocarditis.

Predisposing factors may lead one to the clinical suspicion that the infection is caused by a specific organism. For example, *S. viridans* is the usual infecting organism following oropharyngeal manipulations, although the enterococcus and other relatively penicillin-insensitive streptococci may occur. Staphylococcal infections, in addition to being suspected following cardiac surgery, are also said to be the most frequent cause of endocarditis in young males without known preexisting heart disease. Gram-negative infections may follow genitourinary illness or surgical manipulation. Drug addicts characteristically develop staphylococcal or fungal endocarditis on right-sided cardiac valves. Pneumococcal endocarditis may occasionally complicate pneumococcal meningitis or pneumonia. The fact that a patient has been on preceding antirheumatic prophylaxis does not protect him from endocarditis nor does it mean that the organism is necessarily penicillin resistant.

CHOICE OF ANTIBIOTIC.   The sensitivity of the organism must be determined. If it is highly sensitive to penicillin, a treatment schedule similar to that for *S. viridans* may be employed, although it is usual to add streptomycin intramuscularly for at least the first 2 weeks (Table 1). For enterococci, ampicillin and streptomycin are given in combination for two to four weeks, and then, depending on progress, either ampicillin is given alone or the synergistic combination is continued. Staphylococci should always be regarded as insensitive to penicillin until proved otherwise, and initial treatment should be started with large doses of a penicillinase-resistant penicillin such as methicillin or oxacillin.

NEGATIVE BLOOD CULTURES.   It is usual in this situation to assume that the organism is atypical or relatively insensitive to penicillin and two antibiotics are used. Penicillin, 20 million units intravenously daily, is given together with intramuscular streptomycin for a minimum of 2 weeks, the therapy being changed if the cultures later become positive and indicate the use of another combination of antibiotics. In a case following cardiac surgery the high probability of a penicillin-resistant staphylococcal infection causes one to use a penicillinase-resistant penicillin as the initial treatment.

Depending on the organism and its sensitivity and on the patient's progress, other antibiotics may be used. Consultation with an infectious disease specialist is highly desirable at an early stage.

Other Medical Therapy.   The child is put on bed rest, usually with bathroom privileges, for the first week. If no embolization has occurred, he may be ambulated gradually, provided that good control of the intravenous management is being maintained.

Anticoagulant therapy is now rarely if ever used; it would only be considered if major pulmonary emboli continued to appear after institution of therapy. *Antipyretic drugs* should be avoided unless shaking chills and fever above 103° F. are causing great discomfort and do not respond to tepid sponging; in such cases aspirin or Tylenol in the usual pediatric doses may be used. *Sedatives and analgesics* should be used sparingly, because every effort is necessary to avoid complicating drug fevers. Nevertheless, occasionally a nocturnal sedative is indicated during the first week to ensure a good night's sleep, and a tranquilizer or sedative may be desirable in the young or very apprehensive patient prior to changing the site of the intravenous needle. Darvon* or morphine sulfate is very rarely necessary for pain in pulmonary emboli; if it is necessary, however, such therapy should be discontinued at the earliest possible time for obvious reasons.

Oxygen is used only if respiratory distress or severe congestive failure is present. *Anticongestive measures,* including digitalis, diuretics and a low salt diet, may be necessary if there is evidence of congestive failure.

Fluid and electrolyte intake should be carefully monitored, particularly to avoid massive overloading with sodium or potassium ions in patients on large doses of intravenous penicillin.

---

*Manufacturer's precaution: Safety of Darvon in children has not been established.

TABLE 1. Antibiotics Used in Management of Bacterial Endocarditis

ORGANISM	DRUG OF CHOICE AND DOSE*	SECOND CHOICE*
Streptococcus viridans (penicillin-sensitive)	Penicillin G 10 million u./day I.V. for 3 weeks 10 million u./day orally for 1 more week (optional) Usual dose 35 to 40 ml./kg./day I.V.	Erythromycin (max. 2 gm.) 50 mg./kg./day I.V. 2 weeks 50 mg./kg. orally 2 weeks +streptomycin (max. 2 gm.) 50 mg./kg./day I.M. 1 week 25 mg./kg./day I.M. 3 weeks *or* Cephalothin (Keflin) 20 mg./kg./day I.V. every 6 hours (max. dose 500 mg.) 20 mg./kg./day I.M. 2 weeks +streptomycin
Enterococci, penicillin-resistant *Streptococcus viridians*	Ampicillin 200 to 400 mg./kg./day I.V. for 4 to 6 weeks +Streptomycin 25 mg./kg./day I.M. for 2 to 4 weeks	
Pneumococci, gonococci, Group A beta streptococci	Penicillin G 10 million u./day I.V. for 4 to 6 weeks	
Staphylococci Penicillin-sensitive	Penicillin G 12 million—20 million u./day I.V. for 4 to 6 weeks +Gentamicin, 5 mg./kg./day I.V. for 2 to 4 weeks	Vancomycin 30 mg./kg./day I.V.
Penicillin-resistant	Methicillin, oxacillin or cephalothin 8 to 12 gm./day I.V. for 6 weeks (300 to 400 mg./kg./day) +Gentamicin for 2 to 4 weeks	Vancomycin
Coliforms, Pseudomonas	Ampicillin, streptomycin, penicillin— depending on sensitivity tests	Gentamicin } being Carbenicillin } evaluated
Fungal (Candida, etc.)†	Amphotericin B 1 mg./kg./day I.V.	

*The efficacy of the dose employed should be monitored by serial tube dilution studies.
†Also treat associated bacterial infection.

*Probenecid** in doses of 250 to 500 mg. every 6 hours orally may be given to ensure higher penicillin blood levels if oral or intramuscular penicillin therapy is being used. It is not essential if satisfactory bactericidal serum levels can readily be maintained without its use.

Corticosteroids may have to be given under three special circumstances: (1) In the presence of circulatory collapse. (2) If the endocarditis is complicated by failure and the nephrotic syndrome, steroids may be helpful in the relief of edema. (3) In very rare situations, the use of penicillin together with corticosteroids allows one to continue penicillin therapy in a patient sensitive to that drug. The new penicillin, such as cephalothin (Keflin), or lincomycin* may be used if they do not show cross-reaction. In some instances desensitization is indicated.

Complications. Anemia should be treated with small packed cell transfusions to maintain a hemoglobin of at least 10 gm. in acyanotic patients and between 12 and 14 gm. in those with cyanotic heart disease in whom the previous hemoglobin is known to be 15 gm. or more. Persistent anemia after the first 10 days of therapy is a poor prognostic sign. Megaloblastic anemia, which is very rare, responds poorly to vitamin B_{12}, and again small packed cell transfusions with very careful cross matching may be needed.

*Manufacturer's precaution: Probenecid is not recommended for children under 2 years of age.

*Manufacturer's precaution: Until further clinical experience is obtained, lincomycin is not indicated in the newborn.

In an effort to prevent *embolization,* most patients are kept at bed rest for the first week of therapy or longer if emboli are continuing. If small pulmonary emboli develop, they may be treated symptomatically and usually resolve without any residual effects. Fortunately, massive emboli are rare. Systemic arterial emboli may need surgical intervention. Cerebral emboli are treated by bed rest, oxygen, respiratory supportive measures and physiotherapy.

Renal complications, including a nephrotic-like syndrome, usually respond as the congestive failure and infection come under control. Occasionally, as previously discussed, steroids may be needed for a few days or weeks.

Persistent or recurrent fever is a particularly troublesome complication. In most patients with endocarditis, defervescence occurs after three to seven days on therapy, and simultaneously a marked improvement in appetite and general well-being is noted. However, after the second week, a low-grade fever may recur; this may indicate continuing infection, thrombophlebitis, drug reaction or local inflammatory response to intramuscular injections. With careful clinical monitoring and adequate checks of bactericidal blood levels, it is usually possible to continue with the already planned course of therapy.

Assessment of Progress. Marked improvement in the clinical state, appetite, vigor and general appearance, together with defervescence, usually indicates that effective therapy has been instituted. Blood samples should be obtained after three to four days, and the serum should be bactericidal in dilutions of 1:8 in broth and preferably as high as 1:16 or more. If bactericidal levels are only obtained at high concentrations, an increase or change of antibiotics is indicated. With some enterococci or staphylococci, for example, penicillin doses of 50 million units a day or more may be needed intravenously before adequate levels are attained. An increase in hematocrit and reticulocytosis is also a favorable sign, as is the return of the sedimentation rate to normal, although continued elevation of the sedimentation rate is sometimes seen in patients who otherwise are making excellent progress.

Role of Surgery. *Noncardiac surgery,* such as removal of chronically infected teeth, is usually undertaken about one week after defervescence and establishment of satisfactory bactericidal blood levels. Clearly an abscessed tooth or an area of acute osteomyelitis may require early surgical intervention.

Cardiac surgery in the presence of active infection appears to be and is a heroic measure. Nevertheless, it must not be forgotten that the earliest therapeutic successes in the pre-antibiotic era were obtained by surgical ligation of an infected patent ductus arteriosus. Today surgical intervention is indicated as follows:

1. In endocarditis and mediastinitis following cadiac surgery, particularly in patients with a prosthetic outflow patch or a homograft. Intensive appropriate antibiotic coverage for at least a week but not more than two weeks should usually precede surgery. Removal of the infected outflow patch, direct approximation of the right ventricular myocardium, topical application of antibiotic, adequate wound drainage and postoperative maintenance of endocarditis therapy for at least another two weeks can lead and have led to cure in very ill subjects. Vacillation and reliance on medical therapy alone can lead and have led to cardiac rupture, death from massive pulmonary emboli and other disasters—all modern variations on the ancient medical maxim that infection will not be cured if a foreign body is present. The intracardiac patch used to repair a ventricular septal defect is fortunately very rarely infected, being obviously much less exposed than the mediastinum during prolonged open heart procedures. Occasionally removal of infected sutures used to repair either an atrial defect or a ventriculotomy has been necessary and successful.

2. Occasionally *progressive cardiac failure* may continue owing to aortic or tricuspid valve involvement in a case of bacterial endocarditis without prior cardiac surgery. Under heavy antibiotic coverage, removal of the infected valve and replacement by a prosthesis has been successfully undertaken and this measure should undoubtedly be considered in a patient not responding well to adequate therapy.

3. *Aneurysm formation,* whether in the area of a ductus, a ventriculotomy site or other situations, is a clear indication for emergency cardiac surgery for two reasons: it is almost impossible to sterilize the aneurysm, and the risk of rupture is a real one.

4. *Infection on a prosthetic valve* carries a grave prognosis and repeat surgery may offer the only slim hope of cure.

Psychological Support. The best psychological support in this very trying illness is afforded by a skilled and amiable resident pediatrician capable of performing venipuncture and the maintenance of prolonged intravenous therapy with minimal trauma. Other support at consultant level is afforded by a frank discussion with the parents within

24 hours of admission concerning the necessary delay in establishing a firm diagnosis, the need for venipunctures and the minimal 4 week duration of therapy.

As the days wear on, a consistent and reliable source of information to parent and child is needed (preferably one resident and one consultant), particularly in large teaching institutions where the Tower of Babel syndrome may develop, the nurse saying cultures are negative, the intern, positive, and so forth. The social worker may be valuable in exploring with the parents the implications of prolonged hospitalization, the admitting office in advising on insurance and the possibilities of financial assistance, and the Child Life or similar program in supplying occupation and interest.

As soon as the child feels well enough, usually within a week of starting therapy, school contacts should be resumed and every effort made to ensure that he will graduate with the rest of his class. If therapy is successful and the staff skilled, informed and cheerful, psychologic problems are few. If it is unsuccessful, the rare and special skills needed in the management of incurable and refractory disease are called for, a subject too large for this brief article.

Discharge and Follow-up. The child is usually discharged 7 to 10 days after cessation of therapy, provided that no complications are present. Activities should be moderately limited (no sports) until a return visit to the hospital is made 2 to 4 weeks later. If at that time the child is clinically well, afebrile and without evidence of recurrence of anemia or other suspicious signs, a blood culture is drawn as a precaution and the child allowed to return to his usual level of activity. Anticongestive measures are continued as appropriate, particularly in those with aortic valve involvement who warrant closer follow-up than others. Normal annual check-ups can usually be resumed.

Prophylactic antibiotics should be restarted in rheumatic subjects 4 to 6 weeks after discharge. They are not used in congenital cardiac patients after one attack of endocarditis, though we have empirically and perhaps unreasonably recommended them after two or more attacks.

Elective cardiac surgery should be postponed for at least 6 months after discharge to allow complete healing of myocardial and renal lesions. The desirability of surgery should then be reviewed again on its merits without undue emotional pressure because of the infective episode, because recurrences, though they do undoubtedly occur, are quite rare in less than 3 to 5 years, and because a patient who is a bad operative risk prior to endocarditis is clearly not a better one after it.

Elective cardiac catheterization should also, in the author's view, be postponed for 6 months or more for similar reasons and because alarming and prognostically highly inaccurate hemodynamic findings may be obtained.

PROPHYLAXIS

Suggested Treatment Schedules (American Heart Association and American Dental Association Protocol)

Day of Procedure. Give procaine penicillin, 600,000 units, supplemented by 600,000 units of crystalline penicillin intramuscularly 1 to 2 hours before the procedure.

Intramuscular penicillin is more reliable. However, because of practical considerations, some dentists and physicians rely on oral penicillin when the full cooperation of the patient is assured. If oral penicillin is to be employed, four doses (every 4 to 6 hours) of at least 0.25 gm. of alpha-phenoxymethyl penicillin (Pen-Vee K) or 0.25 gm. of alpha-phenoxyethyl penicillin (phenethicillin), or 500,000 units of buffered penicillin G should be given during the day of the procedure. In addition, an extra dose should be taken 1 hour before the procedure.

For Two Days After Procedure. Give procaine penicillin, 600,000 units intramuscularly each day. In selected instances, 0.25 gm. of alpha-phenoxymethyl pencillin (Pen-Vee K) or 0.25 gm. of alpha-phenoxyethyl penicillin (phenethicillin) or 500,000 units of buffered penicillin G, four times daily by mouth on each day, may be used for those patients in whom full cooperation is anticipated and ingestion is assured.

Contraindications to this Regimen. The main contraindication is sensitivity to penicillin. All patients should be carefully questioned for previous history suggesting penicillin sensitivity. If such a history is obtained, even if equivocal, penicillin should not be given. Under such circumstances, erythromycin should be used in a dose of 250 mg. by mouth four times daily for adults and older children. For small children, a dose of 20 mg./lb./day divided into three or four evenly spaced doses may be used. The total dose should not exceed 1 gm. per day.

Instrumentation of Genitourinary Tract, Surgery of the Lower Intestinal Tract and Childbirth. With these procedures, transitory bacteremia due to penicillin-resistant enterococci is apt to occur. The use of penicillin alone in the dose previously suggested cannot be expected to curtail bacteremia due to enterococci, a common cause of bacterial endocarditis.

For these reasons, it is suggested that as an empirical guide, the previously mentioned intramuscular penicillin regimen be used in combination with streptomycin, 1 or 2 gm. intramuscularly on the day of procedure and for each of 2 days following the procedure. In children, streptomycin may be given in a dosage of 50 mg./kg., not to exceed 1 gm. per day. In patients who are sensitive to penicillin, a combination of erythromycin and streptomycin or a broad-spectrum antibiotic combined with streptomycin may be of some use, although it should be emphasized that very little information is available about these antibiotic combinations and their efficacy in preventing bacterial endocarditis due to enterococci.

Staphylococcal Infections

HENRY R. SHINEFIELD, M.D.

The staphylococcus remains an important etiologic agent in diseases acquired both in the community and in the hospital. The therapeutic approach to staphylococcal disease is conditioned by the capacity of *S. aureus* to form deep-seated abscesses and to persist in tissues for a prolonged period of time.

In general, therapy for staphylococcal disease should consist of a sound antimicrobial regimen coupled with surgery and general supportive therapy when indicated. Some staphylococcal infections require no treatment at all, especially minor skin infections such as folliculitis, which occur occasionally in most people. Established abscesses with localized collections of pus should be drained by methods ranging from incision and drainage of a skin abscess to closed under-water drainage of an empyema cavity.

The selection of a drug and its route of administration in the therapy of staphylococcal disease are conditioned by the age of the patient, the severity of the illness and the probable antibiotic resistance of the staphylococcus (Table 1).

ANTIBIOTICS IN SERIOUS DISEASE

Almost every antibiotic has been evaluated for effectiveness in the treatment of disease caused by the staphylococcus. In general, bactericidal drugs administered parenterally should be used in the treatment of serious staphylococcal disease. At present most staphylococcal infections, whether community-acquired or hospital-acquired, are caused by organisms resistant to penicillin. Therefore initiation of therapy should be with a drug other than penicillin. If the organism is sensitive to benzylpenicillin (penicillin G), this is the drug of choice. When the disease is associated with a penicillin-resistant staphylococcus, the semi-synthetic beta lactamase–resistant (penicillinase-resistant) penicillins are the drugs of choice. In this regard the three beta lactamase–resistant penicillin derivatives methicillin, nafcillin, and oxacillin are equal in clinical effectiveness despite some microbiologic differences in vitro.

Untoward reactions are also the same. In addition to toxic or hypersensitive reactions such as fever, skin rash and leukopenia, methicillin nephropathy is seen in about 0.1 per cent of children treated with this antibiotic. Methicillin remains an important drug despite its well documented association with renal reactions. These consist of hematuria and dysuria and usually do not appear until high-dose intravenous therapy has been continued for at least 10 days. In many cases toxic or irritative reactions disappear when the dosage of the drug is reduced and the hydration of the patient improved. In a few cases hematuria represents a hypersensitivity reaction and persists until therapy is changed to a nonpenicillin drug. The other related antibiotics nafcillin and oxacillin may also cause nephropathy. The frequency with which it is seen in patients receiving methicillin may simply be a reflection of greater experience with this antibiotic. Patients receiving any one of this group of antibiotics should be monitored with baseline and weekly or twice weekly urinalysis, BUN, creatinine, white blood cell and differential count.

If the history reveals an immediate reaction to penicillin, such as anaphylaxis, urticaria or diffuse pruritus, it is best to use some other antistaphylococcal agent. Cephalosporins are effective antistaphylococcal agents and can be used in most patients who are allergic to penicillin or one of its semisynthetic derivatives. However, there is cross-reactivity with penicillin in 5 to 15 per cent of these patients. Therefore care should be exercised when administering these drugs to a penicillin-sensitive patient.

Of the available antistaphylococcal cephalosporins, cephalothin and cephapirin have almost identical pharmacokinetic properties and can be used interchangeably. Cephazolin is excreted more slowly than cephalothin and cephapirin, which results in adequate therapeutic cephazolin serum levels, even if the antibiotic is administered only every six to eight hours. It is also less irritating and

TABLE 1. Dosage Schedule of Drugs Useful in the Treatment of Staphylococcal Infections

ANTIBIOTIC	ORAL (FOR MILD TO MODERATE INFECTION) 1 month to 50 kg.	ORAL > 50 kg. or maximum	PARENTERAL (FOR SEVERE INFECTION) > 1 week < 1 month	PARENTERAL 1 month to 50 kg.	PARENTERAL > 50 kg. or maximum
Penicillins					
Benzyl (Penicillin G)	50,000 to 150,000 units/kg./day in four doses	1.6 to 4.8 million units/day in four doses	100,000 to 250,000 units/kg./day IV every 4 hours	200,000 to 400,000 units/kg./day IV every 4 hours	8 to 24 million units/day IV every 4 hours
Phenoxymethyl (Penicillin V)	50 to 100 mg./kg./day in four doses	1 to 4 gm./day in four doses	—	—	—
Methicillin	—	—	200 mg./kg./day IV* every 6 hours	200 to 300 mg./kg./day IV every 4 hours	6 to 12 gm./day IV every 4 hours
Oxacillin	50 to 100 mg./kg./day in four doses	1 to 2 gm./day in four doses	100 mg./kg./day IM or IV† every 4 hours	100 to 200 mg./kg./day IV every 4 hours	4 to 8 gm./day IV every 4 hours
Nafcillin	50 to 100 mg./kg./day in four doses	1 to 2 gm./day in four doses	100 mg./kg./day IM‡ or IV every 6 hours	100 to 200 mg./kg./day IV every 4 hours	4 to 8 gm./day IV every 4 hours
Cloxacillin	25 to 50 mg./kg./day in four doses	1 to 4 gm./day in four doses	—	—	—
Dicloxacillin	12.5 to 25 mg./kg./day in four doses	0.5 to 2 gm./day in four doses	—	—	—
Cephalosporins					
Cephalothin	—	—	60 mg./kg./day IV every 6 hours	100 mg./kg./day IV every 4 hours	6 to 12 gm./day IV every 4 hours
Cephapirin	—	—	Not recommended	100 mg./kg./day IV every 4 hours	6 to 12 gm./day IV every 4 hours
Cephazolin	—	—	Not recommended	50 mg./kg./day IV every 6 hours	3 to 6 gm./day IV every 6 hours
Cephalexin	25 to 50 mg./kg./day in four doses	1 to 4 gm./day in four doses	—	—	—
Cephradine	25 to 50 mg./kg./day in four doses	1 to 4 gm./day in four doses	—	—	—
Others					
Erythromycin (lactobionate or gluceptate)	—	—	10 to 20 mg./kg./day IV every 8 hours; infuse over ½ to 1 hour	10 to 20 mg./kg./day IV every 6 hours; infuse over ½ to 1 hour	1.5 to 4 gm./day IV every 6 hours; 1 gm. diluted in 100 ml.
Erythromycin base (sterate and estolate)	25 to 50 mg./kg./day in four doses	1 to 2 gm./day in four doses	—	—	—
Lincomycin§	30 to 60 mg./kg./day in four doses	1 to 2 gm./day in four doses	15 to 30 mg./kg./day IV every 8 hours; infuse over 1 hour	20 to 40 mg./kg./day IV every 8 hours; infuse over 1 hour	1.2 to 2.4 gm./day IV every 8 hours; 1 gm. diluted in 100 ml.
Clindamycin	10 to 20 mg./kg./day in four doses	600 to 1200 mg./day in four doses	20 to 40 mg./kg./day IV every 6 hours; infuse over 30 minutes	20 to 40 mg./kg./day IV every 6 hours; infuse over 30 minutes	1.2 to 2.4 gm./day IV every 6 hours; 1 gm. diluted in 100 ml.
Vancomycin	—	—	40 mg./kg./day IV continuous drip	40 mg./kg./day IV continuous drip	2 gm./day IV continuous drip
Gentamicin	—	—	7.5 mg./kg./day IM every 8 hours	5 mg./kg./day IM every 8 hours	5 mg./kg./day IM every 8 hours
Kanamycin	—	—	30 mg./kg./day IM every 8 hours	15 mg./kg./day IM every 8 hours	1.5 gm./day IM every 8 hours

*Manufacturer's note: There is as yet no established intravenous dosage of methicillin for infants or children.

†Manufacturer's note: Experience with the use of oxacillin in premature and newborn infants is limited. Caution should be exercised and frequent evaluation of organ system function is recommended.

‡Manufacturer's note: There is no clinical experience available on the intravenous use of nafcillin in neonates and infants.

§Manufacturer's precaution: Until further clinical experience is obtained, lincomycin is not indicated in the newborn.

therefore may be administered intramuscularly. On the other hand, cephazolin is more susceptible to staphylococcal beta lactamase than are the other two cephalosporins.

From the standpoint of clinical effectiveness there is no evidence that any one of the cephalosporins possesses greater staphylococcal activity than the others. Because of renal toxicity another cephalosporin, cephaloridine, should not be used in pediatrics. Cephalosporins should not be used in central nervous system staphylococcal infections because they do not penetrate the blood-brain barrier well nor do they diffuse well into the cerebrospinal fluid. Some cases of endocarditis have responded poorly to cephalosporins despite the fact that the causative *S. aureus* is sensitive to these antimicrobials by in vitro testing. Under such circumstances other suitable bactericidal antistaphylococcal agents should be substituted.

The aminoglycosides kanamycin and gentamicin are effective antistaphylococcal agents. Serious side effects of ototoxicity and nephrotoxicity restrict their use except in special situations. Gentamicin has been useful in some cases of ventriculitis associated with an infected ventricular shunt. Vancomycin, another antistaphylococcal agent, is rarely used in pediatric patients because of the relative frequency of thrombophlebitis, hearing loss and nephropathy. We have used vancomycin with success in patients with serious infection caused by an organism resistant to all other antistaphylococcal antibiotics or in patients allergic to both penicillin derivatives and cephalosporins.

The proven toxicity of chloramphenicol coupled with questionable therapeutic response limits its usefulness in the treatment of staphylococcal disease. It is also doubtful whether the use of multiple antimicrobial agents offers any advantage from the standpoint of either achieving a better therapeutic response or preventing the emergence of a resistant strain of *S. aureus*. Oral administration of any antimicrobial agent in the treatment of serious staphylococcal disease is not recommended because of the unpredictable absorption, the care required to ensure compliance and the necessity of monitoring serum levels.

Antibiotics may be administered by the intravenous route either continuously or intermittently. To ensure delivery of medication and to avoid problems of antibiotic inactivation in intravenous solutions, we prefer to administer the antibiotic intermittently over a 10 to 20 minute period at four to six hour intervals (Table 1).

ANTIBIOTICS IN MILD TO MODERATE STAPHYLOCOCCAL DISEASE

In the treatment of mild to moderate staphylococcal disease, oral medications may be used. Because of better absorption, a phenoxypenicillin such as penicillin V is preferred over penicillin G if the organism is penicillin-sensitive. Cloxacillin or dicloxacillin are the drugs of choice when treating penicillin-resistant staphylococcal disease. They are preferred over oral oxacillin because of the higher serum levels attained with these antibiotics. Erythromycin or lincomycin can be used in allergic patients or if indicated by antibiotic sensitivities. Cephalexin, an oral cephalosporin, can be used in individuals allergic to penicillin. The drug is well absorbed from the gastrointestinal tract. Again caution should be exercised in its use in these patients because of possible cross-allergenicity with penicillin. Clindamycin is an effective antistaphylococcal agent. However, the frequent occurrence of colitis particularly after oral administration limits its usefulness.

The recommended duration of antibiotic therapy as outlined is somewhat arbitrary and is predicated on clinical experience and the established fact that eliminating *S. aureus* from infected or diseased sites is extremely difficult.

Nonspecific agents used in the therapy of disease associated with *S. aureus* include various vaccines, toxoids, gamma globulin and bacteriophage. In controlled observations there is no good evidence that any of these substances is of significant value in the treatment of staphylococcal disease.

SPECIFIC STAPHYLOCOCCAL INFECTIONS

Impetigo. *S. aureus* may cause bullous impetigo. If only a few lesions are present bullous impetigo usually responds to local treatment consisting of artificial rupture of the vesicles followed by cleansing with soap and water or alcohol. Since metastatic dissemination can occur, lack of response to local therapy is an indication for the use of antibiotics. In a patient not allergic to penicillin the drug of choice for oral therapy is a beta lactamase-resistant antistaphylococcal agent such as cloxacillin or dicloxacillin given in the dose described in Table 1. Emphasis is placed on the initial use of a semisynthetic beta lactamase-resistant penicillin because a large number of *S. aureus* strains encountered today are not susceptible to penicillin. If the organism is found to be sensitive to penicillin, therapy should be changed to phenoxymethyl penicillin. Patients allergic to penicillin or one of its derivatives should receive oral erythromycin, lincomycin or oral cephalosporin.

If the disease is extensive, denuding large areas of the body, initially a parenteral anti-staphylococcal agent such as methicillin or naf-cillin should be given. Therapy should be changed to parenteral aqueous penicillin G if the organism is found to be penicillin-sensitive. For patients allergic to penicillin parenteral erythromycin, lincomycin or a cephalosporin can be used. Therapy is continued one to three days after all evidence of infection has sub-sided.

These patients are generally febrile and may experience difficulty with fluid and elec-trolyte and protein balance as well as tempera-ture regulation. Heating or cooling blankets and appropriate fluids should be used when indicated. Hexachlorophene should not be employed to cleanse the large denuded areas since it may be absorbed and produce convul-sions.

Furuncle and Abscess. Furuncles and other skin afflictions are the most common le-sions produced by the staphylococcus. They are frequently self-limited and heal spontane-ously or may require simple drainage. If the lesions are accompanied by systemic symptoms or surrounded by large areas of cellulitis, an-tibiotic therapy as well as incision and drainage is indicated. The choice of antibiotics is the same as has been indicated for bullous im-petigo. The decision in regard to the route of administration depends on the age of the pa-tient, extent of the disease and ability of the patient to tolerate oral medication.

A useful approach in the treatment of re-current furunculosis which does not respond to local hygienic measures and appropriate an-tibiotic therapy utilizes the concept of bacterial interference. Individuals and families with chronic furunculosis may be protected from le-sions by artificial nasal colonization with a strain of S. aureus of low virulence (strain 502 A).* This regimen includes the use of both a topical nasal antibiotic such as neomycin or bacitracin and an oral antistaphylococcal agent such as cloxacillin or dicloxacillin. The anti-biotic is given until the nasal mucosa is cleared of the resident S. aureus, and then the patient is recolonized with S. aureus 502 A. About 80 per cent of individuals with chronic recurrent furunculosis respond to such therapy. Patients with chronic furunculosis not likely to respond to this regimen include those with underlying disease such as diabetes, eczema, acne or an underlying immunologic disorder. Antibiotics alone or efforts to increase host resistance with various toxoids and vaccines have not been consistently successful in curing this disease.

*May be obtained from the author on request.

Metastasis of the staphylococcal infection to areas more vulnerable than the skin such as the liver, lung, kidney and brain may occur. Deep abscesses may also occur as complications of an operative procedure or trauma. Deep abscesses require intensive therapy, which con-sists of drainage of accessible lesions after lo-calization. Care must be taken to remove any associated foreign body to prevent chronic suppuration. Under these circumstances parenteral antimicrobial therapy is mandatory and should be continued for one to two weeks after all clinical and laboratory evidence of in-fection has completely subsided. In the case of brain or lung abscesses this may mean the con-tinuation of antibiotic therapy for as long as 6 to 12 weeks.

Septicemia and Endocarditis. Septi-cemia is defined as symptomatic bacteremia. Staphylococcal septicemia may be secondary to an infection at a primary site in the skin, bone, joint or deep abscess and in turn may be re-sponsible for seeding these same sites causing a secondary abscess. A concerted effort should be made to identify the primary focus of infec-tion since this must be eliminated to effect a cure. In children with deficiency in host resist-ance, septicemia may occur without any obvi-ous primary site. Treatment consists of paren-teral antibiotic therapy. Aqueous penicillin G is the drug of choice if the organism is sensitive to it. Methicillin should be used for treatment of a resistant S. aureus strain. Antibiotic treat-ment should continue for one week after cessa-tion of all signs and symptoms of infection.

Bacteremia may be secondary to staph-ylococcal endocarditis. Operative procedures on the heart and valves and "mainlining" drugs have increased the incidence of this disease. A high proportion of staphylococcal strains caus-ing endocarditis are coagulase-negative. Staphylococcal endocarditis is treated by the parenteral administration of a bactericidal an-tibiotic. Treatment consists of aqueous penicil-lin G if the organism is highly sensitive to penicillin. If the organism is resistant to penicillin, methicillin should be used.

It is important to start intensive therapy rapidly because the staphylococcus quickly de-stroys heart valves with ensuing heart failure. Therapy should be initiated by the intravenous route and parenteral therapy should continue for at least four to six weeks. As in all serious staphylococcal diseases, oral medication should not be used. Some of the coagulase-negative staphylococci causing endocarditis are resistant both to penicillin and methicillin. Under these circumstances vancomycin should be used. If signs and symptoms persist or a relapse occurs in a patient with a prosthesis, it is likely that the only effective way of treating the infection and eradicating the bacteria is to remove the foreign body.

If the patient responds poorly to the beta lactamase–resistant penicillin and the blood culture remains positive, it is possible that the causative organism is a "tolerant" *S. aureus.* These organisms are not killed at the same antibiotic concentration at which they are inhibited; the mean bactericidal concentration (M.B.C.) is significantly greater than the mean inhibitory concentration (M.I.C.) In these cases the specific *S. aureus* should be tested by the tube dilution technique and the M.I.C. and M.B.C. determined in order to select an appropriate antibiotic. Some of these organisms are not only "tolerant" to the beta lactamase–resistant penicillins, but are also cross-"tolerant" with other cell-wall active antibiotics such as the cephalosporins and vancomycin. Under these circumstances an antibiotic which acts by a mechanism other than cell-wall inhibition such as gentamicin should be substituted or added to the therapeutic regimen.

Osteomyelitis.   See page 446.

Septic Arthritis.   See page 444.

Staphylococcal Enterocolitis.   Staphylococci in small numbers can be recovered from the stool in about 10 per cent of normal individuals. When staphylococci are present as the predominant aerobic bacteria in the stool, there may be symptoms of diarrhea which may vary from mild to severe.

The severest clinical form of staphylococcal infection of the intestine is *pseudomembranous enterocolitis.* In this disorder there is necrosis of the mucosa and formation of a pseudomembrane. Fluid loss and shock are a common cause of death in this disorder. Therefore primary attention should be paid to the replacement of fluid and electrolytes. Since infection is in the bowel wall, this staphylococcal disease is best treated with parenteral antibiotic therapy. Methicillin is the drug of choice. The duration of therapy depends on cessation of diarrhea and the elimination of *S. aureus* from the stool, which takes about 7 to 10 days.

Infections of the Central Nervous System.   Neurological procedures using plastic tubes to relieve congenital or acquired obstructions to the flow of cerebrospinal fluid have resulted in a changing pattern of central nervous system staphylococcal disease; as much as 35 per cent of central nervous system staphylococcal disease is secondary to such neurosurgical procedures. Occasionally staphylococcal infection of the meninges or brain follows a primary infection about the face or at a distant site such as the hip or foot.

Aqueous penicillin G is used if the organism is sensitive to penicillin, and methicillin is used for penicillin-resistant organisms. Therapy for meningitis that is not secondary to shunts should be continued for at least 1 week to 10 days after the patient is clinically well and all laboratory data including spinal fluid findings have returned to normal. Average duration of therapy is about three weeks.

With high doses of methicillin we have treated staphylococcal meningitis and brain abscesses successfully without the use of intrathecal medication. It is recognized that some authorities suggest the routine use of intrathecal medication. In view of our results, lack of definitive evidence to support the usefulness of intrathecal therapy and possible untoward effects from the instillation of medication in the subarachnoid space, we would not recommend the routine of intrathecal use of antimicrobial agents in the treatment of central nervous system staphylococcal disease until more data are available.

In cases that complicate neurosurgical procedures, the agent responsible for the infection may be a coagulase-negative staphylococcus rather than a coagulase-positive organism. It is important to determine the antibiotic sensitivity of the organism so that appropriate therapy can be instituted. Some of the coagulase-negative staphylococci are resistant to both penicillin and methicillin, and in these cases the drug of choice is vancomycin or gentamicin.

With infected shunts there is an associated cerebritis with small collections of pus around the insertion of the tube. Therapy with antimicrobial drugs alone usually is not sufficient to cure this type of infection; the foreign body must be removed by a second neurosurgical procedure before the staphylococci can be eradicated. Prior to removal of the shunt an attempt can be made to clear the infection without surgery. Some cases have been reported to respond to local instillation of gentamicin; 1 to 2 mg. of gentamicin is placed in the shunt and flushed retrograde into the ventricle three times every other day.

If ventriculitis persists the shunt must be removed. This is best done under the cover of antibiotic therapy. To eliminate any nidus of infection in the central nervous system, the antibiotic is initiated before and continued for as long as possible following removal of the shunt. The duration of therapy before a new shunt is inserted depends on the clinical condition of the patient. A return of the signs and symptoms of increased intracranial pressure signals the time of surgery. This is usually one to seven days after the infected shunt has been removed.

Diffuse glomerulonephritis may be a complication of coagulase-negative staphylococcal bacteremia which occurs in patients with a ventriculoatrial shunt. The renal disease probably is a result of an immunologic response to the staphylococcal infection rather than direct bacterial embolization of the kidney. Improvement in renal function is noted after removal of the shunt.

Streptococcal Infections

PATRICIA FERRIERI, M.D.

The group A streptococcus continues to be a common and important pathogen for children. Streptococcal infections of the upper respiratory tract or skin generally are uncomplicated in normal children. However the incidence of acute rheumatic fever remains high in certain population groups, particularly in poor and urban children in the United States and in other countries. Although streptococcal skin infections in children may be seen less commonly in private pediatric practices, these infections vary in their severity and complications and are a serious problem in certain areas of the world. Group A streptococcal infections pose challenges in diagnosis and management and continue to stimulate interest and investigation because of their ability to cause nonsuppurative complications: rheumatic fever which follows only pharyngitis, and acute glomerulonephritis which may follow pharyngitis or pyoderma.

STREPTOCOCCAL PHARYNGITIS

Pharygnitis may be caused by group A streptococci, viruses, *Mycoplasma pneumoniae* and other agents. In some studies of acute pharyngitis in children, about 50 per cent of the patients had no causative agent identified, and group A streptococci were isolated in one-third of the children. There is no single physical finding or combination of findings in patients with acute pharyngitis which permits a definitive diagnosis of streptococcal disease. Although a rash suggestive of scarlet fever in conjunction with clinical pharyngitis is supportive of group A streptococcal disease, it is not conclusive evidence. Scarlet fever may present in mild atypical form, and other infectious agents may cause rashes which resemble scarlet fever. Practically, a throat culture is the most direct way of excluding a streptococcal infection.

Unfortunately, streptococci may be isolated from children whose illness is due to other infectious agents, specifically viruses. Children who are chronic or transient carriers of pharyngeal streptococci present other management problems. For these reasons, one must base a diagnosis of true streptococcal infection on a combination of epidemiologic, clinical, and bacteriologic findings.

A throat culture should be obtained with excellent visualization of the posterior pharynx, avoiding contact with the tongue and lips. Processing of the culture can be carried out in a microbiology laboratory or even in the office by physicians with experience in reading and handling culture plates. The presumptive identification of group A streptococci can be made by determining if the beta-hemolytic streptococci are sensitive to a bacitracin disc. This should not be performed on the original plate but on a pure subculture of streptococci to avoid errors of interpretation of mixed bacterial cultures. Non–group A streptococci (e.g., groups C and G) are not commonly associated with infection and lack the ability to induce nonsuppurative complications. There is no rationale for treatment of patients from whom non–group A streptococci are recovered.

It is sound medical practice to withhold antibiotic treatment until the results of the throat culture are known. The disadvantages of treatment without supportive bacteriologic information include unnecessary expense and the possibility of drug sensitization. Even if therapy is delayed for several days for some reason, one can still prevent acute rheumatic fever. There are exceptions when one can initiate treatment before the culture results are known. These include suspected streptococcal infections in patients with a past history of rheumatic fever and/or rheumatic heart disease, patients who are unlikely to return for follow-up treatment, or close contacts of other patients with documented streptococcal infection.

Treatment. The objectives of treatment are to (1) *prevent the nonsuppurative complication* of acute rheumatic fever which can result from infection with many serotypes of group A streptococci. Eradication of group A streptococci from the upper respiratory tract will prevent rheumatic fever. It is unclear if early treatment of pharyngitis can regularly prevent the development of acute glomerulonephritis. Effective treatment can (2) *prevent the development of such suppurative sequelae* as otitis media, mastoiditis, and sinusitis and (3) *reduce the risk of spread* of streptococci to other close contacts in the home or at school. The duration of clinical illness may be shortened only slightly by antibiotic treatment. Successful treatment is dependent on patient and parental compliance, and therefore careful explanation of the objectives of therapy is an essential component of care of patients with pharyngitis.

Penicillin remains the primary drug in the treatment of streptococcal pharyngitis since it has been the most thoroughly evaluated agent in the prevention of rheumatic fever. Many authorities consider a single intramuscular injection of benzathine penicillin G to be the most effective and secure approach to treatment. This drug possesses one of the lowest treatment failures and reduces significant risk of streptococcal spread by 24 to 48 hours after injection. Although many combinations of injectable penicillin exist, there are no advantages of these preparations. The recommended dosage for eradication of group A streptococci must be based on the amount of benzathine penicillin. The recommended dosage of benzathine penicillin is 600,000 units in children under 60 pounds and 1.2 million units in patients over 60 pounds.

Oral penicillin is widely employed in the treatment of pharyngitis, particularly in adult patients. It is less reliable because of common failure by patients to complete a full course of therapy once clinical improvement is noted. If oral penicillin is prescribed, it is critical that the patient receive a full 10 days of therapy to eradicate the streptococci and prevent rheumatic fever. Buffered penicillin G provides less uniform predictable gastrointestinal absorption and therefore phenoxymethyl penicillin is recommended. The latter drug is administered in a dosage of 200,000 units three or four times a day for 10 days in children less than 60 pounds and 400,000 units three or four times a day for those over 60 pounds. Other penicillins with a wider antibacterial spectrum offer no advantages in the treatment of streptococcal pharyngitis.

Erythromycin is a drug of choice in patients with a history of penicillin allergy. This drug has demonstrated safety and efficacy in many treatment studies. The dosage is 40 mg./kg./day in four divided doses, not to exceed a total of 1 gm./day. Treatment with two doses a day appears to compare favorably with three or four doses. There are occasional strains of group A streptococci which are resistant to erythromycin.

Other antibiotics such as lincomycin and cephalexin (an oral cephalosporin derivative) have demonstrated eradication of streptococci when given for 10 days, but they offer no advantages over penicillin, and one can only infer that they are effective in preventing rheumatic

fever. Since 25 to 30 per cent of group A streptococci are resistant to tetracycline, this drug is contraindicated for therapy. Sulfonamides are not recommended for therapy since they will not eradicate the organisms; however, sulfonamides are effective in preventing colonization with streptococci and provide effective prophylaxis of patients with rheumatic fever (see below, Rheumatic Fever Prophylaxis).

Follow-up cultures of patients with pharyngitis have some value, particularly if oral therapy was employed. These cultures can be obtained 7 to 10 days following a course of oral penicillin or 4 to 5 weeks after an injection of benzathine penicillin. If patients are found to have positive cultures, retreatment with intramuscular benzathine penicillin is recommended and will often eradicate the organisms.

RHEUMATIC FEVER PROPHYLAXIS

Patients with a well documented attack of acute rheumatic fever or with rheumatic heart disease require continuous prophylaxis to prevent group A streptococcal infections and the risks of a new attack of rheumatic fever. The most reliable and recommended prophylaxis is an injection of benzathine penicillin, 1.2 million units, given every four weeks. Alternative prophylaxis is oral penicillin G, 200,000 units twice a day, or sulfadiazine or sulfasoxazole in a dosage of 0.5 gm. daily for children under 60 pounds and 1 gm. daily for those over 60 pounds. In patients with penicillin allergy, sulfonamides are recommended.

STREPTOCOCCAL SKIN INFECTIONS

There are several expressions of group A streptococcal infections of the skin. Streptococcal pyoderma is a broad term that includes impetigo contagiosa (a primary superficial infection of the skin) in addition to various secondary infections superimposed on such dermatologic conditions as eczema, scabies, and varicella. The lesions of impetigo contagiosa in a later stage of development possess characteristically a thick amber-colored crust and are pustular. Such lesions may yield pure streptococci or both streptococci and *Staphylococcus aureus* on culture.

Deeper forms of pyoderma include ecthyma, a chronic ulcerated streptococcal infection usually seen on the legs, and which may follow trauma. Deep soft tissue infections due to streptococci may complicate severe burns and wounds.

Erysipelas is seen less commonly and has a red, indurated, expanding plaque of cellulitis with spread in the subepidermal tissues.

Lesions of staphylococcal impetigo are not

commonly confused with streptococcal impetigo when the former are bullous in nature. However, cultures of skin lesions can be helpful in establishing a precise etiology and in directing therapy since primary staphylococcal disease ordinarily does not respond to the therapy usually employed for streptococcal skin infections.

In contrast to patients with pharyngitis, patients with impetigo usually have few complaints. Fever and cellulitis are rare in uncomplicated impetigo, but regional lymphadenopathy may be detected.

There are many approaches to the treatment of streptococcal impetigo. Hygienic measures, local skin care and topical antibiotic agents, such as bacitracin, may be adequate for mild cases of impetigo. If multiple lesions are present or if infection persists, oral or systemic antibiotics are used. Oral penicillin G, oral erythromycin and intramuscular benzathine penicillin are all effective in eradicating streptococci from skin lesions. Dosages of these drugs are similar to those employed for streptococcal pharyngitis. Oral therapy can be employed for 7 to 10 days, but compliance must be stressed to ensure bacteriologic cure comparable to that achieved with parenteral benzathine penicillin. The additional presence of penicillin-resistant staphylococci in streptococcal skin lesions does not interfere with clinical and bacteriologic cure by penicillin G. Because of its long action, a single injection of benzathine penicillin confers protection against early recurrences of impetigo. Erysipelas may require intramuscular or intravenous penicillin therapy, particularly if it is extensive or on the face, if associated with a toxic clinical state, or if present in the debilitated or compromised host.

Acute nephritis is seen commonly in patients with impetigo who have received oral or systemic antibiotics, and it is unclear if early treatment of streptococcal skin infections will decrease the frequency of this nonsuppurative complication. However, if acute nephritis is detected in patients with impetigo, prompt treatment should be given to contacts with skin infections to ensure eradication of nephritogenic streptococci and to prevent transmission to other susceptible individuals.

OTHER STREPTOCOCCAL INFECTIONS

Streptococcal infections in newborn infants are more often due to group B streptococci. Group A streptococcal infections are less commonly seen, but may present as omphalitis, skin or other serious infections. Serious epidemics have developed in newborn nurseries when a group A streptococcal infection has been introduced. These infections should be viewed as potentially life-threatening and treated with parenteral penicillin G. Attempts to identify personnel harboring streptococci and other measures to interrupt spread of the bacteria and acquisition by other infants must be carried out promptly.

Other group A streptococcal infections in children include acute otitis media and sinusitis, which are treated with a usual antistreptococcal regimen. Peritonsillar abscess and acute mastoiditis are serious infections which require intravenous penicillin therapy.

Group A streptococci are commonly associated with acute cervical lymphadenitis. Definitive diagnosis is obtained by aspiration and culture of an affected lymph node. Since *Staphylococcus aureus* alone, or with group A streptococci, may be an etiologic agent, initiation of treatment with a pencillinase-resistant penicillin is warranted.

Perianal cellulitis or vaginitis may be due to group A streptococci. These often pose management dilemmas since streptococcal carriage and symptoms may persist. Parenteral benzathine penicillin or oral penicillin is effective, but it is not unusual to administer more than one course of therapy to eradicate the carriage state.

Other serious group A streptococcal infections include pneumonia, empyema, meningitis, osteomyelitis, and arthritis. These infections should be treated with intravenous penicillin G, 300,000 to 400,000 units/kg./day in 4 to 6 divided doses in older children. The length of therapy is dependent on the clinical response, but generally prolonged therapy is necessary.

Listeria Infections

J. PATRICK HIEBER, M.D.

Listeria monocytogenes, a small grampositive coccobacillus, is a ubiquitous organism recoverable from water, soil, a variety of insect and animal species and man. In the majority of these settings the organism functions as a commensal simply colonizing its host; only rarely does it overcome the defenses of its animal or human host to produce invasive disease. Although human infections have been noted in all age groups, the majority of cases are seen in two age subsets: the neonate and adults over 45 years of age.

The current concept of pathogenesis of neonatal listeriosis is very similar to that recently worked out for neonatal group B streptococcal disease. During gestation the colonized mothers are asymptomatic or may note only vague symptoms of a flu-like syndrome or cystitis at the time of bacteremia. Early in gestation, seeding of the placenta and subsequent disseminated infection of the fetus may result in abortion or stillbirth. Illness in the affected liveborn infant has two distinct forms: early sepsis and a meningitic form with delayed onset. In the early form the infant is gravely ill within hours of birth with manifestations of disseminated disease: shock, cyanosis, jaundice, hypothermia, hepatosplenomegaly, maculopapular rash, pneumonia and meningitis. This presentation may be indistinguishable from that caused by several other organisms, although large numbers of gram-positive bacilli in the Gram-stained meconium of such an infant can be a distinguishing feature. On the contrary, the meningitic form begins with the well-appearing neonate becoming colonized during the peripartum period. After an incubation period of 4 to 21 days, nonspecific symptoms such as poor feeding, irritability and hypothermia herald the onset of purulent meningitis.

In patients beyond the neonatal period, the majority have an associated disease which, along with their age, results in diminished lymphocyte and macrophage mediated host defenses which are crucial for the containment of intracellular organisms such as Listeria, Mycobacteria, Brucella, Salmonella and Francisella. Conditions associated with an increased risk of Listeria infection include: lymphoreticular malignancy, steroid and immunosuppressive chemotherapy, diabetes mellitus and hepatic cirrhosis.

In all age groups, the majority of cases are sporadic. Only occasionally can human disease be linked epidemiologically to exposure to an infected animal. Infection of the neonate by the colonized mother is the only proven instance of human to human transmission.

Although Listeria has been recovered from a wide variety of disease processes including pneumonia, osteomyelitis, endocarditis and abcesses of liver, spleen and other organs, the majority of patients of all ages present with sepsis and/or purulent meningitis. As these syndromes often clinically resemble those caused by other bacterial species, specific diagnosis and therapy depend on Gram stain and culture identification. Morphologic pleomorphism and Gram variability complicate the interpretation of the Gram stain; the organisms are often mistakenly reported as "diphtheroids." The initial recovery of the organism from cerebrospinal fluid may be dif-

ficult; the yield may be increased by preincubation at 4° C. for several days before subculture on blood agar.

Therapy of Listeria infections includes two major components: efforts to improve the host's intrinsic cellular immunity and prolonged intensive antibiotic therapy with a bactericidal drug. The first goal is approached by attempting to obtain maximum possible control of the patient's underlying disease while minimizing the dosage of steroids and other immunosuppressive agents. The initial antibiotic therapy of choice is a combination of parenteral (intramuscular or intravenous) ampicillin, 100 to 200 mg./kg./day, and either gentamicin, 5 to 7 mg./kg./day, or kanamycin,* 15 to 30 mg./kg./day, which provides wide spectrum coverage for other etiologic possibilities and synergistic bactericidal action on the Listeria organism. The route of administration, and precise dosage per kilogram, and frequency of administration are factors which must be tailored to the individual patient, taking into account cardiovascular status, postnatal age and renal function.

Combination antibiotic therapy should be continued until daily cerebrospinal fluid and blood cultures document bacteriologic cure. Parenteral ampicillin therapy is then continued alone for 14 additional days. Relapses after such a regimen have been reported in a small percentage of patients with severe impairments of host defenses. In a recent case of recurrent Listeria meningitis in a child on steroid therapy we achieved a cure with a second 14 day course of both ampicillin and kanamycin. Failure to sterilize the cerebrospinal fluid after 3 to 4 days of ampicillin and aminoglycoside therapy should suggest the possibility of a parameningeal abscess or ventriculitis; the former should be localized and surgically drained and the latter should be treated with daily intraventricular instillation of gentamicin, 2 to 4 mg./dose, without preservatives until sterile.†

In the unusual instances of penicillin allergy or bacterial resistance to ampicillin, alternative antibiotics include chloramphenicol, tetracycline, erythromycin and sulfonamides. These all are drugs of second choice, as they are bacteriostatic rather than bactericidal against Listeria, a distinct disadvantage in the compromised host. In addition they all have

---

*This dose of kanamycin is higher than that recommended by the manufacturer but has been found to be safe and effective.

†The intraventricular use of gentamicin is not mentioned in the manufacturer's instructions.

toxicities that may complicate their use: chloramphenicol (gray syndrome in neonates, reversible and irreversible bone marrow suppression), erythromycin (hepatotoxicity, thrombophlebitis), tetracycline (dysplasia of bones and teeth in children under 6 years of age) and sulfonamides (displacement of bilirubin from albumin in neonates).

Diphtheria

QUELLIN T. BOX, M.D.

The most important component in the treatment of diphtheria is the administration of specific antitoxin as promptly as possible following an adequately considered clinical diagnosis. The mortality rate in diphtheria is directly related to the duration of disease prior to antitoxin therapy. The doses of antitoxin in use have been empirically determined and are probably well in excess of maximally effective amounts. Ranges of 30,000 to 80,000 units are recommended, the higher doses being appropriate for patients with severe involvement and for those diagnosed late in the course of their disease. The entire dose is given initially; repeated doses are not given. Because of the relatively slow absorption of antitoxin from subcutaneous and intramuscular sites, early toxin neutralization is best assured by the intravenous administration of at least half of the dose of antitoxin. Although intramuscular antitoxin may be adequate in milder cases, I prefer to give the entire dose intravenously after the usual tests for serum sensitivity. Available antitoxin is of equine origin.

In case of a positive reaction to an intradermal test with 0.1 ml. of a 1:1000 dilution of antitoxin, desensitization may be undertaken after appropriate preparation is made to ensure adequate management of adverse reactions, especially anaphylaxis. A facility such as a hospital emergency room or hospital ward treatment room fully equipped for conducting resuscitative measures should be used. A syringe is prepared for emergency use with 1 ml. of 1:1000 aqueous epinephrine. A secure intravenous infusion is begun with 5 per cent glucose solution, and baseline observations of blood pressure, pulse and respiratory rate are made. Following is a typical schedule for a serum desensitization procedure, the test doses of antitoxin being given every 15 to 20 minutes:

0.25 ml.	1:100 dilution	subcutaneously
0.5 ml.	1:100 dilution	subcutaneously
0.1 ml.	undiluted	subcutaneously
0.2 ml.	undiluted	subcutaneously
0.5 ml.	undiluted	intramuscularly

The entire dose of antitoxin diluted 1:20 in 5 per cent glucose in water is then given intravenously, beginning with a slow drip for the first 20 minutes, the remainder then being given over a 30 minute period. A reaction occurring at any point in the serum testing or administration of the antitoxin requires that further administration be delayed pending appropriate management of the reaction and reevaluation of the indication for antitoxin therapy as weighed against the nature and severity of the reaction.

Antimicrobial therapy is never used in diphtheria as a substitute for specific antitoxin. Prior to antimicrobial therapy, paired nasopharyngeal and throat swabs are obtained to be cultured for toxinogenic *C. diphtheriae*. Examination of stained direct smears is not advised. Crystalline penicillin G, 250,000 units/kg./24 hours divided every 6 hours intravenously, is given during the acute phase. After the involved mucous membranes are free of necrotic and purulent material, therapy is reduced to 600,000 units daily of aqueous procaine penicillin and continued to a total of 14 days. This therapy has been completely effective in the rapid elimination of infectivity (24 hours or less to achieve negative cultures) and in eventual bacteriologic cure. This regimen is also adequate for treatment of the frequently associated Group A streptococcal infections. For the patient allergic to penicillin, erythromycin lactobionate or erythromycin gluceptate, 20 mg./kg./24 hours divided every 6 hours intravenously, may be substituted for intravenous penicillin. Erythromycin, 40 mg./kg./24 hours divided every 6 hours orally, may be used in place of aqueous procaine penicillin. Cultures are repeated on two successive days after completion of antimicrobial therapy. For any individual with a persisting positive culture, a repeated course of oral antimicrobial agent is prescribed.

All patients with diphtheria should be hospitalized for treatment. Strict isolation procedures are indicated, especially for the acute period, during high-dose penicillin therapy, until the involved mucous membranes are free of necrotic and purulent material. Complete bed rest is indicated until the danger of severe complications is largely over, at least for 14 days. Fluid and electrolyte requirements are met by intravenous infusion until all danger of aspiration has passed and the patient can swallow without difficulty.

Close observation for complications is especially important. Palatal and pharyngeal paralysis may occur early and predispose to pulmonary complications from injudicious feeding attempts. Excessively vigorous or frequent nasopharyngeal or oropharyngeal suctioning may cause significant trauma or hemorrhage. Airway obstruction from desquamating pseudomembrane may require laryngoscopic or bronchoscopic removal. Tracheotomy should be done early for progressive airway obstruction, rather than being postponed until an emergency procedure is required.

Most current mortality in diphtheria is related to carditis. Appropriate cardiac monitoring is required for early detection of conduction disturbances and other manifestations of carditis. The presence of carditis requires intensive cardiac care, preferably in a unit specializing in such care. Emergency cardiac resuscitative equipment and medications, and personnel expert in their use, must be immediately available for the most successful management of severe carditis. Peripheral neuritis, a late-appearing complication, is usually benign and is self-limited, requiring no treatment. Occasional cases may progress in severity until respiratory support is necessary.

Treatment of diphtheria includes the evaluation of all household contacts. If further cases are diagnosed clinically, appropriate treatment is begun immediately. For all household contacts without evidence of diphtheria, erythromycin, 40 mg./kg./day divided every 6 hours orally for 10 days, is prescribed. As with cases, contacts are cultured for toxinogenic *C. diphtheriae* before and after therapy, and treatment is repeated if positive cultures persist. For those who are determined to be adequately immunized, a booster dose of toxoid is also given. For those with inadequate or no immunization, a complete toxoid series is begun. Diphtheria antitoxin is never used prophylactically. Hospital personnel contacts should be adequately protected by routine toxoid immunization. Convalescents from diphtheria are also given a complete toxoid series, since they may not be immune.

Pertussis

MARGARET A. KELLER, M.D.

Pertussis is most commonly caused by *Bordetella pertussis,* less commonly by *Bordetella parapertussis,* and rarely by *Bordetella bronchiseptica.* Appropriate therapy requires meticulous supportive care with prudent management of complications. Although viruses have been associated with pertussis-like syndromes, recent evidence points to the frequent coexistence of *Bordetella pertussis* and viruses, particularly adenovirus. Thus the isolation of adenovirus does not preclude pertussis of classical bacterial etiology.

Mild cases of pertussis may be difficult to distinguish from viral respiratory infection, and nasopharyngeal secretions with fluorescein-conjugated *Bordetella pertussis* antisera can be particularly helpful in such situations. Any child with a clinical picture typical of whooping cough should be isolated and treated as if he had *Bordetella pertussis* infection unless fluorescent antibody stains of nasopharyngeal secretions remain negative. Due to the fastidiousness of *B. pertussis,* a negative bacterial culture alone is not sufficient to exclude the possibility of infection with this organism.

Supportive Care. In general, children less than one year of age should be hospitalized to allow careful nursing supervision. Although isolation is necessary, the patient must be closely observed. Suctioning and oxygen should always be available at the bedside for immediate use following any prolonged paroxysm which leaves the patient with residual obstruction and cyanosis. Routine use of suctioning may stimulate additional paroxysms. Mist tents tend to obscure the patient from nursing observation and are not necessary in uncomplicated pertussis. Their use should be considered only if the patient requires increased oxygenation due to bronchopneumonia or convulsions. Weight loss from vomiting can be a major problem and is best handled by multiple small feedings during the refractory period immediately following a paroxysm. This is also the best time for administration of oral medications. Patients should not be given foods that can be easily aspirated and, if adequate nutrition cannot be provided orally, intravenous fluids may be necessary.

Antibiotics and Immune Therapy. Erythromycin, 50 mg./kg./day orally in four divided doses, has been shown to be effective in eradicating pertussis organisms from the nasopharynx. However, it has no effect on the outcome of the disease when administered in the paroxysmal phase. A five to seven day course of erythromycin is definitely indicated to reduce the risk to contacts and eliminate *B. pertussis* from the nasopharynx. Ampicillin is not effective for this purpose. Longer courses of erythromycin may lead to selection of resistant organisms as etiologic agents for secondary bacterial complications. Since bacteriologic relapse does occur infrequently, a fluorescent antibody study of nasopharyngeal secretions and culture should be obtained 2 to 3 days after erythromycin has been discontinued. Pertussis immune globulin has not been shown to be effective in the paroxysmal stage in well controlled studies. Its use cannot be recommended.

Complications. Uncomplicated pertussis is characterized by the absence of fever and the presence of a normal respiratory rate between paroxysms. The most common pulmonary complications of pertussis are atelectasis and bronchopneumonia. In atelectasis, the right upper lobe and the right middle lobe are the sites most commonly involved. Atelectasis alone without signs of infection does not warrant antibiotic therapy. Supportive therapy supplemented with vigorous chest physiotherapy when the paroxysmal phase has subsided is usually adequate. Only if resolution does not occur within 2 to 3 months should bronchoscopy be considered.

Bronchopneumonia is a complication that necessitates antibiotic therapy. However, presence of the "shaggy heart border" is common in uncomplicated pertussis and in itself is not evidence of secondary bacterial infection. Initial evaluation of bronchopneumonia should include chest radiograph, blood culture, aspiration of pleural fluid if present, and sputum Gram stain with culture. Until definitive bacteriologic results are available, initial antibiotic therapy of bronchopneumonia should be based on the patient's age and previous antibiotic coverage. Intravenous therapy with ampicillin, 200 mg./kg./day in four divided doses, will effectively treat common lung pathogens in young children. However, if the chest radiograph and/or sputum Gram stain suggest possible staphylococcal disease, a penicillinase-resistant penicillin such as oxacillin, 200 mg./kg./day in four divided doses intravenously, should be added. In patients who have received antibiotic therapy prior to the development of bacterial pneumonia, disease due to resistant organisms must be considered. Infants less than 2 to 3 months of age should receive gentamicin, 5 mg./kg./day intravenously or intramuscularly in 3 divided doses, to treat gram-negative bacteria. Appropriate adjustment of antibiotics should depend on results of cultures.

Encephalopathy should be managed with anticonvulsants if seizures are present. When seizures have occurred, careful evaluation of electrolytes, blood sugar, and blood calcium should be made since alkalosis can result from persistent vomiting. Previously unrecognized rickets has been associated with seizures during an attack of pertussis. Therapeutic guidelines for otitis media are not altered by the presence of pertussis, and the reader is referred to the section on otitis media for a detailed discussion. Ulceration of the frenulum requires no treatment.

Reactivation of latent tuberculosis has been reported with pertussis. Any child previously treated for tuberculosis or for a positive tuberculin skin test should be re-treated with isoniazid, 15 mg./kg./day orally in one dose, for 4 months following the attack.

Management of Contacts. At present, there are no controlled studies to prove that treatment with erythromycin of asymptomatic contacts or contacts in the early catarrhal phase will prevent or modify the disease. However, uncontrolled data have suggested such an effect, and erythromycin prophylaxis is recommended for susceptible contacts by the Infectious Disease Committee of the American Academy of Pediatrics. Immunized contacts should receive a booster DPT if they are under 4 years of age. All immunized children under 4 years of age and unimmunized susceptible family contacts with no history of pertussis should receive erythromycin, 50 mg./kg./day orally in 4 divided doses, for 7 days. If the contact case is being managed in the home, prophylaxis can be extended for 10 days. Pertussis immune globulin has not been shown effective in prophylaxis.

Careful attention must be paid to the medical personnel treating a child with pertussis since immunity from vaccination is not permanent and many younger physicians have not had pertussis. The incubation period is 5 to 21 days with most secondary cases occurring within 10 days of exposure. When medical personnel caring for a child with pertussis develop upper respiratory symptoms within 10 days of contact, fluorescent antibody nasopharyngeal smears and cultures must be obtained. Erythromycin should be started until results are known. Hospital epidemics caused by housestaff and nurses have been reported.

Bacterial Pneumonia

JEROME O. KLEIN, M.D.

Effective chemotherapy is now available for all forms of bacterial pneumonia encountered in the pediatric age group. Optimal treatment, however, requires definition of the etiologic agent. The physician must differentiate viral or mycoplasmal from bacterial pneumonia; if the agent is bacterial, he must decide on the probable species. Clinical signs and laboratory values may be of assistance but are not definitive. A major effort must be made to obtain adequate materials for bacteriologic diagnosis; these include sputum, secretions from the posterior nasopharynx and blood (bacteremia is frequent and a positive blood culture for a respiratory pathogen provides an unequivocal etiologic diagnosis). The physician should also consider the following: tracheal aspiration in young children unable to produce sputum; thoracocentesis when pleural fluid is present; and percutaneous lung aspiration in children who are critically ill, who deteriorate while on therapy or who are abnormal hosts with deficient immune mechanisms.

Therapy should be initiated promptly once bacterial pneumonia is diagnosed or strongly suspected. Initial therapy may be guided by the examination of the Gram-stained smear or sputum or tracheal aspirate. If these materials are unsatisfactory or unavailable, other criteria must be used. The relative frequency of respiratory pathogens in the various age groups may provide guidelines for initial therapy for the child with pneumonia who has no significant underlying pulmonary systemic illness or defect in immune function.

INITIAL CHOICE OF ANTIMICROBIAL AGENTS IN VARIOUS AGE GROUPS

Neonatal Pneumonia.   The treatment of neonatal pneumonia is similar to that of other forms of severe neonatal infection, including sepsis and meningitis; initial therapy must include coverage for gram-positive cocci, particularly group B streptococcus, and gram-negative bacilli.

A penicillin is the drug of choice for the gram-positive organisms. If there is reason to suspect staphylococcal infection, a penicillinase-resistant penicillin is chosen. If there is no significant risk of staphylococcal infection, penicillin G or ampicillin is used. The latter drug may provide a theoretical advantage because of greater in vitro activity against some enterococci and some gram-negative bacilli, particularly *Escherichia coli* and *Proteus mirabilis*, when used alone or in combination with an aminoglycoside.

Choice of therapy for suspected gram-negative bacillary infection is dependent on the antibiotic susceptibility pattern for recent isolates obtained from newborn infants. The patterns vary in different hospitals or communities, and from time to time within the same institution. At the present time, a significant proportion of all gram-negative bacilli cultured from newborns at the Boston City Hospital are resistant to tetracycline, streptomycin, ampicillin and cephalothin. Strains of *Pseudomonas aeruginosa* are resistant to all antibiotics except polymyxins, carbenicillin, gentamicin, tobramycin and amikacin. Based on

antibiotic susceptibility patterns of recent isolates of gram-negative enteric bacilli, we now use kanamycin or gentamicin to initiate therapy for severe neonatal infections.

Chloramphenicol has been used infrequently in newborn infants, owing to the association of the gray baby syndrome with high doses of this antibiotic. Perhaps because of the now minimal use in nurseries, chloramphenicol may be effective in vitro against gram-negative bacilli resistant to other antibiotics. Infants with neonatal sepsis due to a strain uniquely sensitive to chloramphenicol should be treated with this antibiotic in an appropriate dosage schedule (Table 1).

Because of the rapid changes in renal function during the first few weeks of life, different dosage schedules for selected antibiotics should be used for infants six days of age or younger and infants one to four weeks of age (Table 1).

The initial therapy should be reevaluated when the results of cultures are available. Duration of therapy depends on the causative

TABLE 1.   Daily Dosage Schedules for Parenteral Antibiotics of Value in Treating Bacterial Pneumonia in Newborn Infants*

ANTIBIOTIC	DOSAGE SCHEDULE ≤ 6 days of age	1 to 4 weeks of age
Penicillin G	50,000 units/kg. every 12 hours	70,000 units/kg. every 8 hours
Ampicillin Methicillin† Nafcillin‡ Oxacillin**	50 mg./kg. every 12 hours	70 mg./kg./dose every 8 hours
Carbenicillin	50 to 75 mg./kg. every 6 hours	100 mg./kg. every 6 hours
Kanamycin§	7.5 mg./kg. every 12 hours	7.5 mg./kg. every 12 hours
Gentamicin§	2.5 mg./kg. every 12 hours	2.5 mg./kg. every 8 hours
Tobramycin§	2 mg./kg. every 12 hours	1.6 mg./kg. every 8 hours
Amikacin§	7.5 mg./kg. every 12 hours	7.5 mg./kg. every 12 hours
Chloramphenicol‖ Premature	12.5 mg./kg. every 12 hours	12.5 mg./kg. every 12 hours
Full term	12.5 mg./kg. every 12 hours	25 mg./kg. every 12 hours

*Intramuscular or intravenous routes are satisfactory except where specifically noted.

†Manufacturer's precaution: There is as yet no established intravenous dosage of methicillin for infants or children.

‡Manufacturer's precaution: There is no clinical experience available on the intravenous use of nafcillin in neonates and infants.

**Manufacturer's precaution: Experience with the use of oxacillin in premature and newborn infants is limited.

§Intramuscular route usually used; intravenous administration over 30 to 60 minutes.

‖Intravenous route only, inadequate absorption from intramuscular sites.

agent. Pneumonia due to gram-negative enteric bacilli or group B streptococcus is treated for 10 days; disease caused by *S. aureus* requires 3 to 6 weeks of antimicrobial therapy according to the severity of the pneumonia.

Pneumonias in Children One Month to Four Years of Age. The vast majority of bronchopneumonias at this age are caused by respiratory viruses. Therefore, if the initial clinical findings are consistent with viral infection and the child can be observed closely, specific therapy may be withheld pending the results of bacterial cultures. *Streptococcus pneumoniae* and *Hemophilus influenzae* are the major bacterial agents of concern. A penicillin is the drug of choice: penicillin for pneumococcal pneumonia and ampicillin for *H. influenzae* infections. When the etiologic agent is unknown but a bacterial pneumonia seems likely, ampicillin should be used to provide coverage for both pathogens. Strains of *Hemophilus influenzae* resistant to ampicillin have been isolated recently in the United States and Western Europe. At present, ampicillin is still appropriate initial therapy for the young child with mild to moderately severe pneumonia. Chloramphenicol administered by the intravenous route should be considered for the seriously ill child who has pneumonia that may be due to *H. influenzae.* Therapy must be reevaluated when results of the cultures and antibiotic susceptibility tests are available (see below, Chemotherapy for Specific Pathogens).

Staphylococcus aureus has been an uncommon cause of acute pneumonia during the past 10 years. However, if clinical signs compatible with staphylococcal disease are present (such as empyema, abscess formation or pneumatoceles), initial therapy should include a parenteral penicillinase-resistant penicillin (methicillin, nafcillin, or oxacillin).

Pneumonia in the Child Four Years of Age and Older. *Streptococcus pneumoniae* is the major bacterial cause of pneumonia in this age group. *Hemophilus influenzae* is uncommon and need not be considered in initial therapy.

Infection due to *Mycoplasma pneumoniae* is frequent in the school-age child, adolescent and young adult. The tetracyclines* and erythromycin are effective in reducing the duration of illness; once the diagnosis is made or strongly suspected, treatment with one of these agents is appropriate.

---

*Manufacturer's note: The use of tetracyclines during tooth development (last half of pregnancy, infancy and childhood to age eight years) may cause permanent discoloration of teeth. This adverse reaction is more common during long-term use of the drug, but has been observed following repeated short-term courses.

CHEMOTHERAPY FOR SPECIFIC PATHOGENS

Pneumococcal Pneumonia. Penicillin G is the drug of choice for all children with pneumococcal pneumonia, except those considered to be allergic to that antibiotic.

For most children with mild to moderately severe disease, an oral penicillin is suitable. Phenoxymethyl penicillin (penicillin V) and phenethicillin provide significant serum antibacterial activity (the peak is approximately 40 per cent of an equivalent dose of intramuscular aqueous penicillin G). Buffered oral penicillin is less satisfactory, since the peak serum antibacterial activity is approximately half that of weight equivalents of penicillin V or phenethicillin, and larger doses are therefore required.

Children who appear "toxic," who have underlying disease or who have complications such as abscesses or empyema require the higher serum and tissue antibacterial activity provided by a parenteral form. Intramuscular aqueous sodium or potassium penicillin G is rapidly absorbed, high peak levels occurring within 30 minutes; the high levels thus attained make this route optimal for treatment of severe pneumococcal disease. However, since the intramuscular preparation is painful, if therapy of any duration is anticipated the intravenous route should be used.

Procaine penicillin G administered intramuscularly attains lower peak levels (approximately 10 to 30 per cent of those achieved with the sodium or potassium salt), but activity is sustained for 6 or more hours. Since the level of antibacterial activity in the serum may be exceeded many fold by oral penicillins, use of parenteral procaine penicillin G is restricted to patients who cannot tolerate the oral form (patients who vomit or who are comatose).

A single dose of benzathine penicillin G provides a low level of serum antibacterial activity for a period in excess of 14 days. Although this salt often has been effective in pneumococcal pneumonia, failures are frequent and it is not recommended.

The dosage schedule listed in Table 2 may be used to initiate therapy. The duration of therapy is dependent on the clinical response but should be continued for at least three days after defervescence and significant resolution of the radiologic and clinical signs.

Staphylococcal Pneumonia. The high incidence of penicillin G–resistant staphylococci in the hospital and in the community requires the use of a penicillinase-resistant penicillin whenever staphylococcal pneumonia is diagnosed or suspected. Later, if the culture

TABLE 2.   Daily Dosage Schedules for Antibiotics of Value in Bacterial Pneumonias of Infants* and Children

ANTIBIOTIC	ROUTE	RECOMMENDED DOSE PER DAY	SCHEDULE
Penicillin G	PO	100,000 units/kg.	4 doses†
	IM or IV	100,000 to 200,000 units/kg.	4 to 6 doses
Penicillin V } Phenethicillin }	PO	100 mg./kg.	4 doses
Methicillin‡	IM or IV	200 mg./kg.	4 to 6 doses
Oxacillin }	PO	100 mg./kg	4 doses†
Nafcillin§ }	IM or IV	200 mg./kg.	4 to 6 doses
Cloxacillin } Dicloxacillin }	PO	50 mg./kg.	4 doses†
Amoxicillin	PO	40 mg./kg.	3 doses
Ampicillin	PO	100 mg./kg.	4 doses†
	IM or IV	200 mg./kg.	4 to 6 doses
Carbenicillin	IM or IV	200 to 600 mg./kg.	4 doses
Cephalothin	IM or IV	200 mg./kg.	4 to 6 doses
Cephalexin	PO	100 mg./kg.	4 doses†
Kanamycin	IM or IV‖	15 mg./kg.	2 or 3 doses
Gentamicin	IM or IV‖	5 mg./kg.	3 doses
Tobramycin	IM or IV‖	5 mg./kg.	3 doses
Amikacin	IM or IV‖	7.5 mg./kg.	2 doses
Chloramphenicol	PO	50 to 100 mg./kg.	4 doses
	IV	50 to 100 mg./kg.	4 doses
Lincomycin**	IM or IV	10 to 20 mg./kg.	2 or 3 doses
Clindamycin	PO	8 to 16 mg./kg.	4 doses
	IM or IV	20 to 40 mg./kg.	4 doses
Erythromycin	PO	20 to 50 mg./kg.	4 doses
	IV	20 to 50 mg./kg.	4 doses
Vancomycin	IV	40 mg./kg.	4 doses

*One month of age and older.
†Schedule at least 1 hour before meals or 2 hours after meals.
‡Manufacturer's precaution: There is as yet no established intravenous dosage of methicillin in infants or children.
§Manufacturer's precaution: There is no clinical experience available on the intravenous use of nafcillin in neonates and infants.
‖Intravenous administration over 30–60 minutes.
**Manufacturer's precaution: Until further clinical experience is obtained, lincomycin is not indicated in the newborn.

and sensitivity data indicate that the organism is sensitive to penicillin G, it should be used because of its greater efficacy and lesser expense.

There are differences among the various penicillinase-resistant penicillins in oral and parenteral absorption, in vitro activity and enzyme degradation. However, clinical trials indicate that all are effective in treating staphylococcal disease when used in appropriate dosage schedules.

Since 1961, laboratories in Western Europe have reported varying proportions of strains of staphylococci resistant to methicillin and cross-resistant to the other penicillinase-resistant penicillins (and some of the cephalosporins). The incidence of these resistant strains has been low (approximately 1 per cent or less) in the United States. However, if a child with staphylococcal disease, given appropriate doses of one of these penicillins, does not respond as expected, resistance to the antibiotic must be suspected and the sensitivity of the causative organism reevaluated. Vancomycin and gentamicin are effective antistaphylococcal agents; one of these drugs may be used for the

patient with pneumonia due to methicillin-resistant *S. aureus*.

The rapid evolution of staphylococcal pneumonia and the frequent association of empyema, pneumatoceles and abscesses demand close observation and meticulous nursing care. The duration of antibiotic therapy is dependent on the initial response, the presence of pulmonary and extrapulmonary complications and the rapidity of resolution of the pneumonic process. A large parenteral dosage schedule should be used for two to three weeks followed by an oral preparation for one to three weeks.

Hemophilus Influenzae.   This organism is susceptible to a variety of antimicrobial agents including the sulfonamides, tetracyclines, aminoglycosides and ampicillin. All have been used with success in infections due to this agent. At present, ampicillin should be considered the drug of choice in young children with mild to moderate pulmonary disease. It provides coverage for both *S. pneumoniae* and *H. influenzae* when there is uncertainty as to the bacteriologic diagnosis, and the high dosage schedule needed for severe forms of disease can be given without concern for dose-related toxicity (Table 2).

Beginning in 1972, strains of *H. influenzae* (both type b and nontypable) resistant to ampicillin have been reported throughout the United States. Because of these strains, recommendations for treatment of life-threatening disease that may be due to *H. influenzae* (meningitis, epiglottitis or severe pneumonia) have been revised. Initial therapy for these patients includes chloramphenicol administered by the intravenous route and a penicillin, penicillin G or ampicillin. The most appropriate regimen is chosen when results of cultures and antibacterial susceptibility tests are available.

The child with mild to moderate pulmonary disease is treated until a period without fever of at least three days and a minimum of ten days. The child with severe disease is treated for at least two to three weeks.

Pneumonia Due to Gram-Negative Bacilli. Initial therapy must be guided by the following factors: the source of infection, underlying disease process (burn, cystic fibrosis), host susceptibility (deficient immune mechanisms) and the antimicrobial susceptibility pattern for gram-negative organisms in the community and hospital. The basis for choice of antibiotic is similar to that outlined for suspected gram-negative bacillary pneumonia in the neonate. The regimen is modified if indicated by the results of the cultures and the susceptibility of the causative organism. Duration of therapy must be tailored to the clinical course and the response to therapy. Pneumonias with minimal pulmonary lesions and symptoms should be treated for at least three days after defervescence. Severe pneumonias should be treated for a period of two to three weeks.

Therapy for the Penicillin-Sensitive Child. If the patient has a significant history of allergic reaction to any of the penicillins, he must be considered sensitive to all of them; alternative antimicrobial agents should therefore be considered.

Cephalosporins have been used with success in the treatment of staphylococcal and pneumococcal pneumonia and may be used as alternatives to penicillin.

Erythromycin, lincomycin and clindamycin are active in vitro against gram-positive cocci and are effective in the treatment of pneumococcal and staphylococcal pneumonias. Since some staphylococci may be resistant to these antibiotics, it is important to test the organism for susceptibility. Clindamycin, a chlorinated analogue of lincomycin, is well absorbed when given by mouth with meals and has greater in vitro activity and produces less gastric reaction than does lincomycin.

Vancomycin and gentamicin may be considered for use in the patient who is allergic to penicillin and who has severe staphylococcal disease.

Tetracycline should not be used in children under the age of eight years because of the frequency of tooth staining. For children over the age of eight years, it may be of value in infection due to *Mycoplasma pneumoniae*. The small proportion of pneumococci and the significant number (approximately 30 per cent) of streptococci resistant to tetracyclines limit their use in infections due to these agents.

Adjuncts to Chemotherapy. Antibiotics are only part of the management of the pediatric patient with pneumonia; supportive measures, including the following, are also of the utmost importance:

1. Maintenance of fluid and electrolyte balance.

2. Humidification provided by "cool mist."

3. Oxygen for severe dyspnea or cyanosis.

4. Maintenance of mouth hygiene.

5. Antipyretics should be used sparingly, since the temperature course may provide a guideline for the therapeutic response.

6. Bronchoscopy is limited to those instances in which a foreign body, tumor or congenital anomaly is considered.

7. Tracheal intubation or tracheostomy may be considered when there is laryngeal obstruction or when the patient is having difficulty clearing tracheal secretions and more efficient suctioning is warranted.

8. Drainage of pleural effusions may be necessary when the accumulation of fluid embarrasses respiration. Single or multiple thoracocentesis may be adequate when the volumes of fluid are small. If larger amounts are present, a closed drainage system with a chest tube under negative pressure should be placed. The tube should be removed as soon as its drainage function is completed, since delay may result in local tissue injury, secondary infection and sinus formation.

9. Intrapleural instillation of antibiotic should be considered in early cases of empyema, particularly if the fluid is loculated and the presence of fibrous adhesions is a possibility. If a chest tube is in place, antibiotics are instilled following irrigation through the tube. In susceptible infections, aqueous crystalline penicillin G, 10,000 to 50,000 units; ampicillin, 10 to 50 mg.; or a penicillinase-resistant penicillin or a cephalosporin, 10 to 50 mg., may be inoculated in 10 ml. of diluent (sterile

water or normal saline) after the tube is clamped. The clamp is maintained for 1 hour and then released for drainage. The instillations should be repeated three to four times each day that the tube remains in place. If thoracocenteses are done, antibiotic is introduced after pleural fluid is aspirated.

10. Because of their capacity to produce moderate or severe local irritation and febrile reactions, local instillation of intrapleural enzymes is a method used sparingly in children. The fibrinolytic activity of streptokinase combined with the effect of thinning of purulent exudate by streptodornase may aid the penetration of antibiotics and the process of tissue repair in the pleural space.

Meningococcal Disease

RALPH D. FEIGIN, M.D.

Neisseria meningitidis, a gram-negative diplococcus, is the cause of meningococcal disease. Illness may follow infection by any of the meningococcal serotypes; disease due to types B, C and D predominate in the United States.

Meningococci may be found in the nasopharynx of normal individuals. Disease occurs when the organisms invade the blood stream (meningococcemia) and then disseminate to other organ systems.

Acute meningococcemia may present as an influenza-like illness associated with fever, malaise, myalgia, and arthralgias. In a brief period of time, however, morbilliform, petechial, or purpuric lesions may be noted and profound hypotension may appear. The presence of hypotension, purpura, thrombocytopenia, and leukopenia frequently presages a fatal outcome.

Meningococcal meningitis follows blood stream dissemination and, in addition to the findings detailed above, vomiting, lethargy, seizures and other signs of meningeal irritation may be observed. The ultimate survival of patients with meningococcal meningitis, in most series, is better than that noted in patients with acute meningococcemia but without meningeal involvement.

Chronic meningococcemia is rare in children. When it occurs, it is characterized by chills, fever, maculopapular lesions, arthralgia and/or arthritis. Erythema nodosum lesions may be observed in both acute and chronic meningococcal disease.

Diagnosis is dependent upon a careful history and physical examination and is established by cultures of blood and cerebrospinal fluid (CSF). Although the nasopharynx should be cultured, isolation of meningococci from this source is but presumptive evidence of infection. Petechial lesions can be smeared to look for the presence of gram-negative diplococci and may be cultured. Blood, CSF and urine also can be evaluated by countercurrent immunoelectrophoresis (CIE) which will permit detection of capsular antigen whether or not the organism is viable.

The patient should be isolated for 24 hours after initiation of therapy.

Therapy.   Crystalline sodium penicillin G, 200,000 units/kg./day, should be provided intravenously in six divided doses. When the etiologic agent is in doubt, ampicillin may be used in a daily dose of 300 mg./kg./day provided in six divided doses intravenously.* Chloramphenicol sodium succinate, 100 mg./kg./day intravenously in four divided doses, provides effective treatment for patients who are allergic to penicillin. Antibiotic therapy should be continued for about seven days in patients with meningococcemia and for at least 10 days in patients with meningococcal meningitis. In some cases in which pericardial effusion, septic arthritis or pneumonia complicates meningococcemia, prolonged therapy may be indicated as dictated by the course of disease.

Circulatory Failure.   Shock frequently accompanies meningococcemia. When circulatory failure ensues, every effort must be made to ensure an adequate circulating blood volume. A central venous catheter should be inserted and urine output monitored. The latter may require catheterization of the bladder. The blood pressure, pulse rate and rhythm, and central venous pressure must be monitored frequently. This will require the rapid infusion of osmotically active fluids such as 5 per cent dextrose in lactated Ringer's, 5 per cent dextrose in normal saline, colloids or whole blood. Fresh whole blood may be particularly helpful in patients who also have disseminated intravenous coagulation. In patients with a high central venous pressure (greater than 11 to 12 cm.) cardiac decomposition may occur and digitalization may be necessary.

If circulatory failure persists, isoproterenol, 0.2 mg. (200 μg.) in 200 ml. of 0.25 per cent normal saline (1 μg./ml.), should be infused. The rate of infusion can be varied from 1 to 5 μg./min.; this rate may be doubled if there is no response as determined by an increase in blood pressure and urine output.

The use of steroids for the treatment of endotoxic shock is controversial. Controlled experiments in animals and selected studies in

---

*This dosage of ampicillin is higher than that recommended by the manufacturer but has been found safe and effective.

man suggest that any benefit from their administration requires massive pharmacologic doses (250 times the normal cortisol secretory rate per day) administered as early as possible. With this in mind, hydrocortisone, 65 mg./kg., also may be infused intravenously over a 15 minute period and repeated once four hours later.

In patients with meningococcal meningitis who develop hypotension, difficulty in the management of shock may be increased, for every effort must be made concomitantly to minimize the development of cerebral edema. The presence of cerebral edema may be suggested by an irregular respiratory effort, a falling pulse rate, hypertension and persistent seizures. In these patients, fluid administration must be minimized where possible and colloid utilized in preference to crystalloid infusates. In these patients hydrocortisone, 65 mg./kg., may be infused over a 15 minute period as for the treatment of shock, but infusion of this steroid does not provide optimal effect with regard to minimizing cerebral edema. For the latter, dexamethasone, 4 mg./kg., administered intravenously is preferred. Cerebral edema also may be treated by use of a 20 per cent solution of mannitol* in distilled water. This should be administered in a dose of 1 to 2 gm./kg. given over 10 to 15 minutes. The procedure may be repeated but attention to fluid and electrolyte balance is critical.

Seizures may be controlled with sodium phenobarbital, 6 mg./kg. administered parenterally. Following this initial dose, anticonvulsant effect may be maintained with phenobarbital, 5 to 7 mg./kg., given in three divided doses. Phenytoin may be provided in an initial dose of 5 mg./kg. intramuscularly or intravenously every 12 hours. When this drug is utilized by the intravenous route, it is important to flush the intravenous line with normal saline prior to, during and subsequent to its administration.

Disseminated Intravascular Coagulation. This complication generally is associated with hypotension. In addition to treatment of the basic disease with antibiotics and supporting the patient in shock as above, heparin, 100 units/kg. may be given by rapid infusion. This dose may be repeated every four hours if necessary. The whole blood clotting time should be kept at 20 to 30 minutes prior to each succeeding dose of heparin.

Prophylaxis. The rate of meningococcal disease among household contacts is greater than that in the community. For this reason household contacts should be examined and

nasopharyngeal cultures obtained. Contacts then may be treated with rifampin.* For adults, 600 mg. twice daily for two days is recommended. For children between 1 and 12 years of age, rifampin should be given in a dose of 20 mg./kg./24 hours in two divided oral doses for two days. In infants between three months and one year of age, rifampin can be provided in a dose of 5 mg./kg./day. Penicillin provided orally for four days does not eradicate the nasopharyngeal carriage of the meningococcus. Prevention of disease, however, can be effected by the use of 1.6 million units of penicillin G provided in four divided doses each day for 10 days.

Minocycline† has proved to be an effective agent for prophylaxis of meningococcal disease, but as many as 35 per cent of those treated develop headache, vertigo, ataxia or other disturbing reactions.

Sulfonamides are not indicated unless the sensitivity of the meningococcus to these agents has been ascertained. If the strain is sensitive to sulfa, sulfadiazine, 1 gm./day for two days, provides effective prophylaxis.

Close contacts also should be encouraged to seek medical attention if they develop malaise, myalgia, arthralgia, fever or other signs which may suggest the development of meningococcal disease. Prophylaxis is limited to household contacts and medical personnel with close personal exposure to the patient.

Infections Due to *Escherichia coli, Proteus, Klebsiella-Enterobacter-Serratia, Pseudomonas* and Other Gram-Negative Bacilli

HARRIS D. RILEY, JR., M.D.

Members of the taxonomic families *Enterobacteriaceae* and *Pseudomonadaceae* as well as other gram-negative coliform‡ bacilli have emerged as significant pathogens, particularly in hospital-associated infections. The *Enterobac-*

---

*Manufacturer's precaution: The use of mannitol in pediatric patients has not been studied comprehensively.

*Manufacturer's precaution: Data are not available for determining the dosage of rifampin for children under 5 years of age.

†Manufacturer's precaution: Use of minocycline during tooth development may cause permanent discoloration of teeth.

‡Coliform is a general term for fermentative gram-negative rods that inhabit the intestinal tract of man and other animals without causing disease. The term has not been strictly defined: some include in it all the enteric bacteria; others limit it to the lactose-fermenting members.

teriaceae, a family of gram-negative rods that can grow in air or in its absence on simple media, are found chiefly as normal flora (or pathogens) in the vertebrate intestinal tract, although some genera are saprophytes or plant parasites. These ubiquitous gram-negative bacilli include a large number of organisms and literally hundreds of species. They are also known as enteric bacilli, enterics, or enterobacteria. These terms are misnomers because these facultative aerobes, including the predominant *Escherichia coli,* enterococci, and various lactobacilli, account for only 0.1 to 1.0 per cent of the cultivable normal human fecal flora. Various anaerobes far outnumber all others. Enteric bacilli and other unofficial terms are, however, applied in medical microbiology to various superficially similar organisms with quite different metabolism, antigenic structure, pathogenicity, ecology, and evolutionary relations. Table 1 shows the principal divisions and groups of *Enterobacteriaceae.*

The enteric bacilli included in the coliform group are *E. coli, Klebsiella, Enterobacter* and several genera previously classified as "paracolon" organisms including *Serratia, Edwardsiella,* and *Citrobacter.* The coliforms (together with *Proteus-Providence* and *Pseudomonas* organisms) are now the predominant bacteria in hospital-associated infections. *Arizona* organisms are often included among coliforms but resemble more closely *Salmonella,* and *Providencia* is discussed with *Proteus.* While in the intestinal tract, these organisms generally do not cause disease (except for *Edwardsiella* and some types of *E. coli*). *E. coli* is normally a bowel organism as are probably some of the *Klebsiella.* However, the *Enterobacter, Serratia* and *Citrobacter*

groups occur infrequently in the normal intestine and are ordinarily free-living saprophytes. These organisms illustrate the difficulty of determining pathogenicity in absolute terms; usually harmless in their normal habitat, they often cause illness when they reach tissues outside the intestinal tract, especially if the host's defenses are impaired.

Advances in medical science have blurred the traditional separating lines between pathogens and nonpathogens. Today physicians must be prepared to consider virtually all microorganisms as having the capacity to produce disease in the human host whose immunologic and antimicrobial defenses are compromised and who enters an environment which is often contaminated. Thus, we now know of infections caused by microorganisms usually considered as nonpathogens until recently, such as *Serratia marcescans, Erwinia* spp., HB bacteria and others.

Other important gram-negative organisms, such as Salmonella, Shigella, *Hemophilus influenzae, Bordetella pertussis, Bordetella parapertussis,* Brucella, *Francisella tularensis, Yersinia pestis,* Bacteroides, *Eikenella corrodens,* and others are covered in other sections of the text.

All too often these organisms are regarded erroneously as contaminants. The natural habitat of many of these organisms is soil and water. *Proteus, Pseudomonas,* and–*Klebsiella-Enterobacter-Serratia* species and certain others, in addition to being present normally in the intestine, may also exist, usually with other organisms, in skin and mucous membrane lesions. They are opportunists and characteristically exhibit their pathogenic potential in per-

TABLE 1.   Principal Divisions and Groups of Enterobacteriaceae*

PRINCIPAL DIVISIONS	GROUPS (GENERA)	DEGREE OF PATHOGENICITY
Shigella-Escherichia	Shigella Escherichia†	Bacillary dysentery Certain types produce diarrheal disease
Edwardsiella	Edwardsiella	Can cause gastroenteritis and other salmonellosis-like diseases
Salmonella-Arizona-Citrobacter	Salmonella	Gastroenteritis, septicemia, enteric fever
Klebsiella-Enterobacter-Serratia	Citrobacter‡ Klebsiella Enterobacter Serratia	Opportunistic "secondary" pathogens
Proteus-Providence	Proteus Providencia	

*Modified from Davis, B. D., Dulbeceo, R., Eisen, H. N., et al.: Microbiology. Edition 2. Hagerstown, Harper & Row, Publishers, 1973, p. 756.
†*E. coli* includes alkalescens-dispar organisms, formerly in *Shigella*
‡Formerly *Escherichia freundii;* includes Bethesda-Ballerup "paracolon" organisms.

sons whose natural defenses against disease are poorly developed, such as the newborn infant, or impaired. These bacteria contain somatic (0) antigens (endotoxin) in their cell walls. The endotoxin is a protein-lipopolysaccharide complex which differs slightly from one species to the next, so that the antigens are immunologically distinct.

These organisms may be responsible for primary bacteremia, urinary tract infections, peritonitis, severe skin and soft tissue infections, wound infections, enteritis, pyarthrosis, meningitis, pneumonia, and other local and systemic infections. Their role in producing infections of the urinary tract is of the greatest magnitude.

Accurate identification of the gram-negative enteric bacilli is imperative. They differ markedly in susceptibility to various antimicrobial agents and also in virulence, which is important for prognosis and for recognizing potential danger to contacts. Moreover, identification is essential for epidemiological investigation of the sources of infection. In some laboratories, these organisms are not differentiated from *E. coli* and are reported as "coliforms." This is potentially a serious error because many of these organisms, such as strains of *Klebsiella-Enterobacter-Serratia,* are, in general, more resistant to antimicrobials. Moreover, their recovery from blood and purulent exudates or from urine is of more serious epidemiologic and prognostic significance.

Attention to infections due to gram-negative enteric bacilli means that one must be prepared for change. In the past few years, infections due to these organisms, formerly considered semisaprophytes, have increased in frequency and have become serious therapeutic problems. These organisms, once thought to have little virulence or to be completely nonpathogenic (including members of the normal flora of man and saprophytes), have been increasingly associated with disease in the developed countries. Endogenous infections (due to indigenous organisms) and nosocomial (hospital-acquired) infections now represent a significant proportion of serious bacterial infections in the United States and other western countries.

Thus, since the mid 1950's, the frequency of staphylococcal, pneumococcal, and streptococcal infections has diminished considerably, whereas the incidence of infections due to enteric bacteria and other gram-negative bacilli of low virulence has increased strikingly. Enteric organisms have always been the most common agents of urinary tract infections but they are now also the predominant etiological

agents in various endogenous and nosocomial infections such as surgical wound infections, hospital-acquired pneumonias, and others. Treatment of such infections is often made difficult by resistance of the organism to most antimicrobial agents and by the presence of other serious disease in the patient.

Coliform bacilli are particularly likely to be acquired in hospitals. Various aspects of the hospital environment, including blankets, mattresses, nasopharyngeal flora of hospital personnel, irrigating solutions, instruments and nebulizing equipment play an important role. The incidence of these infections is also closely related to catheterization and instrumentation of the urinary tract.

The advent and increased use of antimicrobials have definitely increased their prevalence. Many strains of *Proteus, Enterobacter-Klebsiella-Serratia,* and *Pseudomonas* are either naturally resistant to the commonly available antibacterial agents or develop resistance during therapy. A common clinical occurrence is the elimination of sensitive strains of bacteria by antibiotics with replacement by a resistant species. Various studies have shown that a significant decrease in the total number of strains of gram-negative bacilli sensitive to antimicrobial agents has occurred in the last few years. The decrease in proportion of susceptible strains is not associated with changes in colony morphology or with a loss of virulence of the strain for experimental animals.

Another important influence is the status of the host. The defenses of the body against gram-negative bacteria reside primarily in intact body surfaces and in nonspecific mechanisms such as phagocytosis, possibly the properdin system and the natural bactericidal action of human serum against such organisms. The bactericidal antibodies are contained chiefly in the 19 S globulins, which transverse the placenta poorly. For this reason and because the nonspecific defenses against infection of the newborn infant are not as well developed as in later life, serious infections with gram-negative bacilli are more commonly seen during the first few months of life. This is particularly true of premature and low birth weight infants.

In newborn and low birth weight infants, septicemia with gram-negative bacilli is not infrequently accompanied by a pink macular eruption, prominent over the trunk and buttocks, which may become gangrenous in areas. Another accompaniment of these infections in the neonatal period is hepatocellular damage with resulting hyperbilirubinemia and jaundice.

Persons debilitated by other underlying disorders are particularly susceptible to infections with these organisms. Thus, in addition to the neonate and young infant, these infections are particularly likely to occur in patients of any age with serious life-threatening disorders such as leukemia and other types of malignant disease, in those receiving therapy which suppresses natural body defense mechanisms such as cortisone, antimetabolites and radiation, and those with obstructive uropathy, myelomeningocele, cystic fibrosis, diabetes, and burns.

Although the management of infections due to each of these organisms must be individualized, certain generalizations can be made. There are few infections which the physician is called upon to treat that pose as difficult a problem as do those due to gram-negative coliform bacilli. Infections with these organisms are increasing in frequency, particularly as a hospital-associated phenomenon. Although new antibiotics have become available to which certain of these organisms are susceptible, the susceptibility of a given strain is unpredictable and susceptible strains may develop resistance relatively rapidly. Furthermore, most of the antimicrobials which have activity against these organisms are accompanied by a significant risk of toxicity.

The fact that infections due to these organisms are particularly common in postoperative patients and in those debilitated by other disorders or therapies compounds the difficulties by limiting the choice of available therapeutic agents and makes evaluation of antibacterial treatment more perplexing. Patients with pyelonephritis due to these organisms should be thoroughly studied for the presence of obstructive uropathy. Because of the variability in response to therapy, careful bacteriologic study and in vitro susceptibility tests should precede initiation of therapy.

In general, comparatively large doses of the selected antimicrobial agent(s) should be utilized and should be continued for relatively long periods. Infection, especially bacteremia, due to these and other gram-negative bacteria, may be accompanied by clinical shock, secondary to the elaboration of endotoxins. Appropriate supportive therapy for this complication is an important phase of the total management.

Antimicrobial agents of choice against the gram-negative bacilli which are relatively common as a cause of infection are shown in Table 2. The most reliable guide to the choice of an antimicrobial agent is the results of in vitro antibiotic susceptibility tests. However, in many instances, particularly in infants and children, treatment must be initiated after appropriate cultures are obtained but before the results of these studies are known. Table 2 can be used as a general guide in such situations. The choice of a particular drug depends upon many different circumstances: epidemiologic information, particularly whether the infection is community- or hospital-acquired; the clinical picture, including the site of infection and presence of underlying disease; the frequency of resistance to various antimicrobials among various organisms in the local area; and others.

The dose, route of administration, and other details of therapeutic use of the various antimicrobial agents useful in the treatment of infections due to these organisms are listed in Table 3. Since these infections occur frequently in the neonatal and infancy periods, the difference in the pharmacology and metabolism of drugs in patients in these age groups, as well as in patients with impaired renal function, should be recalled. The dosage schedule for newborn and low birth weight infants is also included.

Several new agents with antimicrobial activity against certain strains of gram-negative organisms have become available or are under investigation. These include several different groups of drugs. Among the new aminoglycosides are tobramycin, amikacin, sisomicin, and butirosin. They are bactericidal and, like gentamicin and kanamycin, can produce ototoxicity and nephrotoxicity. Some of the cephalosporins exhibit activity against certain gram-negative bacilli. At the time of writing seven cephalosporin antibiotics are available in the United States. These are cephalexin and cephaloglycin for oral use; cephradine for both oral and parenteral use; and cephalothin, cefazolin, cephaloridine and cephapirin for parenteral administration. Cephacetrile has been approved but not released, and several others are presently under investigation including cephapirin, cepharidine, cephanone, caphacetrile, cefoxitin, cefamandole, ceftezol, cefaclor, and cefuroxime. Carbenicillin and ticarcillin, alone or in combination with other antimicrobials, are active against certain strains of gram-negative bacilli, especially *Pseudomonas aeruginosa, Enterobacter,* indole-positive *Proteus* species, as well as most organisms inhibited by ampicillin.

Tobramycin, an aminoglycoside antibiotic derived from *Streptomyces tenebrarius,* is very similar to gentamicin in properties, antimicrobial spectrum and pharmacology. Its major advantage over its analog, kanamycin, is the increased activity against *P. aeruginosa.* The exact mechanism of action is not known. *P.*

TABLE 2. Selection of Antimicrobial Agents for the Treatment of Infections Due to Gram-Negative Bacilli of Relatively Common Clinical Occurrence*

ORGANISM	DRUG	
Escherichia coli[†]		
Community-acquired	Ampicillin	Cephalosporin[1]
	Kanamycin	Chloramphenicol
	Gentamicin	Tetracycline
Hospital-acquired	Gentamicin	Tobramycin[3]
	Ampicillin	Cephalosporin[1]
	Kanamycin	Carbenicillin
	Amikacin[3]	Chloramphenicol
	Tetracycline	
Enterotoxigenic and	Polymyxin (O)	Ampicillin
enteroinvasive[‡]	Neomycin (O)	Gentamicin (O)
	Kanamycin (O)	
Enterobacter species	Gentamicin	Polymyxin or colistin
	Tobramycin[3]	Chloramphenicol
	Kanamycin	Tetracycline
	Carbenicillin	Amikacin[3]
	Nalidixic acid	
Klebsiella pneumoniae	Gentamicin with or	Tetracycline
	without a cephalosporin	Cephalosporin[1]
	Tobramycin[3]	Chloramphenicol
	Kanamycin	Amikacin[3]
Proteus mirabilis	Ampicillin	Gentamicin
	Penicillin G	Tobramycin[3]
	Cephalosporin[1]	Nalidixic acid
	Kanamycin	
Indole-positive Proteus	Gentamicin	Nalidixic acid
(*P. vulgaris, P.*	Kanamycin	Tetracycline
morganii, P. rettgeri	Tobramycin	Amikacin[3]
	Chloramphenicol	Sisomicin[3]
	Carbenicillin	Cephalosporin[4]
Pseudomonas aeruginosa[†]	Gentamicin[5]	Tobramycin[3]
	Polymyxin or colistin	Sisomicin
	Carbenicillin	Amikacin[3,6]
Serratia marcescens	Gentamicin	Carbenicillin
	Kanamycin	Chloramphenicol
	Trimethoprim-sulfamethoxazole	Nalidixic acid
		Amikacin[3]

*In most instances, drug of first choice is listed first. Susceptibility tests are important in determining therapy for infections due to any of these organisms. However, in many instances, drug of choice depends on susceptibility results.

[†]For treatment of urinary tract infections, see text.

[‡]Indications tentative.

O = Oral administration

[1]Refers to one of the cephalosporins, administered parenterally or orally depending upon drug and nature of infection. See text for further details and information on new cephalosporins.

[3]See text for discussion of indications and use.

[4]Cefoxitin appears to be the most effective cephalosporin.

[5]Combination of gentamicin and carbenicillin is usually synergistic. Both can be used in serious life-threatening infections. Use of carbenicillin alone is associated with emergence of resistant *Pseudomonas* and super-infection with resistant *Klebsiella.*

[6]Synergistic with carbenicillin against many strains.

aeruginosa and *Proteus vulgaris,* on the average, are two- to four-fold more sensitive to tobramycin than to gentamicin. In vitro it is more active than gentamicin against *Proteus mirabilis.* Clinically, its greatest value lies in its use against infections due to *P. aeruginosa* and

Acinetobacter and, to a lesser extent, to other gram-negative enteric bacilli which have developed resistance to gentamicin (and other agents). It is often synergistic both in vitro and in vivo with the beta-lactase antibiotics (penicillins and cephalosporins). It is less active than is

TABLE 3. Daily Dosage Schedule for Antimicrobial Agents*

DRUG		ORAL	INTRAMUSCULAR	INTRAVENOUS	INTRATHECAL	ADULT OR MAXIMUM DOSE
Penicillin G[1]		500,000–2,000,000 u. in 5 doses ½ hr. a.c.	20,000–50,000 u./kg. in 4–6 doses	20,000–100,000 u./kg. in 4–6 doses		20–100 million u./day
	NB, P[2]	50,000 u./kg. in 4 doses	20,000–50,000 u./kg. in 2–4 doses	20,000–50,000 u./kg. in 4 doses		
Chloramphenicol[3]		50–100 mg./kg. in 4 doses		50–100 mg./kg. in 3–4 doses (10% solution)		3–4 gm./day Maximum in child, 2.0 gm./day
	NB, P[2,4]	25a–50b mg./kg. in 4 doses		15a–25b mg./kg. in 2–4 doses (0.5 mg./ml.)		
Tetracycline[5,e]		20–40 mg./kg. in 4 doses	12 mg./kg. in 2 doses	12 mg./kg. in 2 doses (1 mg./ml.)		2.0 gm./day
	NB, P[2]	10–20 mg./kg. in 4 doses	6 mg./kg. in 2 doses	6 mg./kg. in 2 doses (1 mg./ml.)		
Kanamycin[6]		100 mg./kg. in 4 doses	15–20 mg./kg. in 3–4 doses	15–30 mg./kg. in 2–3 doses (2.5 mg./ml.)		Oral, 3–4 gm./day IM, 1.0–1.5 gm./day
	NB, P[2]	50 mg./kg. in 4 doses	15–20 mg./kg. in 2–3 doses			
Neomycin[6,d]		100–150 mg./kg. in 4 doses	10–15 mg./kg. in 4 doses; limit to 10 days			Oral, 6.0 gm./day IM, 1.0 gm./day
	NB, P[2]	50 mg./kg. in 4 doses	4 mg./kg. in 2 doses			
Streptomycin sulfate[7,d]			20–40 mg./kg. in 2–3 doses		1.0 mg./kg. or 20 mg./day (5 mg./ml.)	2.0 gm./day
	NB, P[2]		10–20 mg./kg. in 2 doses			
Sulfonamides[8]		120 mg./kg. in 4 doses	120 mg./kg. (50 mg./ml.) in 4 doses	120 mg./kg. (25 mg./ml.) in 2–4 doses		3–4 gm./day
	NB, P[2,4]	50 mg./kg./daye in 2–3 doses				

Drug	NB, P[2]				
Polymyxin B[9]	10–20 mg./kg. in 4–6 doses 10–15 mg./kg. in 4 doses	2.5 mg./kg. in 4–6 doses 1ᵃ–2ᵇ mg./kg. in 4 doses	2.5 mg./kg. in 3 doses (0.4 mg./ml. 5% dextrose in endocarditis)	<2 yrs., 2 mg./day or every other day >2 yrs., 5 mg./day (0.5–1.0 mg./ml.)	Oral, 500 mg./day Parenteral, 200 mg./day Intrathecal, 10 mg./day
Colistin[9]	15–30 mg./kg. in 4 doses 10–20 mg./kg. in 4 doses	2.5–5.0 mg./kg. in 3 doses 1.0–2.0 mg./kg. in 2–4 doses	1.5–5.0 mg./kg. in 2–4 doses		5.0 mg./kg./day IM
Novobiocin[10]	20–45 mg./kg. in 4 doses 10–15 mg./kg. in 2–3 doses (NB, P[2,4])	15–40 mg./kg. in 2 doses 10–15 mg./kg. in 2–3 doses	15–40 mg./kg. in 2 doses 10–15 mg./kg. in 2 doses		Oral, 2.0 gm./day IM or IV, 1.0 gm./day
Gentamicin[11]	(NB, P[12])	3–7.5 mg./kg. in 3 doses 5(3–7.5) mg./kg. in 2–3 doses[18]		1–2 mg./day	IM, 5 mg./kg./day[11] Oral, 50–100 mg./kg./day
Cephalothin[13]	40–60 mg./kg. in 2–3 doses (NB, P[2])	80–160 mg./kg. in 4–6 doses	80–160 mg./kg. in 4–6 doses or in continuous infusion 20–40 mg./kg. in 4 doses or in continuous infusion		Parenteral, 2–6 gm./day
Ampicillin[15]	100–200 mg./kg. in 4 doses 25–50 mg./kg. in 4 doses	100–200 mg./kg. in 4 doses 50–200 mg./kg. in 2–3 doses[19]	150–200 mg./kg. in 4 doses		Oral, 2–6 gm./day Parenteral, 2–4 gm./day
Paromomycin[9]	50–100 mg./kg. in 4 doses (NB, P[2])				2.0 gm./day
Cephaloridine	50–100 mg./kg. in 3 doses (NB, P[2])	30–100 mg./kg. in 2–3 doses			6.0 gm./day

Continued on next page

TABLE 3.   Daily Dosage Schedule for Antimicrobial Agents* (*Continued*)

DRUG		ORAL	INTRAMUSCULAR	INTRAVENOUS	INTRATHECAL	ADULT OR MAXIMUM DOSE
Nystatin			1,000,000–2,000,000 u. in 3–4 doses 400,000 u. in 4 doses			
Amphotericin B[16]	NB, P²		1 mg./kg. given over 6–8 hr. period			1 mg./kg.
Methenamine mandelate	NB, P²	100 mg./kg. first dose; then 50 mg./kg./day in 3 doses				40 gm./day
Nitrofuran-toin		5–7 mg./kg./day; reduce dosage after 10–14 days to 2.5–5.0 mg./kg./day				400 mg./day
	NB, P²	1.5 mg./kg./day				
Carbenicillin	NB, P²	50–100 mg./kg./day in 4 doses		400–600 mg./kg. in 4–6 doses 300 mg./kg./day		40 gm./day
Cephalexin		25–50 mg./kg./ in 4 doses				12 gm./day
Nalidixic acid		40–50 mg./kg. in 4 doses; reduce to 20–25 mg./kg./day after 2 weeks				4.0 gm./day
Cefazolin	NB, P²		25–50 mg./kg. in 3–4 doses NR	25–50 mg./kg. in 3–4 doses NR		6.0 gm./day
Tobramycin	NB, P²		3–5 mg./kg. in 3 doses 4 mg./kg. in 2 doses			5 mg./kg./day

Drug		Dose	Dose	Maximum daily dose
Cephradine	NB, P²	25–50 mg./kg. in 4 doses / NR	50–100 mg./kg. in 4–6 doses / NR	8 gm./day
Clindamycin	NB, P²	10–25 mg./kg. in 4 doses / Unknown	10–40 mg./kg. in 4 doses / Unknown	4.8 gm./day
Cloxacillin	NB, P²	50–100 mg./kg. in 4 doses / NR		4.0 gm./day
Dicloxacillin	NB, P²	25–50 mg./kg. in 4 doses / NR		4.0 gm./day
Methicillin	NB, P²		200–300 mg./kg. in 4–6 doses / 50–200 mg./kg.[20] in 2–3 doses	12.0 gm./day
Nafcillin	NB, P²	50–100 mg./kg. in 4 doses	100–200 mg./kg. in 4–6 doses / 50–200 mg./kg. in 2–4 doses[20]	12.0 gm./day
Oxacillin	NB, P²	50–100 mg./kg. in 4 doses	100–200 mg./kg. in 4–6 doses / 50–200 mg./kg. in 2–4 doses[20]	12.0 gm./day
Penicillin V	NB, P²	25,000–100,000 u./kg. in 4 doses / NR		6.4 million u/day
Amoxicillin	NB, P²	20–40 mg./kg. in 3 doses / NR		3.0 gm./day
Amikacin	NB, P²	15 mg./kg. in 2–3 doses / Initial dose, 10 mg./kg.[21]	15 mg./kg. in 2–3 doses / Initial dose, 10 mg./kg.[21]	

Continued on next page

TABLE 3. Daily Dosage Schedule for Antimicrobial Agents* (Continued)

DRUG	ORAL	INTRAMUSCULAR	INTRAVENOUS	INTRATHECAL	ADULT OR MAXIMUM DOSE
Ticarcillin	NB, P²		200–300 mg./kg. in 4–6 doses Initial dose, 100 mg./kg.,²²		Oral, 2 gm./day IM, 8.0 gm./day IV, 8.0 gm./day
Lincomycin	30–60 mg./kg. in 4 doses NB, P²	20 mg./kg. in 2 doses	20 mg./kg. in 2 doses		

*Some of these agents may be administered by other routes. For intrapleural, intraarticular, intraperitoneal, ocular, aerosol and topical use, see Report of the Committee on the Control of Infectious Diseases, American Academy of Pediatrics, Evanston, Ill., 1964. Some, such as neomycin, are specifically contraindicated by the intrapleural and intraperitoneal routes.

[1] Phenoxymethyl penicillin or phenethicillin is preferred for oral therapy. Procaine penicillin should not be used in neonates. Sodium penicillin contains 1.5 mEq. of sodium and potassium penicillin-G, 1.69 mEq. of potassium per 1.0 million units. The latter should be avoided intravenously in neonates and in patients with impaired renal function.

[2] Dose for newborn and premature infants. If renal output is reduced, decrease the dose still further.

[3] Should not be used for minor infections or when less hazardous agents are effective. Observe for bone marrow depression.

[4] Avoid during first week of life unless essential. Desirable to follow treatment with serial blood levels to avoid "gray" syndrome.

[5] Any of the tetracycline group of antibiotics may be used. Intensive therapy in young infants may retard bone growth and result in dental change.

[6] With parenteral administration, auditory nerve and renal injury may occur; frequent audiometric and renal tests are essential. Manufacturer's note: The intravenous dose of kanamycin should not exceed 15 mg./kg./day.

[7] Auditory nerve damage can occur.

[8] A soluble sulfonamide should be used. Manufacturer's precaution: Systemic sulfonamides are contraindicated in infants under 2 months of age.

[9] Observe for renal and neural toxic effects.

[10] Severe skin and liver toxicity occasionally occurs. Manufacturer's warning: Use should be avoided in premature and newborn infants because it affects bilirubin adversely.

[11] In general, dose by the intramuscular route should not exceed 5 mg./kg./day for no longer than 7 to 10 days except in serious or life-threatening situations. Observation for vestibular and renal toxicity should be carried out. Desirable to follow therapy with serial blood levels if renal function impaired. The intrathecal use of gentamicin is not mentioned in the manufacturer's instructions.

[12] For neonates, see No. 18.

[13] Doses up to 200 mg./kg./day in infants and children have been utilized without untoward effect.

[14] For intrathecal use, colistin without dibucaine should be used.

[15] In severe infections, may be necessary to increase oral and intramuscular dose as much as 3 times that listed.

[16] Fever, thrombophlebitis, renal, hepatic, and bone marrow damage may occur.

[17] Infants <7 days, <2000 gm., 15 mg./kg. in 2 doses; >2000 gm., 20 mg./kg. in 2 doses. Infants >7 days, <2000 gm., 20 mg./kg. in 2 doses; >2000 gm., 20 mg./kg. in 3 doses.

[18] Dose should be given in 2 divided doses in infants <7 days and in 3 divided doses in infants >7 days.

[19] In infants <7 days, 50–100 mg./kg. in 2 doses; >7 days, 100–200 mg./kg. in 3 doses.

[20] In infants <7 days, 50–100 mg./kg. in 2 doses; >7 days, 100–200 mg./kg. in 3–4 doses. Manufacturer's precaution: The number of instances in which methicillin was administered intravenously to infants and children is not large enough to permit specific dosage recommendations.

[21] After initial loading dose of 10 mg./kg., follow with 7.5 mg./kg. dose every 12 hrs. (can be given IM or IV).

[22] After initial loading dose of 100 mg./kg., dose is as follows: <2000 gm. = 225 mg./kg. in 3 doses during first week of life; 600 mg./kg. in 6 doses after 7 days of age; >2000 gm., 300–400 mg./kg. in 4–6 doses; 600 mg./kg. in 6 doses after 2 weeks of age. Can be given IM or 15–20 minute IV infusion.

[a] Premature.

[b] Full-term.

[c] First dose should be doubled. Do not use sulfonamides in premature infants or infants under 2 months of age.

[d] In general, limit parenteral therapy to 10 days.

[e] Some investigators have found impaired intestinal absorption of tetracycline in prematures and newborns and have recommended a larger dose (100 mg./kg./day) than in children.

NR = Not recommended.

gentamicin against most strains of *Klebsiella, Enterobacter, Providencia,* indole-positive *Proteus* and *Serratia.* Gentamicin-resistant organisms are likely also to be resistant to tobramycin. The toxicity associated with tobramycin R similar to that of gentamicin. Because of greater experience with gentamicin, tobramycin, in general, should be reserved for use in serious *Pseudomonas* infections or in other infections due to susceptible organisms which are resistant to gentamicin and kanamycin.

Amikacin, a semisynthetic derivative of kanamycin, is a new aminoglycoside antibiotic for parenteral administration. It is active against a wide variety of gram-negative bacteria, including *Pseudomonas, E. coli, Proteus, Klebsiella-Enterobacter-Serratia, Providencia* and *Acinetobacter.* Gram-negative organisms can inactivate enzymatically aminoglycosides such as kanamycin, gentamicin and tobramycin. Amikacin is not a substrate for many of these enzymes and, because of this, is not activated to the same degree. However, nonenzymatic mechanisms can confer resistance to amikacin as they do to other aminoglycosides. Strains of gram-negative organisms resistant to amikacin are generally resistant to kanamycin, gentamicin and tobramycin. At present, in most hospital environments, a majority of gram-negative organisms are susceptible to kanamycin, but kanamycin-resistant strains are common. Resistance to gentamicin and tobramycin is still relatively rare, but in situations in which these drugs have been used freely, resistant strains of gram-negative bacilli may be encountered.

Many strains resistant to kanamycin, gentamicin and tobramycin are, at the present, susceptible to amikacin. Studies to date suggest that amikacin is interchangeable with gentamicin and is more active against *Klebsiella, Enterobacter, Serratia, Providencia* and *Proteus rettgeri* than to tobramycin. The toxicity of amikacin appears similar to that of kanamycin. Amikacin has no advantage over kanamycin, gentamicin, or tobramycin for treatment of infections caused by organisms susceptible to these drugs. In order to delay emergence of organisms resistant to amikacin, the drug should be reserved for treatment of serious infections caused by susceptible gram-negative bacteria known or suspected to be resistant to kanamycin, gentamicin and tobramycin.

Sisomicin, another aminoglycoside presently in the investigational stage, shows increased activity against *P. aeruginosa* and indole-positive *Proteus* as compared with gentamicin but, in animals, has slightly more nephrotoxicity. Microbial species among the common *Enterobacteriaceae,* with the exceptions noted, are usually two- to four-fold more sensitive to sisomicin than to gentamicin and two-fold more sensitive to gentamicin than to tobramycin; but all of these differences may fall within the therapeutic ranges of the drugs.

Butirosin, another aminoglycoside in the investigational stage, has experimentally considerably less toxicity than does gentamicin but also less activity against most aerobic gram-negative bacilli including *P. aeruginosa.*

As mentioned, some of the cephalosporins show activity against certain gram-negative bacteria. However, all isolates of the *Pseudomonas* species, most indole-positive strains of *Proteus* and many members of the *Klebsiella-Enterobacter-Serratia* species are resistant to the presently available cephalosporins. In many hospitals, nosocomial strains of *E. coli, Proteus* spp. and *Klebsiella* spp. are resistant. However, most strains of community-acquired *E. coli,* the nonmotile members of the *Klebsiella-Enterobacter* group and indole-negative strains of *Proteus* are susceptible. Several of the new cephalosporins exhibit antimicrobial activity against various gram-negative bacilli. Cefazolin shows increased in vitro activity against *Klebsiella* but this does not appear to be clinically significant, and cephacetile, a parenteral cephalosporin, against *E. coli.* The investigational drugs cefamandole and cefoxitin have greater in vitro activity against strains of indole-positive *Proteus, Enterobacter* and *Serratia* than currently available cephalosporins.

Cefoxitin (actually a cephamycin) is a parenteral preparation which has a more active anaerobic spectrum and in preliminary studies appears active against certain strains of indole-positive *Proteus,* especially *Proteus rettgeri.* Cefamandole, also for parenteral administration, appears to have the advantage of a more active spectrum against some members of the family *Enterobacteriaceae.* Further experience is necessary before definite recommendations can be made concerning the use of the newer cephalosporins, either alone or in combination with other agents, in infections due to gram-negative enteric bacteria.

Ticarcillin, a new semisynthetic penicillin which has recently become available, has antimicrobial activity against a variety of gram-negative bacteria. It is similar to carbenicillin in antimicrobial spectrum but is more active against most strains of *P. aeruginosa.* The improved in vitro activity permits use of doses of ticarcillin lower than those recommended for carbenicillin. The pharmacology and untoward effects in humans are similar to those of carbenicillin. The clinical results to date appear comparable with those for carbenicillin, although resistance and superinfection during therapy have been observed.

There are other new penicillins in the investigational stage which, either alone or in combination with other drugs, show increased activity against gram-negative bacteria. These include azlocillin, mezlocillin, mecillinam, and others.

Trimethoprim-sulfamethoxazole (TMP-SMZ) is a new antimicrobial combination with significant activity against a broad spectrum of gram-positive and gram-negative pathogens. The drugs act in synergy by blockade of sequential steps in folic acid metabolism. The goal for drug concentrations at the site of infection is a 1 to 20 ratio or about 1.0 μg/ml. of trimethoprim to about 20 μg/ml. of sulfamethoxazole. The daily dose for children over 12 years of age and for adults is 320 mg. of trimethoprim plus 1600 mg. of sulfasoxazole given in two doses. The dose for children 6 to 12 years is 40 to 80 mg. of trimethoprim and 200 to 400 mg. of sulfasoxazole every 12 hours; 2 to 6 years, 20 to 40 mg. of trimethoprim and 100 to 200 mg. of sulfasoxazole every 12 hours; and 2 months to 2 years, 20 mg. of trimethoprim and 100 mg. of sulfasoxazole every 12 hours.

Certain combinations of antimicrobial agents, such as gentamicin and cephalosporin, show greater activity against certain bacteria than does either drug alone. Continuous efforts are being made to investigate the antimicrobial spectrum of a wide variety of different groups of antibacterial agents in combination.

We can continue to expect the introduction of still other antimicrobial agents of various classes which possess activity against various gram-negative bacteria.

An important aspect of the total management of patients with infections due to gram-negative enteric bacilli, particularly those that are hospital-associated, is meticulous investigation of the epidemiology of these infections. However, the epidemiology of these infections is complex, and our understanding of their spread in hospitals is relatively primitive. Studies have been hampered by difficulty in carefully typing these organisms and, thus, tracing their travel through the hospital and related environment. It would appear, however, that multiple reservoirs exist and that the various routes of transmission make the control of such infections all the more difficult. Current evidence indicates that one of the major routes of transmission is by passive carriage on the hands of medical personnel—physicians, nurses, technicians, and so on. Meticulous hand washing is, of course, a key feature in control of such infections.

Several studies have shown that the antimicrobial resistance of these organisms is the result of resistance transfer factors (R-factors). These outbreaks may be the predictive forerunners of a new era of hospital-associated infections in this and other countries in which R-factor carrying organisms assume a more prominent role. There is evidence that nosocomial bacilli which carry R-factors may be present for extended periods in the gastrointestinal tract of patients after discharge from the hospital and at distance from the influence of widespread antibiotic usage. Of great importance is the observation that such patients, after they leave the hospital, seem capable of transmitting such organisms to members of their immediate families. This raises the possibility that hospital strains of gram-negative bacilli may become established in the community at large. This pattern of spread of antibiotic-resistant organisms is, with the exception of the intestinal reservoir, identical with that which occurred during the time when staphylococcal infections constituted a public health problem. At present, the great bulk of community-acquired staphylococcal infections are caused by penicillinase-producing strains.

The significance of gram-negative bacteremia cannot be overstated. The annual incidence in the United States is estimated to be 71,000 cases and the mortality rate to range from 24 to 60 per cent of cases resulting in 18,000 deaths per year. In a large municipal hospital the rate of bacteremia per 1000 hospital admissions during 12 selected years from 1935 to 1972 rose progressively. In 1935, it was 7.4 (291 cases); in 1965, 32.9 (1076 cases); and in 1972, 28 (591 cases). Since 1947, the case:fatality ratio has remained fairly steady (35 to 40 per cent).

A comparison of the findings of 1935 and of 1972 points up the increasing importance of sepsis due to gram-negative bacilli. Of the total cases of septicemia in 1935, 84.7 per cent were due to gram-positive pathogens, 11 per cent to gram-negative bacilli and 4.2 per cent to "other" organisms. In 1972, the proportion due to gram-positive pathogens had dropped to 48.3 per cent, wheras that due to gram-negative bacilli had increased more than three-fold to 34.6 per cent. *Candida,* which had not been reported in 1935, accounted for 4.2 per cent of the total in 1972. Moreover, the frequency due to "other" organisms (many of which were gram-negative bacilli including *Providencia,* atypical pseudomonads mimeae (*Acinetobacter, Serratia* and others) rose to 12.9

per cent of the total. Reports since 1972 indicate that incidence of bacteremia and other serious infections due to gram-negative bacilli has continued to increase.

The length of hospital stay for survivors of bacteremia is approximately three times longer (mean 49 days) and three times more expensive (mean $6692) than that of patients who do not experience nosocomial infections.

ESCHERICHIA COLI INFECTIONS

Escherichia coli are gram-negative motile rods normally found as part of the bacterial flora of the gastrointestinal tract. They have the capacity to produce a powerful endotoxin which enters the circulation and induces shock and the clinical pathologic picture of the Shwartzman phenomenon. *E. coli* are serotyped according to their somatic (O), flagellar (H) and envelope (K; L, A or B) antigens. The ability to be typed does not necessarily denote pathogenicity or virulence. The number of infections due to *E. coli* is legion. Because of this, only those clinical entities important because of frequency or severity are considered.

E. coli is now the most frequently encountered species in gram-negative septicemia resulting in bacteremia and in severe shock resembling that produced by intravenous injections with endotoxin in laboratory animals. The disease has been occurring with greatly increased frequency in the very young (especially the newborn), in those over 60 and in patients debilitated by various factors including corticosteroid therapy, immunosuppressive agents and leukemia, surgery or instrumentation of the intestinal, biliary or genitourinary tract. They also precipitate sepsis. This organism is also the most common cause of infection of the urinary tract and is an important agent in diarrheal disease. The incidence of strains of *E. coli* resistant to various antimicrobial agents is increasing in many geographic regions.

Infection in the Neonate. Gram-negative bacilli, particularly *E. coli*, are the commonest cause of septicemia and meningitis of the newborn. In most areas of the United States, *E. coli* and *Klebsiella-Enterobacter-Serratia* account for more than 75 per cent of the cases. It also is a significant cause of pneumonia in this age group and has been shown along with other gram-negative enteric organisms to be a significant cause of otitis media in infants less than six weeks of age. *E. coli* also produces urinary infection often associated with jaundice in infants less than two months of age.

Supportive measures are important in the neonate with a systemic infection irrespective of type or cause. Generally speaking, medication should be administered by the parenteral route because the depressed infant is likely to vomit and aspirate, as well as to ensure that adequate doses are received. Reestablishment and maintenance of body temperature in an incubator are important, and urinary output should be monitored. Intravenous fluid and electrolyte therapy should be provided by standard methods. Complications such as hyponatremia, hypoglycemia or hypocalcemia may mimic septicemia or complicate it. Thus appropriate diagnostic biochemical determinations must be carried out and appropriate replacement therapy instituted.

Antibiotic therapy is of cardinal importance in the management of infections due to *E. coli*. Because of changing patterns of resistance, in vitro susceptibility studies are essential. Kanamycin has been the drug of choice for *E. coli* infections in the neonate. However, in recent years the emergence of kanamycin-resistant strains of *E. coli* has become more frequent and widespread. In many geographic areas, more than 30 per cent of strains are resistant. In hospitals in which the majority of strains of *E. coli* remain susceptible to it, kanamycin should be used. The intramuscular dosage is as follows:

Infants 1 to 7 days of age	
< 2000 gm.	7.5 mg./kg. every 12 hours
> 2000 gm.	10.0 mg./kg. every 12 hours

Infants 8 to 30 days of age	
< 2000 gm.	10 mg./kg. every 12 hours
> 2000 gm.	10 mg./kg. every 8 hours

In many areas, gentamicin is currently the preferred drug for *E. coli* septicemia of the newborn. For infants under one week of age, the dosage is 5 mg./kg./day in equally divided doses every 12 hours. Beyond one week of age, the dose is 5 to 7.5 mg./kg./day in divided doses every 8 hours for both full term and low birth weight infants. Doses are given intramuscularly except to infants with poor circulation. For intravenous administration the dose is diluted in sterile normal saline and infused over a one to two hour period. If there is impairment of renal function, the dosage of either kanamycin or gentamicin must be reduced to avoid potentially toxic serum levels. In the absence of focal complications, treatment is usually maintained for 7 to 10 days.

Ampicillin administered parenterally is effective in infections caused by susceptible strains, especially those which are community-acquired. The daily dose administered intramuscularly or intraveneously for infants 1 to 7 days of age is 50 mg./kg. in two doses, and for infants 8 to 30 days of age, 75 to 150 mg./kg. divided into three doses. A combination of ampicillin with kanamycin or gentamicin has also been successfully used. Other drugs listed in Table 2 may be used if susceptibility studies show the organism to be sensitive. Amikacin and tobramycin appear to be effective, but their use should be reserved for infections in which the infecting strains are resistant to other antibiotics. Two of the newer cephalosporins, cephacetile and cefamandole, show increased activity against E. coli.

Infection in Older Infants and Children. E. coli septicemia, meningitis, pneumonia and other serious life-threatening infections may rarely occur in normal older infants and children. Infections with this organism when they occur in this age group are most often associated with compromised host defense mechanisms such as leukemia or other malignancies, immunosuppressive therapy, congenital or acquired immunodeficiency states, urinary tract manipulation, intravenous catheters, burns, hepatic failure and severe acidosis associated with renal failure. Meningitis due to this organism in otherwise normal children older than 2 months of age suggests the presence of an occult congenital or acquired central nervous system fistula.

General supportive care depends on the underlying problem. Serious E. coli infections in older infants and children should be treated with kanamycin or gentamicin administered parenterally. Ampicillin administered intravenously in a dose of 200 mg./kg./day given at 4 to 6 hour intervals plus kanamycin 15 to 20 mg./kg./day in two or three divided doses or gentamicin, 3 to 7.5 mg./kg./day in three divided doses has also been effective. Other drugs, as mentioned in the preceding section, may be used depending upon the results of susceptibility tests.

Urinary Tract Infection. E. coli remains the most common cause of primary uncomplicated urinary tract infection. The strains are usually quite susceptible to the sulfonamides or to ampicillin. Sulfisoxazole or trisulfapyrimidine,* 150 mg./kg./day in four divided doses for a period of 2 weeks, affords effective therapy in most patients. Ampicillin, 50 to 100 mg./kg./day orally in four divided doses, is

equally effective but not superior. The sulfonamides are still preferred for urinary tract infection of this nature since they are usually effective, and the cost and incidence of associated untoward reactions are low.

Because these drugs are effectively concentrated in the renal parenchyma and urine, favorable treatment response may be observed even when in vitro susceptibility testing shows the organism to be resistant. For this reason, if a favorable clinical response has been achieved after 48 to 72 hours, pyuria has been diminished and the urine sterilized, treatment may be continued with the drug initiated. If this has not been accomplished by this time, it is likely that the organism is resistant.

In recurrent disease the infecting E. coli is likely to be sulfonamide-resistant and antibiotic susceptibility data must be used as guidelines for selecting alternative drugs.

It is most important to ensure that the patient demonstrates both a clinical and bacteriologic cure and that an asymptomatic bacteriologic relapse does not occur. If the repeat urine cultures at 48 to 72 hours are sterile, treatment should be presumed effective. After the two week course of therapy, repeat urinalysis and quantitative urine cultures should be performed within several days, repeated at monthly intervals thereafter for three months and again at six months and a year.

Diarrheal Disease. The association of E. coli with diarrheal disease has been known for years. Numerous outbreaks of diarrhea occurring in nurseries have been investigated and certain antigenetically distinct strains of E. coli have been connected to these epidemics. The 15 to 20 serotypes associated with diarrhea have been termed enteropathogenic E. coli (EPEC). The relationship of these strains to diarrheal disease has been made almost solely on the basis of epidemiologic evidence. The mechanism by which these few serotypes cause diarrhea, among the hundreds of serotypes of E. coli, has not been clear until recently.

Most of the outbreaks of EPEC investigated in the past have been related to epidemics in neonatal nurseries or sporadic cases in infants less than one year of age. However, in single cases of diarrhea, the causal role of EPEC could not be established.

In recent years, the possible pathogenetic mechanisms for the diarrhea associated with E. coli have been elucidated by the demonstration of the toxigenic and invasive properties of some of the strains. Stool isolates of E. coli can be characterized as being: (1) enteropathogenic; (2) enterotoxigenic (ETEC), by

*Manufacturer's precaution: Sulfasoxazole and trisulfapyrimidine are both contraindicated in infants under 2 months of age.

their ability to produce toxins; or (3) enteroinvasive (EIEC), by their capacity to penetrate mucosal cells. It is now known that strains may have none, one, two or all three of these characteristics. Recent evidence also suggests that the intestinal mucosal adherence of some *E. coli* strains may be related to their pathogenicity.

E. coli has been shown to cause diarrhea by two separate mechanisms: enterotoxin production and mucosal invasion. Strains with invasive capacity produce the characteristic findings of bacterial dysentery, namely local inflammation with hyperemia, ulceration and intraluminal exudate composed of polymorphonuclear leukocytes. Enterotoxigenic *E. coli* causes diarrhea by two means: (1) production of an antigenic heat-labile toxin which resembles cholera toxin, in that it activates cellular adenyl cyclase, thereby increasing intracellular cyclic adenosine monophosphate and promoting secretion of sodium and water; (2) production of a nonantigenic heat-stable toxin, the exact action of which is undefined. Heat-labile enterotoxin has been shown to cause diarrhea in humans; heat-stable enterotoxin, although known to be a major cause of diarrhea in animals, has also recently been shown to be associated with diarrheal disease in humans.

ETEC and/or EIEC strains isolated from the stools of patients with diarrhea usually do not belong to established enteropathogenic serotypes. In a substantial number of diarrheal outbreaks, none or only a small percentage of strains of *E. coli* which were enteropathogenic were found to be enterotoxigenic. Other strains have been shown to be toxigenic but not invasive. Diarrheal disease has been produced in volunteers with invasive strains which were nonenteropathogenic and nonenterotoxigenic. Enterotoxin-producing strains of *E. coli* that produce either heat-labile toxins only or both heat-labile and heat-stable toxins have been well described as etiologic agents in persons with severe cholera-like diarrheal disease in Southeast Asia, in children hospitalized with diarrhea, in North American adults visiting Mexico and Africa, and in water-borne outbreaks of diarrheal disease. Strains that produce only heat-stable toxin had been incriminated until very recently only in traveller's diarrhea in adults.

It should be noted that to date, with a few exceptions, enterotoxigenic *E. coli* have infrequently been isolated from children hospitalized with diarrhea in the United States. From the available data, it appears logical to regard enterotoxin production as the most common mechanism of gastrointestinal virulence of *E. coli*. Elaboration of an invasive property is another but apparently much less common pathogenetic mechanism of *E. coli*. Evidence is available which suggests that ETEC and EIEC, in combination, are more likely to cause diarrhea than either alone.

Diarrheal disease due to *E. coli* is primarily characterized by diarrhea; high fever and other manifestations of systemic toxicity are rarely seen in uncomplicated cases. For this reason, the severity of illness may not be appreciated until signs of overt dehydration supervene.

Supportive therapy for *E. coli*–mediated diarrhea, irrespective of pathogenesis, consists mainly of maintaining adequate fluid and electrolyte intake. Patients with evidence of dehydration should be hospitalized and managed with intravenous fluids and electrolyte therapy, details of which are described elsewhere. In these patients, it is important to determine serum electrolyte concentrations since hyponatremia and hypernatremia occur fairly commonly.

Infants who are not dehydrated can be managed as outpatients. The details of management are described in other sections but two points should be mentioned. Homemade salt solutions should not be prescribed because of the risk of inducing hypertonic dehydration. Adsorptive agents that firm up the stool and those that decrease bowel motility have no place for treatment of diarrheal disease in infants and young children. None of these agents is specifically directed toward the primary cause of the diarrhea. None has been shown to decrease the fluid and electrolyte loss across the bowel mucosa in *E. coli* diarrhea, but by decreasing bowel motility they may mask the amount of fluid accumulated in the bowel lumen. They may also allow heavier colonization of the offending organism with greater enterotoxin production in the jejunum.

The effectiveness of antimicrobial therapy in *E. coli* diarrhea is open to some question. Specific antimicrobial therapy appears to shorten the severity and duration of diarrhea. Neomycin sulfate oral solution is the drug of choice in areas where neomycin resistance is not encountered frequently. It is administered in a dose of 100 mg./kg./day divided into doses every 6 to 8 hours for five days. Continuation of therapy for more than five days is not advised because the bacteriologic cure rate is not improved and because neomycin may cause a malabsorptive state. Colistin sulfate oral suspension is the alternative drug of choice and is given in doses of 10 to 15 mg./kg./day every 6 to 8 hours for five days. This dose is higher than that recommended by the manufacturer but has been found safe and effective. Antibiotic susceptibility testing should be performed because when resistant organisms are involved, treatment has resulted not only in failure but also spread of the infection presumably by suppression of competing normal bacterial intestinal flora.

Controlled studies have not been performed to date evaluating the effectiveness of antibiotic therapy in the treatment of diarrhea due to enterotoxigenic and enteroinvasive strains. Because the bacteria remain within the intestinal lumen in ETEC disease, it seems logical to speculate that nonabsorbable antibiotics might be useful in treatment. However, in an outbreak of diarrheal disease due to a strain of *E. coli* elaborating a heat-stable enterotoxin but which did not belong to an enteropathogenic serotype, oral colistin therapy was ineffective in eradicating the organisms from the stools of culture-positive infants and in preventing illness or shortening the carrier state. It is reasonable to presume that drugs effective against these strains in vitro might be beneficial in decreasing the severity and duration of diarrhea in those patients, as it has been shown to be with shigella dysentery. If strains susceptible to ampicillin are involved, this drug should be administered at a dose of 100 mg./kg./day in 4 to 8 divided doses, preferably intravenously.

It is not clear at this time whether older children with *E. coli* diarrhea should receive antimicrobial therapy.

Outbreaks of *E. coli* diarrhea in newborn nurseries can be catastrophic. Such outbreaks can be controlled by use of rapid fluorescent antibody techniques to detect the presence of organisms in the stool, and to follow such infants by segregation of colonized infants and treatment with oral neomycin or colistin in dosages previously mentioned.

Other Infections. A variety of other infections including pneumonia, peritonitis, abscesses and other infections may be caused by *E. coli*. The information in Tables 2 and 3 can be used for selection of antimicrobial therapy pending susceptibility test results. Surgical intervention and supportive measures depend upon the disease. *E. coli,* including nonenteropathogenic strains, has been causally linked to necrotizing enterocolitis in neonates.

PROTEUS-PROVIDENCIA INFECTIONS

Proteus organisms are gram-negative, motile, aerobic bacilli. They are common transients of the intestinal tract, but most species are free-living in water, soil, and sewage. The four species usually associated with human infections are *P. vulgaris, P. morganii, P. rettgeri,* and *P. mirabilis. P vulgaris* commonly occurs in the normal fecal flora of the intestinal tract and produces infections in human beings only when it leaves this normal habitat. *Proteus* species are a frequent cause of urinary tract infections, but can also cause septicemia, either as a primary infection or secondary to a focus elsewhere, infection of the skin and of the middle ear as well as infection in other organs. Because of the striking resistance of *P. vulgaris* and other indole-positive strains to many antimicrobial agents, their numbers tend to increase when the more susceptible coliforms are suppressed. Recently outbreaks of infection due to multidrug-resistant strains of *P. rettgeri* have been described.

The variable, unpredictable response to antibacterial therapy of *Proteus* infections is striking, and prolonged therapy is often necessary. In addition to in vitro susceptibility studies, *Proteus* isolates should always be classified as to species because of the variability in the susceptibility of various species and strains to different antibacterial agents. For example, *P. mirabilis* is usually susceptible to ampicillin (or occasionally to large doses of penicillin G), and it is the drug of choice in most infections due to this species. Many strains of *P. mirabilis* are also susceptible to gentamicin, cephalosporins, and kanamycin. Indole-positive species such as *P. vulgaris, P. rettgeri,* and *P. morganii,* for practical purposes, are always resistant to ampicillin and penicillin G. The drug of choice must be governed by the results of in vitro susceptibility tests as well as the clinical condition of the patient. Many strains are susceptible to gentamicin, kanamycin and tobramycin and these are usually the drugs of choice in infections due to these species. Some strains are susceptible to carbenicillin and certain ones to one of the cephalosporins.

Most strains of *P. vulgaris* are two- to four-fold more sensitive in vitro to tobramycin than to gentamicin. In vivo, however, strains resistant to gentamicin are likely to be resistant to tobramycin. Amikacin and sisomicin show increased activity against most strains of indole-positive *Proteus.* The use of these two agents should be reserved for infections due to organisms resistant to other available agents. Cefoxitin also shows activity against certain strains of indole-positive *Proteus.* Alternate drugs for infections due to susceptible strains are listed in Table 2. Some strains of *Proteus* are moderately susceptible to novobiocin, but this drug has a significant toxicity risk, and the response to therapy is often variable. Although in vitro the infecting organism is rarely susceptible, clinical results in certain refractory infections, especially of the urinary tract, with cycloserine* have been encouraging. This drug is potentially toxic and should be used with caution. The usual dose is 10 mg./kg./day.

Organisms in the genus *Providencia* are closely related to *P. morganii* and *P. rettgeri,* and were formerly known as *P. inconstans* and included with "paracolon bacilli." They are easily differentiated from *Proteus* by their lack of urease. Members of the group have been isolated from human feces during outbreaks of diarrhea but also in normal individuals. They are primarily associated with urinary tract infections but may also cause sepsis and localized infections. Providencia organisms are highly resistant to antibiotics except for carbenicillin and the aminoglycosides; some strains are inhibited by trimethoprim-sulfamethoxazole.

Providencia stuartii has recently emerged as a hospital pathogen in burned patients, appearing first in burn wounds but subsequently as a cause of pulmonary and urinary infection.

KLEBSIELLA-ENTEROBACTER-SERRATIA INFECTIONS

These related genera are now included in a single division. The three genera can be readily identified by biochemical tests and most strains of *Klebsiella* and *Serratia* can be typed serologically. Organisms belonging to this group are gram-negative bacilli, occur as normal inhabitants in the intestinal tract, but less frequently than *E. coli,* and are found more often on grains and plants; in soil, water and sewage. They are facultatively anaerobic and may be motile or nonmotile.

Along with *E. coli,* strains of *Klebsiella, Enterobacter* and *Serratia* are among the most important enteric organisms infecting man. *Klebsiella* predominates in clinical isolates and as a primary pathogen and usually but not necessarily produces more severe illness.

The necessity for differentiating *Klebsiella, Enterobacter* and *Serratia* from each other, and from enteric bacilli, is underlined by their wide differences in antibiotic susceptibility and in pathogenicity. The increase in prevalence and the greater role in morbidity and mortality of infections due to these organisms since the introduction of antibiotics are more striking than with any of the other coliforms. Pyelonephritis is the most common infection due to *Klebsiella-Enterobacter-Serratia.* These organisms may also produce systemic septicemia,

peritonitis, infections of the skin and soft tissue, as well as infection of the biliary system and gallbladder. A particularly disturbing problem with infections due to these organisms is that resistant mutants tend to be selected out rapidly on exposure to antibiotics. The clinical manifestations of infections due to this group of organisms in various body systems are indistinguishable on clinical grounds from those caused by other organisms. *Klebsiella-Enterobacter-Serratia* organisms most frequently arise in hospitals as secondary pathogens in immunologically compromised hosts. The significance of *Enterobacter* and *Serratia* in human infections have been less well clarified than *Klebsiella*–mediated infection, but all are increasingly important pathogens, especially as opportunistic invaders in the compromised host.

About two-thirds of all *Klebsiella* infections are hospital-acquired. Whereas *Klebsiella pneumoniae* is generally regarded as the most important "human" pathogen in the *Klebsiella* group, it probably accounts for less than 3 per cent of all cases of primary bacterial pneumonia. It and other *Klebsiellae* have become increasingly important causes of hospital-associated infections. The endemic *Klebsiella* infections which occur day-to-day generally involve a large number of different capsular serotypes, but, during specific outbreaks, one capsular type is usually responsible. Outbreaks have been described which are associated with a contaminated common source such as inhalation therapy machines, hand cream bottles, and other equipment used in hospitals. A two-stage phenomenon has been characterized in which patients, after hospitalization, developed intestinal colonization by *Klebsiella* and the same multiply-resistant organisms then were etiologic for those who developed clinical infections. The susceptibility of *Klebsiella* to cephalothin sharply distinguishes this organism from *Enterobacter* and *Serratia,* which produce a cephalosporinase.

Enterobacter species are frequently isolated from sputum (after antibiotic therapy), urinary tract, blood and wound infections and are usually opportunistic in character. *Enterobacter* frequently coexists with *E. coli* and other coliforms and has become an increasingly important cause of nosocomial infections. In 1970 to 1971, an outbreak of *Enterobacter cloacae* or *Enterobacter agglomerans* (Erwinia) septicemia occurred in 378 patients in 25 American hospitals due to microbial contamination of intravenous products manufactured by one company. The patients presented with the syndrome of persistent gram-negative bac-

---

*Manufacturer's precaution: Safety and dosage of cycloserine have not been established for pediatric use.

teremia which was refractory to appropriate antimicrobial therapy. Improvement occurred only after discontinuation of intraveneous therapy or the replacement of the entire intravenous administration system. Antiseptics and disinfectants, particularly aqueous quaternary ammonia compounds, may become contaminated with *Enterobacter* species, as well as with other gram-negative bacilli, and, if used to cleanse hospital equipment or for skin asepsis, result in bacteremia or "pseudobacteremia" (presence of bacteria in blood cultures without infection).

E. hafnia has been associated with gastroenteritis.

Serratia marcescens has been used by bacteriologists for years as a "test" organism for demonstration purposes because the brightened pigment of some strains is so easily observable. However, in recent years it and other members of the *Serratia* group, including nonpigmented strains, have been isolated with increasing frequency from human patients with hospital-associated infections. Extended outbreaks of nosocomial *Serratia* infections have now been described. These organisms in many of these outbreaks have been resistant to available antimicrobial agents and the selective pressure of antibiotic use in the hospital seems to play an important role in allowing them to become important hospital pathogens. A major site of infection has been the Foley-catheterized urinary tract, but other sites have been the primary focal point. Control of such outbreaks have been difficult.

Klebsiella-Enterobacter-Serratia organisms have variable susceptibility to antimicrobial agents and must be tested in vitro. Frequently, however, antimicrobial therapy must be instituted before results of antibiotic susceptibility tests are available. An aminoglycoside antibiotic, such as gentamicin, kanamycin or tobramycin (the choice depending upon the susceptibility patterns of organisms in the local area), is usually the drug of choice with certain exceptions. For example, many strains of *K. pneumoniae* are susceptible to cephalothin and some strains of *Enterobacter* are inhibited by carbenicillin. Trimethoprim-sulfamethoxazole inhibits some strains of *Serratia*. In contrast to *Klebsiella* and *Enterobacter,* almost all strains of *Serratia* are resistant to the polymyxins. For serious *Klebsiella* infections, it is usually desirable to add a cephalosporin. Other drugs for treatment of infections due to members of the *Klebsiella-Enterobacter-Serratia* group, depending upon susceptibility results, are shown in Table 2.

PSEUDOMONAS INFECTIONS

The *Pseudomonas* group is composed of gram-negative, motile rods which are nonfermenters and occur widely in soil, water, sewage and air. *P. aeruginosa* is the member of the genus most commonly pathogenic for human beings. *Pseudomonas* occurs in several antigenic types and several phage types which are equally pathogenic. Because of its ability to form a pigment which colors inflammatory exudate blue or green, the epidemic spread of *P. aeruginosa* in hospital wards has long been recognized. It is found in small numbers in the intestinal tract and on normal skin, particularly when other coliforms are suppressed. *P. pseudomallei,* the agent of melioidosis, and *P. mallei,* the cause of glanders, are now also classified in this genus. Other members of the genus *Pseudomonas,* such as *P. maltophilia, P. cepacia* and others, may occasionally be pathogenic for man but less is known about the epidemiology of these organisms.

P. aeruginosa is ordinarily a pathogen only when introduced into areas devoid of normal defenses or when participating in mixed infections. It is observed most frequently in hospitalized patients. Since the widespread clinical use of antibiotics, this organism has been found with increasing frequency as the cause of infections of the blood, urinary tract, meninges, heart valves, eye and skin. Fatal septicemia due to *P. aeruginosa* has been noted in small epidemics and is particularly prevalent in patients treated with antimetabolites and radiation and in those with extensive burns.

Infants and patients in other age groups debilitated by other diseases, particularly if accompanied by a leukopenia, such as leukemia, appear to be particularly susceptible to infection with *P. aeruginosa.* It is a common cause of pulmonary infections in patients with cystic fibrosis. The necrotic skin lesions produced by *Pseudomonas* infections have a fairly typical discoloration which allows them to be suspected clinically. *Pseudomonas* meningitis occurs secondary to infected lumbar puncture, head injury, myelomeningocele and chronic mastoiditis. The organism has been recovered from a variety of sources in the hospital environment. Pyelonephritis due to *P. aeruginosa* often has its genesis from introduction of the organism into the urinary tract by catheters or in irrigating solutions. It may also cause troublesome and serious eye infections.

P. aeruginosa is resistant to the more commonly used antimicrobial agents and therefore assumes prevalence and importance when more susceptible bacteria of the normal flora are suppressed. Although most strains of *P. aeruginosa* are susceptible to the polymyxins, these agents have been relatively ineffective in eradicating bacteremia and deep-seated tissue infections. Gentamicin and other amino-glycosides and carbenicillin are usually more effective but the polymyxins still have a place in selected infections, particularly in urinary tract infections or in bacteremias arising from the urinary tract. In other instances, the organism may be eradicated but the ultimate results are often unsatisfactory because of the poor host defenses in debilitated patients.

Carbenicillin is effective against susceptible strains but some 20 per cent of strains are resistant to it. It must be given in relatively large doses intravenously. During prolonged therapy with carbenicillin, organisms initially susceptible may become resistant. Most strains of *Pseudomonas* are inhibited by gentamicin but recently an increasing number of strains have been found to be resistant. Presumptive therapy for systemic *Pseudomonas* infection is a combination of gentamicin and carbenicillin. The two drugs appear to act synergistically in vitro, and coadministration may delay emergence of *P. aeruginosa* resistant to carbenicillin.

Tobramycin has been found to be two to four times more active against Pseudomonas than is gentamicin. It is particularly valuable in treatment of infections due to gentamicin-resistant strains. When tobramycin is used in combination with carbenicillin, higher antibacterial serum titers are achieved than with either agent alone. For neonates, the dose is 2 mg./kg./day in two equal doses every 12 hours and, for infants and children, 3 to 5 mg./kg./day in divided doses every 8 hours.

Ticarcillin, a new semisynthetic penicillin similar to carbenicillin, has activity against *Pseudomonas* organisms and, as further experience is gained, may prove to be a useful agent in treatment of such infections.

Amikacin inhibits many strains of *P. aeruginosa* and has been shown to be an effective agent in many infections due to this organism. It may be used alone or in combination with carbenicillin. At the moment, its most valuable use is in the treatment of *Pseudomonas* infections due to strains resistant to gentamicin or to other agents. *Pseudomonas* is a preeminent opportunist and the vast majority of infections caused by it occur in hospitals, particularly those housing patients with serious diseases. Since 1961 *P. aeruginosa* bacteremia has increased and the respiratory tract has become an increasingly important source of infection.

The use of gentamicin, carbenicillin and colistin has not changed the outlook of *Pseudomonas* bacteremia. A polyvalent vaccine has proved useful in burned patients and further attention needs to be given to immunoprophylaxis. At the present time, control of the underlying disease condition contributes most toward survival of patients with bacteremia and other serious *Pseudomonas* infections.

The pseudomallei group of the genus *Pseudomonas* consists of *P. mallei* and *P. pseudomallei*. The former is the cause of glanders, a severe infectious disease of horses that can be transmitted to man. Human infections can usually be treated with sulfonamides.

Melioidosis, due to *P. pseudomallei*, is a disease resembling glanders in man and occurs chiefly in Southeast Asia but perhaps also in the Western hemisphere. It has been observed in Americans who have returned from Vietnam. The clinical manifestations range from a relatively benign pulmonary infection to a rapidly fatal septicemia, characterized by multiple abscesses in every organ system except the gastrointestinal tract. Latency and recrudescence are common. *P. pseudomallei* is susceptible to many antibiotics in vitro. Tetracycline, chloramphenicol or gentamicin, alone or in combination, may be the treatment of choice. Trimethoprim-sulfamethoxazole may be effective.

Outbreaks of nosocomial bacteremia due to *P. cepacia* secondary to contaminated antiseptic and disinfectants used in cleaning equipment or in skin asepsis for intravenous infusions have been described. Certain other pseudomonads may cause infections in humans. These include *P. fluorescens*, *P. maltophilia*, and *P. putida*. Less frequent are *P. acidovorans*, *P. alcaligenes*, *P. putrefaciens*, *P. pseudoalcaligenes*, *P. testosteroni*, *P. dimunita*, and *P. mendocina*. These organisms vary widely in their antimicrobial susceptibility and treatment should be guided by in vitro susceptibility tests.

AEROMONAS INFECTIONS

Organisms of the *Aeromonas* group are found in natural water sources and soil and are frequent pathogens for cold-blooded marine and fresh water animals. The most important members are *A. hydrophilia* and *A. shigelloides*. They may easily be mistaken in the laboratory for *E. coli*.

Aeromonads have been associated in man with septicemia, pneumonia and moderate to severe gastroenteritis. Their recognized incidence in serious human disease has been steadily increasing and many more cases are probably misdiagnosed as being due to coliforms. The organisms have also been isolated from urine, sputum, feces and bile without evident pathogenic significance.

Aeromonads are resistant to penicillin and ampicillin. Most strains are susceptible to gentamicin, the tetracyclines and colistin.

NONCHOLERA *VIBRIO* INFECTIONS

Vibrios are curved, motile, gram-negative bacilli, with a single polar flagellum. Of the 34 species described, *Vibrio cholerae* is the major pathogen; it and related vibrios produce cholera in man. Certain additional members of the genus *Vibrio* cause disease in man and animals, whereas others are found commonly in the normal flora of man. This group of vibrios, similar biochemically and morphologically to the cholera vibrio, but not agglutinated by cholera polyvalent O antiserum, is commonly referred to as noncholera vibrios; they are agglutinated by their homologous antisera. These vibrios may cause mild diarrhea, frank cholera-like disease, or sepsis.

Vibrio parahaemolyticus,* a marine organism, resembles the cholera vibrio in many respects but grows best in the presence of 2 to 6 per cent sodium chloride. It appears to be pathogenic only for man and the organisms are not found in the feces of asymptomatic persons. It is found with increasing frequency in cases of "food poisoning" in various countries, including the United States, where sea foods are regularly consumed. In Japan it accounts for about half of the cases of bacterial food poisoning. The gastroenteritis is infectious rather than toxic. *V. parahaemolyticus* infections of the extremities, eyes, and ears, as well as the blood stream have recently been recognized in the United States. These usually occur in persons cut or scratched by the sharp edges of clams or oysters embedded in the sand of marine shore areas.

Vibrio fetus infections occur in cattle, sheep, and goats, resulting in abortions and sterility in infected herds. Human infections due to *V. fetus*, unknown before 1947, are recognized with increasing frequency in infants, pregnant women (in whom it is associated with abortion), and elderly persons. In the great majority of cases the organism is isolated from the blood stream, but it has also been recovered from the placenta, synovial fluid, and spinal fluid.

So-called related vibrios, morphologically similar to, but serologically distinct from, *V. fetus*, may occasionally cause disease in man.

Noncholera vibrios are inhibited by a variety of antibiotics. Gentamicin is the drug of choice against infections due to *V. parahaemolyticus* but ampicillin, tetracycline, chloramphenicol, cephalothin and kanamycin are frequently effective. Most strains of *V. fetus* are inhibited by tetracycline, chloramphenicol, ampicillin, streptomycin and kanamycin.

YERSINIAE INFECTIONS

The genus *Yersiniae* (family *Enterobacteriaceae*) consists of three species: *Y. pestis*, the causative agent of plague (which will not be considered here); *Y. pseudotuberculosis*, and *Y. enterocolitica*. The two latter organisms are relatively large gram-negative coccobacilli capable of producing disease in man. There is an extensive animal reservoir including mammals (rabbits, pig, cow, mouse, chinchilla) and birds, and occasional cases of animal-to-human transmission have been inferred. Acquisition from contaminated water has been suggested, and the coexistence of positive cultures for both *Yersinia* (*Y. enterocolitica*) and *Salmonella* in several instances also supports a common source for both organisms. Although originally considered as rare causes of human infection, they have been recognized with increasing frequency, especially those due to *Y. enterocolitica*, in both Europe and the United States. The *Yersiniae* may be misidentified as atypical coliform organisms.

Clinical infection with these two organisms takes one of two forms: gastrointestinal and systemic varieties. Acute mesenteric lymphadenitis or enterocolitis is usually a benign process which may mimic acute appendicitis or various types of diarrheal disease. The organism can be isolated from the enlarged mesenteric lymph nodes. The septicemic form which resembles typhoid or paratyphoid fever occurs particularly in patients with underlying disease such as nutritional deficiencies and blood dyscrasias. Abscesses may develop in various organs. The mortality may reach 50 per cent.

Y. pseudotuberculosis, originally designated as *Pasteurella pseudotuberculosis*, is a gram-negative motile (at 22 to 26°C.) bacillus that grows readily in the usual culture media. It has antigenic relationships to the salmonellae. The organism has frequently been cultured from a wide variety of animals, is excreted in the feces of an infected animal and may be spread by skin contamination or oral ingestion. The mode of human infestation has not been clearly defined.

In humans, *Y. pseudotuberculosis* may cause one of two clinical pictures. Generalized infection may occur with high spiking temperature

---

*Initially named *Pasteurella parahaemolytica*.

and septicemic foci in the liver and spleen. The diagnosis is established by blood culture. This form is very severe and, if untreated, may cause death in 10 to 20 days. Mesenteric lymphadenitis, which is a less serious form, clinically may resemble acute appendicitis with the acute onset of abdominal pain, fever and lymphocytosis. At exploratory laparotomy the appendix is normal but there is enlargement of the mesenteric lymph nodes, which show abscess formation, occasionally inflammation of the terminal ileum and cecum with exudate in the peritoneal cavity. *Y. pseudotuberculosis* infections as well as those due to *Y. enterocolitica* may be accompanied by primary pulmonary hilar adenopathy and erythema nodosum. Disease in man may also clinically resemble regional enteritis and other diseases associated with enlarged ileocecal lymph nodes and terminal ileitis such as tuberculosis, amebiasis, actinomycosis, and ulcerative colitis; tularemia, cat-scratch disease, lymphogranuloma inguinale, and certain viral infections. The lack of human case reports of this disease from this country is probably due to the fact that few surgeons have considered this diagnosis or obtained appropriate cultures in patients with the clinical picture of mesenteric adenitis and appendicitis.

Specific treatment of mesenteric lymphadenitis due to *Y. pseudotuberculosis* has not been necessary since the disease is a self-limited one. Antibiotic therapy is suggested, however, for patients with sepsis or prolonged elevation of serologic titers. The causative organism is sensitive to the tetracyclines, chloramphenicol, and streptomycin in vitro, and these drugs are usually effective clinically. Kanamycin (and perhaps other aminoglycosides), ampicillin, and cephalothin are also active in vitro.

Y. enterocolitica is a gram-negative bacillus which has in recent years manifested a spectacular spread as a human pathogen. Its role in disease is not yet clearly delineated but it has been incriminated in a variety of disorders including diarrheal disease (enterocolitis), terminal ileitis, acute mesenteric adenitis, arthritis, erythema nodosum and septicemia.

It was first recognized as a pathogenic invader in the chinchilla and the hare, but it has since been isolated from a wide spectrum of the animal kingdom. Geographically, it initially seemed to be confined to Scandinavia, Belgium, and France, but now it is being recognized throughout the world.

The most frequent isolations are from children, over half of whom are less than 2 years of age. The clinical picture depends on the age of the patient. Infants and young children less than 4 years of age characteristically have a diarrheal syndrome, whereas older children usually develop acute lesions of the terminal ileum or acute mesenteric lymphadenitis resembling appendicitis or regional enteritis. Adolescents and adults may present with enteritis and fever. In patients with the diarrheal form, abdominal pain, vomiting and fever are frequent. The stools may be bloody and contain mucus and neutrophils. In addition, arthralgia, arthritis of various joints, and a variety of rashes, usually erythematous but including erythema nodosum, can be observed. The extraintestinal manifestations are more frequent in older children. The course of the disease is usually self-limited (three days to three weeks), although chronic diarrhea may occasionally ensue. A septicemic-typhoid–like disease has been observed in individuals of any age with a serious underlying disease.

Most of the cases so far have been of diarrhea in children with about half of the total in infants and children less than 2 years of age. Infection can be spread from person to person directly. Infections with *Y. enterocolitica* have also been associated with other pathogenic organisms, with a hospital outbreak, and with a familial occurrence.

The diagnosis is bacteriological by culture of the organism from feces, mesenteric gland, appendix, or serum, and by determination of the antibody level. Human sera in Europe and Japan have usually yielded antibodies to serotypes 3 and 9, whereas in the United States, type 8 has been involved; in South Africa the sera were type 3. The antibody test is very specific, and a high titer is found within eight to nine days. A positive test may persist for several months. There is mounting evidence that *Y. enterocolitica* is far more prevalent than previously suspected. If a patient presents with symptoms suggestive of an infection with this organism, the clinician should request specific laboratory investigation for it.

Y. enterocolitica is usually susceptible to the tetracyclines, streptomycin, chloramphenicol, neomycin, kanamycin, gentamicin, the polymyxins, and nalidixic acid, but insensitive to penicillin and ampicillin. However, the efficacy of antibiotics in the treatment of this disease has not been clearly established.

INFECTIONS DUE TO OTHER GRAM-NEGATIVE BACILLI

Other Enterobacteriaceae

There are certain other members of the Enterobacteriaceae which sometimes cause infection in man. *Arizona* organisms are coliform organisms which also belong to the Enterobacteriaceae family. As mentioned previously, these organisms more closely resemble Salmonella. However, nosocomial infections due to members of this group, notably *Arizona hinshawii*, have been described.

Edwardsiella. The recently (1965) established genus, *Edwardsiella*, includes a group of motile, lactose-negative organisms which resemble salmonellae in some biochemical features and sometimes in pathogenicity for man. They ferment only glucose and maltose. *E. tarda* has been isolated from a variety of mammals and reptiles. It is occasionally found in the intestinal tract of man, especially in acute gastroenteritis, and it can produce serious septic infections. However, man is likely only an accidental host. Tetracyclines, chloramphenicol, kanamycin* and ampicillin are drugs of choice.

Citrobacter. The *Citrobacter* group is composed of Enterobacteriaceae previously designated as *Escherichia freundii* and the Bethesda-Ballerup of "paracolon" organisms. The majority of strains form hydrogen and are delayed lactose fermenters. They are differentiated from salmonellae by various biochemical reactions and growth characteristics.

The Bethesda-Ballerup portion of the group has been extensively studied and an antigenic scheme established. Members of the Bethesda-Ballerup subgroup have been associated with diarrhea in man but they are not considered true enteric pathogens.

Citrobacter strains occur infrequently in normal feces. They have been recovered from urinary tract infections in various septic processes. Drugs of choice are polymyxin B or colistin, gentamicin,* kanamycin and chloramphenicol. Some strains are susceptible to tetracycline.

Other Gram-Negative Bacilli

Acinetobacter. Organisms† in the genus *Acinetobacter* (formerly *Mimeae*) are widely distributed in nature (water, soil, milk). They are also carried on the skin and in the gastrointestinal, genital, and respiratory tracts of up to 25 per cent of healthy individuals. In the last decade there has been a steady increase in their incidence in a variety of infections, often hospital-acquired, including meningitis, septicemia, and wound, genital, and urinary tract infections. Virulence of *Acinetobacter* organisms appears to be low, and they are mainly opportunistic pathogens in patients with burns or with immunologic deficiency. However, severe primary infections (meningitis, septicemia) do occur in children and young adults in apparently good health.

The organisms are nonmotile, plump, paired gram-negative rods ("diplobacilli"). In the stationary phase they often appear as diplococci, easily mistaken for *Neisseriae*. They are obligately aerobic but oxidase-negative.

Acinetobacter lwoffi (previously *Mimi polymorpha* and *Achromobacter lwoffi*) neither ferments nor oxidizes carbohydrates, whereas *Acinetobacter anitratus* (previously *Herellea vaginicola* and *Achromobacter anitratus*) utilizes glucose oxidatively and produces acid from 10 per cent (but not from 1 per cent) lactose-containing medium. These organisms are frequently antibiotic-resistant and antibiotic susceptibility tests are required as a guide to therapy. Drugs likely to be effective are kanamycin, gentamicin, tobramycin, polymyxins and sometimes the tetracyclines.

Moraxella. Moraxellas* are similar to *Acinetobacter* but are oxidase-positive and highly susceptible to penicillin. They are primary animal parasites, most commonly present on the mucous membranes. Most of these organisms do not utilize carbohydrates.

M. osloensis and *M. nonliquefaciens* (collectively, *Mima polymorpha* var. *oxidans* in the American clinical literature) are members of the normal flora of man and also are opportunistic pathogens. They have been isolated in pneumonia, septicemia, otitis, urethritis, and rarely, meningitis. Because of their microscopic appearance and positive oxidase reaction, they are easily confused with *Neisseria gonorrheae* and *N. meningitidis*. Their etiological significance in mixed cultures is uncertain. *M. lacunata* (the Morax-Axenfeld bacillus) is a rare cause of conjunctivitis and corneal infections.

Alcaligenes.* *A. faecalis* fails to ferment or oxidize any of the usual carbohydrates; it is usually motile. It may occasionally be confused on initial isolation with other nonlactose fermenters, chiefly *Salmonella* or *Shigella*. It may be encountered in feces or in sputum as a harmless saprophyte, but it has also been associated with serious infections. Since it is durable, the organism has been involved in contamination of irrigating fluids and intravenous solutions, causing epidemics of urinary tract infections and postoperative septicemia. These organisms are not uniformly sensitive to any antibiotic; tetracycline and chloramphenicol are usually the most effective.

Flavobacterium. Flavobacteria* are

---

*Other aminoglycoside antibiotics may also be effective but clinical experience to date is limited.
†Also nonfermenter.

---

*Also "nonfermenter."

widely distributed in soil and water and are encountered as opportunistic pathogens in man. The members of this heterogeneous group are usually oxidative but may be fermentative, form a yellow pigment (hence the name), are oxidase-positive, and usually are nonmotile.

F. meningosepticum has high virulence for the newborn, especially low birth weight infants, in whom it has caused outbreaks of septicemia and meningitis with a very high mortality rate. While these infections are usually attributed to contaminated hospital equipment and solutions, recent isolation of *F. meningosepticum* from the female genitalia suggests this possible source. The organism also occurs in postoperative bacteremia of adults, in whom the illness is much milder. Other flavobacteria may be recovered from the sputum of grossly debilitated patients, but their etiological role is uncertain.

Infants with fatal meningitis due to flavobacteria sometimes have body temperatures below normal, where adults with flavobacterial septicemia usually have high temperatures and recover rapidly. Since many strains of *F. meningosepticum* cannot grow at 38°C., it has been suggested that body temperature is an important factor in the response of infants with flavobacterial meningitis. The organism has an unusual antibiotic susceptibility pattern for a gram-negative bacillus. It is usually susceptible in vitro to erythromycin, novobiocin, and rifampin, and to a lesser degree to chloramphenicol and streptomycin, but is resistant to gentamicin and polymyxins.

Streptobacillus moniliformis. *Streptobacillus moniliformis,* the cause of one type of rat-bite fever, is carried by many rats presumably as a saprophyte. The organism is an aerobic gram-negative bacillus. It may assume a minute L form which is filterable and resistant to penicillin. In old cultures, especially in solid media, it forms chains with swellings resembling yeast buds, hence the designation "moniliformis."

Streptobacillary rat-bite fever has an incubation period following an infectious rat bite ranging from 2 to 7 days. The local lesion is not distinctive and may be overlooked even when fever erupts. In contrast to spirillary rat-bite fever, the streptobacillary form has a greater tendency to produce a maculopapular rash, arthralgia, arthritis, subcutaneous abscesses, endocarditis and erythemia nodosum. When *S. moniliformis* infects man by the respiratory or alimentary tract instead of by rat bite, the resulting condition is referred to as Haverhill fever. The incubation period is short, often less than 5 days with abrupt onset of fever, chills, headache, vomiting, myalgia and arthralgia and a maculopapular rash. Recurrent cycles of fever are characteristic and at times large metastatic subcutaneous abscesses may appear. Arthritis is prominent. Organisms may be recovered from any of the infected parts.

The organism may be cultured in vitro or recovered by animal inoculation with patient's blood or material from an abscess or an affected joint. A rise in titer of specific agglutinins is also helpful.

Penicillin-G is the treatment of choice but streptomycin and tetracycline are also therapeutically effective. The wound should be immediately cleansed with soap and water. Tetanus prophylaxis should be carried out by standard methods.

Calymmatobacterium (Donovania) granulomatis. Granuloma inguinale is an indolent, ulcerative disease caused by a gram-negative bacillus which is antigenically similar to, but not identical with, *Klebsiella pneumoniae* and *K. rhinoscleromatis.* It is usually transmitted during sexual intercourse but is not highly communicable. The initial lesion commonly appears on or about the genitalia, beginning as a painful nodule. It soon breaks down, forming a sharply demarcated ulcer which spreads by direct extension and often destroys large areas of skin in the groins and about the anus and genitalia. In Wright-stain smears of scrapings from the lesions, the encapsuled causative organism, *C. granulomatis* ("Donovan bodies"), can often be seen within the pathognomonic large mononuclear cells. Granuloma inguinale can be treated successfully with tetracyclines, chloramphenicol or streptomycin. Penicillin G is not effective.

Bartonella bacilliformis. *Bartonella bacilliformis* is a gram-negative, very pleomorphic, motile organism which causes in humans two different clinical manifestations of the same geographically restricted bacterial disease.* The collective designation of the two syndromes is Carrion's disease. The infection is limited to the mountainous areas of the American Andes in tropical Peru, Colombia and Ecuador and is transmitted by the sand fly Phlebotomus.

Bartonella grows on semisolid nutrient agar containing 10 per cent rabbit serum and 0.5 per cent hemoglobin. After about 10 days of incubation at 28° C., some turbidity develops in the medium, and rod-shaped and granular organisms can be seen in sustained smears.

---

*Recently cases of anemia with *Bartonella*-like bodies have been reported from Southeast Asia.

Oroya fever is characterized by the rapid development of severe anemia due to blood destruction, enlargement of the spleen and liver and hemorrhage into the lymph nodes. Masses of Bartonella fill the cytoplasm of cells lining the blood vessel, and endothelial swelling may lead to vascular occlusion and thrombosis. The mortality of untreated Oroya fever is about 40 per cent. The diagnosis is made by examining stained blood smears and blood cultures in semisolid agar media. The initial stage of infection is frequently complicated by *Salmonella* superinfection and *Salmonella* is responsible for many of the deaths. In those who recover, convalescence is slow and blood cultures may remain positive for many months.

The severe anemic stage of the disease may be followed in two to eight weeks by a cutaneous stage (verruga peruana). Verruga peruana is a vascular granulomatous skin lesion which occurs in successive crops, lasts for about one year and produces little systemic reaction and no fatalities. *Bartonella* can be seen in the granuloma. Blood cultures are often positive but there is no anemia.

Penicillin, streptomycin, and chloramphenicol are dramatically effective in Oroya fever and greatly reduce the fatality rate, particularly if blood transfusions are also given. Control of the disease depends upon the elimination of the sand fly vectors. Insecticides, DDT, insect repellents and elimination of breeding areas are of value. Prevention with antibiotics may be useful. Chloramphenicol should be used when the patient is also suffering from secondary *Salmonella* infection.

Others. There are a few other gram-negative bacilli which very rarely cause human infection but have been reported to do so. The type of infection they cause is variable but may be bacteremic or localized in various organ systems. Selection of antimicrobial therapy should be based on in vitro susceptibility test results. The agents which are usually effective are listed.

Actinobacillus actinomycetemcomitans (HB group)	Tetracycline Streptomycin Chloramphenicol
Actinobacillus lignieresii	Kanamycin
Bordetella bronchiseptica	Tetracycline Polymyxins Chloramphenicol
Chromobacterium	Kanamycin or Gentamicin Tetracycline Chloramphenicol
Comamonas terrigenia	Chloramphenicol Tetracycline
Erwinia (now classified as *Enterobacter agglomerans*)	Gentamicin Chloramphenicol Colistin Kanamycin
Hemophilus aphrodilus (HB group)	Penicillin-G Gentamicin Cephalothin Chloramphenicol Tetracycline

Infections Due to Anaerobic Cocci and Gram-Negative Anaerobic Bacilli

JOSEPH W. ST. GEME, Jr., M.D.

Renewed interest in these important bacteria has arisen during the past several years, spurred on by improved and more consistently employed methods for their isolation. The most important pathogens are anaerobic and microaerophilic streptococci, *Bacteroides fragilis* and *melaninogenicus,* and *Fusobacterium nucleatum.* Although some infections are produced by solitary anaerobic pathogens, many of these infections represent mixtures of several aerobic and anaerobic organisms.

Bacteremia. Approximately 10 per cent of all bacteremic illness is caused by anaerobic organisms which gain access to the bloodstream from abdominal foci of infection. The great majority of these serious infections are caused by *B. fragilis,* 90 per cent of which are resistant to penicillin. Mortality rates of 30 per cent or more in the past have been reduced to 15 per cent by vigorous treatment of shock and acidosis with colloid, vasoactive drugs, sodium bicarbonate and careful monitoring of pulse, arterial pressure, central venous pressure, respiratory rate and urinary flow. Either parenteral chloramphenicol sodium succinate (Chloromycetin; 50 to 100 mg./kg./day intravenously in four doses for older infants and children, 2 to 4 gm./day in four doses for larger adolescents) or clindamycin (clindamycin phosphate; 10 to 40 mg./kg./day intravenously or intramuscularly in four doses for older infants and children, 1 to 2 gm./day intravenously or intramuscularly in four doses for larger adolescents) may be used to terminate the *B. fragilis* bacteremia.

Bacterial endocarditis is caused by anaerobic or microaerophilic streptococci in 4 per cent of cases. These infections can be treated by large doses of penicillin (penicillin G, crystalline, 100,000 to 400,000 units/kg./day intravenously or intramuscularly in four to six doses for older infants, children and adolescents).

Anaerobic bacteremia occurs in the newborn. If *B. fragilis* is isolated, the current therapeutic regimen of penicillin and aminoglycoside antibiotic must be modified.

Abdominal Infection. Perforations of the gastrointestinal tract predispose to peritoneal and pelvic suppuration. These infections are caused by a mixture of aerobic organisms, such as *E. coli, Klebsiella pneumoniae,* Proteus species, *Pseudomonas aeruginosa* and enterococci, and anaerobic organisms, such as *B. fragilis,* Clostridia species and peptostreptococci. Less serious infections complicate lower small bowel perforations, such as a ruptured appendix, because the microbial population of this region of the gut is 1000-fold less than that of the colon. Although preliminary data suggest that clindamycin may be preferable to penicillin or ampicillin (150 to 200 mg./kg./day intravenously or intramuscularly in four doses for older infants and children, 8 to 12 gm./day intravenously or intramuscularly in four doses for larger adolescents), periappendiceal abscesses are managed effectively by surgical drainage and combined treatment with penicillin and kanamycin (15 mg./kg./day intramuscularly in three doses for older infants and children, 1 to 2 gm./day intramuscularly in three doses for larger adolescents).

Respiratory Infection. Aspiration pneumonitis usually represents a mixed bacterial infection with anaerobic organisms outnumbering aerobic pathogens. Lung abscesses are also mixed infections caused ordinarily by *S. aureus, K. pneumoniae* and beta hemolytic streptococci as solitary or multiple aerobic pathogens and complicated in treatment by the presence of a significant population of anaerobic streptococci, and occasionally *B. melaninogenicus* and *F. nucleatum.* Because *B. fragilis* is rarely isolated from lung abscesses, these serious pulmonary infections can be treated with penicillin (50,000 to 100,000 units/kg./day intravenously or intramuscularly in four to six doses) and either methicillin (200 to 300 mg./kg./day intravenously or intramuscularly in four to six doses for older infants and children, 8 to 12 gm./day intravenously or intramuscularly in four to six doses for larger adolescents)* or an aminoglycoside antibiotic, such as kanamycin or gentamicin (5 to 7 mg./

kg./day intramuscularly in three doses), for the staphylococcal and Klebsiella species, respectively. Adequate hydration and vigorous postural tracheobronchial toilet are also critically important elements of treatment.

Chronic sinusitis is also caused by similar pluralistic aerobic and anaerobic infections. In 25 per cent of cases, pure cultures of anaerobic streptococci can be recovered. These chronic infections should also be treated with penicillin and adequate medical decongestants or, if necessary, surgical drainage.

Cerebral Infection. About 30 per cent of all brain abscesses are caused by anaerobic streptococci, regardless of the nature of predisposing factors such as cyanotic congenital heart disease, chronic mastoiditis or chronic sinusitis. Mixed infection with aerobic pathogens also occurs. Treatment consists of surgical drainage, large doses of parenteral penicillin for the anaerobic infection and the appropriate antibiotic for the aerobic bacterium if a mixed infection is detected.

Cutaneous Infection. Serious ulcerative, necrotizing and crepitant cellulitis, fasciitis and myositis can occur as a result of mixed infection in the skin and deeper tissues with staphylococci and coliform organisms on the one hand and anaerobic streptococci and bacteroides species on the other. Methicillin, penicillin and chloramphenicol or clindamycin in the usual doses constitute specific antimicrobial treatment.

General Therapeutic Principles. With the exception of bacteremia, when thinking of anaerobic bacterial disease one must design treatment for mixed infection. Penicillin is the antibiotic of choice for the vast majority of anaerobic infections, since *Bacteroides fragilis* is an uncommon pathogen in most tissues and organs. *Bacteroides fragilis* species, a major cause of pure bacteremia and resistant to penicillin, must be treated with chloramphenicol or clindamycin. Clindamycin has produced some cases of pseudomembranous colitis, and continued surveillance of this new antibiotic will be necessary. The cephalosporins are less effective than penicillin, and the aminoglycosides, tetracyclines and erythromycin are of no value in the eradication of an anaerobic pathogen. One must treat anaerobic infections with surgical drainage and the resection of necrotic tissue. This precept of therapeutic management cannot be emphasized enough.

---

*There is as yet no specific recommendation for the use of intravenous methicillin in infants and children.

Hemophilus Influenzae Infections

SYDNEY ROSS, M.D.,
WILLIAM RODRIGUEZ, M.D., Ph. D.,
and WAHEED KHAN, Ph.D.

Hemophilus influenzae is an extremely important cause of a broad spectrum of mild, moderate and severe infections in infants and children. The incidence of these infections is greatest between the ages of three months to three years. The mild to moderate infections include otitis media, bronchitis and cellulitis; serious infections are sequelae of septicemia with resulting localization in diverse sites producing meningitis, pyogenic arthritis, osteomyelitis, obstructive epiglottis and pneumonia.

MENINGITIS

H. influenzae, type b, is the most common cause of meningitis in the United States, accounting for approximately 65 per cent of cases. The most frequent occurrence is in children under five years of age, with the peak incidence in the 9 to 12 month age group.

Conventional laboratory diagnostic methods include Gram stain and culture of the CSF together with glucose and protein determinations. Recently, other diagnostic methods including LDH, limulus lysate, CIE (counterimmunoelectrophoresis), lactic acid and latex agglutination tests on the CSF have been used successfully as ancillary parameters in the rapid diagnosis of meningitis. Results with these five methods are generally available within one hour after lumbar puncture is performed. Three of the five procedures can be done at the bedside. The importance of these newer diagnostic methods is particularly apparent in partially treated cases where sterilization of the CSF may follow antecedent therapy. Since these newer methods (excluding lactic acid) depend on either endotoxin production or breakdown products of bacteria (metabolites or enzymes), they are less susceptible to alteration by prior antibiotic therapy.

The recent emergence of ampicillin-resistant *H. influenzae* has altered the therapeutic approach. Our recent experience in the greater Washington area has shown a 9 per cent incidence of resistant strains of *H. influenzae* (including both typable and nontypable organisms). In other geographic locations, a lesser incidence of resistance has been reported; however, each community should continually monitor its *H. influenzae* isolates for possible increasing incidence of ampicillin resistance. The American Academy of Pediatrics has recently recommended that a drug effective against ampicillin-resistant *H. influenzae* be used in areas where such strains have been isolated. Specifically, the Academy's recommendations for *H. influenzae* meningitis are as follows: (1) ampicillin, 400 mg/kg/day, in combination with chloramphenicol sodium succinate, 100 mg/kg/day, both given intravenously as initial antibiotic therapy; (2) discontinuation of either antibiotic after the results of antibiotic susceptibilities are obtained; (3) antibiotic therapy for at least seven days after defervescence or 10 to 14 days of total treatment with no change in dosage or mode of administration during the entire treatment period; and (4) intrathecal administration of antibiotics should be avoided.

Carbenicillin in a daily dose of 400 mg./kg. intravenously has also proved to be effective antibiotic therapy in our hands. As previously noted, the drug is more resistant than ampicillin to the degradative effects of beta lactamase. Thus far, we have treated 60 patients with ampicillin-sensitive *H. influenzae* meningitis with carbenicillin with a 5 per cent mortality rate; that mortality rate is similar to that previously encountered with ampicillin or chloramphenicol. Further experience is needed, however, before we would recommend it as a possible substitute modality of therapy.

Repeat lumbar punctures should be performed 24 and 72 hours after initiation of therapy and within 24 hours after therapy is discontinued. CSF smear, culture, chemistries, colony count, tests for antigen (CIE), endotoxin (limulus lysate) and enzymes or metabolites (LDH, lactic acid) should be done on each repeat lumbar puncture. The rapid return to normal of these various parameters suggests a good prognosis, whereas tardy normalization connotes guarded outlook.

Serum electrolytes are monitored at least once daily during the initial three days. Serum and urine osmolality as well as urine electrolytes are performed to detect inappropriate ADH secretion if indicated.

Daily head circumference measurements and transillumination of the skull on appropriate patients are done routinely. The use of radioisotopes and the computerized axial tomography scan is reserved for patients with delayed resolution or with a rapidly changing clinical picture including continuous fever, convulsions, signs of increased intracranial pressure or abnormal head growth.

The diagnosis of cerebral edema may be made on the basis of unconsciousness, hypertension, bradycardia, opisthotonus, respiratory irregularity and/or increased CSF pressure of

300 mm. of water or greater. In this situation, mannitol* in a dose of 1.5 gm./kg. over a 30 minute period, is given intravenously and may be repeated in 6 to 12 hours if necessary. In addition, Solu-Cortef (5 mg./kg.) is given in single intravenous dose followed concurrently by dexamethasone in a dose of 10 mg./m² intravenously initially and 20 mg./m² in 24 hours in six hour divided doses. Dexamethasone is continued until evidence of cerebral edema is no longer present.

Subdural taps are performed if a strong suspicion exists of *clinically significant* subdural collection of fluids based on clinical observation. A brain scan may confirm such suspicions. If positive and clinically significant, subdural taps should be repeated on a one to three day schedule until dry, or approximately two to three weeks. Persistence of significant effusions in spite of repeated subdural taps may suggest the necessity of a temporary external free-flowing drain. Failure of this measure constitutes an indication for a subdural-pleural shunt.

Convulsions during the acute phase are managed with diazepam† intravenously in a dose of 0.2 mg./kg. and phenobarbital or phenytoin. These drugs should be used as prophylactic anticonvulsants after hospital discharge if a recurrent convulsive state persists.

Supportive care includes one to one nursing care with constant monitoring of cardiovascular, respiratory, thermoregulatory, and neurological parameters. This intensive nursing care should continue at least until the patient is in a stable condition. This care is of particular importance if the white blood cell count on admission shows a leukopoenia. Usually, intravenous fluids are maintained at two-thirds of normal requirements. Supervening complications of septic shock are handled in a fashion similar to gram-negative endotoxic shock. It is important to remember that vasopressors are not indicated. It is also important to remember that a central venous pressure line may be indicated in the severely ill child.

ACUTE EPIGLOTTITIS

This infection is characterized by a rapid onset of croup, prostration and fever with associated respiratory distress. The hallmark is the presence of a large, cherry-red epiglottis which can obstruct the ingress and egress of air, producing marked obstructive symptoms. Lateral neck films are helpful in making the diagnosis prior to laryngoscopy.

Therapy initially consists of quickly establishing an airway by tracheostomy or nasotracheal intubation. Continuous physician supervision is of prime importance, at least until establishment of the airway. This constitutes an emergency measure and it is important not to temporize. Antibiotic therapy should be started immediately consisting of a combination of ampicillin, 150 mg./kg./day, and chloramphenicol sodium succinate, 100 mg./kg./day intravenously in a six hour divided dosage schedule. Either of these antibiotics can be deleted, depending on the susceptibility of the *H. influenzae* strain which is frequently isolated on blood culture. Antibiotic therapy should be continued for 7 to 10 days.

SEPTIC ARTHRITIS

Pyogenic arthritis is not uncommonly due to *H. influenzae,* type b, in infants and young children. Aspiration generally yields yellow-green pus with the causative organism readily identifiable on smear and culture. Conservative therapy with an appropriate antibiotic generally suffices; however, in cases of septic arthritis of the *hip* joint, surgical drainage is indicated concomitantly. Antibiotic therapy may be employed as follows: (1) ampicillin, 200 mg./kg./day intravenously in a six hour divided dosage schedule for 10 to 14 days; (2) if the organism is ampicillin-resistant, use chloramphenicol sodium succinate, 100 mg./kg./day intravenously for 10 to 14 days, *or* cefamandole,* 100 mg./kg./day intravenously for 10 to 14 days; and (3) since there is good extravasation across synovial membranes after parenteral administration, it is not necessary to instill these antibiotics into the joint space.

ACUTE OSTEOMYELITIS

Infrequently, *H. influenzae,* type b, is a cause of acute osteomyelitis. Treatment consists of either ampicillin or chloramphenicol in doses indicated for meningitis for at least four weeks. Surgical drainage may be necessary.

SOFT TISSUE CELLULITIS

Soft tissue cellulitis, particularly of the face and neck in young children under two years of age, should raise suspicion of *H. influenzae,* type b, as a possible causative organism. In approximately 50 per cent of instances of *H. influenzae* cellulitis, the lesion has a bluish or

---

*Manufacturer's note: There is as yet no established dosage of mannitol for children.

†Manufacturer's precaution: Safety and efficacy of injectable diazepam have not been established in the neonate.

---

*Cefamandole is an investigational drug not yet approved by the Food and Drug Administration.

purplish-red hue. High fever and bacteremia are frequently present together with accompanying upper respiratory symptoms. The differential diagnosis would include streptococcal erysipelas, insect bites and trauma. Therapy consists of either ampicillin 200 mg./kg./day, chloramphenicol sodium succinate, 100 mg./kg./day, or cefamandole,* 100 mg./kg./day, intravenously in a six hour divided dosage schedule for 5 to 7 days.

OTITIS MEDIA

Nontypable *H. influenzae* constitutes one of the major etiologic agents in middle ear disease in infants and children. The incidence of ampicillin resistance among nontypable strains varies geographically. Our monitoring in the Washington area has yielded a rate of 9 per cent resistant strains. More recently, Schwartz (unpublished data) has found a 16 per cent incidence of nontypable resistant strains isolated on tympanocentesis over a 12-month period during 1976 in the Fairfax, Virginia area; this represented a ten-fold increase over the previous year. Since the vast majority of practicing pediatricians (96 per cent) do not or cannot perform a myringotomy in office practice, middle ear fluid is rarely available for culture. In the absence of aspirated middle ear fluid for diagnostic purposes, a nasopharyngeal swab cultured in 5 per cent sheep's blood agar (for pneumococcus and beta hemolytic group A streptococcus) and Filde's or Levinthal's media (for *H. influenzae*) may give some indication regarding the causative organism in the middle ear if the microorganisms show growth on the plate; pure (90 to 100 per cent) or heavy (70 to 90 per cent) growth are consonant with the etiological agent in the middle ear (Schwartz, unpublished data).

There are several modalities of therapy for otitis media: (1) ampicillin, 75 to 100 mg./kg./day; (2) amoxicillin, 40 to 50 mg./kg./day; (3) phenoxymethyl penicillin, 50 mg./kg./day, *plus* sulfisoxazole (Gantrisin), 100 mg./kg./day; (4) erythromycin, 40 mg./kg./day, *plus* sulfisoxazole (Gantrisin), 100 mg./kg./day; and (5) cephalexin, 100 mg./kg./day. All these alternative modes of therapy are given orally for 10 to 14 days. If a treatment failure ensues with ampicillin, the possibility of a resistant strain of Hemophilus should be considered and alternative therapy initiated.

---

*Cefamandole is an investigational drug not yet approved by the Food and Drug Administration.

Tetanus

DEXTER S. Y. SETO, M.D.

Tetanus is an acute infection caused by the anaerobic spore-forming bacterium *Clostridia tetani* and is clinically manifested by neuromuscular dysfunction. This results from an exotoxin (tetanospasmin) which is produced by the organism at the site of infection, which is transported and affects the central nervous system.

The objectives of therapy are to provide optimal support care until the tetanospasmin that is fixed to the nervous tissue has been metabolized, to neutralize circulating toxin, and to remove the source of tetanospasmin. The best results follow aggressive and intensive coordinated efforts by medical, nursing, and anesthesiology personnel at experienced centers.

SPECIFIC THERAPY

Neutralization of Toxin. Tetanus antitoxin in sufficient quantity will prevent unbound toxin from reaching the central nervous system, but will have no effect on toxin already fixed to nervous tissue. There are two antitoxins available, human tetanus immune globulin (TIG) and equine or bovine antitoxin (TAT). TIG is preferable because it is associated with less side effects and it produces higher and more persistent titers of antitoxin. An injection of 4 to 5 units/kg. provides a plasma level of 0.01 to 0.02 units/ml. for 4 or more weeks. A dose of 3000 to 6000 units intramuscularly is recommended, although the optimal therapeutic dose has not been esablished. Several studies have suggested that smaller doses may be equally effective. Although it is recommended that part of the dose be infiltrated locally around the wound, there is no evidence to support that this is effective.

If TIG is not available, TAT should be given in a single dose of 50,000 to 100,000 units, divided equally between intramuscular and intravenous injections. Appropriate testing for hypersensitivity should first be done and if necessary, desensitization performed. Repeated doses of either TIG or TAT are not necessary.

Following recovery from clinical tetanus the patient should complete an active immunization schedule because tetanus is a nonimmunizing disease.

Eradication of the Infection. Thorough debridement of the wound should be done, all devitalized tissue excised, foreign bodies removed and the wound left open. The wound should also be irrigated with a 3 per cent hydrogen peroxide solution. This should be done only after the patient has received sedation, TIG, and antimicrobial therapy. Extensve surgical excision is usually not necessary.

Antibiotic therapy is effective in reducing the quantity of spore forms of the organism, thereby indirectly terminating further toxin production. It is also effective in controlling secondary infections. Penicillin G, 100,000 to 300,000 units/kg./day intravenously in divided doses, should be used for 10 to 14 days. The tetracyclines are also effective in those patients who are allergic to penicillin, but should not be used in infancy and early childhood because of their effects on bone growth and dentition.

SUPPORTIVE THERAPY

Sedation and Muscle Relaxation. Sedation is essential to prevent convulsions and to minimize muscle spasms. A number of sedatives and tranquilizers have been used alone and in combination depending on the severity of the problem. These drugs should be used with caution since they have depressive effects on vital functions and toxic effects, especially in neonates.

In mild to moderately severe tetanus, phenobarbital is effective at 2 to 3 mg./kg./day in divided doses every 6 hours. To stop seizures, the dose may be increased to a total of 10 to 15 mg./kg., and is slowly given intravenously, with one-half the dose given immediately, and one-fourth dose given every 5 minutes until the seizure stops. Phenobarbital should be given either orally if possible or intravenously.

Chlorpromazine (Thorazine) has been used alone or with phenobarbital. The usual dose is 2 mg./kg./day in divided doses every 6 hours orally or intramuscularly. Unless absolutely necessary, it is not recommended for use in infants.

Diazepam (Valium) has two useful actions, muscle-relaxant and tranquilizer. It can be used orally, intramuscularly or intravenously at 0.1 to 0.8 mg./kg./day in divided doses every 6 hours.* In moderate to severe tetanus, it is usually combined with either phenobarbital or chlorpromazine. Since diazepam potentiates the effect of phenobarbital, the dose of phenobarbital should be reduced. Because injectable diazepam has been shown to interfere with the binding of bilirubin to albumin, this injectable preparation should not be used in the neonate or jaundiced patient.

When the disease is severe and not responding to sedatives and muscle relaxants, the treatment of choice is neuromuscular

---

*Manufacturer's note: Safety and efficacy of injectable diazepam in the neonate have not been established.

blockade with D-tubocurarrine to produce paralysis. Suitable facilities and personnel are crucial since nasotracheal intubation (neonate) and tracheostomy (older child) are necessary to provide for artificial ventilation with an intermittent positive pressure respirator. Sedation with diazepam is essential with this approach.

Another drug that may be used primarily for its muscle relaxant effect is methocarbanol (Robaxin), found to be useful in patients suffering severe muscle spasms.

Other Supporting Measures. Maintenance of an airway and oxygenation is of prime importance. Recurrent spasms of the pharynx, glottis, and respiratory muscles may lead to excessive accumulation of secretions in the oropharynx. If gentle suctioning, sedation and positioning of the patient are not effective in preventing pooling of secretions, either nasotracheal intubation (neonate) or tracheostomy (older child) should be performed.

Satisfactory hydration can be maintained by intravenous fluids containing maintenance electrolytes and 5 per cent glucose. In mild cases oral or nasogastric tube feedings (especially in neonates) are sufficient for nutrition. If nasogastric tube feedings are used, the tube should be removed, left out for 6 to 10 hours, and changed daily to avoid esophageal irritation. Because of the risk of aspiration of food or gastric contents, both types of feedings should not be used until spasms are under control.

The patient should be turned frequently to avoid pressure sores and pulmonary stasis. External stimuli that might trigger paroxysmal spasms can be minimized by a quiet room and infrequent examinations.

The physician should be aware of potential complications and be prepared to administer appropriate care when necessary. These complications include aspiration pneumonia, atelectasis, pulmonary emboli, gastric ulcers, skin infections, decubitus, urinary retention, and catheter-related urinary infections, intramuscular hematomas, and compression fractures or subluxation of the vertebrae, most commonly the thoracic vertebrae. These complications can be minimized by proper aseptic technique in the use of the respirator equipment, adequate humidification, gentle suctioning of secretions, care in feeding and appropriate use of antibiotics.

PREVENTION

Because *Clostridia tetani* spores are widely distributed in the environment and naturally acquired immunity does not occur, active immunization is a universal requirement regardless of age.

The term tetanus-prone injuries usually applies to compound fractures, gunshot wounds, burns, crash injuries, wounds with retained foreign bodies, deep puncture wounds, wounds contaminated with soil or feces, and wounds unattended for more than 24 hours. Another type of wound that has been recently recognized as being responsible for 13 per cent of reported cases of tetanus is that of a subcutaneous abscess in drug addicts who are "skin poppers" (drug users who give themselves subcutaneous rather than intravenous injections).

Active Immunization. Tetanus toxoid is available in both fluid and adsorbed forms. Comparative tests have shown that the adsorbed toxoid is superior in inducing high antitoxin titers and achieving durable protection. There is very little difference in the induction of antibody responses to booster doses of either fluid or adsorbed toxoid to be of any clinical importance. Therefore, adsorbed tetanus toxoid is the choice for both primary and booster immunization. Three preparations that are available are (1) diphtheria and tetanus toxoid and pertussis vaccine (DTP), (2) tetanus and diphtheria toxoids, adult type (Td), and (3) tetanus toxoid (T). All preparations contain comparable amounts of tetanus toxoid, but the diphtheria component in the adult type (Td) is only about 15 to 20 per cent of that contained in the standard DTP.

Primary Immunization. In children 2 months through 6 years, DTP is recommended intramuscularly on three visits at 2 month intervals, with a fourth dose 1 year after the third injection. Ideally, the series should begin at 2 months of age. In school children and adults who have not been previously immunized, a series of three doses of Td is recommended, with the second dose 4 to 6 weeks after the first, and the third dose 6 to 12 months after the second. In those children who have been only partially immunized, the schedule for their appropriate age can be finished irrespective of when the last immunization was given.

Booster Doses. Children 3 through 6 years should receive one injection of DTP intramuscularly, preferably at the time of school entrance. Thereafter the recommended dose of Td should be given every 10 years. If a dose is given sooner as part of wound management, the next routine booster is not needed for 10 years from that time.

Prophylaxis in Wound Management. Tetanus has not been reported in individuals with adequate primary immunization. After four doses of tetanus toxoid, antitoxin persists at protective levels for at least 5 years, and an ability to respond promptly to a booster injection persists for a longer time. This amnestic response also develops in those persons who have previously received at least two doses of tetanus toxoid.

Passive protection with TIG or TAT should be reserved only for patients with tetanus-prone wounds, who have had less than two previous injections of tetanus toxoid, or when the wound has been unattended for more than 24 hours. The currently recommended prophylactic dose of TIG is 250 units for wounds of average severity. When tetanus toxoid and TIG are given concurrently, separate syringes and separate sites should be used. If TIG is unavailable, TAT may be used in doses of 3000 to 5000 units. Its use should be preceded by careful screening for sensitivity.

In wound management it is unnecessary to use booster injections of tetanus toxoid more than every 5 years. If tetanus immunization is incomplete at the time of a wound, the remainder of the recommended series should be given. More frequent booster doses are not indicated and may be associated with increased incidence and severity of reactions.

Other Control Measures. Wounds should be cleansed and debrided as indicated. Tetanus neonatorum may be abolished by immunization programs for adolescent girls and women of childbearing age, better training of midwives, and immunization of nonimmune pregnant mothers where the incidence of tetanus neonatorum is high.

Shigellosis

ERWIN NETER, M.D. *and*
ERIKA BRUCK, M.D.

Shigellosis refers to any infection caused by the members of the genus *Shigella*. With rare exceptions the infection is localized in the intestinal tract. Only infrequently do shigellae cause disease elsewhere, such as urinary tract infection, bacteremia, and so on. Shigellosis is essentially a disease of man, but may be encountered in primates. This is in striking contrast to salmonellosis, an infection of numerous animal species.

Shigellae may cause subclinical, mild, or severe infection and, in the absence of underlying disease, is rarely fatal in this country. Colonization of the intestine resulting in the carrier state, without preceding illness, is seen rather infrequently. It is of interest to note that at the present time, in the United States, shigellosis has become less common than even a few years ago. For 1973 and 1974 some 22,000 cases were reported to the Center for Disease Control and for 1975 only about 16,000. In our experience, a decrease in frequency of bacteriologically proved shigellosis is particularly evident when contrasted with increased frequency of salmonellosis. Clearly, in the absence of bacteriologic examination, many mild cases remain unrecognized. However, outbreaks of serious illness have been encountered elsewhere even in recent years, notably the epidemic of Central America. Shigellosis plays a greater role in less developed countries of the world. Of the members of the *Shigella* group, *S. sonnei* is encountered far more frequently in the United States than the other members, *S. flexneri*, *S. boydii* and *S. dysenteriae*. Contrariwise, *S. flexneri* has been the predominant organism in other parts of the world, notably Asia.

Antimicrobial Therapy and Prophylaxis. Past experience has provided evidence that in shigellosis suitable antimicrobial agents are effective as therapeutic agents, both clinically and bacteriologically. In addition, they have been used successfully for prophylaxis. The therapeutic efficacy of antibiotics in shigellosis is in striking contrast to their failure in localized *Salmonella* gastroenteritis. In the absence of significant underlying diseases, chemotherapy is not needed in mild cases of shigellosis, since the infection is usually self-limited and recovery takes place promptly. When the disease is severe, suitable chemotherapeutic agents may be used.

Generally, nonabsorbable drugs, such as neomycin, polymyxin B and others, are either ineffective or less effective than absorbable drugs. Absorbable sulfonamides, tetracyclines, chloramphenicol, and ampicillin have been used with favorable results. The selection depends upon the susceptibility of the pathogen, the severity of the illness, and the age of the patient. Thus, identification of the infecting microorganism and its susceptibility are important guidelines for the physician. If the strain is susceptible to ampicillin, this antibiotic is often selected. Recent evidence suggests that trimethoprim-sulfamethoxazole may be of value, notably when the infecting strain is resistant to other available antibiotics. However, at this time, this drug is not as yet approved in the United States for the treatment of shigellosis in children.

Previous double-blind studies have revealed that with susceptible strains of shigellae, ampicillin treatment is superior to sulfonamides (J. Pediat., 70: 970, 1967). So far as the cephalosporins are concerned, cephalexin may be effective clinically but cephaloglycin is not. Several recent studies have indicated that sulfamethoxazole-trimethoprim promises to be a clinically effective drug combination, particularly when dealing with strains resistant to ampicillin and other antimicrobial agents (Antimicrob. Agents Chemother., 5:439, 1974; Chemotherapy, 20:113, 1074). In one such study (Scand. J. Infect. Dis., 4:231, 1972), pediatric tablets containing 20 mg. of trimethoprim and 100 mg. of sulfamethoxazole were used in two divided doses per day, for an average of 7 mg. of trimethoprim and 35 mg. of sulfamethoxazole per kg. per 24 hours. The effectiveness of this treatment has been shown also by others. The drug combination, recently approved in this country for the treatment of urinary tract infection of children, is available as tablets (80 mg. of trimethoprim and 400 mg. of sulfamethoxazole) and as suspension (40 mg. of trimethoprim and 200 mg. of sulfamethoxazole).

Nonspecific and Supportive Therapy for Dysentery. As in other forms of infectious diarrhea, drugs which claim to decrease peristalsis and thereby the number or the amount of evacuations are not indicated. None of these drugs have been proved to decrease the loss of fluid and electrolytes, and some authors believe they even may prolong the colonization of the intestine by the pathogenic microorganisms.

Loss of fluid and electrolytes is usually small or moderate in shigellosis; however, occasionally severe dehydration, acidosis, and even shock may occur, especially on the first day or two of the illness. In these cases, oral intake should be stopped and intravenous fluid therapy is necessary. The volume should be 2400 to 3000 ml. per square meter of body surface area on the first day; the fluid should contain glucose, preferably 100 gm. per liter, and electrolytes, including potassium and phosphate, in an osmolar concentration about half isotonic or slightly above (not counting the glucose). Any of the commonly used solutions fulfilling these criteria is effective. Parenteral fluid therapy is rarely required for more than 24 or, at most, 48 hours. Watery diarrhea usually subsides promptly when oral intake is stopped. When feeding is resumed, bland food with low roughage should be used at first before gradual resumption of a full diet. Milk intolerance caused by lactase deficiency is not encountered in shigellosis which affects primarily the colon rather than the small intestine.

Although feces may contain blood in the early stages of *Shigella* dysentery, blood loss is rarely serious enough to cause anemia; no therapy is required for this problem. In fact, extensive blood loss should warrant a search for causes of bleeding other than shigellosis.

Typhoid Fever

JORGE B. HOWARD, M.D.

With the advent of modern sanitation the incidence of typhoid fever in the United States has drastically decreased. In other areas of the world, or in localized epidemic situations, considerable numbers of patients harboring *Salmonella typhi* are still encountered. The acute septicemic form of the disease is still suspected in children with prolonged fever, frontal headaches, anorexia, irritability, cough, characteristic brown-coated tongue, and when on physical examination associated splenomegaly or rose spots are found.

The microorganism is initially found only in the blood or bone marrow, and as the disease progresses can also be isolated from urine or stools. Rising serial agglutination titers against the H and O antigens of *S. typhi* can aid diagnosis.

Specific Treatment.   If the patient is able to tolerate oral medication, treatment is started with chloramphenicol palmitate at a dose of 50 mg./kg./day in four doses.* This dose can usually be reduced to 25 mg./kg./day after the child has been afebrile for at least two days. In the presence of shock, delirium, severe vomiting and/or dehydration, intravenous treatment should be initiated with chloramphenicol sodium succinate, 50 mg./kg./day.* Once the patient is well enough to tolerate oral medication, this route can be used for the remainder of the treatment period. Because erratic peak blood levels have been reported, chloramphenicol sodium succinate should not be used intramuscularly.

Fever usually responds slowly to treatment. The patient's toxic condition usually abates before his fever does. Defervescence occurs three to five days after treatment is started. The total duration of treatment should be at least 14 days.

Blood dyscrasia associated with chloramphenicol therapy has been rare in typhoid fever. Nevertheless, all patients receiving chloramphenicol should have hemoglobin, reticulocyte and white blood cell counts twice weekly. If bone marrow depression becomes a problem, an alternative drug is used.

S. typhi strains resistant to chloramphenicol have emerged in several parts of the world, particularly in Southeast Asia and the Indian subcontinent. In patients returning from these areas, alternative antibiotic therapy should be considered. Other antibiotics used include ampicillin, 100 to 200 mg./kg./day in four doses, intravenously, intramuscularly or orally, or oral amoxicillin, 60 to 100 mg./kg./day in three divided doses.* A recent addition is trimethoprim-sulfamethoxazole.† Excellent clinical response is obtained with trimethoprim, 10 to 12 mg./kg., and sulfamethoxazole, 50 to 60 mg./kg., divided into two or three doses and administered orally or intravenously. With these drugs, as with chloramphenicol, treatment is continued for at least 14 days.

In the pediatric age group, carriers of *S. typhi* are infrequent. Our practice is to re-treat these patients for periods of up to 21 days with either oral ampicillin, 200 mg./kg./day, or trimethoprim-sulfamethoxazole, 60 to 100 mg./kg./day. If after this treatment they still continue to eliminate bacteria in the stool, an intensive search for a sequestered site is begun.

Supportive Therapy.   Except under unusual circumstances, in the United States most children with typhoid fever should be hospitalized for isolation and adequate nursing care. Salicylates and acetaminophen derivatives should be avoided for treatment of pyrexia because they can produce marked hypothermia. When it is necessary to reduce the fever, tepid sponge baths or an ice mattress is used.

Bed rest should be strict for the first 10 days of illness, after which ambulation may be introduced gradually. Strenuous exercise and competitive sports should be forbidden for a month following the illness.

The diet must be bland but well balanced with a high protein and calorie content. Spicy foods and those with residues or high fiber content are not advisable. A generous fluid intake is allowed, especially during the febrile period. If vomiting and dehydration occur, standard methods of intravenous fluid and elecrolyte replacement and maintenance are used. Constipation and fecal impaction are relieved by enemas. Because of intestinal friability, cathartics can be dangerous.

In severely toxic, delirious patients steroids can be life-saving. Our choice is to use prednisone, 2 mg./kg./day, for 3 or 4 days. The majority of patients with typhoid fever do not require steroids and their routine use in febrile patients is not justified.

---

*This dosage of chloramphenicol is higher than that recommended for newborn infants.

*This dosage of amoxicillin is higher than that recommended by the manufacturer, but has been found to be effective.

†This use of trimethoprim-sulfamethoxazole is not mentioned in the manufacturer's instructions. Trimethoprim-sulfamethoxazole is not recommended for infants under two months of age.

Treatment of Complications. Complications usually appear in the third or fourth week of illness and become more frequent in untreated patients or in those in whom therapy is started late in the course of the disease. Relapses are heralded by a recrudescence of fever and toxicity after treatment has been discontinued, and should be handled as the initial episode.

The most severe life-threatening complications are gastrointestinal hemorrhage and intestinal perforation. When severe intestinal hemorrhage becomes a problem, parenteral fluid therapy and transfusions may be necessary. If, in spite of adequate supportive therapy, the clinical condition continues to deteriorate, a surgeon should be consulted. Management of intestinal perforation is difficult and controversial. High mortality rates after operative intervention may justify conservative treatment with blood pressure and hydration support and intensive antibiotic therapy to control the peritonitis.

Acute hepatitis and acute pneumonia associated with *S. typhi* infection respond well to antibiotics. Acute cholecystitis may result from typhoid; if gallstones are present cholecystectomy should be performed.

Preventive Therapy. Hospitalized patients represent the risk of contagion to other patients and hospital personnel; thus strict isolation procedures should be followed. Especially important is the disposal of excreta. Modern hospital flush toilets will suffice, but in lieu of them, bed pans and excreta should be treated with a disinfectant.

As typhoid fever has become an uncommon disease in the United States, vaccination is indicated only for travelers or those living overseas in typhoid endemic zones. Two vaccines are currently in use: a heat-killed phenol preserved form and an acetone inactivated form. (Acetone inactivated vaccine is more effective, but it is not available in the United States.) Both are from 70 to 90 per cent effective, but neither is effective when large numbers of organisms are ingested. Vaccination should be considered for family members of a typhoid carrier, persons living in an area in which there is an outbreak of typhoid fever, and those who plan to move to a typhoid fever endemic zone. Children under 10 years of age receive two doses of 0.25 ml. subcutaneously, one month apart. Adults and children over 10 should receive two doses of 0.5 ml. with one month interval. Booster injections if required are administered every one to three years. Paratyphoid A and B vaccines are no longer marketed in the United States.

Each case of typhoid fever should be reported to public health officials so that the source of infection can be sought.

Salmonellosis

JORGE B. HOWARD, M.D.

Salmonellosis, other than typhoid fever, is common in the United States, the actual number of cases reported to the Center for Disease Control having increased steadily in recent years. Man usually acquires the disease through contact with Salmonella-infected domestic animals, food, eggs or milk products.

Salmonella infections in man produce several well differentiated syndromes. Bacteremia and septicemia are occasionally encountered, there being no pathognomonic signs or symptoms that would permit a diagnosis prior to the blood culture results. Treatment of this type of infection is the same as that of typhoid fever.

Gastroenteritis. Salmonella gastroenteritis is often heralded by diarrhea of acute onset, nausea, vomiting, headaches and stomach cramps from 4 to 48 hours after consuming contaminated food. If dehydration is present or impending, fluid and electrolyte therapy is mandatory. Usually antibiotics are not necessary because the disease resolves spontaneously within 4 to 7 days. Coupled with the apparent lack of efficacy against symptoms, antibiotics seem to increase the likelihood of a prolonged Salmonella carrier state.

Certain types of patients are prone to complications: infants less than six months old, gastrectomized patients, those with a chronic or debilitating disease and individuals receiving immunosuppressive therapy. When Salmonella are isolated from the gastrointestinal tracts of these patients, oral or parenteral chloramphenicol or ampicillin should be used until symptomatic relief is achieved. Treatment is then discontinued even though stool cultures may still be positive. As in the case of chronic stool carriers of *Salmonella typhi*, treatment with trimethoprim-sulfamethoxazole has been claimed to be effective in one report, but further experience is needed. At the time of this writing trimethoprim-sulfamethoxazole has not been approved for treatment of Salmonella infections in the United States.

In the majority of cases a soft, bland, low residue diet is all that is required. For relief of stomach cramps one or two doses of paregoric may be used. Infants with prolonged diarrhea may develop lactose intolerance. In such cases a lactose-free formula should be given.

Parents of children who are asymptomatic excretors of Salmonella in their stool should be advised to use careful handwashing and personal hygienic measures.

Extra-intestinal infections. Occasionally Salmonella can produce localized infections in the central nervous system, joints, bones, urinary tract or cardiovascular system.

Salmonella meningitis should be treated with chloramphenicol sodium succinate, 100 mg./kg./day, or ampicillin, 200 to 300 mg./kg./day, for 14 to 21 days.* Patients with sickle cell anemia are prone to Salmonella osteomyelitis. When the diagnosis is made, treatment with ampicillin plus appropriate surgical procedures to drain the pus as well as general supportive measures will hasten recovery.

Because high concentrations of ampicillin are found in the urine, a dose of 50 mg./kg./day can be used safely for treatment of uncomplicated Salmonella urinary tract infections.

In extra-intestinal Salmonella infections, selection of antibiotic, route of administration and length of treatment are dictated by antibiotic susceptibilities, type of illness and rapidity of response to antimicrobial therapy. Antibiotic therapy should be continued for 5 to 7 days after clinical signs of infection have disappeared.

---

*This dosage of ampicillin is higher than that recommended for newborn infants.

Brucellosis

ROBERT-GRAY CHOTO, M.D.

Brucellosis is a worldwide disease acquired from domestic (cattle, sheep, goats, swine, kennel-raised beagles) and other animals (reindeer, moose and yaks). Synonyms are: undulant fever, Mediterranean fever; Rock fever; neopolitan fever; Cyprus fever and mimic disease.

The infecting organism is a gram-negative, noncapsulated, nonsporulating pleomorphic aerobic bacillus—Brucella sp. *B. melitensis* with three types found in caprine animals; *B. arbotus* with nine types in bovines; *B. suis* with four types in swine are the major causes of disease in man. Three other species pathogenic to man are found in wild bovines, canines and the desert wood rat.

Brucellosis is an occupational disease of livestock farmers, abattoir workers, veterinarians and laboratory personnel. Brucella sp. do not grow in aged cheese. Man to man transmission is unknown except for transfusion of blood from infected donors. The incubation period is 6 to 21 days. Sexual transmission is known to occur in animals but is not known to occur in man. The 20 to 50 year age group is the most frequently infected with brucellosis; males outnumber females 6:1. Dissemination is hematogenous with primary localization in tissues rich in reticuloendothelial cells (Table 1).

Brucellosis is a disease with multiple complaints and a paucity of physical findings—none pathognomonic. Symptoms (see Table 1)

TABLE 1. Clinical Factors Related to Brucellosis

Mode of Transmission	*Dissemination To:*
Unpasteurized milk from infected animals	Liver
Handling of fresh contaminated animal products	Spleen
Oral and cutaneous skin abrasions	Bone marrow
Inhalation of heavily contaminated barnyard dust	Lymphoid tissue
Transfusion of infected blood	Meninges
	Endocardium ⎫
	Kidneys ⎬ less frequent
	Male genitalia ⎭
Symptoms	*Physical Findings*
Undulant fever (101 to 104°F)	Lymphadenopathy
Malaise	Hepatosplenomegaly—rarely with jaundice
Somatic aches and pains	Orchitis (rare)
Irritability	Epididymitis (rare)
Reactive depression or	Skin granulomas with or without ulcerations (rare)
acute psychoses	Conjunctivitis (rare)
Laboratory Findings	Arthritis (rare)
Blood cultures	Meningitis (very rare)
Agglutination titer greater than 1:160	Focal endocarditis (very rare)
Sedimentation rate not elevated	
Brucella skin test induration >7 mm.	

are usually worse in the afternoon and the clinical appearance is out of proportion to the multitude of complaints. In endemic areas for *B. melitensis*, up to 50 per cent of the cases have osteomyelitis with granulomas or focal sarcoid-like granulomas in liver and spleen biopsies. In *B. suis* granulomas tend to suppurate.

Diagnosis depends on a good history of exposure, positive blood cultures and an agglutination titer greater than 1:160. Differential diagnoses include typhoid fever, miliary tuberculosis, acute influenza, acute endocarditis and infectious mononucleosis.

Once the diagnosis of brucellosis has been established by positive blood cultures (may take 5 to 30 days on Albimi broth and agar), agglutination titers greater than 1:160 and/or demonstration of intracellular organisms in a biopsy, the treatment of choice is tetracycline. (see Table 2 for alternatives). In acutely ill patients, institution of antimicrobial agents may precipitate a Herxheimer reaction. A short course of glucocorticoids may help avert this reaction and does not need tapering. Hydrocortisone, 5 mg./kg./day orally, or prednisone, 1 mg./kg./day orally in 3 divided doses, may be given for 3 to 5 days. Suppurative granulomas must be surgically drained.

Treatment with penicillins, cephalosporins, and erythromycins has been very unsatisfactory. Animal vaccines are not indicated for human disease. Other therapeutic modalities are under active investigation including co-trimoxazole (Septra, Bactrim), levamisole as well as a human vaccine. Relapses are less frequent with combinations of antimicrobial agents such as tetracycline plus streptomycin. Repeat treatment is indicated if positive blood cultures persist or recur.

Tularemia

DAN M. GRANOFF, M.D.

Children suspected of having tularemia should be hospitalized and antibiotic therapy initiated on the basis of a presumptive clinical diagnosis. Tularemia is probably the only disease for which streptomycin, when used as a single drug, is the antibiotic of choice. Unfortunately, there is little modern pharmacokinetic data available for the use of this drug in children, and our current dosage schedule is based on anecdotal clinical experience, limited drug studies performed nearly 30 years ago, and extrapolation of information obtained from adults. The recommended dosage is 30 to 40 mg./kg./24 hr. Depending on the severity of illness, it should be administered intramuscularly in divided doses every 8 to 12 hours for 6 to 10 days. The maximum daily dose for a child should rarely exceed 1 gm.

When streptomycin is initiated early, lymph nodes may continue to swell for one to two days, but the patient's overall clinical condition will rapidly improve, with fever resolving within 24 to 36 hours. Since response to intramuscular therapy is prompt, intravenous streptomycin is rarely required, and is best avoided because of the greater likelihood of toxicity. In an occasional patient with hypotension, intravenous therapy may be desired, and 7.5 mg./kg. of streptomycin can be mixed with 30 ml. of 0.9 per cent saline and infused slowly over 30 to 40 minutes. This dose is repeated every 6 hours.

There is relatively little clinical experience in the treatment of tularemia with other aminoglycoside antibiotics such as kanamycin and gentamicin, but they are probably equally effective. There may be some advantage in using one of these agents when the clinical course of tularemia is complicated by impairment of renal function, since laboratory determination of serum antibiotic levels is generally more available for gentamicin. The *initial* dose of gentamicin is 2 mg./kg. given in-

TABLE 2. Treatment of Brucellosis

TREATMENT	DOSAGE	DURATION
Children		
Tetracycline*	28 to 30 mg./kg./day orally in 4 divided doses	21 days
Streptomycin	25 to 40 mg./kg./day I.M. in 2 divided doses	21 days
Chloramphenicol†	50 mg./kg./day orally	21 days
Triple sulfonamides‡	15 mg./kg./day orally in 4 divided doses	21 days
Adults		
Tetracycline	2 gm./day orally in 4 divided doses	21 days
Streptomycin	1 to 2 gm./day I.M. in 2 divided doses	21 days

*Manufacturer's precaution: Use of tetracycline during infancy and childhood to age 8 years may cause permanent discoloration of the teeth.

†May be substituted for tetracycline in children under age 8 to avoid dental staining. Hematopoetic monitoring is advised with this drug.

‡May be used in place of chloramphenicol and in combination with tetracyclines and streptomycin.

tramuscularly or intravenously in a manner similar to streptomycin. Subsequent doses will depend on the serum creatinine level or the extent of impairment of creatinine clearance. Peak gentamicin serum levels (30 minutes after administration) of 5 to 10 μg./ml. are therapeutic and safe. These levels can best be achieved by changing the amount given or by altering the interval of administration.

Tetracycline* or chloramphenicol can be used in the rare patient who cannot tolerate aminoglycoside therapy. They are bacteriostatic agents which are less effective than streptomycin and are associated with a higher frequency of relapse. Oxytetracycline (40 mg./kg./24 hr.) is probably the preferred tetracycline, as it may carry less risk of causing discoloration of teeth. Chloramphenicol (50 to 100 mg./kg./24 hr.) is equally effective, but is not usually used because it causes a rare, irreversible aplastic anemia. Therapy with these agents should be administered for 10 to 14 days. In case of recrudescence, which can occur as late as 10 to 14 days after discontinuing medication, treatment should be repeated.

Person-to-person transmission of tularemia rarely, if ever, occurs. Patients do not ordinarily require isolation, but care should be exercised and gloves worn when changing dressings or tending to draining wounds. In patients with the ulceroglandular form of disease, aspiration of pus from infected lymph nodes may be helpful in diagnosis but is usually not necessary for treatment. Should draining fistulae persist after suitable antimicrobial therapy, total surgical excision of infected tissue is usually curative. When the cornea is involved in oculoglandular disease, some authorities recommend local application of 1 per cent atropine ophthalmic solution (1 drop/day). It is also wise to obtain consultation with an experienced ophthalmologist, because corneal ulceration and scarring can occur.

Tularemia is prevented by keeping children away from infected animals. Gloves should be worn when dressing or handling game, and the meat should be thoroughly cooked. Avoidance of contact with ticks and other arthropod vectors is important in prevention. A live, attenuated *Francisella tularensis* vaccine is available from the Center for Disease Control. Although not yet licensed for general use, it is effective in preventing the severe typhoidal form of disease and is primarily used in laboratory workers.

---

*Manufacturer's precaution: Use of tetracycline during infancy and childhood to age 8 years may cause permanent discoloration of the teeth.

Plague

ROBERT-GRAY CHOTO, M.D.

Plague is an acute and fulminant infection caused by *Yersinia pestis* (formerly *Pasteurella pestis*), an aerobic gram-negative, nonsporulating pleomorphic bacillus. Plague is primarily a disease of rodents, with foci all over the world. In the United States epizootic foci are found in over 100 counties generally west of the 100° longitude. Although there have been no major outbreaks, individual cases from these counties have been on the rise. A recent outbreak of plague occurred in Puerto Rico (September 1975 to February 1976) and over 1600 cases were reported.

The disease is transmitted to many by the rat flea *Xenopsylla cheopis* and from man to man as well as rat to man by the human flea *Pulex irritans*. Prevention of plague has been achieved through rat control programs and defleaing of home environs. The individual cases in the United States are usually among young adults (<25 years) and males predominate by a 2:1 ratio.

Clinical manifestations include high fever (104°F or more) of sudden onset, with chills, headaches, delirium, vomiting, cough, dyspnea with or without cyanosis and extreme prostration.

After inoculation by a flea bite, the organisms multiply locally, forming a pustule or vesicle at the site. The vesicle is rarely seen at the time of examination. Spread is both by lymphatics to the local nodes which swell and suppurate (bubonic plague), and hematogenously, resulting in petechiae and hemorrhage of serous membranes (septicemic plague). Disseminated intravascular coagulation is a frequent complication. A rapidly fatal pneumonia characterized by cough, dyspnea, hemoptysis and a cor pulmonale-like picture is called the pneumonic plague.

Plague responds readily to the tetracyclines, streptomycin or chloramphenicol. Treatment should be initiated as soon as the clinical diagnosis is made without waiting for confirmatory blood, sputum and bubo cultures. Dosages are summarized in Table 1.

Cough droplets and bubo exudates are highly infectious and patients should be isolated for 24 to 48 hours after initiation of therapy. Supportive care should be maintained with adequate intravenous fluids. In septicemic plague, acute cerebral edema may result and urea or mannitol may be indicated. Contacts of plague need only to be observed except for contacts of pneumonic plague who should receive prophylactic tetracycline.

Table 1. Methods of Treatment for Plague

AGE	TETRACYCLINE*	OR	CHLORAMPHENICOL†	OR	STREPTOMYCIN‡
Under 12	12 to 15 mg./kg. I.V. in 4 divided doses for 24 hr.; then same dose orally for 9 days		60 to 100 mg./kg./day I.V. in 4 divided doses for 3 days; then 50 mg./kg./day I.V. or orally in 4 divided doses for 7 days		20 to 40 mg./kg./day I.M. in 4 divided doses for 10 days
Over 12	500 mg./day orally in 4 divided doses not to exceed 3 gm./day for 10 days		Same		Same
Adults	0.75 to 1 gm. I.V. loading dose followed by 500 mg. orally every 6 hr. for 10 days		1 gm. I.V. loading dose; then 500 mg. I.V. or orally every 6 hr. for 10 days		1 gm. I.M. loading dose; then 500 mg. I.M. every 12 hr. for 10 days.

*Manufacturer's note: Use of tetracycline during infancy and childhood to age 8 years may cause permanent discoloration of the teeth.

†The incidence of chloramphenicol-induced aplastic anemia is approximately 1:40,000 to 1:100,000.

‡Streptomycin is the most effective (bactericidal) drug for plague and may precipitate a Herxheimer reaction.

Tuberculosis

ROSA LEE NEMIR, M.D.

Once tuberculosis is diagnosed, essential data are an estimate of the duration of infection, previous records of tuberculin tests, radiographic study, a history of known exposure, or record of previous tuberculosis in family members. A history of BCG vaccination should be sought. Recent tuberculin conversion or known exposure to active disease directs a search for evidence of hematogenous dissemination and requires more frequent medical observations.

All children and adolescents with positive tuberculin reactions who have not previously had chemotherapy should receive treatment. The duration and extent of disease determines the length and choice of therapy, whether single or multiple drugs. Uncomplicated primary tuberculosis and recent tuberculin convertors usually require only one year's treatment; all hematogenous manifestations of disease (miliary, meningitis, pleural effusion, bone and joint disease) require longer therapy, in some instances as long as two years. Chronic cavitary disease may take even longer. Two or more drugs are always used when there is evidence of active disease.

Ambulatory care with frequent supervision of therapy and without hospitalization is now satisfactory for most patients. Most tests needed prior to antimicrobial therapy may be obtained in an office or clinic. Hospitalization is required for patients acutely ill with meningitis, miliary, pleural or pericardial effusion, or bone and joint disease. Patients with cavitary tuberculosis (usually adolescents), even though asymptomatic, should receive initial treatment in a hospital. This affords an opportunity to obtain cultures for acid-fast bacilli and resistance studies on the organisms cultured. Sometimes bacilli seen on smear may not be viable, as is suggested by negative cultures on the same specimen. In other instances the bacilli may be other than *Mycobacterium hominis*.

ANTIMICROBIAL THERAPY

Single drug therapy, namely with isoniazid, is used to prevent tuberculous infection or to prevent development of disease when untreated and apparently quiescent infection exists. Evidence for the latter may sometimes be found in radiologic calcifications in lungs or nodes or by history. A third use is treatment of a recently discovered tuberculin positive patient with a normal chest roentgenogram.

Double or multiple drug therapy is used for all seriously ill patients with tuberculosis such as miliary, meningitis, pleural or pericardial effusion, skeletal disease, cavitary lung disease and superficial lymph node infection. Multiple drug therapy combines different modes of attack against tubercle bacilli, especially important when the disease is active and bacilli are rapidly multiplying. The use of two drugs decreases the likelihood of the emergence of resistant strains of acid-fast bacilli. This occurs more often when the exposure is to adults with positive sputum and when irregularity in taking medications exists. For such exposed children, double therapy is a safeguard. Active primary tuberculosis with parenchymal or nodal lesions with or without the complication of endobronchial disease should have multiple drug therapy for at least 6 to 9 months, completing the one year treatment on isoniazid alone.

Isoniazid (INH). INH has a combined bactericidal and bacteriostatic action and readily penetrates caseous lesions. The drug is absorbed rapidly and crosses the blood-brain barrier, producing effective drug levels in the spinal fluid. Within a few hours after medication, high levels are obtained. Obviously INH is the drug of first choice unless sensitivity or some intolerance factor exists.

The dosage for children is 10 to 20 mg./kg./day, usually not to exceed 300 mg. daily (exceptionally 500) given once a day. Tablets (50 or 100 mg.) are preferable to liquid or syrup INH in which 5 ml. contains 50 mg. The pills may be crushed and given in a spoonful of fruit such as banana or apple sauce or fruit juice. From 50 to 70 per cent of INH is excreted in urine within 24 hours. A chemical test for its presence in the urine may help in monitoring patient compliance.

Adverse effects of INH are uncommon and consist of symptoms of hypersensitivity such as fever, various types of skin rashes (maculopapular, purpuric, urticarial), peripheral and optic neuritis (reversible), convulsions and hepatotoxicity. The latter is uncommon in our experience, although transient elevation of serum glutamic oxaloacetic transaminase or serum glutamic pyruvic transaminase may occur during the early weeks of INH therapy, returning to normal usually within 6 to 8 weeks or when the medication is discontinued. Neuritis in children and adolescents is rare. As a preventive, pyridoxine, 25 to 50 mg. daily, is recommended only for the adolescent patient. This pill must be distinguished from the INH tablet, which it resembles.

Drug interaction with phenytoin (Dilantin) may produce increased central nervous system symptoms, excessive sedation and incoordination. Patients receiving this drug or phenobarbital require careful watching and occasional reduction of the dosage of phenytoin. Epileptic patients with tuberculosis require close observation and occasional readjustment of all medications.

Para-aminosalicylic Acid (PAS). This drug, usually as NaPAS, is valuable as a secondary therapeutic agent to accompany INH. It is never used as the sole agent, although it is bacteriostatic, suppressing the growth and multiplication of tubercle bacilli in many tissues of the body, including caseous lesions. It is quickly (1½ hours) absorbed into the blood and serous fluids, but at much lower concentrations into the cerebrospinal fluid. PAS, when combined with other agents such as INH or streptomycin, has an increased bacteriostatic effect and also delays the emergence of bacilli resistant to the primary chemotherapeutic agent. The blood level of free INH is increased when PAS is also given because of competition for acetylation in the liver.

PAS, sold in powder form, granules and solutions of the sodium salt for parenteral administration, is commonly given orally in tablets of 0.5 gm. The daily dosage of 200 mg./kg. to a maximum of 8 to 12 gm. is divided into three doses to sustain therapeutic blood levels.

Adverse effects of PAS are predominantly gastrointestinal, such as nausea, abdominal distress and anorexia. Much less frequently symptoms of hypersensitivity occur, usually early in therapy, producing fever, joint pains and skin rashes (papular, scarlatiniform or urticarial). These symptoms clear quickly when PAS is discontinued or a large dose is reduced. The latter has been the writer's experience with a number of children when the daily dose of 300 mg./kg. was reduced to 200 mg./kg. Children tolerate PAS well, with fewer complaints of gastrointestinal discomfort than adults. Adolescents complain more often. All should take PAS only after meals.

Precaution in prescribing PAS is advised for patients with kidney disease, because of high concentrations of aminosalicylic acid excretion in the urine, and patients in whom gastric ulcer is suspected, a rare occurrence in pediatrics.

Streptomycin. Streptomycin is still a first line drug used in multiple therapy (*never alone*) and usually the third drug for a short period only, especially in adults with extensive disease. In children, severe meningitis and miliary disease are the chief indications for addition of streptomycin. Its action is both bacteriostatic and bactericidal, as it interferes with protein synthesis of tubercle bacilli. Intracellular penetration is relatively low. Unlike INH, streptomycin does not prevent the development of disease once the infection has been introduced. A moderately effective level is found in body fluids including the cerebrospinal fluid when there is meningitis. Most of the drug is excreted in the urine within a short time. Tubercle bacilli rapidly develop resistance when streptomycin is used alone. The addition of a second drug, usually INH, delays but does not completely prevent the appearance of resistant bacilli. Streptomycin, obtainable in vials of 1 gm., must be given intramuscularly, in doses of 20 to 40 mg./kg. daily, maximum 1 gm. daily.

The adverse effects of streptomycin are primarily neurotoxic. Eighth nerve effects are seen less frequently in children than in the aged and older patients. Children are less disturbed by the vertigo due to vestibular damage. Less frequent is tinnitus and loss of hearing, especially to high frequency levels. Either of these findings should lead to reevaluation of therapy and usually withdrawal of streptomycin from the regimen. Rarely hypersensitivity occurs, producing fever and dermatoses.

Ethambutol. This highly effective drug has wide usage in the treatment of adults in place of PAS, unpopular in this age group because of the gastrointestinal symptoms. In adults, ethambutol is used in treatment failures and certain extrapulmonary diseases, in advanced cavitary and chronic pulmonary disease and in atypical mycobacterial infections. There is little published data supporting its use in children, where fear of the optic neuropathy and the difficulty of monitoring visual acuity and color appreciation are limiting factors. This drug, however, can be used in adolescents if PAS is unacceptable or if hypersensitivity occurs. Ethambutol acts by delaying the multiplication of bacteria through interference with RNA synthesis. Resistance develops very slowly, and when given in combination with other drugs, ethambutol delays the appearance of bacterial resistance. EMB tablets of 100 or 400 mg. are given orally and rapidly absorbed and excreted in the urine.* The dosage is 15 mg./kg. given once daily.

Adverse effects of ethambutol are few and uncommon at low dosage levels. Optic neuritis affecting visual acuity and loss of ability to perceive the color green may occur, so that visual tests are required before treatment is begun and monthly monitoring thereafter. The visual tests include the use of a Snellen eye chart, visual fields and green color vision. Obviously limitations exist in the very young patient and when difficulty in communication exists. The writer has not needed to use ethambutol in children and has infrequently given it to adolescents who object to taking PAS.

When a multiple drug regimen is needed for extensive disease as for miliary or meningitis in older children, ethambutol may be the third drug.

*Manufacturer's precaution: There is as yet no established dosage of ethambutol for children under 13 years of age.

Rifampin. This remarkable new drug, a derivative of *Streptomycin mediterranei,* has been used extensively in adults in many parts of the world and recently in the United States, in combination with other antituberculous agents, with consistently excellent results. The second drug is usually INH or ethambutol (adults) with or without streptomycin. The special indications are treatment failures, infections due to bacilli resistant to other therapeutic agents, and extensive severe disease in which immediate control of infection is essential. During the past six years the writer has administered rifampin to children with gratifying success and without toxic manifestations. However, experience with patients under five years of age is universally limited. Rifampin must always be used in conjunction with one or more antituberculous drugs, *never as a sole agent* because of rapid emergence of drug-resistant strains of mycobacteria or of whatever infecting agent is responsible for the disease.

Rifampin's effective action against mycobacteria is by inhibition of DNA-dependent RNA polymerase. The medication, as 300 mg. capsules, may be given once daily, preferably 45 minutes before breakfast or 2 hours after a meal. The dosage is 10 to 20 mg./kg., not to exceed 600 mg. daily. In the United States smaller capsules for children are unavailable. The present 300 mg. capsules may be divided by pharmacists. Elimination is through the bile and urine, producing a deep orange to reddish color in the latter. Similar discoloration may be seen in sweat, tears, saliva, sputum and stool. In infants diapers stained by an orange-reddish color may cause concern to the uninformed. Patients and parents should be forewarned.

The drug is absorbed into all body tissues, including bone. It crosses into the spinal fluid only when there is infection and crosses the placenta freely. Its teratogenic effect is unknown.

Adverse effects of rifampin are uncommon. The toxicity is chiefly hepatic. Abnormal liver function may occur, usually transient, and therefore periodic monitoring (weekly in the beginning) by serum enzyme studies, alkaline phosphatase and bilirubin is necessary. Occasionally jaundice develops, which recedes when the drug is discontinued. Leukopenia and thrombopenia have been reported; therefore weekly blood counts and tests for prothrombin time are advised for six to eight weeks and as indicated thereafter.

Other Drugs. Kanamycin, like streptomycin, affects the eighth cranial nerve and is also nephrotoxic. Viomycin* in addition to these toxic manifestations occasionally produces skin rashes and plasma electrolyte disturbance. Capreomycin,† a product of *Streptomyces capreolus*, in its action resembles the two preceding antibiotics and is used as a secondary drug, especially when strains of bacilli resistant to the standard therapeutic agents emerge. Toxic reactions are transient nephrotoxicity, hearing loss and vertigo. All three of these antibiotics are given intramuscularly.

Cycloserine‡ is a moderately effective drug, given orally in doses of 5 to 15 mg./kg. divided in two daily doses with a maximum dosage of 500 mg./day. It is neurotoxic and may occasionally lead to convulsions. It has definitely limited application and is to be given only to older children when other secondary drugs such as PAS or ethambutol cannot be used or tolerated.

All these secondary drugs are usually given in conjunction with INH and occasionally also with other drugs to prevent emergence of resistant strains of AFB or to treat such strains already cultured. The writer has never had the need to prescribe pyrazinamide or ethionamide.

Now with the apparent and almost certain addition of the much more effective rifampin, use of these drugs in the pediatric regimen becomes of very little importance.

ADRENOCORTICOSTEROIDS

Corticosteroids are not essential in the panel of required medication for tuberculosis. These steroid hormones are used occasionally for their anti-inflammatory action, which is associated with decreased formation of granulation and fibroblastic tissue as in meningitis, pleurisy with effusion and endobronchial lymph node disease; for marked hypersensitivity reactions produced by antituberculous drugs; and rarely for their systemic effect to reduce fever and malaise in severely ill patients. When corticosteroids are given, the patient must be receiving INH or other antituberculous drugs.

Patients without active disease and with only a positive reaction to tuberculin (even though previously treated), who are being given corticosteroids for other diseases, should receive INH. In this case, INH alone, usually

---

*Manufacturer's precaution: Safety of viomycin for children has not been established.

†Manufacturer's precaution: Safety of capreomycin for infants and children has not been established.

‡Manufacturer's precaution: A safe dosage of cycloserine has not yet been determined for pediatric use.

300 mg. daily, is adequate and should be continued several weeks after cessation of hormones.

PRIMARY TUBERCULOSIS

A recently infected patient needs more frequent observations than one whose infection has existed for some time, because hematogenous dissemination may be prevented by early continuous treatment. The patient whose infection is of long standing has passed this early hematogenous stage without developing disease such as miliary or meningitis, but most likely has scattered encapsulated small foci of living bacilli. These constitute a threat of future disease.

Positive Tuberculin Without Evidence of Disease.   These patients should have treatment for one year with INH, 10 mg./kg./day as one dose, maximum 300 mg. daily. Periodic radiographic review of the chest during this period is advised.

Positive Tuberculin With Evidence of Disease.   When the diagnosis of tuberculosis is established, all patients require treatment for 1 year with two drugs: INH, 10 to 20 mg./kg./day, maximum 300 to 400 mg. daily, and PAS, 200 mg./kg./day in three or four doses, maximum 8 to 10 gm. Two drugs are used to prevent the emergence of resistant bacilli and because the addition of PAS increases the effective level of INH. If there is good progress in recovery, frequently INH alone may be used for the last 4 to 6 months of the year's therapy.

Bacteriologic cultures are important not only to verify diagnosis but as a guide in therapy by sensitivity studies. Rarely, atypical mycobacterial infection or other infections mixed with *M. hominis* are found. Symptoms of drug intolerance or sensitivity occur early, so that frequent observations early in therapy are advised. Serial radiographic studies are essential to measure progress.

Primary Tuberculosis Complicated by Endobronchial Tuberculosis.   Occasionally bronchopulmonary nodes produce total or partial obstruction of segments or lobes of a lung, resulting in endobronchial disease. Two mechanisms are involved: (1) direct pressure on bronchi by enlarged nodes or by granulation tissue and (2) caseous material or polyp formation within the bronchus. Two drugs, INH and PAS, are used. It is well known that segmental collapse or atelectasis may continue unchanged for many months despite double drug therapy. Addition of streptomycin is definitely not advantageous. However, many patients treated in the early months of endobronchial involvement do show improvement by the addition of prednisone, 1 mg./kg./day for four to six weeks, maximum daily dose 60 mg. Steroid hormone therapy requires close observation and this is best done, in the beginning at least, in a hospital.

When symptoms of dyspnea, cyanosis or mediastinal shift occur, bronchoscopy by an endoscopist, experienced in care of young patients, is advised. Suction and removal of extraneous material within the bronchus are of therapeutic and diagnostic value. These patients are sometimes immediately improved following the addition of corticosteroids. In those patients with early endobronchial disease without these symptoms, improvement may be determined by radiographic and bronchoscopic findings within several weeks. Preliminary studies on the value of the *addition* of rifampin to the therapy for endobronchial disease, reported from France, are not definitive. They suggest that rifampin used early in the disease offers the best likelihood for improvement. Data are not available for determining the dosage of rifampin for children under five years of age.

In all instances of primary or recently diagnosed tuberculosis, the source case must be diligently sought as an aid in control of disease and in management of the patient. The contact case may be infected by resistant strains of acid-fast bacilli.

Cavitary Tuberculosis. In rare instances caseation and liquefaction occur within the parenchymal primary focus, resulting in early cavitation. This finding does not alter the two-drug regimen for primary tuberculosis. In adolescent patients, cavitary disease of the lung is not uncommon (see below).

Pleural Effusion. Pleural effusion most frequently occurs during the active phase of disease, some months after the onset. Pleural biopsy is sometimes used to establish the diagnosis when it is inclusive and not clarified by the usual cytologic tests and bacteriologic cultures, including examination of pleural fluid smears for bacilli.

The treatment consists of INH and PAS as for primary tuberculosis, but is continued for 18 to 24 months, after the first year, on INH alone. Streptomycin is not indicated. When corticosteroid therapy is given using prednisone, 1 mg./kg./day to maximum of 60 mg., the pleural fluid may be absorbed within two or three days. Hormone therapy is unnecessary and has no advantage unless excessive fluid produces respiratory embarrassment and the patient is toxic. Preliminary observation for 48 hours of antimicrobial therapy is advised before this addition. Long-term studies of pulmonary function do not indicate benefit from the addition.

Miliary Tuberculosis. This is a serious complication of primary tuberculosis, not only because of lung lesions but because of the possibility of accompanying tuberculous meningitis. Spinal tap on such patients clarifies this issue at the outset and may be needed during the disease if the patient fails to improve or develops signs of central nervous system involvement. In the past, triple drug therapy was customary; streptomycin was added to INH and PAS for the first weeks, not longer than four weeks. More recently, however, the use of rifampin with INH, thereby eliminating the more toxic streptomycin, has given good results in adults and is the writer's choice in children. Our experience with rifampin is limited, but in several instances rifampin and INH together were effective in clearing miliary lesions within weeks. Rifampin may be replaced by PAS within five or six months, continuing double drug therapy for one year and INH alone in the second year.

EXTRAPULMONARY COMPLICATIONS

Meningitis. This once universally fatal disease can now almost always be cured if early diagnosis is made. To obtain optimal results, meningitis should be considered a medical emergency and immediate energetic treatment instituted. Actually, tuberculous meningitis is becoming infrequent in the United States, probably because of the extensive use of chemoprophylaxis as well as other public health measures. The most powerful combination and least toxic drugs are isoniazid and rifampin. Their success in treatment of meningitis is reported from the European continent and elsewhere. The dosage and duration of therapy are the same as for miliary tuberculosis. Both INH and rifampin are given orally (INH may be given parenterally when necessary); no intrathecal therapy is necessary.

The addition of streptomycin for a short period may be considered for severely ill patients. If signs of spinal fluid blockage or increased intracranial pressure occur, prednisone should be added and continued for several weeks. Recovery from meningitis is variable. Patients treated early usually respond promptly, but those with advanced disease showing neurologic complications may improve slowly over many months, although some patients are left with neurologic sequelae. Spinal fluid cytology and chemistry are valuable guides to treatment and evaluation of progress. The physiotherapist should be consulted to prevent contractures. General management includes careful attention to electrolyte balance.

Bone and Joint Disease. The common sites of tuberculous involvement are vertebrae (frequently multiple), hip, knees, small bones of the hands and feet, and rarely skull and mastoids. The disease is a result of hematogenous foci implanted during the primary infection, and symptoms may occur six months or years later, occasionally being precipitated by trauma. Diagnosis without symptoms occasionally results from radiologic bone survey in patients with hematogenous tuberculosis.

Early in the disease, medical therapy with appropriate antimicrobials produces good results. If there appears to be surrounding abscess formation, surgical procedures may also be required. A sufficiently long preliminary period of antimicrobial therapy should precede the final decision concerning the use of surgical therapy. Recession of what appeared to be abscesses has been seen.

Triple drug therapy has been the medical treatment for some time; namely, INH, PAS, and streptomycin. Rifampin, however, penetrates bone tissue, is a highly effective antituberculous microbial and is therefore recommended as a second drug instead of PAS with INH. The writer has had four patients successfully so treated (two vertebra, one hip and one ankle). Streptomycin may be used for a period (2 months) to enable study of bacilli isolated for possible drug resistance and to allow time for better evaluation.

Major surgical procedures such as spinal fusion are rarely required, and immobilization and the use of heavy casts is seldom necessary for any length of time. Light support given early in treatment is needed. Orthopedic consultation and guidance is recommended early in therapy with the assistance of physiotherapists and other members of the rehabilitation team. Ambulation with support, not bed rest, is encouraged unless there are other complications of disease. Antimicrobial therapy should be continued for two years, but the last two to six months may require only INH, depending on the rate of healing.

Tuberculosis of Superficial Lymph Nodes. Enlarged superficial lymph nodes in a tuberculin positive child may be due to intercurrent infection, actively multiplying *Mycobacterium hominis* or infection by so-called atypical mycobacteria. Cervical nodes and those around the face are the most frequently involved. Treatment consists of a short period of broad spectrum antibiotic combined with antituberculous therapy until diagnosis is clarified. This requires throat culture and tuberculin testing with antigens for human and atypical mycobacteria.

Medical treatment using double drug therapy produces a slow response. INH, 15 to 20 mg./kg./day, and PAS as described for primary or miliary tuberculosis are given. Early in treatment, the swollen nodes may become soft and inflamed, then recede without surgical intervention. The return to relatively normal size requires many months after medical therapy is begun.

Surgical removal of the presenting infected node may be required because rupture is imminent or because of continued failure to improve. Infection of deep underlying nodes makes the operation tedious and often leads to removal of more than one node. The operation is preceded and followed by antimicrobial therapy for a total of 12 to 16 months. Opinions differ concerning indications for immediate surgery; the writer gives preference to medical treatment. Scars resulting from surgery and occasional surgical complications are among the factors to be weighed. Rifampin as a second drug appears to be valuable, but more experience is needed for final evaluation. The tonsils are rarely the initial cause of these tuberculous nodes. The infection is usually hematogenous, so tonsillectomy is not indicated because of lymphadenopathy alone.

Renal Tuberculosis. This results from hematogenous spread during the primary infection, although symptoms and signs of disease usually occur many years later after damage to the kidney has occurred. Evidence of kidney infection during phases of hematogenous disease such as miliary and peritonitis may be obtained by culture for acid-fast bacilli and urine examination, and still more rarely, by intravenous pyelography. Tuberculous genitourinary tract disease is rare in children. Epididymitis, a still greater rarity, may accompany kidney infection. Treatment is with two antimicrobials as for other hematogenous disease. However, longer treatment is necessary, at least two years and usually three or four years.

Symptoms and radiographic findings may require the initial addition of streptomycin for several months. The powerful combination of INH and rifampin has not yet received adequate trial in this rare form of childhood tuberculosis, but it has been used effectively in adults. Progress of disease may be observed by serial pyelograms, at the beginning of treatment, six months later and thereafter yearly for a time guided by review of pertinent findings.

Occasionally, rapidly growing atypical

mycobacteria are grown from urine. These are contaminants and require no therapy.

Tuberculous Peritonitis. This uncommon development of hematogenous tuberculosis resembles tuberculous pleural effusion in treatment with regard to choice and duration of medication and the rare optional use of adding corticosteroids. If the peritoneal fluid produces abdominal discomfort and respiratory distress after several days of antimicrobial therapy, relief may be obtained by the addition of prednisone.

TUBERCULOSIS IN ADOLESCENTS

The adolescent is peculiarly vulnerable to spread of tuberculous disease following infection. Rapid progression in those untreated is common experience. Recently on the pediatric service of Bellevue Hospital, hemoptysis was the first symptom of recent tuberculous infection in a number of youths. Obviously prompt antituberculous therapy is essential for the tuberculin positive adolescent, particularly if tuberculin conversion is recent.

The choice of treatment with INH alone or with a second drug depends on the probable duration of infection, presence of symptoms or findings of disease, radiographic findings, and presence of other chronic diseases such as diabetes.

Patients whose infection is over a year's duration (by knowledge of known positive tuberculin, calcification in the lung, or history of old exposure) will do well on INH alone (maximum 300 to 400 mg. daily) for 1 year. Patients with recent tuberculin conversion and negative roentgenograms also may be given INH alone for 12 to 16 months, but require closer observation and radiographic evaluation.

Patients with pulmonary parenchymal lesions, especially with cavitation, require double drug therapy for 18 to 24 months. Occasionally streptomycin is added briefly. The writer's choice when cavitation is present is INH and rifampin, the latter for six or more months, replaced by PAS if tolerated or by ethambutol* for the completion of therapy. We treated a number of such patients on the children's chest service and clinic at Bellevue Hospital with most rewarding results and without toxic reactions. The length of combined therapy depends on the extent of disease, response to therapy and absence of other disease. The pos-

sibility of pregnancy must be considered because of its effect on the tuberculosis and its relation to the request for radiologic study.

Patient compliance to medication is essential, and in our experience at Bellevue Hospital, the most difficult to achieve in this age group. Monitoring by urinary excretion of INH shows 70 per cent compliance for each visit. More frequent visits and longer counseling periods are recommended, thus allowing extra time for education. In female adolescent patients, this should include discussion of the unfavorable influence of pregnancy on active or recent tuberculosis. This aspect of education is a serious responsibility of the therapeutic team.

INFANTS BORN OF TUBERCULOUS MOTHERS

Concern for the newborn infant of a tuberculous mother is due to the seriousness of the disease at this age more than to the frequency of the infection. The mother may infect the infant in utero, during birth, or by dissemination of infected particles from her respiratory tract and inhaled by the infant. All infants of these mothers should be given tuberculin tests at four to six weeks and again at three months. Breast feeding of these infants must be evaluated in terms of the activity of the disease state in the mother.

Congenital Tuberculosis. Despite the frequency of tuberculosis in the past, only a little over 300 cases of congenital infection have ever been described. The route of infection is by the bloodstream from mother to fetus or by infected amniotic fluid. The infant has no evidence of disease for some weeks following delivery. Many mothers are not themselves obviously ill. It therefore becomes important to examine the placenta macroscopically and microscopically, to examine the amniotic fluid by smear for bacilli and by culture, and to culture cord blood. These observations must be made in all instances of recent infection in the mother, even though she is under treatment, and is recommended but not crucial in those having had extensive but treated tuberculosis in the past.

Congenital tuberculosis requires triple drug therapy continued for approximately three years, depending on the therapeutic response; the third drug, usually streptomycin, is discontinued at three or four months.

Newborn Infants Infected at Birth. Primary tuberculosis in the lung develops as usual following the inhalation of infected particles from the mother or attendant in home or nursery. However, the infant more quickly

---

*Manufacturer's precaution: There is as yet no established dosage of ethambutol for children under 13 years of age.

succumbs to hematogenous lesions and more easily develops endobronchial disease because of small caliber, softer bronchi.

Antituberculosis therapy as for congenital tuberculosis is required. Cultures for acid-fast bacilli, especially from the mother or responsible adult, should be obtained and tested for sensitivity to therapeutic agents. Protection of these infants from other infections is mandatory. The usual immunizations against infectious disease, sometimes delayed in the sick infant, must not be forgotten, especially the protection against measles.

PREVENTION OF TUBERCULOSIS

Chemoprophylaxis. Chemoprophylaxis is used to prevent disease in tuberculin positive patients when (1) existing infection is quiescent but untreated (previously discussed), (2) when other diseases coexist, or (3) when alterations in physiology, metabolism or immunity threaten the patient's health balance. Some instances of the latter two groups are:

  Corticosteroid or other immunosuppressive therapy, and cancer chemotherapy requiring INH coverage, continuing for 6 to 12 weeks after discontinuance of therapy.
  Surgical procedures requiring anesthesia (4 weeks usually)
  Rubeola vaccination or infection (during and for 6 weeks after)
  Pertussis
  Variola
  Reticuloendothelial diseases, such as leukemia and Hodgkin's disease
  Severe viral pulmonary infection, especially influenza (optional)
  Diabetes (early in disease and when unstable, individualized thereafter)
  Pregnancy—following delivery, 6-12 weeks in some patients. Review of mother's medical history is essential.

Chemoprophylaxis to prevent initial infection is essential for members of a household in which a patient with active tuberculosis resides. Prophylactic INH therapy, 10 mg./kg./day to a maximum of 300 mg., is given to the exposed persons. Possible tuberculin conversion is determined by retesting three months later. Short-term therapy adjusted to the circumstances may ensue. Ample evidence exists for the efficacy and safety of this therapy. Sometimes newborn infants of tuberculous mothers are thus protected for a short period, such as three months, allowing time to evaluate the mother's health and infectiousness.

The advantage of chemoprophylaxis is effectiveness with little or rare toxicity, low cost and immediate protection—which, however, ceases with discontinuance of INH.

BCG Vaccination. Protection by BCG vaccine is immunologic and of variable duration, thereby differing from INH prophylaxis. There is no need for the routine use of BCG vaccination in the United States. Indications are (1) infants whose heavily infected environment and exposure to source cases difficult to control place them at high risk. Vaccination of these infants who are not yet infected is desirable. This means separation from the source case until a tuberculin test can be performed at the end of the incubation period (six to eight weeks). (2) Infants of tuberculous mothers in certain high risk areas. (3) Infants and children who are to live any length of time overseas, in areas of high incidence such as Asia, Africa and South America; BCG vaccination is given to these patients two or three months before departure.

The advantage of BCG vaccination is longer protection (possibly five to seven years) by a one-time procedure, not constant medication. A small scar at the vaccination site develops. The chief disadvantage (apart from occasional regional lymphadenitis and suppuration) is interference with tuberculin test readings. Periodic tuberculin testing following vaccination, with careful recording of the induration, is recommended.

BCG protects but does not always prevent disease, hence the importance of changes in tuberculin reactions. In the children's chest clinic of Bellevue Hospital, among the BCG vaccinated patients from South America, Hong Kong and elsewhere, some are clearly superinfected as judged by excessive tuberculin reactions of more than 15 mm. induration. These require INH, either singly or combined.

Two methods of BCG vaccination are used, the intradermal injection in the deltoid area of the appropriate dosage (usually 0.1 ml. of vaccine, obtainable from Eli Lilly and Co.) and the multiple puncture disc method, sometimes using two sites. The latter may be found in patients from overseas, especially the Far East, a helpful observation in those who often fail to report their vaccination.

ATYPICAL MYCOBACTERIAL INFECTIONS

The prevalence of mycobacteria resembling *M. hominis* is well recognized. In children they produce disease primarily in superficial lymph nodes, chiefly cervical, submaxillary and occasionally parotid. "Epidemics" of swimming pool granulomas from various parts of the world, as well as single individual case reports, include children. *Mycobacterium marinum* are grown from these skin lesions.

Nonphotochromogenic mycobacterium (Battey) is associated with severe pulmonary disease in adults. This occurrence is very rare in pediatric practice. Rarely, reports of bone disease, bacteremia or associated lung infection appear in the pediatric literature.

Differentiation of acid-fast bacilli is made by microbiologic and chemical tests. Most strains of atypical mycobacteria are resistant in varying degrees to antituberculous microbials. Triple drug therapy (and occasionally a fourth agent) for *severe* infection is indicated, using high dosage INH (20 mg./kg./day to a maximum 500 mg.). For superficial lymph node disease alone, two drugs are effective. Addition of streptomycin does not appear beneficial. Experience with rifampin is limited. Surgical removal of nodes when indicated is less complicated than for infections due to *M. hominis*. Whether treatment is medical alone or combined with surgical removal, the medications are continued for one year.

Swimming pool granulomas may be diagnosed by biopsy and culture and treated with several drugs. The addition of rifampin to the regimen seems worthwhile, based on reports of its effect in animals infected with Group I organisms. The writer has seen impressive improvement within some weeks in two patients.

Infections by atypical mycobacteria are noncontagious; often only one member of a family is infected. Isolation and restriction of the child's activity are unnecessary. Positive tuberculin skin reactions to antigens of atypical mycobacteria often are found without evidence of disease. No treatment is required. Unlike human tuberculosis prophylactic therapy for tuberculin positive reaction to atypical mycobacteria antigens is not advised.

Leprosy

CALVIN C. J. SIA, M.D.

The therapy of choice for all varieties of leprosy is sulfone therapy. The parent drug, dapsone (4,4'-diaminodiphenylsulfone, DDS, DADPS, "parent sulfone") is the drug of choice based on therapeutic efficacy, cost and ease of administration. Dapsone is given initially in small doses, with the effective dosage reached only after a suitable period of time and increments made cautiously in borderline disease. In using this drug one is cautioned to be aware of sulfone sensitivity and drug resistance with long-term therapy. Blood cell counts and urinalysis should be performed periodically. For the child, the following dosage is recommended:

> First month: 10 mg. twice a week
> Second month: 20 mg. twice a week
> Third month: 25 mg. twice a week
> Fourth month: 50 mg. twice a week
> Thereafter: 100 mg. twice a week

In indeterminate or tuberculoid leprosy (closed), treatment should be given for at least 2 years, or at least 1 year after all clinical signs of activity have disappeared. In lepromatous and borderline leprosy (open), treatment is continued for at least 4 years, or at least 2 years after all clinical signs of activity have ceased, and the acid-fast bacillary material is no longer seen on skin smears. The term clinical activity refers to any extension of existing lesions or the appearance of new lesions, the persistence of redness or elevation of the lesions, or an increase in signs of peripheral nerve damage.

In attempting to reach optimal dosage, sulfone blood levels may be obtained monthly. A good therapeutic level has been about 0.5 mg./ml.

Because of difficulty of ensuring consistent dosage of oral sulfone in children over a 2 to 4 year period, an injectable sulfone,* acedapsone (diacetyl-diamino-diphenyl sulphone, DADDS, Hansolar) has been used in recent years with apparent success. The treatment program has been :

> Age 6 years or over: 1.5 ml. (225 mg.) IM every 75 days.
> Age 6 months to 5 years: 1.0 ml. (150 mg.) IM every 75 days.

This allows the certainty of maintaining a low, consistent blood level of DDS in treatment with five intramuscular injections of acedapsone per year.

In patients harboring dapsone-resistant strains of *Mycobacterium leprae,* clofazimine (Lamprene, investigational) and rifampin are used, as is the case also for complications of leprosy, particularly lepromatous leprosy. In severe exacerbations, corticosteroids are also used. There is no "routine course" in the use of these drugs. Clofazimine and corticosteroids are used initially in high doses. The clofazimine "loading" dose may be 300 mg./day for 2 to 4 weeks, then reduced to 100 to 200 mg./day until the symptoms (such as neuritis) subside. The time required may vary from two weeks to 36 months. Prednisone may be given initially at 40 mg. daily, halving this after 4 to 5

---

*Injectable sulfone has not yet been approved by the Food and Drug Administration.

days. Thereafter, reduction is stepwise at weekly intervals to 10 mg./day, and prednisone is terminated with 10 mg. on alternate days for 2 weeks or more. Reduction of dose is always based upon absence of pain and reduction in size of nerves. Rifampin has been used at 150 mg./day for 6 to 18 months; it is rapidly bactericidal against *M. leprae.**

Physical rehabilitation plays a large role in the total care of the child with developing deformities and contractures. Physical therapy, early orthopedic care and plastic surgery should also be considered in the overall care.

Infections with Atypical Mycobacteria

EDWIN L. KENDIG, JR, M.D.

It has been established that human disease can be caused by mycobacteria previously considered to be harmless. These organisms, called atypical (unclassified, anonymous) mycobacteria, may be the cause of a disease process simulating tuberculosis. Chronic suppurative lymphadenitis is the usual form of this disease in children, but other systems (such as bones, skin and lungs) may be involved.

The usual antituberculosis drugs are utilized in treatment, but these agents are not always effective; they are more effective in group I and much less effective in groups II, III and IV infections. In the treatment of group III infections, authorities have advised the use of drug combinations, often four drugs—one injectable and three oral. In fact, all treatment consists of at least two drugs used concomitantly. The results of susceptibility studies will determine the antimicrobial agents to be utilized.

Isoniazid, 20 mg./kg./day, should be given orally in a single dose, or in two divided doses (maximal daily dosage of 500 mg.), and paraaminosalicylic acid (PAS), 200 mg./kg./day orally in three or four divided doses (maximal daily dosage 12 gm.). If the organism is even partially sensitive, medication should be continued for one year. (For side effects of isoniazid see the Chapter on Tuberculosis.)

Streptomycin, 20 to 40 mg./kg. (maximal daily dose 1 gm.), in a single intramuscular daily dose, is continued until clinical improvement is noted, and the drug may then be administered three times each week. The duration of treatment depends on the course of the disease, but if treatment is prolonged, the patient should be carefully watched for possible damage to the eighth cranial nerve.

Ethambutol, in a suggested dosage of 20 mg./kg./day, is given orally for four to six weeks and 10 to 15 mg./kg./day thereafter in a single daily dose. The drug appears to be an effective and relatively safe agent, although use in pediatric patients under 13 years of age is experimental. It is well tolerated, and there have been few reports of allergic reactions. So far, the drug has been used mainly in adults, and with larger dosage a few instances of retrobulbar neuritis with resultant loss of vision have been noted. At the recommended dosage and with precautions that include monthly studies of visual acuity, visual fields and tests for color vision, there appears to be much less danger of this side effect. The drug should be discontinued if there is more than a two-line loss of visual acuity as measured on a Snellen eye chart, if there is contraction of the visual field or if there is loss of color vision.

Ethionamide, also available for use in combination with one or more drugs, is administered orally in a suggested dosage of 10 to 20 mg./kg. (dosage in children has not been established). It is given in two or three divided doses (maximum daily dose of 750 mg.). The drug may be hepatotoxic.

Kanamycin, given intramuscularly in a dosage of 10 to 15 mg./kg., is similar to streptomycin and may have all the toxic effects of streptomycin plus renal toxicity.

Reports suggest that rifampin possesses significant activity against certain strains of atypical mycobacteria. Suggested dosage is 10 to 20 mg./kg. (maximum daily dose of 600 mg.).

Prompt excision of suppurative lymph nodes is the most important part of the therapeutic approach. Since there is a tendency toward early and complete liquefaction of affected lymph nodes, these nodes should be completely removed as soon as possible. In adults with pulmonary disease who have localized lesions which have not responded to chemotherapy and are in satisfactory general condition, pulmonary resection is the treatment of choice. They should continue to receive the same antimicrobial therapy as previously outlined. There have been a few reports of pulmonary disease in children, but such involvement in this age group must be rare.

Skin lesions caused by *Mycobacterium marinum (balnei)* must often be excised and the patient is always given the same antimicrobial therapy.

Patients with clinical disease caused by the atypical mycobacteria should not be treated in a tuberculosis sanatorium.

---

*This use of rifampin is not mentioned in the manufacturer's instructions.

Syphilis

IRIS F. LITT, M.D.

The recent marked increase in the incidence of syphilis in this country is reflected in the pediatric age group. The number of cases of congenital syphilis diagnosed in children under 1 year of age in 1970 was 300 in spite of the fact that syphilis is one of the most readily preventable of congenital infections. Because it is still quite susceptible to appropriate therapy, prompt diagnosis is vital.

If syphilis is suspected in a neonate, because of the finding of a large placenta, nephrotic syndrome, bullae of palms and soles or other rash, hepatomegaly or jaundice, treatment should be initiated immediately. Aqueous procaine penicillin G in a dose of 100,000 units/kg. should be administered intramuscularly daily for 10 days.

If there is no clinical evidence of syphilis in the newborn whose VDRL test is positive in a titer equal to or higher than that of an already treated mother, it is appropriate to perform an IgM-FTA test and treat if this is positive, rather than waiting several months to observe the VDRL titer.

Acquired syphilis in the child under 2 years of age is best treated with a single dose of 50,000 units/kg. of benzathine penicillin G administered intramuscularly. This is increased to a single dose of 100,000 units/kg., not to exceed 4.8 million units, in the older child. Penicillin allergy in children with acquired syphilis is an indication for treatment with 3 gm./day of tetracycline orally for 10 to 15 days.*

Follow-up care should include performance of a VDRL at 3-month intervals for 1 year. The discovery of a venereal disease in a prepubertal child should always prompt investigation into the possibility of sexual abuse.

For discussion of management of the adolescent with syphilis, see p. 797.

Leptospirosis

LEONARD C. MARCUS, V.M.D., M.D.

To be effective, antibiotic therapy must be initiated within the first four days of clinical illness. Afterwards, there is a marked decline in response and some contend that antibiotics are of no value after that time. Therefore treatment must be based on clinical judgment and initiated immediately after blood has been drawn for culture and serologic confirmation. Adequate early antibiotic treatment may suppress specific antibody response because the antigenic stimulus is removed by killing the organisms. Although serological confirmation may be masked, the course of antibiotic therapy should be completed if there is satisfactory clinical response.

The antibiotic of choice is penicillin or ampicillin. For an adult, give 600,000 units of crystalline penicillin G every four hours for seven days or 750 mg. of ampicillin every six hours for one week. Children should receive proportionate doses.

The severity of illness varies with the serotype of the infective organism and the susceptibility of the host. Severe cases, in which there is a threat of renal failure or significant hepatic damage, obviously require hospitalization, parenteral antibiotics and supportive care. Mild cases may be treated at home with oral medication, if there is adequate supervision to ensure prompt notification of any adverse change in condition. Because of the variable severity of leptospirosis, clinical judgment should be used in modifying therapy, such as switching from parenteral to oral medication or reducing the frequency of penicillin to every six hours if there is adequate improvement after several days of treatment.

A Herxheimer reaction, characterized by increased fever, drop in blood pressure and transient exacerbation of symptoms, often occurs at the start of effective penicillin therapy. Although distressing to the patient, it subsides spontaneously and is not a contraindication to continuation of treatment.

Some clinicians recommend the tetracyclines as alternative drugs, 2 to 4 gm./day in 4 divided doses to adults. However, there is little proof that these drugs are beneficial and many clinical reports indicate they are ineffective. Chloramphenicol is of little or no value.

The most common serious complication of leptospirosis is renal failure, manifested by progressive uremia, hyperkalemia, confusion and clinical deterioration. This should be treated by peritoneal dialysis or use of the artificial kidney.

Hemorrhagic manifestations may be due to thrombocytopenia and should be treated with transfusion of platelets. If there is evidence of disseminated intravascular coagulopathy, heparin should be used. Appropriate supportive care is given for other possible complications such as hepatic failure or shock.

An ophthalmologist should be consulted if

---

*Manufacturer's note: Use of tetracycline during infancy and childhood to age 8 years may cause permanent discoloration of the teeth.

there is uveitis. Such consultation is not necessary if the eye lesions are limited to conjunctival congestion, since this will clear without topical therapy as the systemic infection is controlled.

Rat-Bite Fever

LEONARD C. MARCUS, V.M.D., M.D.

There are two forms of rat-bite fever: one caused by an aerobic, gram-negative, pleomorphic, filamentous rod, *Streptobacillus moniliformis (Actinobacillus muris)*, and Sodoku fever caused by a spirochete, *Spirillum minor*. Both infections can be severe, requiring hospitalization, especially streptobacillary rat-bite fever,* which may be complicated by endocarditis. Most cases of rat-bite fever due to either organism respond favorably to high doses of penicillin (1 million units per day for two weeks for an adult), but it may be necessary in some cases to also treat with 1 gm. of streptomycin per day for at least one week. Endocarditis due to *S. moniliformis* should be treated with 12 to 15 million units of penicillin daily plus 0.5 to 1 gm. of streptomycin per day for three to four weeks.

S. moniliformis can produce L forms which lack cell walls and therefore are penicillin-resistant. L forms are likely to occur with inadequate penicillin treatment. Therefore a full course of high-dose penicillin should be completed, and some cases may require treatment longer than that recommended above by one or two weeks.

Pneumocystis carinii Pneumonitis

WALTER T. HUGHES, M.D.

Pneumocystis carinii pneumonitis occurs almost exclusively in patients with a serious underlying disease which has compromised the host's resistance to infection. The infection is primarily a diffuse alveolitis, with interstitial edema which results in a severe compromise in pulmonary function and alteration in acid-base profile. Hypoxia with low arterial oxygen tension (PaO_2) is always present, carbon dioxide retention rarely occurs, and the arterial pH is usually increased. The infection remains limited to the lungs even in fatal cases.

Successful management requires early diagnosis, specific antimicrobial therapy and intensive supportive management. The procedure required to obtain material for diagnostic studies is needle aspiration of the lung, lung biopsy, or endotracheal brush catheter technique. Pneumothorax is a complication of these procedures, and management demands attention to this hazard. Also, optimum treatment of the primary disease should be maintained.

Specific Therapy. Two drugs are available for the treatment of *Pneumocystis carinii* pneumonitis: trimethoprim-sulfamethoxazole and pentamidine isethionate. The drugs are equally effective but trimethoprim-sulfamethoxazole has significantly less toxicity and is commercially available.

Trimethoprim-sulfamethoxazole is administered orally in the dosage of 20 mg. of trimethoprim and 100 mg./kg./day of sulfamethoxazole.* The daily dose is divided into four parts and given at 6 hour intervals. A total course of 14 days is required for most cases. The preparation is available as a tablet (80 mg. of trimethoprim and 400 mg. of sulfamethoxazole) and as a suspension (40 mg. of trimethoprim and 200 mg. of sulfamethoxazole per 5.0 ml.). The adverse and toxic side effects are essentially those of sulfonamides. Although uncommon, the reported adverse effects include transient maculopapular rash, nausea, vomiting, diarrhea, agranulocytosis, aplastic anemia, megaloblastic anemia, hemolytic anemia, methemoglobinemia, Stevens-Johnson syndrome, allergic reactions, toxic nephrosis and drug fever. Folic acid deficiency has occurred but only rarely. This is reversible by the administration of folinic acid, 10 to 25 mg. daily.

Pentamidine is the drug of second choice because of the high frequency of adverse effects. Manufactured under the name Lomidine by May and Baker, Ltd., Dagenham, England, the drug is investigational and available in the United States only through the Center for Disease Control. Physicians may obtain the drug to treat specific cases by calling the Parasitic Disease Drug Service at 404-633-3311, ext. 3676; at night the number is 404-633-2176.

Pentamidine is administered as a single daily dose of 4 mg./kg. intramuscularly for 10 to 14 days. If improvement is apparent after 5

---

*Streptobacillary rat-bite fever is often referred to as Haverhill fever, but this term was originally used to describe infection resulting from ingestion of milk contaminated with *S. moniliformis* and some restrict its definition to such nonbite-associated conditions.

---

*Manufacturer's precaution: Trimethoprim-sulfamethoxazole is not recommended for infants under 2 months of age.

days of treatment, the dosage may be reduced to 3 mg./kg./day. The total dosage should not exceed 56 mg./kg. Intramuscular injections should be given deeply into the anterolateral aspect of the thigh. Each 100 mg. of the drug should be dissolved in 1 ml. of sterile distilled water. Filtration of the drug in solution through a Millipore filter (0.22-micron pore size) immediately before injection is advisable to ensure sterility for the immunosuppressed host.

Adverse effects of pentamidine include the following: induration, abscess formation and necrosis at injection sites; nephrotoxicity; hypoglycemia or, rarely, hyperglycemia; hypotension; alteration in liver function; tachycardia; hypocalcemia; nausea and vomiting; skin rash; anemia; hyperkalemia; and thrombocytopenia.

Since the mode of transmission of *P. carinii* is unknown, it is advisable to isolate the patient from other individuals at high risk for this infection.

Supportive Measures. OXYGEN. Oxygen should be administered by mask as needed to maintain the PaO₂ above 70 mm. Hg. The fraction of inspired oxygen (FiO₂) should be kept below 50 per cent if possible, to avoid oxygen toxicity, since oxygen therapy is usually required for relatively long periods of time.

VENTILATION THERAPY. Assisted or controlled ventilation is indicated in patients with arterial oxygen tension less than 60 mm. Hg at FiO₂ of 50 per cent or greater. Patients with acutely elevated Pco₂, without pH changes, and with or without hypoxemia should be considered candidates for ventilatory therapy.

WITHHOLD IMMUNOSUPPRESSIVE CHEMOTHERAPY. Patients receiving immunosuppressive drugs should have these discontinued if the status of the primary disease permits. Corticosteroids are of no benefit and may be deleterious to the course of the pneumonitis.

INTRAVENOUS FLUIDS. Fluid and electrolyte quantities are calculated by the patient's needs, but the solution should contain 5 or 10 per cent glucose to aid in the prevention of hypoglycemia during pentamidine therapy. Metabolic acidosis must be corrected.

ANTIBIOTICS. Bacterial pneumonia or sepsis may occur in association with *P. carinii* pneumonitis. In the seriously ill patient with marked neutropenia (absolute neutrophil count less than 1000/cu. mm.) or evidence of bacterial infection, antibiotics should be given. Oxacillin, 100 mg./kg./day, and gentamicin, 5 mg./kg./day, are administered intravenously until the results of cultures are known.

NUTRITION. Efforts should be made to improve the nutritional status of the patient by dietary means even during the acute stage of the disease. Multivitamins should be given empirically. The value of intravenous alimentation has not been determined.

ANEMIA. Give blood transfusion if hemoglobin level is less than normal. The hemoglobin content must be sufficient to result in an arterial oxygen content of 15 to 20 ml./100 ml. of blood at an arterial oxygen tension of 100 mm. Hg.

PNEUMOTHORAX. Pneumothorax may be a complication of diagnostic procedures. If the pneumothorax is less than 15 per cent with no adverse effect on respiration, close observation is adequate. If the pneumothorax is more extensive, insertion of a thoracotomy tube with a water seal drainage system is necessary.

Parameters to Monitor. *Serum immunoglobulins* at the onset of the illness. Administer immune serum globulin (165 mg./ml.), 0.66 ml./kg. if the immunoglobulin G level is below 300 mg./100 ml.

Roentgenograms of chest daily until clinical evidence of improvement. If needle aspiration of the lung, lung biopsy or endotracheal brush catheter technique has been used as a diagnostic procedure, chest roentgenograms should be made at 30 minutes, 4 hours and 12 hours after the procedure to detect pneumothorax.

Hemoglobin, white blood cell count and differential, and platelet estimate.

Body weight, intake and output daily.

Arterial blood gases: measure pH, Pco₂, Po₂, and base excess or deficit initially and as often as necessary, based on severity of clinical course.

Serum electrolytes: measure sodium, chloride, potassium and carbon dioxide content every 3 days or more frequently if indicated.

Total serum proteins, albumin and globulin: every three days. Hypoalbuminemia may occur.

Blood pressure, pulse and respiratory rate every 4 hours, or more frequently if the condition is critical.

For patients receiving pentamidine: *blood urea nitrogen and urinalysis* every 3 days. If the BUN exceeds 30 mg./100 ml., withhold pentamidine for a day or two; *blood glucose* 4 to 6 hours after each injection of pentamidine. Administer glucose if value of blood glucose is less than 40 mg./100 ml.; *serum glutamic oxaloacetic transaminase (SGOT)* every 3 days; withhold pentamidine for 1 to 2 days if evidence of hepatic toxicity exists; and *serum calcium and phosphorus* every 3 days. If the serum inorganic phosphate level becomes increased and the calcium level becomes decreased from normal values on the basis of renal insufficiency, give calcium lactate, 15 to 20 gm./day, or calcium carbonate, 5 to 8 gm./day orally. The diet should be low in phosphate, and 25,000 to 50,000 units of vitamin D is given orally. For patients with renal impairment and receiving trimethoprim-sulfamethoxazole, the dosage should be regulated on the basis of serum drug levels. Measurement of serum levels of the sulfonamide is adequate. The level of free sulfonamide should be maintained with peak values between 100 and 150 μg./ml. measured 2 hours after the oral dosage.

Expected Course. Fever, tachypnea and pulmonary infiltrates usually persist with little change for 4 to 6 days. If no improvement is apparent after a week of therapy, concomitant or secondary infection most likely exists. These infections have included bacterial pneumonia or sepsis, systemic candidiasis, aspergillosis, cryptococcosis, histoplasmosis and cytomegalovirus inclusion disease as well as other viral infections. Recurrent *P. carinii* pneumonitis may occur several months after apparent recovery in 10 to 15 per cent of cases.

Measles (Rubeola)

JAMES D. CHERRY, M.D.

Measles is an acute communicable disease characterized by cough, coryza, conjunctivitis, fever, Koplik's spots, and an erythematous, maculopapular confluent exanthem. Prior to the present vaccine era, measles epidemics occurred yearly in the winter and spring. At the present time with widespread use of measles vaccine the epidemiology of measles has changed so that its seasonal nature has been somewhat disrupted and the occurrence of illness is frequently sporadic or characterized by many focal mini-epidemics. In addition, the occurrence of measles in previous vaccine recipients ("vaccine failure") is on occasion mild, causing difficulty with differential diagnosis. In other instances a severe but atypical illness is noted. This "atypical measles" occurs following natural measles exposure in children who previously received an immunization regimen which included killed measles vaccine and is characterized by abrupt onset of fever followed by an exanthem with a peripheral distribution.

PREVENTION

Active Immunization—Live Attenuated Measles Virus Vaccine (Schwarz and Moraten Strains). Attenuated measles vaccines are prepared in chicken embryo tissue cultures. Vaccination produces a mild or inapparent noncommunicable infection which induces active immunity in 95 per cent of recipients. Vaccine-induced antibodies persist for many years and although reinfection with illness has been noted on occasion in apparently successfully immunized children, it does not presently appear that waning immunity is of significant epidemiologic importance. Symptoms associated with measles immunization are minimal and are limited to fever, mild malaise, and occasionally a faint rash occurring approximately one week post immunization.

RECOMMENDATIONS FOR USE. In general live measles vaccine should be administered at 15 months of age. Children who have not received vaccine during infancy may be immunized at any age and adults who have not had natural measles should also be immunized. When measles is endemic or epidemic in a community, all children 6 months of age and over should be immunized. In children who were initially vaccinated before 12 months of age, a second vaccination should be administered at 15 months of age or prior to the next measles season, since the likelihood of long-lasting protection in children vaccinated during the first year of life is far from optimal.

PRECAUTIONS. Ideally tuberculin testing should be carried out prior to measles immunization and children with positive tuberculin tests should be on chemotherapy prior to immunization.

Measles vaccination should be deferred during febrile illnesses or when interference from another viral infection might cause measles vaccine failure. Measles immunization should also be postponed for eight weeks in persons who have received whole blood, blood plasma or immune serum globulin because these products may contain sufficient measles antibody to neutralize the vaccine virus.

CONTRAINDICATIONS. Live measles vaccine should not be administered to pregnant women or to persons with diseases or therapeutic programs associated with impaired cell-mediated immunity. These conditions include leukemia, lymphoma or other generalized malignancies; primary immunologic disorders; therapy with steroids, radiation, antimetabolites or alkylating agents.

Reimmunization with Live Measles Vaccine. At the present time there is no evidence that booster doses of measles vaccine are necessary in children who had an antibody response following primary immunization. However, many children who initially were immunized improperly are not presently protected against measles and therefore should be reimmunized. Children in the following categories should be revaccinated: all children who received primary measles immunizations before a year of age; all children whose initial vaccine regimens included a killed measles virus vaccine; and children in whom the original immunization may not have been performed in an optimal manner (the administration of too much concurrent immune serum globulin, suspicion of improper storage of vaccine, and the possibility of concurrent other viral infection which prevented initial vaccine virus infection).

Quarantine and Disease Containment. Prior to the widespread use of measles vaccines, quarantine measures were widely practiced but largely ineffective in preventing the spread of measles. However, today, disease containment is practical because the widespread use of measles vaccine has reduced the general number of susceptible young children, which in turn has decreased the rapidity of epidemic development. Today epidemic measles generally involves a greater age range of the population (cases in adolescents and young adults are frequent), and progression of disease from one age group to another is slower than epidemics that involve one uniform largely susceptible population.

Containment is a vital part of the measles prevention policy in the United States today. Measles is a reportable disease throughout the United States and compliance is the obligation of all physicians. Following early reports of sporadic measles, health department workers can organize local immunization clinics so that disease can often be contained in a small geographic area rather than developing into a widespread epidemic.

Passive Immunization—Immune Serum Globulin (Human). In the present vaccine era there should be little need for passive immunization. However, in instances where a known susceptible child has had definite exposure to measles, immune serum globulin (human) should be administered in a dose of 0.25 ml./kg. If this is performed within five days of exposure, prevention of infection and disease can be expected. The administration of immune serum globulin later in the incubation period may modify illness but will not prevent it. The use of immune serum globulin is particularly important in those children who have not been immunized because of the contraindications mentioned above. In these children immune serum globulin should be administered when measles is epidemic in the commu-

nity in which they reside. Dosage should be repeated every four weeks until the epidemic subsides.

Treatment

Uncomplicated Measles. There is no specific treatment for uncomplicated measles. During the febrile period of illness, activity is discouraged and fluids are maintained by the liberal provision of soft drinks and ices. Fever may be controlled with aspirin, 75 mg./yr. of age every 4 to 6 hours; the maximum dose is 2.4 gm./day. Cough is frequently distressing and can be managed by judicious use of common antitussives. Room humidification is also useful in controlling the cough and generally can be expected to make the patient more comfortable. As the fever disappears a gradual return to normal activity is indicated. However, measles infection is associated with considerable damage to the ciliated epithelium of the respiratory tract and therefore too early resumption of normal activities and exposure to other children and their bacterial pathogens can be associated with severe secondary infection.

Atypical Measles. The most important aspect of therapy of atypical measles is proper diagnosis. Frequently children with atypical measles are erroneously diagnosed as having Rocky Mountain spotted fever or other septic conditions, and their workup is associated with extensive blood cultures, other diagnostic procedures and vigorous antibiotic therapy. Careful attention to a history of prior administration of killed measles vaccine should clarify the diagnosis and prevent the unnecessary trauma associated with extensive diagnostic and therapeutic procedures.

In atypical measles chest roentgenograms should always be obtained because the pneumonia is frequent and much more extensive than the clinical findings would indicate. Activity should be discouraged in the acutely ill patient and follow-up chest roentgenograms should be used as a guide to the resumption of normal activity. In some children pulmonary abnormalities have persisted for a considerable period of time.

Complications of Measles. OTITIS MEDIA. Otitis media is the most frequent complication of measles. The infectious etiology of otitis media in measles is no different from that in other children of comparable ages without measles (*Hemophilus influenzae, Streptococcus pneumoniae,* and *Streptococcus pyogenes* in children less than four years of age and *Streptococcus pneumoniae* and *Streptococcus pyogenes* in older children). The following treatment is recommended: for children less than four years of age either ampicillin or amoxicillin,* 75 mg./kg./day orally in four divided doses for a minimum of 10 days. For penicillin-allergic children cephalexin, 50 mg./kg./day orally in four divided doses for a minimum of 10 days, can be administered. In children four years of age and older penicillin V, 75,000 units/kg./day orally in four divided doses for a minimum of 10 days, should be administered. In penicillin-allergic children either cephalexin, 50 mg./kg./day orally in four divided doses, or erythromycin, 30 mg./kg./day in four divided doses for a minimum of 10 days, can be administered.

Laryngotracheitis. The management of laryngotracheitis due to measles viral infection is similar to that in other patients with croup due to other viral etiologies. The mainstay of therapy is the administration of humidified air and a concerted effort to relieve the apprehension of the patient. Corticosteroids are contraindicated in measles and antibiotics are indicated only if there is laboratory or clinical evidence of secondary bacterial infection. Nebulized saline with or without racemic epinephrine, administered either by intermittent positive pressure or simply by a face mask and compressor, may be useful in achieving acute relief of severe inspiratory obstruction. Recent reports would seem to suggest that racemic epinephrine may bring temporary relief in some children not responding to therapy with saline alone. The judicious use of a single dose of a sedative (phenobarbital, 2 mg./kg./dose, or chloral hydrate, 7 mg./kg./dose) to allay anxiety can be extremely useful. Tracheostomy is rarely necessary in measles croup but its consideration should not be overlooked in the child with severe obstruction who does not respond to an adequate trial with the above measures.

Pneumonia. Pneumonia is a common complication of measles and is the leading cause of death. Pneumonia may be a manifestation of primary viral infection or it may result from a superimposed bacterial infection. Primary measles viral pneumonia is more common than generally appreciated but fortunately in most instances it is relatively mild. Primary measles viral pneumonia is usually interstitial in distribution, but occasionally considerable lobar involvement is noted by roentgenograph. The differential diagnosis between primary viral and superimposed bacterial disease cannot be made with certainty. Since the diagnosis of viral pneumonia in many instances is uncertain, most cases should be treated with antibiotics.

Bacterial pneumonia in measles is due to common organisms that cause pneumonia in children without measles. These organisms include *Streptococcus pneumoniae, Hemophilus influenzae, Streptococcus pyogenes,* and *Staphylococcus aureus.* The differential diagnosis between staphylococcal pneumonia and other pneumonias can in almost all instances be made radiologically (the presence of pleural fluid and pneumatoceles) and therefore antibiotic therapy need not be tailored for staphylococcal disease unless the roentgenograms suggest this illness. If pleural fluid is present, thoracentesis is mandatory prior to therapy.

Therapy for nonstaphylococcal pneumonia in children less than four years of age should employ ampicillin or amoxicillin. A cephalosporin can be used in penicillin-allergic children. In children four years of age and older penicillin is the drug of choice and a cephalosporin can be employed in penicillin-allergic patients. In relatively mild illnesses oral therapy (similar to that described for otitis media as above) is adequate. In more severe cases hospitalization is indicated and therapy should be parenteral. The dose of parenteral ampicillin is 100 mg./kg./day in six divided doses and the dose of penicillin G is 150,000 units/kg./day in six divided doses. In allergic children cefazolin, 50 mg./day in four divided doses, is indicated.

Staphylococcal pneumonia should be treated with either oxacillin or nafcillin, 150 mg./kg./day in four divided doses.* In staphylococcal pneumonia empyema fluid should be removed either by repeated thoracentesis or by the insertion of a chest tube and continuous drainage. In young children continuous drainage is preferred.

Encephalitis. Measles encephalitis is particularly severe with a significant mortality and a neurologic residual rate of at least 50 per cent. The incidence of overt encephalitis is approximately one per 1000 cases of measles. The course of measles encephalitis is unpredictable and the treatment is symptomatic and supportive. Trained nursing care is essential. Careful attention to fluid and electrolyte balance is necessary. In prolonged states of coma

---

*This dosage of amoxicillin is higher than that recommended by the manufacturer but has been found safe and effective.

*This dosage of nafcillin is higher than that recommended by the manufacturer but has been found to be safe and effective.

parenteral hyperalimentation is indicated. Seizure control should utilize standard anticonvulsive agents: phenobarbital, 6 mg./kg./day in three or four divided doses, or phenytoin, 6 to 8 mg./kg./day in two or three doses. Diazepam, 0.2 mg./kg./dose intravenously, 2 minute infusion, may be useful in the acute therapy of seizures.* Controlled studies have shown that corticosteroids in relatively low dosage offer no benefit. In severe intractable seizures or other evidence of cerebral edema the use of intravenous mannitol, 1.5 to 2 gm./kg. of a 20 per cent solution in 30 to 60 minutes,† or high-dose dexamethasone, initial loading dose of 0.2 mg./kg. intravenously or intramuscularly followed by a maintenance dose of 0.5 mg./kg./day in four divided doses, would appear to be indicated. In occasional circumstances respiratory arrest is a problem and artificial ventilators should be used to tide patients over until normal respirations occur.

Appendicitis.   Acute abdominal pain is an occasional occurrence in primary measles and may be caused by generalized mesenteric adenitis due to measles virus or to appendicitis. In appendicitis there is evidence of measles viral involvement of the appendix. However, therapy should be similar to that in other cases of appendicitis; removal of the appendix is indicated as measles appendicitis perforates with a frequency equal to that in patients without measles virus.

Rubella (German Measles) and Congenital Rubella

JAMES D. CHERRY, M.D.

RUBELLA

Rubella is an acute communicable disease of children and young adults characterized by low grade fever, mild malaise, headache and an erythematous maculopapular discrete rash. Prior to the present vaccine era rubella was an epidemic occurrence. Disease appeared predominantly in the winter and spring with major epidemics approximately every 7 years. Since the introduction and widespread use of rubella vaccine the epidemiology of rubella has changed. Major epidemic disease has not occurred since 1964. However, in spite of this lack of a major epidemic spread of virus many local epidemics of rubella have occurred and continue to occur. At the present time disease is most prevalent in teenagers.

Prevention

Active Immunization—Live Attenuated Rubella Virus Vaccine.   At the present time there are two attenuated rubella virus vaccines available for use in the United States (HPV77 strain grown in duck embryo tissue culture and Cendehill strain grown in rabbit kidney tissue culture). Vaccination can be expected to produce antibodies in 95 per cent of those immunized. Immunization of young children has been associated with only minimal lymphadenopathy. Vaccination of adolescents and adults has on occasion been associated with transient arthralgia, arthritis and lymphadenopathy. The vaccine associated arthritis and lymphadenopathy have on occasion been marked.

RECOMMENDATIONS FOR USE.   Live rubella virus vaccine is recommended for all children 15 months of age or older. A prior history of rubella is an unreliable index of immunity; all children regardless of history should receive rubella immunization. Pregnant women should not be given live rubella virus vaccine, as infection of the fetus with the attenuated virus may take place and there is a potential risk to the fetus.

Vaccination of adolescent girls and women of childbearing age is important for the prevention of congenital rubella. These persons should have their blood examined for rubella hemagglutination-inhibiting (HAI) antibodies, and those without demonstrable antibody should be immunized if they agree to prevent pregnancy for a period of three months after immunizaton. Vaccination of adolescent or adult males has not been considered a major priority. However, the immunization of known susceptibles in these age groups can be helpful in controlling outbreaks of rubella in circumscribed populations.

CONTRAINDICATIONS.   Live rubella virus vaccine is contraindicated in pregnancy and in altered immune states such as immunodeficiency, leukemia, lymphoma, generalized malignancy, or therapy with steroids, alkylating drugs, antimetabolites and radiation. Rubella vaccination also should not be performed during febrile illnesses or in situations in which viral interference from another agent might preclude a "take" from the rubella immunization. Rubella immunization should also be deferred for eight weeks following the administration of blood products including immune serum globulin.

---

*Manufacturer's precaution: The safety and efficacy of injectable diazepam have not been established in the neonate.

†Manufacturer's precaution: Dosage requirements of mannitol for patients 12 years and under have not been established.

Passive Immunization. The use of immune serum globulin (human) for the prevention of rubella has been controversial for many years. It is my opinion that its use is clearly indicated under certain circumstances. The specific indication for immune serum globulin is for the prevention of rubella in a woman thought to be susceptible to rubella who is in the first 20 weeks of pregnancy. If an exposure can be clearly documented as an exposure to a specific single person with rubella and the immune globulin is given within 72 hours of that exposure, prevention of both maternal disease and congenital infection is likely. On the other hand, if the exposure was more general in nature (a school teacher exposed to a child or children in the school setting), it is likely that the person was actually exposed a considerable period of time prior to her realization of that exposure. Therefore administration of immune globulin will probably be too late (well into the incubation period of her disease and after viremia), and congenital infection is unlikely to be prevented. The dose of immune serum globulin (human) for the prevention of rubella during pregnancy is 20 ml. intramuscularly.

Quarantine and Disease Containment. Patients with rubella should not have contact with susceptible persons until the rash has disappeared. Rubella containment is a vital part of the prevention policy in the United States today. Rubella is a reportable disease and compliance is the obligation of all physicians and other health professionals. Rubella reporting enables public health workers to organize vaccination programs so that small outbreaks of disease can be prevented from developing into major epidemics.

Management of the Exposed Pregnant Woman

Ideally all pregnant women should have blood drawn for rubella serology at their first visit to their obstetrician. If this has been done and serum antibody to rubella is present no further concern is necessary. If the initial serum showed no rubella antibody and a subsequent exposure to a person with rubella can be documented to have been within 72 hours, 20 ml. of immune serum globulin (human) is administered immediately. If exposure was more than 72 hours before seeking medical attention, immune globulin is not to be administered because it will contribute to confusion in regard to the further diagnosis of rubella and further therapy (termination of pregnancy). If prior to exposure serum antibody information is not available, an immediate blood specimen is obtained and the rubella HAI antibody titer

is determined. If an antibody titer to rubella is found (HAI titer ≥ 8) no further concern is warranted. If no titer is detectable (HAI titer <8), serum immune globulin (human) is given if the exposure was within the preceding 72 hours. In susceptible rubella-exposed women careful clinical observation for the occurrence of fever, lymphadenopathy or exanthem is carried out for a four week period. A second serum specimen is submitted for rubella antibody examination six to eight weeks after the initial specimen. If a rubella antibody titer rise is noted, there is a considerable risk for fetal infection and malformation, and the woman should be advised and therapeutic abortion contemplated.

Management of the Pregnant Woman with an Exanthem Thought to Be Rubella

In this circumstance if previous rubella serology is available it is extremely useful. If previous serum antibody (HAI titer ≥ 8) had been noted, the mother is reassured that the present illness is not likely to be rubella. If, on the other hand, previous serology revealed no rubella antibody (HAI titer <8), a second serum specimen is collected two to three weeks after the disappearance of the rash and examined for rubella antibody. If titer rise occurs, it is highly likely that congenital infection occurred and that anomalies may result; the woman should be counseled in regard to therapeutic abortion.

If a previous serum rubella antibody titer is not available an immediate serum should be collected immediately and again two to three weeks later. These serums should be examined as paired specimens for rubella HAI antibody and, if facilities are available, examined for specific rubella IgM antibody. If rubella titer rise is demonstrated or the presence of rubella IgM is noted, it must be assumed that an acute rubella viral infection has occurred and the patient is advised of the risk of congenital infection and the possible role of therapeutic abortion.

Treatment

Uncomplicated Rubella. No specific therapy is necessary or indicated in uncomplicated rubella. However, it is important that the affected patient understand that he or she is contagious and that transmission of infection to a pregnant woman could have serious consequences.

Complications of Rubella. ARTHRITIS. Joint manifestations associated with rubella are transient, generally subsiding in one to two weeks. Occasionally in adults symptoms can be quite severe, and when weight bearing joints are affected rest is encouraged. Symptoms readily respond to aspirin therapy; corticosteroids are not indicated.

ENCEPHALITIS. Encephalitis is a rare complication and the overall prognosis in regard to both morbidity and mortality is good. In contrast to measles, rubella encephalitis is rarely associated with seizures and usually manifests as somnolence and stupor. Care is supportive with adequate maintenance of fluids and electrolytes.

THROMBOCYTOPENIA. Occult thrombocytopenia is not infrequent in rubella but symptomatic disease is fortunately rare. Thrombocytopenia is usually self-limited; however, on occasions severe bleeding has occurred. Splenectomy is not indicated and there is little evidence that corticosteroid therapy is of specific benefit in rubella-infected patients.

CONGENITAL RUBELLA

Congenital rubella infection occurs following maternal rubella viral infection in the first 20 weeks of pregnancy. The frequency of congenital involvement and to some extent the severity are inversely related to the gestational age at the time of maternal infection. The risk of fetal infection exceeds 50 per cent with maternal infection during the first two months of pregnancy. The diagnosis of congenital rubella is a possibility if any one of the following signs is noted: intrauterine growth retardation, cataracts, microophthalmia, retinopathy, deafness, heart disease, thrombocytopenia, hepatosplenomegaly, metaphyseal rarification of long bones, psychomotor retardation, jaundice, dermatoglyphic abnormality, glaucoma, myocardial damage, hepatitis, generalized adenopathy, hemolytic or hypoplastic anemia, spastic quadriparesis and immunologic abnormalities. A maternal history of possible rubella or rubella exposure early in pregnancy should also alert the physician to be on the lookout for congenital infection. Congenital rubella can be verified by: isolation of rubella virus from the nose, urine or cerebrospinal fluid, or tissues obtained at biopsy; the presence of hemagglutinating-inhibiting antibody in the serum of infants 6 months of age; or the identification of specific rubella IgM antibody in serum of a neonate.

Prevention

At the present time in the United States congenital rubella must be considered a totally preventable disease. Prevention can be assured if those who care for children both in the public and private sector of health care delivery insist upon rubella immunization of all children. In addition serologic screening programs should be available both publicly and privately so that known susceptible women of child-bearing age can be immunized.

Management of Children with Congenital Rubella

Isolation Procedures. Although rubella viral infection in congenital rubella occurs early during the gestational period, the infection persists throughout in utero life, and most babies with congenital rubella are still actively infected at the time of birth. Babies with congenital rubella are contagious and therefore should be placed in isolation. Room isolation and urine precautions are the major necessities. The isolated baby should only be cared for by persons known to be seropositive for rubella (HAI antibody titer ⩾8). Since rubella viral shedding has been known to occur for a year or more in some babies, isolation of infants with congenital rubella is continued for this duration unless repeated viral cultures are proved to be negative.

Following discharge from the hospital no special precautions are necessary in the household setting. However, the parents are advised of the potential risk to pregnant visitors.

The Neonatal Period. As noted above the clinical manifestations of congenital rubella are varied and in many infants no symptomatology is manifest during the first few months of life. In these apparently asymptomatic infants, no particular management problems are encountered. In other neonates the symptomatology of the continued viral infection is readily apparent and frequently severe. In these infants the following findings are important: pneumonia, thrombocytopenia, eye disorders, heart defects, hyperbilirubinemia, and hepatosplenomegaly.

Although purpura and petechiae secondary to thrombocytopenia may be impressively severe in these infants, true hemorrhagic difficulties have not been a major problem. Corticosteroid therapy would not seem to be indicated. Careful evaluation of the eyes is important. Of immediate concern is the search for corneal clouding, as this likely indicates infantile glaucoma. Cataracts and retinopathy also are searched for carefully. Infants with glaucoma are referred immediately for ophthalmological evaluation and therapy. Children with cataracts and/or retinopathy also should be referred, but therapy in the former is best delayed until a later age.

Respiratory distress secondary to extensive viral involvement is managed in a fashion similar to other neonatal respiratory disease. This includes assisted ventilation and careful attention to arterial blood gas pressures and pH. Although jaundice secondary to congenital rubella infection rarely in itself is severe, standard criteria for the treatment for hyperbilirubinemia are followed. Hepatosplenomegaly may be marked in some instances but in itself is of no therapeutic concern.

Cardiac evaluation is similar to that for affected nonrubella infants. Specifically, congestive cardiac failure is treated vigorously and in malignant conditions (patent ductus arteriosus, coarctation of the aorta), life-saving surgery is contemplated.

Long-Term Problems. DEAFNESS. Hearing disability is the most frequent abnormality following congenital rubella infection; over 80 per cent of infected infants have some degree of hearing disability. In many instances deafness is the only clinical manifestation of congenital rubella and because of the difficulty in making this diagnosis in early infancy, diagnosis is frequently delayed. However, early diagnosis of deafness and the institution of proper educational programs are the single most productive aspects in the long-term management of children with congenital rubella. All too frequently ill advised medical advice has delayed appropriate diagnosis and therapy. In all instances when a mother has a suspicion that her child is deaf, an evaluation with specific audiometric testing is carried out. All too frequently general practitioners, pediatricians, and even otolaryngologists believe that hearing cannot be tested in young infants. This concept must be vigorously discouraged; at proper centers the severely deaf child can be recognized in virtually all instances.

Following the diagnosis of deafness, the child is referred immediately to a training program. Information about training programs as well as publications for parents and teachers can be obtained from the Alexander Graham Bell Association for the Deaf, Inc., 1537 35th Street, N.W., Washington, D.C. 20007. The John Tracy Clinic, Inc., 806 West Adams Boulevard, Los Angeles, Calif. 90007, is an important source of information on preschool deaf children. Severely deaf children should be enrolled in an education program before or during the second year of life and fitted with a proper auditory amplification device. Although deafness in congenital rubella is sensorineural, it is surprising that conduction defects are also noted in older children. In these instances other aspects of otolaryngologic care may be indicated.

EYE PROBLEMS. All children with eye problems (cloudy cornea, glaucoma, cataracts, retinitis, strabismus) are referred at an early age for ophthalmological evaluation. Glaucoma needs immediate attention. Cataract surgery is left to the discretion of the ophthalmologist, but in general is well deferred until after the end of the first year. Retinopathy, although frequently impressive on ophthalmoscopic examination, rarely causes much in the way of visual defect. Management of strabismus is similar to that in children without rubella. Information about available schools and services for infants with eye problems due to congenital rubella can be obtained from the American Foundation for the Blind, Inc., 15 West 16th Street, New York, New York 10011.

HEART PROBLEMS. Congenital heart disease secondary to in utero rubella infection is managed similarly to heart disease in children without rubella. It is important that these children be referred to cardiac centers where sophisticated diagnostic techniques and facilities for cardiac surgery for correctable lesions are available.

MUSCULOSKELETAL PROBLEMS. Isolated musculoskeletal defects are relatively uncommon in congenital rubella. However, when the symptomatology would indicate, referral to a cerebral palsy clinic is useful both for specific therapeutic modalities and for the camaraderie of group therapy for the children as well as the parents.

CENTRAL NERVOUS SYSTEM PROBLEMS. Mental retardation has been considered a major part of the rubella syndrome and is believed to occur in about one-third of children infected in utero. However, a careful analysis of the data suggests that many infants who have been labeled retarded are really children with auditory and/or visual defects who have not had proper diagnosis and training for their handicaps. No child with congenital rubella should be labeled as being mentally subnormal until extensive audiologic and ophthalmologic investigation and perhaps specific therapy have been performed. Probably less than 5 per cent of all children with congenital rubella have central nervous system defects that preclude normal development.

IMMUNOLOGIC DEFECTS. A small number of children with congenital rubella have been noted with specifically low levels of serum IgG. These infants have systemic continued viral infection and in general do poorly. Although outcome studies are not available, it would seem prudent to administer immune serum globulin (human), 0.66 ml./kg. every four weeks, to these infants.

MULTIPLE HANDICAPS. All too frequently children infected in utero with rubella virus suffer from one or more of the handicaps mentioned above. The care of these infants and children requires many different resources and modalities of therapy. Frequently it is the physician who is called upon to coordinate both the diagnostic and long-term educational efforts which are necessary for the optimum progress of an affected child. In addition to the Alexander Graham Bell Association for the Deaf, Inc., The John Tracy Clinic, Inc., and the American Foundation for the Blind, Inc., the following agencies may be helpful to the physicians or parents of children with congenital rubella: United Cerebral Palsy, Research and Educational Foundation, Inc., 66 East 34th Street, New York, N.Y. 10016; National Easter Seal Society for Crippled Children and Adults, 2023 West Ogden Avenue, Chicago, Ill. 60612; National Association for Retarded Citizens, Research and Demonstration Institute, 2709 Avenue E East, P.O. Box 6109, Arlington, Texas 76011; Bureau of Education for the Handicapped, Office of Education, 400 Maryland Avenue, S.W., Washington, D.C. 20202; Office for Maternal and Child Health (Title V, Social Security Act), Bureau of Community Health Services, Department of Health, Education, and Welfare, 5600 Fishers Lane, Rockville, Maryland 20857.

Varicella and Herpes Zoster

ANNE A. GERSHON, M.D.

Varicella and herpes zoster are both caused by the same agent, varicella-zoster (V-Z) virus. Varicella occurs when susceptible individuals are exposed to the virus. Herpes zoster is seen in persons who have previously recovered from varicella. It rarely if ever occurs following exposure to V-Z virus and seems to result from reactivation of latent V-Z infection.

VARICELLA (CHICKENPOX)

Symptomatic Treatment. Since varicella is commonly a mild self-limited disease in children, therapeutic aims usually are to treat symptoms such as fever and itching. Antipyretics, oral antihistamines, baking soda baths, and calamine lotion applied to skin lesions are most often used. To minimize secondary bacterial infection of skin lesions the patient's fingernails should be cut short, and daily bathing is advised.

Complications. BACTERIAL SUPERINFECTION. The most common sites for bacterial superinfection are the skin and the lungs. Skin infections may progress from superficial to deep, resulting in cellulitis; on occasion deep vein thrombosis or gangrene may develop. Bacterial infection of the skin which appears to be progressive should be treated vigorously with warm soaks and appropriate antibiotics, usually penicillin or a penicillinase-resistant semisynthetic penicillin. If cellulitis is present blood cultures should be obtained, and if an extremity is involved it should be elevated. Deep seated infections or gangrene due to staphylococci or group A beta-hemolytic streptococci require protracted intravenous antibiotic therapy as well as surgical management. If deep vein thrombosis is present anticoagulants should be considered. "Bullous varicella" represents a form of the staphylococcal scalded skin syndrome and should be treated as such.

Superinfection of the respiratory tract may be due to *Hemophilus influenzae*, pneumococcus, or staphylococcus. Pneumonia following varicella in an otherwise normal child should be regarded as bacterial until proved otherwise, and should be treated vigorously with broad-spectrum antibiotics until the infecting organism can be identified.

ENCEPHALITIS. Encephalitis is an unusual complication of varicella in normal children and is often self-limited. Two types have been described: cerebral, which is usually associated with seizures and change in mental status; and cerebellar, which is usually associated with ataxia. Cerebellar involvement carries a better prognosis than the cerebral form. Varicella encephalitis may occur just prior to or up to two weeks after the onset of varicella. It should, of course, be distinguished from other types of viral or toxic encephalitis, and bacterial meningitis should be ruled out. There is no specific therapy for varicella encephalitis.

OCULAR LESIONS. Ocular lesions may occur in varicella. They are usually superficial and heal spontaneously. No specific therapy is recommended, but for severe cases an ophthalmologist should be consulted.

MISCELLANEOUS. Miscellaneous complications such as Reye's syndrome, thrombocytopenia, and hepatitis are rare following varicella. Such entities should be treated as in any other patient with these manifestations.

Varicella in the Immunocompromised. Varicella may be severe or fatal in immunocompromised patients; for example, persons receiving chemotherapy or radiotherapy for malignant disease, persons who have undergone organ transplantation, persons with congenital or acquired defects in cell-mediated immunity, and persons receiving high doses of steroids for any reason. Infants born to women with the onset of varicella 4 days or less prior to delivery may also develop severe varicella.

Children at high risk to severe varicella should be passively immunized against the infection promptly following exposure to varicella or herpes zoster (see below). During the potential incubation period of varicella, it is advisable to taper steroid dosage to physiologic levels and to withhold chemotherapy and radiotherapy even if passive immunization has been given.

Two types of severe varicella have been observed in high-risk children. One is rapidly fatal with high fever and disseminated intravascular coagulation. The other is initially indolent but new crops of vesicles continue to develop for up to two weeks. Eventually dissemination of virus may result in pneumonia, encephalitis and/or hepatitis. Treatment for varicella pneumonia manifested by dyspnea, hypoxia, and bilateral fluffy pulmonary infiltrates is oxygen and respiratory assistance if necessary; blood gases should be monitored closely. Steroids are of unproven value in varicella pneumonia but they may be tried. Antiviral chemotherapy may also be given (see below).

Passive Immunization Against Varicella. This may be accomplished by several methods. Most efficient is administration of zoster immune globulin (ZIG) which is prepared from plasma of persons convalescing from zoster and contains high titers of antibody to V-Z virus. ZIG is unlicensed; it may usually be obtained from the Center for Disease Control in Atlanta, Georgia for high-risk susceptible patients who have been closely exposed to varicella or herpes zoster. ZIG should be administered within 72 hours of exposure, intramuscularly, at a dose of approximately 1.25 ml./10 kg. of body weight. ZIG at this dosage usually modifies but does not prevent varicella in high-risk patients. Modified varicella is usually manifested by mild disease—few lesions, little or no fever, and a prolonged incubation period. Subclinical infection detected serologically following ZIG has also been observed. For the names and telephone numbers of the consultants at the Center for Disease Control who dispense ZIG when it is indicated, see the Red Book or the Report of the Committee on Infectious Diseases of the American Academy of Pediatrics.

When ZIG is unavailable, standard immune serum globulin (ISG) may be tried for modification of varicella. At best ISG contains one-tenth the V-Z antibody titer of ZIG; therefore a large dose, 0.6 to 1.2 ml./kg. intramuscularly, must be used. Generally the greater risk of the patient, the larger the dose employed. In certain areas of the United States it may be possible to have batches of ISG titered in advance for V-Z antibody content. Approximately 40 per cent of available lots of ISG have V-Z antibody titers which are one-tenth the potency of ZIG; 60 per cent contain less than this concentration of V-Z antibody and are therefore not clinically useful for passive immunization of high-risk susceptible persons against varicella.

Zoster immune plasma (ZIP) may also be used for passive immunization against varicella. ZIP is obtained from otherwise normal individuals convalescing from herpes zoster. It may be given intravenously to high-risk exposed susceptible persons; usually 10 ml./kg. is used. Its use carries the risk of subsequent development of hepatitis. While serum obtained from persons convalescing from varicella (VIP) would seem a logical alternative to ZIG and is sometimes used in place of ZIP, its efficacy for this purpose is unproved.

Antibody to V-Z virus in the form of ZIG, ISG and ZIP has been thought to be of little use for treatment of severe varicella. This is because cell-mediated immunity seems to be of predominant importance in recovery from varicella. Recent evidence, however, suggests that specific antibody may participate in viral clearance (antibody-dependent cellular cytotoxicity). Whether this mechanism plays a role in recovery from varicella is unknown, but since administration of specific antibody to persons with severe varicella carries minimal risk, it should probably be given as ZIP to such patients.

Antiviral Therapy. Of the antiviral drugs available, all of which are unlicensed and investigational, iododeoxyuridine (IDUR) and cytosine arabinoside (Ara-C) have lost favor in recent years because of their toxicity. These antiviral drugs interfere with synthesis of viral DNA, but they also inhibit host DNA synthesis. One of the most unfortunate toxic effects of these drugs is that they cause immunosuppression which further impedes recovery.

Recently, adenine arabinoside (Ara-A) has received attention because while it too acts against both viral and host DNA, it seems to be relatively nontoxic to the patient at therapeutic levels. While the efficacy of Ara-A for treatment of severe varicella is unproved, it should probably be used to treat severe life-threatening varicella. Ara-A is given intravenously in a dose of 10 mg./kg./day over a 12 hour period usually for one week. Since Ara-A is an investigational drug it must be obtained on a research protocol by contacting the manufacturer (Parke, Davis & Company, Detroit, Michigan). Other unlicensed drugs which have been used to treat severe varicella but whose efficacy is unproved include levamisole, transfer factor, and interferon.

There is some rationale for treatment of severe varicella with white blood cells of a normal person convalescing from varicella or herpes zoster as a source of cell-mediated immunity. However this type of therapy carries potential risk because of the possibility of graft versus host reaction due to transfused lymphocytes.

HERPES ZOSTER (SHINGLES)

This syndrome is not uncommon in children who have already had chickenpox. It is usually mild and self-limited, requiring no specific therapy. Some persons with herpes zoster, especially those who are immunocompromised, will develop disseminated infection resembling chickenpox with several to many vesicular lesions. This disease is usually self-limited, requiring no specific therapy, particularly in the immunologically normal host. Even immunocompromised individuals with disseminated zoster usually have detectable serum antibody to V-Z virus and therefore treatment with ZIG, ISG or ZIP is not indicated. Treatment of severe disseminated zoster with Ara-A should be considered. This drug seems to promote recovery from zoster, especially when therapy has been instituted early.

Postherpetic pain, common in older adults convalescing from zoster, is rare in children.

Ocular lesions due to zoster are often deep seated and difficult to treat. An ophthalmologist should be consulted for this complication. Facial zoster is often associated with some degree of encephalitis, and abnormal cerebrospinal fluid. However this complication is usually self-limited and requires no further treatment.

Topical IDUR 5 per cent solution in 100 per cent dimethylsulfoxide has been found to hasten the healing of zoster. This medication, however, is not available in the United States. Topical IDUR 0.1 per cent is available but it has been of no value in topical treatment of zoster and it should not be used. Topical Ara-A similarly has not been helpful for treatment of zoster.

VARICELLA VACCINE

A live attenuated varicella vaccine has been developed in Japan. This vaccine has been given without obvious side effects even to immunocompromised high-risk susceptible children. However this vaccine is not available in the United States.

Smallpox

C. HENRY KEMPE, M.D.

There is no specific therapy for smallpox at present. Penicillin and the broad-spectrum antibiotics, however, are highly effective in preventing the secondary bacterial complications that frequently occur during and after the pustular phase of the disease. Procaine penicillin, 400,000 units a day intramuscularly, or any one of the tetracycline preparations* in dosages ranging from 25 to 50 mg./kg./day, is indicated, especially if started in the pustular phase, on approximately the sixth or seventh day of the disease. This can reduce the bacterial complications involving the lungs, bones and skin.

Vaccinia immune gamma globulin has a place in the prevention or modification of smallpox in persons known to have been exposed, if it is given in the incubation period or in the pre-eruptive phase of the disease.

A related compound, 4-bromo-3-methyl-isothiozole-5-carboxaldehyde-thiosemicarbazone, has been tested in therapeutic trials in hospital patients. There is some slight indication that the drug may reduce the mortality rate in the severe types of smallpox in vaccinated patients, but has little effect in severe cases in unvaccinated patients.

The mild or discrete case of smallpox requires little except strict attention to oral and skin hygiene, fluid intake and routine analgesia. Fingernails should be cut short to prevent scratching, and antipruritic colloid baths in the scabbing period after the 12th day of the disease tend to minimize discomfort.

Severe discrete or confluent cases should be treated like serious thermal burns (see section on Burns). In most cases of severe smallpox, severe dehydration results because of the pain associated with swallowing. Intravenous fluid therapy may be difficult in the face of massive skin involvement. Fluid requirements increase as with any febrile illness, and fluid loss from the skin may be considerable. Oliguria and eventual renal insufficiency may further interfere with the patient's recovery.

---

*Manufacturer's note: Use of tetracyclines during tooth development (last half of pregnancy, infancy and childhood to age eight years) may cause permanent discoloration of teeth. This adverse reaction is more common during long-term use of the drugs but has been observed following repeated short-term courses.

The use of intensive parenteral fluid therapy or the early institution of feeding through a polyethylene stomach tube holds promise. Boiled skimmed milk with added carbohydrate (10 per cent) supplies calories and fluids through the critical 10 days of the early eruptive period. With the use of intensive fluid therapy and prophylactic use of antibiotics, mortality rates in the pediatric age group can be reduced to between 10 and 30 per cent.

All local applications to the skin and baths are to be discouraged. It is important, however, to attempt to clean the eyes with warm normal saline solution to prevent matting and to decrease the chances of permanent involvement of the sclera. There is no evidence that corticosteroids are of value in the treatment of this condition.

Hemorrhagic smallpox is virtually universally fatal, and no treatment has been successful to date. Specific clotting deficiencies, particularly factor V and platelets, suggest intravascular clotting and the possible therapeutic employment of heparin. Should a shock-like state develop, plasma, hydrocortisone or prednisone may be helpful. Currently under study are early use of N-methylisatin beta-thiosemicarbazone and the intravenous use of heparin or dextran. Oxygen and, when indicated, digitalis are of value.

Complications and Prognosis. Bacterial complications include sepsis, pneumonitis, osteomyelitis and septic arthritis. Iritis, corneal ulceration and severe conjunctivitis may lead to decrease in visual acuity, depending on their severity.

The prognosis of hemorrhagic smallpox is virtually hopeless. The prognosis for survival in children suffering from confluent smallpox is also extremely grave. Children suffering from modified smallpox or discrete smallpox due to previous successful vaccination have a good prognosis, especially if they receive optimal supportive therapy.

Control Measures. ISOLATION. Strict hospital isolation is required until all scabs have disappeared.

CONCURRENT DISINFECTION. All articles associated with a smallpox patient must be sterilized in high pressure steam or, alternatively, by boiling them before removing from the patient's room.

TERMINAL DISINFECTION. Thorough disinfection of the patient's room is required, and the wall and ceiling should be painted.

VACCINATION. All contacts should be promptly vaccinated or revaccinated and observed for 16 days from the last day of exposure. Vaccination *after* contact usually does not protect against smallpox unless accompanied by vaccinia immune gamma globulin. Vaccination, to ensure protection, must be done *before* exposure to smallpox. It is important to ignore a history of recent vaccination if exposure has occurred unless there is definite evidence of the formation of a recent scar to show that vaccination has, indeed, been successful.

N-Methylisatin Beta-Thiosemicarbazone. Marboran (Burroughs Wellcome), 1.5 to 3 gm. orally twice a day for two days, decreases smallpox after known intimate exposure regardless of vaccination status. In more than 1100 household contacts given the drug by mouth, three mild cases of smallpox occurred. In a comparable group of contacts who did not receive the drug there were 78 cases of smallpox and 12 deaths. The drug was effective even when given more than six days after contact. The material frequently causes emesis, and it is desirable to administer antiemetics prophylactically. Potential damage to liver and bone marrow should be watched for. Marboran, an investigational drug, is not yet approved by the Food and Drug Administration.

VACCINIA IMMUNE GAMMA GLOBULIN. Vaccinia immune gamma globulin given soon after exposure (12 to 24 hours) to close contacts of patients with smallpox may prevent or modify the disease in the contact. Dosage is a single intramuscular injection of 0.12 to 0.24 ml./kg.

Vaccinia immune gamma globulin is available commercially from Hyland Laboratories, Costa Mesa, California (714-540-5000) or from Center for Disease Control, Atlanta, Georgia (daytime, 404-633-3311); night, 404-633-2176) or from a regional consultant.

References

Bauer, D. J., et al.: Prophylaxis of smallpox with methisazone. Am. J. Epidemiol., *90*:130, 1969.
Public Health Service Advisory Committee on Immunization Practices: Smallpox vaccination of hospital and health personnel. Morbid. Mortal., *25*:9, 1976.

Vaccinia

Smallpox Vaccination

C. HENRY KEMPE, M.D.

Indications for Vaccination. Children should no longer be vaccinated routinely. Selective vaccination is advised for travelers to areas where smallpox still occurs, for health personnel, and in the presence of an epidemic. Since the endemic situation is a changing one it is suggested that a telephone call be made to the local Health Department or to the Center for Disease Control in Atlanta, Georgia, for the latest information. For certain travelers, WHO requires revaccination every three years. In areas of the world where smallpox is endemic, *yearly* successful vaccination is required to give solid protection.

Contraindications to Vaccination. Childhood eczema is an absolute contraindication to vaccination. The presence of a sibling with eczema in the family of the child to be vaccinated also is an absolute contraindication to vaccination because serious secondary vaccinia infections are likely to occur. If vaccination is desired in this situation, the sibling with eczema must be placed in a separate household and must have no contact with the vaccinated child for at least 15 days.

Infants and children who have had many repeated bacterial infections or who have failed to thrive should not be vaccinated. Children suffering from dysgammaglobulinemia have a high mortality rate after smallpox vaccination.

Further contraindications include all forms of leukemia, lymphoma and malignancy as well as other blood dyscrasias, as well as patients who are receiving corticosteroids or antimetabolites for x-ray therapy.

Method of Vaccination and Care of Lesion. To minimize the risk of unnecessary complications, the following practices are recommended.

AGE FOR PRIMARY VACCINATION. In nonendemic areas, primary vaccination need not be done. Otherwise, there are no conclusive data indicating the exact period when complication rates are minimal. The presence of some transplacental maternal immunity, provided the mother has been vaccinated, may be desirable in modifying the primary vaccination reaction, and therefore vaccination may be carried out in the first months of life. Vaccination of newborn infants has been carried out without complications. In such cases in endemic areas, revaccination should be carried out after an interval of six months. If primary vaccination is delayed for several months, children who are at increased risk, such as those suffering from the Swiss type of agammaglobulinemia, will have been readily identified by their clinical course and will, therefore, not become a casualty of smallpox vaccination.

SITE FOR VACCINATION. Primary vaccination and revaccination are best performed on the outer aspects of the upper arm, over the insertion of the deltoid muscle or behind the midline. Reactions are less likely to be severe on the upper arm than on the lower extremity or other parts of the body. With proper technique, resultant scars are small and unobtrusive.

PREPARATION OF THE VACCINATION SITE. With clean skin, the best preparation is none at all. The use of chemical skin cleaners may leave a residue that contains virus-inactivating material, whereas vigorous physical cleansing of the site may create minute abrasions, which then can become the site of second vaccinia eruptions, with resultant involvement of a comparatively large skin area.

VACCINATION TECHNIQUE. Regardless of age, routine primary vaccination should be carried out with no more than three pressures made with the side of a needle. These pressure points should be as close as possible, and carried out at only one site. With the highly potent vaccines currently in use, numerous pressures are not necessary and should not be utilized in a nonimmune person. When children and adults are to be revaccinated after a lapse of more than five years, the same small number of pressures should be used. For revaccination within a five-year period, in persons known to have had a major reaction, the full complement of 30 strokes can safely be used.

VACCINATION REACTION. The terminology for the reactions after vaccination or revaccination should follow that recommended by the Expert Committee on Smallpox of the World Health Organization. A successful primary vaccination is one that on examination after 7 to 10 days presents a typical jennerian vesicle. If this is not present, vaccination must be repeated with fresh vaccine, applying a few more strokes of the needle. The successful revaccination is one that on examination one week (six to eight days) later shows vesicular or pustular lesions, *or* an area of definite palpable induration and congestion surrounding a central lesion; this lesion may be a scab or an ulcer. These reactions are termed *major reactions;* all others should be called *equivocal reactions.* A major reaction indicates virus multiplication with consequent development of immunity. An equivocal reaction may merely represent an allergic response, which could be elicited by inactive vaccine or poor technique in someone who had been sensitized by earlier vaccination, or the equivocal reaction may result from sufficient immunity to prevent virus multiplication.

Because the allergic response cannot be readily differentiated from the one due to true immunity, another vaccination should be performed using a different lot of vaccine if there is a possibility that it is of weak potency, and the procedure should be completed with an additional number of pressures. The site should be examined one week later; if the result is again equivocal, revaccination is repeated, using a full 30 pressures. For the sake of expediency, an equivocal reaction to revaccination with a minimal insertion may be followed by vaccination at two sites, not less than 2 inches apart, using known potent vaccine. This method makes a third return unnecessary in most instances.

In summary, successful smallpox vaccination consists in the production of a major reaction. When potent vaccine and good technique are used, the repeated inability to produce a major reaction can be assumed to be due to solid immunity from previous immunization.

Complications of Smallpox Vaccination.
ERYTHEMA MULTIFORME. A generalized maculopapular eruption may occur at the height of the vaccinia reaction. There is no systemic reaction in addition to those of an uncomplicated vaccination. Lesions are usually not pruritic, although the reaction is an allergy to the vaccinia virus. Treatment is reassurance and any oral antihistiminic. The rash disappears in two to four days.

ECZEMA VACCINATUM. Infants suffering from eczema are peculiarly susceptible to infection with vaccinia virus, and this complication accounts for the largest number of childhood deaths from serious complications of smallpox vaccination. Such children should, therefore, never be vaccinated, even though their lesions appear to be dry, unless they are likely to be exposed to smallpox. They must also be carefully guarded against exposure to siblings and other children who have been vaccinated and who may, in turn, infect them.

Lesions first occur in the area of eczema three to four days after exposure. Soon new crops arise in areas of the skin previously uninvolved. Patients are febrile and toxic for five to 15 days.

Affected children should be treated as if they were suffering from severe thermal burns. The use of oxygen, blood, plasma and electrolytes, as well as penicillin, is indicated (see the discussion under Burns).

Evidence suggests that there is a primary defect in the production of specific antibodies against the vaccinia virus. The use of passively administered antibodies in the form of vaccinia immune gamma globulin has proved to be a valuable adjunct in the specific therapy of this complication. The dose of vaccinia immune gamma globulin is 0.6 to 1 ml./kg., and it is given once or twice intramuscularly. In serious cases the investigational drug N-methylisatin beta-thiosemicarbazone (Marboran) should be used in doses of 200 mg./kg. orally at once, followed by 50 mg./kg. every 6 hours for no more than three days.

GENERALIZED VACCINIA. Generalized vaccinia in children not suffering from skin disorders is seen when viremia happens to occur during primary vaccination, giving rise, in turn, to a generalized skin eruption, each lesion simulating a primary vaccination.

Lesions usually continue to appear in crops over a four- to six-day period after the onset of the disease, which frequently coincides with the height of the primary vaccination reaction (8 to 14 days after vaccination).

The mortality rate of generalized vaccinia in the absence of eczema is much lower, because this complication occurs more frequently in children over two years of age.

The *treatment* is identical to that for eczema vaccinatum.

PROGRESSIVE VACCINIA (VACCINIA NECROSUM; PROLONGED VACCINIA). This extremely rare complication of vaccination is characterized by a complete inability to make specific antibodies against the vaccinia virus. This results in progressive spreading of the primary vaccination take, and eventually most of the arm as well as the rest of the body becomes involved with necrotizing lesions. The systemic reaction is usually mild during the first six weeks of the disease, but progressively increases in the subsequent weeks and eventually leads to death four to six months after onset.

This complication is certainly very frequent in children suffering from either the Bruton or the Swiss type of agammaglobulinemia. But in four instances the quantitative gamma globulin levels were normal even though a qualitative effect (dysgammaglobulinemia) existed.

The logical course of treatment is the provision of large amounts of antivaccina antibodies in the form of vaccinia immune gamma globulin, given in doses of 0.6 to 1 ml./kg. intramuscularly every 8 to 10 days until lesions are entirely healed. Large amounts of high titer serum from adults recently successfully vaccinated or repeated exchange transfusions from such donors have been successful in the Bruton type capable of delayed hypersensitivity response. But even a single blood transfusion can cause a fatal graft-versus-host reaction in the athymic lymphopenic patient, and blood must never be used in such patients.

If antibody therapy does not result in immediate improvement, therapy with Marboran should be instituted. The oral dose is 200 mg./kg. at once, followed by 50 mg./kg. every 6 hours for three days. After a rest of three days, an additional three-day course should be given. The disease has been promptly arrested in approximately half the patients treated to date.

POSTVACCINATION ENCEPHALITIS. This is a rare complication of smallpox vaccination with an incidence of less than 1 per 100,000 vaccinations.

Encephalitic symptoms usually develop at the height of the primary vaccination reaction and not later than the 15th day after vaccination.

The mortality rate is 25 per cent, but there is usually eventual physical recovery of those who survive. Behavioral disorders are frequent. It is thought by many that this complication occurs more commonly after the age of three, and because it is almost exclusively associated with primary vaccination, most physicians prefer early vaccination. The mortality rate, on the other hand, appears to be much higher in the younger child. The complication can be markedly decreased by simultaneous administration of 2 ml. of vaccinia immune gamma globulin intramuscularly into the thigh at the time of primary vaccination.

Vaccinia Immune Gamma Globulin. Human vaccinia immune gamma globulin (VIG) is distributed through the Center for Disease Control, Atlanta (see p. 620) and is also available commercially from Hyland Laboratories, California (see p. 620).

References

Kempe, C. H.: The end of routine smallpox vaccination in the United States. Pediatrics, *49*:1489, 1972.

Herpes Simplex Infections

ANNE A. GERSHON, M.D.

There are two types of herpes simplex virus (HSV), designated types I and II. While these two viruses share some antigens, infection with one type does not protect against infection with the other type. Like other herpesviruses, HSV becomes latent in the host following primary infection. The site of latency is sensory ganglia such as those of the cranial or sacral nerves.

Herpes Gingivostomatitis. This common condition is usually seen in young children but occasionally occurs in adolescents. The gums and buccal mucosa are tender and swollen; often small painful ulcers are present. The gums are friable and sore, the breath is fetid and fever commonly occurs. This condition heals spontaneously within several days, so treatment is symptomatic. Antipyretics and analgesics may be given. Painting the lesions with a small amount of viscous Xylocaine several times daily may decrease pain and enable the patient to take fluids. Occasionally treatment with intravenous fluids for a few days is necessary in young babies who become dehydrated due to poor intake.

Recurrent Herpes. HSV may recur locally on the skin and mucous membranes which are innervated by the sensory nerves in which HSV is latent. Recurrence occurs despite serum antibody and lesions tend to appear repeatedly in the same general area. Occasional patients may be debilitated by severe recurrent HSV lesions, but most have only minor symptoms.

Several treatments have been suggested for recurrent herpes, but none have proved efficacious. Administration of steroids and repeated smallpox vaccinations, once used by some, are potentially dangerous and are contraindicated. A killed HSV vaccine was employed experimentally several years ago, but this preparation has not proved useful. Topically applied ether has been suggested as a means to hasten healing of herpetic lesions, but its efficacy is also unproved. Treatment of HSV lesions with a photoactive dye such as neutral red followed by exposure to light seemed to facilitate healing and discourage recurrences, but when this mode of therapy was subjected to double blind study, it was found to be of no value. In addition there is a theoretical risk that photoinactivation of HSV may unmask the oncogenic characteristics of this virus, possibly making this therapy harmful; therefore this treatment is now to be discouraged. Probably the safest and best way to treat recurrent herpes is to recommend avoidance of recognized precipitating factors such as sunlight or stress.

It has been suggested that persons with recurrent HSV infections have subtle immunologic defects which lead to their disease, but as yet, no such defects have been identified in persons subject to recurrent herpes. A prompt cell-mediated response to HSV, however, has been found during recovery from these infections.

Eczema Herpeticum. Children with eczema are prone to develop severe primary or recurrent HSV infection of the skin. Primary infections tend to be worse than recurrent infections. Treatment is symptomatic and should aim for maintenance of adequate hydration, control of fever, and prevention of bacterial superinfection. As the lesions these patients experience may resemble an extensive burn, the usual local therapy for burns is often helpful, such as application of silver sulfadiazine or nitrofurazone cream to the skin. Since in addition there is evidence that some of these compounds inactivate HSV in vitro, they may play a dual role in therapy for eczema herpeticum.

Herpetic Keratitis. Patients in whom this disease is suspected should be referred to an ophthalmologist. Treatment with topical iododeoxyuridine (IDUR) 0.1 to 0.5 per cent, or topical adenine arabinoside (Ara-A) should be given. Instillation of steroid drops into the eye of a patient with herpetic keratitis is contraindicated.

HSV Encephalitis. This condition, usually caused by HSV I and manifested by fever, headache, personality change, seizures, coma and eventually death or brain damage, is rare in the pediatric age group. The reason encephalitis occurs in certain persons is unknown; some encephalitic patients have a history of recurrent facial herpes, whereas others have not. Treatment is supportive and includes intravenous fluids and, if necessary, maintenance of respiration. The laboratory diagnosis of HSV encephalitis is difficult since it is unusual to recover HSV from cerebrospinal fluid. Usually a brain biopsy and culture must be performed. For documented cases of HSV encephalitis, the experimental antiviral drug adenine arabinoside, 15 mg./kg./day intravenously, may be used. The efficacy of this drug for herpes encephalitis is unproved. Nevertheless this syndrome is usually severe enough to warrant antiviral chemotherapy. Further information concerning use of Ara-A must be obtained on an individual basis from the manufacturer (Parke, Davis & Company, Detroit, Michigan).

Additional Neurologic Disease Due to HSV. HSV II causes meningoencephalitis which is usually less severe than the encephalitis caused by HSV I. This disease is usually self-limited and requires no specific therapy. Rarely, transverse myelitis may occur following infection with HSV I or II, which also is usually self-limited. Both of these neurologic syndromes may occur following or during an attack of genital herpes.

HSV in the Immunocompromised Host. These patients seem to have less severe infections due to HSV than due to varicella-zoster virus for reasons that are not understood. For the rare occasion when an immunocompromised patient develops disseminated infection due to HSV, use of Ara-A should be considered (see previous section).

Neonatal Herpes. This condition most often develops when infants are born vaginally to mothers who have genital herpes. After an incubation period of several days, the infant may develop skin vesicles, eye involvement, and/or widespread disseminated HSV infection with hepatitis, pneumonia, and encephalitis.

Pregnant women near term with genital herpes are best managed by cooperation of the obstetrician, pediatrician, and clinical virologist.

Several approaches to prevent, modify or treat HSV of the newborn have been devised. The simplest is to deliver infants of infected mothers with intact membranes by cesarean section. This approach is effective even if the membranes have been ruptured for up to four hours, but after this interval infection may not be prevented. Amniocentesis is helpful to decide whether an infant is already infected with HSV, since if HSV is recovered from amniotic fluid, cesarean section is no longer indicated. Following birth by cesarean section, infants born to women with genital herpes are kept in isolation and are not handled by the mother until her genital lesions have healed.

While specific antibody was at one time thought to have little bearing on the subsequent course of infants born to women with genital herpes, this view is changing. Experimental evidence suggests that specific antibody given promptly after HSV infection of newborn mice modifies the course of their disease. Infants born to women with recurrent HSV infection, who have detectable titers of antibody to HSV, experience milder disease than infants born to mothers with primary HSV infections. Similarly it is unusual for women with recurrent facial herpes to infect their infants. Thus there may be some rationale for administration of antibody to infants born to women with documented genital herpes. This form of therapy would seem to be of greatest benefit to infants whose mothers have membranes ruptured 4 to 24 hours prior to delivery and who were delivered vaginally despite active maternal genital herpes. However, no information on an effective dose of antibody is available, so a specific recommendation concerning the use of antibody for this condition cannot be made at this time.

Once HSV infection of the newborn has occurred, it is important to assess the extent of the infection. If only the skin is involved, most investigators advise no specific therapy because these infants usually thrive. Occasionally untreated infants with mild central nervous system involvement have also done well. In contrast, infants with moderate to severe central nervous system invasion or eye involvement should probably receive antiviral therapy although it is experimental. Iododeoxyuridine (IDUR) and cytosine arabinoside (Ara-C), once recommended for this purpose, have now been dicarded because of their toxicity. The drug now most often used is the experimental antiviral compound Ara-A at a dose of 10 mg./ kg./day intravenously. Preliminary studies on treatment of newborns infected with HSV have suggested that Ara-A is of benefit to these infants if it is given early in the course of the disease.

Mumps

JOSEPH W. ST. GEME, Jr., M.D.

Mumps virus is a member of the paramyxovirus family, including the parainfluenza viruses, and spreads via the respiratory tract. Subclinical primary infection occurs in 30 per cent or more of susceptible individuals. Infection is uncommon in the preschool child while the major overt manifestations of illness occur in school-age children. Subsequent spread of subclinical and overt infection within families may involve 80 to 90 per cent of susceptible individuals. Peaks of infection occur during the spring with abundant illness during the winter and summer as well. Males incur infection more commonly than females. Adults, only 5 to 10 per cent of whom remain susceptible, develop more significant illness than children.

The incubation period is 17 to 21 days. Viremia has been detected on rare occasions at the immediate onset of symptoms when virus is also shed in the saliva and the oropharynx. Maximal shedding of virus with concomitant intensification of contagiousness is observed during the few days which precede and follow the onset of illness. The limit of salivary shed of virus and potential contagiousness is one week before and after the onset of parotid swelling. Viruria endures for 10 days after the initial symptoms. Infection is systemic and virus is distributed to all organs of the body.

Uncomplicated mumps is managed very simply with rest, liquids, bland diet, and occasional analgesic-antipyretic therapy for general discomfort and high fever. The dose of aspirin is 60 mg./kg./day given in four to six divided oral doses. Acetaminophen can be given in a dose of 30 mg./kg./day in three to four divided oral doses, although for salicylate-equivalent effect twice this dose may be required.

Complications. MENINGITIS AND ENCEPHALITIS. Mumps virus is the most common invader of the central nervous system. Although the great majority of mumps virus infections of the CNS are benign episodes of aseptic meningitis, perhaps 10 to 20 per cent of cases are encephalitic with convulsions and significant alteration of the sensorium. Unique neurologic sequelae include acute cerebellar ataxia, transient paralysis, diffuse infectious neuronitis, sudden coma, aqueductal stenosis, and diabetes insipidus. Neurologic symptoms may rarely precede parotid swelling. Very frequently aseptic meningitis occurs without obvious parotitis. Approximately half of all cases of mumps have cerebrospinal fluid pleocytosis and half of these individuals may manifest some evidence of neurologic illness. In some cases the CSF glucose content may be decreased, which is atypical for viral infections of the CNS.

Diagnostic lumbar puncture may relieve headache. More severe cases may require conservative parenteral fluid therapy, 1200 to 1500 ml./m², plus replacement of inordinate fluid loss due to persistent emesis. Otherwise, rest, oral fluids, and analgesic-antipyretic therapy will suffice. Hospitalization is not mandatory if the CNS infection is unremarkable and one can be assured that the cause is mumps.

ORCHITIS. Approximately 10 to 20 per cent of adolescent and postpubescent individuals experience testicular swelling, ordinarily unilateral in nature. Sterility is unusual, although testicular atrophy may occur in 10 to 50 per cent of cases. Despite the fact that 20 to 30 per cent of all cases of orchitis have some element of bilaterality, the subsequent mild atrophy is insufficient to produce frank sterility.

Large doses (20 ml.) of mumps hyperimmune gamma globulin have been demonstrated in the past to reduce the incidence of significant orchitis by threefold. Currently, hyperimmune globulin is not recommended for the prevention of orchitis. The issue deserves further study. Although there are many anecdotal reports of dramatic therapeutic effect, controlled studies of steroid treatment of orchitis have demonstrated only the suppression of fever.

Bed rest, analgesics, ice packs, and gentle support of the engorged testis constitute the essential therapeutic stratagem. Incision of the enveloping tunica albuginea represents extraordinary management of the most severely involved testis.

PANCREATITIS. Mild, essentially asymptomatic pancreatitis may be more common than suspected. Biochemical diagnosis may be made by the determination of elevated serum lipase values. Parotitis precludes the usefulness of serum amylase determinations. Severe pancreatitis with marked abdominal pain and vomiting is unusual. Since this complication is transient, absolute bed rest, sedation, and parenteral fluids constitute adequate treatment. It is important to note that on rare occasions diabetes mellitus may follow mumps.

MYOCARDITIS. Although the cause of myocarditis is seldom well identified, the group B coxsackie viruses, influenza virus, and mumps virus are important pathogens. Electrocardiographic abnormalities have been identified in 15 per cent of patients with mumps. There is some clinical and experimental support for the hypothesis that fetal mumps virus infection may result in myocarditis and, as an occasional consequence of the reparative process, the chronic cardiomyopathy characterized by endocardial fibroelastosis. Significant myocarditis should be managed with bed rest, anticipation, cardiac monitoring, fluid and salt restriction, diuretics, and occasionally the careful use of digitalis. The role of steroid therapy remains controversial.

OTHER COMPLICATIONS. Sensorineural deafness, thrombocytopenia purpura, arthritis and thyroiditis are rare sequelae of mumps virus infection. Thyroiditis may be followed by hypothyroidism. In the few reported cases of migratory arthritis, salicylate therapy has not been effective.

Prevention. PASSIVE IMMUNIZATION. Large doses of regular commercial gamma globulin (0.4 ml./lb.) convert clinical illness into subclinical infection, similar to the observations with measles and infectious hepatitis. Since the geometric mean titers of mumps virus neutralizing antibody in mumps hyperimmune gamma globulin are six-fold higher than that of regular gamma globulin, an equivalent modifying dose of hyperimmune globulin is 0.07 ml./lb. It is reasonable to predict that lots of gamma globulin with high titers of neutralizing antibody, if administered early in the incubation of mumps, should modify or prevent mumps virus infection. There are insufficient data to confirm such a prediction. The primary target for this form of immunotherapy is the adult male. In this regard there is the need to develop more satisfactory techniques for the rapid detection of the susceptible adult.

ACTIVE IMMUNIZATION. Parenteral administration of live attenuated mumps virus vaccine induces antibody in 95 per cent of recipients and provides apparently complete and sustained immunity against natural mumps. With very few exceptions even low levels of antibody seem to protect. Vaccine may be administered successfully alone or in combination with other live, attenuated viruses, such as measles and rubella. Unfortunately, vaccine administered early in the incubation of mumps does not modify nor prevent subsequent natural infection. Live, attenuated mumps virus infection suppresses tuberculin delayed hyper-

sensitivity, so tuberculin skin testing should be performed prior to administration of vaccine. The vaccine induces both neutralizing antibody and cellular immunity to mumps virus, the latter ascertained by skin testing with inactivated viral antigen. There is no place in current practice for the use of killed mumps virus vaccine.

Detection of Immunity. HUMORAL IMMUNITY. Neutralizing antibody is the best measure of immunity to mumps. Less immunologically specific antibodies, such as complement-fixing and hemagglutination-inhibiting antibody, may reflect prior infection with other antigenically related paramyxoviruses, notably the parainfluenza viruses. Mumps virus reinfection may occur rarely with low serum neutralizing antibody titers of 1:2 or 1:4. These infections are usually subclinical and remain so because the early viral multiplication of reinfection very likely induces a prompt anamnestic rise in serum antibody. The application of the minimal amount of mumps virus skin test antigen achieves the same immunologic result. The adult at risk should be skin tested. If positive, nothing more need be done; if antibody titers are low, they will rise. If skin test is negative, one potential therapeutic alternative is the administration of vaccine which has been studied carefully and is of no value. The other alternative is the administration of 0.07 ml./lb. of mumps hyperimmune gamma globulin which is of theoretical value but has been inadequately studied.

In consideration of reinfection, it should be pointed out that parainfluenza viruses, group A coxsackie viruses, echoviruses, and lymphocytic choriomeningitis virus have been shown to be occasional causes of parotitis. Recurrent bacterial parotitis and ductal stones should also be considered when dealing with a second episode of parotid swelling.

CELLULAR IMMUNITY. Cellular immunity may persist after humoral immunity has waned. The mumps virus skin test reagent (Lilly, if still available) is not generally satisfactory because of inconsistent antigenic potency from lot to lot. However, extensive skin test reactions in the adult, well beyond 15 mm. of erythema, are accurate in the detection of satisfactory immunity. One is looking for the low percentage of adults, perhaps 5 to 10 per cent, who are not immune. Unfortunately, the skin test antigen is unreliable in the school child and adolescent because of frequent false positive and false negative reactions, a reflection of inadequately standardized lots of antigen and immunologic cross-reactivity with the parainfluenza viruses.

Influenza

PAUL F. WEHRLE, M.D.

Since the clinical symptoms and signs of influenza may closely resemble those of other acute respiratory illnesses, the epidemiological nature of the disease is of considerable importance to the clinician. During the winter months, if there is substantial school absenteeism and respiratory illness is prevalent among older individuals also, the clinical diagnosis of influenza may be made with greater confidence. In the older child, complaints of aching, substernal discomfort and frontal headache resembling that of an acute sinusitis are helpful clinical signs, although bacterial causes should be excluded by careful evaluation. Antimicrobial therapy is not indicated unless specific bacterial complications are recognized or suspected. Active prophylactic immunization against influenza using currently available inactivated vaccines is recommended for infants and children more than six months of age if chronic health problems or debilitating disease is known. For those between six months and three years of age the vaccine should be given in reduced dosage in accordance with package insert recommendations.

For fever, myalgia and general discomfort, aspirin is preferred in doses of 30 to 65 mg./kg./day in six divided doses. For the accompanying bronchitis, mist or steam, and an expectorant cough medication (such as saturated solution of potassium iodide, 0.1 to 0.3 ml in cold milk or juice three or four times daily) may be useful. Amantadine hydrochloride (Symmetrel) may be considered for prophylaxis in unimmunized children or in treatment of prolonged illness when susceptible A influenza strains are prevalent. The package insert must be consulted for dosage and warnings.

Complications. Complications are usually bacterial in origin and result from direct extension of organisms such as *H. influenzae,* streptococci, pneumococci or staphylococci from the upper respiratory tract to involve sinuses, middle ear, or respiratory tract. When these complications are recognized, ampicillin, 100 mg./kg./day in four divided doses, or a penicillinase-resistant oral penicillin may be required. Encephalopathy is a rare complication, and examination of spinal fluid is required to exclude bacterial CNS disease.

Active Immunization. Routine influenza immunization has been customarily recommended only for those patients, irrespective of age, with underlying health problems or for those of advanced age. With major shifts in the antigenic structure of the influenza virus expected (such as swine influenza strains in 1976-77), recommendations for immunization of healthy individuals above three years of age have been suggested. Specific dosage recommendations and information regarding a requirement of more than a single dose for younger age groups are subject to official recommendations prior to the advent of the influenza session.

Conditions suggesting that influenza immunization may be indicated are: (1) cardiac disease, especially if there is evidence of cardiac insufficiency; (2) chronic bronchopulmonary disease, such as cystic fibrosis, chronic asthma, chronic bronchitis, bronchiectasis or limited respiratory function due to other causes; (3) chronic metabolic disease; (4) chronic renal disease; and (5) chronic neurological disorders, particularly those involving ventilatory function.

When major shifts in antigenic structure occur, as with swine or perhaps other strains to be expected in the future, more than a single dose of vaccine may be required for those without prior experience with these antigens. Consequently, even though the vaccines currently are more potent and of greater purity, specific recommendations regarding dosage and indications should be reviewed annually. Since these vaccines are prepared from virus grown in embryonated eggs, they should not be administered to persons clearly hypersensitive to egg protein.

Rabies

STANLEY A. PLOTKIN, M.D.

Rabies is a zoonosis transmitted to man by the bites or scratches of infected animals. Since replication probably occurs in skin and muscle before the virus attaches to and ascends the neural axons, it is possible to prevent disease by immunization after exposure.

Many unnecessary vaccination series are done which might be avoided by attention to the following: (1) A history revealing that the biting animal is under surveillance, has been previously vaccinated, belongs to a domestic species, or inflicted the injury on provocation. A bite by a wild animal (if provoked) or by a bat always requires vaccination as does, of course, the identification of rabies fluorescent antigen in the brain of any biting animal. (2) Frequent consultation with local health officials as to the occurrence of animal rabies. For example, in New York City and Philadelphia, vaccination after the bite of a stray dog would not be advised. Two examples representing extremes would be the urgent immunization required by a camper after an unprovoked attack by a skunk; or in contrast, the lack of immunization required by an individual bitten while feeding a squirrel in a nonenzootic geographic area.

Local Treatment. Much folklore surrounds the care of rabies virus infected wounds. Copious irrigation with any solution, such as soapy water, is the most important step in order to mechanically remove virus. In addition, many substances may be used for antiviral activity, including 70 per cent alcohol and 1 per cent benzalkonium chloride (10 times the usual concentration).

Passive Immunization. There has been clear experimental and clinical demonstration that antiserum given together with vaccine increases survival from rabies. Two forms of antiserum are available: one of equine origin (Lederle) and a human rabies immune globulin (Cutter). The dose of equine antiserum is 40 units/kg., whereas the dose of human rabies immune globulin is 20 units/kg. With either antibody preparation, half the dose is infiltrated around the wound. Equine serum is attended by at least a 20 per cent incidence of allergic reactions, and for that reason human rabies immune globulin is preferred, although there is no evidence that human rabies immune globulin is more efficacious in the prevention of rabies. Human rabies immune globulin can be obtained from local distributors of Cutter Laboratories in Dallas (214/631-6240).

Although administration of antiserum in a single dose is advisable as soon as possible after the bite, it should be given no matter how much time has elapsed between exposure and the decision to immunize.

Active Immunization. A vaccine prepared in duck embryo (Lilly) is available. In all cases, and particularly when antiserum has been given concurrently, we advise 23 subcutaneous doses of vaccine: 2 per day for 7 days, 1 per day for the second 7, and 1 each on the 24th and 34th days following the first injection.

Serious systemic allergic reactions to vaccine are likely in about 1 per cent of cases, and severe local reaction in 10 per cent to 30 per cent. Steroids should not be used for controlling these reactions, as they may depress the host's defenses to rabies. Neurologic reactions to duck embryo vaccine are rare.

If severe reactions prevent completion of a course of duck embryo vaccine, an unlicensed vaccine (Wyeth) prepared in human fibroblast cell culture may be obtained from the Rabies Investigations Unit of the Center for Disease Control, Atlanta (404/633-3311). The new vaccine, which is considerably more antigenic than duck embryo and contains no animal protein, is given in four weekly intramuscular injections. Antiserum may be used concurrently with the human cell culture vaccine and all four doses should be given regardless of the number of doses of duck embryo vaccine the patient had received previously. This new vaccine may receive a United States license in 1977. Table 1 offers guidelines for decisions regarding rabies immunization, but no table can cover all situations, and authorities should be freely consulted.

TABLE 1.   Postexposure Antirabies Guide*

ANIMAL	ANIMAL'S CONDITION AT TIME OF EXPOSURE†	TREATMENT
Wild Skunk Fox Raccoon Bat	Regard as rabid	Serum and vaccine
Domestic Dogs Cats	Healthy Escaped (unknown) Rabid or suspect rabid	None‡ Serum and vaccine§ Serum and vaccine"

*These recommendations are only a guide. They should be used in conjunction with knowledge of the animal species involved, circumstances of the bite or other exposure, vaccination status of the animal, and presence of rabies in the region.

†An exposure is considered to be by bite, by scratch with claws or by contamination with saliva of mucosal surfaces or skin that has been cut or abraded.

‡Begin serum and vaccine at first sign of rabies in biting dog or cat during holding period (10 days).

§May be unnecessary if rabies is nonexistent in local area.

"Discontinue vaccine if fluorescent antibody tests of animal are negative.

Prophylactic Vaccination. Antibodies may be elicited in those likely to be exposed subsequently to rabies, such as veterinarians. For duck embryo vaccine, the schedule of inoculations is 0, 28, and 180 days, whereas for human cell culture the schedule is 0, 7, and 21 days. The latter vaccine appears to be virtually 100 per cent reliable in producing antibodies.

Treatment of Rabies. The survival of one or possibly two patients with human rabies has reawakened interest in occasional observations of survival of animals and in neuropathological data showing little destruction of neurons. Thus it has been suggested that if a patient survived the acute encephalitis of rabies, he might recover. Previously, sedation of the patient was the only therapy advocated. Although even sophisticated attempts at therapy have failed to save patients with rabies, it is now mandatory to transport these patients to a medical center in which the full range of respiratory assistance equipment is available.

Included in the treatment of a patient with rabies are suction to prevent pooling of secretions, maintenance of fluid balance by the intravenous route, control of seizures and throat spasms by anticonvulsants and sedatives and, above all, a clear airway and good oxygenation by tracheostomy and endotracheal intubation if necessary.

Large doses of rabies antibody and of interferon have been advocated but their efficacy is uncertain.

Although it is prudent to isolate the patient because of possible virus excretion in the saliva, human to human transmission of rabies has seldom if ever been documented.

Infectious Mononucleosis

JAMES C. NIEDERMAN, M.D.

Infectious mononucleosis is an acute disease caused by the Epstein-Barr (EB) virus. This agent is ubiquitous throughout the world and on the basis of morphology and genome structure is a herpesvirus. Socioeconomically deprived groups have high rates of EBV infection early in life, but little clinical infectious mononucleosis; higher socioeconomic groups have lower levels of childhood EBV infection, but high rates of clinical disease when primary infection occurs in the 15 to 25 year age group. Characteristic clinical features include: (1) fever, sore throat and lymphadenopathy; (2) an increase in relative and absolute numbers of lymphocytes and monocytes (usually greater than 50 per cent and including more than 10 per cent atypical lymphocytes); (3) transient appearance of heterophil antibody; (4) development of specific and persistent EB virus antibody; and (5) abnormalities of hepatic function.

Most cases of infectious mononucleosis are mild or moderate in severity. During a prodromal period of 3 to 5 days, headache, malaise and fatigue are common. In over 80 per cent of cases, frank clinical features include fever, sore throat and cervical adenopathy. Irregular fever may be present for 7 to 10 days and subjective symptoms usually persist for 2 to 3 weeks. During the febrile period, rest in bed with bathroom privileges is advisable, and limited activity is recommended if sore throat, headache, excess malaise and anorexia are present. Isolation techniques are not necessary. Most patients recover uneventfully in 2 to 3 weeks, with gradual increase of activities to normal levels.

Gargling and irrigation of the throat with warm saline or glucose solutions are useful for pharyngitis and membranous tonsillitis. Aspirin, 1 gr. or 60 mg. per dose per year of age, up to 10 gr. or 0.60 gm. every four hours, usually controls pharyngeal discomfort and headache. Occasionally, codeine may be necessary for relief of these symptoms. In toxic patients who have severe exudative pharyngotonsillitis which makes airway obstruction a potential hazard, corticosteroid therapy is employed and a tracheostomy set should be readily available. Prednisone or its equivalent in other steroid preparations may be utilized. An initial dose of prednisone, 10 to 15 mg. four times daily, is decreased gradually and usually discontinued after a period of 7 to 10 days. Corticosteroids in full doses have been used in treating other severe complications, which include central nervous system involvement, thrombocytopenic purpura, hemolytic anemia, myocarditis and pericarditis.

Antibiotics have no effect on uncomplicated cases of this disease, and gamma globulin does not prevent or modify illness. If the throat culture is positive for hemolytic streptococci, a full course of oral penicillin, 200,000 to 400,000 units four times daily over a 10 day period, or an equivalent amount of erythromycin or parenteral penicillin should be administered.

Splenomegaly develops in approximately one-half of patients with infectious mononucleosis; these patients should be cautioned about heavy lifting, abdominal trauma and vigorous athletics until splenomegaly has subsided. Although extremely rare, splenic rupture is one of the few potentially fatal complications of this disease. Severe abdominal pain is unusual in infectious mononucleosis except in the presence of splenic rupture, which necessitates immediate splenectomy.

Although hepatic enlargement is detectable in only about 10 per cent of patients, serum transaminase, cephalin flocculation and thymol turbidity values are elevated in many patients for several weeks. Mild jaundice develops in approximately 5 per cent of patients, and requires only bed rest until the serum bilirubin returns to a normal level. No special diet is indicated.

In rare instances, patients may experience symptoms for several months, and their laboratory abnormalities are slow to resolve. In these cases, atypical lymphocytes persist and heterophil antibody titers may remain elevated for months after onset of acute illness. During this time, only symptomatic therapy is indicated.

Acute Infectious Lymphocytosis

RICHARD B. GOLDBLOOM, M.D.,
F.R.C.P.(C)

This benign syndrome has a single constant characteristic—a marked increase of mature lymphocytes in the peripheral blood—associated with mild, transient and variable symptoms. Ultimately, the condition may prove to encompass several viral infections that share a common hematological response.

In some outbreaks, many children with characteristic hematological features have been asymptomatic. Some have shown mild respiratory symptoms, slight fever, diarrhea or aseptic meningitis (with and without paralysis). The "pertussis syndrome," in which *Bordetella pertussis* has not been isolated, has also been described, and adenovirus has been recovered from some of the patients. In other instances, evidence for an association with enterovirus infections has been found.

The total peripheral leukocyte count is markedly elevated, usually to levels from 25,000 to over 100,000/mm³, with mature lymphocytes accounting for up to 95 per cent of the total. The bone marrow is normal. The lymphocytes are indistinguishable from those seen in normal blood smears, and some evidence suggests that the proliferation involves T-cells and null cells.

Because the disorder is benign and self-limited, no treatment is ordinarily required. Special isolation precautions are not usually indicated, but until the etiology is better understood, it would seem prudent to avoid unnecessary exposure of pregnant women or debilitated or immunosuppressed children to suspected cases.

Cat-Scratch Disease

SIDNEY KIBRICK, M.D.

This disease is almost always self-limited and benign. There is no specific treatment. Antibiotics have no effect and the value of steroids is unproved. Fever, malaise and local pain lasting from days to several weeks are common and may be treated with aspirin or other analgesics.

The adenopathy characteristic of this disease usually subsides within one or two months but may persist much longer. Adenitis which has not progressed to suppuration by six weeks generally tends to subside, although slowly. This regression may be hastened by warm moist compresses.

The suppurating, fluctuant node is most simply treated by closed aspiration, using an 18- or 19-gauge needle and local anesthesia. When pus is thick, saline instillations may facilitate this process. Generally only a few aspirations are necessary. This procedure not only relieves the pain but also provides material for preparation of skin test antigen. Incision for biopsy or drainage is more commonly followed by formation of sinus tracts and chronic drainage than closed aspiration, and is therefore not recommended.

Surgical excision of the involved nodes is advised for the following cases: (1) those not responding to repeated closed aspirations; (2) those with chronic draining sinuses; (3) patients with persistent, painful, disabling adenopathy; and (4) those in which a biopsy is needed to rule out malignancy or some other serious disorder.

This disease is not transmitted from man to man; therefore, isolation of patients is not necessary.

Cytomegalovirus Infections

JAMES B. HANSHAW, M.D.

Congenital Infection. Approximately 90 per cent of congenital cytomegalovirus infections are asymptomatic; the remaining 10 per cent may have mild to severe, even fatal, cytomegalic inclusion disease. Although several drugs such as cytosine and adenosine arabinoside have been used experimentally in patients, there is no evidence that these drugs have any lasting effect on the progression of the disease. The arabinosides and 5-iododeoxyuridine (IUDR) can induce a diminution in virus excretion in some patients. However, in view of the possible toxicity of these compounds and their unproved efficacy, they cannot be recommended.

Most infants with symptomatic infection do not require therapy. Exchange transfusion is rarely necessary for indirect hyperbilirubinemia. Neonatal sepsis, an unusual complication of cytomegalic inclusion disease, is due to enteric organisms or a streptococcal infection. Thus, the therapy would not be different from that used in other newborns with sepsis (p. 531). Since congenital cytomegalic inclusion disease may be a cause of spastic quadriplegia, mental retardation and obstructive hydrocephalus, long-range measures dealing with these chronic problems must be planned on an individual basis.

Acquired Infection. Until recently, clinically apparent disease due to cytomegalovirus infection had not been recognized except in patients with primary or iatrogenic immune deficiency. It is now known that infections in previously healthy individuals may result in a variety of abnormalities, including an infectious mononucleosis–like illness (cytomegalovirus mononucleosis), infectious polyneuritis, hepatomegaly with abnormal liver function tests and pneumonitis. The latter manifestation is more often associated with a deficiency of cellular immunity such as that induced by corticosteroid therapy in homotransplantation. In such instances the pneumonitis may be benefited by a temporary reduction of immunosuppressive therapy. Some young adult patients with cytomegalovirus mononucleosis have persistent fatigue over months—rarely for more than a year. The patient may require 15 or more hours of sleep per day. Although satisfactory controlled studies have not been done, it would appear that improvement is often correlated with extended periods of bed rest. Conversely, attempts to increase activity level frequently result in clinical relapse.

PREVENTION. Cytomegalovirus mononucleosis may occur in previously healthy young adults or following the transfusion of fresh blood. The greater number of transfusion units, the higher the probability of cytomegalovirus transmission. Because of the lability of cytomegalovirus, this complication of transfusion can be diminished significantly by using citrated blood that has been stored for more than 72 hours.

Although there is no available vaccine for the prevention of cytomegalovirus infection, there are live virus vaccine trials currently under way in this country and abroad.

Mycoplasma Infections

RICHARD H. MEADE, III, M.D.

Infections caused by *Mycoplasma pneumoniae* are mainly of the respiratory tract and include otitis media, pharyngitis, bronchitis and pneumonia. They are commonly mistaken for either bacterial or viral diseases since the clinical features of one or the other may be all that can be recognized. They can, in addition, be complicated by secondary viral (adenovirus) or bacterial invasion (*Hemophilus influenzae*) which may be the cause of renewed temperature elevations, by the appearance of new areas of pulmonary consolidation, and even by the development of bacteremia. Other types of mycoplasma infection occur but are uncommon; these include lymphocytic meningitis and

focal encephalitis. Migratory polyarthritis in children of 11 to 17 years of age has also been described. Skin lesions consisting of red macules or of vesicles resembling chickenpox have occurred in company with oral mucosal vesicles and with pneumonia. Pleural effusions of small to large dimension occur in up to 20 per cent of children with mycoplasma pneumonia. Infections have been proved by evidence of specific antibody in children ranging upward in age from 2 months.

In whatever site, the infection is treated best with erythromycin ethyl succinate either in liquid suspension, or tablets for children old enough, 25 to 50 mg./kg. daily divided into four doses. While higher blood levels are obtained with erythromycin estolate, no additional therapeutic effect has been demonstrated. Treatment should be given by mouth except for the child who is so sick that hospitalization is required because of the extent of a pneumonia and its association with headache, nausea, vomiting and cyanosis. Such severe forms of mycoplasma pneumonia are uncommon in children but occur and require intravenous erythromycin, 50 to 100 mg./kg. daily, in doses at 6 hour intervals (up to a maximum of 4 gm. daily). The duration of antibiotic therapy for all respiratory infections is one week. By that time the temperature should have been normal for at least 5 days. The x-ray in patients with pneumonia will show improvement but may remain abnormal for periods up to 2 or 3 weeks.

Clindamycin has been reported unsuccessful in the treatment of mycoplasma pneumonia and is not recommended. Tetracyclines, including demethylchlortetracycline, tetracycline and doxycycline, have been used for a number of years for pulmonary infection and generally have been as successful as erythromycin. The latter is preferred in children who are subject to dental discoloration, and for the particularly sick patient. Tetracycline can be used for adolescent children if it is preferred, or if erythromycin is associated with gastrointestinal discomfort and cannot be tolerated.

Neither tetracycline nor erythromycin can be depended on to prevent the patient from shedding mycoplasma in oral secretions, nor are they capable of preventing relapse or recurrent infection although both are uncommon problems. Dissemination of infection from a patient receiving therapy has not been established so that no special isolation procedures are required. Within any family dissemination has already occurred by the time the diagnosis is made. Relapse, though uncommon, is a clinical problem since recurrent fever and signs of pneumonia must be distinguished from secondary viral infections needing no antibiotic, or secondary bacterial infections requiring a different antibiotic.

Most children with mycoplasma infection require little other treatment. Pain from otitis media, or the headache associated with pneumonia, can be reduced with either salicylate or acetaminophen preparations. The cough associated with pneumonia if loose and productive should not be suppressed. A dry, harassing cough that keeps the patient awake and causes more severe headache should be controlled. Preparations containing codeine phosphate, such as glyceryl guaiacolate and pheniramine maleate, are effective and should be used.

Viral Pneumonia

ROBERT H. PARROTT, M.D.

The first step in the management of "viral" pneumonia is to assess the likelihood that indeed the infection is nonbacterial or nonmycoplasmal in origin. Most pneumonia in infants and young children is due to viruses; the most common causative agents are the respiratory syncytial virus (RSV), parainfluenza viruses 1, 2, and 3, influenza viruses A and B and adenoviruses. In fact, some signs of pneumonia occur in a third of infants and children undergoing first infection with RSV and parainfluenza viruses. However, the clinical spectrum of viral pneumonia is broad and, practically, cannot be differentiated clinically or roentgenographically from that due to *Streptococcus pneumoniae*, *Hemophilus influenzae* or other offending bacteria in the absence of a positive bacterial blood culture.

Rapid viral diagnosis usually is neither practical nor available. Some helpful clinical or epidemiologic hints follow: pneumonia due to RSV and parainfluenza viruses follows a 2 to 3 day "prodrome" of rhinitis and cough and is likely to occur under the age of two; when there is an excess of bronchiolitis in infants in the community, RSV is a likely cause of pneumonia. When there is an outbreak of croup in infants in the community, parainfluenza or influenza viruses may also be causing pneumonia. If multiple children and adults in a family have "colds" at the time of pneumonia in an infant, one of the viral agents is a likely cause. A peripheral white blood cell count over 20,000/cu. mm. strongly suggests a bacterial cause.

Antibiotic treatment is not necessary in viral pneumonia and should not be used if viral etiology is clear. However, because it is usually impossible to be sure about the etiology, the following courses of action are suggested for a child with pneumonia at any age beyond the newborn.

Mild or early signs of pneumonia (slight tachypnea, fever, occasional rales): take a white blood cell count, nasopharyngeal and blood cultures and have reliable parents observe the child at home with advice to watch for increasing respiratory rate or distress and to bring the child back to the doctor as necessary. A follow-up examination is indicated in 10 to 14 days.

Diffuse rales or some signs of respiratory distress: take a white blood cell count, nasopharyngeal and blood cultures and a chest x-ray. Treat presumptively for pneumococcal pneumonia (the most likely treatable cause) pending results of culture and of the antibiotic "therapeutic trial." Procaine penicillin G, 100,000 to 600,000 units for the first 24 hours, is suggested. If blood cultures show pneumococci or other bacteria, turn to page 555 for the treatment of bacterial pneumonia. Nasopharyngeal cultures may be suggestive of etiology if there is a pure culture but *S. pneumoniae* and *H. influenzae* organisms are found regularly in the nasopharynx of normal children.

Very rapid defervescence and improvement after 24 hours of penicillin might also suggest pneumococcal etiology and be an indication for further antibiotics. However, if fever and mild symptoms continue and there is no laboratory evidence for bacterial etiology, penicillin can be stopped and the child can be observed at home with advice to watch for signs of distress. A follow-up examination including chest x-ray is indicated in 10 to 14 days.

Moderate to severe respiratory distress and/or toxicity: admit to hospital for cultures, supplemental oxygen and close observation for respiratory failure and consideration of the potential need for ventilatory assistance. Antibiotics may be used as for *S. pneumoniae*, *H. influenzae* or *Staphylococcus aureus* pending results of cultures and/or of the antibiotic "therapeutic trial." Ampicillin and oxacillin should cover this spectrum and can be used for 24 to 48 hours while awaiting culture results and clinical progress. If blood cultures show bacteria, turn to page 555 for the treatment of bacterial pneumonia. Particularly in the hospitalized infant or child, antibiotics can be stopped after 48 hours if there is no evidence for bacterial infection.

Forty per cent humidified oxygen should

be administered by tent or by mask and/or nasotracheal tube if necessary to maintain saturation at 80 to 90 per cent. Frequent blood gas measurements may be indicated.

After initial hydration, maintenance hydration and electrolytes are given intravenously; dehydration is also assessed and corrected. Avoid overhydration. Because of difficulty with breathing and excess respiratory secretions, oral feeding is avoided or limited for the first day or two. Careful suctioning to remove secretions is helpful. We no longer tend to provide a highly humidified atmosphere unless there is evidence of drying of the upper respiratory secretions. There is a danger of bacterial infection with the prolonged use of mist tents. Also, ultrasonic or jet nebulizers must be used with caution because small particles may actually increase airway resistance. Under any condition the child should never be lost from sight because of dense mist.

For the *newborn* with pneumonia, hospitalization is almost always indicated. All of the above mentioned respiratory viral agents may produce pneumonia in the newborn, but so may agents not usually associated with respiratory tract disease such as the herpesviruses and cytomegaloviruses, *Pneumocystis carinii* and fungi such as Candida. Antibiotics in the therapeutic trial should cover gram-negative organisms and Group B streptococcus.

In *school-aged and adolescent children* the likelihood that pneumonia is due to the common respiratory viruses decreases and *Mycoplasma pneumoniae* joins the bacterial agents as top etiologic probabilities, along with certain adenoviruses. Erythromycin should be considered in a "therapeutic trial."

The roentgenographic signs of viral pneumonia take several weeks to clear. Clinical and x-ray follow-up is indicated in 10 to 14 days in most cases, but particularly if the pneumonia has been moderately severe or if coughing or ronchi persists. Atelectasis is an occasional sequela.

Viral Hepatitis

SAUL KRUGMAN, M.D.

Viral hepatitis is caused by at least two viruses that are morphologically and immunologically distinct: hepatitis A virus and hepatitis B virus. The two types of hepatitis have the following distinctive features: the incubation period for viral hepatitis, type A, is 15 to 50 days, and for type B, 50 to 160 days. Regarding age incidence, type A usually occurs in children and young adults, and type B occurs at any age but predominantly in adolescents and adults. Transmissibility of hepatitis A virus is chiefly by close contact, but also by parenteral exposure, and of hepatitis B virus chiefly by inoculation of contaminated blood or blood products, and also by close contact. Immunity is homologous following type A and type B hepatitis, but neither confers immunity against the other.

The detection of specific antigens associated with type A and type B hepatitis was followed by the development of specific tests for the diagnosis of these diseases. The use of these tests has revealed the occurrence of hepatitis caused by neither type. The agent or agents responsible for "non A non B" hepatitis have not been characterized as yet.

Prevention of Viral Hepatitis, Type A. Since the infection is spread chiefly via the fecal-oral route, procedures designed to block this intestinal-oral pathway should be used for control. These measures include scrupulous handwashing, proper sterilization of food utensils, fly abatement and exclusion of potentially infected food handlers. Although close contact is the most common mode of transmission of type A hepatitis, common source epidemics stemming from contaminated food, milk and water supplies may also occur.

The efficacy of human immune serum globulin (ISG) for the prevention or modification of viral hepatitis type A has been well established. It is recommended for children and adults who have had an intimate exposure to a person with the disease. It is also indicated for persons living in the same household, because they are likely to have direct or indirect contact with the infectious virus. On the other hand, the routine use of ISG for children and adults in schools, offices and factories is not warranted; spread of the disease is unlikely under the conditions in these open facilities. However, in institutions for mentally retarded children and in other closed areas where hepatitis is endemic, ISG is indicated for new admissions and new employees. The dose is dependent upon the type of exposure; a proposed schedule is shown in Table 1.

PREVENTION OF VIRAL HEPATITIS, TYPE B. Contaminated blood, blood products and needles are the most common sources of hepatitis B virus infection. The most common mode of transmission is the parenteral route, but the virus can infect via the oral route. Blood obtained from commercial donors carries a 10- to 15-fold greater risk of causing hepatitis than blood obtained from volunteer donors. The indications for administering blood or blood products should be carefully assessed to be

TABLE 1.   Recommended Dose of Standard Immune
Serum Globulin

TYPE OF EXPOSURE	TOTAL DOSE (ml.)

Type A hepatitis
  Single or short term
    (< 2 months)
	0.5 (up to 50 lb.)
	1.0 (50 to 100 lb.)
	2.0 to 3.0 (over 100 lb.)

Prolonged or continuous* (> 2 months)	1.0 to 2.0 (up to 50 lb.) 2.0 to 3.0 (50 to 100 lb.) 5.0 (over 100 lb.)
Type B hepatitis	1.0 to 2.0 (up to 50 lb.) 5.0 (50 to 100 lb.) 5.0 to 10.0 (over 100 lb.)

*Repeat once after 5 months if exposure continues.

sure that the potential advantages of the transfusion warrant the potential risk of transmitting hepatitis.

The following precautions are indicated for the screening of blood donors: (1) reject persons whose blood contains HBsAg; (2) reject persons who are suspected of being addicted to narcotics; (3) reject those who have received blood or who have had contact with a patient with hepatitis within the past 6 months; and (4) reject donors whose blood was previously suspected of causing hepatitis. The World Health Organization Expert Committee on Viral Hepatitis has recommended that "volunteer blood donors need not be excluded on the basis of a previous history of hepatitis alone or on the finding of anti-HBs *provided that* (a) they have had no attack of hepatitis during at least the previous year and (b) their blood has been found negative for HBsAg by a very sensitive test."

The use of disposable equipment is indicated if feasible. Equipment which cannot be discarded should be thoroughly cleaned and sterilized. The virus can be inactivated by boiling for at least 10 minutes, autoclaving at 15 pounds pressure or being subjected to dry heat at 170° C. (338° F.) for 30 minutes.

The efficacy of ISG for the prevention of type B hepatitis will be dependent upon at least two factors: (1) the amount of protective antibody that is present in the particular preparation, and (2) the dose of virus that is present in the transfused units of blood or the accidental needle stick. The higher the antibody content and the lower the dose of virus, the more likely the chances for protection. Recent studies have shown that lots of immune serum globulin prepared since 1972 have higher antibody titers than those prepared prior to that time,

when testing of blood for HBsAg was not mandatory.

The efficacy of hepatitis B immune serum globulin has been confirmed by various controlled studies. The antibody titer of this preparation is 10,000 times or more higher than that of standard ISG. HBIG was recently licensed for use; it is indicated primarily for persons accidentally inoculated with a contaminated needle. HBIG is also indicated for infants born of mothers whose pregnancies were complicated by hepatitis B infection. The dose of HBIG is dependent upon the antibody titer of the particular preparation, and the recommended dose is listed in the package insert.

Treatment.   There is no specific treatment for children with type A or type B viral hepatitis. The disease is generally so mild that bed rest is unnecessary after the acute stage. The return to activity is usually gauged by the child's desire. The diet is also determined by the patient. When anorexia is present, food is rejected; liquids such as broths and fruit juices should be offered. A normal diet is recommended when the appetite returns. Corticosteroids and other drugs are not indicated for children with uncomplicated hepatitis.

FULMINANT HEPATITIS.   Sudden onset of mental confusion, emotional instability, restlessness, coma and hemorrhagic manifestations may progress to a fatal outcome within 10 days. Under these extraordinary conditions the following measures should be considered: (1) corticosteroid therapy; (2) withdrawal of protein from the diet; (3) oral neomycin, 25 mg./kg. every 6 hours, to suppress the bacterial flora of the intestinal tract; (4) laxatives and cleansing enemas; and (5) exchange transfusion.

Hepatitis B Infection During Pregnancy. Mothers who have acute viral hepatitis, type B, or an asymptomatic HBsAg carrier state during pregnancy may infect their newborn infants. Infection may occur in utero or during the perinatal or postnatal period. Signs of infection (antigenemia) in the infant may be detected from 2 weeks to 6 months after birth. Consequently, periodic samples of blood should be obtained at monthly or more frequent intervals to be tested for HBsAg. Breast feeding is contraindicated because it is usually associated with ingestion of infectious virus present in the serum exuding from the mother's cracked nipples. It is recommended that HBIG, if available, or standard ISG be given intramuscularly shortly after birth. (See Table 1 for recommended dose.)

Enteroviral Infections

PETER ECHEVERRIA, M.D.

Polioviruses, coxsackieviruses and echoviruses are grouped together as enteroviruses because they are commonly found in the human intestine. These viruses are characterized by small size (20 to 30 mμ.), a ribonucleic acid core, resistance to inactivation by ether (absence of a lipid membrane) and resistance to inactivation by acid (pH 3 to 5). Most enteroviral infections are either asymptomatic or result in nonspecific symptoms including low grade fever, coryza and transient macular rashes.

Distinct clinical syndromes, initially associated with certain types, are now recognized to be caused by many of the enteroviruses. Paralysis, one of the more serious consequences of enteroviral infection, is usually due to one of three polioviruses, although muscle weakness occasionally follows coxsackie and echovirus infections. Epidemic myalgia, aseptic meningitis with or without an encephalitic component, pericarditis, and pleurodynia have been associated with both coxsackie and echoviruses.

Herpangina and hand-foot-mouth disease are usually due to coxsackie A viruses. Coxsackie B virus infections have been implicated in myocarditis, orchitis, and more recently in pandemics of conjunctivitis occasionally associated with radiculomyelitis. Both coxsackie A and B viruses have been isolated from a generalized disease of the newborn which includes myocarditis and meningoencephalitis. Although gastrointestinal symptoms frequently accompany enteroviral infections, there is little evidence for enteroviruses as an etiologic agent in uncomplicated pediatric diarrhea.

Enteroviral infections occur most frequently between May and October in the United States. Transmission is primarily by the fecal-oral route, although the respiratory route is possible. Type specific immunity develops in the course of the infection.

A trivalent oral vaccine is the only currently recommended vaccine against poliomyelitis. No vaccines are available for the other enteroviruses. Antiviral agents are not helpful in the treatment of enteroviral infections. Therapy is supportive and includes adequate hydration (intravenous fluid is rarely necessary) and antipyretics. Life-threatening complications and sequelae are rare except in poliomyelitis, myocarditis and generalized disease of the newborn.

Aseptic meningitis is the most commonly recognized enteroviral infection. Aseptic meningitis caused by these viruses is usually a benign self-limited disease (see p. 636).

Coxsackie B types 1 to 5 and coxsackie A-9 viruses have been isolated from infants with acute myocarditis frequently accompanied by meningoencephalitis. This disease is charcterized by sudden pallor, dyspnea, lethargy and tachycardia and may proceed rapidly to death. The prognosis of enteroviral infections in the newborn infant is not as grim as previously thought, but is more serious than infections in the older child. The symptoms are similar to those of bacterial sepsis and the true etiology may become apparent only at autopsy.

Mothers frequently have a history of an enteroviral infection during pregnancy; however, the route of infection of these infants is unclear. Epidemics of enteroviral infection have occurred in newborn nurseries. At present there are no antiviral agents that are helpful in treating this infection and therapy is supportive.

Infants who enter the hospital with aseptic meningitis or other enteroviral infections should not be admitted to a neonatal special care unit but preferably to an older age ward where the consequences of secondary spread are less dangerous.

Herpangina is a distinct clinical entity usually caused by coxsackie A viruses. Children develop high fever, sore throat and occasionally vomiting. Vesicles and punctate ulcers are present on the tonsils, uvula, pharynx, and soft palate. Herpangina is frequently confused with herpetic stomatitis, which involves the gums and buccal mucosa and is more confluent. Treatment is symptomatic. Soft food and liquids are well tolerated; frequently cold drinks or ice cream decrease the symptoms. Viscous Xylocaine may be helpful for the older child. Antipyretics frequently are necessary.

Hand-foot-mouth disease is probably a clinical entity distinct from herpangina and is characterized by similar vesicles on the buccal mucosa and tongue and less frequently on the soft palate and uvula. A maculopapular rash appears simultaneously or several days later on the hands and feet. The rash rapidly becomes vesicular and involves the palms and soles and interdigital spaces. This disease is frequently confused with atypical measles and Rocky Mountain spotted fever. Coxsackie A-16 was initially implicated with the syndrome, but a variety of other coxsackie A viruses have subsequently been isolated from children with this condition.

Pleurodynia, or devil's grip, is characterized by the onset of acute severe paroxysmal chest pain, headache, fever and myalgia. Chest pain is pleuritic and aggravated by deep breathing or coughing. A pleural friction rub is present in one-fourth of the patients. Coxsackie B viruses were first implicated in this syndrome but other enteroviruses have been associated as well. Older children and adults may be more likely to develop pleurodynia, whereas younger children are experiencing an epidemic of aseptic meningitis. Treatment is symptomatic. Pericarditis occasionally occurs with pleurodynia or alone. Treatment with aspirin is usually adequate; the value of steroids is questionable. Rarely, children develop signs of cardiac tamponade and require pericardiocentesis. Chronic constrictive pericarditis may be a sequela of enteroviral pericarditis.

Myocarditis has been associated with enteroviral infections in older children as well as infants in the neonatal period. Since treatment is supportive and no clear evidence of the value of steroids has been demonstrated, it is imperative that other causes of acute myocarditis such as rheumatic fever and collagen diseases be considered, and appropriate therapy instituted promptly if warranted.

Poliomyelitis is rare in the United States, although cases still occur in unvaccinated children. All children with paralytic poliomyelitis should be hospitalized during the acute phase of disease. Careful monitoring is essential since respiratory and pharyngeal paralysis may occur insidiously. Bed rest is also important since exercise during the acute phase may result in increased paralysis. Urinary retention, urolithiasis and contractures may complicate management. Physical therapists and orthopedists should become involved in the management early so appropriate care and follow-up can be given for the child's affected muscles.

It is important to determine whether a non-polio enterovirus, rather than a wild or vaccine strain of poliovirus, is responsible for a case of paralytic disease for medicolegal as well as for public health reasons. Viral isolation should be attempted in all children with paralytic disease. Throat, stool and cerebrospinal fluid specimens should be collected early in the disease and shipped under the appropriate conditions to a diagnostic virology laboratory. Serum specimens collected at the onset of the disease and two to three weeks later are collected for antibody determinations.

All hospitalized children with enteroviral infections should be isolated. Viruses are present in large quantity in the stool and are relatively resistant to drying. Nosocomial infections with enteroviruses have been described and may cause significant morbidity and death, especially in infants.

Acute Aseptic Meningitis

ALEX J. STEIGMAN, M.D.

Acute aseptic meningitis is a clinical and laboratory syndrome often regarded simply as viral meningitis, although there are causes other than viruses. When a virus is successfully identified in this syndrome, it is most often an enterovirus (nonparalytic poliomyelitis, echoviruses, Coxsackieviruses) or mumps virus. Less commonly identified are lymphocytic choriomeningitis virus, herpes simplex virus and others. These are systemic infections with a viremic phase; involvement of the nervous system is an important complication. In the majority of cases reported to the health authorities the precise etiology is not readily determined.

Detailed history, physical examination and study of the cerebrospinal fluid are essential in order to exclude partially treated pyogenic or tuberculous meningitis. For the child who has been receiving prior antibiotic therapy and is now being evaluated, it is prudent to consider the patient initially as having partially treated pyogenic meningitis. History of symptoms, recent exposures, past immunizations, age, season of year, and local epidemic events, together with the cerebrospinal fluid findings, assist in determining whether to continue antibiotics or to alter the regimen until a diagnosis of aseptic meningitis can be made with confidence.

Although a mild degree of encephalitis of subclinical degree probably accompanies many patients with aseptic meningitis a good prognosis should initially be entertained and expressed to the parents.

The direct management of the patient concerns symptomatic relief for headache, excessive fever, nausea or vomiting and muscle spasm. The withdrawal of spinal fluid for diagnosis often relieves the headache. Drugs which must be avoided are opiates, phenothiazine derivatives, diazepam, and similar agents which may produce misleading signs and symptoms.

In view of the fact that the two most commonly recognized viral causes of this syndrome are mumps and the enteroviruses (mumps in the absence of parotitis and enteroviral disease without rash or other clues), patients should be isolated during the early acute phases of their illness.

Management includes the responsibility for collecting appropriate viral specimens so that an etiologic diagnosis can be made, if possible, which may bear on the long-term prognosis as well as give guidance to those responsible for establishing control measures in a community. Mumps is one of the few conditions in which a single blood specimen tested for antibody to viral or soluble mumps antigen may be diagnostic. A patient whose aseptic meningitis is due to mumps will often be found to have an elevation in serum amylase levels.

Early complications are infrequent and include brief periods of acute hypertension which rarely require intervention; also the inappropriate antidiuretic hormone (ADH) syndrome may occur requiring fluid and electrolyte adjustment.

In all cases careful assessment should be conducted several weeks after apparent recovery which should include neuromuscular examination to assure that areas of muscle atrophy are not overlooked. It is imperative that a TEST FOR HEARING be done at this time especially in the case of those whose illness was due to or presumed to be mumps. If mumps is determined as the cause the parents should be so advised in order to avoid anxiety following exposure to mumps in later life.

Encephalitis Infections—Postinfectious and Postvaccinal

M. L. WEIL, M.D.

Postinfectious and postvaccinal encephalitides represent an increasingly diverse group of neurological diseases with multiple etiologies. The classical concept of this group of illnesses is confined to those complications of acute infectious diseases, usually viral, which result in focal perivenous demyelination of the nervous system. Occurrence of a similar pathological picture in experimental allergic encephalitis and neurinitis as well as after immunization of humans with material derived from mammalian nervous tissue suggests that hypersensitivity plays a major role in this process. A broader concept is required since the varied pathogenesis of these diseases includes not only acute and delayed hypersensitivity to brain and foreign proteins, but also a variable role for protective antibody and direct viral involvement. An early accurate diagnosis becomes imperative as an increasing number of antiviral substances and an increasing number of agents to modulate the immune system become available. The temptation to use unproven remedies should be resisted in favor of a carefully designed, approved protocol. Clear evidence for the efficacy of alterations in the immediate or delayed immune response is still needed.

A limited number of specific chemo-therapeutic agents may help control continuing infections. Only specific therapeutic agents of proven efficacy should be used. (See sections on vaccinia, herpes simplex, herpes zoster, and mycoplasma.)

Supportive measures should be utilized as indicated. Hypoxia of the nervous system due to asphyxia or hypoperfusion should be prevented. Cerebral or spinal cord edema may require the use of osmotic diuretics such as mannitol or urea (1 to 2 gm./kg. intravenously) or steroids (dexamethasone, 6 mg./m² intravenous initially, then 4 mg./m² every 4 to 6 hours; or methylprednisolone). This may prevent brain herniation. Hypoventilation with attendant hypoxia and hypercarbia may require assisted ventilation. The comatose patient should be assured an adequate airway. Tracheostomy is utilized early when indicated by impaired swallowing or prolonged coma.

Persistence of infection within the nervous system may result in central or peripheral nervous system symptoms weeks or years after initial improvement. This has been described for measles, rubella, herpes simplex, varicella, syphilis, and vaccinia. Persistent mumps virus infection of the ependyma may result in hydrocephalus. Proper chemotherapy, if available, requires that the exact etiologic agent be established. Some cases of postinfectious polyneuritis (Landry-Guillain-Barre syndrome) have resulted from mycoplasma infections which should be treated with erythromycin. As of this writing, no controlled study of long-term modulation of the immune system with suppression (cyclophosphamide, steroids) or enhancement (interferon, transfer factor, isoprinosine, levamisole) has demonstrated consistent benefit for chronic viral or demyelinating processes.

Postinfectious encephalomyelitis, which occurs more often than encephalitis, may be associated with perivenous demyelination similar to that seen after immunization with mammalian nervous tissue. It usually occurs in children over two years of age. Encephalopathy with cerebral edema and congestion represents the major postinfectious or postvaccinal reaction in children under two, but may occur in all age groups. It must be distinguished from encephalopathy with fatty infiltration of the viscera (see Reye's Syndrome). Acute hemorrhagic leukoencephalitis may be benefited by large doses of steroids but controlled studies are lacking.

Active immunization against rabies has been associated with perivenous demyelination. This complication is most often seen with rabbit spinal cord vaccines, especially when used with live attenuated rabies virus. Vaccine made from suckling mouse brain produces an increased incidence of ascending paralysis of the Landry type. Neurological complications occur much less frequently with duck embryo vaccines.

Neuritic involvement comprises about one-third of the neuroparalytic accidents in rabies immunization. Such involvement is localized primarily to nerve roots, particularly those of the radial and sciatic nerve, as well as cranial nerves III and X. Ascending paralysis and transverse myelitis also occur. Disturbances of autonomic function which may result can lead to major problems with bowel and bladder function, as well as the rapid evolution of trophic ulcers. Steroids or immune suppression have not been of benefit although symptoms may develop in association with the appearance of dermal hypersensitivity to the vaccine.

The occurrence of postpertussis immunization encephalopathy is not related to the number of doses. In some reports reaction has been slightly more frequent when pertussis vaccine is administered to brain-injured children. Other authors have not confirmed this. It is recommended that children with clear brain damage in an area with decreased prevalence of pertussis not be given pertussis vaccine. This will avoid an increased incidence of encephalopathy or seizures. The association between pertussis immunization and massive infantile myoclonus with or without hypsarrhythmia suggests that this form of encephalopathy may be postvaccinal in some individuals. (See appropriate section for possible benefit from early use of steroids or ACTH.)

Tetanus toxoid and typhoid vaccine have been reported to cause local neuritides, most often in the C5-6 region. No remedy is known, although there is often spontaneous improvement.

The use of hyperimmune serum for therapy or passive prophylaxis is described for rabies, tetanus, diphtheria and other diseases. Allergic neuritis, usually involving motor more than sensory systems, may occur most often after an interval of 7 to 12 days. Males are affected nine times more often than females. This type of neuritis may respond to antihistamines, steroids or ACTH. Epinephrine may be of benefit if urticaria is present.

Psittacosis

PHILIP A. BRUNELL, M.D.

Psittacosis is spread principally by psittacine birds which are sold as pets. Quarantine regulations have decreased the magnitude of the problem, but state regulations vary, and latent infection in some birds sold in pet stores still poses problems in control of the spread of disease. Almost all of the reported cases are found in pet bird dealers, owners or breeders.

The illness is characterized by high fever and pulmonary involvement. Systemic symptoms such as anorexia, lethargy and malaise constitute a significant part of the disease; headache is common.

When the diagnosis is made, treatment should be started with generous oral doses of doxycycline, 5 mg./kg./day up to a maximum of 200 mg./day in divided doses. The patient should feel better and the temperature should decline within 3 to 4 days. At this time 2.5 mg./kg. of doxycycline once daily should be given for at least 10 days. This should be considered a minimum course of therapy, since latent infections may be established with recurrences. The small risk of tooth staining from such a course of therapy should not dissuade one from adequately treating this serious infection. Gastric irritation resulting from doxycycline administration can be reduced by giving the medication with food.

If oral therapy cannot be tolerated, doxycycline hyclate in the same dosage used for oral administration should be given intravenously. If tetracyclines are given either orally or parenterally, cautions relating to side effects should be scrupulously observed.

Cough is a very distressing part of the illness. The patient's environment should be adequately humidified. Hard candies, lollypops, cough drops or a demulcent cough mixture are helpful. If cough interferes with sleep codeine or codeine derivatives should be given prior to retiring to assure an adequate night's sleep. A single dose of 0.5 mg./kg. or 15 to 20 mg./m² of codeine is used. Codeine should also be used for intractable coughing during the waking hours, especially if coughing or emesis associated with it interfere with oral feedings. It should not be used in place of adequate humidification and demulcents. During the latter part of the illness potassium iodide, 5 mg./kg./dose, given in milk or fruit juice three times daily, may be useful in liquifying secretions.

Hospitalized patients should be isolated, since there are documented cases of person to person spread, some of which can be traced to hospital exposure.

Rickettsial Infections

WILLIAM E. LAUPUS, M.D.

Arthropod-borne rickettsial infections in the United States are best exemplified by Rocky Mountain spotted fever, the most commonly recognized rickettsial illness. The Center for Disease Control Reports for 1976 recorded 892 cases, of which almost half occurred in the South Atlantic States region. Underreporting is frequent in endemic areas where the prevailing practice is to treat otherwise unexplained headache and febrile illness with tetracycline if a history of tick exposure is elicited.

Q fever and endemic murine typhus are much less frequently seen. The therapy and supportive management of all three rickettsial infections are similar.

Specific Therapy. Tetracycline and chloramphenicol are considered equally efficacious. I prefer chloramphenicol sodium succinate intravenously in children beyond the fourth febrile day if significant manifestations (headache, spiking fever, rash, prostration) of the disease are present. Initially, chloramphenicol should be given intravenously in the amount of 100 mg./kg./day in 4 equally divided doses. The total course should be 10 days and the total daily dose need not and should not exceed 2 gm./day. The response to therapy is not dramatic, fever usually defervesces over 2 or more days and recovery requires several days to 2 or more weeks. As soon as the patient is afebrile and taking oral fluids well, chloramphenicol may be given orally in the usual dose of 50 mg./kg./day in 4 equally divided portions.

Parents should be advised of the potential toxicity of chloramphenicol and of the precautions which will be taken to recognize bone marrow toxicity. The physician should inquire whether chloramphenicol has been administered to the child for other illnesses. Bone marrow depression is less likely when no earlier exposure to the drug exists. Complete blood counts should be done every two days (or daily if white blood count is below 7000/cu. mm.); the chloramphenicol should be replaced with tetracycline if the white blood count decreases to below 5000/cu. mm. or the polymorphonuclear cell count becomes less than 30 percent.

In children who are mildly to moderately ill, I have used orally administered tetracycline, 50 mg./kg./day in 4 equally divided doses for 7 to 10 days. The total daily dose should be limited to 2.0 gm. All of the tetracyclines appear to have similar effectiveness. If the patient is less than 8 years of age, permanent discoloration of the teeth and enamel hypoplasia are possible but unlikely complications from a single course of tetracycline.

Transmission. Rodents are the natural hosts for rickettsia rickettsii, the etiologic agent of Rocky Mountain spotted fever, which is transmitted to man by the wood tick, *Dermocentor andersoni*, and the dog tick, *Dermocentor variabilis*. The tick attaches itself to exposed areas of the skin, burrows with its mouthparts and feeds on the liberated blood; in the process, the rickettsiae are released locally from the tick's salivary glands and establish the human illness.

Clinical Recognition. The illness commences with headache, fever and diminished appetite after an incubation period of 1 to 7 or more days. The headache persists and becomes more severe, the fever and prostration increase, and muscle pains, periorbital and facial edema, and disorientation frequently appear over the next 4 to 5 days. In most children a scattered, macular, light pink rash develops over the wrists and ankles, spreads to the trunk, palms and soles, and becomes petechial. Hematuria, thrombocytopenia, intravascular coagulopathy, shock, avascular necrosis, myocarditis, and heart failure may develop during the illness. The fatality rate in untreated cases may be 40 percent; however, recently effective therapy has lowered mortality to 5 percent. Fatal cases are usually recognized late in the course of the disease when vasculitis and intravascular coagulopathy are severe.

Therapy of Complications. Thrombocytopenia may or may not be accompanied by other signs of consumption coagulopathy. Though rarely necessary, the platelet deficit may be lessened temporarily by platelet or whole blood transfusions. Intravenous heparin, 50 to 100 units/kg. intravenously every 4 to 6 hours, appears to decrease or stop the progression of the coagulopathy but probably does not change mortality or morbidity. Corticosteroids appear to be of little or no value.

Avascular necrosis, probably a "purpura-fulminans" manifestation, may involve large areas of gangrenous skin and subcutaneous tissue as well as terminal portions of digits. Appropriate therapy will include heparin as above. Dextran infusions have also been credited with arresting the progression of the lesions.

An adequate blood volume should be maintained by judicious administration of oral and parenteral fluids. Overhydration should be avoided, particularly when myocarditis is suspected.

Central nervous system vasculitis may be manifested by delirium, confusion, stupor, coma and convulsive seizures. Cerebrospinal fluid may show increased pressure, protein and cell count. Phenobarbital sodium intravenously in a dose of 4 mg./kg. will usually control the seizures.

Tick Removal. The process of rickettsial transmission from the tick to child probably requires several hours; hence, in endemic areas prompt removal of ticks before they become engorged with blood is one of the best means of preventing infection. Picking off or crushing the tick has the disadvantage of leaving the infected mouth parts buried in the skin. Expert removal calls for sufficient irritation to the tick to cause release of the mouth parts. Coating the tick with clear nail polish or petrolatum or touching it with a hot match head is usually successful in loosening its hold and after a few minutes the tick is removed easily with forceps.

Vaccine.   The killed rickettsial vaccine is rarely used in children because of the short duration of protection afforded by the vaccine. Prophylaxis is better accomplished in endemic areas by twice daily inspection of children for ticks and prompt removal of those found.

Chlamydial Infections

MARC O. BEEM, M.D.

The chlamydiae indigenous to man are known by the species name of *Chlamydia trachomatis*. These organisms are obligate intracellular parasites that, with the exception of strains causing lymphogranuloma venereum, are only capable of parasitizing epithelial cells which appear in certain areas of the body, such as the uterine cervix, male urethra, rectum, conjunctiva and respiratory tract.

Except for those parts of the world where endemic trachoma persists, the chief reservoir of *C. trachomatis* infection is genital. Although infection may be spread by indirect routes, transmission usually occurs by direct contact. It is by direct contact that organisms originating in the cervix of an infected mother are transmitted to the infant during parturition. Such natal transmission has long been known to result in conjunctival colonization and disease. Recently it has been shown that respiratory tract colonization also occurs with equal and perhaps even greater frequency than conjunctival colonization. This, in turn, may be associated with disease of the respiratory tract. Although the details of the respiratory component of these infections are not yet completely defined, enough is known to indicate that they must be taken into consideration in the management of natally acquired chlamydial infection.

Conjunctivitis presenting between days 4 and 12 is usually the earliest clinical evidence of chlamydial colonization. Affecting one or both eyes, chlamydial etiology can be suspected on the basis of time of presentation and Gram's stain of the exudate (mononuclear and polymorphonuclear leukocytes but few or no bacteria). Chlamydial etiology can be established by identification of characteristic cytoplasmic inclusions in epithelial cells or by isolation of the agent in cell culture. When conjunctival bacterial cultures are negative or equivocal (such as a few colonies of *Staphylococcus epidermidis* or diphtheroids), and there is little or no response to topical treatment with polymyxin and aerosporin or neomycin, the presumption of chlamydial etiology is strong. In our experience conjunctival cultures of such infants usually yield chlamydiae.

It is the natural course of events for the inflammation to subside rather rapidly to a chronic phase with only modest amounts of mucopurulent discharge and thickening of the palpebral conjunctiva evidenced by a fleshy, pale appearance and diminished visibility of conjunctival capillary blood vessels. This phase of conjunctival infection may occur in infants in whom no acute phase was recognized.

Respiratory tract colonization occurs in virtually all infants with conjunctival disease and in an additional portion with congenital infection who have escaped conjunctival colonization. In many, perhaps the majority of such infants, there are no evident clinical consequences of this respiratory colonization. Some infants, however, have a mild to moderate degree of nasopharyngeal airway obstruction. Additionally, secretory otitis media may be seen.

Lower respiratory tract disease due to chlamydiae most characteristically presents at 6 weeks of age. These infants have a history of respiratory symptomatology that has slowly increased in severity over a period of one or more weeks. Systemic abnormalities are notably absent: temperatures are normal and there is little or no malaise. Lower respiratory manifestations may include spells of staccato coughing, tachypnea, diffuse inspiratory crepitant rales and no, or only minor degrees of, expiratory wheezing. Chest x-rays show diffuse interstitial infiltrates with patchy areas of airlessness in lungs that are usually quite overexpanded. Some infants may show mild degrees of blood eosinophilia and values for serum IgG and IgM are usually, and for IgA sometimes elevated. These infants invariably shed chlamydiae from their respiratory tracts in high titer and have elevated levels of antichlamydial antibodies as assayed by microimmunofluorescent techniques. Significant serum complement-fixing antibody titers to the psittacosis-LGV group antigen are sometimes found, but this serologic test is relatively insensitive and usually negative. It is our experience that, given the full clinical syndrome, the odds greatly favor this diagnosis in infants under 4 months of age with afebrile pneumonia.

The mainstay of the treatment of natally acquired chlamydial infection is systemic therapy. We have found that erythromycin ethyl succinate (40 mg./kg./day) or sulfisoxazole* (150 mg./kg./day) terminates chlamydial shedding within 4 days, and infants so treated for two weeks have remained culture-negative for chlamydiae over observation periods extending up to one year. Adjunctive therapy of conjunctivitis may include topical applications of sulfacetamide (10 per cent ophthalmic ointment or 30 per cent ophthalmic solution) or tetracycline (1 per cent ointment or solution) every 4 hours for the day or two required for the hyperacute changes to subside. It should be emphasized, however, that such therapy alone will neither effect a permanent resolution of conjunctival infection nor reverse the respiratory component.

Infants with lower respiratory tract involvement may profit from chest physical therapy and postural drainage. The response to systemic antichlamydial therapy is slow but follows a predictable course. The severity of the cough begins to diminish noticeably about day 5. By day 14, clinical recovery is substantially complete, although a few abnormal physical signs may remain in the chest. These and the chest x-ray are usually normal by day 21.

Systemic Mycoses

EDOUARD DROUHET, M.D.

Considerable progress has been made in the treatment of systemic mycoses. Nystatin is still the antibiotic of choice in oral candidiasis. Intravenous amphotericin B is used for septicemia and deep visceral infections caused by Candida, *Cryptococcus neoformans*, Aspergillus, and other opportunistic fungi. New oral and parenteral preparations of amphotericin B are available, and the dosage of this potentially toxic drug can be reduced by using it in combination with other antifungal agents.†

Among chemically synthesized drugs, flucytosine (Ancobon), an antimetabolite, appears to be active against visceral mycoses caused by Candida, Cryptococcus and Aspergillus. Its synergy with amphotericin B has led

to use of the two drugs in combination for these severe infections. New derivatives of imidazole (econazole, miconazole, clotrimazole) are presently being studied, as are combinations of chemotherapy and immunotherapy.

ADMINISTRATION OF ANTIFUNGAL AGENTS

Nystatin. The usual dose is 1 to 1.5 million units per day in infants, 3 to 6 million units per day in older children, administered as the oral suspension or as crushed tablets. These doses may be doubled or tripled without risk for long periods of time. Nystatin is the best tolerated of the orally administered polyenes, but even in high doses diffusion into the bloodstream is slight or nonexistent.

Amphotericin B. The oral dose is 100 mg./kg/day. Absorption is low and variable. The parenteral form produces the most rapid and reliable results. Gradually increasing dosages, beginning at 0.1 mg./kg./day in 250 ml. of 5 per cent dextrose in water and ending at 1.0 mg./kg. every other day, provide serum concentrations between 1 and 3 μg./ml. The minimum inhibitory concentration in vitro is below 1 μg./ml. Premedication an hour before the injection with an antihistamine and aspirin, and use of 25 mg. of hydrocortisone in the perfusion solution, reduces the severity of side effects, which are fever with shaking chills, headache, nausea, vomiting, and muscle and joint pains. Renal toxicity characterized by azotemia appears later, usually only after the dose exceeds 1 mg./ml. on alternate days. Hypokalemia must be prevented by administration of a potassium preparation. The injection is given over a 6 to 8 hour period, and the infusate should be protected from light during its administration.

Flucytosine (Ancobon). An antimetabolite, flucytosine is not toxic to human cells and has a marked selective antifungal activity against *Candida albicans* and *Cryptococcus neoformans*. Some strains exhibit primary resistance, so that an in vitro test for sensitivity is required prior to treatment, and secondary resistance may arise, so that the drug is started at high doses. Capsules are given at a dosage of 100 to 200 mg./kg./day divided into four doses. Nausea and vomiting may be reduced or avoided if the capsules are given a few at a time over a 15-minute period. The capsules may be crushed for administration to infants and young children. Injectable flucytosine is supplied as 1 per cent solution in 0.9 per cent sodium chloride and is administered in the same dosage as the oral form by giving three or four injections per day. The high salt content of this solution requires precautions in children with cardiac or renal insufficiency.

---

*Manufacturer's note: Sulfisoxazole is contraindicated in infants under 2 months of age.

†The oral form of amphotericin B is not mentioned in the manufacturer's official directive.

Specific dosages of flucytosine are as follows:

Candidiasis: gastrointestinal or urinary tract, 100 mg./kg./day for 15 to 21 days; bronchopulmonary, 100 mg./kg./day for 30 days or more; septicemia, 100 to 150 mg./kg./day for 20 to 30 days; endocarditis, 200 mg./kg./day for up to two months.

Cryptococcosis: meningeal, 200 mg./kg./day for two to four months; systemic or localized, 100 to 150 mg./kg./day for 60 to 90 days.

Aspergillosis: 150 to 200 mg./kg./day for two months or more.

This agent must be used with caution in patients with bone marrow depression caused by disease or drugs.

Imidazole Derivatives. Clotrimazole has been used orally in infants at doses from 60 to 100 mg./kg./day and produces inhibitory serum levels, but enzymatic degradation occurs within a few weeks. Nausea, vomiting, and diarrhea occur soon after therapy is started in 30 per cent of patients, and depression, disorientation and hallucinations are reported later. For these reasons its use is not recommended.

Preliminary results with oral econazole and miconazole in children with gastrointestinal, urinary tract, and chronic mucocutaneous candidiasis and bronchopulmonary aspergillosis are favorable and show better tolerance than in adults. Oral administration of 50 to 100 mg./kg./day in four doses gives effective blood levels.

CANDIDIASIS (MONILIASIS)

Gastrointestinal Candidiasis. Gastrointestinal candidiasis due to progressive spread of Candida from the oral mucosa is no longer a serious problem: it responds rapidly to oral nystatin in a daily dose of 1 to 1.5 million units in infants, 3 to 6 million units in children. These doses may be double or tripled without any risk for long periods of time. Despite a bitter taste, the oral suspension or crushed tablets are indicated. Nystatin works on contact with the fungus, and the entire digestive tract must be coated in order to obtain the best results.

Amphotericin B, 100 mg./kg./day orally for 5 to 10 days, also cures gastrointestinal candidiasis, including forms that are resistant to nystatin, and the oral agent also has some effect on mucocutaneous candidiasis.

In addition to the classic form of thrush with whitish granular lesions, there is a dry, red, painful erythematous lesion that precedes the whitish deposit. Candidiasis may be detected in the laboratory at this stage by the abundant presence of organisms on direct examination. Esophageal involvement is diagnosed clinically by dysphagia and radiographically by irregular folds of the mucous membrane with a sinuous outline and a heterogeneous areolar appearance. Colitis in the newborn is marked by diarrhea with severe dehydration that may be fatal unless treatment is rapidly instituted. In children the diarrhea and severe vomiting resemble the symptoms of pyloric stenosis. Invasion of the mucous membrane, the submucosa and the muscle layers of the intestinal wall by Candida organisms may lead to perforation. Anal involvement is usually accompanied by gluteal erythema and diaper rash, requiring the addition of topical therapy with nystatin, amphotericin B, 1 per cent crystal violet or imidazole derivatives.

Bronchopulmonary Candidiasis. A respiratory form of candidiasis is seen in newborn and particularly in premature infants whose mothers had vaginitis. Prophylactic treatment of all prematures bearing more than 50 fungal colonies by oral or rectal swab has reduced the incidence of the clinical disease. When it occurs it can be severe, requiring intravenous amphotericin B (0.1 to 0.2 mg./kg./day) or oral flucytosine (150 mg./kg./day in four doses). Bronchial thrush, characterized by localized patches on the trachea and bronchi, responds well to aerosol spray of nystatin, amphotericin B or oral flucytosine.

Candida Septicemia. Delay in instituting treatment for gastrointestinal candidiasis can allow the organisms to spread to other organs. For candida septicemia arising in this manner, give nystatin or oral amphotericin B. If fever is not reduced in 48 hours, use intravenous amphotericin B in a dose that increases from 0.2 mg./kg./day to 0.5 mg./kg./day by 0.1 mg./kg. each day, or use oral flucytosine, 100 mg./kg./day in four doses. Treatment must continue for at least a week after interruption of the fever and the finding of negative blood cultures.

Septicemia of other than gastrointestinal origin, not accompanied by thrush or other gastrointestinal lesions, is marked by fever that is refractory to antibacterial antibiotic therapy. Usually the fungus enters through an indwelling catheter. Removal of the catheter should result in clearing of the infection within 48 hours. If fever persists, give intravenous amphotericin B in progressively increasing doses or oral flucytosine as outlined in the preceding paragraph, and continue therapy for at least a week after signs of the infection disappear.

Candida Endocarditis. In the past only surgical excision of the mycotic growths allowed survival of patients with this serious fungal infection. Combining intravenous amphotericin B, starting at 0.2 mg./kg./day and progressing to 1.0 mg./kg. on alternate days, with oral flucytosine, 200 mg./kg./day in four doses, has brought about medical cure of candida endocarditis. The treatment must be continued for several weeks or even months after cultures become negative.

Other Acute Candidal Infections. URINARY TRACT. Oral amphotericin B will pass into the urine, and a dose of 200 mg./kg./day is effective against minor forms of urinary tract candidiasis. Severe forms require oral flucytosine, 100 to 200 mg./kg./day in four doses.

Peritoneal or Pleural Candidiasis. Oral flucytosine is the agent of choice. Resistant infections will respond to intraperitoneal or intrapleural amphotericin B,* 5 to 10 mg. in 10 ml. of distilled water, or 10 to 20 ml. of a 1 per cent solution of flucytosine.

Meningeal Candidiasis. Oral flucytosine is again the agent of choice, in a dosage of 150 to 200 mg./kg./day. Alternatively, amphotericin B may be given intrathecally (see below under Cryptococcosis for dosage and methods of administration).

Chronic Mucocutaneous Granulomatous Candidiasis (Monilial Granuloma). Progressively higher doses of amphotericin B up to 1 mg./kg. every other day and then continuing at that dosage for two months has given good but often temporary results in this chronic form of candidiasis, which probably has an associated immunologic defect. High doses of flucytosine, 200 mg./kg./day, also give good results, but after two months resistant organisms appear and relapses are subsequently seen. In order to avoid development of strains resistant to flucytosine as well as the toxicity associated with high doses of amphotericin B, a combination of these agents is recommended, with the continuing dose of amphotericin B limited to 0.5 mg./kg. every other day. In a preliminary study, econazole, 100 mg./kg./day in four doses, appears to give good results.

CRYPTOCOCCOSIS (TORULOSIS)

Cryptococcus neoformans infects only patients with diseases of the reticuloendothelial system or leukemia being treated with corticosteroids and immunosuppressive therapy. Its manifestations are meningitis, meningoencephalitis, pulmonary disorders often associated with cough, low-grade fever, and radiological modifications (pseudocysts,

pneumonic infiltration, miliary lesions), cutaneous lesions (acneiform papules and ulcerations of the face and extremities), and bone and joint abscesses. Intravenous and intrathecal amphotericin B cures about 80 per cent of cases of disseminated cryptococcosis. The initial intravenous dosage is 0.2 mg./kg./day, which is increased by 0.1 mg./kg. each day until 1.0 mg./kg. every other day is being given. Treatment is continued for two months, although sterilization of cryptococcal foci is accomplished in 10 to 14 days. For meningitis, give 10 to 15 intrathecal injections of amphotericin B* on alternate days or twice a week, depending on the state of the patient and acceptance of medication. Adult intrathecal therapy is initiated with a dose of 0.1 mg. and is increased to a dose of 0.5 mg; a total dose of 2 mg. is necessary. Three to 5 ml. of cerebrospinal fluid is withdrawn, and the antibiotic is dissolved in it prior to slow introduction of this solution into the intrathecal space.

Oral flucytosine, 200 mg./kg./day in four doses, diffuses rapidly into the central nervous system, but resistance is observed in many cases, even more frequently if lower doses are used initially. Combined therapy with intravenous amphotericin B is now recommended to abort development of fungi resistant to flucytosine and to avoid toxic effects associated with high doses of amphotericin B. The schedule calls for high doses of oral flucytosine (200 mg./kg./day) plus progressively increasing intravenous doses of amphotericin B. Intrathecal amphotoericin B is not necessary. Treatment is maintained for at least a month after sterilization of cryptococcal foci and disappearance of the clinical manifestations.

ASPERGILLOSIS

Aspergillus molds grow in the respiratory tract of patients under treatment with corticosteroids or immunosuppressive agents; the organisms may also grow on previously existing bronchial lesions or pulmonary cavities, though this is rare in children. Allergic aspergillary bronchitis is marked by brown mucus plugs in the expectorate, transient pulmonary infiltrates seen on chest x-ray, eosinophilia and low-grade fever. Treatment consists of amphotericin B, 5 mg. every 6 hours as an aerosal spray, or oral flucytosine, 150 mg./kg./day.†

The intraperitoneal, intrapleural, or intrathecal use of amphotericin B is not mentioned in the manufacturer's official directive.

*In seriously ill patients suffering from funal meningitis or infection of the central nervous system, the intrathecal administration of amphotericin B is indicated, with a view to rapidly controlling the infection.

†Amphotericin B is not available commercially as an aerosol spray.

Localized bronchopulmonary aspergillosis, known as "aspergilloma" or "fungus ball," usually appears in cavities left when tuberculosis is cleared rapidly by modern drugs, more rarely in congenital cysts. Surgical excision (lobectomy) is the treatment of choice. Medical therapy can be tried (see below).

Invasive bronchopulmonary aspergillosis results from a massive inhalation of spores, which are very widespread in earth, hay and seeds. It may require the presence of an immune deficiency, for it is seen most commonly in boys with familial granulomatous disease and in children undergoing corticosteroid or immunosuppressive therapy. Management of both forms of bronchopulmonary aspergillosis is with intravenous amphotericin B in progressively larger doses up to 1 mg./kg. every other day, or high-dose oral flucytosine, 150 to 200 mg./kg./day, or the combination of moderate doses of amphotericin B (up to 0.5 mg./kg. on alternate days) with flucytosine. The combined therapy is recommended to avoid toxicity and development of resistant strains.

Aspergillary endocarditis or meningitis, or renal, peritoneal or hepatic aspergillosis, is treated similarly with amphotericin and flucytosine.

PHYCOMYCOSES

Two types of mycoses caused by Phycomycetes species are to be distinguished. Mucormycoses are produced by invasion of cosmopolitan filamentous fungi of the Mucor, Rhizopus and Absidia genera, and they involve the lungs, meninges and other deep organs. Like other fungus infections these are principally seen in children with severe diabetes or other prolonged metabolic disturbances, or those undergoing long-term corticosteroid therapy. Intravenous amphotericin B must be administered urgently, but surgical excision of the foci of infection is usually necessary. Subcutaneous phycomycoses are caused by Basidiobolus and Entomophthora species and are tropical diseases. They respond irregularly to intravenous amphotericin B, corticosteroids and iodide; flucytosine is ineffective.

OTHER SYSTEMIC MYCOSES

Less common species of fungi that can produce deep-seated mycoses include Alternaria, Cephalosporium, Fusarium, Cladosporium, Phialophora, Cercospora, Geotrichum, Helminthosporium, and Paecilomyces. Their sensitivity to antifungal agents must be tested in vitro. Generally amphotericin B is effective; whereas flucytosine is active only against Cladosporium and Phialophora.

Histoplasmosis

WALTER T. HUGHES, M.D.

The management of histoplasmosis is limited to some extent by the toxicity of the single drug available for treatment. Currently, only progressive or life-threatening forms are treated. When a safe, promptly effective and easily administered drug becomes available, less extensive forms of the disease may benefit from treatment. The following classification generally serves as a guide for the treatment of histoplasmosis with amphotericin B.

Asymptomatic infection is recognized in endemic areas by conversion from nonreactive to a reactive histoplasmin skin test. Subsequent mineralization may be demonstrated in hilar lymph nodes or lung parenchyma by a chest roentgenogram. The patient may have had minor, nonspecific respiratory symptoms. This form of the infection is self-limited and requires no treatment. Fortunately, the majority of cases are in this category.

Acute pulmonary histoplasmosis is manifest as signs and symptoms of acute pneumonitis with one or more pulmonary infiltrates detected by chest roentgenogram. The infection usually subsides within 2 to 8 weeks without treatment. Except in the rare case with overwhelming pneumonitis seriously impairing pulmonary function, acute pulmonary histoplasmosis does not require treatment with amphotericin B. All patients with acute pulmonary histoplasmosis, especially those less than 4 years of age, should be observed closely for signs of extrapulmonary dissemination.

Disseminated histoplasmosis involves deep organs including the liver, spleen, intestine, lungs, lymph nodes, bone marrow, adrenal gland, central nervous system, bone and kidneys. Untreated, as high as 80 per cent of cases end fatally. Therefore, all patients with disseminated histoplasmosis must be treated with amphotericin B.

Chronic pulmonary histoplasmosis occurs infrequently in children. This is a chronic cavitating granulomatous process with fibrosis and loss of lung volume. This infection is usually progressive and requires treatment with amphotericin B.

Histoplasmosis in immunodeficient states. In patients with active histoplasmosis receiving immunosuppressive therapy for malignancy, organ transplants or other chronic diseases, and in children with congenital immune deficiency disorders, progressive infection and dissemination are likely to occur. These patients should be treated with amphotericin B.

Histoplasmosis involving the heart and great

vessels. In addition to endocarditis associated with disseminated histoplasmosis, both acute and chronic stages of pulmonary histoplasmosis may be associated with symptomatic involvement of the heart and great vessels. Pericarditis with effusion, recurrent atrial flutter associated with contiguous involvement of the mediastinum, obstruction of the superior vena cava due to a fibrocaseous mass and chronic fibrous mediastinitis have been reported. When these are active with viable organisms, treatment with amphotericin B is required.

Amphotericin B therapy. (see page 646). The average course of therapy is one month. With extensive infection responding slowly to treatment, courses as long as two to three months may be required. A few cases of disseminated histoplasmosis have been cured with less than one month of amphotericin B therapy; however, sufficient data are not available at this time to justify a recommendation for less than a month of treatment.

In children, a complete blood count, blood urea nitrogen, creatinine, sodium and potassium levels should be measured every three days. All patients should receive a potassium-rich diet and if necessary oral potassium supplements to provide a total potassium intake of 3 mEq./kg./day. Fresh fruits, fruit juices, sweet milk, carrots, beets, asparagus, lima beans, potatoes and bran cereals are potassium-rich foods.

Isolation of infected patients is not necessary since man-to-man transmission does not occur. However, isolates of *Histoplasma capsulatum* in culture may be hazardous to laboratory personnel and should be handled in a bacteriologic hood.

Other drugs. Sulfadiazine or triple sulfonamides have been used in some cases of histoplasmosis with varying degrees of success. However, controlled studies in humans have not been done. Amphotericin B is the drug of choice, and sulfonamides should be used only in patients who cannot take the preferred drug. Some experimental evidence suggests that rifampin in combination with amphotericin B may provide an enhanced therapeutic effect, but confirmatory clinical studies are yet to be done.

Coccidioidomycosis

HARRY T. WRIGHT, Jr., M.D.

Coccidioidomycosis, a noncontagious disease caused by the fungus *Coccidioides immitis,* is acquired almost exclusively in the semi-arid areas of South America, northern Mexico, and the southwestern United States. It usually occurs as a primary disease limited to the respiratory tract, but can disseminate to any organ or tissue except the gastrointestinal tract. The infection is believed to confer immunity.

Most coccidioidal infections in children have the clinical manifestations of a common cold, influenza or pneumonitis, and frequently are accompanied by allergic skin manifestations such as erythema multiforme, erythema nodosum, or a nondescript maculopapular rash. Uncomplicated primary infections in children are treated symptomatically and with bed rest until temperature and sedimentation rate are normal. Antihistamines may be useful for the allergic skin manifestations.

When the disease disseminates, the serum complement-fixing antibody titer usually rises above the dilution of 1:32. With dissemination and without treatment, the prognosis changes from almost zero mortality to a 50 per cent mortality rate in Caucasians and 85 per cent mortality rate in Negroes, but dissemination of disease in children is rare, probably occurring in less than 1 per cent of the cases.

Candidates for Specific Therapy. Disseminated disease which is characterized by multiple abscesses, sinus tract formations, sepsis and malnutrition should be treated with bed rest, supportive measures, antibiotics for intercurrent infections as well as specific antifungal therapy. Specific antifungal therapy is also indicated in the presence of a rising complement-fixing antibody titer above the dilution of 1:64, coccidioidal osteomyelitis, coccidioidal meningitis or a worsening clinical state. Patients with acquired or congenital immunodeficiency states, underlying malignant disease or diabetes are also at risk.

All patients with severe primary pulmonary infections, continuous fever for more than a month, pregnant women, and certain non-Caucasians (Filipinos, orientals, American blacks, and Mexican-Americans) should be treated with specific antifungal therapy.

Untreated infants have a high mortality rate, and a short course of amphotericin therapy is indicated (15 mg./kg. total).*

Specific treatment is indicated as prophylaxis in patients about to have surgical treatment of coccidioidal lesions such as lung abscess, lung cavity, empyema, or a coccidioma (coin lesion). Specific treatment is indicated also in patients with coccidioidomycosis com-

---

*Manufacturer's warning: Under no circumstances should a daily dose of 1.5 mg./kg. of amphotericin B be exceeded.

plicating a noninfectious disease requiring corticosteroids, antimetabolites, or irradiation therapy.

Amphotericin B Therapy. Amphotericin B is the most effective agent available for the treatment of coccidioidomycosis, but only small amounts of the antibiotic are absorbed from the gut, and parenteral therapy is essential. The intrathecal administration of amphotericin B is necessary in coccidioidal meningitis because the blood-borne drug fails to achieve fungistatic concentrations in the cerebrospinal fluid.*

INTRAVENOUS ADMINISTRATION. The intravenous administration of amphotericin B is by the following protocol.

1. The patient is hospitalized for therapy.

2. Intravenous therapy is started in a small peripheral vein using a small gauge (22 or 23) needle.

3. Two solutions are hung by the bedside and connected with a "Y" type administration set in such a way that these solutions may be alternately clamped off. The starting solution is 5 per cent dextrose in water. The desired dosage of amphotericin B is added to 500 ml., or more, of 5 per cent dextrose and water. The maximal concentration should not be greater than 10 mg./100 ml. Saline or other electrolytes must not be used in solutions containing amphotericin B.

4. After the needle is securely in place and functioning well with the 5 per cent dextrose solution, switch to the amphotericin B solution and run at a rate which is tolerated by the patient.

5. The "cut-off" technique may minimize febrile reactions and phlebitis. The amphotericin B drip is cut off and the starting solution is allowed to flush through the needle and vein for 3 to 5 minutes two or three times each hour. During this cut-off period, the amphotericin B solution is re-suspended by inverting and shaking the bottle to avoid settling and an undesirable high concentration of drug in the neck of the bottle. If a febrile reaction occurs, the amphotericin B infusion may be discontinued temporarily, and the starting fluid may be allowed to run in place of the amphotericin B. The amphotericin B is infused again, after a period of rest, and is started at a slower rate.

6. Additives to the amphotericin B suspension include heparin sodium (10 to 20 mg.), which may prevent or lessen phlebitis, and hydrocortisone succinate (25 to 50 mg.),

which will frequently minimize the fever and chills. Some clinicians favor controlling side effects by slowing the rate of the infusion rather than by adding additional medications to the amphotericin B suspension.

7. Premedication which may be helpful includes acetylsalicylic acid, acetaminophen, and/or diphenhydramine hydrochloride, given one half hour prior to infusion and repeated in 2 hours if side effects persist.

8. Electric blankets and hot water bottles may be helpful when chilling occurs.

In children, the medication is usually given over a 6 to 8 hour period. The initial daily dose should not be more than 1 mg., but the dose can be increased thereafter by daily increments of 0.2 mg./kg./day until an optimal dose of 1 mg./kg. (not to exceed 50 mg./day) has been achieved. The dose is maintained at this level in accordance with renal toleration. Administration is usually daily until the optimal dose is reached and is then given every other day.

The total dose and duration of therapy are not established, and indeed vary with the individual and from infection to infection. Total dosage can usually be kept under 1 gm., with small children (50 kg. or less) frequently requiring no more than 0.5 gm. total. Two means for calculating dosage are in use: (1) serologic monitoring in which coincident with effective therapy there will be a fall in the titer of complement-fixing antibody to less than 1:32 or a fourfold decrease from the highest pretreatment titer; and (2) bioassay of the antifungal activity of the serum 1 to 2 hours after completion of an infusion. The dose is adjusted to achieve a concentration twice that of the minimal inhibitory concentration with the *Coccidioides immitis* strain causing disease. Attempts to correlate drug dosage with blood levels have not found great practical application, and the total dose concept, while admittedly arbitrary, still works best from a clinical point of view. The largest dosage of drug will be required in patients with severely disseminated disease, and the smallest in those with primary pulmonary infections in which the danger of dissemination is considered to be significant. Since the danger of permanent renal damage increases with dose, the maximum total dose (adults) is 4 gm.

A decision to terminate intravenous therapy is usually based on initial indication for treatment, accumulated dosage of amphotericin B, degree of renal toxicity, rate of clinical improvement, and stabilization or decline of the complement-fixing antibody titer.

INTRATHECAL THERAPY. Survival has

---

*The intrathecal use of amphotericin B is not mentioned in the manufacturer's instructions.

been significantly enhanced in cases of coccidioidal meningitis by the direct instillation of amphotericin B into the cerebrospinal fluid (CSF). Mortality will approach 100 per cent within a year's time without treatment. Three routes for access to the CSF have been utilized:

Cisterna magna. This is the most effective route of administration since it permits maximum concentration of amphotericin B at the base of the brain where meningeal infection is most severe. Arachnoiditis is not usually a problem with this approach and the procedure is apparently safe except for auditory toxicity.

Lumbar. Treatment may be started at this site to "condition" the patient for tolerance of cisternal therapy later. Prolonged administration by this route will usually produce an adhesive arachnoiditis due to the sluggish circulation of cerebrsopinal fluid. This problem may result in a complete or partial transverse myelopathy. The Froin syndrome, saddle area pain, and bladder disturbances frequently precede this complication.

Ventricular. Injection into a lateral ventricle through an Ommaya reservoir is frequently preferred because it is easier and somewhat better tolerated. Injection of amphotericin B then is easily carried out in the ambulatory or homecare patient. Medication administered by this route is better distributed along the entire CFS circulation provided there is no interfering block between the ventricles and subarachnoid space. Complications include secondary infection, placement errors, therapeutic failures when the valve is in the uninfected lateral ventricle, and adhesion of cerebral tissue to the device.

Freshly made dilutions of drug in sterile distilled water, without preservative, in a concentration of 0.25 mg. amphotericin B per ml. are used for all intrathecal administration. The starting dose is 0.2 ml. of the above dilution or 0.05 mg. This dosage is increased slowly to 1 ml. (0.25 mg.) of drug.

Premedication is essential to minimize the associated problem of headache. Codeine should be given one half hour before the procedure and repeated in two hours if the headache persists. If nausea becomes severe antiemetics such as dimenhydrinate are given intramuscularly. A corticosteroid for antiinflammatory effect is also recommended.

Medication is injected into the CSF every other day or three times per week during the acute phase of disease, decreasing gradually in frequency as the CSF cell count decreases and the patient improves. It is desirable to continue occasional injections indefinitely in view of the high rate of relapse in coccidioidal meningitis.

Most clincans will continue therapy for months, years, or even a lifetime, but with gradually decreasing frequency, depending on the clinical situation and the CSF findings.

The duration of therapy is guided by the determinations of CSF cell count, protein and complement-fixing antibody titer. The antibody titer is the most sensitive indicator of suppression. Several months of continued intensive intrathecal therapy are usually necessary to reach the stage of suppression. By that time usually the patient has been discharged to outpatient care, which will consist of a continued regimen of cisternal or ventricular injections given once or twice weekly. The patient is treated with the expectation that the meningeal infection will be suppressed, until sufficient immunity develops to arrest the disease.

If serological reversion continues during the period of outpatient care, intensive therapy may be stopped in two to three months. It is not certain that final cure is possible, and careful follow-up is necessary once treatment has been discontinued. This requires monthly examination of CSF since abnormal CSF changes can be detected before clinical symptoms appear.

LOCAL THERAPY. In coccidioidal osteomyelitis it has been recommended that drug be dissolved into a 10 per cent solution which may be infused into the surgically exposed bone or joint by simple drip and suction for a period of 8 to 12 days.* Draining sinuses can be similarly treated. Skin lesions respond well to wet dressings or 5 per cent amphotericin ointment.

Toxicity of Amphotericin B. Systemic reactions from amphotericin B are essentially dose related. Local irritation to veins is best minimized by adjusting the concentration of amphotericin B to less than 0.1 mg./ml. and the pH to a range of 5.0 to 7.4.

Anemia, and sometimes thrombocytopenia, occur in up to 75 per cent of patients. This is the result of a direct suppression of erythropoiesis and platelet formation through the direct interaction between erythrocytes, platelets, and amphotericin B. Although transfusion may be of temporary benefit, iron therapy is of no value and withholding amphotericin B usually corrects the anemia.

Nephrotoxicity is extensive, involving both tubular and glomerular damage with azotemia and hypokalemia being invariable accompani-

---

*This use of amphotericin B is not mentioned in the manufacturer's instructions.

ments of its use. Creatinine clearance is a better monitor of renal damage than the usual urea nitrogen level. If renal function is normal at the initiation of therapy and the total dose does not exceed 4 gm. (in an adult), fewer than one-half of the patients will have permanent renal damage. The prominent injury is tubular, and clinically significant hypokalemia necessitating potassium supplementation, detectable hyposthenuria, and a diminished capacity to excrete acid are manifestations of such tubular injury. The histologic study of kidneys severely compromised or rendered nonfunctional by amphotericin B reveals necrosis and calcification of the convoluted tubules. The extent and severity of renal injury must be assessed by renal function studies and hematological tests performed before, twice weekly during, and at least monthly for three months after treatment.

Surgery. Surgical excision or drainage of local coccidioidal lesions should be carried out to obtain healing and to eliminate potential sources for dissemination. Excisional surgery is occcasionally required in children with persistent pulmonary cavitation following recovery from the primary pneumonitis. There is a fairly high incidence of rupture of, or significant hemorrhage from, cavities, and surgical excision (usually with amphotericin B coverage) is recommended when cavities have persisted for more than a year and are more than 2 cm. in diameter. Other criteria for removing cavities include enlargement under serial observation, persistent hemoptysis, secondary infection, or extension to involve the visceral pleura.

Extrapulmonary lesions, sometimes requiring surgery, include cutaneous, osseous and articular coccidioidomycosis.

Alternative Therapy. Because of the limitations of amphotericin B, alternative modes of therapy have been sought.

Miconazole is a synthetic imidazole drug shown to be effective in murine coccidioidomycosis. This drug has been used experimentally in treating teenagers and adults but no reports of its use in children have come to the author's attention. Up to 3.6 gm./day of miconazole were given for up to 3 months. The results of these studies indicate that some patients with chronic coccidioidomycosis, who had failed to respond to amphotericin B therapy, responded to intravenous miconazole therapy. Other patients were not benefited by miconazole therapy. Side effects were generally uncommon, minor and transient except for phlebitis; however, reversible thrombocytosis and anemia due to miconazole therapy have been reported.

Immunotherapy with transfer factor in disseminated coccidioidal osteomyelitis and arthritis has been reported resulting in, or coincidental with, clinical improvement. In patients who have a demonstrated immune defect, and in whom transfer factor has been administered, it would appear that about one-third show improvement, one-third show no change, and about one-third continue to deteriorate.*

Prevention. Vaccines of killed whole cells of *Coccidioides immitis* have been injected intramuscularly in human subjects to determine the safety and tolerable dose of vaccine and immunological responses. The vaccines irregularly induced antibody or delayed hypersensitivity to coccidioidin antigen. It would appear that vaccines resulting in more consistent immunologic stimulation are needed to be effective; however, it is possible that the spherule vaccine may be protective despite absence of detectable antibody or sensitivity to coccidioidin. Further investigations are essential.

Visceral Larva Migrans

THOMAS A. VARGO, M.D.

Visceral larva migrans is a disease found in young children who have eaten dirt contaminated by the ova of the common dog round worm, *Toxocara canis,* or less frequently, the ova of the cat ascarid, *T. cati.* In the intestinal tract the ova hatch into larvae. The larvae do not mature in humans, but are still able to migrate to most organs and tissues for periods of months or years. Visceral larva migrans is frequently a clinically benign disease with its main manifestation being a pronounced and persistent eosinophilia. However, if the larvae invade the lungs, brain, or heart, they may cause serious illness including pneumonitis, seizures, myocarditis and even death.

With rare exceptions, the only way that humans become infested with *Toxocara* is by eating soil containing the ova. Thus, the first step in the treatment of visceral larva migrans is to stop children from eating dirt. The author has treated one young girl with visceral larva migrans who had improvement following thiabendazole therapy (see below), but she expired when she had a relapse that was due to eating dirt.

All dogs periodically should be checked for worms and dewormed with piperazine or whatever medication the veterinarian feels is appropriate. This is especially important in pregnant and nursing dogs, as larvae that were

---

*The use of transfer factor in the United States is investigational.

previously dormant in the bitches become mobile during pregnancy.

Animal excreta should be removed from the yard. If *Toxocara* are present, the soil should be tilled and promptly turned over as the ova remain infective for months to years. No specific medical therapy appears necessary in mild cases of visceral larva migrans.

In those patients who are minimally to moderately ill, e.g., those with fever and mild to moderate respiratory symptoms, there are no definite recommendations for therapy. In such cases, the author prefers to treat with thiabendazole, 25 to 50 mg./kg./day for seven days, and to repeat the course of therapy one month later. Before using thiabendazole it is recommended that the package insert and/or other literature be consulted as this drug has not been officially approved for use in the treatment of visceral larva migrans. Diethylcarbamazine, 10 to 15 mg./kg./day, has been used instead of thiabendazole, but it also has not been approved for treatment of visceral larva migrans.

Corticosteroids (prednisone, 2 mg./kg./day) for 7 to 10 days are given to patients with severe forms of visceral larva migrans such as those seriously ill with cardiac, pulmonary, or central nervous system involvement. The author has seen a child seriously ill with myocarditis due to visceral larva migrans who had rapid and complete improvement following corticosteroid therapy.

All children with visceral larva migrans should be evaluated by an ophthalmologist. Toxocaral involvement of the eye may present as endophthalmitis or a solitary retinal granuloma, and has been confused with retinoblastoma. These changes have occurred months or years after the initial infestation.

The long-term sequelae in children who have had cardiac or CNS involvement are not known. If feasible, children with myocarditis or seizures are examined by a cardiologist or neurologist for recommendations and long-term follow-up. Heart failure or convulsions are treated as mentioned in other sections of this book.

It is emphasized that available medical therapy may be inadequate and that prevention of this disease is possible. The incidence of visceral larva migrans and its potentially serious, even lethal, complications can be minimized by educating physicians, public health officials, parents, and lay people about the hazards confronting the child who eats dirt. Public health measures should be directed at the elimination of sources of contaminated soil, periodic deworming of pet animals, and proper disposal of animal excreta.

Parasitic Infections

JERROLD A. TURNER, M.D., *and* JAMES SEIDEL, M.D.

The most important factors which must be considered in the treatment of parasitic infections are (1) the accuracy of the diagnosis, (2) the potential toxicity of the drugs employed, and (3) follow-up examinations to ensure cure or, in some cases, adequate reduction in parasite load.

Accurate diagnosis is essential to the selection of appropriate chemotherapeutic agents. The laboratory must have personnel experienced in the identification of these organisms, for diagnosis is frequently dependent upon the demonstration and recognition of the parasite or ova. In order to recover organisms, it may be necessary to collect several specimens. In some situations, specialized laboratory examinations may be necessary.

Many of the drugs used in the treatment of parasitic diseases may have serious side effects. A thorough knowledge of the drug is important in order to weigh its toxicity against the effects of the parasitic disease. If the physician is unfamiliar with the parasitic disease or the drugs used in treatment, consultation may be helpful. The parasitic Disease Drug Service of the National Center for Disease Control* provides valuable information and will supply certain drugs, which are otherwise unobtainable, for specific infections.

The following discussion of treatment has three major sections. The first section deals in some detail with the most common parasitic infections encountered within the United States. Drug regimens listed first under each organism are considered the treatment programs of choice. Treatment of less common parasitic diseases is outlined in the second section in tabular form. The third section is an alphabetical listing of the recommended drugs which includes the preparations, toxicity, contraindications and precautions. All drug doses noted in the text are oral unless otherwise specified.

COMMON INTESTINAL AND GENITOURINARY PARASITIC INFECTIONS

Multiple infections with several species of intestinal parasites are frequent. When several different drugs are required to treat the different species of pathogenic parasites, there is

---

*Parasitic Disease Drug Service, Bureau of Epidemiology, Center for Disease Control, Atlanta, Ga. 30333. Telephone (404) 633-3311, ext. 3677 or 3496 during working hours and (404) 633-2176 at other times.

often confusion as to the order in which treatment should be administered. If the patient is symptomatic and it is possible to determine which organism is responsible for the symptoms, it is logical to treat for that infection first. For example, a patient may have hookworm infection, giardiasis and amebiasis. A history of bloody diarrhea and the demonstration of colonic ulcers would indicate therapy for the amebiasis first. If the patient is treated with metronidazole for his amebiasis, the giardiasis may also respond. Finally, treatment would be directed to the hookworm infection.

If the patient is without symptoms, the sequence of treatment is usually not very important. It is generally wise to avoid overlapping or concomitant drug regimens because of problems in sorting out untoward side effects, should they occur. Usually the shorter courses of 2 or 3 days' duration may be given first and the longer courses of medication later. For example, a patient with asymptomatic ascariasis and amebiasis would receive a short course of either pyrantel, piperazine or mebendazole for the ascariasis followed by a three week course of diiodohydroxyquin for the amebiasis. Ascariasis in combination with other asymptomatic infections usually should be treated first to avoid any potential problem with migration of the ascarids which may be provoked by drugs used for other infections. The development of mebendazole has simplified the treatment of multiple infections with intestinal nematodes because of its broad spectrum. It has been found effective in ascariasis, hookworm infection, trichuriasis and enterobiasis.

Entamoeba histolytica Infection (Amebiasis).   The diagnosis of intestinal amebiasis should be based on the demonstration of characteristic morphologic features of the organism in permanent-stained preparations of feces, or in scrapings or biopsy material obtained at proctosigmoidoscopy. Repeated courses of amebicidal drugs for symptoms of colitis are justifiable only if the organism can be demonstrated. Serologic testing is of greatest value in the diagnosis of hepatic amebiasis by differentiating pyogenic abscess from amebic abscess. It is of less value in intestinal infection because of false negatives and persisting antibody related to previous infection. It cannot be used to follow the results of therapy.

INTESTINAL AMEBIASIS. *Asymptomatic* ("cyst passer," "carrier"). Diiodohydroxyquin, 30 to 40 mg./kg. divided into three doses daily for 21 days (maximum single dose 650 mg.). A 2 week course of chloroquine may be administered concomitantly to eliminate the possibility of later development of an hepatic abscess. If follow-up is adequate, the addition of chloroquine and its potential toxicity may be avoided.

Amebic colitis.   Metronidazole, 35 to 50 mg./kg. daily divided in three doses for 10 days, *or* a combination of tetracycline, diiodohydroxyquin and chloroquine given as follows: tetracycline hydrochloride, 10 to 20 mg./kg. divided into four doses daily for 5 to 7 days (maximum single dose 250 mg.); diiodohydroxyquin, as in "asymptomatic" above; and chloroquine, 10 mg. of base/kg. (maximum 600 mg. of base) divided into four doses daily for 2 days, then 5 mg. of base/kg. (maximum 300 mg. of base) divided into two doses daily for 12 days. Tetracycline is not recommended for children under 14 years of age.

Follow-up.   Both kinds of patients should have a series of three fecal examinations 1 month following completion of treatment, or earlier if symptoms persist.

HEPATIC AMEBIASIS (hepatic abscess). Needle aspiration of an abscess is indicated if there is a palpable mass or persistent localized tenderness over the liver or in the intercostal spaces, or if there is a massive abscess with marked elevation of the right hemidiaphragm. Aspiration should also be considered if signs and symptoms fail to respond to chemotherapy.

Chemotherapy.   Metronidazole as for colitis *or* a combination of emetine hydrochloride, 1 mg./kg. daily intramuscularly for 10 days (maximum 65 mg. daily) (alternate: dehydroemetine,* 1 to 1.5 mg./kg. intramuscularly daily for 10 days; maximum *total* dose 1.0 gm.) *and* chloroquine, 10 mg. of base/kg. (maximum 600 mg. of base) divided into four doses daily for 2 days, then 5 mg. of base/kg. (maximum 300 mg. of base) divided into two doses daily for 28 days.

Follow-up.   There should be continued clinical improvement. Retreatment or a change in drug regimens would be indicated if there were a recurrence of symptoms. Abnormalities on hepatic scans may persist for as long as a year after successful therapy.

Giardia lamblia Infection (Giardiasis). *G. lamblia* may be difficult to find in fecal specimens even on repeated examinations. Many consultants recommend examination of duodenal contents by duodenal intubation, duodenal capsule (Enterotest) or biopsy with impression smears.

G. lamblia infections should always be treated even if asymptomatic because of the potential pathogenicity of the organism.

---

*Use of dehydroemetime is still investigational in the United States, but the drug may be obtained from the Parasitic Disease Drug Service.

Chemotherapy. Quinacrine, 7 mg./kg. divided into three daily doses taken with meals (maximum dosage 100 mg.) for 7 days, *or* furazolidone* 5 mg./kg. in four divided daily doses for 5 days, *or* metronidazole, 10 to 15 mg./kg. in three divided doses daily (maximum dosage 250 mg.) for 7 days. (Note: when used for giardiasis, metronidazole is considered investigational).

Follow-up. The patient should have at least three fecal examinations 1 month after completion of therapy or earlier if symptoms persist. In selected cases, it may be necessary to use one of the duodenal sampling techniques (see above) to be completely sure of eradication of the parasite.

Trichomonas vaginalis Infection (Trichomoniasis). Trichomoniasis is most frequently sexually transmitted. Reinfection by sexual partners has often been mistakenly interpreted as a persistent infection which is refractory to treatment. Infection may also be transmitted to the infant from the mother during delivery and may be acquired by contact with contaminated fomites such as towels.

Chemotherapy. Metronidazole, 250 mg. three times a day for 10 days for adults. Because of reports of carcinoma developing in experimental animals, there has been controversy about the liberal use of metronidazole in this common infection. In children and young adolescents who are not sexually active, topical medication and douches to lower the vaginal pH may be preferred.

Follow-up. Clinical improvement and failure to demonstrate the parasites on wet films from the vagina. Sexual partners with proven trichomoniasis should receive simultaneous treatment with metronidazole.

Taenia saginata Infection (Taeniasis Saginata, Beef Tapeworm Infection). Specific diagnosis is dependent upon the examination of gravid proglottids from stool. Ova or *T. saginata* and *T. solium* have identical morphology.

Chemotherapy. Niclosamide† in a single dose chewed thoroughly after a light meal. Children weighing 25 to 75 lb. should receive 1 gm.; more than 75 lb., 1.5 gm. Adults should receive 2 gm. No preparation is necessary. An alternate is quinacrine, 5 mg./kg. (maximum 200 mg.) every 10 minutes for four doses with sips of sodium bicarbonate solution, followed in 1 hour by a saline purgative. The patient should be restricted to a clear liquid diet the

day prior to treatment with quinacrine, and a saline purgative should be administered the night prior to treatment.

If oral quinacrine therapy fails, the patient may be retreated, after the preparation noted above, by administering the same total dose of quinacrine in 50 to 100 ml. of water through a tube placed in the third portion of the duodenum. The tube may be left in place, and the saline purgative is administered 1 hour after the quinacrine. Quinacrine therapy should be administered only when the patient has a fully developed worm as evidenced by the continued passage of proglottids.

Follow-up. Fecal examinations for ova and proglottids should be done 1 month and 3 months after treatment if the scolex was not recovered immediately after treatment. The patient should also be instructed to observe for proglottids. Retreatment can be given if proglottids reappear.

Taenia solium Infection (Taeniasis Solium, Pork Tapeworm Infection). Eggs of *T. solium* are infectious for humans and may produce cysticercosis. Therefore, a person infected with *Taenia solium* is a public health hazard and should receive treatment early. *Chemotherapy* is niclosamide as for *T. saginata*. There is a theoretical risk of releasing eggs into the gut lumen and causing cysticercosis during niclosamide administration. There has never been a documented case of cysticercosis resulting from niclosamide therapy, but the patient should be informed of this theoretical risk. Quinacrine as for *T. saginata* is an alternative therapy. *Follow-up* as for *T. saginata*.

Diphyllobothrium latum Infection (Diphyllobothriasis, Fish Tapeworm Infection). *Chemotherapy* as for *T. saginata*. Follow-up as for *T. saginata*.

Hymenolepsis nana Infection (Hymenolepiasis Nana, Dwarf Tapeworm Infection). *H. nana* infection is probably the most prevalent tapeworm infection, particularly in the pediatric age group. As it is transmitted by the fecal-oral route, all family members and household contacts should be examined.

Chemotherapy. Niclosamide is administered as follows: for children weighing 25 to 75 lb., 1 gm. on the first day followed by 500 mg. for an additional 6 days. For children weighing more than 75 lb., 1.5 gm. followed by 1 gm. daily for 6 days. For adults, 2 gm. daily for 7 days. An alternative is quinacrine as for *T. saginata*. Repeated courses may be necessary.

Follow-up. Fecal examinations at 2 weeks and 3 months following therapy.

Ascaris lumbricoides Infection (Ascariasis, Roundworm Infection)1 Ascariasis should always be treated because of potentially

---

*Manufacturer's precaution: Furazolidone should not be administered to infants under one month of age.

†Niclosamide is not available commercially in the United States but it may be obtained from the Center for Disease Control.

serious complications of obstruction of the small intestine or bile duct. Ascarids also may be vomited and aspirated causing fatal laryngeal obstruction. This infection cannot be transmitted directly between individuals, because eggs require a period of development in the soil.

Chemotherapy.   Mebendazole should be used when ascariasis is associated with either *Trichuris trichiuria* or hookworm infections. Experience with this drug is, as yet, limited, but it appears very effective and no significant side effects have been reported. It is given in the same dosage to all age groups (100 mg. twice a day for 3 days). Other effective drugs are pyrantel pamoate administered in a single 11 mg./kg. dose of the base (maximum of 1 gm.) *or* piperazine citrate, 75 mg./kg. with a maximum of 3.5 gm. given once daily for 2 consecutive days. Comparable doses of other piperazine salts may be given.

Treatment of complications.   Medical treatment of intestinal obstruction caused by a bolus of ascarids is usually successful if the vascular supply to the bowel has not been compromised. In addition to the usual modalities of nasogastric suction and intravenous fluids, piperazine in a dosage of 75 mg./kg. (maximum 3 gm.) is administered by nasogastric tube. The tube is flushed with a small amount of saline and then clamped for 2 hours. Then, nasogastric suction is resumed. This procedure is repeated every 8 hours. Lack of response to medical therapy, the development of multiple fluid levels and marked abdominal distention or rectal bleeding are indications for surgical intervention. At laparotomy if the circulation to the bowel is adequate, the bolus of worms may be "milked" from the small intestine into the colon without performing an enterotomy.

Follow-up.   Fecal examinations 2 to 4 weeks following treatment.

Enterobius vermicularis Infection (Enterobiasis, Pinworm Infection).   This infection is ubiquitous and highly prevalent in children. Prevalence rates of 75 per cent in school children are not unusual. Although the infection is common, symptoms of anal pruritus, restlessness and vaginal irritation are infrequent. There are several effective drugs available, but reinfection is almost unavoidable. The most beneficial component of therapy is education of the patient and the parents concerning the life cycle of the parasite, the prevalence of infection and the frequent exposure to reinfection. Misconceptions about enterobiasis may lead to wasted efforts and inappropriate feelings of guilt and inade-

quacy when vigorous adherence to extraordinary cleaning and hygiene recommendations fails to prevent reinfection.

Contrary to many textbooks and pharmaceutical company literature, there is no evidence that exceptional hygienic measures are at all effective in preventing reinfection. Therefore, there is no justification for recommending anything more than normal household and personal cleanliness. Even simultaneous treatment of all family members can only reduce exposure to reinfection in the home for a brief period. Reinfection from sources other than the home still plays a major role. Except in unusual circumstances initial treatment and retreatment should be directed only to the symptomatic individual.

It should be emphasized that there are other causes of pruritus which may occur in association with enterobiasis or may develop incidentally in someone with a previous history of pinworm infection. Symptoms persisting after treatment require confirmation of continued infection by the use of cellulose tape swabs.

Animals are not reservoirs of pinworm infection, and the misconception that household pets are responsible for transmission of pinworm infection should be dispelled.

Chemotherapy.   Mebendazole has recently been approved for use in enterobiasis. It has the advantage of a uniform dose (a 100 mg. single-dose chewable tablet) for all ages. As yet no untoward side effects have been reported. Alternatively pyrantel pamoate, 11 mg./kg. (maximum 1 gm.), may be given in a single dose, *or* pyrvinium pamoate, 5 mg./kg., may be given in a single dose. Piperazine citrate has also been used, but requires a 7 day course.

Follow-up.   If symptoms clear with treatment, no follow-up is necessary. Recurrence of symptoms after 6 weeks may indicate reinfection. If retreatment of an individual is frequently required after confirmation of reinfection by positive swabs, simultaneous treatment of all family members every 2 weeks for a total of three doses may be tried.

Ancylostoma duodenale or Necator americanus Infection (Hookworm Infection).   Hookworm anemia is associated only with relatively heavy hookworm infections and results from gastrointestinal blood loss caused by the parasites. The manifestation is also more common in individuals with marginal or deficient iron intake. The infection is not directly transmissible from one individual to another.

Chemotherapy.   Mebendazole, 100 mg. twice a day for 3 days, *or* bephenium hydroxynapthoate, 100 mg./kg. (maximum 10 gm.) divided into two doses for 1 or 2 days, *or* tetrachloroethylene, 0.12 ml./kg. (maximum 5 ml.) in a single dose.*

Follow-up. Fecal examination 2 to 4 weeks after completion of therapy. If eggs are rare in fecal concentrations, there is usually no need for retreatment.

Trichuris trichiura Infection (Whipworm Infection). *T. trichiura* is a parasite of the colon and may cause severe bloody diarrhea in heavy infections. Most infections seen in the United States are light and are asymptomatic. In light infections, intestinal symptoms are frequently the result of some other abnormality rather than caused by the whipworm. *Trichuris* eggs become infectious only after a period of development in the soil. Therefore, direct transmission of infection is impossible.

Chemotherapy. Mebendazole, 100 mg. twice a day for 3 days for all age groups.

Follow-up. Repeat examinations 2 to 4 weeks following completion of therapy.

Strongyloides stercoralis Infection (Strongyloidiasis). Strongyloidiasis always requires treatment, and follow-up should indicate a complete eradication of the parasite. *Strongyloides* has the capability of producing internal autoinfection and therefore, if untreated, may persist for the life of the host. Fatal infections have occurred in individuals whose immune mechanisms have been impaired, particularly in association with high doses of corticosteroids.

Strongyloidiasis is not always easy to diagnose, and frequently special techniques of fecal concentration (Baermann, Harada-Mori) may be necessary to recover larvae from the stool. Examination of duodenal contents by intubation or by the use of a duodenal capsule (Enterotest) may also detect elusive infections.

Chemotherapy. Thiabendazole, 50 mg./kg. divided in two doses daily for 2 days (maximun daily dose 3 gm.).

Follow-up. Repeat stool examinations or special techniques, as indicated (see above), 1 month after treatment. Eosinophilia, which is frequently present with this infection, should return to normal.

BLOOD AND TISSUE PARASITES

Plasmodium Infections (Malaria). The treatment of malaria may be divided into different categories: (1) chemosuppression (prevention of clinical malaria attacks by inhibiting the development of red cell infection); (2) treatment of the clinical attack (elimination of the red cell infection which is producing the symptoms); and (3) radical cure (prevention of relapses from infection persisting in the liver cells in *P. vivax*, *P. malariae* and *P. ovale* infections).

The treatment of malaria has been complicated by the emergence of strains of *P. falciparum* which are resistant to chloroquine and other synthetic antimalarials. This resistance has been reported from Brazil, Columbia, Venezuela, Guyana, Panama, Thailand, Cambodia, Malaya and South Viet Nam.

Chemosuppression. All species except chloroquine-resistant *P. falciparum* may be suppressed with chloroquine, 5 mg. of base/kg. given once weekly (maximum dose 300 mg. of base or 500 mg. as phosphate once weekly). Medication should be started 2 weeks prior to arrival in an endemic area and continued for 6 weeks after departure from the area. If the patient has been infected while on suppressive doses of chloroquine, clinical attacks of *P. vivax*, *P. malariae* or *P. ovale* could develop some weeks or months after stopping the chloroquine.

Treatment of clinical attack. All species except strains of chloroquine-resistant *P. falciparum* should respond to chloroquine phosphate, 10 mg. of base/kg. (maximum 600 mg. of base) followed by 5 mg. of base/kg. (maximum 300 mg. of base) in 6 hours; 5 mg. of base/kg. (maximum 300 mg. of base) 18 hours after the second dose, and then 5 mg. of base/kg. (maximum 300 mg. of base) 24 hours after the third dose. If oral chloroquine cannot be administered, chloroquine hydrochloride may be substituted in the dosage 5 mg. of base/kg. intramuscularly (maximum 250 mg. of base in a single dose and not more than 10 mg. of base/kg. or 500 mg. of base in 24 hours).

Prevention of relapses in P. vivax, P. malariae and P. ovale infection. Primaquine phosphate 0.3 mg. of base/kg. (maximum 15 mg. of base) in a single dose daily for 14 days. Treatment with primaquine is not necessary in *P. falciparum* infections or in infections acquired by transfusion or by use of contaminated hypodermic needles.

Treatment of chloroquine-resistant P. falciparum infection. Chemosuppression for these strains should be advised only under unusual circumstances of exposure. Suppression has been successful in adults under military field conditions using dapsone, 25 mg. daily,* in addition to chloroquine and primaquine.

---

*Tetrachloroethylene is available in the United States only as a veterinary preparation (Nema worm caps).

*This use of dapsone is not included in the manufacturer's indications.

P. falciparum infections acquired in areas where resistance has been reported may or may not be chloroquine-resistant. If the patient is not seriously ill and has no complications, chloroquine may be tried as described for sensitive strains. If there is no clinical response or if the level of parasitemia fails to fall within 12 hours, the patient should be treated as for chloroquine resistance. Seriously ill patients from areas of chloroquine resistance should be begun immediately on the combination of quinine sulfate, 25 mg. of the salt/kg. divided into three doses daily for 14 days (maximum 600 mg. of salt every 8 hours), plus pyrimethamine, 0.9 mg./kg. (maximum 50 mg.) divided into three doses daily for 3 days, plus sulfadiazine* 40 mg./kg. (maximum 2 gm.) divided into four doses daily.

If the patient is unable to take oral medication, quinine dihydrochloride may be administered by slow intravenous infusion, 10 mg. of the salt/kg. diluted to 0.5 mg./ml. in normal saline and administered 1 ml./minute every 8 hours (maximum 600 mg. of salt every 8 hours) until oral medication can be tolerated. Cardiac monitoring is recommended if the patient receives intravenous quinine. If there is any degree of renal impairment, frequent quinine blood levels must be determined.

Pneumocystis carinii Infection (Pneumyocystis Pneumonia). See p. 608.

Schistosoma mansoni Infection (Schistosomiasis Mansoni, Bilharziasis). *Chemotherapy.* Stibophen† intramuscularly for five days weekly as follows: for patients weighing 7 to 15 kg., give 1 ml. dosages up to 20 to 25 ml. total dose. For those weighing 15 to 30 kg., each dose is 2 ml. to a total of 40 to 50 ml. For patients 30 kg. and above, give 4 ml. doses up to 80 to 100 ml. total. Alternatively stibocaptate may be used, 10 mg./kg. once or twice weekly for a total dose of 50 mg./kg. for children. For adolescents and adults the dosage is reduced to 8 mg./kg. at the same schedule for a total dose of 40 mg./kg.‡

Follow-up. Fecal examinations and possible rectal biopsy for detection of viable ova 6 months after treatment.

Schistosoma hematobium Infection (Schistosomiasis Hematobium, Bilharziasis). *Chemotherapy.* As for *S. mansoni.* *Follow-up.* Urine concentrations for ova and

possible rectal biopsy for ova 6 months after treatment.

Schistosoma japonicum Infection (Schistosomiasis Japonicum, Bilharziasis). *Chemotherapy.* Antimony potassium tartrate intravenously on alternate days as follows: 7 to 15 kg., 2, 3, 4, 5, 6, 7 ml., continuing at 7 ml. on alternate days for a total of 10 days; 15 to 30 kg., 4, 6, 8, 10, 12, 14 ml., continuing at 14 ml. on alternate days for a total of 10 days; 30 kg. or above, 8, 12, 16, 20, 24, 28 ml., continuing at 28 ml. on alternate days for a total of 10 days. *Follow-up.* As for *S. mansoni.*

Clonorchis sinensis or *Opisthorchis sinensis* Infection (Oriental Liver Fluke Infection, Clonorchiasis). Infections seen in the United States are rarely of clinical significance. Although chloroquine will temporarily suppress egg production, it does not effect a cure. There is currently no available effective chemotherapy.

Echinococcus granulosus Infection (Hydatid Disease). The treatment is strictly surgical. Hydatid cysts usually require chemical treatment in situ during surgery to render the cyst contents noninfectious. Major hazards of surgery are the spread of hydatid tissue and acute allergic reactions in response to spilled hydatid cyst contents.

Cysticerosis (Infection with Larvae of *Taennia solium*). Cysticerci may occur in many different tissues but are usually detected clinically only if they involve the subcutaneous tissues or the central nervous system. There is no effective chemotherapeutic agent. Surgical removal of subcutaneous lesions produces an effective cosmetic result. When the central nervous system manifestations are related to hydrocephalus, this may respond to neurosurgical procedures for shunting cerebrospinal fluid into the vasculature or peritoneal cavity. Occasionally CNS cysticerci may be accessible to surgical removal.

Toxocara canis or *T. cati* Infection (Toxocariasis, Visceral Larva Migrans). See p. 648.

Ancylostoma braziliense Infection (Cutaneous Larva Migrans, Creeping Eruption). *Chemotherapy.* Thiabendazole, 50 mg./kg. (maximum 3 gm.), divided into two doses daily for two days. Topical application of the suspension has been successful in some cases. *Follow-up.* Repeat courses may sometimes be necessary, depending upon the clinical response.

ANTIPARASITIC DRUGS

Amphotericin B (Fungizone). *Preparation.* Supplied in vials of sterile lyophilized powder providing 50 mg. of amphotericin B

---

*Manufacturer's precaution: Sulfadiazine is contraindicated in infants under 2 months of age.

†Stibophen is an approved drug but is no longer manufactured in the United States. Some supplies may still be available.

‡Stibocaptate is not available commercially in the United States but it can be obtained from the Center for Disease Control.

Less Common Parasitic Infections

DISEASE	DRUG REGIMENS	FOLLOW-UP
Dientamoeba fragilis infection (dientamoeba diarrhea)	Diiodohydroxyquin, 30 to 40 mg./kg. (maximum 1.95 gm.), divided into three doses daily for 21 days. *or* Tetracycline hydrochloride, 10 to 20 mg./kg. (maximum 1 gm.), given in four divided doses for 5 to 7 days. Not recommended for children under 14.	At least 3 negative fecal examinations 1 month after treatment.
Balantidium coli infection (balantidiasis)	Diiodohydroxyquin or oxytetracycline in doses as above for tetracycline in *Dientamoeba* infections.	At least 3 negative fecal examinations 1 month after treatment.
Trypanosoma cruzi infection (American trypanosomiasis, Chagas' disease)	Children aged 15 and under. Acute infection: Nifurtimox,* 25 mg./kg. daily divided into four doses for 15 days; then 15 mg./kg. daily divided into four doses for an additional 75 days. Chronic infection: Initial 15 days as for acute infection; then 15 to 18 mg./kg. daily in four divided doses for an additional 105 days. Contraindicated in children under 1 year of age. Adults. Acute and chronic infection: Nifurtimox* begun at 5 to 7 mg./kg. daily divided into four doses gradually increasing in 2 mg./kg. increments biweekly until 15 to 17 mg./kg. is being given daily. Duration of course, 90 to 120 days.	Acute: thick blood smears and, where applicable, xenodiagnosis 1 to 2 months after treatment. Triple concentration method may also be utilized. Follow for serologic response and observe for electrocardiographic changes.
Trypanosoma gambiense infection (African trypanosomiasis, sleeping sickness)	Early infection without CNS involvement: Pentamidine,* 4 mg./kg. IM daily for 10 days (maximum 300 mg./day) *or* Suramin sodium,* 50 mg. IV as a test dose, then 10 to 15 mg./kg. (maximum 1 gm.) IV on days 1, 3, 7, 14, and 21. Not recommended for children under 6 years.	Thick blood smears and triple concentration method 1 to 2 months after treatment.
	CNS disease, Melarsoprol,† 3.6 mg./kg. given in increasing IV doses over 3 consecutive days (maximum initial dose 54 mg.) and alternate with 1 to 2 weeks' rest, for a complete course in 3 to 6 weeks.	No adequate laboratory test. Follow clinical course. Cerebrospinal fluid examination for parasites, elevated protein and cells.
Trypanosoma rhodesiense infection (African trypanosomiasis, African sleeping sickness)	Early infection:* Suramin sodium, test dose 50 mg. IV, then 10 to 15 mg./kg. (maximum 1 gm.) IV, given on days 1, 3, 7, 14 and 21. Not recommended for children under under 6 years.	Thick blood films and triple concentration method, 1 to 2 months after treatment.
	CNS disease: Melarsoprol* as in corresponding stage *T. gambiense* infection.	Cerebrospinal fluid examination as in *T. gambiense* infection.
Leishmania donovani infection (visceral leishmaniasis, kala azar)	Sodium stibogluconate,* 10 mg./kg. (maximum 600 mg.) IM for 6 to 10 days.	Clinical response. Buffy coat blood films, bone marrow aspiration for smear and culture 1 month after treatment if persistent infection is suspected.

Continued on next page

Less Common Parasitic Infections—*Continued*

DISEASE	DRUG REGIMENS	FOLLOW-UP
	Amphotericin B given on alternate days by IV infusion, 0.25 to 1.5 mg./kg./day in a 0.1 mg./ml. dilution, beginning with a low dosage and increasing as tolerated.	
	Strains acquired in the Sudan: Pentamidine,* 2 to 4 mg./kg. IM for 10 days.	
Leishmania tropica infection (cutaneous leishmaniasis, oriental sore) and *Leishmania braziliensis* infection (mucocutaneous leishmaniasis espundia)	Sodium stibogluconate,* 10 mg./ kg. day (maximum 600 mg.) IM for 6 to 10 days. *or* Pyrimethamine,† 0.5 mg./kg. daily for 2 weeks; repeat if necessary after 1 week rest. Supplemental folinic acid should be given in young children.	Smear and culture of lesion.
Naegleria and *Hartmanella* infections (primary amebic meningoencephalitis)	Amphotericin B§ may be effective tried intrathecally and intravenously in combination with high dose sulfadiazine.	Follow clinical course. CSF examination for presence of amebae on wet mounts, and improvement of CSF abnormalities.
Fasciola hepatica infection (sheep liver fluke infection, fascioliasis)	Dehydroemetine,* 1 mg./kg. daily for 10 days. *or* Bithionol,* 12.5 to 50 mg./kg. divided into two doses, given on alternate days for 10 to 15 doses.	Three fecal examinations 1 month after treatment.
Fasciolopsis buski infection (giant intestinal fluke infection)	Tetrachloroethylene** capsules given on an empty stomach 0.10 to 0.12 ml./kg. (maximum 5 ml.) in a single dose.	Three fecal examinations 1 month after treatment.
Heterophyes heterophyes infection and *Metagonimus yokogawai* infection	Tetrachloroethylene** as in *Fasciolopsis* infection.	Three fecal examinations 1 month after treatment.
Paragonimus westermani infection (lung fluke infection, paragonimiasis)	Bithionol,* 30 to 50 mg./kg. divided into two doses given on alternate days for 10 to 15 doses. Not recommended for children under 8 years of age.	Repeat fecal and sputum examinations 1 month after treatment.
Dipylidium caninum infection (dog and cat tapeworm infection, dipylidiasis)	Niclosamide* tablets chewed thoroughly with a light meal as described for *Taenia saginata* in text. *or* Quinacrine as described for *Taenia saginata* infection in text.	Repeat fecal examinatin 1 week and 1 and 3 months after treatment for eggs and proglottids.
Trichinella spiralis infection (trichinosis, trichiniasis)	The efficacy of antihelminthic treatment is questioned. Thiabendazole, 50 mg./kg. (maximum 3 gm.) divided into two doses daily. Duration of course determined by the clinical response. Corticosteroids may be necessary with symptoms of myocarditis or meningoencephalitis.	Clinical response
Trichostrongylus species infections	Thiabendazole, 50 mg./kg. (maximum 3 gm.) divided into two doses daily for two days.	Repeat stool exams 2 to 4 weeks after treatment.

Less Common Parasitic Infections—*Continued*

DISEASE	DRUG REGIMENS	FOLLOW-UP
Capillaria phillipinensis infection	Thiabendazole, 50 mg./kg. (maximum 3 gm.) divided into two doses daily for 30 days. Then 15 to 18 mg./kg. (maximum 1 gm.) daily for 6 months.	Multiple fecal examinations for several months after completion of treatment.
Angiostrongylus cantonensis infection (eosinophilic meningoencephalitis)	Trials of specific therapy are not conclusive. Thiabendazole as for *Trichinella* infections may be tried.	Clinical response.
Wuchereria bancrofti infection and *Brugia malayi* infection (filariasis)	Diethylcarbamazine, 6 mg./kg. divided into three doses daily for 21 to 30 days.	Blood smears and Knott concentration of blood for microfilariae 2 to 4 weeks after treatment. Note: If parasites have been acquired in areas other than the Pacific Islands it is necessary to obtain blood at night for examination for microfilariae.
Onchocerca volvulus infection (onchocerciasis)	Diethylcarbamazine, 12 to 25 mg. in single dose daily on days 1, 2 and 3, then 25 to 50 mg. on days 4, 5 and 6, then 50 to 100 mg. on days 7, 8 and 9, then 100 to 150 mg. for the next 12 days; suramin sodium beginning after the course of diethylcarbamazine, 50 mg. IV test dose, then 10 to 15 mg./kg. (maximum 1 gm.) IV weekly for a total of five doses. For ocular involvement concomitant treatment with topical corticosteroids.	Repeat skin snips or skin shavings for microfilariae 3 to 6 months after treatment or sooner if symptoms recur.
Loa loa infection (loaiasis)	Diethylcarbamazine as in filariasis.	Thick blood smears and Knott concentrations 2 to 4 weeks after treatment.
Dracunculus medinensis (dracontiasis, dracunculiasis, guinea worm infection)	Metronidazole, †† 90 mg./kg. (maximum 2.25 gm.) divided into three doses daily for 5 days. The worm requires manual extraction which is facilitated by the drug treatment. This drug is considered investigational for use with this infection.	Clinical response.

*Available in the United States only from the Center for Disease Control.

†This use of pyrimethamine is not listed in the manufacturer's instructions.

§Intrathecal use of amphotericin B is still considered investigational and not listed in the manufacturer's instructions.

**Tetrachloroethylene is available in the United States only as a veterinary preparation (Nema Worm Caps).

††This use of metronidazole is not mentioned in the manufacturer's indications. Also, this dosage is higher than that recommended for children.

and 41 mg. of sodium desoxycholate with 25.2 mg. of sodium phosphate as a buffer. The powder should be reconstituted by adding to the vial 10 ml. of sterile water for injection USP, *without a bacteriostatic agent,* to make a 5 mg./ml. solution. This is further diluted, one part amphotericin solution in 50 parts of 5 per cent dextrose solution to make a final concentration in the infusion solution of 0.1 mg. of amphotericin/ml. The pH of the dextrose should be above 4.2.

Administration. Therapy is usually initiated with 0.25 mg./kg./day and gradually increasing as tolerated to a maximum dose of 1.5 mg./kg./day. It is given in a slow intravenous infusion, usually over a period of 6 hours. Alternate-day therapy is reported to be better tolerated. The drug may be given intrathecally, but this must be done cautiously and the dose should not exceed 0.5 mg. thrice weekly except in unusual circumstances.* Administration into the basal cistern is sometimes easier than into the lumbar area, where arachnoiditis commonly develops.

Toxicity. Nausea, vomiting, fever and phlebitis at the site of administration are common. Some degree of impairment of renal function nearly always occurs. Other effects

---

*Intrathecal use of Fungizone is not mentioned in the manufacturer's instructions.

are anaphylaxis, hypokalemia, convulsions, hypotension, anemia and cardiac arrhythmias.

Contraindications and precautions. Renal function should be monitored. The patient may have side effects reduced by pretreatment with antinausea and antipyretic drugs. In patients who have shown hypersensitivity reactions to the drug, it should be used only in life-threatening situations. In patients with pre-existing renal disease, the possible benefits of therapy must be balanced against its toxic effects.

Antimony Potassium Tartrate (Tartar Emetic). *Preparations.* Crystalline powder containing 36.5 per cent trivalent antimony or supplied in ampules as a 0.5 per cent solution.

Administration. Intravenously by a fine needle to avoid extravasation. It must be given slowly.

Toxicity. Common toxic effects are nausea, vomiting, severe coughing and itching during or after intravenous administration, pneumonitis, arthralgias, myalgias, bradycardia, ECG changes (T-wave depression, increased Q-T interval, fusion of S-T segment and T-wave), abnormal liver function, headache and mild rash. Less common are hepatitis, hemolytic anemia, thrombocytopenia and an anaphylactoid reaction associated with urticaria, laryngeal edema and collapse. This compound is considered to be the most toxic of the antimonials.

Contraindications and precautions. Myocarditis, hepatitis or severe liver disease or concurrent bacterial or viral infection. Treatment should be stopped if arthralgias or rashes persist or if there is progressive proteinuria.

Bephenium Hydroxynaphthoate (Alcopara). *Preparation.* Supplied in 5 gm. packets for oral use only.

Administration. Drug may be more palatable if mixed with fruit juices, chocolate milk or carbonated beverages. Food should be withheld for 2 hours after administration.

Toxicity. Occasionally nausea, vomiting and mild diarrhea.

Contraindications and precautions. Conditions which may be aggravated by vomiting are relative contraindications. Patients should be warned of bitter taste.

Bithionol (Lorothidol). *Preparation.* Supplied in 500 mg. gelatin capsules. Available only through the Parasitic Disease Drug Service, Bureau of Epidemiology, Center for Disease Control, Atlanta, Ga. 30333. Telephone (404) 633-3311, ext. 3677 or 3496 during working hours and (404) 633-2176 at other times.

Administration. Must be given in 500 mg.

increments. Capsule should not be opened but may be placed in fruit or cereal to facilitate swallowing.

Toxicity. Side effects are common, but rarely require cessation of treatment. Complaints of diarrhea and abdominal cramps should be anticipated but generally subside after 2 or 3 days. Nausea, vomiting, urticaria and other skin eruptions, dizziness, headache and excessive salivation are less common. Rare cases of toxic hepatitis, albuminuria and cardiac arrhythmia have been reported.

Contraindications and precautions. Known sensitivity to bithionol. It is not recommended in pregnancy or in children under 8 years of age.

Chloroquine Phosphate (Aralen Phosphate, Roquine), Chloroquine Hydrochloride (Aralen Hydrochloride). *Preparation.* Supplied in 250 mg. tablets of diphosphate salt (500 mg. salt = 300 mg. base) and as the hydrochloride for parenteral injection in 5 ml. vials containing 40 mg. base/ml.

Administration. Tablets of the diphosphate salt are scored and should be carefully sectioned to provide the dosage required. The tablet or sections may be pulverized and mixed with fruit or cereal to make it more palatable. Chloroquine hydrochloride is given as an intramuscular injection.

Toxicity. Side effects are largely dose-related. Low doses such as those employed in malaria chemosuppression rarely produce symptoms. Treatment of clinical malaria may occasionally be accompanied by gastrointestinal symptoms, headache and pruritus. High doses—500 mg. or more per day—may result in lichenoid skin eruption, nervousness, insomnia and rarely toxic psychosis. Retinopathy may occur, especially with doses totaling more than 100 gm. (rarely used in parasitic infections). Neuromyopathy, ototoxicity and possible fetal abnormalities may occur.

Contraindications and precautions. Relative contraindications are liver disease and hematologic or neurologic disorders. Used in pregnancy only for hepatic amebiasis or for malaria chemosuppression when the risk of malaria outweighs hazards of possible fetal damage. Should be given with caution to patients with psoriasis or glucose-6-phosphate dehydrogenase deficiency. Children are extremely susceptible to overdosage and adverse effects of parenteral chloroquine. Sudden deaths after parenteral administration have been reported. A single dose should not exceed 5 mg. of base/kg. (maximum 250 mg.).

Dehydroemetine Dihydrochloride. Available only through the Parasitic Disease

Drug Service, Center for Disease Control. *Preparation.* Supplied in 2 ml. ampules containing 30 mg./ml.

Administration. Given as a deep intramuscular injection.

Toxicity. T-wave abnormalities and prolongation of Q-T interval are common; S-T segment depression is less commonly seen. ECG changes revert to normal 10 to 15 days after cessation of therapy. Hypotension of varying degrees is common. Aching, tenderness, stiffness and weakness of muscles in the area of the injection site (without redness or swelling) may occur. Diarrhea and nausea may occur. Vomiting is less frequent. Polyneuritis with transient paralysis has been recorded. Neurasthenia may be common and may persist for as long as 2 months.

Contraindications and precautions. Pre-existing cardiac abnormalities, either of myocardium or cardiac conduction system, are relative contraindications, as are pre-existing muscular or neurologic disorders. If these conditions exist, another drug such as metronidazole should be used for amebiasis. Patient should remain at bed rest during therapy and gradually resume activity over a period of several weeks after therapy.

Diethylcarbamazine Citrate (Hetrazan, Banocide, Notezine). *Preparation.* Supplied in 50 mg. tablets.

Administration. Scored tablets sectioned to provide the appropriate dose. Medication should be taken after meals.

Toxicity. Frequently headache, malaise, weakness, joint pains, anorexia, nausea and vomiting occur, but subside as treatment is continued. Mild to severe reactions may occur in response to death of parasites; reactions consist of fever, leukocytosis, eosinophilia and localized inflammation of skin, lymph nodes and lymphatics—and inflammation of the eye in onchocerciasis.

Contraindications and precautions. No strict contraindications. Reactions to death of parasites noted under "Toxicity" should be anticipated. Mild reactions may be controlled with antihistamines, but more severe reactions may require systemic corticosteroid administration. When eye involvement is present in onchocerciasis, an ophthalmic steroid solution should be used.

Diiodohydroxyquin (Diodoquin,* Yodoxin). *Preparation.* Supplied as 650 mg. tablets.

---

*This drug is no longer marketed as Diodoquin but is available as diiodohydroxyquin from several manufacturers.

Administration. Tablets should be given with meals. For administration to young children a suspension may be made by pulverizing the tablets and mixing them with cherry syrup to give a suspension containing 200 to 400 mg./5 ml. The suspension should be shaken thoroughly before usage and must be made up fresh weekly.

Toxicity. Furunculosis (iodine toxicoderma) and generalized dermatitis of varying degrees. Abdominal discomfort, diarrhea, anal irritation and pruritus. Headache and hypoesthesia of hands and feet.

Contraindications and precautions. Hypersensitivity to iodine or to any 8-hydroxyquinoline compound. Severe neurologic damage including optic atrophy, optic neuritis and peripheral neuropathy (subacute myelo-optic neuropathy) has occurred with prolonged high doses of other 8-hydroxyquinoline compounds. Therefore, recommended doses and duration of therapy with diiodohydroxyquin should not be exceeded. Protein-bound iodine levels may be raised, may persist for months, and are unrelated to thyroid function.

Emetine Hydrochloride. *Preparation.* Supplied in ampules containing 20, 30 or 60 mg./ml.

Administration. Deep subcutaneous or intramuscular injection.

Toxicity. Similar to dehydroemetine, but side effects more common and more severe.

Contraindications and precautions. As for dehydroemetine.

Furazolidone (Furoxone). *Preparation.* Supplied as 100 mg. tablets and as a suspension containing 3.33 mg. per ml. (50 mg. per 15 ml.) with kaolin and pectin.

Toxicity. Nausea, emesis and headache may occur. Rarely hypersensitivity reactions have occurred, manifested by hypotension, urticaria, fever, arthralgia and a vesicular erythematous rash. A disulfiram-like reaction associated with ingestion of alcohol has been reported rarely. Hemolysis may occur in individuals with glucose-6-phosphate dehydrogenase deficiency. Experimental data indicate potential enhancement of amphetamine and tyramine sensitivity associated with monoamine oxidase deficiency after 5 days of treatment.

Contraindications and precautions. There is inadequate information to determine the effects of the drug in pregnancy. Monoamine oxidase inhibitors and foods containing tyramine such as broad beans, aged cheese, beer and wine should not be taken while receiving furazolidone. The drug is also contraindicated in infants under 1 month of age. As furazolidone is excreted in breast milk, lactating mothers should not receive the drug while nursing. Known sensitivity to furazolidone is a contraindication. Alcohol should be avoided when taking the drug and for a 4 day period after treatment.

Mebendazole (Vermox). *Preparation.* Supplied as chewable tablets of 100 mg.

Administration. It may be necessary to crush the tablets and mix with food when administering to small children.

Toxicity. Abdominal pain and diarrhea have occurred transiently during expulsion of massive numbers of worms.

Contraindications and precautions. Should not be used in pregnant women and should be used with caution in children under 2 years of age.

Melarsoprol (Mel B, Arsobal). Available only through the Parasitic Disease Drug Service, Center for Disease Control. *Preparation.* Supplied as a 3.6 per cent solution in propylene glycol in 6 ml. ampules. Refrigerated storage is necessary.

Administration. Drug is given by the intravenous route, slowly and carefully to avoid extravasation.

Toxicity. Abdominal pain, nausea, vomiting and diarrhea may occur. Reactive encephalopathy may occur in a significant percentage of patients. It is more likely to occur in debilitated patients and may also be associated with higher than normal doses of melarsoprol. Other neurologic manifestations include a transient worsening of the neurologic findings as therapy begins. The patient may also exhibit confusion, speech abnormalities, restlessness, and movement disorders.

Contraindications and precautions. Melarsoprol should not be used in early (hemolymphatic) untreated trypanosomiasis. Because of the serious nature of trypanosomiasis, pregnancy and age do not limit the use of the drug. Severely debilitated patients should receive a course of suramin prior to use of melarsoprol. Graduated dosage of melarsoprol should be used in the debilitated or somnolent patient.

Metronidazole (Flagyl). *Preparation.* Supplied as tablets of 250 mg.

Toxicity. Side effects are more common with high doses used in treatment of amebiasis. Gastrointestinal reactions are most common and may consist of anorexia, nausea and occasionally vomiting, diarrhea, epigastric distress or abdominal cramping. A metallic taste is frequently reported. Headache, dizziness and vertigo may occur. There have been rare reports of incoordination, ataxia, paresthesias,

and numbness of extremities. Irritability, depression and insomnia may also occur. ECG may show T-wave flattening. Urticaria, erythematous eruptions and pruritus have been reported. A moderate leukopenia occasionally occurs but returns to normal following completion of therapy. Oral or vaginal overgrowth of *Candida* may occur. Dark urine, which probably represents a metabolite of the drug, has been seen in patients receiving high doses. Rare instances of dysuria, incontinence, polyuria, cystitis, pyuria, dyspareunia, fever, decreased libido, proctitis and nasal congestion have been reported.

Contraindications and precautions. History of blood dyscrasia, organic disease of the central nervous system and known sensitivity to metronidazole. It is contraindicated in first trimester of pregnancy. Drug should not be used in the second and third trimesters of pregnancy unless the benefits to the patient clearly outweigh potential risks to patient and fetus. It should be used in trichomoniasis under these conditions only if previous topical treatment has failed. Patients taking the drug should avoid alcohol because of reports that flushing, abdominal cramps and vomiting may occur. Leukocyte counts with differential counts are recommended before and after therapy.

Niclosamide (Yomesan). Available only through the Parasitic Disease Drug Service, Center for Disease Control. *Preparation.* Supplied as chewable tablets of 500 mg.

Toxicity. Nausea, vomiting and abdominal discomfort may occur rarely, and isolated reports of dizziness, fever and urticaria have been noted.

Contraindications and precautions. Inadequate information is available to assess the hazards in pregnancy. It is not recommended for pregnant women and children under 2 years of age.

Nifurtimox (Bayer 2502). Available only through the Parasitic Disease Drug Service, Center for Disease Control. *Preparation.* Supplied as 100 mg. scored tablets.

Toxicity. Gastrointestinal symptoms are common and may consist of anorexia, weight loss, abdominal pain, nausea and vomiting. Neuropsychiatric symptoms are less frequently seen but may necessitate stopping therapy. Convulsions, headache, drowsiness, nervousness, vertigo, insomnia, paresthesias, disorientation and memory impairment have been recorded. Skin rashes have developed occasionally during therapy.

Contraindications and precautions. Pregnancy and in children under 1 year of age.

casionally occur during treatment of falciparum malaria but is usually associated with inadequate therapy.

Sodium Stibogluconate (Pentostam, Solustibosan). Available only through the Parasitic Disease Drug Service, Center for Disease Control. *Preparation.* Supplied as a 33 per cent solution containing 100 mg. of pentavalent antimony per ml.

Toxicity. See antimony potassium tartrate. This compound is less toxic than an equivalent amount of antimony in the trivalent form.

Contraindications and precautions. See antimony potassium tartrate.

Stibocaptate (Astiban, TWSb). Available only through the Parasitic Disease Drug Service, Center for Disease Control. *Preparation.* Supplied in ampules as 0.5 gm. crystalline powder.

Administration. Given intramuscularly or intravenously following addition of sterile distilled water to make a 10 per cent solution.

Toxicity. See antimony potassium tartrate. Stibocaptate is considered the least toxic of the trivalent antimonials.

Contraindications and precautions. See antimony potassium tartrate.

Stibophen (Fuadin). *Preparation.* Supplied in 5 ml. ampules as a 6.3 per cent aqueous solution containing 8.5 mg. trivalent antimony per ml. with 0.1 per cent sodium bisulfite.

Administration. The drug is administered intramuscularly and a test dose of 1.5 ml. is given intramuscularly. If no untoward effects develop, the full regimen can begin 24 hours later.

Toxicity. See antimony potassium tartrate. Stibophen has intermediate toxicity among the trivalent antimonials.

Contraindications and precautions. See antimony potassium tartrate. The patient should have platelets checked at intervals to detect thrombocytopenia. Stibophen is an approved drug but is no longer manufactured in the United States. Some supplies may still be available.

Suramin Sodium (Antrypol, Naphuride sodium, Bayer 205). Available only through the Parasitic Disease Drug Service, Center for Disease Control. *Preparation.* Supplied in ampules containing 1.0 gm. of powder.

Administration. Solution should be prepared immediately prior to use by addition of 10 ml. of sterile distilled water. Suramin should not be used if it has been in solution longer than 30 minutes.

Toxicity. Immediate reaction consisting of nausea, vomiting, loss of consciousness and seizures may occur with full intravenous dose in certain sensitive individuals. Proteinuria is common but is not an indication for stopping therapy unless it is progressive or other parameters of renal function are abnormal. Fever of a minor degree is not unusual. Cutaneous lesions (rashes, localized edema and itching) may occur. Blepharitis, conjunctivitis, photophobia and lacrimation may occur in treatment of both trypanosomiasis and onchocerciasis.

Contraindications and precautions. Suramin should not be used in pregnancy or in children under age 6. A test dose should be given; if an untoward reaction occurs, suramin should not be used. It should never be used alone to treat African trypanosomiasis involving the central nervous system. Melarsoprol should be given in cases of early Rhodesian trypanosomiasis if the response to suramin is not favorable and prompt.

Tetrachloroethylene. *Preparation.* Supplied in soft gelatin capsules of 0.2, 1.0 and 2.5 ml. Tetrachloroethylene for veterinary use may be used with safety in areas where the drug is otherwise unobtainable.*

Toxicity. Epigastric burning sensation, abdominal cramps, nausea and vomiting may occur. Headache, vertigo, inebriation and, rarely, loss of consciousness apparently result if the drug is absorbed.

Contraindications and precautions. Severe anemia and dehydration should be corrected prior to treatment. Very young, severely ill children and patients with liver disease probably should use another drug. Alcohol should be avoided before treatment and for 24 hours after treatment.

Tetracycline (Achromycin, Panmycin, Sumycin, etc.). See oxytetracycline.

Thiabendazole (Mintezol). *Preparation.* Supplied as a flavored suspension, containing 125 or 250 mg./5 ml., pediatric drops containing 100 mg./ml. and as chewable 500 mg. tablets.

Toxicity. Common side effects are anorexia, nausea, vomiting and dizziness. Diarrhea, epigastric distress, pruritus, weariness, drowsiness, giddiness and headache have occurred infrequently. Rare side effects are tinnitus, hyperirritability, numbness, abnormal sensation in eyes, blurring of vision, xanthopsia, hypotension, collapse, perianal rash, transitory rise in SGOT, cholestasis and parenchymal liver damage, hyperglycemia, malodorous urine, crystalluria, hematuria and

---

*Tetrachloroethylene is available in the United States only as a veterinary preparation (Nema worm caps).

appearance of live *Ascaris* in mouth or nose. Rare hypersensitivity reactions may consist of fever, facial flushing, chills, conjunctival injection, angioedema, anaphylaxis, skin rashes and erythema multiforme. Fatal episodes of the Stevens-Johnson syndrome have been recorded.

Contraindications and precautions. Known hypersensitivity to thiabendazole. Patients with hepatic or renal disease should be carefully monitored.

Toxoplasmosis

JACK S. REMINGTON, M.D.

Therapy of human cases of toxoplasmosis presents inherent problems. Acute cases available for careful study have been relatively few, and the diagnosis has often been made too late to institute treatment under controlled conditions. Evaluation of treatment is difficult because of variation in severity and outcome of the disease. The parasite is not always eliminated by specific therapy, and cure in humans is apparently related to the strain of the parasite involved and to the time during the course of infection when treatment is initiated. At present specific therapy is beneficial only against the proliferative form of Toxoplasma and will not eradicate the encysted form of the parasite.

Specific Therapy. Pyrimethamine, a substituted phenylpyrimidine antimalarial drug (in the form of Daraprim), produces not only survival, but also radical cure of animals given experimental infection. The suggested dosage of pyrimethamine in human patients is 1 mg./kg./day in two doses orally, with a maximum dose of 25 mg./day. A dose of 2 mg./kg. to a maximum of 50 mg./day has been used, but with a proportional increase in toxicity. The dose is usually doubled (2 mg./kg.) during the first day or two of treatment, however.* As the half-life or pyrimethamine is 4 to 5 days, a number of authorities administer the above dosage only every 2, 3 or even 4 days.

Pyrimethamine and sulfadiazine act synergistically against Toxoplasma with a combined activity eight times that which would be expected if their effects were merely additive. Comparative tests have shown that sulfapyrazine, sulfamethazine and sulfamerazine are of a similar order of activity to sulfadiazine. All the other sulfonamides tested (sul-

---

*This dosage of pyrimethamine is higher than that recommended by the manufacturer, but has been found safe and effective.

fathiazole, sulfapyridine, sulfadimetine, sulfisoxazole) were much inferior. It would appear logical to use multiple sulfonamides for treatment of toxoplasmosis, because additive effect with less toxicity would be expected. The usual dosage of sulfadiazine or triple sulfonamides is 100 to 150 mg./kg./day in four equal doses by mouth in addition to pyrimethamine. The optimal duration of treatment has not been determined.

Toxicity of Pyrimethamine. Both pyrimethamine and the sulfonamides are potentially toxic drugs. Most physicians are familiar with the untoward reactions to sulfonamides: crystalluria, hematuria and hypersensitivity. Pyrimethamine is a folic acid antagonist which produces reversible and usually gradual depression of the bone marrow. Although toxicity is dose-related, absorption of the drug is not uniform in all patients, and side effects are seen more frequently in patients who absorb the drug best. Platelet depression with its associated bleeding tendency is the most serious consequence of toxicity. Both leukopenia and anemia may occur as well. Less serious side effects are gastrointestinal distress, headaches and a bad taste in the mouth. *All patients treated with pyrimethamine should have a peripheral blood cell and platelet count twice a week.*

Folinic acid (in the form of leucovorin-calcium) has been used to facilitate return of circulating platelets to normal. No data are available on the use of leucovorin-calcium in young children. We usually employ 5 to 10 mg./day in older children and adults. The parenteral form (Calcium Leucovoran Injection, Lederle Laboratories) may be ingested. This substance, which in contrast to folic acid does not appear to inhibit the action of pyrimethamine on the proliferative form of Toxoplasma, may be used in conjunction with this drug to allay toxicity.

Congenital Toxoplasmosis. If congenital toxoplasmosis is diagnosed, children should receive specific therapy whether the infection is clinically apparent or asymptomatic. Even in what often appears clinically to be an acute fulminant disease with multiple organ involvement, early instigation of therapy may prevent further tissue invasion and destruction by the proliferative form of the parasite, allowing regeneration and healing of tissues which have not been irreparably damaged. There are insufficient data to allow for proper evaluation of treatment in the asymptomatic infected infant. However, most investigators consider that treatment of such infants should be undertaken in the hope of preventing late untoward sequelae. A minimum of 6 to 8 weeks of therapy is recommended, and some workers recommend that therapy be continued for a year.

Our knowledge of the treatment of congenital toxoplasmosis is meager. Because pyrimethamine has not been used extensively in young infants, the best course to follow is unknown. In the face of an extremely high mortality rate in cases of clinically apparent fulminant infection, and because of the serious sequelae which may develop in asymptomatic infants, it seems desirable to treat even very young infants.

In infants with the severe form of the congenital infection, corticosteroids have been recommended such as prednisone or methylprednisolone in a dose of 1 to 2 mg./kg./day by the oral route, to be given until the inflammatory process (such as chorioretinitis, high CSF protein) has subsided. If spiramycin (not available in the United States) can be obtained, a regimen using this drug has been recommended (Remington, J. S ., and Desmonts, G.: Toxoplasmosis. *In* Remington, J. S., and Klein, J. O. (eds.): Infectious Diseases of the Fetus and Newborn Infant. Philadelphia, W. B. Saunders Co., 1976, p. 302).

Acquired Toxoplasmosis. Whether the child with an active acquired infection should be treated depends on the nature of the clinical illness. This form of toxoplasmosis may range from acute fatal illness with meningoencephalitis and pneumonia to an essentially asymptomatic infection. Unfortunately, because the diagnosis is often made late in the disease, only a few patients have been studied extensively, and little is known of the efficacy of treatment of the acquired infection. Patients presenting with the more severe form, and especially immunologically compromised patients, must be treated to prevent extensive tissue damage or a fatal outcome. We recommend treatment for 4 to 6 weeks. In the benign form of toxoplasmosis, which closely simulates infectious mononucleosis clinically, specific treatment is usually not necessary. In most such cases which have been treated it is not possible to distinguish between a therapeutic response and a spontaneous remission.

Ocular Toxoplasmosis. The greatest experience with chemotherapy has been obtained in cases of ocular toxoplasmosis. Since it is difficult to reach a definitive diagnosis of this disease, evaluation of the therapy must be based on statistical studies, which, in general, have been encouraging.

Because of the potential hazards associated with the use of corticosteroids, these drugs are best given only in cases of retinochoroiditis with involvement of the macula, maculopapillary bundle or optic nerve. If the lesion appears in other areas of the retina, scarring usually occurs without significant loss of vision, and the potential toxicity of corticosteroids, as well as the possibility of their causing spread of organisms or breakdown of quiescent foci, probably contraindicates their use in this situation.

The daily dosage of prednisone in children is 1 to 2 mg./kg. by mouth up to a maximum of 75 mg./day. The equivalent dosage of another corticosteroid may be given. Chemotherapy is used concomitantly as previously outlined. The dosage of corticosteroid may be tapered gradually when the lesion appears well demarcated and pigmentation has begun. Hypersensitivity appears to play a predominant role in the pathogenesis of relapses of ocular toxoplasmosis, and in such cases corticosteroids should be used in addition to chemotherapy (at least sulfonamides).

Cholera

MARY M. EICHHORN ADAMS, Ph.D., *and* NORBERT HIRSCHHORN, M.D.

The clinical picture of cholera is similar to that of other severe diarrheal diseases. Indeed, cholera in children resembles what was known as cholera infantum in the western world during the early decades of the twentieth century. Cholera infantum, which is still seen in developing countries, probably has several different etiologic agents: enteric viruses, enterotoxigenic bacteria, and some species of *Shigella.* The mortality rate of cholera infantum in the United States was 80 per cent during the 1920's; this figure decreased to about 30 per cent in the 1930's when treatment by intravenous infusion of saline was introduced. These mortality rates resemble those of cholera; in recent epidemics in Asia about 50 per cent of untreated victims of cholera died. Fortunately, however, a simple method of treatment, which is applicable to all severe diarrheal diseases, makes it possible for most patients, both children and adults, to recover from cholera.

The physiological changes that lead to death of persons with cholera are all attributable to loss of water and electrolytes from the body. The massive outpouring of fluid from the intestine is effected by the action of the exotoxin of *Vibrio cholerae* on the cells of the intestinal mucosa. Thus the major goal of successful therapy is replacement of water and electrolytes. Eradication of *V. cholerae* by administration of a suitable antibiotic is a useful adjunct to fluid therapy. Treatment based on these principles has been in use for about 10 years and has drastically reduced the mortality rate among victims of cholera. Even under primitive conditions 98 to 99 per cent of properly treated children survive, and the survival rate for adults is even greater.

Clinical Picture. The signs characteristic of pediatric cholera are those of shock (due to loss of sodium chloride and water); acidosis (due to loss of bicarbonate); and potassium depletion. The predominant symptom is severe watery diarrhea (up to 200 ml./kg./day) lasting 3 to 5 days; however, tetracycline therapy reduces the stool volume within 24 hours and can stop fluid loss in 48 hours on the average. Experience has shown that a careful and continuous clinical assessment of the child's condition is the best method for estimating the fluid volume deficit and determining treatment.

The dehydration caused by cholera and other diarrheal diseases is classified as mild, moderate, or severe according to the following criteria. *Mild dehydration,* characterized by thirst, slightly decreased skin turgor, sunken eyes, and tachycardia, indicates a fluid loss of about 5 per cent of body weight. Children with this degree of fluid loss will have good peripheral pulse and normal sensorium. It should be noted that it is possible for a child to have a fluid loss of up to 5 per cent of body weight and yet, except for thirst, not have any obvious signs of dehydration. *Moderate dehydration* is manifest by obviously decreased skin turgor, flattened veins in the neck, tachycardia, and hypotension. The sensorium remains normal. The fluid loss of the moderately dehydrated child is 5 to 8 per cent of body weight. *Severe dehydration* is indicated by the signs that accompany moderate dehydration as well as by cyanosis, stupor or coma, and absent peripheral pulses. The amount of fluid lost is 10 to 12 per cent of body weight; such a large loss may occur within a few hours after the onset of diarrhea, and death may be imminent if rehydration is not rapidly effected.

In assessing the degree of dehydration in infants, one should remember that a fat baby may not have a noticeable loss of skin turgor. In such cases, the status of the neck veins, color of the skin, and fontanelle, if it is open, are useful indicators.

Therapy. Once the diagnosis of cholera is made and the child's condition is assessed, therapy with intravenous or oral electrolyte solutions and an antibiotic should begin immediately. The initial estimated deficit should be replaced within 4 hours. Experience gained during the cholera pandemic of the early 1970's proved that all but the severely dehydrated child who is unable to drink can be treated by orally administered fluid. The rationale of cholera therapy is to replace the water and electrolytes lost in the stool. The osmolarity of choleraic stool is similar to that of plasma. Hence the concentrations of electrolytes that should be present in solutions used for intravenous or oral therapy are roughly those found in plasma (Table 1). There is considerable latitude in levels of electrolytes that may be present. This fact permits the use of any one of several preparations that have proved effective. Of solutions suitable for intravenous therapy, Ringer's lactate is probably the most widely available of the commercial products. Because its potassium content is low, Ringer's lactate must be supplemented either by addition of 10 mEq. of potassium chloride per liter to the intravenous solution or by oral administration of potassium hydrogen citrate, 4 mEq./kg./24 hours given in 4 divided doses.

TABLE 1.   Concentrations (in mEq./liter) of Electrolytes in Stool of Children with Cholera Compared with the Concentrations in Solutions Used for Intravenous or Oral Therapy

MATERIAL	Na	CL	K	BASE*
Stool (mean values)	101	92	27	32
Ringer's lactate†	128	109	4‡	28
Dacca 5/4/1§	132	99	14	47
NAMRU-2‖	90	64	15	45
WHO oral solution**	90	80	20	30

*Stool base is bicarbonate; suitable bases for rehydration fluids are bicarbonate, lactate, or acetate.

†Also contains calcium, 3 mEq./liter.

‡This amount of potassium is inadequate and must be supplemented (see text).

§Also contains glucose, 10 gm./liter. From the Cholera Research Laboratory, Dacca, Bangladesh.

‖Also contains glucose, 20 gm./liter; calcium, 2 mEq./liter; and magnesium, 2 mEq./liter. NAMRU-2= Naval American Research Unit No. 2 (Taipei).

**Also contains glucose, 20 gm./liter, required for intestinal absorption of electrolytes and water.

In addition to electrolytes, glucose *must* be added to solutions used for oral therapy, 20 gm./liter of the oral solution. Oral administration of glucose is required to promote intestinal absorption of water and electrolytes. Glucose given intravenously does *not* promote salt and water absorption by the intestine. The only purpose of its use in the intravenous fluid is to prevent hypoglycemia.

The World Health Organization (WHO) has recommended a single *oral* glucose-electrolyte solution that can be used for treatment of children or adults. This solution contains the following solutes (in gm./liter):

sodium chloride, 3.5; potassium chloride, 1.5; sodium bicarbonate, 2.5; glucose, 20. A packet containing all the ingredients to be added to one liter of water is available from UNICEF under the name "Oralyte." Alternatively, a solution roughly equivalent to the WHO formulation can be made with use of United States Standard (cooking) spoons for measurement of crushed, dry chemicals.The amounts of each (in level teaspoonfuls/900 ml. of solution) are as follows: sodium chloride, 0.5; potassium chloride, 0.25; sodium bicarbonate, 0.5; glucose, 4.0.

A solution suitable for *intravenous* use can be made by mixing together 500 ml. of 0.9 per cent sodium chloride, 500 ml. of 5 per cent glucose in water, 50 ml. of 1 M sodium lactate *or* 1 M sodium bicarbonate, and 8 ml. of 2 M potassium chloride. If one wishes to use dry chemicals, the following solids (grams) can be added to one liter of water: sodium chloride, 4 to 5; potassium chloride, 1; sodium bicarbonate, 4 *or* sodium lactate, 5.2; glucose, 10. Because sodium bicarbonate will decompose if the solution is boiled, any solution for intravenous use containing bicarbonate should be sterilized by a method other than autoclaving.

The child who is severely dehydrated and unable to drink should be rehydrated with a volume of intravenous solution that is roughly equal to the amount of water lost. A 10 kg. child would require one liter of polyelectrolyte solution. The first half of this should be given over 1 to 2 hours, and the balance in the next 2 to 4 hours. During intravenous administration of fluids, the child should be observed carefully; disappearance of signs of dehydration, maintenance of stable body weight and cardiovascular status, and return of urinary output are adequate indicators of the degree of hydration attained. Mildly puffy eyelids and full rosy cheeks in a previously thin child are signs of full hydration.

As soon as the patient can drink, intravenous therapy should be supplemented by drinking of the oral glucose-electrolyte solution. The solution recommended by the World Health Organization is hypotonic with respect to plasma; if given in amounts equal to 1.5 times the volume of stool lost, it supplies enough water to replace that lost through evaporation or in the urine. By ad libitum drinking of the glucose-electrolyte solution, which is more palatable if warmed to body temperature, a patient will often adjust his intake of fluid to compensate for the amount lost through diarrhea. However, with a child who is too young or too weak to help himself, the medical attendant or parent must make certain that a sufficient amount of liquid is taken. After rehydration is complete, the patient's appetite often returns; light foods and fluids can be given in addition to the glucose-electrolyte solution. Administration of the latter should continue, however, until diarrhea has ceased.

Because the goal of therapy is to replace the fluid and electrolytes lost on a 1:1 basis (with allowances for evaporative and urinary losses), it is useful to keep a record of the volume of stool as well as of the volume of fluid administered. The intake-output balance should be calculated every few hours, and the amount of fluid to be given during the subsequent time period should be adjusted accordingly. Use of a cholera cot facilitates measurement of stool volume and aids sanitation. Such a cot can be improvised by cutting a hole just above the middle of the mattress or canvas of a bed or cot. A bucket is placed beneath the hole, and a calibrated "dip stick" is used for measurement of the volume of stool in the bucket. In the absence of a cholera cot, a bedpan can be used. Any type of diaper can be used for an infant; weighing of the diaper before and after use will provide a rough measurement of the amount of stool. Ideally, urine should not be mixed with stool; an older child can be asked to use a bedpan or urinal, but with an infant, separation of urine and stool is not possible.

After the initial volume deficit has been replaced, fluid therapy should be continued until diarrhea ceases (2 to 3 days with antibiotics). Once the child can drink enough liquid to compensate for his losses, intravenous therapy is discontinued. A child with serious to profuse diarrhea should then drink about 10 to 15 ml. of fluid/kg./hour; those with mild diarrhea can drink less (5 ml./kg./hour). Oral fluid is given at these rates for the first 4 to 6 hours; thereafter, the volume taken by mouth should equal 1.5 times the amount lost in the stool during the previous time period.

Frequent bedside evaluation of the child's state of well being (with emphasis on signs of hydration), coupled with ad libitum drinking of the glucose-electrolyte solution, is often a satisfactory method of judging fluid needs and is used when measurement of stools is not practical.

There is no reason to withhold food or milk from a child during oral (or intravenous) fluid therapy. In fact, it is desirable to feed the child within the first 24 hours of therapy. A child who is inclined to eat can be given food that is easy to digest and suitable for his age, such as bread, banana, rice, or fish. It is probably best to avoid use of cow's milk for the duration of illness if other foods can be used. However, breast milk is recommended for the infant who is still nursing.

Antibiotics. Three antibiotics have proved effective in eradicating *V. cholerae*: tetracycline, furazolidone, and chloramphenicol. Tetracycline is almost always available and is the drug of choice. Although all three drugs have some toxicity for children, adverse reactions are rare because of the brief duration of therapy.

Unless the patient is unconscious the antibiotic should be given by mouth. The dosages of antibiotics recommended for children are as follows: tetracycline,* 25 to 50 mg./kg./day in divided doses for two days; furazolidone,† 5 mg./kg./day in divided doses for three days; chloramphenicol, 50 to 75 mg./kg./day in divided doses for three days.

The efficacy of antibiotics in treatment of cholera has been proved; both the duration of diarrhea and the total volume of fluid lost can be reduced by 50 per cent or more. Thus use of an antibiotic is a valuable adjunct to fluid therapy for cholera.

Complications. Children are more likely to be affected by complications of cholera than are adults. Hypokalemia, which rarely causes ill effects in older patients, may produce cardiac arrhythmias, ileus, hypotension, and cardiac arrest in children with cholera. However, hypokalemia can be avoided or corrected by administration of intravenous or oral fluid containing an adequate amount of potassium.

Overhydration, unless extreme, is not harmful provided that an adequate amount of potassium is given and acidosis is corrected. However, in children with uncorrected acidosis or preexisting heart disease, overhydration may result in pulmonary edema. Signs of excessive volume replacement are, in order of appearance, puffy eyelids, distended neck veins, a slow full pulse, and cardiac failure. Careful and frequent bedside observation of the child, with particular attention to these indicators, offers the best method for prevention of any untoward effects of overhydration.

Manifestations of central nervous system dysfunction (stupor, coma, convulsions) occur in about 10 per cent of children with cholera and are often due to hypoglycemia. The hypoglycemia can usually be avoided or corrected by addition of glucose (1 to 2 per cent)

to the intravenous fluid or by earlier feeding. Persistent hypoglycemia is unusual, but hypoglycemia may recur if administration of glucose is discontinued. If hypoglycemia persists despite administration of glucose, the child's prognosis is poor.

Immunity and Prevention. Adequate sanitation is the surest means to prevent cholera, but it may be difficult or impossible to provide in some parts of the world; therefore a vaccine that induces long-lasting immunity to cholera is needed. The vaccine now available is made of killed *V. cholerae* and is given parenterally; it affords fairly good protection but only for a few months. The current goal of vaccine development is oral immunization with a live, attenuated vaccine strain of *V. cholerae*. It is hoped that such a vaccine will confer longer lasting and more complete protection than that provided by the killed *V. cholerae* vaccine.

Immunization Practice

SHIRLEY L. FANNIN, M.D., F.A.A.P.

Routine immunization is a standard part of the well child care delivered by most physicians. Recommended immunization schedules in the United States are made by two major groups, the American Academy of Pediatrics and the United States Public Health Service's Advisory Committee on Immunization Practices (ACIP). Many prominent scientists, expert in various aspects of vaccine production and usage, belong to both groups. The variations found in their recommendations are based on target population considerations.

A physician must know several things about immunizing agents before using them: What is the composition of the agent? Who should be immunized? Who should not be immunized? How must the immunizing agent be handled and administered? What are the risks versus benefits of the agent?

The best guide for answering most questions concerning composition, contraindications, and relative risk versus benefits may be found on the package insert accompanying the immunizing agent. This should be read by the physician before using any new or unfamiliar agent.

The immunizing principle in most vaccines is an infectious agent or a viral or bacterial antigen. Vaccines may vary from highly purified components of these agents to crude suspensions of the whole agent. Many vaccines, therefore, contain not only the immunogenic agent but various other components, such as antibiotics, stabilizers, pH indicators and ex-

---

*Manufacturer's warning: Permanent discoloration of teeth may occur when tetracycline is administered to children under 8 years of age.

†Manufacturer's warning: Do not administer furazolidone to infants under 1 month of age.

traneous infectious agents. These extraneous components may cause difficulty in an individual patient with hypersensitivities or allergies.

Immune serum globulin (ISG) is the major source of antibodies for passive immunization. It is prepared from plasma that has been obtained from specifically immunized persons or from populations known to have appropriate plasma levels of the desired antibodies. It is a concentrated preparation containing 16.5 ± 1.5 gm. of gamma globulin (principally ISG) per 100 ml. and is given only by the intramuscular route. The product label usually specifies standardization with reference to content of antibody against a certain disease; for example, measles immune serum globulin contains at least 4000 units of measles antibody per milliliter.

Indications for Immunization. Vaccines and antibody preparations are administered as protection against either an immediate or a distant threat of infection. The objectives are to prevent diseases, modify illness, or prevent complications.

As a general rule, only healthy individuals who are free of infection should receive vaccines. The obvious exceptions are those with a mild afebrile upper respiratory illness which does not contraindicate routine immunization, children with cerebral injury who should be protected against the usual childhood diseases, and persons with diabetes, chronic respiratory disease, or cardiovascular disease who should receive influenza vaccine. In contrast, immune serum globulin or animal serum globulin containing specific antibodies is frequently administered to persons with specific diseases or defects (immunosuppressed patients, immunodeficiency disease, or leukemia) or even specific infection (shingles).

Contraindications for Use of Immunizing Materials. Immunization has some hazards for certain individuals eve though it may be totally safe for the remainder of the population. General precautions to be observed:

1. Presence of a febrile infection is a contraindication to the use of immunizing agents.

2. Immunizing agents should not be administered during the incubation period of a communicable disease. An exception is the use of live measles vaccine in exposed susceptible persons within 48 hours after exposure. This may prevent the natural disease.

3. Most live virus vaccines should not be given to pregnant women. The exception is polio virus vaccine during an epidemic of the disease when its administration to pregnant women is both permissible and recommended.

4. Use of live virus vaccines should be avoided in persons with immune deficiency diseases, in those receiving immunosuppressive therapy, and in patients with lymphatic malignancies.

5. Egg-sensitive individuals should not receive vaccines derived from chick embryo cultures or from viruses grown in chicken eggs.

6. Persons allergic to dog dander or other canine antigens should not receive vaccine derived from dog kidney.

7. Persons known to be sensitive to animal serum should receive this material only if it is absolutely essential and if a desensitizing regimen is used. Such a desensitizing regimen would include the presence of a physician and availability of epinephrine, resuscitative instruments, and other measures to treat shock immediately.

How to Use Immunizing Agents. The decision on whether to administer an immunizing agent early or late is based on several considerations: presence of disease in the community; accessibility to the patient; immune competence of the patient; and the patterns of medical care in the population concerned. Recommended schedules for routine immunization of a pediatric population generally reflect medical practice in the community. The Academy of Pediatrics' recommendations use an idealized well baby schedule as a framework for accomplishing infant immunization, thus the 2, 4, 6, and 18 month recommendations for infant DTP immunization. The Public Health Service's recommendations are geared to the population least likely to receive constant pediatric care and most likely to be exposed early to conditions promoting the spread of these early childhood diseases, thus the recommendation to begin immunization at 6 weeks of age.

Knowing when and how to vary an immunization schedule for the maximum disease prevention benefit of the patient is paramount in understanding immunization practice.

How to use immunizing agents includes not only the consideration of the dose and route of administration, but also the appropriate handling of the vaccine. The package insert is the best guide for the user of the vaccine. It details appropriate storage, idiosyncrasies of handling the material, as well as the dose and route of administration. The instructions on the package insert must be followed exactly. There are many more children who are inadequately immunized because of improper handling of the vaccine than there are because of an intrinsic defect in the vaccine.

Side Effects of Immunizing Mate-

rials. Side effects have been noted during the development and use of almost all the common immunizing agents. Some are purely idiosyncratic and unpredictable; others are common enough to be anticipated with each use of the specific immunizing agent.

DIPHTHERIA TOXOID. Diphtheria toxoid usually has few side effects. However, it has been noted that severe local reactions tend to appear with increasing age. Therefore, the dosage of diphtheria toxoid is decreased to 1/14 or 1/15 the childhood dose after 6 years of age.

PERTUSSIS VACCINE. Fever, local induration, irritability and lethargy are common side effects and increase with multiple doses. Most side effects appear within 6 hours after vaccine administration and may last for 24 hours. Severe reactions are uncommon and vary from encephalopathy to shock. Central nervous system symptoms (stupor, coma, and convulsions) predominate. Also described are high pitched screaming episodes which last for hours. Most severe reactions occur within 24 to 48 hours, but some have been noted as late as one week following vaccine administration. Thrombocytopenia is also a rare observation.

TETANUS TOXOID. Side effects are unusual; however, in persons receiving frequent immunizations with this toxoid, an Arthus reaction may occur.

LIVE MEASLES VIRUS VACCINE. In about 15 per cent of children receiving measles vaccine, a febrile illness with or without a generalized morbilliform rash may occur 7 to 10 days following vaccination. Progressive and lethal subacute sclerosing encephalopathy is a remote possibility following vaccination, but this reaction is much less frequent than when following the natural disease. A generalized fatal reaction from the vaccine virus may occur in children with immunologic deficiencies in the cell-mediated immune system.

LIVE RUBELLA VACCINE. Five to 10 per cent of children receiving this vaccine may have arthralgia as a side effect. In a much smaller number of this group, arthritis will develop within 1 to 7 weeks. The incidence of arthralgia is much higher, up to 40 per cent among adolescents and adults, especially females. In the majority of cases the joint symptoms are transitory and without signs of joint disease. In a few cases the symptoms have been confused with rheumatoid arthritis. In only rare cases have symptoms persisted. About 1 or 2 children of every 10,000 immunized may have a painful neuropathy affecting both upper and lower extremities. This side effect may occur as long as 10 weeks after immunization.

LIVE MUMPS VACCINE. This vaccine is without serious side effects.

ORAL TRIVALENT POLIO VACCINE. This vaccine is usually without side effects. There is a minimal risk of paralytic polio directly attributable to the vaccine virus, especially types I and III. This risk is approximately 1 in 9 million according to the most authoritative estimates. This paralysis may affect either the person vaccinated or a close contact such as a susceptible family member.

INFLUENZA VACCINE. Febrile reactions within 6 hours after vaccination are so frequent that routine use of this vaccine in healthy children is not recommended. Associated with the fever can be malaise, muscle and joint aches, headache and fatigue. As many as 8 to 10 per cent of children under three years of age may be at risk for central nervous system reactions manifested as convulsions. With each new influenza vaccine produced, the incidence and type of side effect varies. The most current information on side effects is available in the package insert accompanying the vaccine.

For recommended schedules for active immunization, see Table 1.

PASSIVE IMMUNIZATION

Immune Serum Globulin

Standard Immune Serum Globulin (Gamma Globulin). VIRAL HEPATITIS, TYPE A(HB_sA_g NEGATIVE). For household contacts, ISG should be given as soon as possible after known exposure. Its prophylactic value decreases as time increases after exposure. The use of ISG more than five to six weeks after exposure is not indicated. ISG is not routinely recommended for other contacts but special groups should be evaluated on an individual basis, such as nursery schools, day care centers, and so on. Dosage guidelines for ISG prophylaxis of viral hepatitis, type A, for acute exposure are: up to 22 kg., 0.5 ml.; 22 to 45 kg., 1.0 ml.; and over 45 kg., 2.0 ml. Within limits, larger doses of ISG provide longer lasting but not necessarily more protection.

MEASLES. Live measles vaccine can usually prevent disease if administered within 48 hours of exposure. For susceptible infants and children exposed more than 48 hours, 0.25 ml./kg. (0.1 ml./lb.) of ISG should be given, followed by live measles vaccine 3 months later unless contraindicated. If exposure was more than 6 days ago, ISG will have little if any effect and is therefore generally not recommended. Measles is considered communicable during the prodrome (usually 4 days) and during the 4 days after the onset of rash.

Specific Immune Serum Globulin

Tetanus Immune Globulin (TIG): 250 units are used for wound prophylaxis; 3000 to 6000 units for therapy. (See Wound Management below.)

Vaccinia Immune Globulin (VIG): For severe, generalized vaccinia, eczema vaccinatum, vaccinia necrosum, ocular vaccinia, accidental exposure with extensive skin disease to vaccinia. Available commercially.

Pertussis Immune Globulin: Value not established.

Mumps Immune Globulin: Value not established.

Rabies Immune Globulin (HRIG): Recommended for postexposure rabies prophylaxis instead of animal serum.

Zoster Immune Globulin (ZIG): An investigative product; may prevent or modify varicella-zoster infections if given promptly within 72 hours of exposure. Must be obtained through the Center for Disease Control, Atlanta, Georgia.

Hepatitis-B Immune Globulin: For those exposed parenterally to hepatitis B and in those exposures related to renal dialysis units, HBIG, recently licensed for use, has proved of value.

Note that any type of immune serum globulin may cause biological false positive STS and TPI tests for syphilis. Smallpox vaccination may cause a false positive STS. These agents should, therefore, be used with caution while a diagnosis of syphilis is being considered.

Antitoxins

Diphtheria Antitoxin (equine origin): 10,000 units for unimmunized contacts only if daily observation not possible; 20,000 to 120,000 units for therapy. Screen for horse serum allergy before use.

Botulism Antitoxin (equine origin): Trivalent (A,B,E) antitoxin preferable for therapy. Bivalent (A,B) antitoxin also available. Screen for horse serum allergy before use of either trivalent or bivalent antitoxin. May be obtained through the local health department.

Tetanus Antitoxin (equine or bovine origin) or tetanus immune globulin (TIG) is preferable. The dose of TIG is 250 units at a site separate from Td (tetanus-diphtheria). Animal antitoxin, equine or bovine, dosage is 3000 to 5000 units.

Rabies Antiserum: Human rabies immune globulin (HRIG) is preferable.

Wound Management

Available evidence shows that complete primary immunization with tetanus toxoid provides long-range protective antitoxin levels. Additionally, protective antitoxin develops rapidly in response to a booster dose in persons who have previously received at least two doses of tetanus toxoid. Therefore, passive protection with TIG or antitoxin need be considered only when the patient has had less than two previous injections of tetanus toxoid or when the wound has been unattended for more than 24 hours.

Table 2 is a conservative guide to active and passive tetanus immunization at the time of wound treatment or debridement. It presumes a reliable knowledge of the patient's immunization history.

Combined tetanus-diphtheria toxoids (Td or DTP in children less than 7 years old) should be used instead of tetanus toxoid. If passive immunization is used, TIG is preferable to animal antitoxin because of longer protection and freedom from side reactions. For wounds of average severity, 250 units should be administered at a site separate from that used for accompanying Td. If TIG is unavailable, equine or bovine tetanus antitoxin may be used with proper precautions against serum sensitivity. The recommended dose of the latter products is 3000 to 5000 units.

Simultaneous Administration of Different Vaccines and Antibody Preparations

1. Inactivated (killed) vaccines can be given simultaneously at different sites (DTP, Td, typhoid, cholera, and so on).

2. Live virus vaccines may only be given in licensed combinations, such as M-R, M-M-R, or in instances where studies have shown adequate antibody response after simultaneous administration: (a) licensed combinations (pre-combined) measles-rubella virus vaccine, live, or measles-mumps-rubella vaccine, live; (b) polio vaccine and any one of the live virus vaccines or approved combinations; (c) smallpox and yellow fever vaccines; and (d) measles "Schwarz" strain and rubella "Cendehill" strain may be administered at separate sites. Other single antigen measles and rubella strains have not been tested at present for simultaneous administration.

3. Inactivated (killed) vaccines can be given simultaneously at separate sites with a live vaccine or approved live vaccine combinations.

4. When live virus vaccines are not given simultaneously, they should be given at least 2 weeks apart. Interference between live viruses is most likely to occur in the interval of 2 days to 2 weeks. The exception to this is smallpox and yellow fever vaccine. Studies have shown no interference between these vaccines even

TABLE 1. Common Immunizing Agents

AGENTS	PRIMARY IMMUNIZATION SCHEDULE	BOOSTER SCHEDULE	COMMENTS AND CONTRAINDICATIONS*
Diphtheria and tetanus toxoids and pertussis vaccine (DTP)	For children 2 months through 6 years: First: 0.5 ml. IM 2 months Second: 0.5 ml. IM 4 months Third: 0.5 ml. IM 6 months Fourth: 0.5 ml. IM 1 year later	Fifth dose DTP: 0.5 ml. IM at time of school entrance. (Many physicians elect not to give DTP after 4 years of age.)	If history of severe reaction, pertussis vaccine may be given separately at reduced dosage. Under 1 year of age, preferable site is anterolateral thigh. After last booster, use adult Td at 10-year intervals.
Tetanus and diphtheria toxoids, adult type (Td)	For children 7 years and older and adults (if no primary series of DTP): First: 0.5 ml. IM Second: 0.5 ml. IM 4 to 6 weeks later Third: 0.5 ml. IM 6 months to 1 year later	0.5 ml. IM every 10 years for life. (Consider booster for direct exposure to diphtheria on an individual basis.)	Preferable for children 7 and older because of sensitivity to pertussis antigen and high-dose diphtheria toxoid. Adsorbed toxoids superior to fluid in efficacy for both primary and booster immunizations. Use Td instead of tetanus toxoid for wound management.
Influenza virus vaccine (inactivated)	Adults: 0.5 ml. subcutaneously or IM as specified by manufacturer. Begin in September and complete by mid-November. Children: Not routinely recommended for healthy children. See manufacturer's package insert.	Yearly booster of vaccine prepared for current flu season.	Recommended for older persons, particularly those over age 60 years, and for persons of all ages with chronic debilitating conditions, including cardiovascular and respiratory disease, neoplasms and chronic metabolic disorders. May be considered for persons with other chronic diseases or for persons providing essential community services if sufficient quantities available. Contraindication: Allergy to vaccine components.
Measles virus vaccine, live, attenuated	15 months or over: 0.5 ml. subcutaneously	Not established	Fever and rash may occur 5 to 12 days after vaccination. Comments: Persons previously immunized only with killed measles vaccine or those immunized before 12 months of age should be reimmunized with live measles vaccine. Those who received ISG or measles immune globulin (MIG) with live measles vaccine should be individually evaluated for reimmunization. Contraindications: Altered immune states, including leukemia, lymphoma, and generalized malignancy; radiation, steroid, alkylating agent or antimetabolite therapy; severe febrile illness; untreated active tuberculosis; dysglobulinemia; pregnancy; hypersensitivity to vaccine components.
Rubella virus vaccine, live	For children 15 months to puberty: 0.5 ml. subcutaneously. Should be given in special circumstances to postpubertal females when: susceptibility has been established by HI test, pregnancy is ruled out at time of immunization, and reliable precautions are taken against pregnancy for at least 2 months following immunization. May also be useful in adolescent or adult males in preventing or controlling outbreaks in circumscribed population groups.	Not established	Comments: Rash, arthralgia, or transient arthritis can occur following immunization. Arthralgia more frequent after administration to adult females. Contraindications: Pregnancy, altered immune states, including leukemia, lymphoma, and generalized malignancy; radiation, steroid, alkylating agent or antimetabolite therapy; severe febrile illness; allergy to vaccine components.
Measles and rubella virus vaccine, live (M-R)	For children 15 months to puberty: 0.5 ml. subcutaneously	Not established	Contraindications: See measles virus vaccine and rubella virus vaccine.

Vaccine	Dose and schedule	Revaccination/booster	Contraindications and comments
Measles, mumps and rubella virus vaccine, live (M-M-R)	For children 15 months to puberty: 0.5 ml. subcutaneously	Not established	See measles virus vaccine, rubella virus vaccine, and mumps virus vaccine.
Mumps virus vaccine, live	Recommended for all susceptible individuals over 15 months of age: 0.5 ml. subcutaneously. Can be given to susceptible postpubertal males within 48 hours of exposure, however, efficacy not determined.	Not established	Contraindications: Altered immune states, including leukemia, lymphoma, and generalized malignancy; radiation, steroid, alkylating agent or antimetabolite therapy; concurrent illness; hypersensitivity to vaccine components.
Poliovirus vaccine, live, oral, trivalent (Sabin vaccine, TOPV)	For children 6 weeks through 18 years: First: 1 dose orally 2 months; Second: 1 dose orally 4 months; Third: 1 dose orally 12 months later. If circumstances do not permit the optimal interval between the second and third doses, the third dose may be given as early as 6 weeks after the second.	A dose of TOPV recommended at time of school entry. Need for additional boosters not established.	Contraindications: Altered immune states, including leukemia, lymphoma and generalized malignancy; radiation, steroid, alkylating agent or antimetabolite therapy. Not recommended routinely for adults in the United States. Unimmunized adults at special risk because of possible exposure to a case, or travel to endemic areas, should be immunized with TOPV as indicated for children. Booster doses are not necessary for frequent travelers.
Typhoid vaccine (inactivated)	6 months through 9 years: First: 0.25 ml. subcutaneously; Second: 0.25 ml. subcutaneously 4 weeks later. 10 years or older: First: 0.5 ml. subcutaneously; Second: 0.5 ml. subcutaneously 4 weeks later	.25 to 0.5 ml. subcutaneously or 0.1 ml. intradermally every 3 years.	Recommended for persons *chronically* exposed to case or carrier, or to community outbreak; travel to highly endemic areas; high-risk laboratory workers. Intradermal boosters yield fewer systemic reactions. Do not use acetone-killed or dried vaccine intradermally.
Smallpox vaccine (live vaccinia virus)	Primary immunization: 12 months or older: Bifurcated needle recommended. (Dried vaccine must be reconstituted.) Sites: Outer aspect of arm over deltoid or triceps; *not* over scapula nor on thigh. After inoculation, wipe off excess vaccine with dry sterile gauze. No dressing needed. Primary vaccination successful if a typical vesicle appears within 6 to 8 days. Revaccination successful if vesicle or induration around a central lesion (which may be an ulcer or crust) appears within 6 to 8 days. If unsuccessful, repeat with reliable vaccine lot.	All persons on exposure to case. Revaccination every 3 years if indicated.	Not to be given routinely in the absence of special indications. Vaccination recommended only for persons traveling to endemic countries and for special laboratory workers. Not recommended for other groups. Avoid vaccination during pregnancy. Contraindicated when patient or household member has eczema or other forms of chronic dermatitis, when patient has agammaglobulinemia, generalized malignancy, leukemia or lymphoma, or is receiving radiation, steroid, alkylating agent or antimetabolite therapy.
New Vaccines Meningococcal polysaccharide vaccines			Vaccines for Groups A and C meningococcal infections are presently available for use. Evidence implies that the only effective use of these vaccines would be during outbreaks of type A or C infections. The supply available for outbreak control can be released only through the Center for Disease Control. The use of the vaccines for household contacts of isolated cases is not generally recommended. Surveillance and antibiotic prophylaxis are still the recommended approaches to household contacts of meningococcal disease. Immunization of persons traveling to and remaining in countries where epidemics are in progress may benefit from immunization, but the risk of a United States traveler acquiring the disease has been negligible in past epidemics.

*See package insert for details.

TABLE 2.   Guide to Tetanus Prophylaxis in Wound Management

HISTORY OF TETANUS IMMUNIZATION (DOSES)	CLEAN, MINOR WOUNDS		ALL OTHER WOUNDS	
	Td	TIG	Td	TIG
Uncertain	Yes	No	Yes	Yes
0 to 1	Yes	No	Yes	Yes
2	Yes	No	Yes	No*
3 or more	No†	No	No‡	No

*Unless wound more than 24 hours old.
†Unless more than 10 years since last dose.
‡Unless more than 5 years since last dose.

when administered in the 2 day to 2 week period.

5. Immune serum globulin (ISG) may depress antibody response to inactivated vaccines and may completely block antibody responses to live vaccines. ISG peaks 2 days after administration and has a half-life of 20 to 25 days. ISG may be administered as soon as 2 to 3 weeks after the administration of a vaccine, but should not be given simultaneously with live or killed vaccines. ISG given as long as 3 months before certain live virus vaccines, such as measles, may block antibody formation. Whole blood transfusions may have a similar effect because of the immune globulins it contains.

19

Allergy

Allergic Rhinitis

SHELDON C. SIEGEL, M.D.

Allergic rhinitis affects approximately 15 per cent of children and ranks high among the most common problems that pediatricians and family practitioners face. Although often considered a trivial illness, it is associated with a significant morbidity. The local discomfort and general malaise produced by the illness account for a huge annual expenditure for symptomatic medication and for considerable absenteeism from school and work. The most recent data from the National Health Survey reveal that in over 75 per cent of the patients afflicted, the symptoms were severe enough to require one or more physician visits in a single year. Furthermore, allergic rhinitis frequently contributes to sequelae such as hyperplastic rhinitis, nasal polyps, acute or chronic sinusitis and otitis media. Customarily its onset is in early childhood and persists throughout life.

The diagnosis is usually established by the characteristic symptom complex and physical findings. In addition to the symptoms of nasal stuffiness and rhinorrhea, early morning paroxysmal sneezing and itching of the nose, palate or pharynx are especially characteristic of this disorder. The nasal mucous membranes have a typical pale to bluish, moist, glistening and boggy appearance. The finding of eosinophilia in the nasal secretions of peripheral blood is particularly helpful in confirming the diagnosis. Corroborative skin tests or radioallergosorbent (RAST) tests with suspected allergens aid in determining whether specific IgE antibodies are present and in assessing whether immunotherapy may be indicated.

Allergic rhinitis may be seasonal or perennial, the former usually due to pollen or mold aeroallergens. Appropriate management obviously requires that it be differentiated from nonallergic causes of nasal congestion and rhinorrhea. Vasomotor rhinitis is the most common disorder mistaken as allergic rhinitis. Other conditions include rhinitis medicamentosa, deviated nasal septum, infectious rhinitis and nasal congestion due to drugs—rauwolfia derivatives, estrogen, and cromolyn. During pregnancy certain patients may be afflicted with symptoms of marked nasal congestion which usually resolves after termination of the pregnancy. Nasal congestion is also found in patients with hypothyroidism.

Successful management of seasonal and perennial allergic rhinitis depends upon three basic treatment approaches: avoidance of suspected allergens, pharmacologic therapy, and immunotherapy (hyposensitization).

AVOIDANCE THERAPY

When possible, the removal of allergens from the patient's environment or a patient's exposure to an allergen constitutes the simplest and most effective form of treatment. For example, if a patient is sensitive to a household pet, removal of the pet from the home is usually mandatory. Household items such as upholstered furniture, mattresses or rug pads may also contain animal danders and may be difficult to eliminate. When patients are sensitive to feathers or kapok, substitution with a "nonallergic" material such as foam rubber or Dacron may be helpful and is preferable to covering them with dust-proof encasings. However, old foam rubber can become moldy and should be discarded when this occurs.

When house dust is a causative factor, measures to decrease dust exposure, especially in the patient's bedroom, should be undertaken. Encasing of mattresses and box springs with plastic or airtight covers, elimination of rugs and dust-collecting items such as books, toys and chenille spreads, removal of upholstered furniture, cleaning furnace filters and maintenance of adequate humidity will all help to reduce dust concentrations. Detailed instructions as to the preparation of a dust-free bedroom can be obtained in any standard allergy text or from pharmaceutical firms manufacturing allergy extracts.

There is now ample evidence that some house dust mite species (particularly *Dermatophagoides pteronyssinus* and *D. farinae*) are a major allergenic component in house dust, although not all house dust–sensitive patients are mite-sensitive. These house dust mites are ubiquitous organisms throughout the world. The only effective method of controlling them are those same measures which are useful in decreasing house dust concentrations.

In homes with forced air heating or cooling systems, the installation of an efficient, centrally installed electrostatic precipitator or laminar-flow impingement high efficiency particulate air (HEPA) filter system will materially help in reducing dust and aeroallergens from the home. Generally, air filtering room units, irrespective of type or make, are relatively inefficient and ineffective in materially reducing exposure to air-borne allergens. In addition, some may generate irritant levels of ozone. Units which generate negative ions are also promoted as being beneficial for patients with allergic rhinitis; however, it has not been established that negative ions are of value in preventing or treating this disease.

Although molds are difficult to eliminate from a patient's environment, patients highly sensitive to these allergens may benefit from receiving detailed instructions as to likely sources of these offenders, as well as measures for treating the home for elimination of molds. Clothing stored in damp closets with poor circulation, attics, sealed-off rooms, indoor plants, shower stalls, basements, home foundations, air conditioners, humidifiers, and vaporizers are common indoor sources of mold growth. To avoid excess outdoor exposure to fungus spores, the patient should be advised against mowing the lawn, raking leaves, clearing brush, and working with mulch piles or stored farm products. For molds growing under a home, spraying with a Bordeaux mixture (5 lb. bag obtained from a nursery, mixed with 20 gallons of water) will reduce mold growth. Controlling mold growing on walls or molding inside a home can be accomplished by cleaning with 1 to 2 cups of kerosene in a pail of warm soapy water, by using Lysol or Zephiran, by spraying with X-14 Mildew Remover (calcium hypochlorite, 4.8 per cent), or by painting with fungus-inhibiting paints which are available in most commercial paint stores. Trioxymethylene powder and crystals of paradichlorobenzene will help to eliminate molds in limited areas of the home. Reducing humidity in closets by keeping an electric light on in the closet or by the use of silica gel, activated alumina or calcium chloride will also help to inhibit mold growth.

Although expensive and often impractical, removal of the patient to an area relatively free of the offending seasonal pollens may be especially helpful. For example, ragweed-sensitive patients will obtain substantial relief of symptoms by vacationing in northern coniferous areas or the Pacific Coast during the peak pollinating period (the last week in August and the first week in September). A brochure entitled "Hay Fever," published by the Allergy Foundation of America (801 Second Avenue, New York, N.Y. 10017), provides a list of those other areas in the United States where ragweed pollen may be avoided. During the pollinating season, avoidance of excessive exposure to the offending pollens can also be minimized by avoiding long automobile rides in the country, avoiding fields overgrown with grasses and weeds, keeping bedroom windows closed, and using air conditioners with adequate filters.

PHARMACOLOGIC THERAPY

The use of appropriate pharmacologic agents can be of great benefit to the patient with allergic rhinitis. The five major classes of drugs that have proved useful in the management of allergic rhinitis are antihistamines, sympathomimetics, anticholinergics, the corticosteroids and cromolyn sodium.

Antihistamines. These compounds are the most effective for controlling symptoms of nasal itching and sneezing and constitute the major type of drug currently used for the treatment of allergic rhinitis. They are thought to act as competitive inhibitors for histamine at receptor sites on reactive cells. To be effective, they must be given prior to histamine release and attachment of histamine at the receptor sites. Accordingly, chronic use during pollen seasons or persistently for patients with perennial allergic rhinitis is the best method of administration.

On the basis of their chemical structure, the antihistamines have been classified into five groups (Table 1). Patients failing to respond favorably or developing decreasing response

TABLE 1.   Classification of Antihistamines

DRUG (GENERIC AND TRADE NAME)	MANU-FACTURER	PREPARATIONS AVAILABLE	DOSAGE
ETHANOLAMINES			
Diphenhydramine (Benadryl) (Bax) (SK) (Fenyhist)	Parke-Davis McKesson SKF Mallard	Capsules: 25 and 50 mg. Elixir: 10 mg./4 ml. Injection: 10 and 50 mg./ml.	5 mg./kg./day in 3 or 4 divided doses Children over 10 kg.: 12.5 to 25 mg. 3 or 4 times a day
Carbinoxamine (Clistin)	McNeil	Tablets: 4 mg. Repeat action: 8 and 12 mg. Elixir: 4 mg./5 ml.	0.4 mg./kg./day in 3 or 4 divided doses Children 1–3 yr.: 2 mg. 3 or 4 times a day Children 3–6 yr.: 2–4 mg. 3 or 4 times a day Children over 6 yr.: 4 mg. 3 or 4 times a day
ETHYLENEDIAMINES			
Tripelennamine (Pyribenzamine)	CIBA	Tablets: 25 and 50 mg. Delayed action: 50 and 100 mg. Elixir: 37.5 mg./5 ml.	5 mg./kg./day in 3 or 4 divided doses Children: not to exceed 300 mg./24 hr.
Methapyrilene hydrochloride (Histadyl)	Lilly	Pulvules: 25 and 50 mg. Syrup: 20 mg./5 ml. Injection: 20 mg./ml.	5 mg./kg./day in 3 or 4 divided doses Children over 6 yr.: 25 mg. 3 or 4 times a day
ALKYLAMINES			
Chlorpheniramine maleate (Chlor-Trimeton)	Schering	Tablets: 4 mg. Repeat action: 8 and 12 mg. Syrup: 2 mg./5 ml. Injection: 100 mg./ml.	0.4 mg./kg./day in 3 or 4 divided doses Children over 6 yr.: 2 mg. 3 or 4 times a day Infants: 1 mg. 3 or 4 times a day
(Teldrin) (Histaspan) (Cosea) (Histex) (Drize M) (Allerbid Tymcaps)	SKF USV Alcon Mallard Ascher Amfre-Grant	Spansules: 8 and 12 mg. Spansules: 8 and 12 mg. Spansules: 8 and 12 mg. Sustained release capsules: 12 mg. Sustained release capsules: 8 mg. Sustained release capsules: 8 mg.	Long acting preparations: Children 6–12 yr.: 8 mg. A.M. or P.M. Children over 12 yr.: 8 mg. twice a day
Brompheniramine maleate (Dimetane)	Robins	Tablets: 4 mg. Repeat action: 8 and 12 mg. Elixir: 2 mg./5 ml. Injection: 10 and 100 mg./ml.	0.4 mg./kg./day in 3 or 4 divided doses Children over 6 yr.: 2 mg. 3 or 4 times a day

TABLE 1. Classification of Antihistamines (Continued)

DRUG (GENERIC AND TRADE NAME)	MANUFACTURER	PREPARATIONS AVAILABLE	DOSAGE
PIPERAZINES Cyclizine hydrochloride (Marezine)	Burroughs Wellcome	Tablets: 50 mg.	3 mg./kg./day in 3 divided doses Children over 6 yr.: 25 mg. 3 or 4 times a day
PHENOTHIAZINES Promethazine (Phenergan)	Wyeth	Tablets: 12.5 and 25 mg. Syrup: 6.25 mg./5 ml. Fortes syrup: 25 mg./5 ml. Suppositories: 25 and 50 mg. Injection: 25 and 50 mg./ml.	2 mg./kg./day in 3 or 4 divided doses Children over 6 yr.: 6.25 to 12.5 mg. three times a day
(Lemprometh) (Remsed)	Lemmon } Endo }	Tablets: 25 and 50 mg.	
MISCELLANEOUS Cyproheptadine hydrochloride (Periactin)	Merck, Sharp & Dohme	Tablets: 4 mg. Syrup: 2 mg./5 ml.	0.25 mg./kg./day in 3 or 4 divided doses Children over 6 yr.: 4 mg. 2 or 3 times a day, not to exceed 16 mg./day. Periactin should not be used in newborn or premature infants.
Hydroxyzine (Atarax)	Roerig	Tablets: 10, 25, 50 and 100 mg. Syrup: 10 mg./5 ml.	2 mg./kg./day in 3 or 4 divided doses Children over 6 yr.: 50 to 100 mg. in divided doses
(Vistaril)	Pfizer	Capsules: 25, 50 and 100 mg. Suspension: 25 mg./5 ml. Injection: 25 and 50 mg./ml.	Children under 6 yr.: 50 mg./day in divided doses

(tachyphylaxis) to an antihistamine of one group may have a good response to a drug from another group. Because of the large number of these drugs available, physicians should familiarize themselves with a few drugs from each group. The dosage of representative agents of each group is also given in Table 1.

A major limitation to the use of the antihistamines is their side effects, especially drying and sedating effects. Because of their drying effects they have in the past been considered undesirable in the patient who has both asthma and allergic rhinitis. Recent evidence suggests that they can be used in most patients with asthma without having any adverse effects on the course of their disease.

Sympathomimetic Drugs. Sympathomimetic drugs with primarily alpha-receptor activity are effective vasoconstrictors of vessels of the mucosal surface and, when used topically as nose drops or sprays, reduce nasal congestion. Prolonged topical administration of these agents results in progressively severe nasal obstruction owing to a rebound recongestion phenomenon (rhinitis medicamentosa). Accordingly, except for short-term circumstances, these topical agents are contraindicated for the treatment of allergic rhinitis. Administered orally, these agents are less effective. Phenylephrine, ephedrine, isoephedrine, phenylpropanolamine, and cyclopentamine are the more commonly used oral agents; most often they are used in combination with various antihistamines. Selective preparations and dosages are given in Table 2.

Anticholinergics. Atropine and other pharmacologically related drugs often relieve rhinorrhea. However, the desired therapeutic responses can rarely be obtained without concomitant side effects—drying of mouth, drying of secretions, tachycardia, and blurring of vision. Consequently they are not usually prescribed except in combination with an antihistamine and a sympathomimetic. The isopropamide iodide in Ornade (chlorpheniramine maleate, phenylpropanolamine hydrochloride, isopropamide iodide) is effective in drying secretions, but is available only in capsule form. It should not be used for children under 6 years of age, nor in patients for whom iodides are contraindicated. In older children who cannot swallow capsules, the spansules can be emptied from the capsule and the drug administered with a food such as applesauce.

Corticosteroids. Although these agents have a profound beneficial effect on allergic rhinitis, they are rarely indicated for the treatment of this condition. The established side effects and complications of oral corticosteroid therapy far outweigh the beneficial effects that may be desired in a disease with a negligible mortality. Nevertheless, their use for short periods of time, 1 or 2 weeks, during the height of a pollen season can be beneficial; the risk of administering these agents under these circumstances is minimal because of the self-limiting nature of the problem.

Topical nasal corticosteroids also usually produce excellent results in most patients with allergic rhinitis. One such preparation, available as a water-soluble dexamethasone, is delivered by a Freon-propelled aerosol unit (Turbinaire). At the recommended dose of 2 puffs in each nostril three times a day (0.08 mg. of dexamethasone per actuation), sufficient hormone is absorbed to cause systemic effects. Thus this preparation, as with systemic corticosteroids, is best limited for temporary use during the height of the pollen season and for weaning patients off topical sympathomimetic drugs. Newer topical corticosteroid agents (beclomethasone dipropionate,* triamcinolone acetonide and flunisolide), which are still under investigation in the United States of America and not available commercially, have been reported to be highly effective in the management of allergic rhinitis without producing any systemic side effects. However, with the long-term usage of these agents, hemorrhagic areas in the nasal mucosae and blood-tinged secretions have been reported. If initial reports are confirmed, these preparations, when approved by the Food and Drug Administration, will be extremely useful for selected patients.

Cromolyn Sodium. The administration of intranasal cromolyn sodium in powder form (10 mg. in each nostril) or as a 2 per cent solution administered three times daily has also been shown to be effective in some patients in alleviating symptoms from allergic rhinitis.† The only adverse effects which have been noted are irritation of the nasal mucosa due to the preservatives in the solution or due to the mechanical effects of the insufflated powder. Although the powder form in the United States has been approved only for the treatment of asthma, in recalcitrant cases unresponsive to other forms of treatment, the author has had patients use cromolyn sodium as they

---

*Beclomethasone dipropionate is available commercially as Vanceril.

†Manufacturer's warning: The use of cromolyn sodium is not recommended for children under 5 years of age.

TABLE 2.   Antihistamine and Sympathomimetic Combinations

TRADE NAME	CONTENTS	MANUFACTURER	PREPARATIONS AVAILABLE	DOSAGE
Actifed	2.5 mg. triprolidine 60 mg. pseudoephedrine	Burroughs Wellcome	Tablets	Children over 6 yr.: 1 three times a day
	1.25 mg. triprolidine 30 mg. pseudoephedrine/5 ml.		Syrup	Children over 6 yr.: 1-2 tsp. three times a day Children 1-6 yr.: ½ tsp. three times a day
Co-Pyronil	15 mg. pyrrobutamine 25 mg. methapyrilene 12.5 mg. cyclopentamine	Dista	Pulvules	Children over 6 yr.: 1-2 every 4 to 12 hours
	7.5 mg. pyrrobutamine 12.5 mg. methapyrilene 6.25 mg. cyclopentamine/5 ml.		Suspension	Children over 6 yr.: 1-2 tsp. every 4 to 12 hours
Demazin	4 mg. chlorpheniramine 20 mg. phenylephrine	Schering	Repetabs Tablets	Children over 12 yr.: 1-2 tablets twice a day
	1 mg. chlorpheniramine 2.5 mg. phenylephrine/5 ml.		Syrup	Children over 6 yr.: 1-2 tsp. every 4 hours
Dimetapp	12 mg. brompheniramine 15 mg. phenylephrine 15 mg. phenylpropanolamine	Robins	Extentabs	Children over 12 yr.: 1 twice a day
	4 mg. brompheniramine 5 mg. phenylephrine 5 mg. phenylpropanolamine/ 5 ml.		Elixir	Children over 4 yr.: 1 tsp. 3 or 4 times a day Children 1-4 yr.: ½ tsp. 3 or 4 times a day

Novahistine Fortis / Novahistine Melet	2 mg. chlorpheniramine 10 mg. phenylephrine	Dow	Tablets, capsules and chewable	Children 6-12 yr.: 1 every 3 or 4 hours
Novahistine elixir	2 mg. chlorpheniramine 18.75 mg. phenylpropanola-mine/5 ml.	Dow	Exlixir	Children over 6 yr.: 1 tsp. every 4 hours not to exceed 4 doses
Novahistine LP	4 mg. chlorpheniramine 20 mg. phenylephrine	Dow	Long-acting tablet	Children over 6 yr.: 1 tablet
Novafed A	8 mg. chlorpheniramine 120 mg. pseudoephrine	Dow	Capsule	Children over 12 yr.: 1 capsule twice a day
Pyribenzamine ephedrine	25 mg. tripelennamine 12 mg. ephedrine	CIBA	Tablets	Children over 12 yr.: 1 tablet every 4 hours
Rondec	2.5 mg. carbinoxamine 60 mg. pseudoephedrine/ tablet or 5 ml.	Ross	Filmtab and chewable tablets	Children over 6 yr.: 1 tablet 4 times a day
			Syrup	Children over 6 yr.: 1 tsp. 4 times a day
	1 mg. carbinoxamine 30 mg. pseudoephedrine per ml. (dropperful)		Drops	Children under 6 yr. 1-3 mo.: ¼ ml. 4 times a day 4-6 mo.: ½ ml. 4 times a day 7-9 mo.: ¾ ml. 4 times a day 10-17 mo.: 1 ml. 4 times a day

would snuff, sniffing the contents of a half-capsule (10 mg.) into each nostril, with good results in older children.

IMMUNOTHERAPY

When environmental control measures and drug therapy prove to be inadequate for controlling symptoms, consideration should be given to a course of immunotherapy. Although first described in 1911, it has only been in recent years that its effectiveness in the management of ragweed and grass pollinosis has been firmly established by well controlled studies, supported by immunologic in vitro data. Evidence of its efficacy with other specific allergens is not as well proved and difficult to assess; nevertheless, when patients are unresponsive to other approaches to therapy, immunotherapy is worth a trial when it can be reasonably demonstrated that the patient is sensitive to these allergens by history, skin testing, RAST, or inhalation challenge. In addition to establishing a causal relationship to the allergen in question, other factors must be considered in determining whether immunotherapy should be undertaken. Among these are the age of the patient, the severity and duration of the symptoms, response to other less costly and involved therapy, the presence of concomitant asthma, incidence and severity of complications, and the nature of the allergen or allergies involved.

The details and rationale of the methodology of this form of therapy are beyond the scope of this article and can be found in all standard allergy texts. Basically the technique consists of repeated injections of gradually increasing doses of aqueous extracts made from the offending allergenic substances (pollens, fungi, dust, danders, insect antigens). Optimal results are achieved by administering the highest dose of extract that is safely tolerated. Initially the injections are usually given once or twice a week. Once the highest tolerated dose has been reached, the interval between this maintenance dose is gradually lengthened up to 6 week intervals. The duration of therapy depends on the response of the patient.

In recent years numerous modifications of the conventional aqueous extracts as well as the method of administering the antigens have been proposed. Most extract alteration has been designed to increase the dosage of antigen employed with the use of fewer injections. For this purpose aqueous extracts which have been alum precipitated are now commercially available and their use appears promising. These extracts must be distinguished from ex-

tracts made with the organic solvent pyridine and then alum precipitated. These latter extracts contain little antigen, and their clinical effectiveness needs further clarification.

A number of other techniques of immunotherapy have been advocated for the treatment of allergic rhinitis and other allergic disorders. These controversial methods include the use of low dosages of antigen, titration neutralization, and sublingual desensitization. These procedures are not supported by basic or controlled clinical research, nor is their therapeutic validity substantiated.

Bronchial Asthma

HENRY LEVISON, M.D., F.R.C.P. (C)

Asthma is characterized by an increased responsiveness of the airways to various stimuli, and manifested by slowing of forced expiration; the degree of severity may alter spontaneously or as a result of therapy. The term asthma may be modified by words or phrases indicating its etiology, factors provoking attacks, or its duration. (This is the definition of asthma now recommended by a Joint Committee of the American Thoracic Society and the American College of Chest Physicians.) Pathologically, there is hypertrophy of bronchial smooth muscle, submucosal edema, and hypersecretion of viscous mucus.

Since airway obstruction in asthma is reversible, continuous disability in asthmatic patients is never acceptable. Bronchial asthma is an extremely variable disease and treatment must be tailored to the needs of each patient; thus, treatment plans must take into account differences in pathogenetic mechanisms, drug metabolism, and tolerance for individual classes of drugs. Patients with seasonal disease and clearly identifiable immunopathogenic mechanisms may benefit from hyposensitization. This type of patient, as well as those exposed to immunogenic materials at their work, may also benefit from environmental control or change in occupation.

Patients with mild infrequent (once or twice a year) episodes of asthma can be treated with bronchodilators intermittently, although recent studies unequivocally show that defects in ventilatory function may persist after recovery from acute asthmatic episodes. More important, residual peripheral airway obstruction may adversely affect the lung's response to asthmogenic stimuli, a fact evidenced by most asthmatic patients' benefit from continuous bronchodilator therapy even in the absence of symptoms. With these considerations in mind, some generalizations regarding the care of patients with chronic asthma can be made.

GENERAL MEASURES

Education of the patient and his family as to the characteristics of asthma and the futility of sporadic medication in comparison with continuous prophylaxis will pay dividends in compliance with instructions. Continuing support and reassurance are important. Environmental control may imply complete avoidance of certain allergens or measures to minimize exposure to them. Self-control over emotional upheaval, and avoidance of irritants, such as tobacco smoke, strong odors, temperature extremes, wind, dust, or cold drinks, may be valuable adjuncts in selected patients. Physical fitness and ideal body weight are also desirable.

METHYLXANTHINES (PHOSPHODIESTERASE INHIBITORS)

Theophylline is a xanthine derivative which produces bronchodilation by increasing the intracellular concentration of cyclic AMP and by inhibiting the enzyme (phosphodiesterase) responsible for the metabolism of cAMP. These drugs can be given as tablets or suppositories or by injection. Substances that inhibit phosphodiesterase can reverse bronchoconstriction or prevent it. They share a common pathway with the β-sympathomimetic drugs, which have a similar ability to produce bronchodilation. However, phosphodiesterase inhibitors are said to be capable of producing relief where *beta* stimulants have failed, possibly because intracellular receptors remain responsive when desensitized. Severe asthma may become relatively refractory to these xanthine derivatives, but the refractoriness may be overcome with corticosteroids.

Table 1 lists anhydrous theophylline equivalents of representative formulations. The usual recommended oral dose of anhydrous theophylline or its equivalent is 6 mg./kg. every 6 hours. The maximum dose should not exceed 900 mg./day or 24 mg./kg./day, whichever is less, for children up to 9 years of age. Over the age of 9 years the maximum dose is 900 mg./day or 19 mg./kg./day (the lesser of the two). Using sustained-release theophylline (see Table 1) the dosage interval is 8 hours. Therapeutic levels of theophylline between 10 and 20 mg./liter of plasma should be sought; much of the failure attributed to this class of drugs is the result of inadequate levels.

The half-life of theophylline given orally or intravenously varies: in infants, from 18 to

TABLE 1. Anhydrous Theophylline Equivalents of Representative Theophylline Formulations

BRAND NAME	STRENGTH	EFFECTIVE "FREE" THEOPHYLLINE (*per cent*)
Liquids		
Elixophyllin	5.3 mg./ml.	100
Elixophyllin—pediatric suspension	20 mg./ml.	100
Slo-phyllin GG	10 mg./ml.	100
Quibron	10 mg./ml.	100
Somophyllin	18 mg./ml.	85
Choledyl elixir	20 mg./ml.	64
Theophyl-225	7.5 mg./ml.	100
Tablets		
Theolair	125 mg./tablet	100
Theolair	250 mg./tablet	100
Slo-phyllin	100 mg./tablet	100
Slo-phyllin	200 mg./tablet	100
Theophyl	225 mg./tablet	100
Aminophylline	100 mg./tablet	80
Aminophylline	200 mg./tablet	80
Choledyl*	100 mg./tablet	64
Choledyl*	200 mg./tablet	64
Rectal Solution		
Somophyllin	60 mg./ml.	80
SUSTAINED-RELEASE PRODUCTS		
Gyrocaps		
Slo-phyllin	60 mg.	100
Slo-phyllin	125 mg.	100
Slo-phyllin	200 mg.	100
Tablets		
Theo-Dur	100 mg.	100
Theo-Dur	300 mg.	100

*Erratic absorption.

24 hours; in children, from 3 to 5 hours; and in adults, from 2.9 to 9.5 hours; there is great individual variation due to variable metabolism. The drug is metabolized by the liver, and renal clearance plays a minor role in its elimination (unchanged theophylline = <10 per cent of total urinary metabolites). Recently it has been shown that liver disease, congestive heart failure and smoking are major factors determining the disposition rate of theophylline.

The side effects of theophylline are dyspepsia, nausea, vomiting, headache, dizziness and, occasionally, palpitations. Many of the liquid preparations are in an alcohol base, which may contribute to gastrointestinal upset. If gastrointestinal side effects occur, they can often be overcome by introducing a smaller dose of theophylline and increasing it up to the recommended dose. Thoughtful selection and careful titration of dose to the severity of symptoms, tolerance and metabolic requirements in individual cases are imperative. The oral route is preferred; theophylline can be given as a rectal solution to treat an acute episode, but rectal suppositories are unreliably absorbed and frequently irritating.

β-ADRENOCEPTOR STIMULANTS

Adrenergic receptors can be divided into two classes, α and β; the latter are of two types, β-1 and β-2. The α-receptors mediate arterial constriction, β-1 receptors mediate cardiac response, and β-2 receptors mediate relaxation of the circular bronchial muscle and the arterial tree.

Adrenergic agents in common use are listed in Table 2. They all stimulate β-receptors, but the relative effects on β-1 and β-2 receptors can vary. The agents that directly stimulate β-1 and β-2 receptors equally are epinephrine and isoprenaline (isoproterenol); epinephrine also stimulates α-receptors. Those that selectively stimulate β-2 receptors by direct action are salbutamol, terbutaline, isoetharine and metaproterenol. Ephedrine has now been superseded by the newer selective β agents. A number of oral bronchodilators combine theophylline with ephedrine but the combination may cause a higher incidence of adverse effects than theophylline alone without a corresponding benefit, and is more costly.

Methods of use and dosages of the β-stimulating agents are listed in Table 3. *These drugs are most efficacious when inhaled.* When using inhaled preparations on an outpatient basis, patients should receive explicit instructions in their use and be instructed to seek a physician's advice if they require more than the recommended daily dose. In an acute exacerbation if the inhaled drugs are not available, subcutaneous aqueous epinephrine (1:1000), 0.01 mg./kg. to a maximum of 0.3 mg., should be given.

CROMOLYN SODIUM: DISODIUM CROMOGLYCATE

This drug is chemically related to chromone khellin, a muscle relaxant used as an antispasmodic for renal colic. Its effectiveness depends upon its ability to inhibit the release of histamine and SRS-A from sensitized mast cells. The drug is a prophylactic agent: it will not reverse bronchoconstriction once this has occurred. Disodium cromoglycate cannot be taken by mouth or injection; it is inhaled as a powder from a Spinhaler, a method that depends on the patient's ability and willingness to cooperate. The usual prophylactic dose is 1 Spincap (20 mg.) four times daily, but patients who experience exercise-induced asthma attacks only, can prevent them by inhaling the drug 10 minutes beforehand.*

Patients for whom disodium cromoglycate is prescribed, especially those who are steroid-dependent, may be able to reduce or eliminate their steroid requirement. Studies have also shown no significant difference in rates of therapeutic benefit in patients who receive the full dosage and those maintained on a reduced regimen. The only unwanted effect of disodium cromoglycate is the transient irritation of the throat and larynx which occurs just after an inhalation. This can be overcome by administering a bronchodilator aerosol immediately before the cromolyn.

CORTICOSTEROIDS

In most instances, continuing dyspnea despite the full use of theophylline, β-stimulants and disodium cromoglycate can be relieved by the systemic administration of corticosteroids. However, even small doses of steroids may give rise to numerous unwanted effects.

Several mechanisms have been postulated for the mode of action of corticosteroids in allergic diseases. In vivo and in vitro studies have virtually excluded the possibility that steroids inhibit the production of antibodies or interfere with the antigen-antibody interaction that occurs in type 1 reactions. Experimental data strongly suggest that steroids modify symptoms of bronchial asthma by one or all of the following: (1) interference in the production of histamine; (2) a direct vasoconstrictor effect; (3) relaxation of bronchial smooth muscle; and (4) the potentiation of catecholamines.

In children, prednisone, 0.5 mg./kg., daily on alternate days is usually well tolerated. In some patients alternate-day therapy is inadequate for satisfactory control of symptoms. With alternate-day therapy, untoward side effects are absent in many cases, and even with relatively high doses the integrity of the adrenal-pituitary axis is maintained, and side effects are minimal. Attempts to reduce the

TABLE 2.   Receptor Activity of Adrenergic Drugs in Common Use

DRUG	ALPHA	BETA-1	BETA-2
Phenylephrine	+	–	–
Epinephrine	+	+	+
Ephedrine	+	+	+
Isoproterenol	–	+	+
Isoetharine	–	±	+
Metaproterenol	–	±	+
Terbutaline	–	±	+
Salbutamol	–	–	+

*Manufacturer's precaution: Cromolyn sodium is not recommended for children under 5 years of age.

TABLE 3.   Beta-Adrenergic Bronchodilators

| DRUG | FORMULATION AND DOSAGE | | |
	Metered Aerosol	*Nebulizer**	*Oral Preparation*
Isoproterenol (Isuprel)	75 μg./puff; 1 puff up to 4 times daily for ages 6 to 14 years. Over age 14, 2 puffs 4 times daily.	0.5 per cent solution; 0.25 ml. up to 4 times daily. After age 8, 0.5 ml. 4 times daily.	Poor oral absorption
Metaproterenol (Alupent)	750 μg./puff; 1 puff up to 4 times daily for ages 6 to 14 years. Over age 14, 2 puffs 4 times daily.	2 per cent solution; 0.25 ml. up to 4 times daily. After age 8, 0.5 ml. 4 times daily.	2.5 mg./kg./dose up to 3 times daily.
Salbutamol (Ventolin)	100 μg./puff; 1 puff up to 4 times daily for ages 6 to 14 years. Over age 14, 2 puffs 4 times daily.	0.5 per cent solution; 0.25 ml. up to 4 times daily. After age 8, 0.5 ml. 4 times daily.	0.05 mg./kg./dose up to 3 times daily.
Terbutaline (Bricanyl)†	250 μg./puff; 1 puff up to 4 times daily for ages 6 to 14 years. Over age 14, 2 puffs 4 times daily.	0.5 per cent solution; 0.25 ml. up to 4 times daily. After age 8, 0.5 ml. 4 times daily.	0.05 mg./kg./dose up to 3 times daily.
Isoetharine (Bronkosol)	340 μg./puff; 1 puff up to 4 times daily for ages 6 to 14 years. Over age 14, 2 puffs 4 times daily.	1.0 per cent solution; 0.25 ml. up to 4 times daily. After age 8, 0.5 ml. 4 times daily.	Poor oral absorption

*All solutions made up to 2 ml. with normal saline.
†May be given subcutaneously, 0.03 to 0.05 mg./kg./dose.

systemic effects of these drugs have resulted in the introduction of a steroid aerosol (beclomethasone dipropionate), which contains the surface-active poorly absorbed corticosteroid. This agent, whose mechanism of action is not fully understood, provides relief from asthma without depression of the hypothalamic-pituitary axis, even after several years' use in the recommended doses. A drawback is the container, a pressurized canister that can be used only by children who can activate the spray. The usual dosage is 100 μg. four times daily.

The only unwanted effect of steroid aerosol *in the recommended dosage* is fungal infection of the tongue, pharynx and larynx. This occurs in about 5 to 10 per cent of patients, the incidence rising with increasing dosage. The incidence can be reduced by washing out the mouth with water after inhalation or by administering an antifungal agent such as amphotericin B (0.1 mg. of amphotericin B in 1 ml. of distilled water) simultaneously. Fungal infection of the lung has not been reported. Patients should be warned not to exceed the recommended dosage; larger doses of steroid aerosols interfere with adrenal function. Furthermore, this form of therapy is useless during acute attacks. Prednisone should be reinstituted immediately, orally or intravenously.

OTHER DRUGS

Several new drugs in use in other countries are not yet commercially available in the United States.

Parasympatholytic Agents. Recognition that the parasympatholytic nervous system participates in the antigen-antibody reaction has supported the use of atropine and atropine-like drugs. Atropine compounds have been used in asthmatic subjects in England for many years, and atropine has been given by inhalation experimentally in the United States. The bronchodilator effect is slightly longer after inhalation of an aerosol of atropine methylnitrate (SCH 1000) than after isoproterenol, and is even greater with both combined. SCH 1000, which is marketed as a metered aerosol, has been used in Britain and the United States and is now undergoing large scale clinical testing. The dosage is one puff (20 μg.) to be inhaled four times daily. This drug does not alter the blood gases or heart rate or cause dryness of the mouth. Preliminary studies in our laboratory indicate that the inhalation of 40 μg. of SCH 1000 produces bronchodilation comparable to that of salbutamol.

MOBILIZATION OF BRONCHIAL SECRETIONS

Dehydration, a characteristic of moderate to severe asthma, should be corrected as quickly as possible. Simple hydration with clear fluids at room temperature is probably the most effective way to liquefy and mobilize secretions. Antihistamines, although useful in some cases, may accentuate local respiratory tract dehydration if given before fluid replacement. Expectorants have been advocated to facilitate removal of secretions by reducing their viscosity and render cough more productive, but there is no convincing evidence clinically or by indices of respiratory function that they do this.

EXERCISE-INDUCED BRONCHOSPASM

Exercise is a well-recognized cause of acute airway obstruction (treadmill testing causes exercise-induced bronchospasm in approximately 70 per cent of patients with asthma). In some patients, this is their only disability and it may severely restrict life-style. Exercise-induced bronchospasm can be prevented by the inhalation of 1 capsule of cromolyn 10 to 30 minutes before exercise or the inhalation of two puffs of a β-agent 30 minutes before exercise; oral β-agents are relatively ineffective and need to be administered 1 to 2 hours prior to exercise.

STATUS ASTHMATICUS

This is difficult to define but usually refers to acute respiratory difficulty not responsive to the usual outpatient bronchodilator regimen (inhalation of a β-agent or subcutaneous administration of epinephrine). The minimal investigations required in managing a patient in status asthmaticus are a chest radiograph for detection atelectasis, pneumonia, pneumothorax or pneumomediastinum and arterial blood gases to monitor therapy.

Therapy.   Hypoxia is usual, requiring an oxygen concentration of 25 to 30 per cent or more to provide physiologic levels of arterial oxygen tension.

These patients may be dehydrated because of diminished intake and excessive loss of fluids. In general, it is recommended that they receive 1¼ times usual maintenance requirements. In some cases the chest radiograph shows left atrial enlargement and signs of pulmonary interstitial fluid accumulation, and overloading with fluid should be avoided.

Metabolic acidosis should be corrected with sodium bicarbonate as soon as possible, since it appears to reduce the therapeutic efficacy of bronchodilators. A simple formula for determining the dose of bicarbonate in mEq is $0.3 \times$ body weight in kg $\times$ base deficit, given slowly and monitored with repeated blood gas determinations.

STEROIDS.   The usual dosage is 3 to 4 mg./kg. of hydrocortisone, or 1 mg./kg. of methylprednisolone given intravenously every 4 to 6 hours. Methylprednisolone has the advantage of producing less salt retention, and its dosage is readily interchanged with an oral preparation of prednisone, which most patients require as their condition improves after status asthmaticus.

THEOPHYLLINE.   The recommended dose is 5 mg./kg. intravenously as a bolus given over 20 minutes every 6 hours. Alternatively, aminophylline can be given intravenously in a loading dose (6 mg./kg. over 20 minutes) and then 1 mg./kg./hour. With the latter method, blood levels of theophylline must be monitored.

β-ADRENERGIC BRONCHODILATORS.   Inhaled salbutamol should be given every 4 hours; if it is not available, metaproterenol or isoproterenol can be given (see Table 3). The majority of patients benefit from this form of therapy. However, a small percentage remain severely ill, with arterial CO_2 tension rising above 60 mm. Hg. In such cases isoproterenol should be given intravenously, but with extreme caution because the agent affects β-1 receptors and thus has considerable cardiac effects, necessitating continuous monitoring of the electrocardiogram and blood pressure. A constant infusion pump is used to infuse isoproterenol, and an arterial line must be inserted for continuous measurement of arterial O_2 and CO_2 tensions and pH. The dosage is 0.1 μg./kg./min. initially, and this is doubled every 15 minutes until bronchospasm is broken or any limiting factor is reached. During this time intravenous theophylline is discontinued.

In our institution the limiting factors of isoproterenol infusion are a pulse rate greater than 200 beats per minute, cardiac arrhythmias (such as ventricular tachycardia, ventricular fibrillation and frequent ventricular atopic beats), or progressive deterioration clinically or in blood gas levels, despite therapy. Most patients respond to a dose of 0.8 μg./kg./min. If the patient's condition continues to deteriorate, artificial ventilation will be required. (It is not within the scope of this article to describe the management of the patient with status asthmaticus who requires artificial ventilation.) As soon as a patient's condition responds to intravenous isoproterenol, the dose should be reduced slowly and the infusion discontinued by 24 hours. Salbutamol, a more specific β-2 agonist, is now available as an intravenous preparaton. It is less likely to produce cardiac arrhythmias but still requires careful cardiac monitoring and continuous measurement of arterial O_2 and CO_2 tensions and pH. Salbutamol should be given intravenously in a dose of 2.5 to 7.5 μg./kg./hr., which may be given as a continuous infusion or as a bolus over 10 minutes. Antibiotics are not indicated in status asthmaticus unless there is clinical or radiological evidence of infection.

Serum Sickness

VICTOR C. VAUGHAN, III, M.D.

Serum sickness is a prototype of disease due to the protein complexes formed by antigen and antibody (immune complex disease). It was first delineated early in this century when animal sera were commonly used in the treatment of such illnesses as diphtheria and tetanus. Immune complex disease is now more commonly the result of immunologic reactions to drugs than to sera, probably most often to penicillin; it also includes arthritides associated with rubella, hepatitis A and B, adenoviruses, vaccinia, variola, Hodgkin disease, insect stings and other conditions. Immune complex disease is responsible for some manifestations of systemic lupus erythematosus and periarteritis nodosa.

Two pathophysiologic processes predominate in serum sickness, which seems to depend upon a reaction occurring under conditions of antigen excess for some of its manifestations and upon previous exposure to the antigen for other features in some patients. The first process is the formation of antigen-antibody complexes; the second process involves the release of histamine and other chemical mediators from host cells through the interaction of these cells with antigen or complexes. The first of these reactions predominantly involves IgG and IgM antibodies; the second involves IgE.

The clinical features of serum sickness depend upon the interrelation of these two processes. It seems likely that the increased vascular permeability due to reaction with IgE is necessary for the movement of immune complexes into those tissues where they will cause their characteristic clinical effects. The immune complexes are predominantly responsible for fever, adenopathy, arthritis, nephritis, rare manifestations of serum sickness in the central nervous system and peripheral nerves, and for the swelling at the site of injection (Arthus phenomenon). Immune complexes fix complement in involved areas. The chemical mediators dependent upon IgE are responsible for urticaria, angioedema, and other manifestations of the immediate type of hypersensitivity.

The onset of serum sickness typically occurs about 7 to 10 days after the injection of a relatively large amount of foreign antigen under conditions of antigen excess. When the formation of antibody to this antigen begins, the concentration of the antigen begins to fall, reaching very low levels at about the time symptoms begin and free antibody first appears in serum, after which the titer of antibody rises rapidly. Serum sickness is typically ushered in by swelling at the site of the injection of serum if this has been intramuscular or subcutaneous, by urticaria and often angioedema, and then by the occurrence of fever, adenopathy, and swelling, tenderness, and inflammation of joints. The renal disease prominent in some animals is generally inconspicuous in man, there being generally only some proteinuria and perhaps microscopic hematuria. Central nervous system symptoms or a peripheral neuropathy of the Guillain-Barré type may rarely occur. All these reactions are generally reversible, sequelae being very unusual.

When there has been previous experience with the provocative antigen, the timetable of events may be considerably accelerated, to a day or two or less, or antibodies of the IgE variety may cause the onset of the reaction to be explosive, as in the case of anaphylactic shock.

The diagnosis of serum sickness is predominantly clinical, resting upon a history of exposure to serum or to drugs, upon clinical manifestations, and upon typical findings in blood and urine. The serologic diagnosis of serum sickness is easier for the illness precipitated by animal sera than for that precipitated by drugs. Inasmuch as serum sickness due to drugs is probably dependent upon complexes of drugs with normal serum proteins, the verification of the basic immunologic mechanisms is not so easy as when foreign proteins are involved.

The treatment of serum sickness is suggested by the clinical findings in the individual instance. In the case of patients receiving drugs which may be responsible for manifestations of serum sickness, it will generally be expedient to discontinue their administration, and to find effective substitutes if necessary.

For those manifestations mediated by the wheal and flare response to IgE antibodies, which are often the most conspicuous signs and symptoms in acute serum sickness, administration of epinephrine, ephedrine, and antihistaminics will be the most useful measures. Epinephrine is likely to give the most rapid relief, and ephedrine may sometimes be used effectively to maintain relief from urticaria or angioedema once a response has been initiated by epinephrine. The concomitant use of antihistaminics, such as diphenhydramine, is usually also helpful, and is sometimes more effective than use of epinephrine and its analogs.

For the clinical effects of deposition of immune complexes in involved tissues there is no specific therapy, the effects being generally spontaneously reversible in a few days' time. Aspirin in the usual dosage is often highly effective for the relief of fever and tenderness and swelling in joints. Corticosteroids will abate the inflammatory reaction that takes place at the site of deposition of immune complexes in affected tissues. Prednisone, 1 to 2 mg./kg./day, may be given for severe manifestations and will generally be required for a few days only.

The prognosis for recovery from serum sickness is very good. The duration of illness will depend upon the rapidity with which the offending antigen is removed from the body. In the case of repository penicillin, symptoms may last for some weeks; more often the duration of serum sickness is less than a week. When the cause of symptoms or signs due to a serum sickness type of immune response is not identified, continued exposure to antigens or drugs may produce prolonged clinical manifestations. Drug fever may be a rather common example, often with a few or no other signs of serum sickness.

The prevention of serum sickness is often possible. The use of animal sera in management of illnesses in man ought to be regarded as contraindicated where immune sera of human origin exist. There is no adequate reason now, for example, to use sera of animal origin for the prophylaxis or treatment of diphtheria or tetanus. Normal schedules of active immunization should be kept up to date.

A further measure helpful in prevention of serum sickness is the use of drugs in children only upon adequate indication, as well as their administration by the oral route when possible rather than parenteral, especially in the case of penicillin.

If unusual circumstances demand the use of animal sera, an adequate history of previous exposure or of clinical allergies due to animal products must be taken, and appropriate tests with the proposed serum should be given prior to its administration in order to avoid the possibility of a fulminant immunological response such as anaphylactic shock. In the case of positive immunologic tests to a serum prior to its administration, programs of rapid desensitization may be used if there is no possible substitute. These require the dilution of the serum to 1:20 or more dilute, and the administration of small doses (beginning with 0.05 ml.) every 15 to 20 minutes, doubling the dose each time so long as no reaction occurs, until the required total dose is given. If a reaction occurs and can be controlled with medication, desensitization is resumed, beginning with half the dose which gave the reaction. Analogous schedules of desensitization may be used to permit the administration of penicillin under exceptional circumstances, such as in the case of a patient needing penicillin for the management of bacterial endocarditis. It should be understood, however, that such forms of desensitization are designed to prevent *acute* (anaphylactic or wheal-and-flare) reactions, not serum sickness itself. Those susceptible to serum sickness may continue at risk, under the conditions of antigen excess established.

Angioneurotic Edema

FRED S. ROSEN, M.D., *and*
HARVEY R. COLTEN, M.D.

Angioneurotic edema is a symptom of circumscribed areas of swelling of the subcutaneous tissue. The swelling is never discolored or red, is never painful, and usually does not itch.

HEREDITARY ANGIONEUROTIC EDEMA

Affected individuals are prone to sudden, unheralded attacks of circumscribed subcutaneous edema. The swelling, which may be severe enough to cause remarkable disfigurement of the affected part, evolves very quickly and usually subsides within 72 hours. There is no discoloration, redness, pain, or itching. Despite the undistinguished appearance of the edema, involvement of the mucous membranes of the hypopharynx and larynx may result in untimely death from asphyxiation.

Treatment. Daily administration of methyl testosterone linguets has prevented attacks of angioedema in approximately one third to one half of patients. It must be taken daily in a single dose of 10 to 25 mg. The mechanism of its effect is not known. Methyl testosterone therapy is not recommended for children.

Epsilon-aminocaproic acid has been successful in halting attacks of angioedema.* However, the side effects with chronic administration of this agent are so annoying

---

*This use of epsilon-aminocaproic acid is not mentioned in the manufacturer's instructions.

that its usage has been very limited. An analogue, tranexamic acid, has been found to have fewer side effects, causing only occasional minor gastrointestinal distress. In doses of 1 to 3 gm./day orally, it has proved effective in aborting attacks of angioedema. The drug has not yet been released by the Food and Drug Administration.

Infusions of plasma have been recommended in the therapy of attacks of angioedema. However, this approach is not recommended by us because it has been of questionable value and is not innocuous in the view of several observers who have attempted to use it. It is not possible to raise the level of C1 inhibitor (deficient in the inherited form of the disease) above 7 mg./100 ml., a level under which attacks of angioedema occur, except by infusing very large amounts of plasma. For instance, 100 ml. of plasma would raise the inhibitor level by 1 mg./100 ml. in a 40 kg. child. Fresh plasma contains more substrate for C1 than inhibitor; consequently, its administration early in the course of an attack, prior to the onset of tachyphylaxis, might in fact exacerbate the symptoms. Such an event has been observed.

Epinephrine is useful in controlling swelling in very few patients. Hydrocortisone also provides benefit very rarely in patients. Antihistamines are of no use. Intravenous administration of diuretics, such as meralluride or ethacrynic acid,* is helpful in halting the progression of life-threatening angioedema.

Tracheostomy should be performed without hesitation in patients with laryngeal obstruction. It is frequently life-saving.

NONHEREDITARY ANGIONEUROTIC EDEMA

Nonhereditary angioneurotic edema is generally a benign condition of diverse etiology. Food ingestion, drugs, and insect stings in appropriately sensitive individuals, and psychic or physical factors may precipitate attacks of angioedema. The clinical consequences of angioedema are a function of the site involved; angioedema of the larynx may be fatal if prompt therapy is not instituted. Angioedema secondary to acute infection or to connective tissue disorder must be differentiated, since the diagnostic and therapeutic efforts must be specific for these primary diseases.

In the case of angioedema due to an obvious precipitating event (e.g., insect sting), an etiologic diagnosis by means of history and skin

testing is not difficult. Avoidance of exposure, immunotherapy, and the availability of an emergency kit consisting of aqueous epinephrine, a tourniquet, ephedrine, and an antihistamine (such as diphenhydramine) are generally successful in preventing subsequent episodes of angioedema. The emergency kit should be carried by the patient at all times during periods when exposure to stinging insects is likely.

In angioedema due for example to food ingestion, skin testing is of doubtful value; and if the onset of clinical symptoms is delayed for several hours following ingestion of the offending agent, the history may not be helpful. In fact, it is estimated that in nearly 50 per cent of all cases of nonhereditary angioedema, an etiologic diagnosis is not made.

Accordingly, although elimination of the offending agent is the most successful therapy, symptomatic therapy may be the only available measure. Aqueous epinephrine is of value, particularly in the more severe cases. Parenteral or oral antihistamines or oral sympathomimetics (ephedrine) are also indicated. Maintenance of adequate ventilation in instances of laryngeal edema may require intubation or tracheostomy if the response to epinephrine is not prompt. The role of corticosteroids in the treatment of angioedema has not been rigorously studied, though those agents are frequently employed. In no instance should corticosteroids be considered a substitute for epinephrine in the emergency treatment of severe cases of angioedema.

Allergic Gastrointestinal Diseases

C. WARREN BIERMAN, M.D., *and* DENNIS L. CHRISTIE, M.D.

Gastrointestinal allergy, though usually caused by food, may also be induced by drugs or even by inhaled allergens which are swallowed when cleared by the respiratory tract. Gastrointestinal allergy may be obvious and easily diagnosed or may be subtle and remain unsuspected for months to years. Easily recognized is the IgE-mediated reaction of acute vomiting and diarrhea, uvular edema, flushing, hives and respiratory distress occurring within minutes of ingesting a food. Far more difficult to diagnose are such conditions as allergic "celiac-like" syndrome or protein-losing enteropathy which may be mediated by other immunoglobulin classes and/or by sensitized lymphocytes.

---

*Manufacturer's precaution: Until further experience is accumulated in infants, therapy with the oral and parenteral forms of ethacrynic acid is contraindicated.

Though there is a direct relationship between dose of the offending food ingested and the severity of the reaction in any given patient, the degree of sensitivity varies widely between patients, ranging from anaphylaxis from a sip of eggnog to urticaria after six Easter eggs.

The spectrum of gastrointestinal allergic disease is noted below.

Allergic Diseases Confined to GI Tract
Abnormal motility (vomiting and diarrhea)
Allergic "celiac-like" syndrome
Protein-losing enteropathy
Eosinophilic gastroenteritis
Iron deficiency anemia due to gastrointestinal blood
     loss

Allergic Disease Involving Organs Remote from GI Tract
Acute systemic anaphylaxis
Atopic dermatitis
Allergic rhinitis
Serous otitis 2° allergic rhinitis.
Asthma
Urticaria

Nonallergic Diseases in Which Allergic Factors May Intensify the Disease
Idiopathic pulmonary hemosiderosis with milk precipitins
Chronic ulcerative colitis with milk precipitins
Celiac sprue with precipitating antibody to wheat
IgA deficiency with precipitating antibody to bovine IgM
Chronic pulmonary disease with milk precipitins

Controversial Diseases (Allergy Has Not Been Proved)
Allergic tension fatigue syndrome
Hyperkinesis due to food additives, coloring, natural salicylates
Enuresis

An increasing number of diseases confined to the gastrointestinal tract are now being recognized both in children and adults. In some, small bowel mucosal damage and infiltration of eosinophils occur after challenge with specific foods, and specific allergic mechanisms have been demonstrated.

Since small amounts of ingested food antigens may gain entrance into the systemic circulation, particularly in early childhood, food allergy may be an important factor in diseases remote from the gastrointestinal tract such as infantile eczema, allergic rhinitis, serous otitis, asthma and urticaria. These diseases involving organs remote from the gastrointestinal tract are primary IgE-mediated conditions.

In both children and adults, food allergy may exacerbate nonallergic disorders such as idiopathic pulmonary hemosiderosis, chronic ulcerative colitis, IgA deficiency and wheat gluten enteropathy.

Several disease states, such as the allergic tension fatigue syndrome, hyperkinesis and enuresis, are thought by some to be related to "allergy," but since no allergic mechanism has been identified, these claims remain controversial.

The management of gastrointestinal allergy depends on identification and elimination of the responsible food from the patient's diet. Though corticosteroid therapy appears to benefit patients with eosinophilic gastroenteritis or with protein-losing enteropathy, most patients can be controlled by removal of offending food from their diet. The diagnosis of gastrointestinal allergy is based on a detailed dietary and growth history to identify potentially allergic foods, a family history to determine other relatives who may have had similar symptoms and/or other allergic diseases and a detailed environmental history to identify potential environmental factors which may relate to the child's symptoms.

Physical examination determines the child's nutritional state, growth, pallor and the presence of such allergic manifestations as dermatitis, urticaria, allergic rhinitis, serous otitis or asthma. Laboratory tests further confirm the type and severity of the child's problem. A blood count identifies presence of anemia or eosinophilia. Quantitative immunoglobulins including IgE reveal any gross immune deficiency states as well as hypergammaglobulinemia E, which is often associated with gastrointestinal allergy. Low serum proteins usually mean loss of protein from the gastrointestinal tract secondary to small or large bowel mucosal disease. Precipitating antibodies to milk, wheat or eggs in the serum identify IgG or IgM antibodies to proteins in these foods. Large numbers of eosinophils in nasal secretions help to verify a diagnosis of allergy. Finally, a duodenal biopsy can identify structural changes of the mucosa which are diagnostic of specific diseases.

Trial Diets and Diet Diaries.   The initial approach to management of gastrointestinal allergy rests in the use of trial diets accompanied by a diary on which ingested food and symptoms are recorded. The trial diet in the infant may be performed by removing all foods and substituting a nonmilk formula. In the older infant, toddler and child, trial diets may consist of a milk substitute, one grain, one fruit, one vegetable, and one meat. In the enthusiasm to identify the offending food, the physician must make certain that the diet is adequate so that iatrogenic deficiency disease does not develop. A dietitian should be consulted when food restriction is severe.

Milk Substitutes.   A variety of cow's

TABLE 1.   Cow's Milk Substitutes

PROTEIN	CARBOHYDRATES	PROPRIETARY NAME
Soy	Sucrose, corn syrup	Isomil
	Sucrose	Neo-Mull-Soy
	Sucrose, corn syrup	Nursoy
	Sucrose, corn syrup	ProSobee
	Dextrins, maltose, glucose	Soyalac
	Sucrose, glucose, maltose	Soyamel
	None	CHO-free
Casein	Glucose	Pregestimil
Hydrolysate	Sucrose	Nutramigen
Beef heart	Sucrose	Meat-based formula
Goat's milk	Lactose	

milk substitutes are available (Table 1). It is essential to note the type of carbohydrate available in each formula since some infants will have a disaccharidase deficiency from specific protein-induced small bowel mucosal damage. If sucrose deficiency is present, all soy formulas except CHO-free will continue to cause diarrhea. Several hydrolyzed casein formulas are available. Pregestimil, which contains glucose, may be better tolerated than Nutramigen, which contains sucrose as a source of carbohydrate. Meat base formula prepared from beef heart has limited usefulness in our experience because it may cross-react with some antibodies directed toward the albumin or globulin fraction of milk. A fourth choice, goat's milk, also has limited usefulness because of substantial cross-reactivity of many goat's milk and cow's milk proteins. If goat's milk is tolerated, additional folic acid must be added to avoid megaloblastic anemia due to folate deficiency.

GRAINS.   A single grain that the child has not yet received or one that will not impose a hardship if the child becomes allergic to it should be selected. For instance, wheat is a poor choice for American infants because a wheat-free diet becomes difficult after the second year of life. Rice is a poor choice for infants of Oriental or Filipino extraction because rice is likewise a staple of their diet as is corn for blacks. Rye or rice crackers are readily available for teething biscuits or finger foods.

FRUITS.   Apple is useful as sauce, as juice or as fresh apple. Occasionally allergy to apple may occur but it is infrequent. Bananas may induce allergic sensitization.

VEGETABLES.   Select a vegetable which may be easily puréed to which the child has not yet been exposed. Some vegetables such as legumes should be avoided if the patient is receiving a soy formula, since the induction of allergy to either beans or peas may cross-react with the soy.

MEATS.   Lamb and pork are the most useful meats for initial trial diets. Beef and veal may have proteins cross-reacting with antibodies directed to milk so that milk-sensitive children will probably react to them. Chicken or turkey is best avoided because of potential cross-reaction to egg, which is a highly antigenic food for children.

VITAMINS.   If proprietary formulas are employed, further vitamins need not be given. If not, synthetic multiple vitamins should be added to ensure adequate vitamin intake. Adequate amounts of iron should likewise be included in the diet. If calculated iron intake is insufficient, supplemental iron should also be supplied. It is wise to avoid prepared baby food as much as possible since the added "hydrolyzed vegetable protein" is wheat gluten. Other additives such as flavoring, coloring, and monosodium glutamate may complicate the trial diet by adding further nonessential substances to which the child might react.

Diet Diary.   A diet diary should be employed with the trial diet to provide prospective information concerning the possible relationship of specific foods to symptoms. In the diet diary the mother records the foods ingested, symptoms, and medications administered on a day-to-day basis. An initial trial diet for a four week period provides an important baseline for further dietary changes. If symptoms are controlled, a new food may be added to the child's diet every two weeks, adequate time to be certain that this new food is tolerated. Should the child react, the new food is withdrawn until symptoms disappear, and tried again. If three trials cause similar reactions, the food should be avoided.

In the event that the child fails to improve on this initial approach, one of several possibilities exists. (1) The child still has food in his diet which is causing symptoms. (2) The child is allergic to other factors such as house dust or animal danders which are responsible for continuing symptoms. (3) Nonallergic factors are continuing the symptoms. In a child with atopic dermatitis the continuing dermatitis can be related to a bacterial infection of the skin. In a child with chronic diarrhea, a primary disaccharidase deficiency may be present or bacterial enteritis may be a factor. (4) The parents are not following the prescribed diet restriction. (5) The child's symptoms are not due to food.

Allergy Skin Testing.   Food skin tests may be helpful if the child continues to have symptoms on a restricted diet and appropriate laboratory tests have ruled out other causes of symptoms. Skin tests for common foods and common environmental factors will serve to identify IgE-associated factors which may be of importance in the etiology of the child's symptoms. Selected food skin tests applied by scratch or prick tests and followed up by intradermal tests may help to identify foods to which the child is not allergic. These foods then may be introduced into the diet. Skin tests will also help to identify foods to which the child is immunologically sensitive. They should be avoided. Once symptoms are controlled, foods associated with positive skin tests may be cautiously introduced, one at a time, recording possible reactions on the diet sheet. If there is no reaction the child can be considered immunologically but not clinically allergic to this food. If the child does react, extended food elimination will be necessary.

SPECIFIC PROBLEMS

Chronic Diarrhea. One of the more troublesome symptoms related to food allergy in pediatric practice is diarrhea. Diarrhea can occur immediately after protein ingestion or gradually over several weeks. Gluten, cow's milk and soy proteins have been conclusively demonstrated to cause significant small bowel mucosal disease. All can cause malabsorption of carbohydrate, fat and protein with subsequent failure to thrive or abnormalities in motility with primary water loss but normal growth.

Allergic gastroenteropathy is a term applied to a disease of infants and children who have protein loss from their gastrointestinal tract, peripheral eosinophilia, hypoalbuminemia and edema. Eosinophilic gastroenteritis may be a type of allergic gastroenteropathy mediated by IgE. These patients may have repeated diarrhea following ingestion of a specific protein. A careful dietary history can frequently identify the offending food.

Examination of the child's stool can give useful information. Pus or blood may be due to cow's milk colitis as well as to an infection. Watery stool with a low pH (5.5 or less) and a positive test for reducing substance suggest carbohydrate intolerance. This can occur as a result of a primary disaccharidase deficiency or a secondary one caused by damage to the small bowel mucosa from a specific protein. Large, bulky, oily stools generally mean significant fat malabsorption. Specific disaccharide tolerance tests will give firm evidence that either sucrase or lactase deficiency is present. Small bowel biopsy is indicated in those infants with abnormal screening tests and significant diarrhea.

Treatment of protein sensitivity is initiated by strict avoidance of the offending protein. In the majority of infants, elimination of the protein results in rapid improvement. Pregestimil, a casein hydrolysate formula, appears to be beneficial in those infants with either cow's milk or soy protein sensitivity. Because glucose is the carbohydrate, Pregestimil is also useful when the offending protein has caused a secondary disaccharidase deficiency.

The question of how long to avoid the protein causing the diarrhea remains controversial. Some believe that cow's milk protein sensitivity in the gastrointestinal tract will resolve by age one. However, gluten sensitivity does not spontaneously disappear and therefore a gluten-free diet is indicated for life. For this reason the diagnosis of celiac sprue should be based upon a small bowel biopsy showing a nonspecific flat lesion and a clinical response to a gluten-free diet.

Atopic Dermatitis (Infantile Eczema). When infantile eczema begins between 2½ months and 12 months, 30 per cent will have skin symptoms persisting to adult life, 53 per cent will develop asthma, and many others will develop allergic rhinitis with middle ear involvement. At present the best diagnostic approach to the child with eczema is to look for associated allergic disorders, especially those involving ear and chest, obtain a detailed history to determine food allergy, and pursue a gastrointestinal evaluation for eosinophilic gastroenteritis in the child who falls below the third percentile for weight.

Treat acute dermatitis with wet compresses. Treat chronic dermatitis with conjugated steroid cream or ointment such as triamcinolone acetonide, fluocinoline acetonide, fluorandranolide acetonide (0.1 to 0.1 per cent) or beclomethasone diproprionate (0.01 per cent) applied every 4 to 6 hours. Apply emollients to control dryness. Avoid skin irritants and drying agents. Keep the skin cool to make it less itchy and administer antihistamines such as diphenhydramine (Benadryl), 5 to 10 mg. every 4 hours to aid in reducing pruritus. Treat skin infections promptly and adequately with systemic antibodies.

In addition, the physician should treat specific allergic factors that may have a causal or aggravating relationship to the dermatitis by: (1) eliminating suspected dietary items which can be determined by history; (2) placing the child on a nutritionally complete diet consisting of foods not suspected to cause problems; (3) reintroducing suspected foods one at a time when the child has clinically improved; if the eczema flares up on at least three trials, the suspected food should be eliminated;

(4) rechallenging foods known to have a causal relationship to eczema at 2 to 3 year intervals; and (5) consulting a pediatric allergist if the child fails to respond to this management.

Allergic Rhinitis and Serous Otitis. Allergic rhinitis in infants, preschool and early school-aged children is frequently associated with serous otitis and intermittent conductive hearing loss. They may lead to delayed speech development and learning handicaps or recurrent acute otitis media. A recent study indicated that 51 per cent of allergic children had eustachian tube dysfunction as diagnosed by screening audiometry, pneumatic otoscopy, and tympanometry. In the child with chronic serous otitis or recurrent otitis media, the pediatrician should seek for allergy since, with its diagnosis, a specific therapeutic approach is available.

Treat allergic rhinitis with antihistaminic drugs administered around the clock. Treat serous otitis with topical, long-acting nasal decongestants such as oxymetazoline HCl (Afrin) or xylometazoline HCl (Otrivin). Do not administer more frequently than twice daily for more than 5 days to avoid medication-induced rhinitis. Instruct patient and parent to do middle-ear self-inflation with a Valsalva maneuver or balloon insufflator three times daily. Give a limited trial of nasal dexamethasone spray twice daily for a maximum of 3 weeks for serous otitis if it fails to respond to a one month trial of the measures discussed above. Be certain that parents are not giving infants bottles in bed which may result in reflux of fluid up eustachian tubes. Treat ear infections promptly and adequately with systemic antibiotics.

In addition the physician should treat specific allergic factors that predispose to serous otitis by eliminating suspected foods with the use of a trial diet and eliminating environmental allergens or irritants such as house dust, mold, animal danders, feathers, bedding dust and tobacco smoke.

If after a six week therapeutic trial of medication, dietary and environmental control, serous otitis media with hearing loss persists, the patient is referred to a pediatric allergist for an allergic evaluation and to an otolaryngologist for consideration of tympanostomy tubes. Since surgical therapy is temporary in most cases caused by nasal allergies, it is important to effect proper allergic management while the middle-ear ventilating tubes are in place.

Asthma. Wheezing in infants and toddlers is frequently related to a variety of factors, including infections, allergy to food and/or allergy to inhaled particles and irritants such as tobacco smoke. The infant who wheezes with colds frequently becomes the child who wheezes on specific exposure to allergens. Food allergy is often a major factor in infants and toddlers whose asthma begins early in life. As the child grows older, he or she becomes increasingly allergic to inhaled allergens and food allergy becomes much less important.

Initiate theophylline therapy, 4 mg./kg. every 6 hours, employing an alcohol free, dye-free, sugar-free theophylline preparation. Determine peak and trough serum theophylline concentrations 2 and 6 hours after a dose. Readjust dose and dosing interval on the basis of these blood levels. Initiate a trial elimination diet and diet diary. Pursue active environmental control measures with emphasis on house dust, mold, animal danders, and tobacco smoke.

If after a trial of the above measures, the patient improves, the child's diet is enlarged gradually, adding one food at a time. If, on the other hand, wheezing continues, and such conditions as cystic fibrosis, congenital pulmonary abnormalities and foreign bodies in the lung have been excluded, the child is referred for an in-depth allergic evaluation.

Urticaria. See page 477.

Drug-Induced Disease
Adverse Drug Reactions

MILES WEINBERGER, M.D.

Drug-induced disease has been a long-standing cause of morbidity and mortality. More than 2500 years ago, Hippocrates cautioned physicians not to cause harm with their therapeutic efforts. Oliver Wendell Holmes stated, "if the whole materia medica, as now used, could be sunk to the bottom of the sea, it would be all the better for mankind and all the worse for the fishes." Development of the science of pharmacology has resulted in an even larger selection of potent agents than that which concerned the honorable Mr. Holmes. The increased potential for drug-induced illness, however, is tempered by a magnitude of real benefit that would have astounded our predecessors. The recent development of medical drug specialists, clinical pharmacologists, and the expansion of the pharmacy profession's traditional dispensing role to include drug consultation have been associated with increased attention to the better usage of drugs, identification of drug-induced illness and its treatment, and realistic assessments of benefit and risk.

TABLE 1. Immunologically Mediated Adverse Medication Effects

TYPE	MECHANISM	SYMPTOMS	TREATMENT
I	Reagin-mediated	Anaphylactic shock, urticaria, laryngeal edema, bronchospasm	Epinephrine 1:1000 (subcutaneous) followed by antihistamine; drug may be continued in hospitalized patient if essential and symptoms mild or controlled with above measures.
II	Complement-dependent cytolysis	Hemolytic anemia, granulocytopenia, thrombocytopenia	Discontinue drug immediately; hospitalize; evaluate for other causes; specific treatment is otherwise usually unnecessary but treatment of complications may be required.
III	Toxic-complex disease	Serum sickness–like reactions, exanthematous eruptions, drug fever, arthralgia	Discontinue drug unless essential; antihistamines and/or corticosteroids may relieve symptoms.
IV	Cellular immunity	Contact dermatitis	Discontinue drug, topical corticosteroids may speed resolution (but ingredients in topical corticosteroid preparations may also cause contact dermatitis).

Most adverse drug reactions are the result of predictable pharmacological properties of the drug and its interaction with the patient or other drugs. Other drug reactions, however, are not predictable, i.e., they are idiosyncratic. Immunological mechanisms for some of these reactions have been defined, and classification of drug-induced allergic illness by the appropriate immunologic mechanism has therapeutic implications (Table 1).

While immunological (allergic) reactions to drugs are not readily suspected in advance, drug-drug interactions and drug-disease interactions are more predictable and thus potentially preventable. The risk of drug-induced disease has been shown to increase disproportionately as the number of simultaneously administered drugs increases. Physiologic potentiation for toxicity can occur, bioavailability can be decreased thus negating the potential for benefit, or metabolism of one drug can be altered by the other thus resulting in decreased effect (increased elimination) or increased toxicity (decreased elimination). Many such interactions have been defined.*

Similarly, many interactions have been defined between administered drugs and underlying disease states (Table 2). These include conditions such as liver and renal disease that alter drug elimination mechanisms. The increased risk of certain drug reactions in the newborn is at least partly due to the transient renal and hepatic immaturity seen in the neonatal period. Other adverse drug reactions are the result of congenital metabolic defects, e.g., glucose-6-phosphate dehydrogenase deficiency and Crigler-Najjar syndrome. Anatomical defects such as glaucoma and subaortic stenosis account for other reactions, whereas many go undefined, such as aspirin sensitivity in asthma.

The risk of adverse drug reactions occurring as a result of the pharmacological activity of the drug is thus amenable to prophylaxis and/or treatment by understanding the drug's range of activity, including its potential for interaction with other drugs and physiologically abnormal states. For drugs with narrow therapeutic indices, toxic potential can also be reduced by the assistance of drug level quantitation in body fluids; this has already become routine for digoxin, anticonvulsants, theophylline, salicylates, aminoglycoside antibiotics, lithium, and quinidine.

Unfortunately, not all drug reactions can be neatly classified as either a defined and potentially predictable pharmacologic effect or an allergic reaction with an identifiable immunologic mechanism. Regardless of cause, however, successful treatment first requires identification of the relationship between an illness and the therapeutic agent. This requires an index of suspicion whenever an unusual event occurs during the course of therapy. Vir-

*References for tabulation of drug-drug interactions are found in: Hansten, P. D.: Drug Interactions, Philadelphia, Lea & Febiger, 1971; and Martin, W. E., Alexander, E. W., Hassan, W. E., and Farage, D. J.: Hazards of Medication. Philadelphia, J. B. Lippincott Co., 1972.

TABLE 2.   Selected Clinical Entities Associated with Abnormal Responses to Drugs

CLINICAL CONDITIONS	POTENTIAL DRUG SENSITIVITY	EFFECT	TREATMENT
Asthma	Aspirin	Bronchospasm	Avoid. Use acetaminophen as routine antipyretic in asthmatics.
	Propranolol	Bronchospasm	If necessary to use, treat with therapeutic doses of theophylline.
Crigler-Najjar syndrome	Salicylate	Salicylate toxicity due to decreased conjugation and elimination	Avoid.
Glaucoma	Mydriatics, corticosteroids	Increased intraocular pressure	Identify type of glaucoma and treat appropriately.
Glucose-6-phosphate dehydrogenase deficiency	Primaquine, sulfonamides	Hemolytic anemia	Identify patients at risk and avoid offending drug.
Hypoalbuminemia	Drugs which have high protein binding such as phenytoin	Toxicity because of increased free drug reaching receptors	Treat underlying condition; use protein bound drugs cautiously.
Liver dysfunction	Drugs metabolized by the liver such as theophylline or chloramphenicol	Toxicity due to accumulation with multiple dosing	Use liver metabolized drugs cautiously; measure drug levels.
Newborn	See liver dysfunction and renal insufficiency in this table	Toxicity from multiple dosing because of decreased elimination	Use doses designed for newborns; measure drug levels.
	Drugs which can displace bilirubin from serum protein such as the sulfonamides	Kernicterus	Avoid those drugs in perinatal period.
Porphyria	Barbiturates	Symptoms of hepatic porphyria because of increased porphyrin synthesis	Avoid.
Renal insufficiency	Drugs eliminated predominantly by the kidney such as digoxin or gentamicin	Toxicity due to accumulation with multiple dosing	Use drugs cautiously; measure drug levels.
Subaortic stenosis	Digoxin	Fatal reaction by correcting heart failure and cardiac dilatation with compensatory widening of subaortic muscle ring	Treat underlying condition.

tually all systems of the body have the potential to suffer undesirable drug effects.*

Dermatologic Manifestations. Exfoliative dermatitis, Stevens-Johnson syndrome, and toxic epidermal necrolysis are serious diseases that have been associated with administration of a variety of pharmacological agents. These are life-threatening illnesses requiring intensive supportive measures and are often treated with corticosteroids though without proof of efficacy.

Fixed drug eruptions have been most typically associated with barbiturates, but a variety of other agents have occasionally been implicated. Unlike the more serious reactions mentioned above, these are benign reactions generally requiring no treatment other than discontinuing the drug. A variety of other ill-defined rashes are also seen from a wide variety of drugs; specific therapy other than discontinuing the offending drug is generally not required.

Photosensitivity is induced by many drugs but most typically by demeclocycline, griseofulvin, sulfonamides, and thiazides. A distinction is made between phototoxic and photoallergic reactions with the latter being reagin-mediated (Table 1) and manifested by urticaria, whereas the former is more a sunburn type of rash. An effective sunscreen containing paraaminobenzoic acid in alcohol (PreSun) or similar preparations to prevent the effects of the ultraviolet radiation exposure can be used for prophylaxis if sun exposure is otherwise unavoidable.

Urticaria and anaphylactic-like reactions are classic manifestations of reagin-mediated allergy, but can also occur from drugs with no evidence of immune responsiveness, e.g., aspirin or iodinated contrast media. Treatment, however, is the same as for urticaria, laryngeal edema, bronchospasm, or vascular collapse from true anaphylaxis.

Alopecia is a common manifestation of cytotoxic agents. Usually the necessity of the drug for chemotherapy outweighs the considerations regarding the hair loss. Other drugs cause hirsutism. These include both corticosteroids and anabolic steroids which also cause acne. Phenytoin and chlorpromazine are additional agents associated with hirsutism, whereas iodides are an additional cause of acne. Since there is no indication for chronic

use of iodides, reactions to this drug are avoidable. The drugs that cause hirsutism require caution to assure that the drug is needed and that the administered dose is clinically appropriate. The hirsutism does not necessarily regress with cessation of drug. Drug-induced acne will usually improve if the offending agent is stopped. Conventional acne therapy may be useful if therapy must be continued.

Hematopoietic Manifestations. Suppression of various elements of the bone marrow has been associated with antimetabolites used for immunosuppression and cancer chemotherapy. This is usually reversible with cessation of the drug. Chloramphenicol has been associated with irreversible bone marrow suppression. In addition to discontinuing the drug, vigorous treatment of the aplastic anemia or agranulocytosis may be needed.

Hemolytic anemias by at least two different immune and several metabolic mechanisms can be drug induced. Avoidance of further hemolytogenic drug insults in the injured patient is the most appropriate treatment. Transfusions should only rarely be necessary. Drug-induced megaloblastic anemias can also occur. Folic acid antagonists can cause this but some drugs can impair folate absorption, e.g., phenytoin, primidone, and barbiturates. Iron deficiency anemia has been reported as a result of chronic aspirin therapy with subsequent gastrointestinal blood loss.

Lymphoid tissue proliferation has occurred as a result of long-term therapy with anticonvulsants such as phenytoin. Careful monitoring of blood levels may decrease this risk, and discontinuing the drug, if necessary, will generally allow regression of the lymphoid tissue.

Gastrointestinal Manifestations. Broad spectrum antibiotics are associated with swollen or hairy tongue and diarrhea. Tetracycline can be deposited in developing dental enamel resulting in mottling, discoloration, and enamel hypoplasia. The tongue lesion and diarrhea are rapidly reversible upon discontinuation of the drug but the drug-induced dental defect is permanent. Tetracycline therefore should not be used from the last trimester of pregnancy through 8 years of age.

Many drugs cause nausea and vomiting either centrally or by direct irritation. Digoxin, theophylline, codeine, and erythromycin are common causes of these symptoms. Gastrointestinal toxicity from digoxin and theophylline is generally related to blood level and can be treated by lowering the dose until serum concentrations are within the therapeutic range. If symptoms from codeine and eryth-

---

*Extensive tabulations of reported associations of drugs with clinical manifestations of disease are included in: Cluff, L. E., Caranasas, G. J., and Stewart R. B.:Clinical Problems with Drugs. Philadelphia, W. B. Saunders Co., 1975.

romycin persist, discontinuation of the drug may be necessary.

Liver Manifestations. Cholestatic jaundice has been associated sporadically with a variety of medications including phenothiazines, some macrolide antibiotics (troleandomycin and erythromycin estolate), and anabolic steroids. Discontinuation of medication usually results in gradual clearing of the cholestasis over a few weeks.

Hepatocellular damage has resulted from halogenated anesthetic agents such as halothane. A fatal outcome is not unusual. Careful and strict avoidance of the offending anesthetic agent is subsequently essential.

Respiratory Manifestations. Pulmonary infiltrates can occur from nitrofurantoin, busulfan, and methotrexate. These and methysergide can also result in pulmonary fibrosis. These lesions are not always reversible although some response to corticosteroids is reported. Since onset of symptoms is generally gradual after prolonged therapy, recognition of symptoms and prompt discontinuation of medication are essential before significant irreversible lesions have developed.

Bronchospasm occurs as a manifestation of reagin-mediated allergic reactions, particularly in asthmatics. Asthmatics also demonstrate a variety of unique drug reactions as a function of hyperreactive airway disease. These include histamine and methacholine which induce bronchospasm that can be blocked by prior administration of any of the potent bronchodilators. The bronchospasm from propranolol, a beta-adrenergic blocker, is most effectively blocked by theophylline. Aspirin sensitivity is present to varying degrees in as many as 20 per cent of asthmatics. As a result, asthmatics are best advised to use an aspirin substitute such as acetaminophen for antipyresis and minor analgesia. The only indication for aspirin in an asthmatic would be the unlikely event of the patient's simultaneously requiring aspirin's anti-inflammatory effect for treatment of rheumatic fever or rheumatoid arthritis. The risk of bronchospasm could be examined under these circumstances by serial pulmonary function measurements following a test dose.

Endocrine Manifestations. Corticosteroids can decrease glucose tolerance in individuals with active or latent diabetes mellitus. Insulin can also produce hyperglycemia in a diabetic through a mechanism called the Somogyi effect, which is essentially a reactive hyperglycemia following hypoglycemia. Thiazide diuretics and furosemide can also be diabetogenic resulting in increased glucose levels. The hyperglycemic effects of these drugs, however, rarely require treatment or discontinuation of the required medication. Temporary increases in insulin may be indicated in active diabetics for these drug-induced effects other than the Somogyi effect, which requires reduction in insulin dosage.

Hypothyroidism can be induced by excessive iodide ingestion, as can goiter. Since there is no indication for iodide therapy other than briefly for hyperthyroidism, this reaction is 100 per cent avoidable. Hypothyroidism is also a common outcome of ^{131}I treatment of hyperthyroidism. Lifelong treatment with thyroid and/or follow-up is indicated in these patients to prevent the manifestations of hypothyroid disease.

Corticosteroid therapy results in a symptom complex known as Cushing's syndrome, which is also associated with growth suppression in children and eventually with osteoporosis and vertebral compression fractures. When long-term corticosteroid therapy is essential, the use of single doses of a short-acting corticosteroid administered every other morning effectively minimizes the risks of Cushing's syndrome. While long-term suppression of asthma and nephrosis can be effected with this regimen, rheumatoid arthritis and systemic lupus erythematosus are reported to be more resistant to control in this manner. A new inhaled corticosteroid, beclomethasone dipropionate, has recently been reported as an additional means to use corticosteroids for long-term asthmatic suppression without significant risk of cushingoid changes.

Cyclophosphamide is frequently associated with amenorrhea in women and suppression of spermatogenesis in men. Since this drug is generally used only for serious indications, these complications are generally not avoidable. Anabolic steroids lead to virilization in the female and may cause precocious sexual development in the male. These drugs have very limited indications and should thus generally be avoided.

Renal Manifestations. The potential for nephrotoxicity exists for many drugs. Identification of the drugs at risk with appropriate evaluations of renal function allows discontinuation of drug or dosage adjustment as indicated. Some drugs induce a lesion resulting in the nephrotic syndrome. This has been most commonly associated with the anticonvulsants, trimethadione and paramethadione. Discontinuation of the causative drug usually results in prompt improvement.

Outdated tetracyclines have caused renal tubular dysfunction resembling Fanconi's syndrome, cystinosis with glycosuria, amino-aciduria, phosphaturia, proteinuria, and renal tubular acidosis. Greater stability of current tetracycline preparations and more careful attention to drug expiration dates have decreased the frequency of this problem. Demeclocycline (Declomycin), a tetracycline derivative, has been associated with a lesion resembling nephrogenic diabetes insipidus. Since there is no specific indication for this drug in pediatrics, it should not be used, thus avoiding this risk.

Methysergide (Sansert),* a prophylactic drug for migraine headaches, can induce retroperitoneal fibrosis in about 1 per cent of users, resulting in ureteral obstruction and hydronephrosis. Regression of fibrosis may follow cessation of the drug; corticosteroids may enhance resolution.

Fetal and Neonatal Manifestations. Antineoplastic agents can cause abortions and multiple congenital anomalies. Phenytoin has also been implicated in causing skeletal abnormalities. Coumarin but not heparin crosses the placenta and has caused fatal fetal hemorrhage. Maternal isoniazid has resulted in the birth of infants with psychomotor retardation, convulsions, and myoclonus felt to be caused by the interference of isoniazid with pyridoxine metabolism. Radioactive iodine administered during pregnancy can result in fetal thyroid destruction and hypothyroidism. Neonatal goiter can be caused by iodine-containing drugs and antithyroid compounds such as propylthiouracil and methimazole.

Most of the analgesics and both local and general anesthetics used during delivery have the potential to result in a depressed infant at birth. Kernicterus can result from drugs that displace bilirubin from protein being administered to either the infant or the mother shortly prior to delivery. Such drugs include synthetic vitamin K, sulfonamides, and salicylates.

The infant, because of decreased drug eliminating capacity for many agents, can become toxic more readily than immediately beyond the neonatal period when drug disposition mechanisms rapidly mature. A classic example is chloramphenicol, which results in the "gray syndrome" after 2 to 9 days with abdominal distention, occasionally vomiting, hypothermia, a gray ashen cyanosis, respiratory difficulty, and vascular collapse. This occurs as a result of the neonate's limited ability to conjugate and thus detoxify and eliminate the drug. Prevention is possible by conservative

dosage recommendations (25 mg./kg./day) when use of this drug is essential in the newborn.

The treatment of the whole range of fetal and neonatal manifestations of adverse drug reactions requires minimizing exposure and an understanding of drug activity and metabolism in the neonate. Each drug applied to perinatal medicine should undergo clinical pharmacological investigation that examines disposition mechanisms and metabolism in addition to efficacy.

Metabolic Manifestations. Diuretics cause fluid and electrolyte loss. Potassium loss can be particularly profound with most of the diuretics. Hypokalemia can result in a metabolic acidosis as a result of paradoxical aciduria. These adverse effects should be avoided as much as possible by limiting dosage and duration of diuretics when possible. When prolonged administration is essential, potassium loss should be anticipated and greater than normal potassium maintenance guided by serum potassium measurements may be required.

Excessive amounts of vitamin D can lead to hypercalcemia with weakness, lethargy, nausea, and vomiting. Symptoms may persist for prolonged periods after the drug is discontinued. Thiazide diuretics reduce urinary calcium excretion and can aggravate hypercalcemia in patients with actual or potential hypercalcemia. Hypocalcemia occurs as part of severe drug-induced renal damage. Mithramycin, an antineoplastic drug, produces dose-related hypocalcemia.

Hyperuricemia can be induced by thiazide diuretics and furosemide. More commonly, hyperuricemia results from chemotherapy of lymphomas and acute leukemia.

Acute intermittent porphyria with episodes of abdominal pain, vomiting, constipation, peripheral neuropathy, psychic disturbances, fever, tachycardia, and transient hypertension can be precipitated most characteristically but not exclusively by barbiturates. Porphyria cutanea tarda symptomatica with photosensitivity and superficial erosions, vesicles, and hyperpigmentation in light-exposed areas can also be exacerbated by barbiturates and a variety of other drugs.

Neurologic Manifestations. Heavy metal intoxication is characteristically associated with peripheral neuropathy characterized by numbness, paresthesias, weakness, and distal (stocking and glove) loss of sensation. Such treatment today is limited predominantly to gold therapy for rheumatoid arthritis where the risks must be carefully weighed against the chance of benefit.

---

*Manufacturer's note: Methysergide is not recommended for use in children.

Antituberculous therapy with isoniazid or ethionamide has the potential to cause a peripheral neuropathy that responds well to pyridoxine used either for treatment or prophylaxis.

Certain antibiotics (colistin, polymyxin, and kanamycin) can produce degrees of peripheral nerve damage particularly in the presence of renal insufficiency. Vincristine and vinblastine have been reported to produce paresthesias. Long-term therapy with chloroquine occasionally causes neuromyopathy with proximal muscle weakness of the legs and later the arms. Most of these can be prevented with appropriate drug dosage and/or discontinuation of therapy when possible.

Succinylcholine, normally a short-acting paralytic used at surgery, can result in unexpected prolongation of paralysis in genetically susceptible individuals.

Extrapyramidal symptoms with acute dystonic reactions, akathisia, and parkinsonian symptoms can occur from phenothiazines. With prolonged administration, potentially irreversible tardive dyskinesia may occur.

Seizures are a potential toxic complication from overdosage of many drugs including theophylline, amphetamines, anticholinergics and drugs with the potential for toxic anticholinergic effect such as antihistamines and tricyclic antidepressants. Treatment requires support of adequate ventilation and the use of a rapid acting anticonvulsant by the intravenous route.

Central nervous system depression is a complication to varying degrees of many drugs. Coma, unaccompanied by localizing neurological signs, should always be considered as possibly drug induced. Hypnotics, sedative, and psychoactive drugs are often implicated. Treatment consists of respiratory support and increasing the rate of elimination of the intoxicant when feasible.

Behavioral Manifestations. Anxiety can result from sympathomimetic drugs, excess thyroid, and occasionally in children as a paradoxical response to barbiturates. Tolerance may occur to these effects. Dosage adjustment may also be useful.

Euphoria, elevation of mood, is common with amphetamines and occasionally occurs from corticosteroids. This rarely is of sufficient concern to require treatment or alteration of essential therapy.

Depression is more of a problem occurring after withdrawal of amphetamines or long-term corticosteroid therapy. Rauwolfia alkaloids (reserpine) are also a classic cause of drug-induced depression. This latter drug is rarely needed in pediatrics; other hypertensive medications are more effective and present fewer problems. Withdrawal of amphetamines and corticosteroids is a problem in children, however, and close attention should be given to the potential for the development of depression. Gradual withdrawal and sufficiently frequent visits to provide psychological support are usually adequate measures.

Ocular Manifestations. Posterior subcapsular cataracts that usually do not impair vision can result from systemic corticosteroid therapy, most often in patients with rheumatoid arthritis. These appear to be related to both dose and duration.

Retrolental fibroplasia is a complication of oxygen therapy in the premature. There is no effective treatment once it occurs, but it can be prevented by avoiding ambient oxygen concentrations that result in excessive arterial pO_2's.

Prolonged high-dose therapy with chloroquine and hydroxychloroquine has led to irreversible retinal damage with marked visual impairment. Retinopathy does not necessarily stop progressing with discontinuation of the medication and may even start after cessation of therapy. These drugs should be used with caution.

Optic neuritis is an occasional complication after high-dose or long-term therapy with chloramphenicol, streptomycin, isoniazid, ethambutol, penicillamine, and digitalis. The latter is a rare cause. Optic neuritis induced by isoniazid and penicillamine is reported to be treatable with pyridoxine.

Otic Manifestations. The aminoglycoside antibiotics have all been associated with auditory nerve damage. Avoiding toxic blood levels and/or prolonged administration eliminates this complication. Tinnitus is a complication of high blood levels of quinine and salicylates. Cessation or appropriate dosage adjustment controls these symptoms.

Multisystemic Manifestations. Fevers from drugs can occur as a result of an immune mechanism associated with a drug-induced serum sickness–like reaction. Nonimmune mechanisms are active, however, in the classic Herxheimer reaction and overdosage with amphetamines. Hyperthermia has resulted from phenothiazines.

A syndrome clinically indistinguishable from systemic lupus erythematosus has been induced most commonly by hydralazine but also occasionally as a result of therapy with isoniazid and phenytoin. This is dose-related and thus potentially preventable. Symptoms may persist even after reduction or withdrawal of medication requiring treatment with corticosteroids.

Physical Allergy

RICHARD WYATT, M.D., *and*
MILES WEINBERGER, M.D.

Physical allergy consists of those reactions which appear to be allergic in nature, but are mediated by physical stimuli such as scratching, pressure, vibration, cold, heat, exercise, and sunlight (Table 1). Clinical symptoms are also varied and can consist of localized cutaneous allergic reactions, generalized systemic symptoms, and even life-threatening anaphylactic reactions. Some of these reactions have an established immunological basis with the release of mediator substances including histamine, bradykinin, and serotonin. Although the pathophysiology is not always clear, the entire complex of reactions is referred to as "physical allergy."

MECHANICAL HYPERSENSITIVITY

Cutaneous hypersensitivity manifested by urticaria occurs as a result of three distinctly different forms of trauma which include mild scratching, pressure, and vibration.

Dermographism. Dermographism is the occurrence of urticarial wheals 3 mm. or greater in diameter after a scratch with the use

TABLE 1. Physical Agents Producing Urticaria

I. Mechanical
    Dermographism
      Primary
        Idiopathic
        Allergic
      Secondary
        Cutaneous mastocytosis
        Transient forms
    Delayed pressure urticaria
    Delayed dermographism
    Hereditary vibratory angioedema

II. Thermal
    Cold
      Acquired
        Idiopathic
        Associated with cryoglobulinemia
        Associated with cryofibrinogenemia
        Associated with cold hemolysins
        Transient forms associated with other factors
      Familial cold urticaria
    Heat
      Cholinergic
      Localized heat urticaria
      Familial localized heat urticaria

III. Light
    Solar urticaria
      Probably allergic types
      Associated with abnormal protoporphyrin
        metabolism
      Idiopathic types

of a force of 400 gm. or less. Normal individuals are able to tolerate 1000 gm. or more without wheal formation. The wheals follow the shape of the trauma, but characteristically do not have pseudopods. Approximately 5 per cent of the normal population have this tendency, with an increased incidence occurring among patients with urticarial drug reactions and other forms of urticaria. This is prone to occur when the number of cutaneous mast cells are increased, e.g., in urticaria pigmentosa or diffuse forms of cutaneous mastocytosis. Dermographism also tends to occur in patients following reactions to drugs, especially penicillin, cutaneous exposure to tetrahydrofurfuryl nicotinate (Trafuril), exercise, or exposure to cold in cold-sensitive patients. About 50 per cent of patients are shown to have passively transferable skin-sensitizing antibody for dermographism.

Treatment consists of avoidance of trauma and use of antihistamines. Hydroxyzine (Atarax) is the most potent antihistamine as judged by its ability to suppress histamine-induced wheal formation. The dose for children is 2 to 3 mg./kg./day with larger doses sometimes needed for lack of response. Drowsiness is a common side effect, but normally does not last more than 1 to 2 weeks after initiating therapy. For unusually severe cases, tolerance to trauma is sometimes achieved by daily repeated exposure to rubbing with a brush during bathing in order to induce whealing. Since this is usually impractical, a short course of prednisone for 5 to 10 days at 2 mg./kg./day or up to 80 mg./24 hours may be effective for intermittent, severe incapacitating reactions.

Delayed Pressure Urticaria. This form of urticaria consists of the development of deep painful swelling after the application of pressure to the skin. The lesions occur approximately 4 hours after the stimulus and last 8 to 24 hours. It can be disabling and occur anywhere on the body including the soles of the feet after walking, palms after clapping or manual labor, or even the face after kissing. The patient may have malaise and a "flu-like" syndrome of aches and pains, headaches, and even rigors coinciding with the period of maximum whealing.

A useful diagnostic test consists of hanging a 15-pound weight on the end of a crepe bandage draped over a shoulder, thigh or forearm for 10 minutes. One can expect a lesion to occur anywhere from 2½ to 12 hours after the application of pressure.

The cause is unknown but some investigators stress the close similarity to the Arthus reaction. Others suggest the release of kinins. Recently a case was reported to have occurred in both father and son suggesting a possible familial incidence.

Treatment is largely unsatisfactory with little response to antihistamines, and in only a few patients have systemic corticosteroids appeared to afford any relief. At most, only a change in the timing or depth of the urticaria can be expected from the use of single pharmacological agents.

Hereditary Vibratory Angioedema. In this disease, vibratory stimuli cause a local erythematous, edematous, cutaneous or subcutaneous lesion. There might be accompanying generalized or facial erythema along with a transient headache. The area of the stimulus may remain swollen for hours to days depending on the strength of the stimuli. Lesions are sometimes elicited by frictional stimuli to the skin. The disease is inherited as a mendelian dominant trait and lasts for life, with the severity sometimes decreasing with age.

The nonimmunologically induced lesions seem to be caused by mast cell histamine release, which would account for the generalized symptoms, including flushing.

Patients with this disease may lead a normal life if stimuli which (by history) cause reactions are avoided. This is a mild disease that normally does not require emergency or even routine medical treatment.

COLD HYPERSENSITIVITY

Angioedema, urticaria, hemoglobinuria, gastric hyperacidity, and generalized anaphylaxis occur as manifestations of cold hypersensitivity. Distinct clinical groups can be identified (Table 2).

TABLE 2. Cold Urticarias

Familial (congenital)

Acquired
  Primary or essential
  Secondary to or associated with
    Cryoglobulinemia
    Cryofibrinogenemia
    Cold hemolysin syndrome
    Other factors
      Drugs (penicillin, griseofulvin)
      Foods (port, custards, menthol lozenges)
      Infections
        Viral (measles, chickenpox)
        Bacterial (scarlet fever, focal sepsis)
        Parasitic (Ascaris infection)
      Insect bites
      Serum sickness (horse serum)
      Uterine fibroids
      Hypothyroidism

Cold Urticarias. The development of urticaria typically occurs after exposure to cold air in winter; cold water during swimming, bathing, doing dishes; or with consumption of cold beverages and food. Lesions may consist of localized urticaria restricted to the area of exposure or of mucosal angioedema with respiratory distress occurring after ingestion of cold food. Severe life-threatening generalized anaphylactic reactions during swimming in cold water have occurred.

There are two distinct clinical patterns that exist. A rare familial form that is autosomal dominant occurs shortly after birth and persists for life. There is typically a lag period after exposure of 30 minutes to 4 hours before symptoms appear. Constitutional symptoms may be present consisting of headache, fever, and chills lasting 4 to 6 hours, as well as arthritis with swelling and erythema lasting days.

The essential or acquired form is more common, occurring later in life with a tendency to disappear after a varied amount of time. Localized urticaria is present at the point of contact. Systemic symptoms consist of flushing, headache, nausea, vomiting, dyspnea, cough, gastric hyperacidity or anaphylaxis.

Diagnostic procedures include local cold challenge with an ice cube for approximately two minutes, which results in a wheal at the point of contact occurring only in the essential cold urticaria. Passive transfer with serum is positive in about one-half of the cases of the essential type. Immunoglobulins of both the IgE and IgM class have been implicated as the responsible agent for mast cell mediator release.

Detection of cryoglobulins, along with a history of Raynaud's phenomenon, necrosis, ulceration or mucosal hemorrhages, should alert one to look further for other causes of cold intolerance, e.g., kala-azar, subacute bacterial endocarditis, multiple myeloma, chronic lymphatic leukemia, Weber-Christian disease, empyema, bronchiectasis, rheumatic fever, and others. Cryofibrinogens should be sought when reactions to cold include unexplained bleeding or thromboses. Their presence could indicate collagen vascular disease or malignancy. Symptoms resulting from cryoglobulins or cryoprecipitates are best treated by dealing appropriately with the underlying disease.

Treatment of familiar or essential cold urticaria consists primarily of cold avoidance. Antihistamines may be tried as some patients will respond. In at least one report, cyproheptadine, but not other antihistamines, blocked cold challenges. Cyproheptadine (Periactin), 0.5 mg./kg./day divided 3 times per day is given, with an occasional patient needing larger doses. Some success has been claimed by induction of cold tolerance following repeated daily cold exposure for five minutes in a cold shower or washing with a basin of cold water. The tolerance is thought to be due to depletion of histamine stores in the skin. This method should not be used indiscriminately as the danger of life-threatening reaction is always present. Large intramuscular doses of penicillin G have also been tried although the rationale is not clear. One million units 2 to 3 times weekly for a total of 10 million units have been given with apparent benefit reported after 3 to 4 million units.

Paroxysmal Cold Hemoglobinuria. Cold exposure is followed by the passage of dark urine with free hemoglobin and constitutional symptoms which vary in intensity and time of onset. Rigor usually occurs first, followed by fever, profuse perspiration, weakness, dyspnea, wheezing, urticaria, and generalized anaphylaxis. Jaundice as well as generalized abdominal complaints can occur. Acrocyanosis and Raynaud's syndrome are not uncommon.

Increased cold agglutinins can cause this symptom complex. Cold agglutinins are normally found in 95 per cent of the normal population. Increased levels are found in several diseases such as Mycoplasma pneumonia infection, viral infections, bronchiectasis, alcoholic cirrhosis, congenital hemolytic anemia, lymphomas, and Waldenström's macroglobulinemia.

Donath-Landsteiner biphasic cold hemolysins also cause this syndrome. These IgG molecules react with red cell antigens below 20° C. and activate the first component 0.5 complement. Upon rewarming, the remainder of the complement cascade occurs resulting in hemolysis. This is usually associated with congenital and tertiary syphilis and rarely with viral infections.

Treatment consists of treating the underlying disease after which the urticaria subsides. The urticaria associated with paroxysmal cold hemoglobinuria is reported to respond to avoidance and antihistamines.

HEAT URTICARIA

Localized Heat Urticaria. This disease is associated with a wheal limited to the area of contact, often with surrounding erythema, following exposure to localized heat. With a large enough exposure, systemic manifestations including abdominal cramps, nausea, vomiting, diarrhea, angioedema, flushing, and even anaphylaxis have occurred. This is a rare condition thought to be mediated by the release of histamines, possibly through a heat-activated enzymatic mechanism or simply through disruption of mast cell membranes in the subcutaneous tissue. A useful diagnostic test can be done using a 25 cc. Erlenmeyer flask filled with water at 45° C. or above for 5 minutes. The usual reaction normally is only erythema.

There is a rare familial type of delayed localized heat urticaria which occurs 1½ to 2 hours after heat exposure, reaching a maximum at 4 to 6 hours and persisting for 12 to 16 hours. It is inherited as a dominant genetic factor and has its onset in childhood.

Treatment for localized heat urticaria consists primarily of avoidance of undue heat. Antihistamines have been reported to block heat challenge. Chlorpheniramine, 0.35 mg./kg./day, or hydroxyzine, 2 to 3 mg./kg./day, may be beneficial, with a trial of higher doses if needed and tolerated.

Generalized Heat Urticaria. Generalized heat urticaria or cholinergic urticaria is induced by increase in temperature, exercise, or psychic stimuli. Mild forms occur in up to 15 per cent of the normal adolescents but without severe systemic effects. The lesion is a distinct micropapular urticaria with a large flare that may give the appearance of a generalized flush.

It is speculated that the mechanism may be a neural reflex phenomenon via the cholinergic nervous system. Hypersensitivity to cholinergic stimuli is suggested by the presence of a positive skin test to methacholine or acetylcholine, characterized by wheals surrounded by smaller satellite lesions with considerable erythema. These patients also often have cholinergic-like systemic symptoms occurring with skin lesions including diarrhea, abdominal cramps, syncope, general weakness, and hypersalivation.

Histamine has been suggested to have a role in this disease when it was found to be increased in the blood following exercise lasting 30 minutes. Vibrational stimuli were also found to increase histamine levels. In a patient with atypical cholinergic urticaria with no pruritus or erythema, histamine and bradykinin were normal, but an increase in serotonin was found.

Treatment largely consists of minimizing excessive exposure to triggering stimuli. Some cases respond to the application of cold and exposure to a cool environment. Trials with several different antihistamines should be tried in severe cases before this therapy is abandoned. Anticholinergic agents have not generally been of any benefit.

TABLE 3.   Drugs and Other Agents Associated with Photoallergic Reactions

PHOTOSENSITIZER	PROBABLE MECHANISM OF ACTION
Antiseptics	
Bithionol (bisphenol)	Photoallergic
Tetrachlorosalicylanilide	
Tribromosalicylanilide	
4′, 5 Dibromosalicylanilide	
3, 5 Dibromosalicylanilide	
Hexachlorophene	
Diuretics	
Thiazides and related sulfonamides	Photoallergic
Tranquilizers	
Chlorpromazine	Phototoxic and photoallergic
Sunscreening agents	
Digalloyl trioleate	Photoallergic
Paraaminobenzoic acid	
Antifungals	
Griseofulvin	Photoallergic
N-butyl-4 chlorosalicylamide (Jadit)	
Antihistamines	
Promethazine hydrochloride	Photoallergic
Antibacterials	
Sulfonamides	Phototoxic and photoallergic
Oral hypoglycemic agents	
Chlorpropamide (Diabinese)	
Tolbutamide (Orinase)	Photoallergic
Miscellaneous agents	
Dibromosalicylic acid	Photoallergic
Cyclamates	Photoallergic

LIGHT HYPERSENSITIVITY

Light hypersensitivity manifests itself as unusual dermatological reactions to very small exposure to light which is well tolerated by normal skin. The reactions can consist of urticaria or as more troublesome reactions with erythema, vesiculation, bullae, or papulovesicular eruptions which occur with phototoxic and photoallergic eruptions. The mechanisms are varied and the differential diagnosis can be difficult.

Photoallergic and Phototoxic Reactions. Photoallergic reactions occur when light is absorbed, converting a nonallergic substance into a new compound which is able to act as a hap-ten. With conjugation to a carrier protein, it acts as an antigen which then initiates an allergic reaction. Sulfonomides and chlorothiazides are well known examples of drugs that cause photoallergy. Other examples are shown in Table 3.

Phototoxic reactions have similar skin manifestations and occur upon first exposure when excitation of the photosensitizer occurs upon exposure to certain specific wavelengths of light. This type of reaction occurs in everyone to some extent when exposed to certain compounds such as psoralens, tetracyclines, and coal tar derivatives. Some compounds have the ability to cause both phototoxic and photoallergic reactions.

The most important part of treatment is elimination of the photosensitizing agent or avoiding light with the use of protective clothing and sunscreens discussed below.

Solar Urticaria. Solar urticaria occurs in certain people oftentimes after an extremely brief exposure to light—as short as 30 seconds. The urticaria is accompanied by pruritus and is confined to the area of exposure lasting up to several hours. Systemic reactions including asthma and anaphylaxis can occur with large exposure of body surface. Six distinct types of solar urticaria can be differentiated by their characteristic wavelength and immunological characteristics (Table 4).

Management is often difficult and primarily consists of avoiding the reaction-producing wavelength. Small increasing doses of sunlight may induce tolerance by increasing the horny layer of the skin and by melanin pigmentation. Since wearing protective garments often is not practical, sunscreen preparations were developed. For protection in the sunburn spectra of 2800 to 3200Å, benzoic acid derivatives such as Pabanol and PreSun are used. Sensitivity to light of wavelengths greater than 3200Å is more difficult to avoid since this includes the visible spectra and is not filtered by glass or sunscreens such as the benzoic acid derivatives. Opaque creams such as titanium dioxide (e.g., A-Fil) may be useful to block the longer

TABLE 4.   Classification of Solar Urticarias

URTICARIA TYPE	ACTION SPECTRUM	PASSIVE TRANSFER	REVERSE PASSIVE TRANSFER	MECHANISM
I	2850 to 3200Å	Positive	Positive	Allergic
II	3200 to 4000Å	Negative	Negative	Unknown—no serum factor demonstrable
III	4000Å to 5000Å	Negative	Negative	Unknown—no serum factor demonstrable
IV	4000Å to 5000Å	Positive	Negative	Unknown—probably allergic
V	2800Å to 5000Å	Negative	Negative	Unknown—no serum factor demonstrable
VI	4000Å	Not reported	Not reported	Protoporphyrin (IX) acts as a photosensitizer; immunologic studies not yet reported

wavelength light. Antihistamines, antimalarials (chloroquine) and steroids given systemically have been reported to give partial relief, but on the whole are disappointing.

Anaphylaxis

DOUGLAS C. HEINER, M.D., Ph.D.,
and LOUIS F. KUEHN, M.D.

Anaphylaxis results from an immunological reaction which leads to the release of chemical mediators and results in smooth muscle contraction, vasodilation and increased permeability of small blood vessels in organs such as the respiratory and gastrointestinal tracts. There often is a drop in blood pressure and a picture of shock. One may think of anaphylaxis as being localized or generalized. Positive skin tests are an example of local anaphylactic reactions and these in themselves are rarely dangerous. Generalized or systemic anaphylactic reactions, on the other hand, are potentially life-threatening and require immediate treatment.

The signs and symptoms of generalized anaphylactic reactions in man may include: (1) a slow, rapid or irregular pulse, hypotension, precordial discomfort, congestive heart failure, ventricular tachycardia or cardiac standstill; (2) a feeling of tightness or pain in the chest, and wheezing, dyspnea, cyanosis or respiratory failure; rhinitis, cough and edema of the upper respiratory airways are commonly found; (3) mild to severe abdominal pain, gastric dilatation, vomiting diarrhea or melena; (4) involvement of the central nervous system with agitation of obtunded sensorium, loss of consciousness, convulsions, coma or death; (5) generalized pruritus, profuse sweating, urticaria or angioedema.

Any of the above may occur within seconds or minutes after exposure to an antigen. Rarely does the first symptom begin more than an hour after exposure. On the other hand, symptoms may persist for hours and may recur for 24 to 48 hours, particularly if therapy is discontinued prematurely. Treatment must be instituted without delay and should be individualized because of the variability in severity of clinical manifestations. Principles helpful in the treatment of every case are outlined below for ready reference.

GUIDE TO SEQUENTIAL MANAGEMENT OF ACUTE GENERALIZED ANAPHYLAXIS

1. Clear the airway and establish air exchange as necessary using mouth-to-mouth resuscitation, intubation, mechanical ventilation, and so on.

2. Administer aqueous epinephrine, 1:1000, 0.1 to 0.5 ml. (0.01 ml./kg. or 0.1 ml./20 lbs.) to a maximum of 0.5 ml. intramuscularly or intravenously. This should be given into the heart if there is cardiac standstill, and should be followed by external cardiac massage. The same dose may be repeated at 5 to 20 minute intervals to a total of three doses. Susphrine, 1:200, 0.008 ml./kg. or 0.08 ml./20 lbs. may be used after a demonstrated response to the first dose or two of aqueous epinephrine.

3. If feasible apply a tourniquet above the site of entry of the offending agent (such as insect bite or antigen injection). Half the above dose of aqueous epinephrine is diluted in 2 ml. of normal saline and infiltrated around the site of entrance of the foreign antigen.

4. If anaphylaxis is severe, or if there is incomplete clearing with epinephrine of bronchospasm, airway obstruction, bradycardia or cardiac standstill, give aminophylline (7 mg./kg. or 70 mg./20 lbs.) intravenously slowly over 10 minutes. This may be repeated after 6 hours.

5. Diphenhydramine (Benadryl), 1.25 mg./kg.; chlorpheniramine (Chlor-Trimeton), 0.25 mg./kg.; or promethazine (Phenergan), 1 mg./kg. is given intravenously immediately after the initial dose of epinephrine (or after aminophylline in severe forms of anaphylaxis). Hydroxyzine (Vistaril), 1.0 mg./kg., may be used intramuscularly but not intravenously. The antihistamine should be given every 6 hours for 48 hours to minimize late recurrences of symptoms.

6. Oxygen is given by mask or endotracheal tube if there is clinical hypoventilation or cyanosis, or if the arterial pO_2 is below 70 mm. Hg in room air.

7. Intravenous fluids (half normal saline in 5 per cent dextrose in water) should be started to permit the ready use of plasma volume expanders, fluid and electrolytes, intravenous medications, and so on.

8. If hypotension, heart failure, arrhythmia or anoxia is a problem, continuous monitoring of blood pressure, central venous pressure, electrocardiogram, and frequent blood gas determinations may be essential.

9. For persisting hypotension use an intravenous vasopressor agent such as norepinephrine (Levophed), 4 ml./liter of 5 per cent dextrose, not to exceed a rate of 1 to 2 ml./min., regulating the speed of administration according to the arterial pressure. Plasma (or 5 per cent human serum albumin), 10 ml./kg. up to 300 ml., may also be given intravenously.

10. Corticosteroids: hydrocortisone (Solu-Cortef), 100 mg.; methylprednisolone

succinate (Solu-Medrol), 20 to 40 mg.; or dexamethasone sodium phosphate (Decadron), 4 mg.; should be given intravenously initially and every 6 hours for 2 days in patients with severe anaphylaxis to forestall a recurrence. Oral corticosteroids may be used in place of intravenous once shock is under control and oral fluids are well tolerated. Steroid action is optimal only after 1 to 2 hours, hence these are *not* the drugs of choice for initial therapy.

11. Isuprel (isoproterenol) by intravenous drip, 0.2 mg./100 ml. of 5 per cent dextrose in water, is a useful drug should epinephrine not be available or if the patient is resistant to other therapy. It may be dangerous to use this drug in conjunction with epinephrine because of the synergistic effect of the two in causing tachycardia or arrhythmia. Continuous cardiovascular monitoring is essential when the two drugs are used within an hour of one another or when isoproterenol is given by intravenous drip.

The above outline is designed to permit treatment of the variable clinical pictures one may encounter in human anaphylaxis. The severity and type of symptoms determine the specific approach to therapy. The intravenous administration of epinephrine is preferred when alarming symptoms must be reversed immediately. Intracardiac administration may be lifesaving if there is severe shock or cardiac standstill. Deep intramuscular administration is sufficient in most instances of moderate severity. The subcutaneous route is somewhat less rapid and is recommended in mild reactions. If the patient fails to respond satisfactorily to the initial dose of aqueous epinephrine, the dose may be repeated within a minute or two in life-threatening situations. The minimal lethal dose of epinephrine is probably about 4 mg. or 4 ml. of 1:1000 aqueous solution. This is about six times the recommended therapeutic dose which in turn often causes mild side reactions. In the rare case in which it may be necessary, phenotolamine (Regitine) in a dose of 1 mg. per 20 lbs. up to 5 mg. for adults may be given intravenously or intramuscularly to counteract untoward effects of epinephrine overdosage.

The second most valuable drug in the therapy of severe anaphylactic reactions is aminophylline, an agent which has received too little attention for this purpose. While it is true that mild systemic anaphylaxis can be managed effectively with epinephrine and antihistaminics alone, it is equally true that many lives could be saved if the treatment of severe reactions included early administration of aminophylline in proper dose as well as its subsequent use to prevent and treat relapses.

Anaphylactic reactions following hyposensitization injections with pollen extracts are more likely to occur when the pollen season is at its peak. Injections should be given low enough in the arm to permit the use of a tourniquet to slow absorption in the event any anaphylactogenic dose is unwittingly administered. Tourniquets may also be useful when insect bites are on an extremity.

If there has been a prior systemic anaphylactic response to a bee sting, one should administer epinephrine both systemically and by local infiltration. Bee sting kits are available commercially and should be carried by all persons known to have had systemic reactions to hymenoptera. Hyposensitization of known susceptibles with venom or whole Hymenoptera extracts is recommended when occupational or home situations are such that repeated stings are likely, or if it is unlikely that epinephrine and other therapeutic agents will be immediately available in the event of a sting.

A vigorous approach utilizing a modern intensive care unit may be needed in dealing with cardiac arrest or respiratory failure. Fortunately the patient with anaphylaxis generally has a good prognosis if skilled treatment is promptly undertaken. He will seldom have simultaneous heart disease and is unlikely to have repeated cardiac arrest if the hypoxia of anaphylaxis has not produced irreversible damage to the myocardium.

The more delayed the onset of an anaphylactic reaction following allergen exposure, the milder it is likely to be. The most severe reactions usually begin within a few seconds or minutes of exposure and almost never make their first appearance after 60 minutes unless medication with antianaphylactic effects has previously been given.

Anaphylactoid reactions, according to some authors, are idiosyncrasies which are unrelated to immunologic responses except that potent pharmacologically active chemical mediators are released. Such reactions may be difficult if not impossible to separate from true anaphylaxis on the basis of clinical evaluations. Initially therapy is identical with that for anaphylaxis. Some so-called anaphylactoid responses may actually result from unrecognized cross reactions to sterically similar allergens or hapten-carrier combinations previously encountered. Only sophisticated immunochemical investigations can help to settle this point. Reactions to the initial encounter with radiographic contrast media are an example. They may be violent and instantaneous, and they demand immediate vigorous therapy as outlined above.

Penicillin is probably the most frequently

encountered anaphylactogen due to its inherent allergenicity and the frequency of its use. The busy practicing physician must be constantly aware of the potential problems which can occasionally accompany the injection of penicillin. Epinephrine and other drugs should be readily accessible, and the need for hospitalization of patients with severe symptoms should be kept in mind. Training in resuscitation techniques can be helpful and should be part of hospital education programs.

Anaphylaxis following ingestion of an allergenic food or drug may begin within a minute or two, or may become manifest only after an hour or more has passed. Time may be required for absorption or for conversion to an allergenic metabolic product within the gastrointestinal tract. The size of the molecule, its susceptibility to acid denaturation and proteolytic degradation, gastric emptying time and intestinal mobility, the presence of foods in the gastrointestinal tract and emesis may all play a role. Sublingual or oropharyngeal absorption perhaps accounts for rapid reactions to certain allergens of low molecular weight. Symptoms of anaphylaxis vary widely due to differences in release of pharmacologically active chemical mediators and in the susceptibility of individual organ systems.

Efforts to prevent anaphylactic reactions are as important as an effective plan of treatment. They include an awareness of the potential hazards of antibiotic injections, hyposensitization procedures, intravenously administered radiographic dyes, insect stings and drug therapy. A knowledge of the many signs and symptoms which may be encountered, prompt judicious therapy which is extended for 48 hours, and careful avoidance of the allergen in the future can be life-saving. Unnecessary drugs should be avoided.

Any substance previously known or thought to have caused an anaphylactic reaction in the past should be used again only when essential to the life or well being of the patient, after careful skin tests have been done and a desensitization schedule drawn up. In general, in such cases one should begin with intradermal injections in the forearm of 0.02 ml. of a 1:1,000,000 dilution of the solution to be injected. If there are no local or systemic reactions within 15 minutes, 0.02 ml. of a 1:100,000 dilution is injected into another site on the same forearm. This process of increasing the concentration in 10-fold increments at 15 minute intervals can be continued until either local or systemic evidence of sensitivity is obtained.

Once any reaction suggesting hypersensitivity is observed, all subsequent injections are given in doubling rather than log increments. Subsequent injections can be given intramuscularly (occasionally slowly intravenously) after "covering" the patient with antihistaminics, theophylline and corticosteroids in full therapeutic doses. Epinephrine must be at hand for use if needed, as should the other items comprising an emergency kit. If severe reactions follow any dose, all the indicated measures described above must be taken and additional use of the drug undertaken with extreme caution and only if the life of the patient requires that the drug be given.

An emergency kit should be kept in each physician's office or should be available for immediate use if he deals with patients who might require treatment for anaphylactic reactions of any cause. Suggested contents of a kit are listed below:

Drugs

Epinephrine hydrochloride solution 1:1000, 1-ml. ampules or 30-ml. vials
Injectable antihistamines—two of the following:
  Diphenhydramine (Benadryl), 50 mg.-ampules
  Chlorpheniramine (Chlor-Trimeton), 10 mg.-vials
  Hydroxyzine (Vistaril), 10 ml.-vials (25 mg./ml.)
  Promethazine hydrochloride (Phenergan), 25 mg.-ampules
Injectable aminophylline, 250 mg.-ampules
Water-soluble corticosteroid esters
  Hydrocortisone (Solu-Cortef or Hydrocortone), 100 mg.-vials
  Methylprednisolone (Solu-Medrol), 40 mg.-vials
  Dexamethasone (Decadron), 4 mg.-vials
Injectable adrenergic agents
  Metaraminol (Aramine), ampules or vials (10 mg./ml. or 10-ml.)
  Levarterenol (Levophed), 4-ml.-ampules (2 mg./ml.)
  Isoproterenol hydrochloride, 1 ml.-ampules (1:5000 solution, 0.2 mg./ml.)
Parenteral fluids
  Five per cent dextrose in normal saline
  Five per cent dextrose in water
  Salt-poor serum albumin, 20-ml. vials
Injectable anticonvulsant drugs
  Amobarbital sodium (Amytal), 65-mg. ampules
  Diazepam (Valium), 10 and 50 mg.-ampules
Sodium bicarbonate, 50-ml. ampules (45 mEq.)

Equipment
  Tourniquets
  Intravenous infusion tubing
  Sterile syringes and needles
  Several sizes of airway and endotracheal tubes
  Lifesaving tube
  Ambu bag
  Aspirator or suction bulb
  Surgical instruments for venous cut-down

20

Accidents and Emergencies

Food Poisoning

JAMES M. HUGHES, M.D.

Food poisoning syndromes may be divided into infections and microbial intoxications (illnesses caused by specific pathogens or toxins elaborated by them) and chemical poisonings (illnesses caused by organic or inorganic chemicals which contaminate foods before or during preparation). In the United States, reported outbreaks of food poisoning are most often bacterial infections or intoxications, though chemical poisonings are being recognized with increasing frequency.

Certain general therapeutic measures are applicable to all kinds of food poisoning. As most cases are characterized by varying degrees of vomiting and diarrhea, the severity of fluid and electrolyte abnormalities must be assessed and promptly corrected by either oral or parenteral fluid therapy. In cases where moderate to severe dehydration has occurred, vital signs and urine output should be closely monitored.

Indications for specific therapeutic measures (e.g., antibiotics, antitoxins, antidotes) are determined by the specific pathogen or agent causing the illness. Symptomatic therapy with antidiarrheal compounds (Lomotil, paregoric, Kaopectate) is probably not efficacious and may be deleterious in some situations; antiemetics such as trimethobenzamide (Tigan) or prochlorperazine (Compazine) should not be given to neonates or young infants and are of limited efficacy in older patients. Frequent feedings of small volumes of liquids such as broth, juice, or noncarbonated soft drinks are preferred for patients with vomiting or diarrhea.

The most common documented outbreaks of food-borne infections and microbial intoxications reported in the United States in 1973 to 1975 were staphylococcal food poisoning, nontyphoid salmonellosis, botulism, *Clostridium perfringens* food poisoning, shigellosis, *Bacillus cereus* food poisoning, and *Vibrio parahaemolyticus* food poisoning, in that order. In recent years, food-borne illness due to both enterotoxigenic and invasive *Escherichia coli* has also been recognized. Though not reported in the United States, food-borne outbreaks caused by *Vibrio cholerae* and noncholera vibrios (organisms biochemically identical to but serologically distinct from *V. cholerae*) occur in other areas of the world. Though hepatitis A and trichinosis are also transmitted by foods, management of these illnesses with predominantly extraintestinal manifestations is not discussed.

Organisms that cause food poisoning characterized by gastrointestinal symptoms do so either through the production of enterotoxins or by tissue invasion. A diagnostic clue to pathogenesis may be obtained by emulsifying a drop of methylene blue with an equal amount of stool; the presence of polymorphonuclear leukocytes indicates that tissue invasion with an inflammatory response has occurred, while their absence suggests that the disease is mediated by an enterotoxin.

Staphylococcus aureus, C. perfringens, and *B. cereus* food poisonings are caused by enterotoxins elaborated by the organisms and are usually self-limited; antibiotics and antidiarrheal drugs play no role in therapy. These illnesses may result in severe dehydration in the very young or very old; fluid therapy is the mainstay of treatment. In staphylococcal food poisoning, in which vomiting may be severe, a dose of trimethobenzamide or prochlorperazine may be administered to children over two years of age if necessary. Severe dehydration and death may occur in cholera and noncholera vibrio infection, diseases also mediated by an enterotoxin. Oral or parenteral fluids are the mainstay of therapy. Tetracycline shortens the duration of fluid loss in cholera; the drug may also be of benefit in noncholera vibrio infection.

In contrast to these diseases, the pathogenesis of nontyphoid salmonellosis and shigellosis is characterized by tissue invasion. In nontyphoid salmonellosis manifested by clinical gastroenteritis in the absence of bacteremia, focal infection, and enteric fever, both antibiotics and antiperistaltic drugs are contraindicated since antibiotics neither shorten nor modify the illness, but prolong the carrier state and favor the development of antibiotic resistance, whereas antiperistaltic drugs such as Lomotil and paregoric may delay excretion of the organisms and have occasionally been thought to be responsible for dissemination of the infection.

Though appropriate antibiotic therapy modifies the severity and shortens the duration of symptomatic shigellosis, one should weigh these benefits against the potential risks of antibiotic therapy (especially when the organisms are resistant to less toxic antibiotics such as ampicillin and tetracycline) and the possibility of selection of antibiotic resistant organisms. In making a decision regarding antibiotic therapy for an illness that is usually self-limited, the severity of illness and likelihood of secondary spread of the infection should be considered. Antiperistaltic drugs are contraindicated in shigellosis because they prolong the duration of fever and excretion of the organisms.

E. coli causes diarrheal disease by several different mechanisms. Classical enteropathogenic *E. coli* (EPEC) strains cause disease in infants by an undefined mechanism; outbreaks which occur in newborn nurseries are often a result of person-to-person spread. Two other categories of *E. coli* have been implicated as a cause of food-borne disease. Some *E. coli* cause disease similar to but generally milder than cholera by elaboration of a heat-labile and/or a heat-stable enterotoxin. Therapy of these infections consists of fluids; although appropriate antibiotic therapy might theoretically be of value, these infections are usually self-limited and antibiotic therapy is probably of no significant value. Recent evidence suggests that Pepto-Bismol may be effective in decreasing stool frequency and fluid loss in infections due to enterotoxigenic *E. coli*. Still other *E. coli*

cause disease by tissue invasion resulting in a syndrome analogous to bacillary dysentery; this syndrome appears to be rare in infants, however. Therapy is again supportive and includes fluids; data evaluating the efficacy of absorbable antibiotics in this illness are not available. Antiperistaltic drugs should not be used.

V. parahaemolyticus food poisoning may be caused by a toxin or tissue invasion. The illness is usually self-limited, and fluids are the mainstay of therapy. Antibiotics are probably of little value, and antiperistaltic drugs should not be prescribed.

Botulism is one of the most severe kinds of food poisoning, with a mortality rate of approximately 20 per cent. Patients with suspected or proven botulism are hospitalized in an intensive care unit and intubated at the first sign of respiratory compromise; ventilatory assistance may be required. Specific therapeutic measures include gastric lavage if the patient is seen within several hours of onset, a cathartic if there is no evidence of paralytic ileus, and high colonic enemas with tap water or saline in an effort to remove unabsorbed toxin and *Clostridium botulinum* organisms from the intestinal tract. Administration of trivalent (ABE) botulinal antitoxin parenterally following skin testing for horse serum sensitivity is recommended as soon as the diagnosis is established with reasonable certainty. Although the appropriate dosage is somewhat arbitrary, one vial (containing 7500 units A antitoxin, 5500 units B antitoxin, and 8500 units E antitoxin) is given intravenously and an additional vial intramuscularly. In older children and adults, this dose is repeated once in 4 to 6 hours. Emergency consultation and trivalent antitoxin may be obtained from the Center for Disease Control (404-633-3311, extension 3753 days; 404-633-2176 nights and weekends). The role of oral penicillin and guanidine therapy in botulism remains controversial, and these drugs should probably not be used in cases of food-borne botulism.

Although botulism is more common and more severe in adults than in children, a syndrome of infant botulism affecting children less than 6 months of age has been recently recognized. As botulinal toxin and organisms may persist in these patients' stools after they become asymptomatic, the role of antitoxin therapy in infants is controversial; potential benefits must be weighed against the risks of sensitization or reactions to the horse serum preparation.

Asymptomatic individuals who have consumed foods suspected of causing botulism are given an emetic and/or gastric lavage if they have eaten the food in the past several hours, and a cathartic or high colonic enema if they have eaten the food in the past 48 hours, and are hospitalized for treatment at the first symptom or sign of botulism.

Fish and shellfish poisonings are the most commonly reported chemical poisonings in the United States. In scombroid fish poisoning, an antihistamine provides relief of the characteristic pruritus and urticaria, while bronchodilators (epinephrine or aminophylline) may be required in severe cases accompanied by bronchospasm. Therapy of ciguatera fish poisoning is primarily symptomatic; because of the characteristic painful paresthesias, analgesics may be required. Patients should be observed closely for evidence of respiratory compromise; intubation and ventilatory assistance may be required in severe cases. In these cases, gastric lavage, a cathartic and high enemas are administered in an effort to remove unabsorbed toxin. Therapy of paralytic shellfish poisoning is similar to that of ciguatera except that analgesics are not required.

The second most commonly reported and most serious kind of chemical food poisoning is mushroom poisoning. At least seven different types exist; the most severe is caused by species containing phallotoxins and amatoxins (*Amanita phalloides, Amanita verna, Amanita virosa,* and certain *Galerina* sp.). These patients should be given gastric lavage, a cathartic and high enemas; hypoglycemia may occur and require treatment with intravenous glucose solutions. Thioctic acid, an experimental drug, appears to be an effective antidote in these cases and may be obtained by contacting Dr. Frederic Bartter or Dr. Jerry Mitchell at the National Institutes of Health (301-496-6268 weekdays; 301-656-4000 or 202-244-5562 nights and weekends). Peritoneal dialysis or hemodialysis may benefit patients who develop renal failure. Patients with illness caused by species containing pharmacologically active amounts of muscarine (many *Inocybe* sp. and some *Clitocybe* sp.) may benefit from subcutaneous atropine if they have symptoms and signs of parasympathetic hyperactivity.

Heavy metals such as copper, tin, zinc, and cadmium occasionally cause food poisoning. As these illnesses are characterized by short (5 to 15 minute) incubation periods and vomiting, the responsible agent is usually rapidly eliminated from the gastrointestinal tract, and systemic toxicity is rare. Treatment is symptomatic, and antiemetics are not given because they might cause retention of the toxic ions in the gut with systemic absorption.

Food poisoning usually is a self-limited illness; however, it may be severe in very young, very old, and debilitated individuals. Certain food-borne illnesses (botulism, mushroom poisoning, and paralytic shellfish poisoning) may cause severe illness and death in previously healthy individuals. Effective therapy includes supportive and, in many cases, specific measures; the latter require recognition of the specific etiology of the illness. Equally important in the management of food-borne disease outbreaks is the prevention of additional cases; this goal may be achieved through prompt notification of public health authorities of cases of suspected food-borne illnesses. Public health officials may then identify the responsible food, thereby preventing future cases, and locate other individuals who have already eaten it and are at risk of becoming ill.

Acute Poisoning

FREDERICK H. LOVEJOY, JR., M.D., *and* JOEL J. ALPERT, M.D.

Well over one million poisonings occur yearly in the United States. The majority of poisonings occur in the pediatric age group and are generally self-limited. The outcome, however, is age related. For example, because adolescent poisonings are often purposeful, the severity of the poisoning in this age group is often greater than in childhood. The last 20 years has seen a reduction in the overall mortality from poisonings, primarily as a result of improved diagnosis, therapy and efforts at prevention. Poison centers provide both the public and professionals with rapid access to information on diagnosis and appropriate therapy. Many particularly dangerous poisons are now less accessible to children as a result of safety packaging.

Nonetheless, acute poisoning remains a major cause of morbidity and hospitalization in children and adolescents requiring familiarity with available means for the identification of an ingested substance and a well grounded understanding of the approaches to management. This chapter is intended to offer a general approach to management as well as a review of a number of specific toxins and their therapy.

IDENTIFICATION

Initial management of the overdosed victim depends upon a clear assessment of the severity of clinical involvement and rapid identification of the ingested substance. Further, for effective management of the acute overdose the physician requires a rapid answer to four critical questions. What was taken? When was it taken? How much was taken? Are there any symptoms that would increase the hazard of the various procedures used to remove the ingested product?

Ingestions generally involve those substances which are commonly available in the home. Table 1, taken from calls to the Boston Poison Information Center for a five month period, lists the most common household products and drugs presently ingested by adolescents and children. With children the ingested product generally is known. In the case of the adolescent overdose, identification is often difficult. For all ages, knowledge of medications and products kept in the home as well as drugs commonly being abused locally will be helpful. The quantity ingested is often difficult to determine especially where liquids are involved. As a useful estimate, a swallow in a young child is equivalent to 2 to 5 ml. If a poisoning occurred with tablets or capsules, it is helpful to know how many were present prior to the incident.

It is important to use the largest estimated amount when recommending therapy. When more than one child is involved, it should be assumed that each child consumed the total amount of ingested agent and both should be treated. Knowing what has not been ingested can also be helpful. Knowing that the product is not a caustic or hydrocarbon and that the child is not seizing or comatose allows one to proceed, even in the uncertain situation, to removal.

The physical condition of the child is determined rapidly over the phone or by direct examination. The state of consciousness and the rate of progression of clinical illness are of critical importance. A grading system based on repeated careful physical examinations is help-

TABLE 1. Drugs and Household Products Most Commonly Ingested by Children and Adolescents*

DRUGS	HOUSEHOLD PRODUCTS
Aspirin	Bleach
Valium	Moth balls
Vitamins	Cologne
Rubbing alcohol	Gasoline
Desitin	Perfume
Fluoride	Ammonia
Acetaminophen	Alcohol
Dimetapp	Shampoo
Dalmane	Lysol
Darvon	Mercury in thermometer
Ex-Lax	Turpentine
Librium	Ink
Chlordane	Cement
Elavil	Matches
Phenobarbital	Chalk

*Descending frequency of ingestion, inhalation or cutaneous exposures from 8240 calls during the five month period from July to November 1976 (Boston Poison Information Center Computer Program).

ful in determining initial severity of the ingestion and its subsequent rate of improvement or worsening over time. A commonly used scale adapted from Matthew and associates is: grade 0—fully awake; grade I—drowsy with response to verbal command; grade II—comatose and unresponsive to verbal command; grade III—comatose and responsive only to deep painful stimuli; grade IV—comatose and unresponsive to painful stimuli, areflexic, with or without respiratory depression. This grading system is also highly useful in assessing response to antidote therapy.

Immediate correction of any compromise of vital function is essential. The priorities to be observed include: provision of a clear airway, maintenance of pulmonary ventilation by mechanical respiratory assistance, evaluation of cardiac function, provision of a secure intravenous route, treatment of shock by fluids and colloid rather than vasopressor drugs, treatment of hyperpyrexia with a cooling blanket rather than use of antipyretic agents, and management of convulsions due to hypoxia and acidosis with effective pulmonary ventilation and treatment of drug-induced convulsions with anticonvulsant agents. The institution of methods to remove a toxin should be considered only after the above procedures have been completed.

Of particular interest on physical examination are the vital signs, the eyes, autonomic nervous system, respiratory, cardiovascular and cutaneous systems as well as the smell and color of all body fluids (vomitus, blood, urine). Qualitative analysis of blood, urine and vomitus will assist in the diagnosis of the poisoning of unclear etiology. Quantitative analysis of blood will assist in a more accurate assessment of the severity of the poisoning. Knowledge of appropriate and available laboratories and their quality are essential.

Signs and Symptoms Suggesting a Specific Poison

Signs and symptoms, though nonspecific, often point to a diagnosis and in certain instances may permit identification of the poison. Most children who ingest a poison are recognized before symptoms develop and a careful history will generally identify what has been ingested. When these circumstances do not hold, a carefully performed physical examination with attention to typical odors and screening tests can help in making a rapid diagnosis. Diagnostic therapeutic trials will further facilitate making a diagnosis. Confirmation is still necessary by definitive laboratory analysis. A partial list of common toxins or groups of toxins is listed, followed by the signs and symptoms these toxins produce.

GROUPS OF TOXINS

Anticholinergic agents—tricyclic antidepressants, antihistamines with anticholinergic properties, atropine and scopolamine drugs, plants.

Caustic agents—acid and alkali detergents, electric dishwasher granules.

Cholinergic agents—carbamate and organophosphate insecticides (malathion, parathion, chlorthion), anticholinesterase drugs (physostigmine, neostigmine), parasympathomimetic drugs (nicotine), mushrooms (muscarine containing), plants.

Drugs causing hypoxia—respiratory depressant drugs, carbon monoxide, cyanide, drugs causing methemoglobinemia (nitrobenzene, analine, acetanilid, nitrites, pyridium).

Drug withdrawal—narcotics, alcohol, barbiturates, amphetamines, methaqualone.

Heavy metals—arsenic, inorganic and organic mercury, thallium, iron, lead.

Narcotic and narcotic-like drugs—heroin, methadone, codeine, morphine, propoxyphene, pentazocine, diphenoxylate hydrochloride.

Sedative drugs—barbiturates, ethanol, methanol, tranquilizers, benzodiazepines, solvents, chloral hydrate, phenols, bromides, benzene, xylene, chloroform, carbon tetrachloride.

Spider bites—black widow, scorpion.

Sympathomimetic and stimulant drugs—amphetamines, cocaine, ephedrine, benzedrine.

Uncouplers of oxidative phosphorylation—salicylates, hexachlorobenzene, dinitrophenol, sodium fluoroacetate.

SIGNS AND SYMPTOMS

Specific drugs are listed when they are a common cause of a particular sign or symptom.

Temperature

Hyperthermia—uncouplers of oxidative phosphorylation, anticholinergic drugs, quinine, boric acid, snake bites.

Hypothermia—sedative drugs in large overdose.

Central Nervous System

Depression and coma—uncouplers of oxidative phosphorylation (salicylates), anticholinergic agents, drugs causing hypoxia, narcotics and narcotic-like drugs, cholinergic agents, metals (arsenic, iron), sedative drugs.

Convulsions—anticholinergic agents (tricyclic antidepressants), sympathomimetic drugs (amphetamines, cocaine), drug withdrawal, narcotics (codeine, propoxyphene), metals (lead), organophosphate and chlorinated hydrocarbon insecticides, drugs causing hypoxia, camphor products, salicylates, strychnine.

Paralysis—food poisoning (botulism), shell fish poisoning, dying back neuropathy (triorthylcresyl

phosphate, malathion, mipafox), heavy metals (thallium), plants (coniine).

Respiratory

Hyperventilation—drugs causing hypoxia, uncouplers of oxidative phosphorylation, sympathomimetic drugs, drug-induced pneumonias (hydrocarbons, talc inhalation).

Hypoventilation—sedative drugs in large overdose, narcotic and narcotic-like drugs, snake bites.

Cardiac

Arrhythmias—anticholinergic agents (tricyclic antidepressants), digitalis-containing drugs, plants, narcotics (codeine, propoxyphene), pesticides (red squill, sodium fluoroacetate), sympathomimetic agents (methylphenidate, amphetamines), phenothiazines, ipecac syrup.

Tachycardia—sympathomimetic drugs, anticholinergic agents, drug withdrawal.

Bradycardia—sedative drugs, narcotic drugs, cholinergic agents, digitalis.

Hypertension—sympathomimetic drugs, heavy metals (inorganic mercury, lead).

Hypotension—sedative drugs in large overdose.

Gastrointestinal Tract

Hematemesis—caustic agents, phenols, fluoride, heavy metals (iron, arsenic), salicylates, theophylline, boric acid.

Abdominal colic—heavy metals (arsenic, iron), black widow spider, drug withdrawal (narcotics), cholinergic agents, snake bites.

Dysphagia—food poisoning (botulism), caustic agents.

Skin

Cyanosis—drugs and household products producing methemoglobinemia, carbon monoxide, sedative drugs in large overdose.

Jaundice—drug-induced hemolytic anemia (naphthalene), hepatotoxic drugs (carbon tetrachloride, acetaminophen).

Increased sweating—cholinergic agents, heavy metals (arsenic, mercury, bismuth), uncouplers of oxidative phosphorylation.

Flush—sympathomimetic drugs, anticholinergic agents, boric acid, carbon monoxide, reserpine, alcohol, snake bites.

Hair loss—heavy metals (thallium, arsenic), radioactive agents (radium, x-ray), chemotherapeutic agents.

Eye Signs

Dilation of pupils—anticholinergic agents, sympathomimetic drugs, psychedelic drugs (LSD, marijuana), drug withdrawal, glutethimide.

Constricted pupils—narcotics and narcotic-like drugs, cholinergic agents, barbiturates, phenothiazines, alcohol, phencyclidine.

Colored vision and scotomata—salicylates, quinine.

Mucous Membranes

Increased salivation—caustic agents, heavy metals (arsenic, thallium, mercury, bismuth), cholinergic agents, organophosphate insecticides, muscarine-containing mushrooms.

Dry mucous membranes—anticholinergic agents, sympathomimetic drugs, narcotic and narcotic-like drugs.

Discoloration—heavy metals (lead, mercury, bismuth, arsenic).

Abnormal Odor on Breath

Alcohol odor—phenols, chloral hydrate, alcohol; acetone—lacquer, alcohol; coal gas—carbon monoxide; wintergreen—methyl salicylate; garlic odor—phosphorus, arsenic; bitter almonds—cyanide; others—hydrocarbons, turpentine, camphor, ether, paraldehyde.

Abnormal Color of Urine

Dark green—phenol, resorcinol; brown or black—antipyrine (after long use); yellow—picric acid; bright yellow changing to scarlet on adding alkali—santonin; orange—Azo Gantrisin, pyridium; blue green—methylene blue; red—warfarin, fava beans.

Rapid X-Ray Diagnosis

Radiopaque particles in gastrointestinal tract—lead, arsenic, iron, chloral hydrate, bismuth, thallium; radiopaque lines in bones—lead, fluoride; stomach—double fluid level hydrocarbons.

Rapid Laboratory Tests

Carbon monoxide (1 ml. blood and 10 ml. of water and 1 ml. of 5 per cent NaOH)—normal blood turns brown; if carbon monoxide level less than 20 per cent, blood turns straw yellow; if greater than 20 per cent pink persists; phenothiazines—2 ml. urine plus 2 to 5 drops 10 per cent ferric chloride solution—light pink to lilac color; salicylates—2 ml. urine plus 2 to 5 drops 10 per cent ferric chloride solution, boiled—burgundy red; chocolate-colored blood failing to turn pink on exposure to air or oxygen for 10 minutes—methemoglobinemia.

Diagnostic Therapeutic Trials

Naloxone hydrochloride for narcotics; atropine for organophosphate insecticides; diphenhydramine for extrapyramidal tract signs from phenothiazines; deferoxamine for iron; physostigmine for anticholinergic agents.

Detailed management of the many drugs and products taken in overdose can be found in various general toxicology texts, drug references and computerized indexes as noted in the reference section of this chapter. An approach to the management of a partial list of common childhood and adolescent ingestions is outlined in Table 2.

PREVENTION OF SYSTEMIC ABSORPTION

The effectiveness of emetics and lavage depends on the promptness with which these procedures are instituted as well as on the pharmacologic properties of the ingested agent. Most drugs are well absorbed from the gastrointestinal tract with peak levels occurring within 2 hours of ingestion; therefore, removal by emesis or lavage is generally useful only in the first few hours following ingestion. After a period of 2 to 3 hours following ingestion, removal is considered only for certain drugs that are slowly absorbed (methyl salicylates, enteric-coated drugs and drugs causing grade III or IV coma) or for drugs that slow gastrointestinal motility and result in delayed absorption (narcotics and anticholinergic agents). The form in which the drug is dispensed influences the rate of absorption. Liquids are absorbed more rapidly than solids, and enteric-coated products are absorbed more slowly and erratically than standard capsules or tablets. A full stomach will also slow absorption.

The degree to which a drug is ionized influences its absorption through lipid membranes. As the amount of nonionized drug increases, its lipid solubility and consequently its rate of absorption increase. Barbiturates, for example, are weak acids (pKa 7.2 to 8.0) and in the acid medium of the stomach exist primarily in the nonionized form and are therefore well absorbed. In the alkaline media of the small bowel a greater proportion of the barbiturate is ionized with less rapid and complete absorption. Knowledge of the pKa of a drug (available in pharmacology texts) is thus an important factor in determining whether a toxin will be primarily absorbed in the acid medium of the stomach or in the more alkaline environment of the small bowel.

Decisions concerning removal of ingested products are among the most common and most critical in the initial management of the acute overdose. The patient's level of consciousness is the most important consideration in this decision. Because of the risk of aspiration pneumonia, emesis should not be induced if the patient is already obtunded or if the onset of action of the ingested product is sufficiently rapid that obtundation may occur at the time of emesis. The presence of convulsions is also a contraindication to removal of a toxin by emesis. The risk of leaving the ingested product in the stomach must always be carefully weighed against the risks involved in inducing emesis and the amount of ingested toxin that can be expected to be recovered by the emetic

TABLE 2.   Treatment of Specific Poisons

DRUG	TOXICITY AND EXCRETION	SYMPTOMS	TREATMENT
Acetaminophen (Tylenol, Tempra, Liquiprin)	Potential hepatotoxicity with ingestions of >15 gm. in adolescent and >5 gm. in child. Hepatotoxicity with serum level >300 μg./ml. 4 hours following ingestion. Major route of excretion—hepatic metabolism	Nausea, vomiting, diaphoresis; 36 to 48 hours following ingestion—jaundice, elevated hepatic enzymes and bilirubin, prolonged prothrombin time; fully reversible or progresses to hepatic failure; renal and myocardial toxicity	Removal with emesis or lavage, activated charcoal (Table 3), support for hepatic failure, treatment of hepatic failure, (cysteamine, methionine, acetylcysteine) (see text)
Acids (Lysol)	Toxicity related to concentration and duration of exposure	Corrosive burns of mucous membranes, mouth, esophagus and stomach; pain in area of burns; circulatory collapse and shock; complications—esophageal and gastric perforation, glottic edema, pulmonary edema, pneumonia, stricture formation of esophagus and pylorus	Emetics and lavage are contraindicated; immediate removal from esophagus with water or milk: neutralization with an alkali not advised; opiates for pain; intravenous therapy for shock; for further therapy see under Alkali
Alkali (Lye, Drano, Saniflush, Clinitest)	Toxicity to esophagus related to concentration and duration of exposure	Corrosive burns of mucous membranes of mouth and esophagus; pain in area of burns; circulatory collapse and shock; complications—esophageal and gastric perforation, glottic edema, pulmonary edema, pneumonia, stricture formation of esophagus	Emetics and lavage are contraindicated; immediate removal from esophagus with water or milk: neutralization with an acid not advised; opiates for pain; intravenous therapy for shock; with evidence of esophageal or gastric burn (clinically, by esophagoscopy or by esophagram), prednisone, 2 to 3 mg./kg./24 hour for 3 weeks and then tapered over 1 week; broad-spectrum antibiotic coverage while on steroids; following therapy, upper gastrointestinal series for evidence of stricture; dilation of stricture if present
Ammonium hydroxide (ammonia)	Toxicity to esophagus related to concentration and duration of exposure	Corrosive burns of mucous membranes of mouth and esophagus; circulatory collapse and shock; complications include esophageal and gastric perforation, glottic edema, pulmonary edema, pneumonia	Emetics and lavage are contraindicated; immediate removal from esophagus with water or milk: neutralization with acid not advised; further therapy as outlined under Alkali

TABLE 2. Treatment of Specific Poisons (Continued)

DRUG	TOXICITY AND EXCRETION	SYMPTOMS	TREATMENT
Amphetamines (Benzedrine, Dexedrine, Dexamyl)	Symptoms when therapeutic dose exceeded. Lethal dose in man estimated at 20 to 25 mg./kg. Major route of excretion—hepatic metabolism; minor route—renal	Nervousness, hyperactivity, mania, psychotic-like state; tachycardia, hypertension, cardiac arrhythmias, hyperpyrexia; convulsions and shock	Emesis or lavage; activated charcoal (Table 3); control of seizures with barbiturates or diazepam; support for cardiovascular and respiratory failure; acidification of urine with ammonium chloride to increase excretion of drug; chlorpromazine; phenoxybenzamine or phentolamine for hypertensive emergencies. (See Table 4 and text.)
Aniline	Induces methemoglobinemia. Cyanosis with methemoglobin levels of greater than 15 per cent; lethargy with levels greater than 40 per cent; potential lethal levels at greater than 70 per cent Major route of excretion—hepatic metabolism	Apathy and headache, cyanosis with dyspnea, hypotension and convulsions, circulatory and respiratory failure, intravascular hemolysis	Emesis or lavage; removal from source of exposure; oxygen; methylene blue (Table 4 and text); transfusion therapy for intravascular hemolysis
Antihistamines and cold medications (Dimetapp, Congesprin, Actifed, Contac, Sudafed, Allerest, Triaminic)	Symptoms when therapeutic dose exceeded Major route of excretion—hepatic metabolism	Excitation, disorientation, drowsiness, coma; anticholinergic syndrome—dry mouth, dilated pupils, fever, flushed skin, tachycardia, absent bowel sounds, urinary retention; hypertension, hypotension; convulsions; arrhythmias; cardiovascular collapse and respiratory depression	Emesis or lavage; activated charcoal (Table 3); vigorous gastrointestinal catharsis; treatment of fever; maintenance fluid therapy; support for circulatory and respiratory failure; treatment of seizures with barbiturates or Valium; treatment with physostigmine. (See Table 4 and text.)
Arsenic	Major toxicity—gastrointestinal, hepatic, renal and central nervous system Major route of excretion—renal	Sweetish metallic taste in mouth; burning sensation in throat; diarrhea, vomiting, dehydration; delirium, convulsions, coma, hyperreflexia, seizures; pulmonary edema; hemolysis; arsenic in gastrointestinal tract—radiopaque on x-ray; toxic effects on liver, kidney and marrow	Emesis or lavage; intravenous hydration; treatment of liver and renal decompensation; transfusion therapy for hemolytic anemia; dimercaprol (BAL) therapy indicated when unknown amount ingested, with symptoms or when toxic levels exist (Table 4 and text)
Atropine (atropine and scopolamine-containing agents)	Symptoms when therapeutic dose exceeded Major route of excretion—hepatic metabolism	Excitation, disorientation, drowsiness, coma; anticholinergic syndrome—dry mouth, dilated pupils, fever, flushed skin, tachycardia, absent bowel sounds, urinary retention; hypertension,	Emesis or lavage; activated charcoal (Table 3); vigorous gastrointestinal catharsis; treatment of fever; maintenance fluid therapy; support for circulatory and respiratory failure; treat-

Poison	Toxicity	Signs and Symptoms	Treatment
		hypotension; convulsions; arrhythmias; cardiovascular collapse and respiratory depression.	ment of seizures with barbiturates or diazepam (Table 4); treatment with physostigmine
Barbiturates (amobarbital, secobarbital, pentobarbital, phenobarbital)	Potentially fatal dose 40 to 50 mg./kg. for short-acting barbiturates, and 65 to 75 mg./kg. for long-acting barbiturates. Blood levels of 3 to 4 mg./100 ml. for short-acting barbiturates and 10 to 15 mg./100 ml. for long-acting barbiturates found with severe overdose (grades III–IV). Excretion of short acting barbiturates—hepatic metabolism. Excretion of long acting barbiturates—renal and hepatic metabolism	Mental confusion, drowsiness, coma; ataxia, vertigo, slurred speech; decreased deep tendon reflexes, decreased response to pain; hypotension, hypothermia; pulmonary edema with short-acting barbiturates; respiratory failure	Emesis or lavage; activated charcoal (Table 3); forced fluid diuresis for long-acting barbiturates; alkalinization of urine for long-acting barbiturates (Table 4); osmotic agents and diuretics for long-acting barbiturates (Table 4); maintenance fluids for short-acting barbiturates; support for respiratory and cardiovascular failure; dialysis for long-acting barbiturates
Bleach (Clorox, Purex, Sani-Chlor)	Major toxicities to intestinal mucosa and central nervous system. Major route of excretion—renal	Irritation and pain to mouth and esophagus; stricture and perforation extremely unlikely; nausea and vomiting; delirium, obtundation and coma; hypotension	Removal with lavage if vomiting has not occurred; removal from skin by flooding with water; support for central nervous system and circulatory failure; treatment as caustic (acid-alkali) not necessary
Boric acid	Fatal dose is estimated at 0.1 to 0.5 gm./kg. Major route of excretion—renal	Bloody diarrhea and dehydration; erythroderma and exfoliation; lethargy, convulsions; jaundice; hypotension; anuria; coma	Removal from skin, with ingestion emesis or lavage, intravenous fluids, treatment of seizures with barbiturates and diazepam (Table 4)
Bromides	Bromides produce toxicity by displacing chlorides from plasma and cells. Bromide toxicity occurs at >50 mg./100 ml. Major route of excretion—renal	Acute ingestion causes nausea, vomiting, paralysis and coma; chronic poisoning causes confusion, ataxia, slurred speech, irritability, delusions, psychotic behavior, stupor	Emesis or lavage; sodium chloride, 5 gm./day in divided doses for 1 to 4 weeks (in adolescent) to hasten excretion; hemodialysis
Camphor (Campho-Phenique, camphor liniment)	Fatal dose for a 1 year-old child is approximately 1 gm. Major route of excretion—hepatic	Headache; burning in mouth and throat; camphor odor on breath; nausea and vomiting; feeling of warmth, excitement, irrational behavior, muscle spasms, convulsions, coma; circulatory and respiratory collapse	Emesis or lavage; activated charcoal (Table 3); treatment of seizures with barbiturates or diazepam (Table 4); support for respiratory and circulatory failure

TABLE 2.   Treatment of Specific Poisons (Continued)

DRUG	TOXICITY AND EXCRETION	SYMPTOMS	TREATMENT
Carbon monoxide	Cellular hypoxia as a result of high affinity of carbon monoxide for hemoglobin. Major route of excretion—respiratory	At 20 per cent carboxyhemoglobin—headache, vertigo, shortness of breath; at 40 to 50 per cent carboxyhemoglobin—coma, cherry-red color to lips and skin, cardiac arrhythmias and ischemia, respiratory failure, irreversible brain damage	Removal of patient from site of exposure to uncontaminated air; 100 per cent oxygen by mask for 30 min. to two hours; with respiratory depression, artificial respiration with 100 per cent oxygen; maintain temperature and blood pressure; recognition and treatment of cerebral edema. (See Table 4 and text.)
Carbon tetrachloride	Toxic dose by ingestion is as low as 3 to 5 ml. Causes injury to liver, kidneys, myocardium, central nervous system. Major exposure—oral or by inhalation. Major route of excretion—hepatic metabolism	Abdominal pain, nausea and vomiting; headache and confusion; obtundation, coma, respiratory depression; circulatory collapse; renal, hepatic and myocardial damage	Emesis or lavage; maintenance hydration; avoid epinephrine and related compounds; respiratory support; management of renal and hepatic damage
Cathartics (mineral oil, Ex-Lax, phenolphthalein, Metamucil)	Generally of low toxicity	Irritation of gastrointestinal tract causing tenesmus, vomiting, diarrhea; rarely hypotension, collapse, coma	With large ingestion, emesis or lavage; milk to decrease gastrointestinal irritation; if severe symptoms, hydration, medication for pain, treatment of shock
Chloral hydrate	Dose greater than 50 mg./kg. causes hypnotic effects. Major route of excretion—hepatic metabolism	Drowsiness, mental confusion, coma, shock, respiratory depression	Emesis or lavage, maintenance fluids, respiratory support
Cyanide	Cyanide exerts toxicity on cellular cytochrome oxidase systems causing cytotoxic anoxia. Severe and rapid onset of toxicity. Routes of exposure include ingestion and inhalation. Survival for 4 hours often associated with recovery	Death in 10 to 15 minutes; bitter almond smell; tachycardia, bradycardia; absence of cyanosis; coma; hypotension; convulsions	Respiratory support with 100 per cent oxygen; removal to uncontaminated atmosphere and removal of contaminated clothing; lavage after antidotes have been given; immediate use of amyl nitrite by inhalation followed by sodium nitrite; sodium thiosulfate (See Table 4 and text.)
Detergents, soaps and cleaners	Variable toxicity	Anionic detergents (Tide, Cheer, Ajax, Top Job, Comet, Windex, Mr. Clean, Lestoil, Joy, Spic n Span, bar soap, bub-	For anionic detergents–supportive therapy; no removal necessary. For cationic detergents: emesis or lavage,

		ble bath, household detergents) cause mild vomiting and diarrhea; cationic detergents (pHisoHex, Zephiran, Diaparene) cause nausea, vomiting, convulsions, coma; electric dishwasher and laundry granules cause caustic burns	support for coma and respiratory failure, and treatment of seizures with barbiturates or diazepam (Table 4). For treatment of dishwater and laundry granule burns, see under Alkali
Digitalis	Toxic symptoms when therapeutic dose exceeded Major route of excretion—hepatic metabolism with biliary and renal excretion of metabolites	Nausea, vomiting, altered color vision, slow and irregular pulse, hypotension, arrhythmias due to increased myocardial irritability	Emesis or lavage; activated charcoal (Table 3); maintenance fluids; potassium; quinidine, Pronestyl, Xylocaine as determined by type of arrhythmias
Ergot derivatives (Sansert, ergotamine)	Toxic symptoms when therapeutic dose exceeded. Low toxicity Major route of excretion—hepatic metabolism	Diarrhea, vomiting; convulsions; hypotension; coma; constriction of blood vessels with numbness, coldness and gangrene of extremities with chronic ingestion	Emesis or lavage; control of seizures with barbiturates and diazepam (Table 4); respiratory and cardiovascular support; vasodilators may be required with chronic ingestion
Ethyl alcohol (ethanol, isopropyl alcohol, cologne, perfume)	Blood level: 0.05 to 0.15 per cent, mild; 0.15 to 0.3 per cent, moderate; 0.3–0.5 per cent, severe; above 0.5 per cent, coma Major route of excretion—hepatic metabolism	Initial excitation, delirium and inebriation; later depression, stupor, coma; alcohol odor on breath; hypoglycemia; slurred speech and muscle incoordination; respiratory failure	Emesis or lavage, glucose for hypoglycemia, maintenance fluids, support for respiratory and circulatory failure, hemodialysis
Fluoride	Of low toxicity with 50 to 200 mg./kg. as the estimated fatal dose. Fluorides act as cellular poisons interfering with calcium metabolism and enzyme mechanisms Major route of excretion—renal	Nausea, vomiting and diarrhea; salivation and irritation of mucous membranes; tremors and convulsions; respiratory failure; complications include jaundice, oliguria, anemia, leukopenia	Emesis or lavage, intravenous fluids, oxygen, support for cardiovascular and respiratory failure, calcium gluconate by mouth as local antidote to bind ingested fluoride (see text)
Hormones (Enovid, Ortho-Novum, Oracon, Norlestrin, Premarin)	Low toxicity	Nausea and vomiting, fluid retention, vaginal bleeding in girls	Emesis or lavage if more than 15 to 20 tablets have been ingested

TABLE 2. Treatment of Specific Poisons (Continued)

DRUG	TOXICITY AND EXCRETION	SYMPTOMS	TREATMENT
Hydrocarbons (kerosene, gasoline, mineral spirits, paint thinner, lighter fluid, barbecue fluid, dry cleaning fluid)	Toxicity to lungs and central nervous system. Major route of excretion—hepatic metabolism	Hydrocarbon smell in mouth and on breath; burning in the mouth and esophagus; vomiting; pulmonary symptoms—cough, fever, bloody sputum, cyanosis, rales, pulmonary infiltrates; central nervous system drowsiness, mild coma, seizures	Removal is not indicated with petroleum distillate hydrocarbon ingestions in children. If very large amounts (>100 ml.) are taken (as in a suicide attempt), in alert patient emesis with ipecac syrup is a safer method of removal than lavage. For pneumonia use of oxygen and antibiotics with signs of superinfection; use of steroids not indicated. Supportive therapy for central nervous system depression and seizures; avoid epinephrine; appropriate support for hepatic, renal, cardiac and bone marrow toxicity
Chlorinated hydrocarbon insecticides (DDT, dieldrin, lindane)	Variability of toxicity among compounds. Routes of absorption include gastrointestinal and cutaneous. Variability of absorption from cutaneous route	Vomiting, excitation, numbness, weakness, incoordination, tremors, seizures, circulatory and respiratory failure	Decontamination of skin, removal with emesis or lavage, gastrointestinal catharsis, support for respiratory or circulatory failure, control of seizures with barbiturates and diazepam (Table 4)
Organophosphate insecticides (parathion, chlorthion, Bidrin, Dimetilan, Sevin)	Major route of excretion—hepatic metabolism with metabolites often pharmacologically active	Blurred vision, sweating, miosis, tearing, salivation, papilledema, cyanosis, seizures, pulmonary edema	Decontamination of skin, removal with emesis or lavage, gastrointestinal catharsis, support for respiratory or circulatory failure, control of seizures with barbiturates and diazepam, atropine sulfate, pralidoxime chloride. (See Table 4 and text)
Carbamate insecticides		Same as for organophosphate insecticides	Decontamination of skin, removal with emesis or lavage, gastrointestinal catharsis, support for respiratory or circulatory failure, control of seizures with barbiturates and diazepam, atropine sulfate. (See Table 4 and text.)
Ipecac syrup	Amounts greater than 30 ml. are potentially toxic	Nausea and vomiting; tachycardia, arrhythmias, hypotension; dyspnea; cardiac, hepatic and marrow toxicity; coma	Removal by emesis or lavage, activated charcoal (Table 4), observation for arrhythmias or heart failure, treatment of hepatic or marrow toxicity
Iron (ferrous sulfate, ferrous	Serum level of >400 μg./100 ml. associated with systemic toxicity. Major toxicities—	Symptoms occur ½ to 4 hours post ingestion; vomiting, diarrhea, melena; drowsiness, lethargy, pallor; metabolic	Emesis or lavage; bicarbonate or phosphates to precipitate iron and prevent absorption; fluid therapy and expand-

Poison	Source / Toxicity and route of excretion	Signs and symptoms	Treatment
(ferrous gluconate, ferrous fumarate, vitamins with iron)	gastrointestinal, central nervous system, liver and vasculature Major route of excretion—renal	acidosis; hepatic damage and coagulation defects; coma and shock; stricture of gastrointestinal tract; iron tablets, radiopaque on x-ray	ers for shock. If (a) shock and coma, (b) serum iron level of greater than 400 μg./100 ml., (c) overdose in lethal range, treat with deferoxamine (Table 4 and text). (d) positive provocative chelation, treat with deferoxamine (Table 4 and text). Hemodialysis or exchange transfusion for renal failure
Lead	Toxicity by ingestion and inhalation. Symptoms with blood level >40 μg./100 ml. Danger of encephalopathy with levels greater than 80 μg./100 ml.	Ingestion causes chronic toxicity, inhalation, acute toxicity; abdominal pain, nausea, vomiting; opaque lead particles on x-ray; lethargy, ataxia; encephalopathy and coma	Emesis or lavage; gastrointestinal catharsis; treatment for renal failure and encephalopathy; calcium EDTA and/or BAL or d-penicillamine therapy (Table 4 and text)
Lomotil (atropine and diphenoxylate hydrochloride)	Toxicity when therapeutic dose exceeded (combined toxicity of atropine and diphenoxylate hydrochloride) Major route of excretion for both drugs—hepatic metabolism	Atropine signs 1 to 2 hours following ingestion occur infrequently; diphenoxylate signs 2 to 5 hours after ingestion; pinpoint pupils; lethargy, coma; respiratory depression; hypotension; convulsions	Emesis or lavage; activated charcoal (Table 3); gastrointestinal catharsis; naloxone hydrochloride (Table 4 and text); ventilatory support for respiratory failure
Mercury Inorganic	Exposure from inorganic mercury found in rodenticides, mercury amalgam, diuretics	Major toxicity to gastrointestinal tract, kidneys, and liver; bloody diarrhea, metallic taste in mouth; abdominal pain; renal tubular damage and anuria; hepatic damage	Emesis or lavage; fluid therapy and transfusion therapy; treatment of liver and renal failure; dimercaprol (BAL) (Table 4 and text)
Organic	Exposure from manufacturing plants and agricultural usage Major route of excretion—renal and gastrointestinal tract	Major toxicity to central nervous system; paresthesias, hypesthesia; weakness, apathy, inability to concentrate, loss of memory; ataxia, tremors, chorea; hearing difficulty; coma, seizures	N-acetyl penicillamine (Table 4 and text)
Methyl alcohol (wood alcohol)	2 tsp. are toxic. Toxic blood level greater than 10 to 20 mg./100 ml. Major toxicities at >50 mg./100 ml. Toxicity caused by methanol and metabolic breakdown products formaldehyde and formic acid. Major route of excretion—hepatic metabolism	Headache and dizziness, nausea and vomiting, visual impairment, metabolic acidosis, coma, cyanosis, hypotension, respiratory failure	Emesis or lavage, monitoring for acidosis and correction with sodium bicarbonate, ethanol therapy (Table 4 and text), hemodialysis in association with ethanol therapy

TABLE 2.   Treatment of Specific Poisons (Continued)

DRUG	TOXICITY AND EXCRETION	SYMPTOMS	TREATMENT
Naphthalene (mothballs, repellent cakes, deodorizer cakes)	Greater than 1 tsp. is toxic Major route of excretion—hepatic metabolism	Nausea, vomiting, abdominal cramps; convulsions; coma; intravascular hemolysis with G6PD deficiency; oliguria and anuria	Emesis or lavage; control of seizures with barbiturates and diazepam (Table 4). For intravascular hemolysis, intravenous fluids and alkalinization of the urine with bicarbonate (Table 4) to prevent precipitation of hemoglobin in tubules. Support for respiratory and circulatory failure; transfusion for anemia
Narcotic analgesics (morphine, codeine, Demerol, methadone, propoxyphene, pentazocine)	Symptoms when therapeutic dose exceeded Major route of excretion—hepatic metabolism	Lethargy, coma; pinpoint pupils; respiratory depression; hypotension; convulsions	Emesis or lavage, activated charcoal (Table 3), gastrointestinal catharsis, naloxone hydrochloride (Table 4 and text), ventilatory support for respiratory failure
Nicotine	Fatal dose of nicotine is about 40 to 60 mg. Swallowed as tobacco, nicotine is less toxic because of poor absorption from the stomach Major route of excretion—hepatic metabolism and renal excretion of metabolites	Nausea and vomiting, tachycardia, hypertension, headache, sweating, convulsions, coma, respiratory failure	Emesis or lavage, activated charcoal, control of seizures with barbiturates and diazepam, support for respiratory failure, atropine for parasympathetic overstimulation. (See Table 4 and text.)
Nitrates and nitrites	Individual susceptibility varies considerably. Ability to cause methemoglobinemia Major route of excretion—renal	Nausea and vomiting, headache, flushed skin, dizziness, hypotension, respiratory failure, coma	Emesis or lavage, oxygen, blood transfusion, methylene blue therapy (Table 4 and text), support for respiratory and circulatory failure
Phencyclidine (PCP, "Angel Dust," Peace Pill)	Widespread use. Passed. Alleged to be THC, LSD, psilocybin and mescaline Major route of excretion—hepatic metabolism with renal excretion of metabolites	*Low dose*—excitation, paranoid behavior, miotic pupils, nystagmus, increased blood pressure, pulse and respiration, slurred speech, drowsiness. *High dose*—decreased reflexes, coma, seizures, opisthotonus, hypotension, respiratory depression	Emesis or lavage; reduction of sensory stimuli; diazepam, 0.5 mg./kg/24 hrs. for control of agitation, opisthotonus; acidification of urine with ammonium chloride to enhance renal excretion (Table 4); support for respiratory and circulatory failure

Substance	Toxicity	Signs and Symptoms	Treatment
Polishes and waxes (Pride, Old English, O'Cedar, Jubilee, Kleer Floor Wax, Bruce Cleaning Wax, Aerowax, Armstrong 1-Step, Pledge Furniture Polish, Stanley Furniture Cream)	Main toxicity is pulmonary, caused by aspiration. Central nervous system signs less severe, secondary to absorption from lungs	Burning of the mouth and esophagus; vomiting and diarrhea; pulmonary involvement—cough, fever, dyspnea, rales, cyanosis, pulmonary infiltrates; infiltrates clear over 1 to 4 weeks	Do not induce emesis for pulmonary involvement: oxygen, moisture, antibiotics when clinical course or sputum examination indicate superinfection; supportive therapy for central nervous system depression and seizures
Psychedelic drugs (LSD, mescaline, psilocybin, STP, DMT)	Duration and intensity of effect varies from drug and from individual to individual. Major route of excretion—hepatic metabolism	Dilation of pupils, tachycardia, mild hypertension, incoordination, visual hallucinations, distortion of sensory perception, exaggerated sense of comprehension	"Talking down" in quiet nonthreatening atmosphere; diazepam, 0.5 mg/kg./24 hours for sedative effect; avoidance of chlorpromazine with STP or DMT
Salicylates (St. Joseph's, Bayer, Bufferin, Rexall, Empirin, Anacin, Excedrin, Congesprin, Ben Gay)	Symptoms at 150 mg./kg. or greater or at serum levels greater than 30 mg./100 ml.; 50 to 80 mg./100 ml., mild symptoms; 80 to 100 mg./100 ml., severe symptoms; greater than 100 mg./100 ml., potentially fatal. Major route of excretion—renal; minor route—hepatic	Vomiting, hyperventilation, fever, thirst, sweating, hypoglycemia or hyperglycemia, prolonged prothrombin time, confusion, delirium, coma, convulsions. In small children, metabolic acidosis; in older children, respiratory alkalosis.	Emesis or lavage; activated charcoal (Table 3); forced fluid diuresis (1 to 2 times maintenance); colloid for volume expansion; glucose for hypoglycemia; sponging for fever; vitamin K_1 for hypoprothrombinemia (Table 4); alkalinization of urine with bicarbonate (Table 4); hemodialysis, peritoneal dialysis or exchange transfusion with (a) levels greater than 100 to 150 mg./100 ml., (b) anuria, (c) heart disease preventing forced fluid diuresis
Strychnine (rodenticides)	Fatal dose for an adolescent is 15 to 30 mg. Toxicity due to increased reflex excitability	Increased deep tendon reflexes with muscle stiffening and opisthotonus; respiratory failure	Emesis or lavage, control of seizures with barbiturates and diazepam (Table 4), prevention of peripheral stimuli and enforcement of quiet, support for respiratory and circulatory failure
Sympathomimetics (Ephedrine, epinephrine, Isuprel, Neo-Synephrine)	Toxic symptoms when therapeutic dose exceeded. Major route of excretion—hepatic metabolism	Nervousness; tachycardia, arrhythmias; dilated pupils; blurred vision; convulsions, respiratory failure; coma	Emesis or lavage, treatment of seizures with barbiturates or diazepam (Table 4), support for respiratory and circulatory failure

TABLE 2.   Treatment of Specific Poisons (Continued)

DRUG	TOXICITY AND EXCRETION	SYMPTOMS	TREATMENT
Thallium	Single doses of 8 to 10 mg./kg. have been fatal in children Major route of excretion—renal	Abdominal pain, vomiting, diarrhea; diaphoresis, hyperpyrexia, salivation; hypotension, hypertension; ataxia, tremors, choreiform movements, paresthesias, coma; peripheral neuropathies; alopecia	Emesis or lavage; vigorous gastrointestinal catharsis; potassium chloride, 5 to 25 gm./day orally to augment rate of excretion; prussian blue (potassium ferric hexacyanoferrate) and Dithiocarb under investigation and of unclear value at this time (see text)
Theophylline (caffeine, aminophylline, slophylline)	Toxicity when serum levels exceed 25 µg./ml. Nausea and vomiting seen between 15 and 25 µg./ml. Major route of excretion—hepatic metabolism	Agitation, restlessness; vomiting, hematemesis; fever; tachycardia and cardiac arrhythmias; convulsions; vasomotor collapse; respiratory failure	Emesis or lavage; enemas for rectally administered overdose; avoidance of sympathomimetics; supportive therapy for dehydration, seizures, arrhythmias and hypotension
Thyroid (Cytomel, Synthroid, desiccated thyroid, Choloxin)	Toxicity when therapeutic dosage exceeded. Thyroxine is about 200 times and triiodothyronine 800 to 1000 times as potent as desiccated thyroid. Long half-life of 6 to 7 days Major route of excretion—hepatic metabolism	Palpitation, rapid pulse; headache; tremors, nervousness, delirium; diaphoresis, hyperpyrexia; vomiting; symptoms may occur up to 1 week post ingestion	Emesis or lavage, supportive care for hyperpyrexia and central nervous system excitation
Tranquilizers (Mellaril, Equanil, Miltown, Placidyl, Doriden, Noludar, Dalmane, Librium, Valium)	Toxicity when therapeutic dosage exceeded Major route of excretion—hepatic metabolism	Sleepiness, weakness, unsteadiness, incoordination, hypotension, cyanosis, respiratory failure, coma	Emesis or lavage, activated charcoal (Table 3) and gastrointestinal catharsis, maintenance of an adequate airway and oxygen, support for respiratory and circulatory failure, supportive therapy during coma
Turpentine and other volatile oils (xylene, benzene, toluene)	Predominant central nervous system toxicity Major route of excretion—hepatic metabolism	Nausea, vomiting; central nervous system excitation, lethargy, coma; pneumonia and pulmonary edema; renal, hepatic and bone marrow toxicity	Emesis or lavage, treatment of seizures with barbiturates and diazepam (Table 4), ventilatory support for respiratory failure, treatment of renal, hepatic or bone marrow failure

Drug		Clinical features	Treatment
Tricyclic antidepressants (imipramine, amitriptyline)	Symptoms when therapeutic dose exceeded Major route of excretion—hepatic metabolism	Excitation, disorientation, drowsiness, coma; anticholinergic syndrome—dry mouth, dilated pupils, fever, flushed skin, tachycardia, absent bowel sounds, urinary retention; hypertension, hypotension; convulsions; arrhythmias; cardiovascular collapse and respiratory depression	Emesis or lavage, activated charcoal (Table 3), vigorous gastrointestinal catharsis, treatment of fever, maintenance fluid therapy, support for circulatory and respiratory failure, treatment of seizures with barbiturates or diazepam (Table 4 and text)
Vitamin A	Of low toxicity with symptoms from ingestion of 200,000 to 300,000 units	Fatigue, anorexia, vomiting, bulging fontanelle, increased intracranial pressure	Emesis or lavage with large ingestions
Vitamin D	Of low toxicity with symptoms from ingestions of 100,000 to 150,000 units Major route of excretion—hepatic metabolism and biliary excretion	Elevation of serum calcium, metastatic calcifications, renal damage	Emesis or lavage with large ingestions; support for renal failure
Warfarin (Dicumarol)	Repeated doses needed to cause symptoms. Only single ingestions that are massive in amount will cause symptoms	Prolonged prothrombin time and clinical bleeding occurring a few days to a few weeks following ingestion	Emesis or lavage following a very large single ingestion, monitoring of prothrombin time, vitamin K_1 (Table 4 and text), transfusion therapy

process. We prefer to use a safe emetic and induce emesis whenever there is the slightest doubt as to potential toxicity.

Mechanical Removal. Mechanical methods of removal of a toxin include the use of a blunt object such as a spoon or toothbrush placed in the posterior pharynx to stimulate the gag reflex and promote vomiting. The success of such a procedure is poor, although it may be worth a rapid try if no other means is available.

Lavage. Gastric lavage is a useful technique for the removal of ingested poisons and is most frequently utilized with adolescent and adult ingestions where the state of consciousness of the patient is more likely to be affected. In animal work it appears to be less effective than forceful emesis, with 35 per cent of a known toxin removed 40 to 45 minutes following ingestion and 15 per cent removed one hour following ingestion. Lavage further requires that the patient first be brought to the hospital setting before therapy is instituted, this delay causing increased time for absorption of the ingested product. In addition, the removal of whole or partially dissolved tablets or capsules is possible only with the use of a large bore oral gastric tube. The commonly used nasogastric tubes (12 to 18 Fr.) are generally more successful with liquids than with tablets. The lavage procedure is uncomfortable and may entail an increased risk of vomiting with subsequent aspiration.

Gastric lavage is the preferred method of removal of an ingested toxin at any age when attempts to induce emesis with ipecac syrup have failed, or when these efforts involve a significant risk to the patient. It is also indicated in the patient less than nine months of age. In the obtunded patient with an intact gag reflex or in the patient who is initially alert but who may become obtunded before emesis is complete, gastric lavage, rapidly and carefully performed, is preferable to ipecac syrup. When the gag reflex is sluggish or absent, lavage should be undertaken only after the patient has been intubated, the risk of aspiration pneumonia being prevented by use of a cuffed endotracheal tube. The lavage tube has the advantage of providing the only route for the administration of activated charcoal in the uncooperative child or the comatose adolescent.

Additional contraindications to lavage include convulsions and the ingestion of caustic products or petroleum distillate hydrocarbons. Caustics reburn the esophagus during the process of vomiting and present only a minimal systemic risk when left in the stomach. Though the initial management of the petroleum distil-

late hydrocarbon ingestion remains controversial, in the pediatric patient one should avoid attempts at their removal (the exception being where very large amounts may be ingested). Small amounts of hydrocarbons aspirated into the tracheobronchial tree are highly toxic both locally and systemically, whereas adverse systemic effects from gastrointestinal absorption are infrequent and of minimal severity.

Chemical Removal. Chemical emesis has been shown to be the most useful technique for removal of ingested poisons. A variety of different methods exist. Copper sulfate and zinc sulfate may cause hepatic toxicity, renal toxicity, intravascular hemolysis and gastrointestinal corrosion and for this reason should not be used. Apomorphine is a rapidly acting, highly effective emetic; it will induce vomiting in essentially 100 per cent of patients in 2 to 5 minutes. Being a narcotic, however, it frequently causes central nervous system depression for 45 minutes to an hour following its use, limiting its widespread use for the routine acute overdose. Naloxone hydrochloride can be used to reverse this transient depression. Apomorphine must also be freshly prepared (when properly stored in a dark bottle it has a shelf life of three weeks).

Ipecac syrup is an effective emetic, inducing emesis in 86 per cent of children with an initial dose. This figure approaches 96 per cent when a second dose is given. It is effective in inducing emesis with all ingested toxins including phenothiazines. Forceful emesis occurs within 15 to 20 minutes removing both tablets and liquids. It rarely causes more than one or two episodes of emesis. The two main alkaloids of ipecac syrup, cephaline and emetine, exert their emetic effect by acting both centrally on the vomiting center in the medulla and peripherally on the gastrointestinal mucosa.

The dose of ipecac syrup for the patient from 1 to 12 years is one tablespoon (15 ml.) of ipecac syrup followed by 100 to 500 ml. of clear fluid (depending on age). It is important that the patient be kept in motion. If emesis has not occurred in 20 minutes, the dose may be repeated. If emesis does not occur in an additional 15 to 20 minutes and removal of the ingested product is still indicated, lavage should be performed. For the patient above 12 years, 30 ml. of ipecac syrup can be given followed by fluid and motion. If emesis does not occur and removal is still desired, lavage rather than additional ipecac syrup is indicated. For children between 9 and 12 months of age, a single dose (10 ml.) of ipecac syrup is given, followed by fluid and motion. If emesis does not occur or in instances in which the child is less than nine months of age, careful lavage is the preferable method of management. The amount of toxin recovered by emesis is inversely related to the time that has elapsed since ingestion occurred. The quantity recovered is relatively small, with only 35 to 40 per cent of an ingested toxin removed when emesis is induced one hour following ingestion.

Ipecac syrup is a remarkably safe emetic. Central nervous system and cardiac toxicity have been seen only when the 30 ml. limit has been substantially exceeded or when the fluid extract of ipecac (which is 14 times as concentrated as the syrup) has been used. Ipecac syrup is an inexpensive drug, available without prescription and has a long shelf life, thereby allowing it to be kept in the home for use at the time of poisoning. It can be administered outside the hospital setting on the advice of a physician or poison center, thereby allowing earlier institution of therapy than if the patient was required to come to a hospital setting. Complete care of the acute poisoning thus must logically also include education as to the importance of ipecac syrup being available in every home with children.

Local Antidotes. During the last decade activated charcoal was "rediscovered" as an adjunct to the more traditional methods of management of the acute overdose. It is an odorless, tasteless, fine black powder that, because of its small particle size and large surface area, binds many organic compounds and creates a stable complex that is highly resistant to dissociation. A partial list of the compounds for which activated charcoal has been shown to be effective is outlined in Table 3. The universal antidote (charcoal, magnesium oxide and tannic acid) is less effective than activated charcoal, and tannic acid is hepatotoxic. Activated charcoal is not effective in preventing gastrointestinal absorption of alcohol, iron, caustics and cyanide.

To achieve optimal binding of a poison, activated charcoal is best used within one hour of ingestion following the prior removal of the toxin by emesis or lavage. Charcoal, being black in color, serves as an indicator of gastrointestinal motility and provides a general indication of the time at which the ingested product has been eliminated from the body. It further is useful when interruption of hepatoenteric circulation of a drug is desired (tricyclic antidepressants and cardiac glycosides). It should not be used prior to or concomitant with ipecac syrup, as the charcoal will bind the emetic and prevent its pharmacologic action.

Charcoal is administered orally in an

TABLE 3. Drugs Absorbed In Vivo by Activated Charcoal

Analgesics and Antipyretics
Acetaminophen (Tylenol)
Acetylsalicylic acid
Mefenamic acid (Ponstel)
Methyl salicylate
Paracetamol (Trigesic)
Propoxyphene (Darvon)
Salicylamide
Sodium salicylate

Barbiturates, Sedatives, and Hypnotics
Barbital
Ethchlorvynol (Placidyl)
Glutethimide (Doriden)
Pentobarbital
Phenobarbital
Secobarbital (Seconal)

Tranquilizers and Antidepressants
Chlorpromazine
Imipramine (Tofranil)
Nortriptyline (Aventyl)

Miscellaneous
Amphetamine
Atropine
Chlordane
Chloroquine (Aralen)
Chlorpheniramine
Digoxin
Hexachlorophene
Isoniazid
Malathion
Nicotine
Phenylpropanolamine
Phenytoin
Propanolamine
Quinine
Scopolamine
Strychnine

amount 5 to 10 times the weight of the ingested product or at a dose of 0.5 to 1 gm./kg. in the child or 30 gm. in the adolescent (Table 4). It should be mixed in 30 to 60 ml. of water and flavored with 5 ml. of cherry syrup to increase its palatability. Because the pediatric patient may refuse to swallow activated charcoal, administration of the drug by nasogastric tube may be necessary. Other antidotes which exert a local effect include: calcium in the form of calcium gluconate, calcium lactate, or milk to minimize the caustic effect of fluoride on the gastrointestinal mucosa and 1 per cent sodium bicarbonate to precipitate iron in the gastrointestinal tract and neutralize its caustic effects.

Gastrointestinal Cathartics. Enhanced elimination of a toxin through the gastrointestinal tract is often essential to prevent its subsequent absorption slowly over time from the small and large bowels. This will be particularly true with drugs that slow bowel mobility such as narcotics, anticholinergic drugs or drugs causing grades III and IV levels of coma. Magnesium sulfate or sodium sulfate is effective in increasing the rate of transit of a toxic product through the gastrointestinal tract, thus minimizing its absorption. The dose for either cathartic is 250 mg./kg. given orally and repeated every three hours until productive of a stool. These drugs should not be used if there is compromise of renal function. Saline cathartics are not recommended because they can be toxic if absorbed.

Additional Routes of Absorption. Many drugs such as insecticides are well absorbed through the skin. Careful attention to thorough washing with soap and water will effectively eliminate continued absorption by this route. Inhalation as a route of absorption can be prevented by removal of the patient to a noncontaminated environment and by the use of augmented concentrations of oxygen as indicated by the clinical condition of the patient. Finally, the rectal route is often forgotten as a route of absorption of various toxins. The removal by enema of medications which have been given rectally in suppository form is a simple and essential method of removal of a toxin.

MODIFICATION OF SYSTEMIC TOXICITY

Pharmacologic Considerations

Once absorbed, the severity and duration of clinical manifestations of an overdose are determined by the toxin's maximum blood level and its half-life. Saturation of albumin-binding sites as well as displacement of a toxic drug from these sites by other drugs will increase the severity of ingestion. Enhanced tissue distribution of a toxin as a result of alterations in serum pH (acidosis with salicylate or long-acting barbiturate intoxications) will also increase toxicity. Clearly in an overdosed patient, close attention must be given to the drug's maximum blood level, its half-life and potential adverse effects from the addition of other drugs as well as alterations in acid base status. It is beyond the scope of this review to discuss these principles in depth.

Systemic Antidotes

Desired characteristics of a systemic antidote include high specificity and efficacy with low incidence of side effects. A limited number of antidotes meet these requirements. Naloxone hydrochloride for narcotics, sodium nitrite and sodium thiosulfate for cyanide, methylene blue for methemoglobinemia, atropine sulfate for organophosphate insecticides and oxygen for carbon monoxide poisoning are generally needed urgently, whereas the remainder can be used once the patient is well stabilized. The amount of antidote needed will be determined by titration to reduce the pharmacologic effect of the toxin. Antidotes should never be used prophylactically. A drug formulary of these antidotes, their indications and suggested doses for children and for adolescents (Table 4) is included to supplement the text and to serve as a rapid reference. The adolescent of 13 and above has reached a state of physiologic and anatomic development which requires the use of adult doses for the majority of drugs and antidotes.

Atropine Sulfate and 2-PAM. Organophosphate insecticides of the anticholinesterase variety act by inhibiting plasma cholinesterase. The attendant rise in acetylcholine levels produces the characteristic muscarinic and nicotinic signs and symptoms of intoxication: miotic pupils, increased salivation and respiratory secretion, bradycardia, vomiting, diarrhea, muscle fasciculations and weakness. Atropine sulfate is a physiologic antidote that reverses the effects of acetylcholine through competition at receptor sites. Atropine is given liberally by the intravenous route in a dose of 0.05 mg./kg. or 2 or 3 mg. for the adolescent, with additional doses at two to five minute intervals (or more frequently if indicated clinically) until muscarine and nicotinic effects have disappeared and cholinergic blockade is achieved (dilated pupils, dry mouth, tachycardia, decreased bowel sounds). Atropine is highly effective for carbamate insecticide poisoning as well. Finally, atropine will block the effect of drugs which exert their toxicity through excessive parasympathomimetic effect (nicotine).

Pralidoxime chloride (2-PAM) is a second antidote utilized for organophosphate insecticides once full atropinization has been accomplished and the patient is stable. 2-PAM is able to specifically break the covalent bond between cholinesterase and the alkylphosphate of the organophosphorus compound. The dose is 0.5 to 1 gm. for the adolescent and 250 mg. for infants given slowly intravenously. With evidence of clinical improvement it may be repeated in 1 hour. Carbamate insecticides are responsive to atropine but are unresponsive to 2-PAM.

Chlorpromazine. Central nervous system excitation and excess motor activity secondary to amphetamine ingestions may be decreased by chlorpromazine given at a dose of 1 mg./kg. by the oral or intramuscular route.

This dose should be reduced to 0.5 mg./kg. if a barbiturate has been ingested along with the amphetamine. If the patient has taken STP (dimethoxy methylamphetamine) or DMT (dimethyltryptamine), chlorpromazine may cause hypotension. In these instances diazepam rather than chlorpromazine is the preferred antidote.

Cyanide Antidotes.   Cyanide, by binding to ferrous iron in mitochondrial cytochrome oxidase systems, inhibits cellular respiration and creates cellular anoxia. The approach to therapy involves oxidizing hemoglobin iron from its ferrous to ferric state (methemoglobin). At this higher valence, methemoglobin has greater affinity for cyanide than does the ferrous iron of the mitrochondrial enzyme systems.

Cyanide poisoning can be fatal within 15 minutes of ingestion. Since speed in initiating treatment is critical there is no time for laboratory corroboration of the diagnosis. A history of exposure to cyanide along with the rapid onset of coma, bradycardia and hypotension is adequate for a clinical diagnosis of cyanide poisoning.

For treatment of cyanide poisoning, a state of methemoglobinemia is created initially by the administration of amyl nitrate given as a broken pearl held in a handkerchief over the patient's nose for a period of 30 seconds out of each minute. A five per cent concentration of methemoglobin is created by this maneuver. A new ampule is used every three minutes until sodium nitrite becomes available.

Sodium nitrite is then given intravenously as a 3 per cent solution at a rate of 2.5 to 5 ml./min. The optimal dose is based on the child's hemoglobin concentration and weight and should result in a methemoglobin level of 25 per cent, a concentration that is both effective and safe (Table 5).

Methemoglobin levels should be frequently determined and their concentration should not exceed 35 to 40 per cent. The main adverse effect from sodium nitrite is hypotension, which is generally transient and responds to volume expanders. In adolescents the dose of sodium nitrite (3 per cent solution) is 10 to 20 ml. given at a rate of 2.5 to 5 ml./minute.

The second part of therapy involves the removal of cyanide from methemoglobin by administration of sodium thiosulfate. This leads to formation of sodium thiocyanate complex which is then excreted in the urine. The pediatric dose of sodium thiosulfate should be based on the patient's hemoglobin concentration and weight (Table 4). Thiosulfate is administered 20 to 30 minutes after sodium nitrite by intravenous infusion at a rate of 2.5 to 5 ml./min. The dose in the adolescent is 50 ml. of the 25 per cent solution. The toxicity of sodium thiosulfate is low.

Should symptoms persist or recur, both sodium nitrite and sodium thiosulfate may be repeated once 2 to 3 hours after the first dose. The second dose of sodium nitrite should be one half the initial dose.

Deferoxamine (Desferal).   Deferoxamine has proved to be a highly effective and specific chelating agent for the treatment of acute iron intoxication. It competes with the beta globulin transferrin for the absorbed iron. The iron then bound to deferoxamine is excreted by the kidneys.

Indications for the use of deferoxamine in iron intoxication include: (1) a serum iron level exceeding the iron-binding capacity (generally > 400 μg./100 ml.), (2) shock or coma, (3) a positive provocation chelation test (deferoxamine at 50 mg./kg. intramuscularly as a single dose producing a burgundy colored urine that indicates a serum iron level exceeding the iron-binding capacity), (4) an ingested dose in the potentially lethal range that has been inadequately removed by emesis or lavage.

The therapeutic dose of deferoxamine is 50 mg./kg. (up to 1 to 2 gm.) given intramuscularly every 6 to 8 hours. The drug may also be given intravenously, but this route has the risk of inducing hypotension (a complication of iron intoxication as well) if the infusion rate exceeds 15 mg./kg./hr. Oral administration of deferoxamine will bind iron remaining in the gastrointestinal tract. The risk of bolus absorption of the chelated iron through the damaged intestinal mucosa with resultant hypotension, however, has resulted in the drug presently being used mainly by the intramuscular route. The necessity for continued therapy can best be estimated by serial serum iron determinations. The return of urine color to normal can also be used as a rough estimate of the rate of lowering of the serum iron and the duration of treatment that will be required. Adverse effects of deferoxamine include rash, pain at the injection site, hypocalcemia and hypotension.

Diphenhydramine (Benadryl).   Extrapyramidal tract signs induced by phenothiazines, including opisthotonus, torticollis, oculogyric crisis, rigidity, dystonia, trismus and tremors, are rapidly reversed with diphenhydramine. These signs are especially common with the piperazine group of phenothiazines including prochlorperazine (Compazine) and trifluoperazine (Stelazine).

These adverse effects are reversed within

TABLE 4. Drug Formulary in Toxicology

SUBSTANCE	INDICATION	ADOLESCENT DOSE	PEDIATRIC DOSE
GENERAL DRUGS			
Activated charcoal	Gastrointestinal decontamination	5 to 10 times the estimated amount ingested or 15 to 30 gm. in 60 to 120 ml. of water. Mix well before use. Give orally or by nasogastric tube	5 to 10 times the estimated amount ingested or 0.5 to 1 gm./kg. mixed with 30 to 60 ml. of water mixed with 5 to 10 ml. of cherry syrup prior to use. Mix well before use. Given orally or by nasogastric tube
Ammonium chloride	Enhanced urinary excretion of basic compounds by acidification of urine	1.5 gm. IV every 6 hours up to a maximum of 6 gm./day. Oral dose 8 to 12 gm. daily	75 mg./kg./dose IV or orally every 6 hrs. up to maximum of 2 to 6 gm./day.
Apomorphine	Induction of emesis	0.07 mg./kg./dose subcutaneously	0.07 mg./kg./dose subcutaneously;
Barbiturates	Control of seizures	150 mg./m²/dose intravenously	5 to 9 mg./kg./dose intravenously;
Dexamethasone (Decadron)	Cerebral edema	10 mg. IV as an initial dose followed by 4 mg. every 6 hours intravenously	0.4 mg./kg. IV as an initial dose followed by 0.1 mg./kg./dose IV every 4 to 6 hours
Ethacrynic acid (Edecrin)	Enhanced urinary excretion	50 mg./dose or 0.5 to 1.0 mg./kg./dose IV every 8 hours	0.5 to 1.0 mg./kg./dose intravenously every 8 hours
Furosemide (Lasix)	Enhanced urinary excretion	20 to 40 mg./dose IM or slowly IV (over 1 to 2 minutes) every 8 to 12 hours	1 to 3 mg./kg./dose I.M. or slowly I.V. (over 1 to 2 minutes) every 8 to 12 hrs.
Glycerol	Cerebral edema	2 gm./kg./day in 4 divided doses orally	3 gm./kg./day in 4 divided doses orally
Ipecac syrup	Induction of emesis	30 ml. orally given with fluids followed by motion	15 ml. orally repeated in 15 mins. if not effective. Given with fluids followed by motion
Isoproterenol (Isuprel)	Hypotension	2 mg. in 1000 ml. of 5 per cent dextrose in water (conc. of 2 μg./ml.). Given IV at rate of 0.1 μg./kg./min. and increased slowly as needed	2 mg. in 1000 ml. of 5 per cent dextrose in water (conc. of 2 μg./ml.). Given IV at rate of 0.1 μg./kg./min. and increased slowly as needed
Levarterenol (Levophed)	Hypotension	4 ml. vial added to 1000 ml. of 5 per cent dextrose in water (conc. of 4 μg./ml.). Give IV at rate of 0.1 to 0.2 μg./kg./min. and increase slowly as needed	4 ml. vial added to 1000 ml. of 5 per cent dextrose in water (conc. of 4 μg./ml.). Give IV at rate of 0.1 to 0.2 μg./kg./min. and increase slowly as needed
Magnesium sulfate (Epsom salt)	Gastrointestinal catharsis	5 gm. or 50 ml. of a 10 per cent solution orally and repeat every 4 hours until productive of stool	250 mg./kg./dose orally and repeat every 3 hours until productive of stool
Mannitol	Enhanced urinary excretion	25 to 50 gm. in a 20 per cent solution IV over 30 min. every 4 to 6 900 gm./day)	1 to 2 gm./kg. in 20 per cent solution IV over 30 min. every 4 to 6 hours (max. 100 gm./day)

Mannitol	Cerebral edema	25 to 50 gm. in a 20 per cent solution IV over 30 min. given every 4 to 6 hours (max. 200 gm./day)	1 to 2 gm./kg. in 20 per cent solution IV over 30 min. given every 4 to 6 hours (max. 100 gm./day)
Metaraminol (Aramine)	Hypotension	10 mg./ml. in a 10 ml. vial. Add 100 mg. to 1000 ml. of 5 per cent dextrose in water (conc. of 100 μg./ml.). Give IV at rate of 5 μg./kg./min. and increase slowly as needed	10 mg./ml. in a 10 ml. vial. Add 100 mg. to 1000 ml. of 5 per cent dextrose in water (conc. of 100 μg./ml.). Give IV at rate of 5 μg./kg./min. and increase slowly as needed
Prednisone	Caustic injury to esophagus	10 to 20 mg./dose IV, IM or orally every 6 hours for 2 to 3 weeks with dosage tapering at end of therapy	2 to 3 mg./kg./day IM, IV or orally every 6 hours for 3 weeks with dosage tapering at end of therapy
Sodium bicarbonate	Enhanced urinary excretion of acid compounds by alkalinization of urine	2 mEq./kg./dose IV during first hour followed by sufficient $NaHCO_3$ to keep urinary pH> 7.5 (generally 2 mEq./kg. every 6 to 8 hours). Additional potassium necessary to accomplish alkalinization.	2 to 4 mEq./kg./dose IV during first hour followed by sufficient $NaHCO_3$ to keep urinary pH > 7.5 (generally 2 mEq./kg. every 6 hours). Additional potassium (3 to 4 mEq./kg./day) necessary to accomplish alkalinization
Diazepam (Valium)	Control of seizures	5 to 10 mg./dose intravenously titrated to control seizures	0.1 to 0.25 mg./kg./dose intravenously titrated to control seizures
ANTIDOTES			
Amyl nitrite pearls (kit from Eli Lilly and Company)	Cyanide poisoning	Inhalation for 30 seconds out of every minute. New ampule every three minutes	Inhalation for 30 seconds out of every minute. New ampule every three minutes
Atropine sulfate	Organophosphate and carbamate insecticides	2 to 3 mg./dose of IV solution (0.4 mg./ml.) every 2 to 5 min. until fully atropinized and then as necessary to maintain atropinization	0.05 mg./kg. of IV solution (0.4 mg./ml.) every 2 to 5 min. until fully atropinized and then as necessary to maintain atropinization
Calcium disodium ethylenediamine tetraacetate (calcium disodium) versenate) (CaEDTA)	Heavy metal (lead) poisoning	1 gm. IM or IV over 1 hour twice a day for 5 to 7 days. Repeat course after rest period. Add procaine for IM use	50 to 75 mg./kg./day IM or IV divided into 2 to 3 doses for 5 to 7 days. Repeat course at 50 mg./kg./day after rest period. Add procaine for IM use
Chlorpromazine (Thorazine)	Amphetamine induced hyperactivity and psychosis	25 mg./dose IV every 6 hours. Reduce dose if barbiturate ingested. Titrate subsequent doses to desired response	1 mg./kg./dose IV every 6 hours. Reduce dose if barbiturate ingested. Titrate subsequent doses to desired response

TABLE 4. Drug Formulary in Toxicology (Continued)

SUBSTANCE	INDICATION	ADOLESCENT DOSE	PEDIATRIC DOSE
Deferoxamine (Desferal)	Iron poisoning	1 to 2 gm. IM every 6 to 8 hours. For severe intoxication IV dose at a rate not to exceed 15 mg./kg./hr. Do not exceed 6 gm. in 24 hours	50 mg./kg. not to exceed 1 to 2 gm. IM every 6 hours. For severe intoxication IV dose at a rate not to exceed 15 mg./kg./hr. Do not exceed 6 gm. in 24 hours
Dimercaprol (BAL)	Heavy metal (arsenic, mercury, lead, gold) poisoning	3 mg./kg./dose IM at 4 to 6 hour intervals for first 5 days, then 3 mg./kg./dose every 12 hours for next 5 to 9 days	3 to 4 mg./kg./dose IM at 4 to 6 hour intervals for first 5 days, then 3 to 4 mg./kg. every 12 hours for next 5 to 9 days
Diphenhydramine (Benadryl)	Phenothiazine extrapyramidal reaction	25 to 50 mg./dose IV slowly, then every 6 hours orally or IV for maintenance	1 to 2 mg./kg./dose IV slowly, then every 6 hours orally or IV for maintenance
Ethanol	Methanol and ethylene glycol poisoning	Ethanol given as a 50 per cent solution IV at a dose of 0.5 to 1.5 ml./kg. every 2 to 4 hours to maintain a blood level between 100 and 150 mg./100 ml. In mild cases, 3 to 4 ounces of whiskey every 4 hours orally	Ethanol given as a 50 per cent solution IV at a dose of 0.5 to 1.5 ml./kg. every 2 to 4 hours to maintain a blood level between 100 and 150 mg./100 ml. In mild cases, 3 to 4 ounces of whiskey every 4 hours orally
Methylene blue	Methemoglobinemia	1 per cent solution given intravenously slowly over 5 to 10 min. at a dose of 10 mg., repeated in 4 hours if needed	1 per cent solution at a dose of 1 to 2 mg./kg./dose intravenously given slowly over 5 to 10 min., repeated in 4 hours if needed
Naloxone hydrochloride (Narcan)	Reversal of narcotic depression	0.4 mg. intravenously repeated every 2 to 3 min. for 2 or 3 doses for initial effect. Continued therapy until narcotic effect no longer present.	0.01 mg./kg./dose IV repeated every 2 to 3 min. for 2 or 3 doses for initial effect. Continue therapy until narcotic effect no longer present
Oxygen	Carbon monoxide poisoning	100 per cent oxygen by inhalation	100 per cent oxygen by inhalation
d-Penicillamine (Cuprimine)	Heavy metal (lead, mercury) poisoning	250 to 500 mg. orally every 6 to 8 hours, depending on severity	For acute therapy 25 to 50 mg./kg./day in 4 divided doses orally for 5 days. For chronic therapy 25 mg./kg./day in 4 divided doses orally (max. 1 gm./day)

Physostigmine salicylate (Antilirium)	Anticholinergic poisoning	2 mg. slowly over 2 to 3 min. IV with repeat in 2 to 5 min. if no effect. Once effect accomplished give lowest effective dose slowly every 30 to 60 min. with recurrence of symptoms	0.5 mg. slowly over 2 to 3 min. IV with repeat in 2 to 5 min. if no effect. Once effect accomplished give lowest effective dose slowly every 30 to 60 min. with recurrence of symptoms
Pralidoxime chloride (2PAM)	Organophosphate insecticide	0.5 to 1.0 gm. IV after initial treatment with atropine, given slowly at a rate of 500 mg./min. and repeated every 8 to 12 hrs. as needed	250 mg./dose given slowly IV after initial treatment with atropine and repeated every 8 to 12 hrs. as needed
Sodium thiosulfate (kit from Eli Lilly and Company)	Cyanide poisoning	50 ml. of 25 per cent solution at a rate of 2.5 to 5.0 ml./min. IV 15 min. after sodium nitrite. May be repeated once	1.65 ml./kg. of 25 per cent solution at a rate of 2.5 to 5.0 ml./min. IV 15 min. after sodium nitrite. May be repeated once
Sodium nitrite (kit from Eli Lilly and Company)	Cyanide poisoning	10 to 20 ml. of 3 per cent solution at a rate of 2.5 to 5.0 ml./min. IV. May be repeated once with persistence or recurrence of symptoms	.33 ml./kg. of 3 per cent solution at a rate of 2.5 to 5.0 ml./min. IV. May be repeated once with persistence or recurrence of symptoms
Vitamin K_1	Hypoprothrombinemia	5 mg./dose intravenously	2 to 5 mg./dose intravenously

2 to 3 minutes by the intravenous administration of diphenhydramine at a dose of 1 to 2 mg./kg. Ataxia and lethargy, which are signs of phenothiazine toxicity, respond less consistently to diphenhydramine. The antidote may be used for both diagnostic and therapeutic purposes. To prevent recurrence of symptoms diphenhydramine should be continued for a 24 hour period at an oral dose of 1 to 2 mg./kg. every six hours. Sedation may be a minor side effect of therapy and excessively rapid infusion may produce hypotension.

EDTA, BAL, d-Penicillamine. These chelating agents are used in the therapy of both acute and chronic heavy metal poisoning. Heavy metals bind to various body proteins (ligands) such as sulfhydryl groups (which are essential for various enzymatic activities) forming an unstable complex. Chelating agents successfully compete with body ligands for the heavy metals. A stable complex is formed between the heavy metal and the chelating agent which is then excreted in urine, feces or both. Desired characteristics of a chelating agent include resistance to metabolic degradation, chelating ability at the pH of the body, sufficiently small molecular size to allow penetration to sites of storage of the toxin, a low affinity for calcium, zinc and other body metals and a capacity to form a complex with the toxic metal that is of low toxicity. A sufficient excess of the chelating agent must be given to assure that the heavy metal is bound rather than simply redistributed in the body. Characteristics of specific chelating agents and their range of effectiveness are reviewed below.

Calcium disodium ethylenediamine tetraacetate (EDTA) (Versenate). Heavy metals such as lead that preferentially bind to oxygen and nitrogen are effectively chelated by EDTA. Because the sodium salt of EDTA will chelate calcium resulting in hypocalcemia, the calcium disodium salt is used. The dose of CaEDTA is 50 to 75 mg./kg./day given in two to three doses. Although the intramuscular route is preferred, the drug may be given by slow intravenous infusion. Use of the oral route is not advised. Since the kidneys offer the only route of excretion for the heavy metal complex, urinary flow must be established before initiating therapy. The duration of therapy is usually 5 to 7 days. When multiple courses are needed a rest interval of at least two days is advisable before reinstituting therapy.

Adverse effects include rash, injection site reactions, fever, hypercalcemia, electrocardiographic abnormalities, Fanconi syndrome and acute tubular necrosis. As these reactions are dose-related, one should monitor through-out therapy serum calcium, phosphorus and BUN as well as obtain frequent urinalyses and electrocardiographic tracings. Reduction or discontinuation of EDTA may be required if these reactions develop.

Dimercaprol (BAL) is used in the treatment of heavy metals that bind to sulfur and phosphorus, the most common being lead, mercury and arsenic. Dosage, duration of treatment and necessity of repetitive courses of therapy depend on the severity of the poisoning. As a general rule, arsenic and mercury require 10 to 14 days and lead 5 to 7 days of therapy. The drug is given by the intramuscular route at a dose of 3 to 4 mg./kg. During the first two to five days when the body burden of heavy metal is at its highest, BAL is given every 4 to 6 hours. This is reduced to every 12 hours during the later days of therapy. Iron should not be administered in conjunction with BAL since a toxic complex is formed. As the liver is the primary excretory pathway for BAL, significantly compromised hepatic function is a contraindication to its use. It may, however, be used in the presence of renal failure.

Adverse reactions are dose-related, becoming frequent when a dose of 5 mg./kg. is exceeded, and include lacrimation, blepharospasm, paresthesias, nausea, vomiting, tachycardia and hypertension. Blood pressure, pulse and neurologic examinations should be performed repeatedly throughout the treatment period.

d-Penicillamine (Cuprimine) may be used for acute poisoning with arsenic and mercury and chronic poisoning with lead, copper and mercury. N-acetyl penicillamine has significant advantages over d-penicillamine for mercury poisoning. d-Penicillamine is given only by the oral route and must be taken on an empty stomach at least an hour and a half before meals. For short term therapy, 25 to 50 mg./kg./day in four divided doses (with a maximum daily dose of 1 gm.) may be given for five days. For chronic therapy, 25 mg./kg./day in two to four divided doses is given. Since the drug is primarily excreted by the kidneys, renal failure is a contraindication to its use. Adverse reactions are dose related. At doses greater than 50 mg./kg./day, rash, fever, nephrotic syndrome, leukopenia, neutropenia, eosinophilia and coagulation defects may be seen. The drug is contraindicated in patients with penicillin allergy.

Ethanol. Methanol, found in antifreeze, paint remover, shellac, solvents and as an inexpensive source of alcohol, causes central nervous system depression, blindness and metabolic acidosis. These findings are thought to be the result of the metabolism of methanol to formaldehyde and formic acid. Both ethanol and methanol are metabolized in the liver by the enzyme alcohol dehydrogenase, with ethanol exhibiting a greater affinity for the enzyme than methanol. The rationale of therapy is to saturate the enzyme with ethanol, thus preventing the metabolism of methanol to its toxic metabolites. Methanol will then be slowly excreted over two to five days by the kidneys.

Ethanol is provided at a dose of 0.5 to 1.5 ml./kg. of the 50 per cent solution given every 2 to 4 hours. It is important to achieve and maintain serum ethanol levels greater than 100 mg./100 ml. until methanol levels have fallen to the nontoxic range (less than 10 mg./100 ml.).

Methanol and its metabolites are highly dialyzable. When methanol levels exceed 50 to 100 mg./100 ml., in the presence of severe acidosis or when retinal edema and hyperemia are noted, dialysis should be combined with ethanol therapy. Ethanol, given as described above for methanol intoxication, is also an effective antidote for ethylene glycol poisoning.

Methylene Blue. Methylene blue is the antidote of choice in the therapy of methemoglobinemia, the latter being induced by many compounds including nitrites, aniline, phenacetin, nitrobenzenes, sulfonamides, chlorates and quinones. The toxicity of methemoglobinemia occurs as a result of the oxidation of hemoglobin iron from its ferrous to its ferric state. This results in reduced oxygen transport capacity and decreased release of oxygen to the tissues. Methylene blue given intravenously as a 1 per cent solution in a dose of 1 to 2 mg./kg. over 5 to 10 minutes reduces iron from its ferric to its ferrous state. This dose may be repeated in three to four hours. Oxygen is given during therapy. As methylene blue is itself toxic (causing vomiting, diarrhea, altered sensorium, chest pain and cyanosis), its use should be reserved for patients with significant methemoglobin levels (above 30 to 40 per cent) or patients with symptoms (dyspnea, cyanosis, altered sensorium). The effectiveness of therapy should be monitored by serial methemoglobin determinations.

Naloxone Hydrochloride (Narcan). This narcotic antagonist is highly specific and effective in the treatment of poisoning resulting from methadone, diphenoxylate hydrochloride (Lomotil), propoxyphene (Darvon), morphine, apomorphine, meperidine (Demerol), pentazocine (Talwin) and codeine. Unlike the previously used antagonists, nalorphine (Nalline) and levallorphan (Lorfan), naloxone is without agonist properties and therefore will not produce respiratory or central nervous system depression even in the patient who has ingested a non-narcotic drug. Naloxone has a wide margin of safety with doses 10 times that recommended being without apparent ill effect. Naloxone may be used as a diagnostic trial as well as for treatment of the narcotic overdose.

The initial dose for narcotic-induced respiratory and central nervous system depression and hypotension is 0.01 mg./kg. given intravenously. The desired effects are seen within 2 to 3 minutes and consist of pupillary dilation, increased blood pressure and respiratory rate, and generally an increase in the level of consciousness. Because the antagonist achieves its effect by competing with the tissue-bound narcotic, the patient with a large narcotic overdose generally requires multiple doses of naloxone (up to three times within 10 minutes) to produce the desired response. Once a favorable response to the antagonist is obtained, the drug should be given as often as is necessary to maintain normal blood pressure and respiratory rate, normal or dilated pupils and an alert sensorium. Frequent careful monitoring of the patient, often for as long as 24 to 36 hours (the exact time being dependent on the half-life of the narcotic), is necessary until the effects of the ingested toxin have passed.

Oxygen for Carbon Monoxide Poisoning. Because of the high affinity of carbon monoxide for hemoglobin, oxygen is displaced from hemoglobin by carbon monoxide with the formation of carboxyhemoglobin. The latter has a decreased oxygen carrying capacity and a diminished ability to release oxygen to the tissues, resulting in tissue hypoxia. High concentrations of oxygen are rapidly effective, displacing carbon monoxide from its binding by hemoglobin. Carboxyhemoglobin levels can be decreased by 50 per cent in 1 to 2 hours with 100 per cent oxygen.

Physostigmine (Antilirium). Physostigmine, a drug with anticholinesterase properties, has been used increasingly in the treatment of poisonings from various anticholinergic agents including belladonna alkaloids, antihistamines, tricyclic antidepressants and certain plants. While having peripheral pharmacological properties similar to those of neostigmine, physostigmine has the added ability to enter the central nervous system, thus exerting central as well as peripheral effects. Physostigmine is capable of reversing signs of central nervous system excitation or depression, hypertension, signs of atropinization (dilated pupils, dry mouth, tachycardia, hyperpyrexia, bladder and bowel atony) and cardiac arrhythmias (sinus, atrial, nodal and ventricular tachycardias). It does not appear to be effective for the control of hypotension or seizures.

The drug may be used as a diagnostic trial in the suspected anticholinergic overdose. Its use should be considered for symptoms and signs thought to present a significant hazard to the patient including cardiac arrhythmias, hypertension, deep levels of coma, and complications secondary to the effects of atropinization. The recommended dose in children is 0.5 mg. and in adolescents is 2.0 mg.

The dose is administered slowly intravenously over 2 to 3 minutes. If no effect is observed, the dose may be repeated at five minute intervals up to a total dose of 2 mg. in children and 4 to 6 mg. in adolescents. Since the metabolism of physostigmine is more rapid than the ingested drug, the antidote may be required as often as every 30 minutes to 1 hour until the patient is free of serious toxic effects.

The use of physostigmine carries two risks. First, if the drug is given too rapidly the patient may develop seizures. Second, inadvertent overtreatment can result in cholinergic crisis, characterized by miotic pupils, salivation, diarrhea and vomiting. This latter effect may be reversed by the administration of atropine at a dose one-half that of the physostigmine.

Vitamin K. Vitamin K_1 is used in the treatment of warfarin and dicumarol toxicity. These anticoagulants are common components of pesticides and exert their effect by inhibiting prothrombin synthesis, thereby producing a hemorrhagic diathesis. Vitamin K_1 given in a dose of 5 mg. orally will reverse this effect. Vitamin K_1 use is generally limited to instances of repeated exposure or to massive overdose from warfarin and dicumarol compounds.

Investigational Antidotes

The antidotes listed below are presently in an investigational status or are of unclear effectiveness. Their use should be considered at the time of an overdose with the status of their efficacy carefully reviewed at that time.

Antidote	Toxin
Thioctic acid (alpha lipoic acid)	Amanita genus of mushrooms
Pyridoxine hydrochloride	Isoniazid
Sodium diethyldithiocarbamate (Dithiocarb)	Thallium
Cysteamine, methionine, acetylcysteine	Acetaminophen

Antisera

Various antisera are available for food poisoning and spider and snake exposures and their use should be considered at the time of the toxic exposure.

Antisera	Source
Antivenom	Black widow spider
Antivenom	Scorpion spider
Antivenom	North American pit viper
Antivenom	Coral snake
Bivalent (A & B) antitoxin	Botulism food poisoning
Trivalent (A, B, & E)	Botulism food poisoning

ENHANCED EXCRETION

Hepatic and Respiratory Excretory Mechanisms. Toxins are usually removed from the body by three major pathways: hepatic, renal or respiratory. The active compounds are converted to inactive metabolites by the liver and then are excreted in the urine or feces, are excreted unchanged by the kidneys, or are removed from the body by the respiratory route. For most agents one pathway predominates: for example, the hepatic route for phenytoin, the renal route for boric acid and bromides and the respiratory route for carbon monoxide. For a few drugs, such as phenobarbital and salicylates, both renal and hepatic pathways are important. Drugs that primarily undergo hepatic inactivation are treated by supportive therapy alone, allowing time for the liver to detoxify the ingested product. For some products taken in overdose, hepatic metabolism may produce metabolites which are in themselves toxic (methanol, fluoroacetate, parathion, heptachlor, nitrobenzene, ethylene glycol, acetaminophen). In these cases the risk of toxicity will persist until the body has excreted not only the parent compound but the relevant metabolites as well.

Forced Diuresis. If the predominant excretory route of the active compound (or metabolite) is the kidneys, forced fluid diuresis may enhance its removal by increasing glomerular filtration, thereby minimizing reabsorption in the distal tubules. Osmotic agents (mannitol or urea) and diuretics (furosemide, ethacrynic acid) also increase glomerular filtration and renal tubular flow, thereby enhancing the renal excretion of toxic compounds (for doses see Table 4).

Ionized diuresis is an additional method of enhancing excretion and is based on the principle that a drug in its ionized form crosses lipid membranes poorly. Thus in the case of weak acids (aspirin, phenobarbital) alkalinization of the urine (to pH 7.5 to 8.0) will increase the proportion of ionized drug passing through the renal tubules, thereby decreasing its renal tubular reabsorption. In a similar fashion urinary excretion of alkaline drugs (amphetamine and strychnine) may be enhanced by acidification of urine (to pH 4.0 to 4.5) with ammonium chloride (for doses see Table 4).

All methods of enhanced excretion carry some risk and monitoring of serum and urinary electrolytes, central venous pressure, electrocardiogram and body weight is necessary. The risks involved with enhanced excretion, though small, must be carefully weighed against the risk of conservative support with maintenance fluid therapy alone.

Dialysis. Infrequently in the adolescent and child, the severity of the ingestion will place the patient at sufficient risk to necessitate removal of the drug more rapidly than can be accomplished by methods of enhanced excretion. Hemodialysis and to a lesser extent peritoneal dialysis and exchange transfusion can effectively and rapidly remove a limited but important number of drugs and/or their metabolites. Dialysis may be considered when the severity of the ingestion requires more rapid removal than normal or enhanced excretion can provide, when normal excretory pathways are compromised (renal or hepatic failure) or when underlying pathology contraindicates forced diuresis (renal disease, congestive heart failure). The need for dialysis is universally agreed upon for a limited number of toxins, for example, methanol and ethylene glycol. For other ingestions the reader is referred to the extensive literature in this area.

PREVENTION

Finally, no therapy for poisoning is complete until the reasons for its occurrence have been explored with the parents or victim and advice for future prevention has been fully outlined and explained. For childhood poisoning the aim should be to make the environment as safe as possible by removing all poisons from the child's access. The use of safety containers, education of the child and family, and follow-through to review with parents potential risks existing in the home for their child are methods of accomplishing this objective. For the adolescent, poisoning should be viewed in the context of experimentation or as a suicide gesture or attempt, and immediate vigorous intervention is indicated to prevent a future recurrence.

Salicylate Poisoning

REGINE ARONOW, M.D.

Factors which may modify the therapeutic approach to salicylate poisoning are the route (ingestion, percutaneous or placental transfer) through which the child received the salicylate, amount and type of preparation (such as 1¼, 5 or 10 grain aspirin tablets, sustained-release 10 grain tablets, oil of wintergreen), acute versus chronic exposure, time since exposure, general health, presence of symptoms and age of the child. The most serious cases of salicylate intoxication in children result from delay in obtaining treatment (over 12 hours), ingestion of oil of wintergreen (4 ml. = 2.9 gm. of salicylate) or the intended therapeutic use of excessive or too-frequent doses over a period of days.

ACUTE INTOXICATION

It is axiomatic that when children accidentally ingest substances 50 per cent of the histories are inaccurate, and estimations of amounts ingested may vary by that much as well. If there is certainty that a dose of less than 100 mg./kg. or ¾ grain/lb. was ingested by a well child with no other salicylate exposure in the previous 24 hours, no specific therapy is generally required except to ensure that the child takes no further salicylate and has an adequate oral fluid intake over the next 12 hours. If no more than six hours has elapsed since a dose of 100 to 200 mg./kg. or ¾ to 1½ grain/lb. has been ingested by a well child and no symptoms are present, emesis should be induced by giving 3 to 6 teaspoons of syrup of ipecac followed by a glass of water. An adequate oral fluid intake must be encouraged for the next 12 hours. However, if a history is obtained of salicylate use in the preceding 24 hours, if new symptoms such as hyperpnea have occurred, or if the child is not well (nausea, vomiting, diarrhea, fever, oliguria or previously diagnosed renal dysfunction), examination by a doctor is mandatory and the following laboratory indices should be obtained: serum salicylate, blood pH, pco_2 or plasma CO_2 content, serum sodium and potassium, BUN, blood glucose, and urine pH and specific gravity.

If the ingestion occurred on a relatively empty stomach, peak serum salicylate levels may occur in 90 to 120 minutes. Salicylate is absorbed throughout the gastrointestinal tract, so that peak levels may be delayed by the presence of food in the stomach, gastric stasis, or distinctive formulations such as delayed release tablets or oil of wintergreen. The asymptomatic patient should be given syrup of ipecac (3 to 6 teaspoons followed by a glass of water) as soon as possible to induce forceful emesis. The symptomatic patient should be lavaged with at least 500 ml. of half-strength saline, as considerable amounts of salicylate can be retrieved for up to 12 hours after ingestion. This should be followed by administration of a cathartic to hasten the excretion of any unabsorbed material in the intestinal tract *or* activated charcoal (10 times the estimated salicylate dose).

If seen within the first four hours following ingestion, most asymptomatic children with serum salicylate levels between 30 and 40 mg./ 100 ml. can be adequately treated in the emergency room with administration of maintenance intravenous fluids and of sodium bicarbonate according to the following protocol. Upon evidence several hours later of an alkaline urine and serum salicylate levels falling below 20 mg./100 ml., the child may be discharged.

Children with gastrointestinal or central nervous system disturbances or hyperpnea, evidence of acid-base derangement, or serum salicylate levels over 40 mg./100 ml. should be admitted to the hospital. If there is evidence of metabolic acidosis and a serum salicylate level above 60 mg./100 ml., the child should be admitted to the intensive care unit so that peritoneal dialysis with 5 per cent salt-free albumin added to the dialysate can be instituted immediately in addition to the administration of sodium bicarbonate according to the protocol and correction of electrolyte and fluid deficits. A pediatric nephrologist should be consulted, as more efficient hemodialysis may be justified when there has been a delay in obtaining therapy; an extremely high level of unbound serum salicylate exists (indicating probable high CSF salicylate levels); severe central nervous system symptoms are evident (convulsions and deepening coma); renal damage is apparent; or independent severe kidney disease has been diagnosed.

Diuretics generally do not increase the excretion of salicylate in the urine and may accentuate disturbances of electrolyte and fluid balance. Acetazolamide can intensify metabolic acidosis and has been shown to influence the salicylate volume of distribution, so that the spinal fluid salicylate level may rise with a falling serum salicylate level.

The younger the child, the more severe the presenting metabolic acidosis may be. The child increasingly over the age of five years may initially have respiratory alkalosis, as do adults. This rather rapidly converts to metabolic acidosis as compensatory excretion of base occurs and interference with intermediary metabolism of the Krebs cycle results in ketosis and an accumulation of organic acid metabolites.

The following is the suggested procedure for the management of acute salicylate poisoning, after preliminary evaluation with laboratory results and after procedures for decontamination of the gastrointestinal tract have been instituted.

1. Start an intravenous infusion with 5 per cent glucose in water. The severity of the dehydration and acid-base disturbance will dictate the need to replace deficits. As soon as adequate urinary output is evident, add 40 to 60 mEq. of potassium in the form of potassium chloride to each liter of intravenous mix. The rate of infusion should be at least 2 to 4 ml./ minute for several hours depending upon the age of the child and the degree of hydration. Adequate potassium replacement is essential in order to effectively alkalinize the urine, and enough fluids are given to maintain a good urinary output.

2. Give 20 to 30 ml. of 7½ per cent sodium bicarbonate (available in ampule form) intravenously over a 3 to 5 minute period.

3. Insert a Foley catheter. Check the pH of the urine with pHydrion paper or a pH meter every 15 minutes. In order for this therapy to be effective, the urine must be maintained at a pH of at least 7. The rate of urinary excretion of salicylate is increased four- to five-fold by raising the urinary pH above 7; then, a 50 per cent reduction in the serum salicylate level usually can be accomplished within 5 hours.

4. Whenever the urine is acid (pH of less than 7), give an additional 10 to 20 ml. of 7½ per cent sodium bicarbonate over a 3 to 5 minute period every 15 minutes. You cannot assume that a given dose of sodium bicarbonate will make the urine alkaline. The urine must be checked with regularity. The alkalinizing therapy should be continued until the salicylate level is below 20 to 30 mg./100 ml. and the child is asymptomatic.

5. The estimated body tolerance for sodium is 250 mEq./m²/day. Since the bicarbonate solution has a high sodium content (each 100 ml. of 7½ per cent sodium bicarbonate contains 88 mEq. of sodium), the potential for sodium intoxication exists with bicarbonate therapy. Far more sodium than is necessary will be administered if the urine is not kept alkaline *constantly*. If the procedures outlined are followed rigidly, it will rarely be necessary to administer a quantity of sodium that exceeds 240 mEq./m²/24 hours.

6. If the physician in charge is not willing or able to follow these directions, he should use some other modality of therapy. Good supportive care with careful monitoring of fluid and electrolyte parameters is critical.

7. In the event of renal shutdown, the alkalinizing approach alone cannot be utilized and one must resort to peritoneal dialysis, hemodialysis or exchange transfusion.

The hyperglycemia that may be evident does not require specific therapy but should correct itself as the salicylate intoxication is relieved. Continue to give 5 per cent glucose intravenously. Occasionally a very young infant may show hypoglycemia which should be treated by a small infusion of 10 per cent glucose.

Hyperpyrexia may be present and can be reduced by a cooling mattress or cautious sponging with tepid water.

Convulsions may be controlled by paraldehyde or intravenous diazepam administered slowly so as not to depress the respiratory rate.

In severe or chronic salicylate intoxication, 5 to 10 mg. of vitamin K_1 or its oxide may be given prophylactically and, if laboratory evidence of impending hemorrhagic phenomena exists, a small fresh blood transfusion may be indicated.

CHRONIC INTOXICATION

In chronic poisoning there is little correlation between serum salicylate level and the severity of illness. The salicylate in the central nervous system compartment is what must be removed. Alkalinization therapy and peritoneal dialysis with 5 per cent salt-free albumin added to the dialysate should be instituted as quickly as possible. Fluid and electrolyte deficits must be corrected. The management described for acute intoxication applies except that relating to actual serum salicylate levels. Anticipate possible renal damage and adverse effects on prothrombin and platelets. A rare patient may exhibit fluid retention suggestive of an inappropriate secretion of ADH. Slow intravenous administration of 20 per cent mannitol, 1 gm./kg., to induce diuresis followed by appropriate fluid restriction may be necessary.*

Consultation should be obtained if the serum salicylate level reaches zero and the patient remains critically ill or acidotic, to determine how long alkalinization and peritoneal dialysis should be continued; or if there is failure to alkalinize the urine of a critically ill child with the described protocol, to consider alternative therapy such as the use of the amine buffer, tromethamine (THAM-E).

Although death usually occurs from respiratory failure, the underlying cause may be selective hypoglycemia of brain tissue, critical CSF salicylate levels having been reached, or cerebral hemorrhage.

---

*Manufacturer's precaution: Dosage requirements of mannitol for patients 12 years and under have not been established.

Acetaminophen Intoxication

REGINE ARONOW, M.D.

The marketplace offers an increasing variety of products containing acetaminophen which are becoming commonplace in homes. Child-resistant packaging has not been mandated for such over-the-counter products, so it can be anticipated that the incidence of accidental ingestions will rise.

Although the action of acetaminophen as an antipyretic and analgesic is similar to that of aspirin, with remarkably few adverse effects when used in therapeutic doses, the problem overdosage may pose involves serious hepatotoxicity and far exceeds that of salicylate poisoning. Injury occurs in the first pass of the drug through the liver, as a result of the formation of an arylating metabolite through the cytochrome oxidase system, in excess of the protective glutathione store.

Initial symptoms can be nondescript or limited to nausea, vomiting, diarrhea, mild abdominal pain, sweating or a pale drawn facies. Hepatic injury, which may proceed to hepatic failure, coma and death, can become evident by laboratory or clinical findings in 24 to 48 hours or may not be evident until day 4 or 5. Also, renal damage, pancreatitis and rarely myocardial necrosis may develop. By this time, acetaminophen is no longer detectable in the blood.

The literature contains many documented cases of acetaminophen poisoning in adults but mentions only one young child. It remains to be established whether children have some unique physiological protection from this kind of poisoning or if there are manifestations not being recognized.

Pharmacokinetic studies reveal that children up through the age of nine years, in contrast to those from 12 years of age to adulthood, conjugate a dose of acetaminophen primarily with sulfate and only to a lesser degree with glucuronide. The critical issue, however, relates to the activity of the mixed oxidase microsomes that convert acetaminophen into the toxic metabolite and the glutathione-dependent detoxification pathway. The developmental aspects of the mechanism in humans have not been defined. Until studies are complete, we must assume pediatric patients are at as much risk as are adults.

Generally 15 gm. of acetaminophen has been a hepatotoxic dose for an adult. Assuming the same relative toxicity on a weight basis, the hepatotoxic dose in a two year old would be 2.1 gm.

SUGGESTED APPROACH TO ACCIDENTAL INGESTION

Consider the ratio 2 gm./10 kg. and calculate the amount that may be hepatotoxic for the weight of the patient involved. Since 50 per cent of our histories are inaccurate and other circumstances may influence the toxicity (adverse effects; previous use of microsome-inducing agent such as phenobarbital or reduced glutathione stores from a low-protein diet), use one half the amount calculated to institute immediate treatment.

1. Any child taking 100 mg./kg. should be referred to an appropriate emergency room with dispatch. (If there is syrup of ipecac available at home, ½ to 1 oz. may be administered followed by a glass of water, and then proceed to the emergency room with a container for the vomitus.) Lavage with at least 500 ml. of half-strength saline; instill 5 gm. of sodium sulfate laxative up to age 10 years, then 10 gm.; clamp tube, wait 15 minutes, instill activated charcoal slurry—10 times the suspected amount of acetaminophen.*

2. Draw base line bilirubin, SGPT, LDH, PTT. Keep in contact with patient daily for at least three days. If serum acetaminophen levels are available, more specific therapy may be indicated.

3. If the patient has symptoms (nausea, vomiting, abdominal discomfort, drawn facies) or if 200 mg./kg. has been ingested, hospitalize. Maintain on intravenous fluids, check laboratory indices daily, and include serum amylase and creatinine clearance. *Treat as impending liver failure.*

4. Even if no symptoms exist, recheck bilirubin, SGPT, LDH and PTT on day 4 or 5.

If over four hours have elapsed it is doubtful that activated charcoal and the laxative will be effective in preventing initial injury. However, a bolus often forms when a large number of pills are ingested, so further injury may be prevented. Because hepatotoxicity occurs on the first pass of acetaminophen through the liver, diuresis has no therapeutic value. It is also potentially dangerous, as acetaminophen has an antidiuretic effect.

With a therapeutic dose, peak blood levels may be reached in 45 minutes with a half-life of one to two hours, and about 30 hours are required to excrete the total dose. Blood levels appear to be the best early prediction of the serious consequences from a given dose. The following ranges are wide and not absolute.

	UNBOUND ACETAMINOPHEN SERUM CONCENTRATION (μg./ml.)	HEPATIC NECROSIS
At 4 hours	> 300	Probable
	120 to 300	Possible
	< 120	Unlikely
At 12 hours	> 120	Probable
	50 to 120	Possible
	< 50	Unlikely

If the actual time of ingestion is unknown, two accurately timed blood levels can be used to calculate the half-life. If it exceeds four hours, it is a bad prognostic sign.

The earlier specific therapy is instituted, the greater the chance to be successful. It is doubtful if any will be effective after 8 hours. Patients surviving the hepatotoxicity do not seem to have residual complications three months later.

Unfortunately, glutathione administration does not build up hepatic glutathione stores, so precursors such as L-cysteine, methionine, or cysteamine are being tried. The latter chemical has seemed to be therapeutic when used by one group of investigators but not so by another. It can cause unpleasant symptoms itself. N-acetyl-cysteine* and methionine used within a few hours of ingestion seem to have a therapeutic effect. Penicillamine, BAL and dithiocarb have also been used. Penicillamine seemed to induce renal complications, so it had a limited trial; BAL had an unsuccessful inadequate trial; and dithiocarb has only been used therapeutically in mice. Steroids have not proved effective and there is little to indicate that any form of dialysis can prevent the hepatotoxicity.

Research on specific therapy is continuing. Regional Poison Control Centers will be aware of the advances, and consultation should be obtained immediately after instituting decontamination of the patient's gastrointestinal tract.

Lead Poisoning

SERGIO PIOMELLI, M.D.

The treatment of lead poisoning in children depends on an exact diagnosis not only of the existing exposure, but also of its degree. Since all children are exposed to lead in the modern environment, they accumulate an ex-

---

*Charcoal may interfere with definitive therapy. Obtain consultation before administering.

*Trials with 20 per cent Mucomyst administered orally are under way in the United States on an IND (Investigational New Drug) protocol.

cess of lead in the body. There are no such entities as "normal body content of lead" or "normal blood lead level," since lead serves no function in the human body, and populations living remote from urbanization and "civilization" have nearly undetectable blood lead levels.

Different individuals are exposed to lead in different amounts. There is a range in body burden of lead from rural children with the lowest level, to urban children with a higher level, to excessively exposed children with a definitely increased level, to children with clinical signs and symptoms of lead intoxication culminating in lead encephalopathy. A spectrum of overexposure to lead exists and all attempts at classification are necessarily arbitrary. The symptoms of lead poisoning are vague and undefined: apathy, hyperirritability, vomiting and abdominal pains. Lead encephalopathy is evidenced by forceful vomiting, lethargy alternating with lucidity, convulsions and coma.

Symptomatic children (with or without overt encephalopathy) require immediate treatment. Asymptomatic children with blood lead levels ≥ 80 μg./dl. require immediate treatment, as they are at an extremely high risk of becoming symptomatic. The management of children with increased body burden of lead is not standardized and the author will describe the therapeutic guidelines used in his clinic.

TREATMENT OF SEVERE LEAD POISONING

Children with overt encephalopathy, symptoms attributable to lead poisoning or blood lead levels ≥ 80 μg./dl. are included in this category. The blood lead level should be measured in a venous blood sample, as micromethods can give falsely high results due to contamination. Do not treat a child solely on the basis of a blood lead level ≥ 80 μg./dl. determined by micromethods unless there is other clear-cut evidence such as an erythrocyte protoporphyrin level ≥ 190 μg./dl., abdominal x-ray showing lead, or clinical symptoms.

In children presenting with encephalopathy, it may not be possible to obtain an immediate blood lead level. In these circumstances, the sample for blood lead level should be drawn and additional presumptive evidence obtained. Measurement of erythrocyte protoporphyrin can be obtained in minutes since the erythrocyte protoporphyrin is invariably elevated in severe lead intoxication, a low erythrocyte protoporphyrin rules out this diagnosis. If the erythrocyte protoporphyrin is elevated, x-rays of the abdomen and the long bones are obtained. It is better to obtain the results of the blood lead level before initiating therapy; however, in extreme clinical severity, it may be safer to initiate therapy immediately, even when in doubt.

The principles of therapy are simple: maintenance of diuresis without overhydration; control of convulsions, if present, with diazepam and paraldehyde; chelation of lead with BAL and Ca Na EDTA. It is extremely important to know that *only* Ca Na EDTA (calcium disodium EDTA) should be used. *Na EDTA (trisodium EDTA) can induce acute hypocalcemia and should never be used.*

Diuresis should be established with intravenous fluids (10 per cent dextrose in water, 10 ml./kg./hr.). After diuresis is established, just enough fluids are given to obtain a urine flow between 350 and 500 ml./m²/day. Care should be taken not to overhydrate in order to prevent excessive intracranial pressure. Spinal tap should not be performed; if it is absolutely necessary to rule out other conditions, no more than 1 ml. of fluid should be withdrawn. Corticosteroids can be given to alleviate increased intracranial pressure; their use should be limited to the most severe cases, as experimental evidence indicates that they may potentiate the renal toxicity of Ca Na EDTA. Convulsions should be controlled initially with diazepam. Before giving diazepam, it is necessary to have an intravenous infusion running and to make sure that intubation and assisted respiration equipment is at hand in case of respiratory failure. Diazepam (Valium), 0.15 mg./kg., is given slowly (over approximately 2 minutes) by syringe; it should not be mixed with any diluting fluid.* If necessary, an additional dose of 0.1 mg./kg. can be given after 20 to 30 minutes. Control of convulsions should be maintained by paraldehyde, 0.15 ml./kg. Barbiturates should be used during the recovery phase.

Chelation therapy should be initiated without wasting any time in giving enemas or cathartics to remove lead from the intestine. Chelation therapy should be started with an intramuscular injection of BAL at the dose of 4 mg./kg. This is followed by alternating, every 4 hours, Ca Na EDTA, 12.5 mg./kg., and BAL, 4 mg./kg. Both medications are given intramuscularly; Ca Na EDTA should be mixed with 0.5 ml. of procaine hydrochloride 2 per cent to reduce pain. In most severe cases, both BAL and Ca Na EDTA can be given every 4 hours. Treatment is continued for a minimum of 5

---

*Manufacturer's precaution: Safety and efficacy of injectable diazepam in the neonate have not been established.

days, to a maximum of 7 days, if enceph-alopathy persists; then treatment is inter-rupted for 48 hours. Blood lead levels should be monitored daily; when the blood lead level falls below 60 μg./dl., BAL is dropped, but Ca Na EDTA is continued; when the blood lead level falls below 30 μg./dl., Ca Na EDTA is dis-continued. It is important to remember that iron should never be given to patients receiv-ing BAL; if severe anemia is present, blood transfusion may be indicated. The erythrocyte protoporphyrin during intense chelation therapy rises, at times rapidly, due to the mobilization of lead; this is no reason to discon-tinue therapy. In the author's experience, a single course is usually inadequate and at least 2 (to a maximum of 4) courses of 5 days each (followed by 48 hours' rest period) are needed. The measurement of urinary lead is quite helpful in deciding whether to give additional courses. These are usually required in children who excrete more than 2 mg. of lead per day during the initial course.

After the blood lead level has been re-duced by the initial chelation therapy, almost invariably a rebound occurs. Thus the physi-cian should not rest under the impression that the problem is solved just because the blood lead level has dropped. A repeat measurement of blood lead level is mandatory 10 to 12 days after the last course of chelation therapy; at this time re-equilibration results in a rebound and the blood lead level is always higher than at the last day of chelation. Most frequently, the blood lead level is between 60 and 50 μg./dl. at this point. Repeated courses of Ca Na EDTA alone are given (50 mg./kg. in a single intramuscular dose for 5 days each, with 9 days interval) until the blood lead level (obtained at least 8 days after chelation) stabilizes below 40 μg./dl., the urinary lead excretion falls below 1 μg. of lead per mg. of Ca Na EDTA given, or the erythrocyte protoporphyrin decreases below 60 μg./dl. These Ca Na EDTA courses may be given on an outpatient basis with medi-cal supervision.

An important recommendation is never to let the child return to the previous lead-containing environment. The apartment must be deleaded or the child relocated. It may be necessary to maintain the child in a convales-cent home until appropriate measures are taken. Recurrences of lead intoxication tend to be of progressively increasing severity. Blood lead and erythrocyte protoporphyrin levels in these children should be monitored every month for the first year after they have stabilized, and every third month thereafter.

MANAGEMENT OF CHILDREN WITH INCREASED BODY BURDEN OF LEAD

Children with increased body burden of lead are usually asymptomatic and are brought to medical attention when detected by screen-ing programs. A scale of severity has been selected to provide a priority sequence on the basis of the results of the screening tests. As discussed above, the "normal" values for blood level and erythrocyte protoporphyrin are theoretical figures, as all children are affected to some extent by environmental lead.

At present, it is suggested that children with blood lead levels ≤ 30 μg./dl. and erythro-cyte protoporphyrin ≤ 60 μg./dl. be consid-ered "normal" (class I). Several investigators feel that these values are rather high and would like to have the values reduced to ≤ 25 μg./dl. for blood lead and to ≤ 40 μg./dl. for erythrocyte protoporphyrin. Children with blood lead levels between 30 and 49 μg./dl. and erythrocyte protoporphyrin between 60 and 110 μg./dl. are considered to have moderately increased body burden of lead (class II); blood lead levels between 50 and 79 μg./dl. and erythrocyte protoporphyrin between 110 and 190 μg./dl. indicate increased body burden of lead (class III); and blood lead levels ≥ 80 μg./dl. and erythrocyte protoporphyrin ≥ 190 μg./dl. indicate severe lead intoxication (class IV).

It must be noted that these criteria are guidelines to interpret the results of screening tests and should not be used as absolute values. Falsely elevated values for blood lead in sam-ples obtained by finger puncture often occur due to contamination; these results should be considered with particular caution and defin-itely rejected as spurious if not paralleled by an elevation of erythrocyte protoporphyrin. On the other hand, levels of erythrocyte pro-toporphyrin and blood lead occasionally do not coincide with the expected range. Because erythrocyte protoporphyrin is a better indi-cator of exposure to lead, children with a greater erythrocyte protoporphyrin than an-ticipated by the blood lead level should be up-graded in terms of risk and thus investigated with a greater urgency. The physician, how-ever, must be aware that erythrocyte pro-toporphyrin may be elevated by iron deficiency anemia and that there are rare individuals with the genetic defect erythropoietic protopor-phyria (a condition which results in increased photosensitivity) who have extremely elevated erythrocyte protoporphyrin levels (≥ 190 μg./dl.). Thus a child should never be treated with chelation on the basis of the results of the erythrocyte protoporphyrin alone.

In our clinic, when patients with suspected increased body burden of lead are detected by screening (erythrocyte protoporphyrin $\geq$ 60 μg./dl. and blood lead level $\geq$ 30 μg./dl.), a careful physical examination, detailed history, confirmatory venous blood lead levels as well as serum iron and total iron-binding capacity are obtained.

If the confirmatory blood lead level is between 60 and 79 μg./dl. (or higher) the child is admitted for a 5 day course of BAL and Ca Na EDTA as detailed above for severe lead intoxication. Decision as to further treatment is based on the daily lead excretion. A note of caution: The EDTA provocative test should not be performed on asymptomatic children with blood lead levels $\geq$ 60 μg./dl., as this may induce convulsions.

If the blood lead level is between 30 and 59 μg./dl., radiological examination of the abdomen and long bones is obtained, but the final decision on treatment is based on the result of the EDTA provocative test. This is done by intramuscular injection of 50 mg./kg. of Ca Na EDTA (maximum dose 1 gm.), followed by collection of urine for 8 hours. This test can be performed on an outpatient basis. The test is considered positive if more than 0.5 μg. of lead is excreted per mg. of Ca Na EDTA received.

The Ca Na EDTA provocative test is positive in the majority of those children; however, chelation therapy is given only to those children with a markedly elevated lead excretion ($\geq$1.5 μg. of lead per mg. of Ca Na EDTA received). These children receive one 5 day course of Ca Na EDTA intramuscularly at a dose of 50 mg./kg./day (maximum 1 gm.). The blood lead is measured 9 or 10 days after the end of chelation therapy; repeated courses are given until the blood lead stabilizes below 40 μg./dl. and the erythrocyte protoporphyrin returns to normal. Urinary lead excretion is monitored during therapy to evaluate its efficacy.

Those children in whom urine lead excretion in the EDTA provocative test is between 1 and 1.5 μg. of lead per mg. of Ca Na EDTA received are treated with oral d-penicillamine at the dose of 20 mg./kg./day in divided doses.* The blood lead and erythrocyte protoporphyrin levels are monitored monthly and the EDTA provocative test is repeated periodically (every 4 to 6 months).

_____
*This use of d-penicillamine is not mentioned in the manufacturer's instructions.

The children in whom urine and lead excretion in the EDTA provocative test is between 0.5 and 1 μg. of lead per mg. of Ca Na EDTA received are not treated, but are followed monthly with tests of levels of blood lead and erythrocyte protoporphyrin; if the elevation of blood lead or erythrocyte protoporphyrin persists, then the EDTA provocative test is repeated.

In all cases, the parents are alerted to the various possible sources of lead exposure, the housing is investigated by a sanitarian, and the sources of lead are removed. The most effective measure is education of the parents, who are usually totally unaware of the possibility of their child being exposed to lead in the house. Despite patronizing statements to the contrary, the cause of lead poisoning is a bad house, not a bad mother. The overwhelming majority of our patients' parents take whatever measures are in their power to remove the source of lead and often transfer their children to the home of relatives until the appropriate repairs are made by themselves, the landlords, or the housing authorities.

Iron Poisoning

SERGIO PIOMELLI, M.D.

Acute iron poisoning usually occurs in small children who ingest medicinal iron (ferrous sulfate). The children are misled by the candy-like appearance of the tablets. Severe toxicity occurs when more than 300 mg. of elemental iron is ingested (more than 4 or 5 tablets). Often, the iron tablets had been prescribed (unnecessarily) for the mother by her obstetrician during pregnancy, and they are discovered by the child in the exploratory activities of the second year of life. The mortality of iron poisoning, which was originally estimated to be as high as 50 per cent, has been greatly reduced by improved modalities of treatment and, probably even more, by the realization that there are many mild cases which often go unreported.

The initial symptoms of acute iron poisoning are vomiting and then diarrhea, often with gastrointestinal bleeding. These symptoms are due to the local irritation induced by iron. Often, most of the ingested iron is vomited before arrival to the hospital. Nevertheless, induction of additional vomiting and gastric lavage should be performed. Later symptoms, which may occur either rapidly or several hours later, consist of hypotension, acidosis, lethargy, shock and coma. Hepatic damage may also occur.

The principles of therapy are simple: removal of the iron from the stomach, countermeasures to treat shock and hypotension, correction of electrolyte imbalance secondary to vomiting and diarrhea, and chelation therapy with desferrioxamine-B only in those cases where iron ingestion has been large enough to give free iron (that is, in excess of the serum iron-binding capacity) in the circulation.

When iron intoxication is suspected, vomiting should be induced immediately with syrup of ipecac (15 ml.), and the vomitus examined for presence of iron tablets. Gastric lavage is not adequate for removal of tablets. If shock is present, appropriate countermeasures should be taken, including use of plasma expanders, blood transfusions and pressor amines. Meanwhile, blood should be drawn for counts, electrolyte levels, rapid (Fischer) iron test, serum iron, blood typing and crossmatching. Radiological examination of the abdomen may reveal residual radiopaque tablets of iron; however, it may fail to do so, if these are dissolved.

After vomiting has been induced, the stomach is lavaged by nasogastric tube with a 3.5 per cent solution of sodium dihydrogen phosphate (half-strength Fleet's enema). Then, 50 ml. of 1 per cent sodium dihydrogen phosphate (one-third strength the previous lavage fluid) is instilled in the stomach.

After these initial measures, and before initiation of chelation therapy, it is best to try to assess the actual amount of iron ingested and absorbed. Of greatest value in this regard is the Fischer test. This is of such importance in the treatment of iron poisoning that it should be available to all pediatric emergency rooms, if possible, in the form of a "kit." The Fischer test detects iron in excess of the serum iron binding capacity. This is a presumptive screening test and should be later confirmed by quantitative measurement of serum iron.

If the test is negative, and the patient does not appear critically ill, it may be better not to start chelation therapy, but to limit treatment to intravenous fluids, correction of dehydration, electrolyte imbalance, and acidosis, and supportive measures.

If the Fischer test is positive (or if unavailable), chelation therapy is started with desferrioxamine-B at the dose of 10 mg./kg./hour by slow intravenous infusion; this dose must not be exceeded. The patient should be monitored carefully for tachypnea, tachycardia, pallor and hypotension, since both desferrioxamine-B and its iron chelate may have a hypotensive effect. Desferrioxamine-B gives to the urine a deep red-brown color only when iron excretion is significant; this color is due to the complex between iron and desferrioxamine-B (ferrioxamine). Thus if no red-brown color appears in the urine within the first two hours, this indicates that no excess iron is present in the circulation. This implies a favorable prognosis and therefore chelation therapy should be interrupted. If the urine turns red, therapy should be continued by intramuscular injections at a dose of 10 mg./kg. every 4 hours until the urine loses its color. It may be necessary to continue therapy for up to 72 hours. It is not advisable to give desferrioxamine-B by mouth.

In extreme cases, early exchange transfusion may be considered.

All patients with suspected iron poisoning should be admitted for a minimum of 24 hours' observation. Patients with proven iron ingestion should be tested radiologically 2 to 3 months later for possible residual stomach or esophageal strictures.

Desferrioxamine-B, 20 mg./kg./day by intramuscular injection, is also useful in the treatment of chronic iron overload in patients with chronic, transfusion-dependent anemias (Cooley's anemia, aplastic anemias).*

Fischer Test for "Free" Plasma Iron. Blood is drawn into a heparinized iron free tube (green top Vacutainer). It is centrifuged for 3 minutes at high speed in a table centrifuge. With iron-free pipettes (or, if unavailable, with plastic syringes) add 0.1 ml. of hydroxylammonium chloride, 0.2 ml. of ammonium acetate buffer, and 0.1 ml. of TPZ chromogen to an iron-free tube and mix. Then, add 0.5 ml. of plasma, mix and observe for 5 minutes for development of blue color. It is useful to have a negative control (normal plasma) and a positive control (normal plasma with added ferric chloride). The control plasmas can be stored in the freezer indefinitely.

Stinging Insect Hypersensitivity

BERNARD A. BERMAN, M.D.

Allergic reactions resulting from the sting of a bee, wasp, yellow jacket, hornet or fire ant, all members of the order Hymenoptera, are a cause of concern because fatalities can, and do, occur. The sting reactions are far more preva-

---

*This use of desferrioxamine-B is not mentioned in the manufacturer's instructions.

lent in late summer, and adults, 30 years of age or older, are bothered more so than are children.

The local reaction from a sting may represent an allergic or toxic response, the usual findings being localized swelling, itching, pain and redness. This type of reaction is commonplace and can persist for several days. Treatment with a variety of topical preparations, including creams, lotions, application of ice, as well as systemic therapy with antihistaminics, are of little or no help in reducing the discomfort and swelling, although antihistaminics may lessen the itch. Short-burst prednisone therapy, up to 30 mg. each day for three consecutive days, is rarely prescribed, but it may have to be used and is often helpful if there is extensive localized swelling.

Since the venoms of wasp, yellow jacket and hornet are occasionally contaminated with bacteria, the initial local allergic or toxic reaction may be complicated by infection, and if so, must be treated accordingly.

Whereas stings which cause local reactions are generally a nuisance and not a cause of concern, it is the systemic allergic response, ranging from pruritus, urticaria and wheezing to dyspnea, nausea, abdominal discomfort, fear, anxiety and collapse, that constitutes a medical emergency. Such a reaction may occur within seconds after a sting, but usually is observed from 15 minutes to 1 hour later, with the majority of patients recovering after appropriate therapy. If a systemic reaction occurs without collapse, treatment is generally successful after the patient receives aqueous epinephrine 1:1000, 0.30 cc. subcutaneously (0.20 cc. for a small child), along with diphenhydramine (Benadryl), 25 to 50 mg. intramuscularly. Epinephrine may have to be repeated once or twice more, but do not exceed tolerance. Aerosolized epinephrine, 1:100, is a useful adjunct for upper respiratory tract obstructive symptoms. If wheezing continues to be a major problem, refer to Asthma for a more detailed discussion of therapy.

When the patient's condition has stabilized, he is discharged with instructions to rest, take Chlor-Trimeton or Fedahist, both over-the-counter preparations, one tablet of either, three times a day for three to four days. Prednisone, 30 mg. a day for four consecutive days, constitutes a safeguard for the potentially hazardous late-appearing systemic reaction, occurring, as it may, two to three days later.

Venoms contain a variety of mediators, some identified, others not. Some of the well known mediators in venom include kinins, serotonin and histamine. Thus should a patient suffer single or multiple stings, and the reaction consist of headache, nausea and light-headedness, this kind of response represents clearly a toxic reaction, and other than rest and reassurance, no specific therapy need be given.

For the rare patient with an anaphylactic reaction, refer to Anaphylaxis.

Immunotherapy is necessary for patients who experience systemic reactions after a sting. Another group who qualify for treatment are children with severe extensive local swelling involving both sides of a joint, or whose swelling spreads to an entire extremity. Treatment is also useful for the child with serum sickness reactions, normally occurring 10 to 14 days after a sting.

Should a patient suffer a systemic reaction, defer skin testing for at least two weeks. Skin testing performed any earlier may result in a false negative reaction because skin-sensitizing reaginic antibodies are exhausted for several weeks after an acute reaction. Intradermal testing, utilizing mixed whole body extract, is standard procedure. Although the immunogens of the various insects possess dissimilar antigens, their common antigenicity is of sufficient magnitude to allow tests with a mixture containing equal parts of bee, wasp, yellow jacket and hornet. The fire ant has as its habitat the southern part of the United States. When the fire ant stings, it secures itself to its victim by its jaws, then proceeds to revolve about the head, inflicting stings in a distinctive circular distribution. For the fire ant, a specific extract is available for both skin tests and treatment.

SKIN TESTING

For skin testing, constantly monitor the patient because systemic reactions have been reported during this procedure. Start skin tests with an initial dose of 0.02 cc. of a 1:100,000,000 dilution and then, every 20 to 30 minutes proceed to the next dose, each being 10 times as concentrated as the previous dose, until a positive wheal and flare reaction or a 1:1000 dilution is reached, whichever occurs first. Tests continued beyond a 1:1000 dilution are usually of no help, because reactions beyond this concentration probably represent an irritant response. There is extremely poor correlation between the severity of the clinical systemic reaction and the dilution of extract expected to provoke a positive skin test. In fact, it is not unusual to observe an occasional patient with negative skin tests even after a severe systemic reaction. Thus it is clear that skin tests are rarely performed for diagnostic purposes, but rather are used chiefly for determining the starting dose for immunotherapy.

IMMUNOTHERAPY

Regarding immunotherapy, the initial dose is calculated at 0.10 cc. of a dilution 10 times less than that which evoked a positive skin test response. Thus if a wheal and flare reaction was observed with a 1:100,000 dilution, the initial dose for immunotherapy would be 0.10 cc. of a 1:1,000,000 whole body extract. If the skin tests are negative up to and including a 1:1000 dilution, start with 0.10 cc. of a 1:1000 mixed whole body extract.

The program for treatment with whole body extract is not dissimilar from treatment programs useful for hyposensitization of the typical patient with pollen hay fever or asthma. The dose of extract is increased weekly until a top tolerated dose is reached, but not to exceed 1.00 cc. of a 1:100 dilution or tolerance, whichever comes first, although some allergists proceed to a dose of 0.20 cc. of a 1:10 dilution. Once a top tolerated dose is attained, injections are administered monthly for the following year, and every six weeks for the second year, then every 8 to 10 weeks indefinitely. Until valid and/or worthwhile in vivo or in vitro tests are available to determine if the patient has lost the potential for anaphylactic reaction to a sting, immunotherapy will have to be administered indefinitely. Treatment schedules must always be individualized and the top dose may have to be adjusted downward, depending on the patient's tolerance.

EMERGENCY TREATMENT PROGRAMS

Individuals who survive an initial systemic reaction risk a similar or even more explosive reaction should they be re-stung. Therefore to lessen the chances of death or severe reactions from an insect sting, it is absolutely essential that an emergency treatment regimen be made available to responsible members of the family, be it the parent, the child, or both. The physician can prepare a kit which contains vials of epinephrine 1:1000, a disposable 1 cc. tuberculin syringe with a 25⅝ inch needle, an antihistaminic tablet, aerosolized epinephrine (Medihaler-Epi), and a tourniquet, the latter to be applied intermittently above the sting site, should it be on an extremity. Commercial kits, with most all of the aforementioned contents, but also a preloaded syringe containing epinephrine, can be purchased directly from Hollister-Stier Laboratories, Inc. Parents are urged to run through a dress rehearsal simulating the program to be followed should the child be stung. The technique of administering epinephrine is the physician's responsibility. The parents and/or the child can practice the injections at home, using saline in place of epinephrine during practice sessions. Epinephrine, being extremely unstable, rapidly loses potency when the color changes from clear to brown. When this occurs, it should be replaced. Whenever possible, try to store epinephrine in a cool, dry location and inspect it regularly for discoloration. The dosages of epinephrine are 0.30 cc. subcutaneously for the older child and 0.20 cc. for those children four years or younger. Should it happen that a child or a parent resists the administration of epinephrine, a suitable but less efficacious alternative would be the use of aerosolized epinephrine (Medihaler-Epi). Because only a minimal amount of epinephrine is absorbed systemically after inhalation, we recommend four to eight whiffs of a Medihaler-Epi followed immediately by ingestion of an antihistaminic agent, either Chlor-Trimeton or Fedahist. One or two tablets of either antihistaminic is a suitable dose, but for those who are unable to swallow tablets, a liquid antihistaminic in proportionate dose is administered.

A useful addition to any emergency kit is one or two dimes. On several occasions these have proved to be life-saving, particularly when pay telephones, usually located in rural areas, require coins for emergency calls to medical facilities.

Use of Emergency Medical Kits

Before a child is assured of some degree of protection from a subsequent sting, at least six to nine months of sustained immunotherapy is needed. Let us presume you are treating a 12 year old child residing in the upper Midwest who, following a sting in late May, suffered a systemic reaction, and a program of immunotherapy was initiated a month later, in June. Should this child be re-stung later in the summer, the chances are that there will be insufficient protection against the sting. Under these circumstances, the potential for a systemic reaction is very real. Thus, should this child be re-stung, he should immediately receive all of the contents of an emergency kit and then proceed to the nearest medical facility for observation.

Now let us presume that the same physician, treating the same kind of patient, begins immunotherapy in June, and one year later, in July, the child is re-stung. It is more than likely that this child possesses sufficient protection from immunotherapy to avert a systemic reaction. The medications in the emergency kit need not be administered immediately after the sting; the child should be observed and instructed to rest, and medications from the emergency kit are to be administered only if the child develops incipient signs or symptoms of an acute allergic reaction. After receiving medication, take the child to the nearest medical facility.

By now, it should be clear that any patient with a history of a systemic sting reaction should always have available, during the stinging insect season, in any locality, medications capable of reversing an acute allergic reaction. A Medic-Alert identification tag is issued to each patient undergoing treatment. The child patient, or parent should carry on his person a letter detailing the emergency treatment program.

INSECT VENOMS

Venoms are still considered experimental preparations and though there is more and more data indicating their superiority over whole body extract, they are currently not available as licensed biological agents for treatment.

PREVENTION OF STINGS

All interested parties of the stinging insect victim should be knowledgeable of the habitat of the offending agent, learn how to lessen the risk of exposure to a sting, and be familiar with bits of important information of their common enemy—the stinging insect. The following summary, compiled by the Insect Committee of the American Academy of Allergy, provides this kind of information.

Prevention about the Home.   Any sort of food attracts Hymenopters. Garbage cans dirty on the outside attract the Hymenoptera. Keeping food covered until the moment of disposal, meticulous cleanliness about the garbage area, and repeated spraying of patio and garbage cans with insecticide tend to keep insects away.

Gardening should be done cautiously. A trowel penetrating a bumble bee's nest, scything or power mowing over a yellow jacket's nest will infuriate the insects. Electric hedge clippers, tractors and power mowers should not be used by persons sensitive to insect stings. Vines, which may conceal hives, may have to be removed from the house.

Personal Methods of Prevention.   Perfumes, hair spray, hair tonic, suntan lotion, and many other cosmetics that attract insects should not be used. Floppy clothing in which insects might become caught, bright colors, flowery prints, and black should be avoided. Light colors—white, green, tan and khaki—are thought neither to attract nor to antagonize stinging insects. Any object, whether touched, sat on, or brushed against, should be inspected for the presence of Hymenoptera. Children should be taught not to pick up a wagon handle or other toy without first looking to see that no insect has alighted on it. Aimless kicking of a dead log, so often done by boys on hikes, sends vibrations through the ground disturbing nearby yellow jackets. Public trash baskets, such as those in state parks, should be avoided.

An insecticide bomb, kept in the glove box of the car, can be used should a stray insect fly in. Shoes should be worn at all times when outdoors except on a hard, sandy beach. (There is one type of wasp that spends most of its life on dune grass.) Sandals are not considered adequate protection, but sneakers are.

Immediate Removal of the Stinger. Among the Hymenoptera, the honeybee alone leaves her stinger (with venom sac attached) in the victim. Since it takes two to three minutes for the venom sac to inject all the venom, instant removal of the stinger and sac will prevent many of the harmful effects of the venom. This can be done with one swift scrape of the fingernail. The sac should not be picked up between the thumb and forefinger because this maneuver merely squeezes in more venom. The hornets, wasps and yellow jackets, which do not lose their stinger, should be brushed off promptly.

Nests and Their Removal. Although some types of Hymenoptera are more combative than others, every type will sting readily if its hive is molested. For this reason, it is important to destroy hives about the home. This should never be done by, or in the presence of, someone allergic to Hymenoptera. Inspection of the premises at weekly intervals during the spring and summer will enable detection of hives. *Wasps* construct open-comb nests under eaves, in carports, behind shutters, in shrubs, and woodpiles; in fact, in almost any protected place. *Yellow jackets* build in the ground, emerging through small holes during the day and returning at dusk. *Hornets* build gray pyriform or football-shaped hives, usually in shrubs or trees, often high or far out on a branch. *Honeybees,* resting in a hollow tree, may nest in areas that are out of reach.

Bites and Bite-Related Infections

LEONARD C. MARCUS, V.M.D., M.D.

Treatment of bites by humans or lower animals involves surgical and medical considerations. The surgical issues involve cleaning and closing the wound. The major medical issues involve the prophylactic and therapeutic

use of antibiotics and prophylactic immunization for tetanus and rabies. Most infections
transmitted by bites can be prevented by
proper early treatment and most can be cured
if appropriate treatment is given.

The care of the bite wound, per se, is basically the same as for any comparable trauma
from a contaminated source. First, the wound
should be thoroughly cleaned and any nonviable tissue removed by debridement. Because
of their antiviral activity, quaternary ammonia
compounds such as 1:100 benzalkonium
chloride (Zephiran) are used if there was possible exposure to rabies. Soap, which neutralizes quaternary ammonia compounds, is
thoroughly rinsed from the wound before the
latter are applied. Care is taken to avoid contamination of quaternary ammonia compounds, and it is best if they are kept in small
sterile containers since they can support the
growth of *Pseudomonas aeruginosa*.

After cleansing and debridement, large
deep bite wounds can be sutured to promote
cosmetic healing. Primary closure of dirty
wounds will favor infection, however, especially in the case of human, monkey or cat
bites. Deep puncture wounds and severe crush
injuries which cannot be adequately cleaned
and debrided should be left unsutured in
order to heal by drainage and second intention. Many surgeons recommend that all bites
inflicted by humans be left unsutured because
of the probability of local infection. If infection
develops in a wound that was sutured, the sutures must be removed to permit adequate
drainage. Although it is often recommended
that potentially rabid bite wounds not be sutured, I know of no definitive study proving
that primary closure promotes the likelihood
of rabies developing. If the wound is potentially disfiguring or disabling, the patient
should be referred to a plastic surgeon, hand
surgeon or other appropriate qualified surgeon for care.

Tetanus prophylaxis should be given for
bites. If the child completed tetanus immunization and received the last tetanus booster
within the previous five years, no booster is
needed. If the child had adequate tetanus immunization 5 to 10 years previously, a single
booster of tetanus toxoid should be given. If
the child never had proper primary immunization or more than 10 years have elapsed since
the last dose of tetanus toxoid, then separate
injections of tetanus toxoid and tetanus immune globulin, human origin, should be given.

Prophylactic immunization for rabies is instituted immediately if the biting animal is
known or is reasonably suspected of being

rabid. Rabies immune globulin of human origin (Hyperab) is given using 20 I.U./kg. Half
the globulin is used to infiltrate the wound
prior to suturing and half is given intramuscularly. Despite its high cost this human globulin
is greatly preferred over equine origin globulin
because of the high incidence of serum sickness with the latter product. At the same time,
a series of injections with duck embryo rabies
vaccine (DEV) is started, either as 21 daily
doses or 14 doses in the first seven days (either
as two separate injections or a double dose
daily) and then seven daily doses. Two booster
doses of DEV should be given on the 10th and
20th day after completing the primary series.
DEV is administered subcutaneously at separate sites, such as on the abdomen, using alternate sites each day.

Local erythema, induration and pain at
the site of DEV injection commonly occur,
usually after the first week of injections. Fever,
malaise, drowsiness and dizziness occur with
some frequency, but severe neurologic reactions are rare. Allergic reactions such as urticaria, bronchospasm and anaphylaxis have
been reported. Side effects are treated with antihistamines and epinephrine. Rarely will they
be severe enough to mandate cessation of
treatment.

The decision to initiate prophylactic
treatment for rabies when the biting animal is
not available for examination or the nature of
the exposure is not certain is problematical and
must be based on probability of risk and levels
of apprehension on the part of the physician,
patient and family versus risks and discomfort
of therapy. Once decision is made to treat, both
serum and vaccine should be given. If there is
valid reason to institute any prophylactic
treatment, then half-way measures should not
be used. If the biting animal was missing initially, but is found and proved nonrabid during the course of treatment, then active immunization should cease.

A human diploid cell vaccine for rabies
has been developed which offers great promise
in that it stimulates protective antirabies antibody production, but has few side effects. At
the time of this writing, it is not commercially
available in the United States.

Because bite wounds can be presumed to
be contaminated with bacteria, prophylactic
treatment with antibiotics, if there is more than
superficial tissue injury, is justifiable. It is helpful to culture the wound prior to antibiotic
treatment, and this should be done without fail
if infection develops despite antibiotic
prophylaxis.

The majority of bacterial pathogens associated with animal bites are sensitive to penicillin in standard doses; for example, 125 to 250 mg. of phenoxymethyl penicillin orally, four times a day for a week, should prevent most infections. However, penicillin-resistant *Staphylococcus aureus* infections can result from bite wounds, especially those of human origin. Therefore a penicillinase-resistant drug such as sodium cloxacillin or cephalexin monohydrate (Keflex) may be more effective prophylactically than penicillin, especially for human bites. However, considering cost and effectiveness, penicillin probably still is the prophylactic antibiotic of choice for animal bites.

Patients who are allergic to penicillin can be treated with a cephalosporin if they are not also allergic to this group of drugs. (Many patients allergic to penicillin have cross sensitivity to cephalosporins). Other alternative drugs for penicillin-sensitive patients are the tetracyclines or erythromycin.

A Gram stain of any exudate in the wound can provide information leading to rational selection of an antibiotic while awaiting culture and sensitivity reports. The empirical choice of prophylactic agents outlined above is appropriate when the patient is presented immediately after the bite, before there is an exudate.

If infection develops while using penicillin, if the pus is not foul-smelling and if gram-positive cocci in clumps are seen, then a penicillinase-resistant drug (such as cloxacillin or cephalosporin) is used. If the pus has no foul odor and gram-negative rods are present, either ampicillin or amoxacillin alone or a cephalosporin and/or an aminoglycoside (such as gentamicin) should be prescribed. If there is crepitation in the wound and a foul odor, there may be anaerobic infection: gram-negative rods may indicate *Bacteroides* infection; gram-positive rods with spores, *Clostridium* spp.; and gram-positive cocci in chains, anaerobic streptococci. Anaerobic infections can be treated with clindamycin or high doses of penicillin while awaiting sensitivity studies.

Patients with severe septic complications such as septicemia, endocarditis, visceral abscesses, septic arthritis or osteomyelitis should be hospitalized, have blood cultures taken and be treated with appropriate parenteral antibiotics.

Pasteurella multocida is a pathogen commonly associated with cat bites and, somewhat less frequently, with dog or other animal bites. Besides local infection of soft tissues, this organism can produce all the septic complications necessitating hospitalization listed above. Although it is a gram-negative rod,

most strains are sensitive to penicillin. The tetracyclines are usually suitable as alternative drugs.

The closely related *Pasteurella pneumotropica* has been isolated from two cases of dog bite (including one person who died with systemic infection) and one cat bite. The tetracyclines are usually effective treatment.

There are certain gram-negative rods, frequently isolated from dogs' mouhs and occasionally from infections resulting from dog bite, not yet classified by genus and species, designated IIj and EF-4. Both of these organisms are sensitive to ampicillin, tetracycline and chloramphenicol. Most strains of IIj are sensitive to penicillin, but most isolates of EF-4 are penicillin-resistant.

Burn Therapy

CHARLES A. PECK, Jr., M.D.,
Lt. Col., M.C., U.S.A.

Thermal injuries may be broadly categorized into minor or major injuries. Patients with minor burns, that is, burns of partial thickness injury involving 10 per cent or less of the total body surface or small full-thickness burns, may be treated as outpatients. This is not a broad nor all encompassing rule and judgment must be exercised, taking into consideration the patient's age, the location of the burn, the circumstances under which the injury was incurred and any associated injuries or disease. If there is any reason to suspect abuse, if the child is less than two years of age, or if for any reason the physician would consider hospitalization, the child should be hospitalized.

MINOR BURNS

These burns usually involve the extremities, but may be isolated to a small truncal burn. The burn wound is cleansed with warm saline and any blebs are debrided. If analgesic is needed, meperidine hydrochloride, 0.5 mg./lb., is given intramuscularly. The wound is then covered with fine mesh gauze in a single layer, and 4 by 4 gauze sponges are applied. It is then wrapped with a gauze dressing, being sure to anchor the dressing well so it will not slide. The patient is given tetanus toxoid prophylaxis. Neither systemic nor topical an-

The opinion or assertions contained herein are the private views of the author and are not to be construed as official or as reflecting the views of the Department of the Army or the Department of Defense.

tibiotics are used and the patient is seen in five to seven days.

At this time, the burn is re-inspected by taking the dressing off layer by layer down to the fine mesh gauze. The fine mesh gauze is left in place and the burn wound inspected through it. If the burn was a superficial partial-thickness burn, the area will already have begun to dry, with areas of crusting around the fine mesh gauze. If it appears that this is the case, and there are no depressions or pockets of fluid collection, 4 by 4 gauze sponges and a gauze wrap are reapplied. If there are areas of deeper partial thickness, small pockets of fluid material will have appeared. These areas of the fine mesh gauze are removed, and a nonadherent impregnated fine mesh gauze is applied along with 4 by 4 sponges and a gauze wrap. The parents are instructed to change the dressing twice daily using clean, not necessarily sterile, techniques, and soaking the burn area for one-half hour prior to changing the dressing to facilitate removal and promote drainage. The dressing is then reapplied in the manner previously described. The parents are instructed to bring the child to clinic in five to seven days.

On this visit, superficial partial-thickness burns are usually healed. The fine mesh gauze is gently separated, and the patient and parents are instructed to protect the area against sunlight and minor trauma. Usually lanolin or cocoa butter is prescribed, to be applied to the area twice daily for two weeks.

The deep partial-thickness burn is reexamined in the same manner. At this stage, reepithelization has begun. Any devitalized tissue is removed sharply, the dressing reapplied and soaks continued for another week. At 17 to 21 days, most of the wound has reepithelized. In areas that have not healed, further debridement is undertaken, and soaks are continued twice daily until healing occurs. In deep partial-thickness burns over joint surfaces, because of scarring and possible contracture, vigorous physiotherapy is taught early in the course of treatment, usually to coincide with the soaks. Again, lanolin or cocoa butter is applied to the healed surface. In special areas such as the neck, padded neck collars may be used early in the course of treatment to prevent contracture.

In almost all instances, children less than two or three years with burns of the hands, face and neck or perineum are treated in the hospital. Full-thickness burns involving areas of two to three inches or greater in small children are also treated in the hospital. Bigger children with full-thickness burns of two to three inches may be treated as outpatients, with separation of the eschar at about three weeks and autografting as an outpatient. Any children who appear to be developing burn wound sepsis as manifested by fever, erythema around the burn wound and unhealthy-appearing granulation tissue are hospitalized. The wound is cultured, debrided and kept open, and silver sulfadiazine is applied. The majority of burns in bigger children may be treated on an outpatient basis; however, larger burns, burns of critical areas and burns in infants should be treated in the hospital.

MAJOR BURNS

Burns of 10 per cent or more of the total body surface are major burns and should, depending on severity of the burn and size of the child, be treated in the hospital. Burns of 25 per cent or more of total body surface should be treated at a burn center. Treatment of major burns may be divided into three areas: first aid, resuscitation and burn wound care.

First Aid. The main goals in first aid treatment are maintenance of an adequate airway, arrest of any external hemorrhage by pressure, splinting of fractures and care of the burn to ease pain and keep the burn wound clean. After assessment, if the burn wound is the major problem, a clean sheet or blanket is placed over the patient. I do not believe ice packs should be applied to the wound unless this can be done immediately, which is usually not the case. Ointments or salves should not be placed on the burn. If the patient is in shock or if transport time is significant (over one-half hour), an intravenous infusion of normal saline or lactated Ringer's solution is started. It is preferable that a plastic catheter be used in an area free of burns. The legs, if at all possible, should not be used.

If transport time to the primary treatment facility is short, no narcotics should be administered. If transport time will be long, medication needed to relieve pain should be given intravenously. Coverage of the burn and assurance of the patient help to allay apprehension and pain. Tetanus toxoid prophylaxis should be given if transport time is long. The patient should not be given anything by mouth until evaluation and triage at the primary treatment center.

After arrival at the hospital, determination is made early in the course as to whether the facility is to be the definitive treatment center or whether the child should receive further care at a burn center. Burns of greater than 25 per cent of total body surface and significant burns of the airway, hands and perineal area should be treated at a burn center. Burns of the incineration type involving 90 per cent or greater of the total body surface, patients with multiple injuries of which the burn is not the primary injury, lack of trained personnel to transport the patient, and inability to obtain an adequate vehicle for transportation are all factors which preclude further transport of the patient. If further transport is believed necessary, it should be done early in the post-burn period.

Treatment prior to transport is a continuation of first aid, that is, ensuring that there is an adequate airway, ensuring proper intravenous infusion into a nonburned area, and insertion of a Foley catheter and nasogastric tube. The patient should be normotensive and normothermic, and results of an ECG and chest film should be normal. Tetanus prophylaxis is administered if not previously done. The burn wounds, if the time of transport is greater than one-half hour, should be gently washed with saline, and a bulky dressing of gauze applied. Washing should not be vigorous, and debridement should not be attempted.

All treatment should be placed on a permanent record which should accompany the patient. A telephone call should be placed to the burn center and the accepting physician so that a smooth transition and continuity of care can be established.

Resuscitation of Major Burns. Fluid resuscitation should be undertaken early in the therapy to prevent hypovolemic shock. A rough estimation of the total fluid requirement during the first 24 hours of resuscitation should be made; I have used Ringer's lactate solution, 3 ml./kg. of body weight times the total per cent of body surface burned, as a gauge for the total requirements for the first 24 hours of therapy. This is altered to ensure a urinary output of 1 to 2 ml./kg./hour and a central venous pressure of about five to six. One-half of the total estimate is given in the first eight hours, the other half divided over the next 16 hours. This, as with all formulas, is only a gauge and the patient should be checked frequently to ascertain the adequacy of fluid replacement. This would include evaluation of serum electrolytes, osmolality, hemogram and daily weights.

Unless there is concomitant blood loss from associated injuries, colloid is not given in the first 24 hours of treatment, but is given as needed during ensuing fluid replacement in the next 24 hours. During this period, only maintenance fluid is given in addition to the plasma requirements. I give albumin at the rate of 1 gm./kg./24 hour period. Usually by 48

to 72 hours, oral replacement may be undertaken and maintenance fluids are continued with colloid replacement as needed until full oral alimentation is achieved.

Care of the Burn Wound. Since its availability, we have been using silver sulfadiazine topical antibiotic and open wound care for major burns. The burn is cleansed with a mild soap and debrided of loose blebs and material. The patient is then placed in bed on clean sheets, and silver sulfadiazine is placed on the burn wound. The gloved hand is used to spread the antibiotic over all the burn surface, about one-quarter inch in thickness. A cradle is placed over the body and heat lamps are used as necessary to maintain normothermia. The cream is washed off the surface twice daily using hydrotherapy, which also permits debridement of loose tissue. Physiotherapy is done especially in areas where the burn involves joint surfaces. Following hydrotherapy, the cream is reapplied. Early in the post-burn period, the cream has a tendency to slide off the wound; in such areas the cream is reapplied as needed. Cultures of the burn surface and the hydrotherapy unit are performed three to four times a week, and areas of full-thickness injury are biopsied and cultured if burn wound sepsis is suspected.

Areas of partial-thickness and full-thickness injury become more apparent during the course of therapy. After two to three weeks, areas with epithelial islands from skin appendages will reepithelize. The area of eschar of full-thickness burns can be separated at about three weeks, and if the underlying surface is clean, autologous skin grafting performed. In larger burns, where there is limited supply of autologous skin, porcine heterograft is applied to the granulating surface, while a portion of the area is covered with autograft which has been meshed. The porcine heterograft is changed every 48 to 72 hours or more frequently to prevent build-up of serum and possible infection. When the donor area is again ready, autologous graft may be reharvested and another area covered.

In selected instances involving less than 10 per cent of total body surface, full-thickness areas are excised and primarily grafted after preparation of the bed, three to four days with porcine heterograft.

SPECIAL CONSIDERATIONS

Respiratory Burns Children with respiratory burns need special attention. They require a mist humidifier, special nasotracheal suctioning, and close monitoring of arterial blood gases. If secretions and sloughed tissue cannot be adequately removed with suctioning, repeated bronchoscopy may be necessary. Progression of the respiratory burn, if severe, may require tracheostomy and usually requires assisted ventilation with a respirator.

Burn Wound Sepsis. This occurs as a complication of burn wound treatment. Below the eschar of full-thickness burns, there develops a significant collection of bacteria which begin to invade the surrounding normal tissue resulting in fever, tachycardia and sepsis. In suspected instances, the burn wound is cultured on the surface and in the depths by biopsy, areas of purulent material are unroofed, and the patient is begun on specific antibiotics depending on the Gram stain and ultimately the culture. Unfortunately, many times either fungal or viral opportunistic organisms for which there are few effective antimicrobials are the causative agents.

Nutritional Factors. One of the basic requirements of a burn patient is increased caloric need. Children are begun on oral alimentation early in the course of burn therapy. If oral alimentation is not possible because of ileus or because the patient will not or cannot cooperate, parenteral hyperalimentation is instituted to ensure positive nitrogen balance and to ensure good wound healing.

ESCHAROTOMY AND FASCIOTOMY

Circumferential full-thickness injuries, especially of the extremities, act as constricting bands and may cause vascular compromise of the distal portion of the extremity. In such instances, escharotomy and release of the band will usually restore circulation. Also, full-thickness burns of the anterior and posterior chest wall may cause restriction of chest wall excursion. This may be relieved by incision of the eschar laterally and inferiorly like a shield to permit better excursion.

COMPLICATIONS

There are multiple complications which may occur throughout the course of therapy. In the early period, the concern is with shock and acute renal failure. This is usually due to inadequate fluid resuscitation. Myocardial infarction and inhalation injury can also occur. Gastrointestinal complications include paralytic ileus, upper gastrointestinal bleeding, pancreatitis, acalculous cholecystitis and duodenal obstruction. Burn wound sepsis has been discussed. Complications of suppurative thrombophlebitis, contractures and pyarthrosis can also occur.

All these complications are life-threatening, especially in debilitated burn patients. Prevention of such problems is the key, but this is not always possible. For that reason, we have made little progress in the salvage of patients with burns of greater than 60 to 70 per cent of total body surface.

CONCLUSION

Thermal injury is one of the most stressful of injuries to the body. The mortality rates for burns of less than 40 per cent of total body surface has been greatly reduced. The mortality rate of those patients with burns of 40 to 60 per cent of total body surface is improving, but in those patients with burns of 75 per cent or greater of total body surface injury, the mortality rate has been altered little.

Near-Drowning (Nonfatal Submersion)

SAMUEL T. GIAMMONA, M.D.

Death by drowning, one of the major causes of childhood mortality, is responsible for 10 per cent of all accidental deaths in the United States, with children being the chief victims (40 per cent under age 4). "Near-drowning" implies recovery, but to prevent a near-drowning accident from becoming a mortality requires an understanding of the pathophysiology of drowning and a plan of therapy. Drowning results in acute asphyxia because laryngospasm occurs when fluid is inhaled into the larynx; 10 to 15 per cent of drowning victims have irreversible laryngospasm without fluid aspiration. Three or four minutes later, laryngeal relaxation allows fluid aspiration (with contained material) into the lungs, which causes ventilation and perfusion inequalities resulting in severe hypoxia and acidosis.

At the site of the accident, the first rescuer should immediately start artificial ventilation which will allow for increased oxygenation. No time should be wasted trying uselessly to remove water from the lung. Within 3 minutes after total obstruction of the airway, arterial oxygen tensions will fall below 15 mm. Hg, a level incompatible with brain cell survival if prolonged beyond 6 to 9 minutes. Mouth-to-mouth resuscitation is the preferred mode of ventilation unless a self-inflating mechanical ventilation bag (Ambu) or hand-operated oxygen valve is immediately available to a trained individual.

When foreign material is visible at the mouth or in the pharynx, turn the patient's head to the side and clean the mouth and pharynx out with fingers, handkerchief or suction (if available). Approach the patient from the side and support the upper airway by inserting the thumb between the teeth, grasping the mandible and pulling it upward forcefully. The head should be tilted at the neck with only moderate extension so as not to buckle the cervical inlet. Occlude the patient's nose if he is a large child, then take a deep breath, place the mouth firmly over the patient's mouth, and blow forcefully (gently in smaller child) into the open mouth (or mouth and nose of infant) watching for the chest to rise. As soon as the chest rises, remove the mouth from the patient and permit him to exhale passively by elastic recoil of the lungs and chest wall. The inflations are to be continued at a rate of 20 per minute for older children or adults and 30 to 40 times a minute for infants. If the chest fails to rise properly, or one hears excessive rumbling in the stomach, improve support of the jaw, improve mouth contact to patient's nose and mouth, and utilize a greater volume and force for the next inflation.

Mouth-to-mouth resuscitation (which provides an oxygen concentration of 15 to 18 per cent) should be continued until spontaneous breathing ensues or until the victim is transported to an emergency facility regardless of the status of the patient. After artificial ventilation has been secured, maintenance of effective circulation should be attempted. External cardiac massage may be given by trained personnel. If no heart beat is noted, closed chest cardiac massage should immediately be started to synchronize (3 breaths per 15 heart beats) with the continued ventilation. An electrocardiogram should be obtained as soon as possible to determine whether electrical defibrillation is required and if arrhythmias are present. Heat loss may be extensive following the submersion accident, and it is vital that hypothermia be corrected by use of warm blankets at the scene and by the use of warming mattress in the hospital setting. Hypothermia with peripheral vasoconstriction will intensify and lengthen the metabolic acidosis in the presence of hypoxia.

All children, regardless of the duration of submersion and degree of hypoxia, should be hospitalized for 24 hours and all necessary resuscitative measures providing maximal oxygenation should be continued until documentation of adequate arterial oxygenation is obtained. At the hospital, if spontaneous breathing has started, supplemental oxygen by mask or tent for 12 to 24 hours may be all that is required as long as vital signs remain stable and normal, all laboratory data including arterial blood gases are within accepted normal range, chest x-ray is unremarkable, ventilation is adequate, and the electrocardiogram is normal.

For the more severely affected victim, one must restore normal arterial blood gases and acid base levels by effective ventilation, oxygenation and use of appropriate electrolytes and fluids. The airway should immediately be examined to determine if suction and artificial airway insertion are needed to maintain airway patency. On occasion, there may be need to perform laryngoscopy or bronchoscopy to remove foreign material such as sand, twigs, or debris contained in aspirated material. Nasogastric aspiration of gastric contents should be carried out to reduce the possibility of vomiting.

Oxygen to restore arterial blood gases to normal (utilizing 100 per cent oxygen until blood arterial gas studies indicate need for less oxygen to maintain adequate arterial oxygen tensions) may be administered by mask, by placement of nasotracheal or endotracheal tube, by intermittent positive pressure ventilation or by complete mechanical volume-controlled ventilation. The mode used may vary in each case. Active measures to reinflate atelectatic lung include clapping, vibration and postural drainage in addition to hyperinflation with positive pressure breathing 15 minutes per hour utilizing a pressure of 25 to 40 cm. of water. Oxygen should be continued at 5 to 15 liters/min. (40 to 100 per cent oxygen) as needed. If respiratory failure is present, mechanical ventilation should be started with a volume respirator giving 1½ to 2 times estimated tidal volumes. Dead space tubing may be added to maintain adequate P_{CO_2} levels. If inadequate oxygenation of arterial blood continues with use of a volume respirator and 100 per cent oxygen, positive end-expiratory pressure (PEEP) will often be a useful maneuver to prevent alveolar collapse. If hypovolemia or shock is present, PEEP may worsen the circulatory status unless blood or colloid is infused initially to restore circulatory blood volume. Succinylcholine (1 to 2 ml. intravenously) or curare may be required to synchronize the patient with the ventilator. All ventilatory and oxygenation procedures should be continued as long as indicated by abnormal arterial blood gases.

If bronchospasm is noted by wheezing and prolapsed expiration, 0.5 ml. of 1:200 isoproterenol diluted in 4.5 ml. of isotonic saline can be given by aerosal every 1 to 4 hours as necessary. Toxicity can be judged by increase or changes in cardiac rate and requires constant cardiac monitoring. Steroids may be necessary to relieve bronchospasm (2 to 5 mg./kg. of prednisone or its equivalent).

More than 80 per cent of victims of nonfatal submersion will demonstrate some radiologic evidence of pulmonary infiltrates associated with leukocytosis and fever, which indicate the body's reaction to the fluid and debris aspirated. These findings do not indicate infection and are best treated by good postural drainage with vibrating and clapping of chest by competent personnel. If fever should recur after 48 hours or blood and sputum cultures indicate infection, appropriate antibiotic therapy is necessary. Prophylactic use of antibiotics to prevent infection has never been documented to be useful in these patients. The use of steroids to decrease inflammatory reaction likewise has not proved useful except in those children with severe bronchospasm.

Although much has been written about the important difference in the body's reaction to the type of fluid aspirated (fresh water versus salt water), it is a clinical fact that adjustments are rapidly made by the body once the victim is taken out of the water, so that by the time the patient arrives at a hospital, the fluid and electrolyte changes are usually corrected, or there are minimal changes in osmolality of the body fluids. No difference is recommended in initial plans for fluid and electrolyte management. Initial therapy should be 10 to 20 ml./kg. of Ringer's lactate. After blood studies are obtained, calculated maintenance fluids at two-thirds normal amounts (80 ml./100 calories metabolized) can be given over the next 24 hours to minimize cerebral edema. The severity and duration of fluid and electrolyte abnormalities have no direct relationship to type of fluid aspirated and must be judged individually on every patient because of the variation produced by the volume aspirated and the delay in correction induced by cardiovascular, pulmonary, or cerebral dysfunction. Blood analysis for hemoglobin, hematocrit, blood electrolytes, total protein, calcium, and blood sugar should be obtained in addition to arterial blood gases.

A major problem in these patients is arrhythmia induced by a combination of factors—hypoxia, hypothermia, metabolic acidosis—which may develop and/or persist as therapy is in progress because of cardiac intracellular trauma or metabolic imbalance which will persist even though arterial blood gases are returning to normal. Therefore constant electrocardiogram monitoring is mandatory. Bradycardia should be specifically treated. If there is no ventricular arrhythmia, isoproterenol (Isuprel) can be given intravenously, starting at 0.1 μg./kg./min., and titrating dosage until there is a desired response. Isuprel mixture is made by diluting 0.2 mg. (stock 0.2 mg./ml. 1:5000) in 50 cc. of 5 per cent dextrose in water or Ringer's lactate (0.004 mg./ml. final concentration). If ventricular arrhythmia is present, atropine sulfate can be given intravenously at 0.01 mg./kg.

If cardiovascular collapse and shock are present, immediate resuscitation with Ringer's lactate (20 ml./kg. in ½ hour), followed by plasma infusion in sea water drowning or whole blood infusion in fresh water drowning, is rational therapy, but each patient's fluid needs must be individually evaluated and treated. If severe metabolic acidosis is present, judicious use of bicarbonates may be warranted (½ the base deficit × weight in kg. × 0.3 = mEq. of sodium bicarbonate or approximately 2.5 mEq./kg.), which may be repeated in an hour or two if needed. Seizures may occur during resuscitation and indicate hypoxic damage or impending cerebral edema. Diazepam (Valium),* 0.3 mg./kg. intravenously, is the preferred drug to stop seizures, but requires close monitoring, as it may precipitate respiratory arrest.

Steroids may be given to combat cerebral edema: 2 to 10 mg./kg. of prednisone or its equivalent; dexamethasone (Decadron) currently is the preferred drug for therapy. The use of deep hypothermia with a single dose of phenobarbital, 10 to 20 mg./kg. or greater, or sodium pentobarbital (Nembutal), 10 to 20 mg./kg., monitored by blood levels, plus repeated high dosage of mannitol,† 1.5 gm./kg., or barbiturates, 2 to 4 mg./kg. every 2 hours intravenously, to lower cerebrospinal fluid pressure is currently being tried for relief of cerebral edema in selected cases at some medical centers. It is now possible to monitor cerebrospinal fluid directly by insertion of a subdural or cerebral ventricular catheter to more precisely regulate dosage of drugs needed to control cerebral edema. The additive effect of barbiturates and hypothermia may eliminate neurological function sufficiently, however, to prevent careful bedside evaluations. These extreme measures must only be used if the physician and facilities allow meticulous, continuous monitoring of the patient. It remains to be

---

*Manufacturer's precaution: The safety and efficacy of injectable diazepam in the neonate have not been established.

†Manufacturer's precaution: Dosage requirement of mannitol for patients 12 years and under has not been established.

demonstrated if this therapy would be beneficial to near-drowning accident victims.

All therapy should be continued for 24 to 72 hours and then gradual reduction in ventilation, oxygenation, circulatory and cerebral support should be attempted until the child's stable normal state is reached. Fortunately, most children without extensive cerebral necrosis make a complete and permanent recovery.

The Injured Child

Evaluation and Management

THOMAS S. MORSE, M.D.

Remember that *saving life* comes first. *Begin* by checking ventilation and circulation.

Is the child breathing? If not, breathe for him. Tilt the head well back, clear the oropharynx, and get air into the lungs, first by mouth-to-mouth resuscitation, then oxygen by mask. Only then insert an endotracheal tube. Select its size by picking a tube that will just fit into the child's nostril. Place it deliberately and carefully. Check to see that air moves freely; if not, suction carefully down the tube. Check to see that both sides of the chest move equally. If not, the tube may be down too far into one bronchus; is it obstructing the other?

Check the chest. If there is an open wound, cover it. For pneumothorax, insert a needle into the anterior axillary line on the side which moves least well, followed by a chest tube. For hemothorax, insert a large needle into the posterior axillary line on the side that moves least well, followed by a chest tube.

Remember, oxygen does not cure anything. If the child needs oxygen, *find* and *treat* the *cause*.

Is the heart beating? If not, massage it *as soon as ventilation is started*. Use the heel of the hand over the lower half of the sternum, or the flat surface of two fingers on infants. Ventilation *and* circulation must be accomplished *together*. It does no good to circulate anoxic blood.

Send for help and emergency equipment.

Breathe at about 20 puffs per minute for a school-age child, 30 puffs for a preschool child, 40 for an infant. Switch to oxygen via an endotracheal tube as soon as feasible.

Massage the heart at 60 to 80 beats per minute. Place a board under the back. If ventilation and massage are adequate (and started early enough), a good pulse will be felt in the neck or groin with each massage, dilated pupils will constrict, and peripheral circulation will improve.

Now the crisis is over. A normal heart beat may be restored simply by pumping oxygenated blood through the coronary arteries. Continue ventilation and circulation.

During the first 5 minutes of ventilation and massage, insert a dependable intravenous needle or do a cut-down on a visible vein in an uninjured extremity. Draw blood only for type and crossmatch. Inject 1 ml./pound of undiluted sodium bicarbonate. (This is supplied by either 44 mEq./50 ml. or 1 mEq./ml.) If bleeding is the obvious cause of arrest, pump in 10 ml./pound of Ringer's lactate or plasma. Dilute 1:1000 epinephrine to 1:10,000 and inject 2 ml. intravenously.

If there is no regular beat after 5 minutes of good ventilation and massage, obtain an electrocardiogram if possible. If this shows asystole, dilute 10 per cent calcium chloride to 1 per cent and give 10 ml. intravenously. Continue ventilation and massage for 2 minutes. Repeat 1 ml./pound of undiluted sodium bicarbonate intravenously, followed by 2 ml. of diluted epinephrine and 10 ml. of diluted calcium chloride. If the EKG shows fibrillation, repeat 1 ml./pound of undiluted sodium bicarbonate and prepare to defibrillate. Remember, the fibrillating heart does not pump blood, and anoxic heart muscle cannot be defibrillated; therefore, continue massage to the moment of defibrillation.

Shock the heart once with 150 watt-seconds. Ventilate 20 seconds; then if fibrillation persists, resume massage. After about 2 minutes, repeat 1 ml./pound of undiluted sodium bicarbonate and shock again with a higher current. Isoproterenol may be used instead of epinephrine. It is supplied in 1 ml. ampules containing 0.2 mg. Dilute 1 to 10 and give 1 ml. of diluted isoproterenol in place of 2 ml. of diluted epinephrine. If a regular beat returns but remains weak, support the circulation with intravenous drip containing 2 mg. of isoproterenol in 500 ml. If fibrillation persists or recurs repeatedly, inject 5 ml. of 1 per cent procainamide hydrochloride (3 ml. of 1 per cent lidocaine may be better).

Most cases of cardiac arrest in salvageable injured children are caused by hypoxia and respond promptly to the above routine. If closed chest massage does not produce adequate circulation (palpable pulse, pupil response), decide quickly whether arrest is caused by exsanguination. If it is, pump rapidly 10 ml./pound of O negative low-titer uncrossmatched blood, plasma or Ringer's lactate in addition to that already given. With exsanguination ruled out or treated as above, if circulation by closed massage is still inadequate, do not hesitate to open the chest.

SHOCK

In freshly injured children, shock is *almost always* caused by *blood loss* (except in burn patients). Immediately after injury, shock in injured children is practically never due to closed head injury, sepsis, or heart failure (unless the heart itself has been injured). A child who has bled into shock has lost at least one-quarter of his total blood volume, or *10 ml. per pound.*

The only difference between reversible shock and irreversible shock is *TIME.* Work quickly.

Lay the child flat with his legs elevated. Stop external bleeding, usually by direct pressure over open wounds. Listen with an ear to the chest to be sure the heart is beating. Feel the peripheral pulse. If it is weak and rapid, the extremities are cool and dry, and blood pressure is low or absent, then the child is in shock.

Insert at least one dependable intravenous needle or do a cut-down on a visible vein in an uninjured extremity; have at least one needle in an arm if abdominal injury is suspected. Draw blood for type and crossmatch only; take other samples later. Pump in 10 ml./pound of lactated Ringer's solution, plasma, or saline. Follow with 1 ml./pound of undiluted sodium bicarbonate. If the above treatment has restored blood pressure permanently to normal, probably no blood transfusion will be needed.

If 10 ml./pound restores blood pressure only temporarily, type-specific crossmatched blood will be needed. Meanwhile, give more plasma or lactated Ringer's solution. Look for continuing blood loss under dressings, into soft tissue around major fractures, or into chest or abdomen.

If 10 ml./pound does not bring systolic pressure even to 70, consider using uncrossmatched O negative blood. Until blood is available, *keep on pumping* plasma or lactated Ringer's solution until systolic pressure is at least 70.

As soon as the emergency phase of treatment of shock is completed, insert a nasogastric tube and empty the stomach. Insert an indwelling urethral catheter. The rate of urine output is a useful guide to adequacy of shock treatment; mimimum is roughly 1 ml./5 pounds/hour.

After these steps, it may be helpful to insert a central venous pressure catheter. If the child is hypotensive and the CVP is low or zero, more replacement is needed. If the CVP is high and the child is still hypotensive, check chest for tension pneumothorax or cardiac tamponade. Stop further intravenous fluid until a cause for the elevated CVP is found, either in patient or equipment. (Be sure to stop assisting ventilation momentarily while measuring CVP.)

If ventilation is adequate and the heart is beating, the most common treatable cause of continued hypotension is that you *still* have not given enough replacement. The other treatable cause is that a major vessel is bleeding internally. The untreatable cause is that the child got too little replacement too late.

The evaluation and management of every injured child must start in the same way and must proceed to this point in the same orderly fashion if life is not to be lost by squandering the few precious moments during which it can be saved by restoring ventilation and circulation. Beyond this point, the order in which the regions of the body are evaluated and treated will vary with the nature of the injury. These body regions are discussed below in a sequence which roughly parallels the descending order of urgency with which the usual injuries of children found therein must be managed.

EVALUATION

Approach every injured child with the attitude that he may have *more than one injury.* Do not let obvious surface wounds distract you from a thorough search for intra-abdominal injuries. Most life-threatening injuries which are missed on initial evaluation of an injured child are in the abdomen. The usual ones are rupture of the spleen or liver, which produces hidden bleeding, or rupture of the intestine, producing peritonitis. Often more than one organ is injured. Blood or intestinal contents in the peritoneal cavity produce pain, tenderness and spasm. If these are present initially, the following procedures are carried out:

(1) Insert a nasogastric tube, check the aspirate for blood, and connect to intermittent suction; (2) measure and record the abdominal girth; with the tube working, increasing girth suggests bleeding; (3) crossmatch whole blood, at least 20 ml./pound; (4) in the absence of head injury, give sodium pentobarbital or secobarbital intramuscularly, 2 mg./pound. This will enable a tense, frightened child to relax in 20 to 30 minutes but will not mask true tenderness. If tenderness persists, explore the abdomen.

Remember: a small perforation of the intestine or a small tear in the spleen may not produce symptoms until hours after injury. *Check* and *check again.*

ABDOMINAL X-RAYS. Obtain these as soon as initial evaluation and stabilization are completed. Take posteroanterior chest, flat and upright, or decubitus films of the abdomen. Check for masses, evidence of free air or fluid, fractures and the position of the nasogastric tube. Small amounts of free air are best seen under the diaphragm on the *chest* film.

SERUM AMYLASE. This is elevated in many children with blunt abdominal injury. Mild elevation is usually insignificant and returns to normal in 3 or 4 days. Elevation above four times the normal level may point to a pancreatic injury or to perforation of the duodenum or jejunum with leak of digestive juices into the peritoneum. Do not let an elevated amylase level deter you from exploring a tender abdomen. More than the pancreas may be injured.

ABDOMINAL PARACENTESIS. This is not done in a child who clearly needs an operation, nor is it indicated in lucid, oriented children with no abdominal tenderness. It is useful, when positive, in doubtful cases, such as in children with head injuries that make evaluation of abdominal findings impossible, and also in children with pelvic fractures, rib fractures or hematuria suggesting renal injuries. These children have an obvious cause of abdominal tenderness, but may have an intra-abdominal injury as well.

Use a plastic percutaneous intravenous catheter. Tap midway between the umbilicus and the midaxillary line, first on the right side and then on the left side. If there is no blood, leave the catheter in place on the left side, infuse normal saline, 10 ml./pound, and allow the fluid to run back out. This will increase the accuracy of abdominal paracentesis from about 70 per cent to about 90 per cent.

INTRAVENOUS PYELOGRAPHY. Every child with hematuria (any red cells at all in the urine) after an injury should be studied by pyelography. If the child has an indwelling urinary catheter, clamp it before the study begins. The best study is the infusion pyelogram. Mix sodium diatrizoate (Hypaque), 1 ml./pound, with an equal amount of saline and infuse rapidly—all within 3 to 4 minutes. Expose the first film just as the last of the contrast material is administered, then take exposures at 5, 10, 20 and 30 minutes, including a lateral at 30 minutes. For interpretation see Kidney, below.

CYSTOGRAPHY. Injection of contrast material via the urinary catheter into the bladder is not necessary if infusion pyelography is done as above.

RADIOACTIVE ISOTOPE SCANS. These may be very helpful on occasion, particularly if the infusion pyelogram shows no function at all on the injured side. (See Kidney, below.)

SELECTIVE ARTERIOGRAPHY. In some centers, arteriography is being extensively used to evaluate kidney, liver and spleen injuries. The difficulty of performing selective arteriography on small children, and the satisfactory results of simpler diagnostic methods, limit practical application to unusual cases.

ABDOMEN

BLOOD LOSS. Unrecognized bleeding is the most common cause of preventable death in abdominal injury. Frequently, an obvious area of blood loss, such as a femoral fracture, is erroneously assumed to be the only area of blood loss. Injured children should not be given blood by slow intravenous drip, because this makes the detection of hidden bleeding very difficult. If blood is to be given, it should be given rapidly in increments equivalent to one-eighth or one-fourth of the blood volume —5 or 10 ml./pound. Each increment is followed by a period of observation, during which changes in pulse rate, blood pressure and hematocrit suggesting blood loss are much easier to interpret than if administration and loss of blood are going on simultaneously.

A child who is in shock following an injury has lost at least 10 ml. of blood per pound of body weight. This amount may be pumped in as fast as it can be without fear of overloading. If this amount restores the blood pressure *permanently* to normal, no further transfusion is needed. If the blood pressure returns to normal and then slips away again, give the same amount rapidly again while making plans to handle the continuing bleeding. If 10 ml./pound of whole blood does not restore the blood pressure even momentarily to normal an operation to stop major hemorrhage is usually necessary. Additional blood should be given at once.

SPLEEN. Emergency splenectomy is the traditional treatment for traumatic rupture of the spleen. The mortality following splenectomy is extremely low. Most early deaths in children with splenic rupture result from injuries to other organs, delay in diagnosis, or inappropriate safeguards to prevent hemorrhagic shock during transport.

Recently there has been a growing appreciation that removing the spleen reduces a child's resistance to infections. While this is particularly true in the first few years of life, deaths from overwhelming sepsis have been reported weeks or months following splenectomy performed at any age. This concern has prompted several centers to study the merits of nonoperative treatment or of "conservative" operations designed to save all or part of the injured spleen. The roles of angiography and radioactive spleen scanning in helping to select patients for these lesser operations or for nonoperative treatment also are being studied. It is too early to conclude from these studies that any mode of "conservative" therapy is safer than prompt, total splenectomy.

LIVER.   Not all liver injuries require operation, but laparotomy carries little risk and should not be withheld if bleeding persists. Hematomas are evacuated, devitalized liver tissue is removed, and bleeding is controlled. Large lacerations are sutured; small ones are left alone. The peritoneal cavity is frequently drained, but common duct drainage by T-tube is usually *not* advisable.

STOMACH.   Mortality is directly related to delay in diagnosis and treatment. Careful cleaning of the peritoneal cavity, use of systemic antibiotics, and simple suture of the perforation give surprisingly good results if done promptly. The usual mistake at operation is failure to look for and repair a second area of gastric perforation which is frequently present on the posterior gastric wall or lesser curvature.

DUODENUM.   Small blow-outs are easily closed. Large ones may tax judgment. Pancreatoduodenectomy may occasionally be necessary, but usually a simpler procedure suffices.

SMALL INTESTINE.   Perforations are usually small and easily closed. These are the usual cause of persistent peritoneal irritation and smoldering leukocytosis and fever in a child whose abdomen does not contain blood. They are frequently multiple, and those at the margin of the mesentery are easily overlooked. Look carefully on *both sides*.

AVULSION OF MESENTERY.   Persistent localized ileus with moderate tenderness will be present, and often paracentesis suggests a small amount of intraperitoneal blood. The bowel will usually remain intact for about 72 hours, even if completely devascularized, so early evidence of perforation is not usually found. Resection and anastomosis before perforation give good results.

COLON.   Perforation of the colon causes the highest rate of mortality and morbidity of all intestinal injuries. Suture only very recent perforations or those distal to a colostomy. Exteriorize most colon perforations.

RETROPERITONEAL HEMATOMA.   The pendulum is swinging toward exploration of retroperitoneal hematomas, especially those near the renal vessels, pancreas and duodenum. Leave alone distal ones, small ones and those which appear completely stable. Before approaching, plan proximal and distal

vascular control and have available at least 40 ml./pound of the freshest whole blood obtainable.

PANCREAS.   Most pancreatic injuries heal without treatment, but devitalized tissue should be removed. Resection of all tissue to the left of the portal vein is well tolerated. Total pancreatectomy is rarely necessary. Serum amylase elevations persisting more than 10 days after injury usually signify a complication such as traumatic pseudocyst. These do not require complicated internal drainage. External tube drainage suffices in children.

DIAPHRAGM.   Ruptures are occasionally missed because they are uncommon. Remember to look at the diaphragm on the chest x-ray. Often the blood supply to the displaced viscera is compromised, making early operation mandatory.

KIDNEY.   Eighty per cent of blunt kidney injuries heal without operation. These yield normal infusion pyelograms or evidence of calyceal compression. The collecting system of the injured kidney may contain less contrast material than its normal counterpart, but all dye which can be seen is in the collecting system and ureter where it belongs.

The most common indication for operation is urinary extravasation, which signifies a major laceration. This is best done 2 to 3 days after injury, when demarcation of devitalized renal tissue has taken place and bleeding from fractured parenchyma is easy to control.

The other indication for operation is vascular injury, and this must be done as an emergency if the kidney is to be salvaged. The infusion pyelogram shows no visualization at all on the injured side, the scan shows no uptake, or the arteriogram shows no flow to the kidney.

URETER.   The ureter is rarely injured by blunt trauma, but may be lacerated by a penetrating injury. The simpler the repair, the better.

BLADDER.   Perforation is often but not always associated with pelvic fracture. Infusion pyelogram or cystogram shows extravasation of urine. Prompt closure and suprapubic drainage is the treatment of choice.

PENETRATING INJURIES.   Children with penetrating abdominal injuries should be surgically explored because the incidence of visceral injury is high and the risk of exploration is very low. The abdomen may be entered via any wound below the nipples.

If penetration through the peritoneum is in doubt and peritoneal irritation is not present, the skin may be closed tightly around a catheter through which 50 per cent sodium diatrizoate (Hypaque) can be injected into the wound. Children showing x-ray evidence of contrast material in the abdomen are candidates for surgical exploration. This maneuver is especially helpful in children with head injuries which make abdominal evaluation difficult.

INCISION. In growing children, a long transverse incision gives good exposure and a far better cosmetic result than does a vertical incision. The latter is frequently preferable in teenagers and adults.

THORAX

The urgent thoracic injuries produce airway obstruction, tension pneumothorax, hemothorax, sucking wounds, flail chest or cardiac tamponade. The major goals in management are to intercept exsanguination and life-threatening infections by prompt surgical closure of significant rents in the heart, major vessels, trachea, bronchi and esophagus; to rid the pleural cavities, mediastinum and pericardium rapidly of space-occupying air, blood or fluid; to reexpand collapsed lungs as quickly and as completely as possible; and to guard against reaccumulation of air or fluid and recurrence of pulmonary collapse.

AIRWAY OBSTRUCTION. If blood is the cause—from pulmonary contusion, bronchial or tracheal injury or aspiration from nose or mouth—gentle suction via endotracheal tube is usually adequate. If stomach contents are the cause, in addition to suction via endotracheal tube, consider bronchoscopy, hydrocortisone 100 mg. every 8 hours for 2 days to minimize inflammatory reaction produced by acid peptic juice, and systemic antibiotics. History and evaluation of aspirated material are important, because x-ray findings may be indistinguishable from those of a pulmonary contusion.

TENSION PNEUMOTHORAX. If there is embarrassed ventilation with an overexpanded hemithorax, shift of trachea and bronchi to the opposite side and a hyperresonant hemithorax with diminished breath sounds, relieve with a needle inserted in the anterior axillary line, followed by a chest tube to underwater seal. If a large amount of air continues to flow from the tube, apply gentle suction. If the lung still cannot be expanded, perform bronchoscopic examination for major tracheal or bronchial injury. If saliva or gastric contents emerge from the chest tube, perform contrast swallow to localize the esophageal perforation, which urgently requires surgical closure and mediastinal drainage. Use a chest tube for all but very small pneumothoraces in children.

HEMOTHORAX. Hemothorax varies in severity from asymptomatic to exsanguination. Major hemothorax produces a shift of mediastinal structures to the opposite side, dullness, and diminished or absent breath sounds. If bleeding into the chest alone has produced shock, urgent operation is needed to repair major vascular injury. In most other cases, bleeding subsides and exploration of the chest is not needed. Place a large chest tube in the midaxillary line to empty the chest and reexpand the lung. Follow the rate of subsequent blood loss. An hourly loss of up to 2 ml./pound, particularly if the rate is slowing, usually will stop without operation. If loss exceeds 15 ml./pound in the first 8 hours, and particularly if loss accelerates, early operation is indicated.

HEMOPNEUMOTHORAX. This is usually due to laceration of pulmonary parenchyma, which will most often heal spontaneously. If one chest tube does not handle both blood and air, insert a second tube.

FLAIL CHEST. A segment of chest wall moves inward on inspiration and outward on expiration owing to multiple rib fractures. Treatment varies with the severity of respiratory embarrassment. Manual stabilization enables cough, which may greatly improve the child temporarily. If ventilation is not excellent, with normal blood gases following external splinting, intubate and support on respirator with positive pressure. Consider elective tracheostomy in severe forms, as a positive pressure respirator may be needed for 1 to 2 weeks.

CARDIAC TAMPONADE. Because this is infrequently seen in injured children, diagnosis is easy to overlook. It is usually but not always associated with a penetrating wound of the heart. The child gives the appearance of having both circulatory and respiratory embarrassment. The pulse is rapid and weak, pulse pressure is narrow, venous pressure is elevated and heart sounds are muffled. It may develop insidiously after initial examination has been performed. Aspirate by placing needle in xiphosternal angle and going upward, outward and backward, all at about 45 degrees of midplanes of chest. In the absence of a penetrating wound, further treatment depends on rapidity of reaccumulation. Those with rapid recurrence of tamponade, and all children with penetrating chest wounds near the heart, should be promptly explored.

After assessing the chest for these urgent conditions, inspect the front and back for surface wounds and palpate all over for fractures, hematomas and subcutaneous emphysema. Obtain emergency chest x-rays, portable ones if necessary. Note any deviations from the expected normal and ask, "How could this abnormal finding *be explained by an injury?*" For example, could a high stomach bubble point to a ruptured diaphragm, or a widened mediastinum indicate a vascular injury rather than a preexisting enlarged thymus? Also note carefully and adjust accordingly the position of nasogastric, endotracheal, CVP or thoracostomy tubes.

NECK AND BACK

All children who complain of neck pain and all children with head injuries should be suspected of having a cervical spine fracture. Move only with manual traction, with the neck slightly extended.

Explore all penetrating injuries of the neck in the operating room. Do not probe neck wounds in the emergency room.

In the conscious child, check arm and leg movement. Ask about pain or paresthesias. Palpate each vertebral spinous process. Spine fractures cause pain when pressure is applied to the spinous process. In the unconscious child, elicit withdrawal from painful stimulus; pinprick fingers and soles.

If weakness suggests a spinal cord injury, give dexamethasone, 3 to 6 mg. intravenously.

Consider all spinal cord injuries *reversible,* and get emergency neurosurgical consultation. Insert a nasogastric tube and a urethral catheter. Protect anesthetic areas from pressure injury.

EXTREMITIES

The urgent problems are uncontrolled bleeding and injuries which compromise blood supply to feet and hands. Direct pressure is usually the safest way to control bleeding. If a tourniquet is used, record the time of application, put it on tight enough to occlude arterial flow, and plan prompt definitive management.

Compound fractures, dislocations and other fractures which impair blood flow require urgent treatment. Splint fractures before moving the patient.

Lacerated arteries in the distal part of leg or forearm usually may be ligated, but arterial lacerations proximal to the bifurcation of brachial and popliteal arteries should be repaired if possible.

Test motor nerve function. Axillary—abduct the arm. Brachioradial—flex the biceps. Ulnar—spread the fingers. Median—touch the thumb to the little finger. Radial—extend the wrist and fingers. Femoral—flex the hip. Sciatic—flex the foot. Check for sensory loss.

Now review the findings, and try to get an accurate history of the accident. With the history in mind, go over the affected areas again.

Accident Prevention

ARTHUR M. GROSSMAN, M.D.

Accidents are the leading cause of injury and death in children, accounting in the United States for 18 million injuries and 50,000 deaths annually. All developed nations report parallel findings.

In view of the seriousness and pervasiveness of injuries and deaths due to accidents, physicians and parents alike need to learn to view accidents in the same way they view diseases. Accidents can be classified; they have causes; and they are frequently preventable.

Since prevention is the best treatment, it is necessary first to classify accidents by their causes and then to show how each can be prevented or at least minimized.

Accidents Involving Transport. To prevent injuries in a moving vehicle, beginning with transporting the newborn from the nursery to home, an infant should be placed in supine position in an approved car restraint on the rear seat of the car, head forward, securely strapped with seat belts. At five months, the infant should be placed erect. At 20 pounds, children should face forward, and at 40 pounds, the child may be placed in the regular automobile safety belt. Even for short drives, the car seat should be used. This program is best initiated at the prenatal level through hospitals or offices which offer pamphlets explaining the details of proper automobile transport. It should be stressed that children are never, but never, to be left alone in a car. Seat belts should be mandatory.

Strollers, buggies and walkers should all have wide, noncollapsible bases. Accidents on skateboards, bicycles, minibikes, and motorcycles usually involve automobiles. Skateboards should be checked for safety (making sure that the wheels turn easily); they should be ridden only on concrete (not on asphalt pavement) and in areas which are free of traffic. Children who are going to use these vehicles should be properly instructed in their use, because serious trauma can result from such accidents. Elbow and knee pads, and helmets are a requirement. Children on bicycles should stay off busy streets and highways. New standards of safety set by the Consumer Products Safety Commission for steering and brake stems, frame strengths, tire reliability, seat design, chain guards, nonslip pedals, and night reflectors must be met. Minibikes are safe only on desert soil. Motorcyclists should always wear shoes, gloves and helmets.

Accidents Involving Falls and Crib Hazards. An infant should never be left unattended, even for a moment, when on a bathinette. This includes never turning one's back on the infant.

Bassinets and cribs should have firm and level mattresses. Crib slats are to be no more that 2⅜ inches apart to prevent the head from becoming trapped between them. The drop rail, when lowered, must be nine inches above the mattress support, and the drop rail clamp should be secured with an accident-proof locking device (U.S. Consumer Products Safety Commission). Half-inch thick carpeting around the crib will prevent most injuries caused by falls from a crib (P.A.S., 50 Union Ave., Irvington, New Jersey 07111).

Stairs should be carpeted whenever possible, with a gate placed at the top and the bottom until the child reaches three years of age.

Windows should be covered outside by firm screens and should have limiting locks. Balconies should have at least a three-foot guard rail and a child-proof screen. Failing the ability to provide these, the door to the balcony should be locked above the child's reach. If the child is to be allowed on the balcony, he or she must be supervised at all times.

Accidents Involving Environmental Hazards. All fireplaces should be screened. Toddlers should be kept away from stoves, appliances and electrical outlets. Safety electric outlet plates are desirable. Boiling liquids and matches should be placed out of reach. Nonflammable night clothing is essential.

Poisons, Drugs, Chemicals and Plants. Drugs should be kept under lock and key. If the mother needs to carry medication with her, she is warned against leaving her purse within reach of the child. She should likewise be warned against leaving any poisons or chemicals under the sink or in other places easily reached by a toddler. Additionally, if the lawn has been sprayed, it is advisable to keep the child away from the area. Since some plants are poisonous if chewed or swallowed, and others may cause allergies, dermatitis or mechanical injury, parents are warned not to allow their children to eat or chew on unidentified vegetation.

Before placing an infant in water, the temperature should be hand tested. Parents should be warned against leaving children alone near any body of water, and neighborhoods should be checked for unguarded pools. Whenever possible, parents are instructed that infants should be taught to swim at the age of nine months. Children should be taught never to swim alone, to avoid swift rivers, and to check depth before diving. (See p. 750 for Near-Drowning.)

Toys. Small children and infants should play only with solid, large stuffed animals, blocks or balls made of nonflammable materials. The parents should be warned against giving the children toys with sharp edges, small loose parts or spring actions (Bureau of Product Safety of the Food and Drug Administration). A child should not run with a stick in his or her mouth.

Tools, Weapons, Missiles and Hand Guns. Sharp instruments and tools should be locked up. Whenever children are throwing darts or shooting bows and arrows, they should be supervised. Young children should not be given toy handguns, rifles, or knives. All handguns and weapons of any sort should be locked up, and ammunition stored separately. To prevent accidental homicide, violent television programs are to be avoided as much as possible. Children, unaware that a real gun is lethal (the movie villain who is shot always gets up to act again), may be encouraged to "play" with a *real* weapon. In this connection, it is absolutely necessary that *all* weapons be kept locked up, out of reach, and unloaded.

Animals. Children should be watched when they are playing with dogs and cats. Infants and large dogs are not to be roommates. Children especially need to be attended when around horses; horses, in addition to bucking, can kick or bite. In snake country, parents as well as children should always wear high shoes and socks. In areas with large insect populations, white, tan or green clothing is recommended, and insect nests should not be touched.

Sports. Before the age of 12 years competitive contact sports are not recommended. When involved in group sports, children should wear sufficient padding and use screened helmets for protection from head, neck and dental injuries.

Zippers. Underpants should always be worn with zippered clothing to protect the genitalia.

Bathroom Areas. Keep medicine cabinets locked. Shower doors should be shatterproof whenever possible. Ordinary glass doors are dangerous.

Pacifiers, Beads and Chains. Pacifiers should be solid, firm rubber and should have no strings or ribbons attached. Beads and chains should not be placed around the necks of infants and children.

Foreign bodies tend to find their way into the various body apertures, most often ears, nose and vagina. Toys or articles given to children should be larger than the diameter of the mouth. Pins, nails, and other small objects should be kept in sealed jars. In a room with crawling infants, sewing or knitting equipment should be on a table out of reach. Peanuts, popcorn and Cracker Jack should likewise be kept out of reach of those under 6 years of age.

Child Abuse.   If a child is seen with repeated injuries or if the history is contradictory, the physician should look for the possibility of child abuse (see p. 808), and this should be reported to a Child Abuse Agency at once.

General Therapeutic Measures.   In the event that an accident does occur, parents should be prepared for emergency treatment and have emergency supplies on hand. Each parent should have readily available the names and telephone numbers of those people who can help: emergency hospital, the family doctor, the fire department rescue squad, the pharmacist, a relative and a responsible friend or neighbor. Medical supplies should be kept in each home according to the physician's recommendation and include: sterile 2″ × 2″ plastic-covered gauze; 4″ roll of gauze bandage; povidone-iodine swab aids; bacitracin ointment or a similar product; ipecac syrup, 1 ounce; activated charcoal, 15 to 20 gm.; roll of ½″ adhesive tape; and sterile petrolatum.

The "Doctor's Home Pediakit" in a child-safety plastic box contains all of these plus several medications for vomiting, pain and convulsions. Instructions for parental first aid emergency treatment are printed on the inside of the box. Informative pamphlets can be obtained from the Children's Hospital Medical Center in Boston, the Department of Health, Education and Welfare, or the American Academy of Pediatrics.

FALLS.   For head injuries see p. 40; for fractures see p. 451.

BURNS.   Advise parents to remove clothing immediately and to apply cold water compresses to burned areas for 10 minutes. For further details see p. 747.

POISONING.   Poisons present the most serious hazard at age 2 to 3 years when the child has become mobile and curious. Immediate treatment should include the identification of the ingested material and a call, if necessary, to the nearest poison center. Routinely have the parent bring along with the child the bottle or container which held the poison or overdose of medicine which may be affecting the child. Parents should be advised to produce emesis (except for hydrocarbons and caustics) by giving up to 3 teaspoons of ipecac syrup followed by 8 oz. of water. If emesis does not occur within 20 minutes, this may be repeated. Following total emesis advise parents to use activated charcoal tablets or powder in a dosage of 15 to 20 gm. See p. 709 for further details on poisoning.

ANIMALS.   For dog bites *get the dog* and report to the authorities. Wash the wound with soap and water and apply Betadine. Check for tetanus booster. If the dog was rabid, see pp. 627 and 745. For snake bites see p. 734.

Choking.   The child should be turned over the knee with head down and struck with the hand over the upper thoracic spine. Parents should be instructed not to remove any object from an aperture unless the object projects at least halfway out.

21

Unclassified Diseases

Histiocytosis X

CAROL CROWLEY M.D., *and*
THOMAS F. NECHELES, M.D.

Histiocytosis X is a term which encompasses a spectrum of uncommon diseases of similar pathology and unknown etiology, including those previously referred to as eosinophilic granuloma of bone, Hand-Schüller-Christian syndrome, and Letterer-Siwe disease. Diseases included under the broad designation histiocytosis X vary from solitary lesions of bone, which have an excellent prognosis, to fulminant syndromes with widespread parenchymal involvement, systemic manifestations, and often a fatal outcome. Whether the varied clinical manifestations of histiocytosis X reflect differing host responses to the same etiologic factors or whether they are caused by entirely different pathogenetic mechanisms is unknown. Physicians treating these diseases should be thoroughly familiar with the entire spectrum of clinical manifestations. Treatment must be determined largely on the basis of the extent and pattern of disease involvement and must be individualized to suit the needs of each patient.

The extent of disease at presentation and the clinical course are, in general, closely related to the age of the patient at the time of diagnosis. The prognosis, in turn, is related to the extent of disease. There may be progression from limited disease to more extensive involvement after treatment has begun; in such instances, therapy must be modified. Solitary bone lesions are seen most often in older children, adolescents, and adults. At the opposite end of the spectrum of histiocytosis X is a syndrome characterized by involvement of multiple bones, skin, the hypothalamic-pituitary axis, lungs, lymph nodes, liver, spleen, and bone marrow, with systemic signs, such as fever and weight loss; this is seen most commonly in infants and very young children. This latter presentation, if untreated, usually leads to death from infection, bleeding, pulmonary failure, or hepatic failure. Syndromes of intermediate severity are seen most often in children between the ages of two and eight. Permanent sequelae, such as bone deformities, diabetes insipidus, growth retardation, and hearing loss, are not uncommon.

Lahey devised a method for staging patients with histiocytosis X (J. Pediat., *60*:664, 1962) which was later modified by Lucaya (Am. J. Dis. Child., *121*:289, 1971). Their staging system is based on the number of organ systems involved with disease. Recent evidence has indicated that parenchymal involvement with functional impairment implies a worse prognosis than does infiltration with preservation of normal function (J. Pediat., *87*:184, 1975). Table 1 is a staging system which takes the latter fact into account and which has provided, in our hands, a useful guide to prognosis and treatment.

TABLE 1. Staging of Histiocytosis X

Stage I	Solitary bone lesion
Stage II-A	Multiple bone lesions
Stage II-B	Multiple bone lesions plus pituitary and/or skin involvement
Stage III	Parenchymal involvement (with or without the above) with normal function
Stage IV	Parenchymal involvement with organ dysfunction

The diagnosis of histiocytosis X, which is usually suspected on clinical and radiologic grounds, must be established by pathological examination of a biopsy specimen from an involved area. Following confirmation of the diagnosis, the extent of disease must be ascertained by: physical examination; chest x-ray and pulmonary function evaluation if indicated; skeletal survey and/or bone scan; liver function studies; blood counts; and bone marrow examination. Only after careful assessment of the status of the particular patient can a treatment regimen be planned.

A solitary bone lesion (Stage I) is treated by surgical curettage, often accomplished at the time of the biopsy. Radiation therapy in low doses (600 to 1000 rads) is useful as an adjunct for large lesions, especially if there is danger of pathological fracture, or if the involvement is in a particularly worrisome site, such as a cervical vertebra. The occasional solitary lesion of soft tissue may be similarly treated by surgery and/or radiation therapy.

Disseminated histiocytosis X (i.e., more advanced than Stage I) requires treatment with chemotherapy. Numerous chemotherapeutic agents, either alone or in combination, have been found to be effective in treating and arresting the progression of disease. The particular regimen selected depends upon the clinical status of the patient and the stage of disease. Whether it is the immunosuppressive, antiinflammatory, or antineoplastic properties of the chemotherapeutic agents which make them useful for the treatment of histiocytosis X is unknown.

Stage II-A and some cases of Stages II-B and III may be successfully managed with a single chemotherapeutic agent. Vinblastine is perhaps the most effective and is well tolerated by the majority of patients. The initial dose of vinblastine is 5 mg./m^2 intravenously weekly. The dose is then increased to the maximum tolerated dose (i.e., the highest weekly dose which can be achieved without allowing the WBC to fall below 3000 or the platelets below 100,000). Weekly vinblastine should be continued for several months to a year following complete remission. If the disease stabilizes but does not resolve completely, or if more lesions appear after chemotherapy is stopped, weekly vinblastine should be continued indefinitely.

Infants and young children with Stage IV histiocytosis X require aggressive therapy with combinations of chemotherapeutic agents. Combinations including a vinca alkaloid (such as vinblastine) with an alkylating agent (such as cyclophosphamide) and prednisone are effective in many patients. Vinblastine may be given in a weekly intravenous dose of 5 mg./m^2; cyclophosphamide can be given initially intravenously, 100 mg./m^2 every other day for five doses; and prednisone 40 mg./m^2 orally daily for two to four weeks and tapered thereafter. If a complete or partial response is achieved, weekly vinblastine is continued for at least a year, and longer if chronic active disease is present.

Children who continue to have progressive disease despite the above regimen may be treated with vincristine and methotrexate, or vincristine and 6-mercaptopurine, or with other alkylating agents such as chlorambucil or nitrogen mustard. Patients who fail to respond to one combination of chemotherapeutic agents often prove to be resistant to other drugs as well, but a trial is appropriate in the face of progressive histiocytosis X.

All of the above mentioned chemotherapeutic agents have significant toxicity and their use in the therapy of histiocytosis X should be carefully considered. Therapy should be undertaken only by physicians experienced in the use of such drugs and closely monitored with frequent blood counts and periodic evaluations of liver and renal function.

Radiation therapy is useful not only in the management of Stage I disease, but also as an adjunct to chemotherapy in children with advanced histiocytosis X. Low doses of radiation therapy (600 to 1000 rads) are useful for palliation of painful bone lesions and to prevent pathological fractures, especially for vertebral lesions.

Certain complications of histiocytosis X can sometimes be ameliorated by radiation therapy. Hypersplenism with pancytopenia due to a massively involved and enlarged spleen can sometimes be corrected rapidly by irradiating the spleen (600 rads). Such low doses of radiotherapy do not impair the immunological function of the spleen. This treatment therefore has a definite advantage over splenectomy, since hypersplenism due to histiocytosis X is most often seen in young children who have significant morbidity and mortality from postsplenectomy infections.

Exophthalmos due to involvement by histiocytosis X of the orbital bones and soft tissues of the retro-orbital region often responds to similar doses of radiation therapy. Diabetes insipidus due to hypothalamic and/or pituitary involvement is frequently refractory to chemotherapy and, in such cases, radiation therapy to this area may be given; despite radiation therapy, the diabetes insipidus may persist and require Pitressin or related drugs for its management. Diabetes insipidus is one of the most common permanent sequelae of histiocytosis X. Similarly, growth retardation due to inadequate secretion of growth hormone by the anterior pituitary, though less common than posterior pituitary failure, is often refractory to therapy and may require growth hormone replacement.

Infections are common in patients with histiocytosis X because of both the nature of the disease and its treatment. Otitis media is most common and may result in hearing loss. Infections must be treated appropriately when they occur. Prophylactic antibiotics are not useful and predispose the patient to opportunistic infections.

With appropriate treatment, about 70 per cent of children with disseminated histiocytosis X and virtually all of those with only bone lesions survive. Their management is a challenge, but a great responsibility, for physicians who care for them.

Amyloidosis

ALAN S. COHEN, M.D., *and*
ALAN RUBINOW, M.D.

Amyloidosis is an extracellular deposition of a fibrous, eosinophilic protein in one or more sites of the body. Characteristically, the Congo red stain produces an apple-green birefringence under polarizing microscopy, and in the electron microscope it appears as fine, rigid, nonbranching fibrils.

In primary amyloidosis, the protein moiety of the fibril consists of portions of or whole immunoglobulin light chains. A unique nonimmunoglobulin protein AA has been isolated from secondary amyloid. The precursor of AA protein appears to be an alpha globulin, SAA (serum AA), found in small quantities in normal serum. High titers are found in chronic infections and inflammatory conditions that predispose to amyloid formation as well as neoplasms and aging. SAA behaves as an acute phase reactant returning to normal levels with control of the disease process.

Amyloidosis during childhood is of the secondary type accompanying chronic inflammatory disorders, i.e., juvenile rheumatoid arthritis, inflammatory bowel disease and familial Mediterranean fever (FMF).

Rational therapy should be directed at (1) decreasing chronic antigenic stimuli producing amyloid; (2) inhibition of the synthesis of the amyloid fibril; (3) preventing extracellular deposition of amyloid fibril; and (4) promoting lysis or mobilization of existing deposits. Eradication or suppression of the predisposing disorder apparently slows the progression of the amyloidosis. Empirical therapy with liver extracts, ascorbic acid in high doses and numerous other modalities have been uncontrolled and of equivocal value. Corticosteroids and immunosuppressive agents are not advocated and indeed experimental evidence indicates that they may enhance amyloid deposition. There is no necessity to discontinue their use if they are effectively controlling the underlying inflammation.

Encouraged by the prophylactic effect of colchicine in acute attacks of FMF, colchicine has been shown to prevent amyloid production in the casein-treated mouse model. Preliminary reports suggest that colchicine therapy may prevent amyloidosis in patients with FMF. The mechanism of its action is unknown. The possible adverse effects of long-term colchicine therapy in children have not been assessed.

Progressive renal failure is a major cause of morbidity and death from amyloidosis. Very carefully selected patients may benefit from hemodialysis and renal transplantation. Despite these encouraging developments, there is no proven specific therapy for amyloidosis. Rigid adherence to supportive and symptomatic therapy is the mainstay of management.

Sarcoidosis

EDWIN L. KENDIG, Jr., M.D.

The cause of sarcoidosis is unknown; there is, therefore, no known specific therapy. Adrenocorticosteroids and corticotropin are the only agents available at present which can suppress the acute manifestations of sarcoidosis. These agents are used only during the acute and dangerous episodes.

Adrenocorticosteroid (or corticotropin) therapy is always indicated in patients with intrinsic ocular disease, diffuse pulmonary lesions with alveolar-capillary block, central nervous system lesions, myocardial involvement, hypersplenism and persistent hypercalcemia. Relative indications for adrenocorticosteroid therapy include progressive or symptomatic pulmonary lesions, disfiguring cutaneous and lymph node lesions, constitutional symptoms and joint involvement, lesions of the nasal, laryngeal and bronchial mucosa, and persistent facial nerve palsy.

Fresh lesions are apparently more responsive than are older ones. Suppressive action is often temporary, but it is beneficial when the unremitting course of such disease will produce loss of organ function. For example, adrenocorticosteroids can reduce the level of serum calcium and may thus help prevent nephrocalcinosis and renal insufficiency and possibly band keratitis. Whether adrenocorticosteroids should be utilized in the treatment of those patients whose disease consists only of asymptomatic miliary nodules or bronchopneumonic patches in the lung fields is debatable.

The initial dose of prednisone or prednisolone is 1 mg./kg./day, and triamcinolone, 0.75 mg./kg./day, in 4 divided doses. A gradual reduction in the level of dosage of adrenocorticosteroid is initiated as soon as clinical manifestations of the disease disappear. A maintenance dose of prednisone, 15 mg. every other day, is continued until the patient has received a 6 months total course of treatment.

Siltzbach reported the frequent occurrence of temporary relapse following the discontinuation of adrenocorticosteroid therapy, but noted that improvement usually follows even if the treatment is not resumed. In the management of ocular sarcoidosis, adrenocorticosteroids in the form of either ointment or drops (0.5 to 1 per cent) are utilized in conjunction with the systemic use of these agents. During the course of such local therapy, the pupils are kept in a state of continuous dilatation by use of an atropine ointment (1 per cent).

Adrenocorticosteroid ointment may also be utilized in the treatment of cutaneous lesions, but only in conjunction with systemic therapy, since better results are obtained with the latter.

Familial Mediterranean Fever

HELEN F. BRICKMAN, M.D., *and*
DEBORAH ZEMER, M.D.

While no effective treatment is available for the acute attack of serositis in an individual with familial Mediterranean fever (FMF), colchicine has been found to be remarkably effective in preventing attacks. For as long as the drug continues to be administered, it markedly reduces the frequency and severity of the characteristic episodes. Enthusiasm for its pediatric use was tempered by the hitherto minimal use of this ancient remedy in children. However, the Israeli experience has shown that 90 per cent of children will be greatly relieved, most of them completely, by the usual adult dosage of 0.5 mg twice daily;* a few may require twice that amount. Compliance is important since a brief lapse in therapy is characteristically followed quickly by an attack.

Adverse side effects have been negligible so far. Indeed, the growth spurt after the institution of colchicine therapy may be impressive in children who did not thrive before. There has however been some concern regarding the eventual effect of prolonged colchicine administration on the reproductive system. An increase in cells with abnormal numbers of chromosomes has been noted in adults receiving colchicine, and one instance of Down's syndrome was observed in a child conceived during colchicine therapy of the parent. But while azoospermia may occur in rats after large doses of colchicine, infertility in males with FMF on therapeutic doses has not been observed; females with FMF have somewhat diminished fertility without any treatment. When colchicine is prescribed for adolescents, it should, if possible, be discontinued in both males and females three months before pregnancy, and during the first trimester in the mother.

Notwithstanding the caution thus imposed, a child with FMF whose life is disrupted by frequent severe disabling episodes of acute polyserositis should receive preventive colchicine. Also, the rare instance of progressive destructive arthropathy presenting in FMF warrants colchicine, which has afforded benefit in a few such cases. However, protracted involvement of the hip joint responds poorly to medical management and requires orthopedic intervention, such as aspiration of the joint to improve arterial flow before much aseptic necrosis of the femoral head has occurred, and prosthetic replacement of the joint when severely affected.

In addition, there has been a preliminary report of a favorable effect of colchicine on the primary amyloidosis of FMF, as well as on experimental amyloidosis. Experience is accumulating to suggest that patients with FMF on colchicine therapy for two to three years are not developing proteinuria. Confirmation that colchicine can prevent or even delay this lethal phenotypic expression of FMF would constitute a major indication for its use.

No other remedies have shown consistent efficacy. Those individuals with FMF who are not taking colchicine should be advised to

---

*This use of colchicine is not mentioned in the manufacturer's instructions.

avoid activities which they have repeatedly observed to trigger attacks, for example, prolonged or intense physical exercise or ingestion of meals high in fat content. During attacks, only nonnarcotic analgesics should be used.

Although unnecessary intervention by the surgeon should be kept to a minimum, an episode of acute peritonitis in an individual with FMF may be difficult to distinguish at its onset from a non-FMF abdominal emergency, to which the FMF population is presumably as prone as any other. Those experiencing frequent such attacks should probably undergo appendectomy. Mechanical ileus due to adhesions should be considered in an abdominal attack persisting longer than six to eight hours. It is hoped that the finding of cryofibrinogenemia in the first few hours of an attack will be found as specific for an acute episode of FMF as a preliminary report suggests, or that some other laboratory aid will be found to fill this diagnostic need.

Genetic counseling is indicated as in other autosomal recessive conditions. Given the restricted ethnic incidence of FMF, such advice should be more easily followed in the North American melting pot than in the Middle Eastern heartland of the disorder. Children with FMF, as with other chronic illnesses, may require extended psychotherapeutic support.

22

Special Problems in the Newborn

Intrauterine Growth Retardation and Postmaturity Syndrome

JEFFREY J. POMERANCE, M.D., M.P.H.

Intrauterine growth retardation is diagnosed whenever birth weight is below the tenth percentile for the respective week of gestation (occasionally 2 standard deviations below the mean is used or approximately the third percentile). Postmaturity syndrome is diagnosed whenever an infant is born after more than 42 weeks gestation (post-term) and exhibits signs of recent weight loss and dehydration.

The etiology of intrauterine growth retardation falls broadly into three categories: nutritional, infectious and genetic. Nutritional causes can be further subdivided with some overlay into (1) maternal disease (chronic toxemia, hypertensive cardiovascular or renal disease, congenital cyanotic or noncyanotic or acquired heart disease, chronic pulmonary disease, malnutrition, chronic illness, sickle cell anemia); (2) placental disorders (infarction, abruption, abnormal cord insertions, tumor, multiple gestation, twin to twin transfusion) and (3) environmental (maternal addiction, maternal cigarette smoking, high altitude, radiation injury). Infectious causes include chronic fetal infection with cytomegalovirus, rubella virus, *Toxoplasma gondii* and *Treponema*

pallidum. The more common genetic causes include trisomies 13, 18 and 21, and Turner's syndrome. In addition, inherited disorders without chromosomal abnormalities occur in infants with intrauterine growth retardation (diastrophic and achondroplastic dwarfs). The etiology of postmaturity almost always involves placental pathology associated with prolonged gestation (infarcts, uteroplacental insufficiency, abruption).

As with other disease entities, prevention is preferable to therapy and both of these entities are preventable, at least in their more severe forms. In intrauterine growth retardation secondary to infectious or genetic causes, the only therapy currently available is interruption of pregnancy. Intrauterine growth retardation secondary to nutritional deprivation and the postmaturity syndrome give rise to a very distinctive pattern of fetal growth. Length and more especially head growth are spared relative to body weight. Ultrasound techniques are available which in experienced hands allow for the precise measurement of the fetal biparietal diameter. Sequential measurements allow for early recognition of intrauterine growth retardation. This information together with the oxytocin challenge test, 24 hour urine estriol (or perhaps serum estriol) and the lecithin: sphingomyelin ratio enable us to ask the fetus, "How are you doing?" and "Would you prefer to be somewhere else?" A well timed exit from the uterus may prevent the more severe symptoms of intrauterine growth retardation or the postmaturity syndrome.

Hypoglycemia is the most frequent problem encountered by infants with intrauterine growth retardation or the postmaturity syndrome. This may occur within an hour or two of birth (especially following fetal distress) and may continue to be a problem for 24 to 48 hours (or occasionally longer) after birth or until oral feedings are well established. Frequent monitoring of blood glucose is therefore required. The first blood glucose estimation should be made within the first hour or two of life. The Dextrostix method in our hands has been satisfactory for screening purposes.

Dextrostix estimations of blood glucose tend to err on the low side, so that a reading of 40 mg./100 ml. or higher may be interpreted as the absence of hypoglycemia. Lower readings should be confirmed by a capillary or venous sample sent to the laboratory. If the blood glucose estimation is less than 40 mg./100 ml. and the infant is active and alert, a 5 or 10 per cent glucose water feeding of 5 to 10 ml. is given either by nipple or gavage. A Dextrostix estimation of blood glucose is then repeated in 15 to 20 minutes. If the infant is manifesting symptoms or if the repeat Dextrostix is not 40 mg./100 ml. or higher (after the initial low Dextrostix has been verified by the laboratory), intravenous glucose is administered. Between 2.5 and 5 ml./kg. of 10 per cent glucose is administered at approximately 1 ml./min. via peripheral vein. Intravenous infusion is then continued with a 10 per cent glucose solution (rarely higher concentrations are needed) at the rate of 80 to 120 ml./kg./day. Gradually oral feedings are begun and the intravenous infusion rate is decreased accordingly. Blood glucose is monitored until the infant has been weaned from intravenous fluids for 12 to 24 hours.

Infants suffering from intrauterine growth retardation may have a significantly greater problem in thermoregulation than if they had been normally grown. Hence the problems associated with "cold injury" may complicate the situation. These infants have decreased amounts of brown (as well as white) fat which presumably predisposes them to poor thermoregulatory responses. Because their body composition and basal metabolic rates differ from those of infants of appropriate weight, the usual tables for the neutral thermal environment do not apply. Incubator settings are best determined by servocontrol with abdominal skin temperature between 36.0 and 36.5°C.

Polycythemia is a relatively frequent finding in infants with intrauterine growth retardation or postmaturity syndrome. The cause is unknown, but chronic intrauterine hypoxia has been suggested. Frequently the polycythemic infant is asymptomatic or at least the symptoms are relatively subtle (lethargy, poor feeding). Occasionally, however, symptoms are blatant and easily recognized (respiratory distress, pleural effusion, cardiac failure, convulsions). Symptoms may be related to increasing viscosity, which rises sharply as hematocrit values reach 70 per cent. When the initial blood is drawn for blood glucose estimation, two capillary tubes are collected for hematocrit determination. If this value is 65 per cent or greater and the infant has symptoms attributable to polycythemia or if the hematocrit is 70 per cent or greater, even in an asymptomatic infant, bloodletting is performed (usually through an umbilical venous catheter). Small aliquots are removed (5 to 20 ml., depending on infant weight) and replaced with plasma until the hematocrit is approximately 60 per cent. Follow-up hematocrits are necessary during the next 24 hours as sequestered red blood cells may emerge and raise the hematocrit to dangerous levels again. Bloodletting is essential even in asymptomatic infants with hematocrits of 70 per cent or greater as initial symptoms may be secondary to spontaneous venous thromboses (frequently cerebral or renal).

Postmaturity syndrome is frequently complicated by the passage of meconium into the amniotic fluid prior to birth. Although the fetus does "breathe" while still in uterus, it is distinctly rare that significant quantities of meconium particles are propelled into small bronchioles and alveoli prior to birth. Therefore, direct tracheal suction performed by a skilled professional at the time of delivery, *prior* to any positive pressure ventilation, all but eliminates the morbidity and mortality of meconium aspiration syndrome.

Prognosis in infants with intrauterine growth retardation depends most upon etiology. Those with infectious and genetic etiologies fare worst, while those with nutritional etiologies as a group fare better. Survival and ultimate outcome depend on the degree of intrauterine growth retardation (or severity of the postmaturity syndrome) and on the adequacy of early postnatal nutrition. The combined effect of intrauterine and early postnatal malnutrition on central venous system development can be devastating.

Birth Injuries

JOSEPH L. KENNEDY, JR., M.D.

The introduction of fetal monitoring techniques and the more common use of cesarean section particularly in breech birth have combined in recent years to make serious birth injury less common. The newer techniques have in themselves contributed some problems. The pediatrician must be intimately familiar with the marks of the normal birth process so that he may offer a worried parent justified reassurance. Attempts at treatment of minor birth injuries are often interfering, and may in fact foster undue parental concern.

Superficial Injuries. *Caput succedaneum and molding* are to be expected in most deliveries. The shape of the infant's head is often of deep concern to the parents. Molding may be marked when the infant is large, the labor long, the mother primigravid, or the membranes ruptured prior to the onset of labor. Parents should be reassured that the head will look normal in a matter of days and that molding is normal and not associated with brain damage. The edema, suffusion and localized intradermal hemorrhage of the presenting part begins to regress within 12 to 24 hours. Within the caput may be found localized abrasions, lacerations from intrauterine scalp sampling, and the puncture marks, sometimes with localized hemorrhage, of the monitoring electrode. These breaks in the skin represent a potential portal of entry for bacteria, particularly when there has been premature rupture of membranes or a long labor. Local treatment with a topical antibiotic cream or powder may prevent abscess or cellulitis.

The caput associated with the use of vacuum extraction may be more marked. Lesions similar to the caput occur not uncommonly with breech delivery. Bruising and edema of the genitalia worry parents; reassurance is usually warranted. Severe intratesticular hemorrhage may, however, produce late fibrotic changes. Hemorrhagic necrosis of portions of the labial or perianal areas results in localized sloughing with healing in 10 to 14 days. No treatment is needed other than careful cleaning of the affected areas. Unusual presentations such as that of face, arm, or leg result in similar localized changes. Extensive enclosed hemorrhage, particularly in the premature infant, may be a significant extravascular source of bilirubin, and rarely a significant source of blood loss. Muscle crush injury with shock, disseminated intravascular coagulation and renal damage has been described.

Lacerations may be caused by amniotomy, episiotomy, fetal blood sampling, fetal incision at cesarean section or by the edge of a forceps blade. Sutures are sometimes required. Topical antibiotic cream or powder may be used to prevent infection. These wounds do well without a dressing.

Superficial forceps injury consisting of erythema with abrasion, superficial drainage and crusting will heal rapidly and without scarring. Dressings are contraindicated. *Deep forceps injury* (subcutaneous fat necrosis) becomes evident between the fourth and eighth day. It heals spontaneously in a matter of weeks. Progression to an abscess is seen rarely. As with other neonatal skin injuries, warm soaks are contraindicated because of the susceptibility of the newborn to water-borne bacterial infection and of the newborn skin to thermal injury. Subcutaneous fat necrosis presumably from trauma attendant to delivery is occasionally seen elsewhere on the body, where it may be confused with a local cellulitis.

Scalp abscess occurs in 5 per cent of infants who have had intrauterine monitoring. Most lesions are small and self-limited. A few have required incision and drainage. Careful cultures always reveal bacteria, usually those of the vaginal flora. Systemic antibiotics are not indicated unless signs of septicemia are present, nor is continued hospitalization required. Large or enlarging lesions should be followed weekly until resolution begins, because there have been a few reports of osteomyelitis and subgaleal abscess. Biparietal scalp necrosis with abscess formation occurs when the widest part of a large fetal head is pressed against the ischial spines during labor. Management is similar.

Tight nuchal cord causes localized cyanosis, edema, suffusion and petechiae above the neck. Similar changes may be seen with face presentation, nuchal encirclement during breech delivery or during vertex delivery with shoulder dystocia, or when ergotrate has been given to the mother before the trunk has been delivered. Localized facial cyanosis alone may be seen in severe congenital hypothyroidism, and in a rare infant who responds to a cold environment primarily by vasoconstriction of the face. The soft tissue lesions require no treatment. Infants with nuchal cord should be watched for respiratory distress, which may occur because of nasal mucosal edema in an infant who is an obligate nasal breather. Nasal obstruction is relieved with an oral airway. Some infants born after partial cord compression become hypovolemic because of sequestration of the infant's blood in the placenta, when flow in the umbilical vein is impeded. Serial monitoring of blood pressure, pulse, respiratory rate and hematocrit should be done in infants with a history of cord compression.

Cephalhematoma is usually unilateral and parietal in location. It is initiated during the birth process and hence is rarely demonstrable within the first few hours of life. Associated linear skull fractures are not rare, but skull x-ray is unnecessary since depressed fractures do no occur in the absence of other trauma, and since the expectant treatment is the same whether or not a linear fracture is present. Resolution of the lesion may take 4 to 10 weeks. It is sometimes accompanied by calcification of the lesion, new bone formation and occasionally by a partial collapse of the swelling. Initially the periosteal stretching may produce local tenderness; it has become customary for this reason to lay the infant's head on the unaffected side. Parents are often very anxious and need a great deal of reassurance that healing will occur without untoward effects. The breakdown of hemoglobin in a large cephalhematoma may cause the serum bilirubin to rise by 3 to 5 mg./100 ml., but can never be the sole explanation for marked neonatal jaundice. Cephalhematoma should never be aspirated because of the danger of introducing infection.

Subaponeurotic hemorrhage occurs rarely after difficult deliveries and vacuum extraction. The premature infant is somewhat more susceptible. Diagnosis is made by the appearance of increasing scalp swelling crossing suture lines, often fluctuant or crepitant, associated with pitting edema. Hemorrhage may be severe enough to cause death in hypovolemic shock. Prompt diagnosis and treatment with blood and plasma expanders may be lifesaving. The milder lesions will regress spontaneously, but, like other enclosed hemorrhages in the newborn, may be associated with some rise in serum bilirubin, and rarely with disseminated intravascular coagulation.

Intracranial Hemorrhage. The exact diagnosis of a neonatal intracranial hemorrhage *(subdural hemorrhage, intraventricular hemorrhage, intracerebral hemorrhage,* or *subarachnoid hemorrhage)* is less important than the immediate management of the affected infant. Diagnosis of hemorrhage is suspected when there is lethargy, hypotonia, seizures, focal neurologic signs, irregular respiration, apnea, fall in hematocrit, metabolic acidosis, bloody spinal fluid, full fontanelle or irritability. The maternal history is usually one of abnormal presentation, prolonged second stage of labor, or difficult delivery, often with oxytocin aug-

mentation. Intraventricular hemorrhage, common in the small sick premature infant, where it may not represent a true birth injury, is rare as a solitary finding in the term infant. Computerized axial tomography (CAT scan) is the best way of diagnosing a lesion amenable to neurosurgical intervention.

Routine tapping of the subdural space in an infant without skull fracture, localizing signs or evidence of increased intracranial pressure is contraindicated since it may in itself cause subdural bleeding. Neurosurgical consultation is advisable if the diagnosis is suspected. In most infants careful observation and symptomatic treatment are preferable to overvigorous diagnostic measures.

Seizures should be controlled with phenobarbital, 10 mg./kg. intravenously or intramuscularly followed by 6 mg./kg./day parenterally in two divided doses. The initial 10 mg./kg. dose may be repeated if necessary. Serum phenobarbital level should be kept in the range of 10 μg./ml. to 25 μg./ml. Phenytoin (10 mg./kg. intravenously) is of little additional help and has a 24 hour delayed onset of action. It should be used only when seizures are severe, prolonged and refractory to treatment. Intravenous diazepam is synergistic with the barbiturates, and the combination of the two drugs has been reported to cause severe respiratory depression. Diazepam should not be used unless artificial ventilatory support is immediately available. Hypoglycemia, hypocalcemia and hyponatremia are common in these infants; a search for these metabolic abnormalities should be made in every infant and appropriate treatment undertaken.

Supportive therapy of the infant with intracranial hemorrhage should include intravenous nutrition, treatment of associated hypoglycemia, monitoring for hypovolemia with appropriate replacement of blood or plasma, and careful attention to fluid balance to prevent aggravation of a seizure disorder by overhydration.

As recovery ensues, electroencephalography may sometimes give helpful prognostic information. CAT scan and monitoring of head circumference daily for 10 days then twice weekly will give early indication of the need for neurosurgical intervention for hydrocephalus.

Skeletal Injuries. *Clavicular fracture* occurs with shoulder dystocia, particularly with large infants and with breech delivery. Diagnosis is made by the obstetrical history and by finding pain, crepitus or angulation on palpation. There is usually only little displacement; healing with palpable callus is evident at 2 to 3 weeks. A figure-eight bandage is unnecessary; simple pinning of the shirtsleeve to the shirt with gentle handling suffices. A follow-up examination should be done at 2 to 6 weeks to identify the rare fracture that goes on to non-union.

Fractures of the humerus, femur, or other long bones are usually associated with difficult breech delivery. Simple fractures of the humerus in good alignment require only immobilization and splinting, with the arm adducted and the forearm flexed at 90°. Poor alignment will require casting. Fractures of the femur do best with immobilization by splint or cast, together with traction. Prognosis for birth fractures is good.

Separation of an epiphysis of the humerus (usually proximal) *or femur* (usually distal) is suspected when there is pain and lack of movement of the affected extremity after a difficult delivery. Diagnosis is confirmed by x-ray at 10 to 14 days, when callus formation will be evident. Treatment is similar to that for fracture. Brachial plexus injury can be associated and should be looked for.

Neuromuscular Injuries. *Brachial plexus injury* is caused by lateral traction of the neck during difficult breech extraction or vertex delivery with shoulder dystocia. When injury is severe or extensive, chest fluoroscopy (or inspiratory and expiratory films) should be done to identify diaphragmatic paralysis. Immediate treatment consists of pinning the arm in abduction, external rotation and supination for 10 to 14 days. After this time physiotherapy is begun with careful passive exercising several times daily. Careful neurologic follow-up is mandatory. The prognosis is generally good except when the damage extends to the lower nerve roots. Diaphragmatic paralysis requires chest physiotherapy during the immediate neonatal period, follow-up x-rays, and careful observation during any intercurrent respiratory infection.

Facial palsy, sometimes associated with brachial palsy but more commonly an isolated finding, is usually resolved in several weeks. It requires no treatment except when the eye is involved. In this instance instillation of 0.5 per cent methylcellulose drops should be made four times daily to prevent corneal ulceration.

Paralysis of the radial, obturator, or external popliteal nerves is uncommon, requires no treatment and resolves spontaneously.

Sixth nerve palsy, usually unilateral, is found not uncommonly at birth. It cause is unknown and it disappears spontaneously by age one month.

Spinal cord injury occurs with difficult breech deliveries, particularly when the fetal neck is hyperextended. The injury is therefore preventable by cesarean section. The management of the woman in labor with a breech presentation should include an x-ray to identify the 5 per cent of infants at risk. Early diagnosis and supportive care should help minimize problems in the infant who is to survive. Diagnosis is suggested by flaccid paralysis with areflexia of arms and legs, diaphragmatic breathing, and urinary retention. Four-hourly Credé maneuver of the bladder will help prevent bladder damage and urinary tract infection. Chest physiotherapy and positioning is useful in the infant with thoracic involvement to prevent atelectasis and pneumonia. X-rays of the spine will occasionally show a fracture or dislocation. The prognosis in general is poor, but an occasional severely affected infant has survived with only minimal residual damage.

Internal Thoracic Injuries. Attempt at amniocentesis may puncture the lung causing *pneumothorax* and sometimes subcutaneous emphysema after birth. Treatment is immediate tube thoracostomy with underwater drainage. Prognosis is good. Some cases of *chylothorax* are thought to be due to injury to the thoracic duct during delivery. Treatment of chylothorax causing respiratory embarrassment consists of repeated needle aspirations.

Internal Abdominal Injuries. Intraabdominal bleeding may occur from rupture of the liver or spleen, the latter usually only when it is enlarged, as with erythroblastosis. Shock, abdominal distention and occasionally a bluish discoloration of the abdomen warrant immediate surgical intervention, with concurrent replacement of intravascular volume with blood, plasma or albumin. More commonly, rupture of the liver results in a *subcapsular hematoma* with gradual deterioration over several days. Infants at risk because of birth history should have careful monitoring of pulse, blood pressure and hematocrit, together with daily gentle palpation of the surface of the liver. The liver or spleen may also be injured by amniocentesis, intrauterine blood transfusion or by vigorous resuscitative efforts at birth.

Injury of the adrenal glands may be hypoxic rather then traumatic in origin. Blood transfusion to restore volume together with prompt surgical intervention may be life-saving in the infant with massive hemorrhage. Milder lesions may be followed carefully. There is no need to administer corticosteroids.

Rupture of the bladder at delivery presenting as ascites is almost totally confined to male infants with bladder neck obstruction. Treatment is of the underlying condition.

Other Birth Injuries. Serious eye injuries are rare. Subconjunctival and retinal hemorrhages are common, unassociated with other bleeding, and require no treatment. Discoloration of the nasal septal cartilage has been recently suggested as a cause of deviation of the tip of the nose. When the deviation is made more marked on depression of the nasal tip, otorhinolaryngologic consultation may be indicated. Skull fractures are rare, and usually of little clinical significance. Small linear fractures are not uncommonly found when multiple serial x-rays are done on infants with cephalhematoma (cf. supra). Linear fractures require no treatment; follow-up should be done at two months, however, to rule out the development of a leptomeningeal cyst. Depressed "fractures" are usually intrauterine spontaneous skull depressions. Neurosurgical repair is indicated for cosmetic reasons since many do not resolve spontaneously. Attempts to elevate the depressed area by applying pressure or suction are contraindicated since further damage may result.

Resuscitation of the Newborn

GEORGE A. GREGORY, M.D.

Asphyxia accounts for approximately 25 per cent of perinatal mortality in North America. Those who survive asphyxia often have cerebral palsy and/or retardation of neurologic and motor development. The relationship of mild perinatal asphyxia to learning difficulties in later life is unclear. If we are to reduce the effects of perinatal asphyxia we must understand and undertake neonatal resuscitation immediately after birth.

There are many causes of perinatal asphyxia. In general, however, it is related to inadequate placental and umbilical artery blood flow prior to or during the birth process.

Assessment at Birth. The Apgar score is still the standard by which infants are evaluated at birth. A score of 0 to 10 is given based on 0 to 2 points for heart rate, respiratory rate, muscle tone, reflex irritability, and color (Table 1). Each variable must be evaluated independently at 1 and 5 minutes of age or the test is of no value. A score of 5 or less at 5 minutes is associated with an increased incidence of intracranial hemorrhage, cerebral palsy, and neurologic deficits. If the Apgar score is 3 or less at one minute and no improvement in the patient's condition with assisted stimulation ventilation, or 6 or less at 5 minutes, arterial blood gases and pH should be measured; for only by measuring blood gases and pH will the often present hypoxia and acidosis be detected. A Pao_2 of less than 50 torr is abnormal and indicative of mismatched ventilation and perfusion, whereas a $Paco_2$ greater than 45 torr indicates inadequate alveolar ventilation. A base deficit of less than -10 shortly after birth indicates a metabolic acidosis and suggests additional asphyxia to that occurring normally during the birth process.

PROCEDURE FOR RESUSCITATION

Establishing an Airway. As the fetal head is delivered secretions are removed from the mouth and nose with a bulb syringe. Failure to do so may result in partial or complete airway obstruction because infants are *obligatory* nasal breathers. Once delivered, if the infant is well, hold him at the introitus until the umbilical artery pulsations cease. Then cut the umbilical cord and transfer the infant to the resuscitation cart. Dry him with a towel to stimulate crying and to reduce evaporative heat loss. Maintain his body temperature between 36 and 37° C. with a servocontrolled infrared heater. Hypothermia may reduce pulmonary blood flow and cause hypoxemia, acidosis, and symptoms similar to those of hyaline membrane disease.

If at 1 minute of age the Apgar score is 8

TABLE 1. **The Apgar Scoring System***

Sign	0	1	2
Heart rate	Absent	Less than 100 per min.	More than 100 per min.
Respiratory effort	Absent	Slow, irregular	Good, crying
Muscle tone	Limp	Some flexion of extremities	Active motion
Reflex irritability (response to catheter in nose)	Absent	Grimace	Cough or sneeze
Color	Blue, pale	Body pink, extremities blue (acrocyanosis)	Completely pink

*Each sign is evaluated individually and is scored 0 to 2 at both 1 and 5 minutes of age. The final score at each age is the sum of the individual scores. (*From* Apgar, V.: A proposal for a new method of evaluation of the newborn infant. *Curr. Res. Anesth., 32*:260–267, 1953, with permission.)

to 10, little resuscitation is required. If it is 5 to 7, the asphyxia is usually mild and responds to vigorous stimulation and blowing warm humidified oxygen over the face. If the Apgar score is 3 or 4, the asphyxia is moderate but usually responds to ventilation with bag and mask and oxygen. If the Apgar score is 2 or less at 1 minute, the asphyxia is severe. Immediately intubate the trachea and ventilate the infant. The adequacy of ventilation is determined by expansion of the chest, a normal heart rate, disappearance of cyanosis, and normal breath sounds and blood gases. The pressure required to ventilate an asphyxiated infant is usually less than 25 cm. of water; rarely are higher inspiratory pressures required. Ventilatory rates of 20 to 50 per minute are usually adequate.

Tracheal Suctioning. Sixty per cent of infants born following meconium staining of the amniotic fluid have meconium below their vocal cords. If the meconium in the amniotic fluid is particulate or "pea soup" in nature, intubate the trachea immediately. Place a paper mask between the endotracheal tube connector and your mouth and suck on the endotracheal tube as it is withdrawn from the trachea. If meconium is retrieved, repeat the procedure a second time before ventilating the trachea with oxygen. If necessary, suction the airways again. Positive pressure ventilation prior to removing meconium from the trachea may result in respiratory failure, a pneumothorax and/or "pushing" meconium into the lung periphery where it cannot be retrieved. If large quantities of blood are present in the mouth at birth, tracheal intubation and suctioning are performed.

Correction of Acidosis. Correct respiratory acidosis by assisting ventilation with a bag and mask or bag and endotracheal tube. *Do not* attempt to correct respiratory acidosis with sodium bicarbonate; this often makes the situation worse in that $Paco_2$ rises if nothing is done to improve ventilation. Metabolic acidosis (base excess less than -10 mEq./liter) is initially corrected by assisting ventilation to raise the pH above 7.2. Repeat the blood gas and pH measurements in 5 minutes. If the base deficit and pH have not improved give sodium bicarbonate.* Care must be taken not to administer sodium bicarbonate indiscriminately or more rapidly than 1 mEq./kg./min., as this may cause severe respiratory acidosis ($HCO_3 + H+ \rightarrow CO_2$

_____

*The volume of sodium bicarbonate required to ¼ correct the base deficit is calculated by multiplying 0.3 × base deficit × body weight (kg.), and dividing the product by 2.

$+ H_2O$) if ventilation is inadequate. To avoid the possible CO_2 increase, assist ventilation during administration of this drug. A sudden increase in cerebral vascular volume, as may occur with more rapid injection of this hypertonic solution or with an increase in $Paco_2$, may suddenly increase intravascular pressure, rupture cerebral vessels and cause intracranial hemorrhage.

Vascular Resuscitation. Blood volume expansion. Infants asphyxiated immediately before or during the birth process are often hypovolemic, hypotensive and acidotic. The presence of hypotension will only be appreciated if arterial blood pressure of every newborn infant is measured in the delivery room. Hypotension in this situation usually means hypovolemia, the diagnosis of which is made when the mean or systolic arterial pressure is less than two standard deviations from the mean (Table 2) or the *intrathoracic* venous pressure is less than 3 cm. of water, the pulse volume is diminished, skin color is pale, and/or capillary refill takes longer than 3 seconds.

Hypovolemia is initially treated with 10 ml./kg. of blood, or 1 gm./kg. of albumin, or 10 ml./kg. of Ringer's lactate, or 10 ml./kg. of plasma. It may be necessary to give even more volume before central venous and arterial pressures return to normal. If one has advance notice of a high-risk delivery, cross-match 0 negative, low titer blood against the mother prior to delivery so that the blood can be given to the infant in the delivery room if necessary. Hypotension may also occur with severe al-

TABLE 2.   Average Systolic, Diastolic and Mean Blood Pressures (Torr) During the First Two Hours of Life in Normal Newborn Infants Grouped According to Birth Weight*

BIRTH WEIGHT	AGE	
	1 Hour	*2 Hours*
1001 to 2000 gm.		
Systolic	49	49
Diastolic	26	27
Mean	35	36
2001 to 3000 gm.		
Systolic	59	57
Diastolic	32	32
Mean	43	41
3000 gm.		
Systolic	70	67
Diastolic	44	41
Mean	53	51

_____

*From Kitterman, J. A., et al.: Aortic blood pressure in normal newborn infants during the first 12 hours of life. Pediatrics, 44:959–968, 1969 with permission.

kalosis (overvigorous assisted ventilation) or maternal intoxication with alcohol or magnesium. These causes of hypotension are usually easily differentiated from other causes of hypotension because the former have normal peripheral color and slightly diminished or increased peripheral perfusion. The blood volume of alkalotic and intoxicated patients may need expanding, but do so cautiously. Hypermagnesemia may be treated by a judicious infusion of 100 to 200 mg./kg. of calcium gluconate while monitoring the electrocardiogram. A pneumothorax and/or pneumomediastinum must always be considered in a hypotensive infant.

Cardiac Massage.   Do closed chest massage if the heart rate is less than 100 beats per minute at one minute of age and fails to increase immediately with stimulation and ventilation. Place the fingers of both hands behind the infant's back and the thumbs over the junction of the middle and lower third of the body of the sternum (Fig. 1). Compress the sternum two thirds of the distance to the vertebral column 100 times a minute and attempt to develop a systolic arterial pressure of approximately 80 torr. This combination of rate and pressure will usually maintain the diastolic arterial pressure at or above 20 torr, which is probably adequate for coronary artery perfusion. During cardiac massage, ventilate the infant approximately 30 times per minute. The effectiveness of cardiac massage is determined by continuously measuring arterial blood pressure through an umbilical artery catheter and examining the pupils. Adequate perfusion and oxygenation are occurring if the pupils are small or midsized.

Drugs.   If the electrocardiogram is flat give 0.1 ml./kg. of a 1:10,000 mixture of epi-

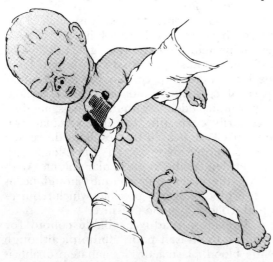

Figure 1.

nephrine and saline while continuing closed chest massage. Repeat this dose as often as necessary to produce a cardiac rhythm. For severe bradycardia give .03 mg./kg. of atropine intravascularly. If atropine does not increase heart rate, infuse isoproterenol (4 mg. in 250 ml. of 5 per cent dextrose in water) until the heart rate increases. At this point rapidly reduce the rate of infusion to keep the heart rate within the normal range. If clinically the cardiac output is still depressed, give 0.25 ml./kg. of a 10 per cent solution of calcium chloride intravascularly. All of these drugs are more effective if the pH is above 7.1. Therefore, assist ventilation and give bicarbonate as needed. Continue resuscitation as long as there is reasonable hope for a neurologically intact child.

Respiratory Distress Syndrome

LOUIS GLUCK, M.D.

All infants with respiratory distress syndrome (RDS) or hyaline membrane disease require therapy for shock, which very often is present at the outset of symptoms and which always develops as infants worsen. Shock in the newborn is characterized by shunting of blood from pulmonary (with patent ductus arteriosus), renal, mesenteric, and skin circulations; with subsequent generalized hypoperfusion of tissues, but increased cardiac output and brain circulation. The hypoperfusion causes inadequate tissue respirations, primarily oxidative metabolism, resulting in lactic acidemia and metabolic acidosis. It is imperative that therapy for shock be instituted as early as possible in the course of RDS, prior to or concurrent with application of any continuous positive airway pressure (CPAP) techniques, since these may worsen shock by decreasing cardiac output, decreasing pulmonary venous return, and decreasing total pulmonary blood flow.

The management is divided into three sections: stabilization and essential supportive care, ventilatory management, and proper follow-up care.

STABILIZATION AND ESSENTIAL SUPPORTIVE CARE

Resuscitation.   All other things being equal, a depressed newborn who develops RDS will be affected more severely than one born with a good Apgar score. Therefore, resuscitation, stabilization, and supportive care of the small newborn baby must be immediate and aggressive. Hopefully, the fetus will have been monitored during labor, so that the condition of the baby at birth and the plan for management can be anticipated before birth. This requires that adequate personnel and equipment be present at delivery. *All* personnel who handle newborns *must* be trained in evaluation, resuscitation, and the delivery of supportive care to the newborn.

Equipment for immediate use must include an anesthesia bag, an adequate assortment of masks to fit any size infant, a variety of airways (both oropharyngeal and endotracheal), a pencil handle laryngoscope and bulb syringes and DeLee traps for suctioning. This equipment must be checked daily and must be in good working order. Proper resuscitation must be instituted whenever necessary for apnea or profound hypoventilation and immediately at birth if a baby is depressed.

Perhaps the most important skill to be learned is the proper use of an anesthesia bag. Aneroid manometers calibrated in centimeters of water pressure must be included on-line, enabling personnel instituting resuscitation with an anesthesia bag to know exactly what pressures they are delivering.

The second most important skill is the proper use of the laryngoscope and endotracheal tube. The laryngoscope blade has a flange to provide oral exposure by displacing the tongue to the left side of the mouth; the instrument itself is designed for right-handed people. With the laryngoscope in the left hand, the blade is inserted into the right corner of the mouth and extended along the right side of the tongue (with the infant supine) to about halfway to the uvula. The blade is swung to the left to move the tongue completely out of the way and then the tip is advanced into the vallecula, the space directly in front of the glottis. The airway should be cleared of secretions. The fifth finger of the left hand pushes slightly upward on the trachea below the larynx to elevate and expose the larynx, while the rest of the left hand holding the laryngoscope pushes directly forward and upward, not levered back, which would obscure vision.

The baby's head during laryngoscopy must not be hyperextended. The larynx in tiny babies is not at the lower cervical segments, but rather at the level of C3 to C4, directly below the base of the tongue. Thus the maneuver described above, of pushing the left hand forward and up with the laryngoscope tip in the vallecula while pressing up just below the larynx, easily elevates the larnyx into view so long as the head is either flat on the pad or bed or even slightly flexed.

Warmth. Low birth weight babies, especially prematures, have a great surface area in relation to their mass, lack adequate fatty sub-cutaneous insulation, and usually are born into cold delivery rooms. Not only is an excessive expenditure of energy required to try to stay warm, but hypothermia also produces severe metabolic acidosis, decreases pulmonary blood flow, and can be profoundly additive and worsen other conditions depressing the neonate (such as drugs or asphyxia).

During the tension of resuscitation of a depressed infant the necessity of keeping the baby warm is frequently forgotten. Right after birth the neonate should be dried, especially to prevent evaporative losses, even as other resuscitative efforts are made. There should be an open radiant heater in the delivery room under which procedures are done; together with drying the baby, this helps maximally to prevent hypothermia. The continuing therapy must include provisions to keep the baby warm. The very small infant even under radiant heat may be kept under a cradle made from transparent plastic wrap (such as Saran) and kept at an axillary temperature of 36 to 37° C.

Specific Management of Shock. The mnemonic VIP stands for ventilation + infusion → perfusion and describes the plan for the management of shock. It is important in the initial stabilization to overventilate the baby somewhat, especially if the infant is depressed and therefore probably has significant metabolic acidosis. Hyperventilation will produce a relative ventilatory alkalosis, and even before the pH rises significantly, the *trend* for pH to rise appears sufficient to open clamped down, nonperfusing pulmonary, renal, mesenteric, and skin blood vessels. Clinically, one usually sees a generalized flush; the baby tends to become pink even though this color may reflect perfusion of blood through skin rather than arterial Po_2.

Infusion should be done with colloid solutions because small babies have low total serum protein (frequently 3 gm./100 ml. or less) and because the rapid distribution from the intravascular space into the extracellular space of crystalloid solutions without colloid may produce edema, without at the same time necessarily correcting the intravascular volume. If CPAP is used the resultant decreased cardiac output may worsen this edema and further deplete the intravascular volume. With CPAP, the circulating volume should be as high as physiologically possible, which requires a high colloid osmotic pressure.

The most readily available colloid for stabilization is salt-poor albumin, although whole blood, plasma, or Plasmanate probably is preferable if available. Normally after the first day, fluids are infused at a rate of from 80 to about 100 ml./kg./24 hours, whereas on the first day this may be as low as 60 ml./kg., although an infant under an open radiant heater will require 80 to 150 ml./kg./day on the first day and 125 to 150 ml./kg./day thereafter unless very carefully wrapped to prevent evaporation. For a particular infant the fluid intake must be individualized. All maintenance fluids should contain salt-poor albumin (1 to 2 gm./kg./24 hours) as well as calcium gluconate, 200 mg./kg./24 hours. Additional salt-poor albumin can be given as needed to correct metabolic acidosis due to volume depletion. This is usually given 1 gm. at a time. Potassium (2 to 3 mEq./kg./24 hours) must be given as the chloride and/or acetate, and the total sodium intake is calculated at 5 mEq./kg./24 hours. Whole blood or packed red cells must be given as frequently as necessary to keep the hematocrit at 45 per cent.

An infant's clinical signs must be observed carefully since therapy in large part is guided by what one sees. Monitoring the heart rate, respiratory effort, skin color, response to stimuli, and general tone—in other words, a continuing recapitulating of the Apgar findings, in the special care unit or nursery—is an excellent clinical way to check on the status of the infant.

Alkalinizing Agents.   The indications for the use of sodium bicarbonate in correcting metabolic acidosis are not clear. There are few instances where volume expansion with colloids and slight hyperventilation do not raise the pH promptly. Potential morbidity from a low pH probably exists where the pH is below 7.2 and if the acidosis is prolonged. If the pH is below 7.2, sodium bicarbonate probably is indicated to hasten correction of the acidosis, remembering that pH is a logarithmic expression, and therefore at a pH of 7.1 there is a several-fold excess of [H+] over that at a pH of 7.2. Sodium bicarbonate is supplied in a concentration of 1 mEq./ml. and should be diluted in half before administration.

The dose of bicarbonate is calculated by multiplying base deficit times body weight in kilograms times 0.3. This should be administered *slowly,* preferably through a central arterial umbilical catheter placed in the abdominal aorta below L3; or a venous catheter placed in the inferior vena cava; and only *half the calculated dose* should be given. If reasonable partial correction has not occurred within 20 to 40 minutes, then the rest can be given, although this seldom is necessary if the stabilization has been done well. In respiratory acidosis sodium bicarbonate is contraindicated and actually may increase the Paco$_2$.

Antibiotics.   There is recent awareness of the fulminant disease in newborns produced by infection with group B beta hemolytic streptococcus. Ordinarily larger infants born at or near term are infected. The signs and symptoms of sepsis and pneumonia with this organism may be similar to those of hyaline membrane disease. Many large infants in the past said to have had hyaline membrane disease may well have had this disease. Initially the x-ray may resemble that seen in early hyaline membrane disease, but frequently fluid both in the interlobar fissure and at the bases of the lungs may help differentiate this from RDS. Because of the potentially fulminant course of this disease, it is our policy to start any baby of 2000 gm. birth weight or more with a clinical picture suggesting RDS on an immediate, rapid intravenous infusion of 250,000 units of crystalline penicillin, to be followed by a minimum of 100,000 units per kilogram every 12 hours.

It probably is best to start all babies with presumed RDS on antibiotics; about 20 per cent of those autopsied with hyaline membrane disease also have significant bacterial pneumonia. It usually is impossible in RDS to differentiate a baby with pneumonia from one without. It is our practice to draw blood cultures (and others as indicated) on neonates with findings of RDS and to institute antibiotics for about three days while awaiting results of cultures. We utilize broad spectrum coverage with an aminoglycoside such as gentamicin plus penicillin or ampicillin.

Nutrition.   For a baby to recover from RDS it is essential that starvation be prevented or minimized. A newborn and especially a premature, requires minimally about 60 calories per kilogram just to prevent weight loss. Glucose may help prevent breakdown of protein for gluconeogenesis. However, only infants who are not breathing hard or rapidly may safely be fed and then by gavage. Babies with retractions and high ventilatory rates are not candidates for oral feeding or for gavage, but can be fed successfully through transpyloric (sometimes called nasojejunal) tubes.

The food of choice without question is breast milk. Recent evidence shows that once birth weight is regained, small prematures then gain at about the same rate as premature infants on cow's milk formulas. Furthermore, the protein in cow's milk qualitatively is vastly different in amino acid composition from that of breast milk. Certain amino acids such as tyrosine and phenylalanine, associated with brain damage in tyrosinosis and phenylketonuria where they are not metabolized properly, may be found in excessively high levels in the blood of babies fed cow's milk. Moreover, Gaull and associates showed recently that human breast milk contains large amounts of sulfurylated taurine, whereas cow's milk contains very little. Taurine is an apparent neurotransmitter and may be essential to brain growth in the fetus. It thus seems essential that human breast milk, preferably from a baby's own mother, be the food of choice.

VENTILATORY MANAGEMENT

Physiologically there are significant differences between infants who weigh less than 1500 gm. at birth and those who weigh more than 1500 gm., in problems of management and in the outcomes of these two groups of babies. Babies weighing more than 1500 gm. at birth appear to have sufficient reserve to withstand various approaches to therapy and a high percentage live. On the other hand, one must be "aggressively cautious" with a tiny baby if the infant is to survive.

The diagnosis of hyaline membrane disease, in addition to the clinical findings (such as rapid respiratory rate, suprasternal and substernal and intercostal retractions, expiratory grunt, shunting, and so on), requires an obligatory oxygen need. Thus, the *initial* therapy around which the stabilization and support described above is provided, is a trial of oxygen for the infant in a hood. A proportion of babies, those with mild RDS, can be managed on hood oxygen alone. However, a significantly high percentage of babies develop ventilatory failure and require some form of ventilatory assistance in addition to oxygen.

Ventilatory failure in an infant is diagnosed by increasing oxygen needs, exceeding 60 per cent FiO_2 while unable to maintain an arterial oxygen concentration (Pao_2) of 50 torr. Other indications for ventilatory assistance, in addition to increasing oxygen demands, include a rising $Paco_2$, which reflects a significant respiratory acidosis usually with hypoventilation, and, of course, apnea.

The prime dictum in ventilatory assistance in RDS is to do no harm; use the mildest possible indicated form of therapy for RDS when there is ventilatory failure. In the experience of the author, once ventilatory failure is established where the infant is not able to oxygenate adequately at an FiO_2 of 60 per cent, mechanical ventilation is indicated for infants who weigh *less* than 1500 gm. Those who weigh more than 1500 gm., however, should be given an initial trial on some form of CPAP. Noninvasive (endotracheal intubation not used) CPAP techniques include nasal prongs, mask CPAP (which may compress the nose unless set up expertly) and continuous negative pressure (CNP) applied externally to the chest wall by bypassing the cycling mechanism of a negative pressure ventilator which is then kept in a constant negative mode. These techniques may be effective in prematures weighing more than 1500 gm., but seldom are effective in those under 1500 gm.

Ordinarily infants weighing more than 1500 gm. are continued on noninvasive CPAP to an FiO_2 of 80 per cent. If a Pao_2 of 50 torr is not maintained, then the baby either may be intubated and put on standard CPAP described originally by Gregory or, more usually, is treated with mechanical ventilation. At the University of California Medical Center, San Diego, we prefer mechanical ventilation for babies weighing less than 1500 gm. who are in respiratory failure (Pao_2 less than 50 torr in 60 per cent FiO_2), and do not first give the infant a trial on CPAP. The mechanical ventilator used in our Infant Special Care Center is a pressure-controlled, continuous flow unit, the BABYbird (although the pressure controlled Bourns ventilator may be utilized similarly). Ventilator settings depend upon the size of the

TABLE 1. Ventilator Settings

	INITIALLY	AFTER INFANT STABILIZES
Peak inspiratory pressure (cm. of H_2O)		
Birth weight < 1500 gm.	18 to 20, up to 25	18 to 20, up to 25
≥ 1500 gm.	20 to 25, up to 35	18 to 25
Positive end expiratory pressure (cm. of H_2O)	2 to 4	2 to 4
Inspiratory time (seconds)	1.0	1.0 to 2.0
Ventilatory rate (cycles/minutes)	20 to 30	10 to 20 or fewer

infant as outlined and described in the table and text below.

The mechanical ventilation of infants weighing less than 1500 gm. is begun with very low inspiratory pressures, usually 18 to 20 cm. of water, and relatively low ventilatory rates, seldom exceeding 20, except where prematures are severely depressed or where it is difficult to initiate aeration. The pressures required to expand the chest during initial stabilization with an anesthesia bag may be as high as 35 cm. of water; however, these are acute insufflations with very short inspiratory time. In transferring such an infant to a ventilator with a one-second inspiratory time, pressures are started at 18 to 20 cm. of water.

With the prolonged inspiratory time and PEEP, lung expansion is relatively easy, with recruitment of collapsed alveoli rather than overexpansion of partly open alveoli as occurs with short burst, high pressure ventilation. Larger babies weighing more than 1500 gm., according to their needs, may be begun on higher pressures and higher rates. *Initial* inspiratory time for all babies is one second, timed by a stopwatch mounted on the BABYbird ventilator. The positive end expiratory pressure (PEEP) necessary to maintain open alveoli need never exceed 2 to 4 cm.; usually 2 cm. of water pressure is adequate and seldom must exceed 4 cm. even in large babies.

After a baby is stabilized, the acidosis is corrected and the infant's oxygenation and general condition have improved, attempts are made to reduce the ventilatory rates and peak inspiratory pressure gradually. The rate is decreased to 20 cycles/minute or less, while at the same time the inspiratory time may be lengthened to 1.5 or a maximum of 2 seconds. During the first two days, especially, the attempt is made to keep total inspiratory time (the ventilatory rate times the inspiratory time) at about 30 seconds per minute. I:E ratios in this ventilatory management are ignored because neonates are encouraged to breathe spontaneously by the intermittent mandatory ventilation plus the continuous flow which maintains a low PEEP. The rate is reduced and then the inspiratory time is brought gradually down as the baby is weaned from the ventilator. As weaning progresses, the infant is encouraged to breathe more of the time as the ventilatory rate is reduced to about 4 cycles per minute. It thus becomes a process of sighing the infant periodically while maintaining some continuous positive distending pressure at very low levels and allowing the baby to heal.

In our experience these ventilatory techniques are followed by little discernible residual lung disease; the course of RDS usually is over within about 72 hours to 5 to 7 days at the longest in the smallest and sickest infants. Experience with this ventilation at our institution furthermore has shown that in infants weighing 1200 gm. or more, one can expect 96 per cent or more of these babies to survive with minimal or no complications.

A significant problem complicating RDS and frequently requiring intervention is patent ductus arteriosus (see also p. 142). This enjoys a high incidence among small premature infants and is characterized clinically by the failure to progress by an infant with RDS who had been getting better, who then stops getting better, and who may begin to require higher FiO_2 or increasing settings on the ventilator to maintain adequate Pao_2. Physical examination may reveal the murmur, bounding pulses, and so on, while the x-ray may show increased vascular markings with shunt vessels and often pulmonary edema and cardiomegaly. When a trial on medical management (fluid restriction and digitalization especially) fails, it has been customary to treat patent ductus arteriosus surgically with ligation.

Recently, pharmacologic intervention with indomethacin has yielded highly encouraging results, where nearly all patent ductus arteriosus close, usually after one dose and almost assuredly by three doses, with very infrequent failures. Indomethacin or similar prostaglandin synthetase inhibitors will likely be included in the pharmacopeia as the drugs of choice in the treatment of patent ductus arteriosus associated with RDS.

The recent suggestion about the use of corticosteroids administered to women in premature labor to accelerate maturity of fetal lung is still controversial at this writing and also may be defined clearly by the next edition. At this writing it is fair to say that steroids appear to be effective, even though too few controlled studies exist, but the dangers and potential long-term problems from their use are presently unclear.

FOLLOW-UP CARE

It is essential to make provisions for adequate follow-up of infants who have had RDS (and, in general, of all high-risk infants). Adequate follow-up is a costly business for which currently there is little governmental or institutional support. Consequently, follow-up programs increasingly have been deemphasized, and relatively few institutions now sponsor adequate follow-up. Moreover, studies by Dr. Charlotte White at our institution show that the average practicing pediatrician who follows those babies on discharge from a tertiary center does not order proper hearing tests or eye tests, or examine infants in enough depth to detect early minimal signs of neurological abnormalities.

The field of perinatal medicine continues to produce a major proportion of individuals with cerebral palsy, brain damage, epilepsy, mental retardation, minimal brain damage, behavior disorders and, at school age, communication disorders, including dyslexia. It is absolutely essential that provisions be made to follow babies physiologically and neurologically, especially during the first 1 to 2 years; to have very early hearing testing; and to evaluate each high risk baby for adequacy of vision very early. Should abnormalities be found it is much easier to rehabilitate a young handicapped infant rather than an older child with significant defects that should have been detected and treated much earlier.

Disorders of the Umbilicus

IRWIN J. LIGHT, M.D.

The umbilical cord, vital for survival of the fetus prior to birth, becomes obsolescent at the instant of birth. Severance of the umbilical cord initiates degeneration resulting a few days later in separation of the stump. Within hours the cord begins to dry and shrink; within 1 to 2 days the stump is dry, firm, and mummified; within 5 to 10 days separation of the stump is complete. Care of the umbilicus through the ages has varied with the time and place. Today's concerns relating to the medical management of the umbilicus are focused mainly on prevention and treatment of infection and hemorrhage, and care of congenital malformations.

ROUTINE MANAGEMENT

After birth the umbilicus is one of the first sites to be colonized by bacteria. From this site pathogenic organisms may be spread to other body sites, may be disseminated to other infants and adults in the nursery by the contaminated hands of infant caretakers, or may produce systemic disease by entering the surgical wound established in the umbilical stump. Today, the importance of aseptic technique in cutting the umbilical cord and the hazards of applying nonsterile substances to the severed umbilical stump are self-evident.

After severance of the cord, attempts are made to maintain a dry uncontaminated umbilical site. Since the growth of microorganisms is enhanced by a moist environment, drying of the umbilical stump is encouraged; application of 70 per cent alcohol to the umbilicus on admission to the nursery and once daily thereafter during the nursery stay is suitable for this purpose. In order to prevent bacterial contamination a succession of potions, poultices, and medicines has been applied to this site over the years, procedures in themselves often responsible for contamination or enhancement of infection. More recently, efforts to minimize colonization by pathogenic bacteria have included the routine application of a wide variety of topical soaps, lotions, ointments, dyes, and powders with or without antibacterial agents. The benefits of these agents have often been unproved; they frequently inadvertently encourage the proliferation of an undesirable bacterial flora, and at times they have toxic systemic effects when applied to the skin of newborn infants. The American Academy of Pediatrics currently recommends a "dry technique" for routine newborn skin care. In nonepidemic periods it is recommended that no antibacterial agents be applied to the skin or to the umbilicus. If an antibacterial agent is required, triple dye [each ml. contains brilliant green (2.29 mg.), gentian violet (2.29 mg.), and proflavine hemisulfate (1.14 mg.) in distilled water] has been used. This is applied to the umbilical site on admission to the nursery and once daily. In infants with indwelling umbilical vessel catheters the topical application of antibiotic ointment to the umbilical site has not been proved effective in decreasing systemic infection.

In nursery epidemics of staphylococcal disease, the infants are the usual reservoir of infection and the umbilicus is the most frequently colonized site. In addition to other conventional control measures, effective elimination of this reservoir may require special management of the umbilical site of all infants. Treatment of the umbilicus with triple dye, antibiotic ointment (bacitracin), or purposeful colonization of the umbilical stump and external nares with a relatively nonpathogenic strain of *Staphylococcus aureus* (502A) may be indicated.

INFECTION

The umbilical stump is frequently colonized with staphylococci, gram-negative bacilli, and streptococci. In the absence of disease, isolation of either of the two former organisms is not a suitable indication for local or systemic antibiotic therapy. Isolation of group B streptococci from the umbilical site in asymptomatic infants is considered by some to be an indication for systemic treatment with penicillin.

Infection at the umbilical site may result in localized omphalitis, cellulitis or abscess; infection may extend by direct spread producing portal thrombophlebitis or peritonitis; or infection may be disseminated by the hematogenous route producing sepsis, pneumonia, or meningitis. Therefore all newborn infants with umbilical infection must be treated with a full course of systemic antibiotics which would include a penicillin and an aminoglycoside as indicated in the treatment for neonatal sepsis.

Typically the omphalitis caused by group A streptococcus is an uncomplicated low-grade indolent granulating infection which fails to heal. Treatment should include systemic penicillin.

In primitive societies even today the necrotic umbilical cord stump, contaminated by dirt and other foreign materials, remains the single most common portal of entry for infection with tetanus bacilli. In addition to the general management and systemic treatment of infants with tetanus neonatorum, attention must be given to the umbilical stump. Debridement of the infected site and cleansing with an antibacterial soap followed by repeated washing with hydrogen peroxide during the next 48 hours are recommended. Neither excision of the umbilicus nor local infiltration about the umbilicus with tetanus antitoxin is recommended.

UMBILICAL GRANULOMA

Following separation of the umbilical stump, delayed healing most frequently results from granulation tissue at the umbilical site. The umbilical granuloma which results will usually disappear after cauterization with silver nitrate. Sometimes a second treatment may be necessary, but if healing does not occur after two to three weeks of treatment, the possibility of a patent omphalomesenteric duct or urachus should be considered.

CONGENITAL MALFORMATIONS

Single Umbilical Artery. A frequent malformation of the umbilical stump occurring in approximately 1 per cent of infants is the presence of two umbilical vessels including one artery and one vein, in contrast to the normal two arteries and one vein. The anomaly itself is not harmful but because of the association with other malformations, recognition of this lesion may provide a useful clue to latent deformities. Unfortunately, after the first few hours of life the dry mummified umbilical cord may make visualization of the umbilical vessels impossi-

ble. Removal of a section of umbilical cord immediately after birth or of dry mummified cord, which is then placed in a bottle containing 3 per cent acetic acid, results in a firm translucent specimen in which the vessels can be evaluated even days later.

Umbilical Hernia. As a result of incomplete closure of the fascia of the umbilical ring, intraabdominal contents may protrude through the anterior abdominal wall. Although the defect is present at birth, herniation frequently does not occur until several weeks after birth. The protruding mass most often contains small bowel and is covered by skin. The hernia is easily reducible; incarceration is rare, and spontaneous closure occurs in most infants.

Since spontaneous closure of the defect is so common, the initial treatment of choice in the absence of small bowel obstruction is reassurance of the parents and observation of the lesion. Strapping is probably of no benefit in hastening the closure of the defect. Although it is agreed that early surgery is not indicated for uncomplicated lesions, surgical opinion regarding the optimal timing of surgery varies depending on the size of the defect and the age of the infant. Elective repair is usually not performed unless the fascial defect is unusually large (greater than 2 cm.) or if the defect persists beyond three years of age.

Omphalocele. Early in fetal life the midgut which extends into the umbilical stalk enters the abdominal cavity which closes anteriorly around these organs. Failure of completion of this process results in a protrusion of the abdominal viscera into the base of the umbilical cord. The protrusion is covered by a transparent membranous sac which may rupture in utero resulting in exposed bowel. After birth, loss of fluid from the exposed intestine can result in hypovolemic shock. Other major congenital anomalies are often present.

The sac should be kept moist with warm saline-soaked gauze dressings, being careful not to allow the infant to become cold as a result of the increased evaporative heat loss. Hypovolemic shock should be treated by the administration of plasma expanders. Since this lesion is a life-threatening surgical emergency, the infant, once stabilized, should be transferred directly to a medical center for further management by a pediatric surgeon. Appropriate surgery can be life-saving but depending on the degree of prematurity, the severity of illness of the infant, associated anomalies, the presence of infection, and the size of the sac, surgery may not be indicated or may be deferred. Under these circumstances, if the integrity of the sac can be maintained, the skin will slowly grow over the sac. This process can be hastened by painting the sac with 2 per cent aqueous Mercurochrome every four to six hours until a tough eschar is formed. The eschar is then slowly replaced by skin. Although merbromin (Mercurochrome) is most commonly used for this purpose, toxicity can occur as a result of absorption of mercury from the surface of the sac. For this reason some surgeons prefer to use silver nitrate or povidone-iodine, although application of these will result in the absorption of silver or iodine respectively.

Patent Omphalomesenteric Duct or Urachus. Persistence of the primitive omphalomesenteric duct can result in a communication between the umbilicus and the terminal ileum. Failure of obliteration of the allantois may result in a communication between the bladder and the umbilicus. Persistence of either of these fetal structures may be recognized as a mass or discharge of mucous, feces or urine from the umbilical site. The diagnosis is confirmed radiologically and the lesion should be repaired by a pediatric surgeon.

HEMORRHAGE

Bleeding from the umbilical vessels prior to birth probably occurs more frequently than is generally recognized. This is most likely to occur as a result of abnormal placental insertion of the umbilical vessels (e.g., vasa previa). Significant maternal vaginal bleeding can occur which may not always be recognized as fetal blood; the placenta may not be examined for the presence of disrupted vessels, and the hematocrit may be normal. In any acute blood loss, time must elapse before hemodilution will result in a decreasing hematocrit. In any infant with poor peripheral perfusion in the delivery room, blood loss with resultant hypovolemia must be considered and immediate treatment with plasma expanders may be life-saving.

Significant blood loss from the severed umbilical vessels after birth is an uncommon occurrence in the normal full-term infant, especially if attention has been paid to securing the clamps or ties on the umbilical stump. In sick or asphyxiated newborn or premature infants, pulsation of the umbilical vessels may be prolonged, thus increasing the risk of bleeding from this site. For infants with significant blood loss, replacement transfusion is indicated. Persisting oozing from the umbilical stump should be considered evidence of a possible defect in hemostasis. The slight oozing that sometimes occurs at the time of separation of the umbilical cord does not require treatment.

Infants of Drug Addicted Mothers

ENRIQUE M. OSTREA, Jr., M.D. *and*
PAUL V. WOOLLEY, Jr., M.D.

Passive addiction can occur in the neonate as a result of the chronic use of drugs by the mother during pregnancy. As a consequence, signs of withdrawal may be noted in the infant soon after birth. It should be noted that passive neonatal addiction can occur with *narcotic* and *non-narcotic* agents. Among the narcotic drugs, the most common form of neonatal addiction is that secondary to heroin and methadone, whereas among the non-narcotic drugs, neonatal addiction has been reported secondary to maternal intake of barbiturates, bromide, ethchlorvynol (Placidyl), diazepam (Valium), chlordiazepoxide (Librium), glutethimide (Doriden) and alcohol. Passive addiction in the neonate to non-narcotic agents can occur even when low therapeutic doses are taken by the mother.

Manifestations of withdrawal (abstinence syndrome) secondary to narcotic and non-narcotic addiction in the neonate are essentially similar. The onset is soon after birth, usually within the first 24 to 48 hours of life. However, withdrawal may occur early, within the first 12 hours if the mother exhibited withdrawal during labor. In contrast, withdrawal from barbiturates, especially phenobarbital, has been reported to occur as late as 1 to 2 weeks after birth. This may be related to the delayed excretion of the drug by the infants.

The withdrawal manifestations can be grouped into major and minor types. The major ones are those which could be life-threatening if unchecked—vomiting, diarrhea, weight loss, irritability (including hypertonicity and high-pitched cry), tremors and tachypnea. The minor manifestations are sweating, fist sucking, sneezing and yawning. Although tremors are frequently encountered in neonatal withdrawal from narcotics, frank convulsions are rare. In contrast, withdrawal from non-narcotics is more likely to involve convulsions.

The diagnosis of drug withdrawal, suspected from the symptom complex presented, is confirmed by maternal history and identification, by chromatographic methods, of the drug or its metabolites in the urine of the mother or the infant. The infant of the heroin addicted mother not infrequently is of low birth weight and may even be small for gestational age. In contrast, the infant of the methadone maintained mother is usually of normal birth weight or heavier, particularly if

TABLE 1.   Assessment of the Clinical Severity of Neonatal Narcotic Withdrawal

	MILD	MODERATE	SEVERE
Vomiting	Spitting up	Extensive vomiting for 3 successive feedings	Vomiting associated with imbalance of serum electrolytes
Diarrhea	Watery stools < 4 times per day	Watery stools 5 or 6 times per day for 3 days. No electrolyte imbalance.	Diarrhea associated with imbalance of serum electrolytes
Weight loss	< 10 per cent of birth weight	11 to 15 per cent of birth weight	> 15 per cent
Irritability	Minimal	Severe but relieved by cuddling or feeding	Unrelieved by cuddling or feeding
Tremors or twitching*	Mild tremors when stimulated	Severe tremors or twitching when stimulated	Convulsions
Tachypnea	60 to 80/minute	80/100 minute	> 100/minute and associated with respiratory alkalosis

*Tremors or twitchings, as opposed to convulsions, were episodic myoclonic jerks which could be abolished by restraint of the involved extremity. (After Ostrea, E. M., et al. J. Pediat., 88:642, 1976.)

the mother is on a high daily dose of methadone. The differential diagnoses of drug withdrawal include sepsis, hypoglycemia, hypocalcemia, hypomagnesemia, meningitis, infectious diarrhea and drug toxicity secondary to maternal use of lithium, chlorpromazine or tricyclic antidepressants such as imipramine (Tofranil).

In view of the scant information available regarding neonatal withdrawal from nonnarcotic drugs, the subsequent discussion deals mainly with neonatal withdrawal from narcotics.

A system for the clinical assessment of the severity of the neonatal narcotic withdrawal is necessary to serve as a guideline for treatment and prognosis. It has been shown that the severity of neonatal withdrawal is directly related to the dose of methadone taken by the mother. However, such a relationship has not been established for heroin. A direct relationship has also been found between the severity of withdrawal and the persistence of withdrawal manifestations, which on some occasions can last for as long as 6 to 8 weeks. The severity of withdrawal is classified as mild, moderate or severe, based on the criteria outlined in Table 1.

In view of the hyperirritability, infants should be swaddled and cuddled more often. The frequency of diarrhea and vomiting is noted, and the infant is weighed three times daily. Temperature and respiratory rates are taken every four hours. Laboratory examinations to detect serum electrolyte and pH imbalance are done, if indicated. It is not necessary to keep the infant in a special, quiet and dark room, as this has not been found to ameliorate the intensity of withdrawal. The use of drugs to treat the withdrawal syndrome is based on the severity of the manifestations: (1) the presence of five or more mild criteria, (2) moderate vomiting, diarrhea or weight loss, or (3) severe criterion.

Both narcotic and non-narcotic drugs have been used: paregoric, 3 to 6 drops every 4 to 6 hours; chlorpromazine,* 2 to 3 mg./kg./day in 4 divided doses; phenobarbital, 3 to 6 mg./kg./day every 6 hours; and diazepam,† 1 mg. intramuscularly every 8 hours. Although these drugs have all been shown to be effective in treating withdrawal manifestations, we prefer

*Manufacturer's precaution: Chlorpromazine should not be used in children under 6 months except where potentially life-saving.

†Manufacturer's precaution: The safety and efficacy of injectable diazepam have not been established in the neonate.

to use a narcotic agent, since its action is more physiologic during an abstinence state. Besides, although the central nervous system manifestations of withdrawal can be successfully diminished by the aforementioned drugs, the narcotic agents seem to be most effective in relieving the gastrointestinal manifestations, especially diarrhea.

Among the narcotic drugs currently used, we prefer tincture of opium U.S.P. (laudanum) instead of paregoric, since the latter contains camphor which is a known CNS stimulant. It should be carefully noted that laudanum comes as a 10 per cent solution and contains 1.0 per cent morphine, whereas paregoric only contains 0.04 per cent morphine. Therefore, to yield a concentration of morphine equivalent to that present in paregoric, laudanum should be diluted 25-fold. At this dilution (0.04 per cent), laudanum can be given at the same dose as paregoric (3 to 6 drops every 4 to 6 hours).

The aim of the treatment with drugs is to render the infant comfortable, but not obtunded. Thus the drug should be titrated starting with the smallest recommended dose until the desired effect is achieved. Once the infant is asymptomatic, the drug can then be tapered slowly until it is completely discontinued. This usually takes from 4 to 6 days. The infant should still be observed for a day or two after the discontinuance of the drug for the possible recurrence of the symptoms (rebound phenomenon). When the infant is discharged from the nursery, the mother should be instructed to anticipate some mild jitteriness and irritability that may persist in the infant for 4 to 6 weeks, depending on the initial severity of the withdrawal.

Breast Feeding

R. M. APPLEBAUM, M.D.

Breast Milk Jaundice. Breast feeding may result in indirect jaundice during the first month or two of life. The incidence is rare—about 1 in 200 breast fed babies. The milk may contain a steroid metabolite of progesterone, pregnane-3 (a), 20 (beta)-diol, which inhibits glucuronyl transferase, an enzyme that conjugates bilirubin. Indirect hyperbilirubinemia occurs about the fifth day of life or toward the end of the first week, and reaches a peak by the second or the third week. Levels of 20 mg. per 100 ml. or more are infrequent, but have been reached during these peaks. The babies appear well and demonstrate only a yellow color of the skin, eyes, and serum. No cases of kernicterus

have been reported and the development of the infant appears normal.

Too often physicians wrongly attribute physiological jaundice occurring during the first week to breast milk. Breast feeding mothers are thus needlessly delayed in going home, while their infants are placed under phototherapy. As a result, mothers separated from their infants develop engorgement, sore nipples and ultimately breast infection due to interrupted and delayed feedings. If breast milk jaundice is strongly suspected by the end of the first week, nursing should be continued as long as peak levels do not exceed 20 mg. per 100 ml. or more. Blood samples can be monitored periodically by the physician. If peak levels do exceed 20 mg. per 100 ml., nursing is interrupted temporarily until a drop below this level occurs, usually 1 to 3 days. During this brief interruption in nursing, the mother may be placed on a breast pump* or taught to manually massage and express the milk from her breasts, while the infant is placed on a supplementary formula. Breast feeding may then be resumed since the bilirubin level rapidly falls below 20 mg. per 100 ml., even though hyperbilirubinemia of about 4 to 5 mg. per 100 ml. may continue and last as long as 1 to 2 months. At times there may be a momentary brief rise following resumption of breast feeding, but this rise is quickly followed by a fall as breast feeding continues uninterrupted. There is a 70 per cent incidence of hyperbilirubinemia with subsequent pregnancies in such cases. In no case should therapy require that the mother-infant nursing bond be permanently disrupted because of this entity.

Breast Feeding and Drugs in Human Milk. All drugs are excreted into the breast milk in varying quantities and over varying periods of time from the moment of ingestion. Fortunately, most drugs are clinically insignificant and pose no hazard to the nursing infant, since less than 1 per cent of the ingested dose is excreted into breast milk, and even less may be absorbed by the infant. Even with a high plasma:milk ratio, a potentially harmful drug can be detoxified and converted to an innocuous metabolite by the breast itself. On the other hand, a low plasma:milk ratio of a less potent drug does not ensure against harmful or annoying side effects, particularly if the mother is taking medication prior to nursing and over an extended period of time for a chronic condition. Then, too, inefficient or efficient enzymatic detoxification systems de-

---

*Loyd-B-Pump, Lopuco, 6117 Parkway Drive, West Laurel, Maryland 20810.

pendent upon age and genetic constitution may determine its ultimate effect on the infant.

In general those drugs that can safely be given are most oral antibiotics, antihistamines, simple cough remedies containing codeine or dextromethorphan in normal prescribed quantities, antipyretics such as aspirin or acetaminophen, psychotropic agents except diazepam (Valium), barbiturates, analgesics (Demerol, codeine, morphine, Darvon, etc.) and insulin in the nursing diabetic mother. Although tetracycline can stain secondary dentition, no known cases have been reported in the nursing infant probably due to low plasma:milk levels, and also because tetracycline itself may be bound to the calcium in the breast milk thereby decreasing its absorption. Chloramphenicol is probably safe since a large percentage of the drug is rendered into an ineffective metabolite in breast milk, but its use should warrant continuous blood studies. The social toxicants, alcohol, caffeine, and nicotine, usually cause no ill effect if ingested or smoked in moderate and nonabusive quantities. Theophylline is probably safe, but is best taken *after* nursing so as to minimize peak levels in breast milk. Cathartics (milk of magnesia, methylcellulose), fecal softeners (dioctyl sodium sulfate), and laxatives such as castor oil and phenolphthalein do not enter the milk in measurable amounts and cause no gastrointestinal symptoms.

Those drugs best avoided in the lactating mother are ergot, atropine, anticoagulants (except heparin), bromides, radioactive iodine and iodides, antithyroid agents such as thiouracil, metronidazole, streptomycin, antineoplastic agents, oral antidiabetic agents, and dihydrotachysterol. Addicts taking heroin and other hallucinogens should not nurse their infants as addiction and withdrawal symptoms may occur.

Other drugs that may be prescribed but must be closely supervised with caution are steroids used longer than short-term for chronic conditions, reserpine, nalidixic acid, lithium carbonide, amphetamines, and antiepileptic medication such as barbiturates and phenytoin for long-term usage. Since little is known about plasma:milk ratios of cardiac drugs such as digitalis and antiarrhythmic agents, their use requires careful observation of the infant. The anthraquinones, frequently used laxatives in the nursing mother (senna, cascara, aloin, rhubarb) rarely cause diarrhea, but gastrointestinal symptoms should be monitored closely. Since little is known about the long-term sexual effects of contraceptives on nursing infants and their questionable quan-

titative and qualitative effect on breast milk, they should be used with reservation by the physician.

The dilemma of drugs and breast feeding could be greatly simplified if the mother were to take no drugs at all, or if the physician were to prescribe only drugs absolutely essential to the welfare of the nursing mother. A physician may find it advantageous to substitute a safer drug for a potentially harmful drug, e.g., ibuprofen (Motrin) where studies show no excretion into breast milk, or aspirin, instead of phenylbutazone (Butazolidin) or its congeners as an anti-inflammatory agent for bursitis, arthritis, and other related conditions. If a potentially harmful drug must be used for a short duration, the mother may pump her breasts manually or use an efficient mechanical hand pump; nursing can be resumed upon discontinuance of medication.

Breast Infection. Any inflammation of the breast or nipple should be reported and treated immediately in order to prevent complications such as breast abscess. Frequently, the first sign reported to the physician is that of a localized area of red "streaking," which may represent a localized obstruction of one or several duct systems and is referred to as "caking of the breast." The physician should not remove the infant from the infected breast; on the contrary, the mother is instructed to nurse twice as frequently at that breast. This enhances the letdown reflex which prevents inspissation of milk, engorgement and further infection. There is no danger to the infant since breast milk has anti-infective properties, and the increased gastric acidity of nursing infants destroys many harmful pathogens which may be ingested. *Gentle* breast massage and manual expression prior to nursing may be used to enhance the letdown, but should be used with discretion if the breast is too engorged and inflamed. The mother should lie in a prone position as much as possible and obtain ample rest. Two or three hot moist washcloths may be placed over the inflamed area, and then covered with a plastic liner (Saran Wrap) to retain heat.

If the mother develops chills, malaise, fever, and systemic manifestations of infection along with more generalized inflammation of the breast (mastitis), an antibiotic may be given every 6 hours for 48 to 72 hours in addition to the above conservative therapy. Most oral antibiotics such as penicillin, erythromycin or ampicillin may be given safely in doses from 250 to 500 mg. every 6 hours without harm to the infant. The mother will usually note marked subjective improvement within 12 to

18 hours with a decline in fever and systemic symptoms. If necrosis and abscess formation follow, often through neglect and procrastination of treatment, incision and drainage must be instituted, and the infant removed temporarily from the breast for a day or two until drainage ceases and healing ensues. The mother may nurse at the opposite unaffected breast or use mechanical means such as massage or a hand pump during this interim in order to maintain emptying at both breasts, while the infant can then be placed on a temporary supplement.

Proper Techniques of Breast Feeding. Prior to breast feeding, the nipples should be gently wiped with sterile water. Benzalkonium (Zephiran), alcohol or other chemical disinfectants may irritate sensitive nipple epithelium. Under no circumstances should nipples, either prior to or following delivery, be "toughened" by frequent abrasive scrubbing or applications of tincture of benzoin. Following each nursing session, a bland emollient such as A&D Ointment or lanolin (preferably unrefined) may be applied sparingly.

It is best for the mother to nurse her infant sitting upright rather than lying on her side. The infant is placed on a double folded pillow inserted on the mother's lap so as to prop the infant to breast height. The head is placed in the crook of the "holding arm" which is pronated and held adducted at a right angle while the hand is cupped about the buttock of the infant. The mother's opposite hand, or "steering hand," is used to "root" the nipple by placing the margins of the areola between the thumb and forefinger (or second and third finger). As the infant "roots" for the nipple, the mother lifts or hikes the infant upward and toward the chest wall, so that the infant's mouth is thrust well upon the areola. This lifting action is essential to pinion and secure the head against the breast with the gaze of the infant looking up and toward the mother's face. The ipsilateral leg (never contralateral) is then flexed so that the knee is against the pillow and back of the infant's head. This serves the dual purpose of supporting the entire weight of the infant and prevents the mouth from rotating off the areola onto the nipple, which would occur if the unsupported holding arm were to supinate and drop from the weight of the infant. The mother's back should be straight and never leaning over the infant, thus relieving strain and tension on the mother's holding arm, neck, and shoulder muscles. The fingers of the opposite "steering hand" indent the areola inward toward the chest wall simultaneously as the infant is lifted upward during engagement of the mouth on the areola, and held in place so that an air space is present between the infant's nose and breast. This prevents air hunger and protracts the nipple to the infant's hard palate which aids in good oral suction and flow of milk. The cheeks should always be flush against the mother's breast signifying good penetration of nipple and areola and assuring an airtight seal with maximum strength of suck.

If the breast is engorged, the mother may express a few cc's of milk prior to nursing to soften the areola and allow for proper engagement of the mouth on this area and not the nipple. The mother should also be taught to break suction properly following feeding in order to prevent tearing of the nipple as the infant is withdrawn. This is done by placing the little finger at the corner of the infant's mouth thereby breaking oropharyngeal suction as air enters the mouth.

Nursing every 3 hours assures more complete emptying of the breasts preventing engorgement and inflammation and allows greater satiety in the infant with 2 extra caloric feedings in a 24 hour period. In hospitals in which rooming-in is the accepted procedure, a self-demand flexible schedule is superior to a rigid time schedule, allowing for timing of feedings with the infant's hunger cycle. The infant should be allowed to nurse for at least 5 minutes on each breast the first day, 10 minutes on each breast the second day and 15 minutes on each breast the third day. Nursing 1 or 2 minutes only leads to engorgement, poor letdown and sore nipples with inflammation. Upon going home, the mother nurses on demand—from 20 to 40 minutes at both breasts or until satiety is reached.

Both breasts are to be used since the letdown allows for "admixing" of the richer fatty "hind milk" in the proximal ducts with the weaker fatty "fore milk" in the distal sinus reservoirs at the second or opposite breast thereby increasing the caloric value of the milk. The mother is instructed to start her next feeding at that breast she left off last, so as to gain this caloric advantage of "admixed residual" left in the distal ducts from the previous feeding and to ensure complete emptying.

Mothers should not receive sedatives at night because they slow milk production and decrease milk letdown. Supplementary feedings of milk or sugar water after meals should be avoided since these extra feedings only detract from the mother's milk production and letdown, and disturb the different action of sucking required at breast feeding versus sucking at the bottle.

Treatment of Sore Nipples. Massage and manual expression prior to feeding often prevent sore nipples during the first few days following delivery. This technique can also be used before birth for a minute or two twice daily in order to enhance nipple protractility and strength of sucking. The hands are first lubricated with massage cream. With the thumbs of both hands in opposition and the remaining fingers tucked under the breast, massage is begun. The thumbs slide downward exerting gentle traction toward the outer edges of the areolar margin. This is repeated 3 to 4 times propelling milk into the distal lactiferous sinuses. Following massage, expression of the milk is accomplished by indenting the thumbs or second and third finger on the areola inward toward the chest wall until drops or a fine spray of milk occurs.

Exposing the nipples to air, sunlight, a heat lamp, or the warmth derived from a 75 watt bulb 2 or 3 times a day for several minutes may give added relief to sore nipples and aid in toughening nipple epithelium. This may be followed with a bland ointment or emollient cream.

If the nipples are excessively sore, rotating the nipple in the mouth may prevent excessive pressure on the same irritated area. The mother may also start feeding on the breast with the unaffected nipple first, thereby allowing the letdown reflex to operate and act as a lubricant to the nipple as the infant is switched to the affected breast. It is important that the mother always lift the infant upward and toward her so that mouth parts are engaged on the areola and not directly on the nipple (see Techniques), since this is a frequent cause of sore nipples and infection.

If the infant has thrush, the mother may have sore nipples from cross infection. The physician may investigate the mother for a possible vaginal yeast infection if persistent thrush and sore nipples are a problem. The application of a nystatin cream to the mother's nipple is frequently of help.

A scab on the nipple from chronic irritation may obstruct nipple pores and cause recurrent obstruction and inflammation of the breast. The mother may use hydrogen peroxide to dissolve the scab and to allow free flow of milk, followed by heat and the use of a bland ointment or emollient cream as previously outlined.

Breast Milk in Therapeutic Situations. The use of breast milk for prevention of gram-negative neonatal sepsis is well established on clinical grounds. Not only does breast milk have antistaphylococcal properties, but may also protect against bacterial gastroenteritis caused by *E. coli, Salmonella* and *Shigella* organisms. The breast fed infant also appears to be well protected against such bacterial diseases as tetanus, whooping cough, pneumonia, and diphtheria and against diseases caused by Coxsackie, adeno, influenza and polio viruses.

This protective effect of breast milk is attributed to the large amount of secretory immunoglobulin (IGA) and to the smaller but significant quantity of IGG and IGM. Other anti-infective properties of colostrum and breast milk are due to the cellular content of colostrum lymphocytes and phagocytosing macrophages, as well as to lysozyme, lactoferrin, interferon, and bifidus growth factor. Infants should be allowed to nurse from mothers who have fever secondary to infectious viral or bacterial agents, since they develop a passive immunity to the infection from mother's milk. An infant removed from the breast may not only be more likely to develop infection, but the mother's condition will most certainly be aggravated by superimposed breast infection secondary to engorgement caused by prolonged and delayed feedings.

Acute necrotizing enterocolitis is a highly lethal disease of the newborn occurring primarily in the premature or low birth weight infant and term infants suffering from severe cardiovascular disease or those who may have allergic diarrhea secondary to milk intolerance. The clinical signs are abdominal distention, bilious vomiting, melena, sepsis, peritonitis, and progressive lethargy with eventual respiratory failure leading to death. Human breast milk has been found curative in many of these infants.

Acrodermatitis enteropathica, a disease characterized by a vesicular dermatitis around the body orifices and distal parts of the extremities with multiple paronychia of the hands and feet and associated diarrhea and other digestive dysfunctions, may occur after weaning the infant from breast milk to a substitute formula. The disease is postulated to be based upon an inborn metabolic error with the original site in the intestinal flora, so that there is an inability to detoxify bacterial products absorbed from the lumen of the intestine. Breast milk has proved to be of help and frequently life-saving in this condition.

In tropical or underdeveloped countries, infants may suffer from marasmus, chronic enteritis, and protein deprivation which may be secondary to improper dilution and improper hygienic preparation of milk formulas because of poor socioeconomic reasons. Breast feeding should be encouraged among the mothers living in underpriviledged areas in order to endow the infant with the maximal nutritive benefits derived from the high biologic protein that only breast milk can inexpensively provide, along with its added anti-infective benefits.

Allergy to milk other than human breast milk may be an important cause of symptoms in the infant ranging from mild dermatological to gastrointestinal and respiratory symptoms and, infrequently, vascular shock. Many allergists recommend that breast milk be given to the infant with a strong family history of allergy. Protection may be provided by secretory IGA, which protects against potentially harmful macromolecular absorption of food antigens introduced early in the infant's life, thereby preventing later allergic sensitization.

Because of these conditions and others, many neonatal centers now have or are developing human breast milk banks. It is best for the mother to supply her own fresh breast milk, if feasible, since bottle preparation of bank breast milk entails autoclaving the milk and then freezing which may destroy both immunoglobulins and protective cells. It is also best for banked breast milk to be pumped through plastic tubing and stored in plastic containers, since breast milk cells may adhere to glass. (Information on regional and local milk banks which supply frozen or human fresh milk may be obtained by writing to La Leche League, Int., a nursing mothers' organization, 9616 Minneapolis Avenue, Franklin Park, Illinois 60131.)

Prematurity, Cesarean Section, and Multiple Births.   Because of its anti-infective factors and the nutritional benefits derived from its increased digestability and ease of absorption and assimilation of high quality protein, fat, and carbohydrate, breast milk is often used for the premature infant in order to supply ample calories for rapid growth and development. If the infant is placed in an Isolette for an undetermined time, the mother may extract fresh breast milk by means of an electric breast pump* and feed her infant in this manner when the sucking response is too weak. A mother may maintain her milk supply in this manner for many weeks as long as each breast is emptied every few hours by mechanical means. As the infant gains weight and strength and ability to suck, the mother may arrange her time to nurse during hospital hours, so as to resume full nursing at the time of discharge.

---

*Egnell breast pump, 16 Forest Lane, Cary, Illinois 60013.

Following cesarean section, infants can be brought to their mothers when they have reacted. The mother need not lie on her side in typical nursing fashion, but instead the infant may be placed on a pillow beside the supine mother with his legs under her right arm while feeding at the right breast and vice versa. In other words, the infant nurses from behind to relieve undue pressure on the mother's abdominal sutures. The mother may nurse the infant from the front in the usual manner after healing occurs. It is particularly important that the infant nurse every 3 hours around the clock in order for the mother to maintain adequate milk supply and letdown secondary to complete emptying of the breasts, and to offset sluggish basal metabolism with poor milk yield secondary to the effects of anesthesia required at the time of surgery.

In those cases of multiple births, the routine described under prematurity may be followed if the infants are too weak to suck. Supplementation with glucose water or mother's milk per bottle may be necessary until infants are ready to nurse. The infants should be brought simultaneously at feeding time rather than separately as this proves to be too exhausting to the mother. Each infant is placed at the same breast since milk production and letdown become accustomed to the strength of sucking of that respective infant. The infant lies on a pillow or cushion placed under each arm as the mother sits in a large armchair or hospital bed. The babies may nurse from behind as mentioned above. Nursing time may vary from 20 to 30 minutes every 2 to 3 hours. Supplementation is usually not necessary because the milk supply quickly meets the caloric requirements of both infants, usually by the second week.

Contraindications, Indications, and Diet of the Nursing Mother.   In general, there are few contraindications to nursing. These may be due to chronic contagious diseases such as tuberculosis or *severe* maternal heart disease, renal disease, starvation, or other chronic debilitating factors in which the increased stress of lactation would prove detrimental to the mother's health. Infants nursing from mothers who suffer from poor diet and inadequate nutrition can grow and thrive at the expense of the mother's system and metabolic pool for several months, at which time milk yield will diminish, finally leading to poor growth in the infant. A diabetic mother who is well managed may nurse successfully without difficulty, and insulin given to the mother is not ingested by the infant through breast milk. If the mother must take potent drugs for chronic conditions over long-term usage (see Drugs and Breastfeeding), this too may be a contraindication. Infants with severe cleft lip or palate deformities may have a difficult time nursing, but the mother may extract her milk by means of a breast pump or manual expression, and supplement the infant's diet in this manner. Some infants with *severe* neurological defects may suck poorly and require partial or complete supplementation. Infants with cardiac problems thrive very well at the breast.

Most mothers can and should be encouraged to nurse by their physician if they are well motivated to do so and are eating a well balanced diet. No mother should be coerced into nursing her infant. Nursing mothers should be encouraged to continue to take their prenatal vitamin supplement during lactation in order to supply increased calcium, iron, and vitamins A and D required for lactation. Nursing mothers require an additional 500 kilocalories or more per day, but will not gain weight because of increased metabolism required for lactation; appetite suppressants or diets may cause more harm than good.

Feeding of the Premature Infant

EKHARD E. ZIEGLER, M.D.

Nutritional management of the premature infant must be considered in the context of total medical care. Nutritionally desirable goals may be practically unattainable. Ideally, nutritional management of the newborn premature infant leads to prompt restoration of the type of nutrient flow that continuously reached the fetus until birth intervened. As a result, under ideal circumstances growth continues with little or no interruption. In practice, this goal cannot be achieved and some compromise must be accepted. Since it appears reasonable to consider premature birth an undesirable interruption of normal growth, every attempt should be made to permit resumption of the growth pattern that would have occurred in utero under normal conditions. This point of view provides a frame of reference from which nutrient requirements may be derived and against which results of nutritional management may be measured.

Advisable Intakes of Nutrients for Growing Premature Infants. In estimating nutrient requirements of the growing premature infant, it has been assumed that growth (both in rate and composition) should resemble that of the fetus in utero. Advisable intakes (Table 1) have been derived from estimates of requirements by adding a safety factor of 20 per cent.

The advisable intakes are applicable to nutritional management of *growing* premature infants. A relatively high percentage of the requirements for many nutrients including calories is accounted for by the quantities incorporated into newly synthesized tissue. Therefore, in the case of the nongrowing (such as the sick) premature infant, intakes amounting to only small fractions of the advisable intakes may be adequate. Notable exceptions are calories, water and electrolytes. Because of limitations in intestinal absorption, requirements for certain nutrients are less when nutrients are provided parenterally than when provided enterally, and are less when absorption is very efficient (such as calcium from human milk) than when it is poor (such as calcium from formulas).

Advisable intakes of nutrients have been expressed per 100 calories because it is desirable for optimal utilization that calories and specific nutrients be provided in more or less fixed relation to one another. In addition, this method of expression facilitates comparison of advisable intakes with formula composition.

Advisable intakes are presented in Table 1 for three gestational age and body weight

TABLE 1. Advisable Intakes of Nutrients and Composition of Feedings

	ADVISABLE INTAKES			COMPOSITION OF FEEDINGS					
	1000 gm. 26 to 28 Weeks	1500 gm. 29 to 31 Weeks	2000 gm. 32 to 34 Weeks	Human Milk	SMA	Similac 20	Enfamil	Similac 24	Enfamil Premature Formula
Calories (kcal./kg./day)	130	130	130						
Protein (gm./100 kcal.)	2.8	2.6	2.4	1.5	2.2	2.3	2.2	2.7	2.8
Na (mEq./100 kcal.)	2.5	2.3	2.0	1.0	1.0	1.5	1.8	1.7	1.8
K (mEq./100 kcal.)	2.0	1.8	1.6	1.4	2.1	2.7	2.7	3.2	2.9
Cl (mEq./100 kcal.)	2.3	2.0	1.7	1.5	1.5	2.2	2.2	2.6	2.4
Ca (mg./100 kcal.)	160	160	160	45	66	77	82	100	160
P (mg./100 kcal.)	100	100	100	18	50	59	68	77	80
Mg (mg./100 kcal.)	8	7	6	4	8	6	7	7	10
Essential fatty acids (gm./100 kcal.)	0.5	0.5	0.5	0.5	0.7	1.2	2.3	1.2	1.2

categories. It will be noted that advisable intakes for several nutrients decrease with advancing maturity, that is, approach those for the full-term infant. Actually, nutritional management of the infant weighing more than 2000 gm. may be the same as that of the full-term infant. Infants who are small for gestational age (small for dates) have higher requirements for calories per unit of body weight than infants whose weight is appropriate for gestational age. Whether the same holds true for other nutrients is not yet known. A reasonable approach would be to provide a caloric intake of 140 to 150 kcal./kg./day (or more, if necessary) and to provide all other nutrients in proportion to the caloric intake, the proportion being that indicated by the gestational age of the infant.

Advisable intakes for vitamins are indicated in Table 2. Vitamin E is known to be poorly absorbed and therefore a relatively large dose (30 I.U./day) is recommended. Vitamin K is not included in Table 2 because it should be given at birth, and thereafter the amount present in formula is adequate.

Because of the possibility that administration of iron may be associated with an enhanced rate of red cell destruction, neither iron supplemented formulas nor other supplements of iron are recommended during the first 8 weeks of life. Iron stores may be relied upon to supply iron required for hemoglobin synthesis during that period. In view of this delay in introduction of iron supplements and because of uncertainties regarding the availability of iron, an intake of 7 mg./day is recommended beginning at 8 weeks of age.

Provision of Nutritional Support. PARENTERAL. Body stores of energy and specific nutrients are less in the premature than in the full-term infant. Failure to provide nutritional support soon after birth is therefore more serious. In the case of infants with birth weights less than 1500 gm., it is now common practice to administer water and glucose in-travenously within 2 hours of the time of birth. Sodium, chloride and, when renal function has been established, potassium are also administered. The goal is to replace ongoing energy expenditures and losses of nutrients and to support immature homeostatic mechanisms. Estimates of requirements for these purposes must take into account medical and environmental factors. At the same time, parenteral alimentation is to be viewed as a temporary measure, and failure to meet requirements for growth for a few days may not be serious. Every effort should be made, however, to meet maintenance requirements.

When introduction of enteral feedings must be delayed, a source of nitrogen should be included in the intravenous regimen beginning at 2 to 4 days of age. Protein hydrolysates or amino acid mixtures should be provided in a proportion of approximately 0.1 gm. for each gram of glucose (2.5 gm./100 kcal.). This is the same proportion that is commonly employed in solutions for total parenteral nutrition. These solutions may be infused into peripheral veins of premature infants at concentrations of glucose not exceeding 12.5 gm./dl. Even in the nongrowing infant receiving only maintenance energy intakes, this regimen will result in diminution of the net loss of nitrogen. Fat emulsions may be administered intravenously to provide additional energy and essential fatty acids. The latter may also be provided in the form of safflower oil applied to the skin (1 to 2 gm./day). Total parenteral nutrition using central venous catheters is rarely indicated.

Monitoring is an essential part of parenteral alimentation. Serum concentrations of at least glucose and electrolytes and serum osmolality must be determined regularly, and urine must be monitored for presence of glucose and for osmolality. If fat emulsions are administered intravenously, plasma lipid determinations must be performed and close attention must be given to serum bilirubin concentrations.

ENTERAL ALIMENTATION. Administration of calories and nutrients by peripheral vein, even with the use of fat emulsions, is unlikely to achieve intakes that will permit growth. Introduction of enteral feedings should therefore be considered as soon as the infant's condition permits. While maintenance requirements for water, calories and electrolytes continue to be provided parenterally, enteral feeding may be attempted in a cautious manner.

A method employing slow infusion into the stomach by nasogastric tube has proved satisfactory, especially for very small and sick infants. With this technique as currently em-

TABLE 2.   Advisable Intakes of Vitamins*

Vitamin A	500	I.U.
Vitamin D	400	I.U.
Vitamin E	30	I.U.
Thiamine	0.2	mg.
Riboflavin	0.4	mg.
Niacin	5.0	mg.
Vitamin B$_6$	0.4	mg.
Folic acid	60	μg.
Vitamin C	60	mg.

*Concurrent use of two or more commercially available vitamin preparations may be necessary in order to achieve these advisable intakes.

ployed, a small volume (such as 3 ml./hour) is infused at a steady rate over a period of 3 hours using a mechanical pump. When not contraindicated because of other considerations, right decubitus position is favored because it enhances gastric emptying. After 3 hours the infusion is stopped and one hour later gastric content is aspirated. The infant is carefully observed for abdominal distention and for change in respiratory status. If the aspirate amounts to more than 20 per cent of the volume infused, no further infusion is usually given for 8 to 12 hours. With smaller aspirates, intragastric infusion may be continued, alternating 3 hour periods of infusion with 1 hour rests.

If well tolerated, the rate of infusion may gradually be increased, such as an increase of 0.5 to 1.0 ml./hour every 6 hours. When feedings are well tolerated, periods of infusion may be prolonged, such as to 6 hours with a subsequent 2 hour rest, or bolus feedings may be tried, using a volume half that administered during the previous 3 hours of continuous infusion.

Choice of Feeding.   Table 1 presents the composition of human milk and of several commercially prepared formulas. It is apparent that in a number of instances nutrient content of feedings (expressed per 100 kcal.) is less than the advisable intakes. Human milk falls short of advisable intakes for several nutrients, notably protein, sodium, calcium and phosphorus. However, other properties such as high digestibility and several possibly protective properties make human milk seem an attractive feeding to many neonatologists. If human milk is fed to growing small premature infants, monitoring for signs of nutritional deficiency should be carried out with particular care.

Among the commercially prepared formulas, Enfamil Premature Formula and Similac 24 appear to provide nutrient intakes that are in better agreement with advisable intakes than are those of the other feedings. The fat of Enfamil Premature Formula consists partially of easily absorbed medium-chain triglycerides. It seems probable that all formulas provide adequate amounts of trace minerals. Formulas based on soy isolates have not been extensively evaluated in premature infants and their use is therefore not recommended. Formulas containing whey proteins and casein in a ratio of 60:40 (such as SMA) are preferred by some neonatologists. However, despite certain theoretic advantages of employing this mixture of proteins, evidence of beneficial effects on performance of premature infants has so far been unimpressive.

It is probably good practice to begin with calorically dilute feedings, such as 40 kcal./dl. (12 kcal./oz.), prepared with sterile water. If feedings are tolerated, concentration may be increased stepwise to 80 kcal./dl. (24 kcal./oz.).

With adequate fluid intakes, especially in a growing infant, renal solute load is of no concern. However, when fluid intakes are restricted or when the infant does not grow, urine osmolality or specific gravity should be monitored regularly. Urine concentrations exceeding 300 mOsm./liter of water (specific gravity 1.012) should be avoided.

During the first eight weeks of life, formulas without added iron or with iron content less than 2 mg./liter are recommended. Supplemental vitamins should be provided because of specific requirements (such as for vitamin E) and because advisable intakes of several other vitamins exceed the quantities provided by the relatively small volumes of formula consumed by premature infants.

Monitoring Nutritional Status.   Daily measurements of weight constitute the single most valuable index of nutritional performance. Whether it is desirable for a premature infant to exceed the rate of weight gain of the fetus remains uncertain, although it should be noted that most premature infants go through a period of relative undernutrition, and catch-up growth should therefore be expected.

Measurements of length and skinfold thickness are difficult to perform and, unless they are done by specially trained personnel, such measurements are not recommended for routine use.

Serum concentrations of urea reflect recent protein intake. While it is safe to state that concentrations below 8 mg./dl. reflect inadequate protein intake, it is impossible to identify an upper limit of normal. Serum concentrations of albumin represent a sensitive index of protein nutritional status and should be determined regularly. Decreasing serum concentrations of albumin strongly suggest inadequate protein nutritional status.

Elevations of serum alkaline phosphatase activity and roentgenographic evidence of inadequate bone mineralization are not uncommon among premature infants more than 2 months of age. These abnormalities generally disappear over a period of about 6 months and their long-term significance is uncertain; however, careful monitoring of progress is desirable until the findings return to normal.

23

Special Problems in the Adolescent

Emotional Problems of Adolescents

GORDON HARPER, M.D., *and*
JULIUS B. RICHMOND, M.D.

The *development tasks* of adolescence are: (1) shifting one's primary emotional investment from family to the world outside; (2) integrating (that is, making one's own) one's maturing sexual capacity; and (3) identity formation, deciding who one is in the world. The emotional problems of adolescents derive from these three related developmental tasks.

It should be emphasized that working with adolescents is not a task for every physician. The demands and frustrations which adolescents impose on their physicians (and on their parents and their friends), their extremes of self-indulgence and asceticism, of sloppiness and strictness (with self and others), mean that not every doctor will be comfortable working with them. At the same time, adolescents need to feel that those they deal with genuinely like them, so that liking the work (and the patients) without dissembling is important. Physicians accordingly should select themselves on the basis of their own tastes and training for this kind of work or refer patients to those who enjoy it more. Some physicians may have had specialized training in adolescent medicine or work in a clinic specialized in the medical care of adolescents.

SHIFTING EMOTIONAL TIES: SEPARATION PROBLEMS

The shift in the balance of emotional ties from family to the world outside the family, which occurs gradually throughout adolescence, is a process of separation for both parents and adolescent. When the separation is difficult for either, the pediatrician may be called on to arbitrate many kinds of parent-child turmoil. These episodes are always trying, but are less perplexing once seen in terms of loss: parents feel they are losing a child they are not ready to give up; the teenager is losing the stage in life when he could be openly dependent at a time when he does not feel completely comfortable being on his own. The family must change to accommodate the new needs of the adolescent, neither overcontrolling when the adolescent needs to experiment with his own independence, nor abdicating when he needs to know what and whom he can count on. Teenage rebelliousness is the behavior most frequently complained of; over-compliance, especially when the child has not developed a satisfying life outside the family, is a more serious symptom, but all too acceptable to most families.

For most patients, treatment consists of education of parents and adolescents about the developmental issues of adolescence. For some adolescents, the pediatrician has a role in promoting activities outside the family; for most, such promotion will hardly be necessary.

Dealing with the adolescent separately in medical matters, not just through his parents, conveys concretely the message that the adolescent can now begin to deal with those outside the family on his own.

In more severe cases, adolescent school phobia or intense mother-child (especially mother-daughter) struggles over sleep, diet, hygiene, or physical symptoms indicate more serious problems. School phobia in adolescence can carry a poor prognosis for future psychological development; prompt efforts to return the child to school as well as psychiatric consultation are indicated. Intense mother-child struggles in early adolescence call for pediatric efforts to decrease the intensity of this regressive relationship: offering guidelines about what can be expected of an adolescent, or about how parents decide what can be expected of *this* adolescent; exploring whether the mother can back off in her efforts to find out or to control the child intrusively; discovering the child's interests apart from the relationship with the mother; involving the father in parenting; or promoting other activities for the mother to compensate for the felt loss of her child. In some cases such efforts will succeed in promoting easier separation; in many, psychiatric consultation and/or referral will be necessary.

SEXUAL MATURATION: FEELINGS AND THE NEED FOR FACTS

Sexual maturation provides the adolescent with new energy, wishes, and anxieties. The energy lies behind the private excitement over dirty jokes of the preadolescent and his same-sex peers; the early adolescent's intense same-sex friendships and cautious interest (often in the safety of friends) in the other sex; and the mid and late adolescent's developing interest in individual heterosexual relationships. The anxieties focus on one's own maturation and the adequacy of one's own genital equipment, and on the consequences of sexual activity, from fantasies and wet dreams to masturbation, sex play, and intercourse. Despite the increase in adolescent sexual activity in some groups in parts of the country, by and large adolescents continue to keep themselves very poorly informed about sex. Anxiety and lack of information lead many adolescents to bring sexual questions to the doctor, but often in the disguised form of physical complaints. Any vague physical complaint by an adolescent, especially when it concerns appearance or localizes to the pelvic area, offers an opportunity for gentle exploration of the adolescent's ideas, experiences, and feelings about sexual matura-

tion and activity. Telling an adolescent that every adolescent is concerned about the adequacy of his or her sexual development, and that all people at some point are anxious about the fantasied consequences of universal activities like masturbation can produce great relief. Sex education regarding hygiene, fertility and contraception, and venereal disease can be started in the same setting.

IDENTITY FORMATION: LOOKING INSIDE AND FINDING ONESELF

The inner and outer demands to define oneself in one's own eyes and in the eyes of those one defines as important require the adolescent to take stock of himself. He must somehow integrate his endowment and his current abilities with the real-life opportunities to develop his capacities and exercise his abilities. This developmental phase is difficult for adolescents who are uncertain about themselves, their origins, or their futures—which is partly why depression is a major problem in adolescence (see below). For the adolescent with handicap or with chronic illness, the need at this time to look both back and forward can renew all the feelings (for himself and for the family) associated with the onset or discovery of the handicapping condition. Depression "coming from nowhere" for such adolescents and their families can usefully be linked to and understood and discussed in the context of this developmental issue.

DEPRESSION

There has been increasing interest in the past decade in depression in adolescents (and children). New knowledge of the genetics and biochemistry of depression in adults, and new evidence for the efficacy (in adults) of the tricyclic antidepressants underlie this interest. The diagnostic problem in this age group is the mix of symptoms one sees. The "classic" picture of depressed mood, psychomotor retardation, altered vegetative function (sleep, appetite, and sex), and self-critical ideas is seen in only a minority of depressed adolescents (and in even fewer depressed children). It is more common to see a dysphoric state (which may be irritability or apathy as well as depression) and a falling off in any or all of the areas in which adolescents function: family, school, and peers. Thus, fights at home, academic or disciplinary problems at school, or frustrations in or withdrawal from peer relations may be the most conspicuous symptoms.

Other depressive symptoms include drug experimentation or antisocial behavior. While these activities usually occur in the peer setting, in which a given adolescent may be no more depressed than others, they may be recognized as depressive symptoms when the depressed adolescent is "doing it on his own," in the absence of a sanctioning peer culture; when he consistently leads the way in possibly dangerous behavior; or when he manages to harm himself, or consistently risks doing so, in the same escapades which others manage to pull off safely. Scapegoating by peers (or within the family), a possible cause of depression, may also be a depressive symptom: the depressed adolescent either invites the scapegoating or fails to protect himself once scapegoated. Many psychophysiological symptoms in adolescents will make sense only when seen in the context of an unacknowledged depression.

Some depressed adolescents are on steroid therapy, which may precipitate or exacerbate depression, even psychotic depression. While such patients are few, both among the depressed and among those taking steroids, assessment of depression includes consideration of the possible role of licit as well as illicit drugs. If implicated, steroids should be withdrawn.

Treatment begins with recognition that the adolescent previously labeled as having a poor attitude, or as being lazy or selfish, is in fact depressed; such a diagnosis in itself can be therapeutic for child and family. Next the physician must review with the patient and family recent events, especially changes not previously recognized to be significant losses. The extent of depression in other members of the family must be assessed; the symptomatic adolescent may not be the most depressed member. Adolescents sustain losses of important people when grandparents or parents die; losses of familiar places and friends with a family move, or a separation milestone such as going away to school or college; losses of a phase of life which felt more congenial as they enter the uncharted years of physiological puberty and psychosocial adolescence; and the loss of childhood innocence as they see some of the realities of adult life. The meaning of the losses must be reviewed with the patient and when relevant with his parents. Extra time and a chance to talk are appropriate responses to the depressed adolescent's isolation and discouragement. Environmental manipulation at home or at school (talk with teachers or guidance staff; a change of school may be indicated) may be the most therapeutic intervention.

A trial of antidepressant medication may be undertaken if symptoms are seriously interfering with life and have continued a month or more. A positive family history for affective illness will make one more inclined to treat pharmacologically. To use medication, the pediatrician *must* have a therapeutic alliance with the patient. That is, he and the patient must be able to agree on some symptom, distressing to the patient and for which he seeks relief, and which antidepressant medication might plausibly help. Without such agreement, the drug gets caught in the adolescent's "them-versus-me" struggles for autonomy, and the negative effect of that interaction will outweigh any therapeutic benefit. This kind of medication cannot be prescribed without the patient being seen in person, nor can the physician leave to the parent the job of telling the adolescent patient about the medication and its purpose.

Imipramine (Tofranil)* and amitriptyline (Elavil)† are the drugs most often used; most pediatricians have more experience with imipramine because of its use in enuresis. For both drugs, 150 to 300 mg. per day is the dose for adult-sized adolescents, with smaller patients getting proportionately smaller doses. Because of the buildup of tissue levels, a single evening or bedtime dose is adequate; it may also help with sleep problems. Because of the autonomic side effects, many patients do better building up to the full starting dose (say, 150 mg.) over 3 days. The patient (and parents) must be told several things: the therapeutic effect can take 10 to 21 days to occur; the drug should not be stopped (nor higher doses tried) prematurely. Autonomic side effects (dry mouth, blurred vision, constipation, orthostatic hypotension) will be noted and will be troubling. Most will be transient and will be gone by the time therapeutic benefit occurs; they can be taken as a sign the drug is beginning to work. Others (especially dry mouth) may be longstanding as well as annoying.

Indications for psychiatric consultation and/or referral include: (1) suicidal talk or behavior; (2) severe symptoms: total social withdrawal, intractable family fighting, serious psycho-physiological symptoms, or expressed feelings of hopelessness; (3) patient's inability to make a therapeutic agreement with the pediatrician with regard to whatever mode of treatment; and (4) failure of symptoms to respond over a month or so of pediatric care.

---

*Manufacturer's precaution: Administration of imipramine in pediatric conditions other than enuresis or in children younger than 6 years of age is not recommended.

†Manufacturer's precaution: In view of the lack of experience with the use of amitriptyline in children, it is not recommended at the present time for children under 12 years of age.

ANOREXIA NERVOSA

Anorexia nervosa is increasing, if not in true incidence at least in visibility and popular awareness. The diagnostic criteria are weight loss of 20 to 25 per cent without evidence of physiological basis in an adolescent or young adult with some distortion of body image, misperception of body size, or delusional ideas about appetite. There are 5 to 10 times as many females affected as males. In some early adolescent patients with a chronic course, cessation of weight gain may occur without frank weight loss. About half the patients still growing at onset of the illness will suffer some slowing of linear growth, with poor prognosis for catch-up.

There are many variably associated features such as primary or secondary amenorrhea, dehydration with bradycardia, increased motor activity, and covert vomiting or gorging on food or water. The pituitary-endocrine axis is slowed, especially with regard to thyroid and sex hormones, but this is probably secondary to hypothalamic dysfunction, reflected among other things in poor temperature homeostasis.

The cause of the hypothalamic disorder remains obscure. A connection with the affective disorders is plausible because of the salient disturbances in anorexia nervosa of regulation of mood, self-esteem, and appetite; but relevant data on the natural history, genetics, and biochemistry in this disorder and in other adolescent affective disorders are not available.

A strikingly consistent psychosocial picture is seen in these patients, characterized psychologically as overly accommodating and perfectionistic but with underlying ambivalence, especially toward mothers, and failure to develop satisfying autonomy. Marital schism, often latent, may be associated, and the boundaries in family roles between parents and the sick child blurred. In the social field around these patients one notes unusual patterns of doctor-doctor and family-doctor interaction (as on referral and in subsequent communications) marked by intense affect, especially around issues of caring for the patient (caring well or poorly, parents' caring, medical care, nursing care), and frequent splitting among those concerned with the patient—family, doctors, nurses, teachers.

The patients move stiffly with excessive use of extremities and voluntary breath holding, but may loosen up with recovery. As a group they are artistically gifted, but their drawings tend to be mechanical or stiff, like their own movements.

While there is disagreement as to the relative physiological, psychological, and familial contributions to this complex disorder, observers from different psychological perspectives agree that anorexia nervosa is a massive "holding action" in which the body is made to serve the psychological need of slowing down development, when growing up appears foreboding, impossible to manage, or lethal. The words of Marlowe's Faustus as the designated hour of his doom approached, "Lente lente currite noctis equi" (Go slow, go slow, ye racing steeds of night) epitomize the wish of this group of patients to see developmental time stop.

Treatment must be directed to the weight disorder (often presenting with crises of inanition and/or dehydration); to the patients' fear of loss of the ability to manage their own appetites, body, and growing up; and to the family's frequent disarray in the face of such a serious illness. Because of the tendency to split, an explicit alliance and close working together among all professionals and with the patient's family are prerequisites for any treatment. Hospitalization is often required. Given an appropriate alliance, the weight disorder can be treated on pediatric wards, giving Sustacal 240 cc. (= 240 calories) or 480 cc. 4 to 6 times daily on each day the patient's weight does not rise by 0.1 kg. over the previous in-hospital maximum weight. Antidepressants may be useful for treatment of manifest mood disorder. Weight gain alone, without commensurate psychological progress, does *not* constitute recovery from anorexia nervosa. In the view of most physicians who have treated these difficult patients, the psychological work with patient and family requires psychiatric collaboration.

Obesity at Adolescence

ANDREA M. MARKS, M.D., *and*
MICHAEL I. COHEN, M.D.

Most clinicians are not often faced with the rare massively or morbidly obese adolescent weighing more than two times his or her ideal weight. Similarly, there is little concern for the teenager eager to lose 5 or 10 pounds prior to summer vacation. It is, however, that large middle group of adolescents weighing more than 20 per cent above ideal weight but less than two times the ideal weight that demands our attention. Virtually all such obese adolescents have no identifiable endocrine disturbance to account for their excessive fatness. The obese teenager usually has been of normal height, and among girls there is a significant trend toward advanced height age, accelerated bone maturation, and early sexual maturation and menarche. Multiple factors are likely to be causative in obesity and the resultant physiologic, psychologic and social stigmata are equally variable and multifaceted.

Obese teenagers are subject to decreased glucose tolerance and sensitivity to insulin, elevations in serum cholesterol and triglyceride concentrations, hypertension, and excessive strain on joints and supporting tissues. Additionally, they are the objects of strong prejudice in our society, and have been shown to suffer to a greater degree than their leaner peers from passivity, anxiety, depression, low self-esteem, rejection and progressive withdrawal. These disturbances are also more prevalent in obese adults who had the onset of their obesity during childhood or adolescence. Our goals in therapy are therefore twofold: to assist patients in weight reduction, as well as to encourage them to achieve greater socialization and normalization in their lives. Since sustained weight loss is often difficult if not impossible to achieve, the second goal may in fact become the critical therapeutic objective.

CHANGES DURING ADOLESCENCE

Adolescence is a period of dramatic physical and emotional change. The earliest signs of puberty are usually breast budding in the female and testicular enlargement in the male. Shortly thereafter, inches grown during the height spurt will account for approximately 15 per cent of the final adult height. Strikingly, body poundage normally doubles during adolescence. This is largely accounted for by accelerated muscle growth in the male, as contrasted with enhanced adipose tissue growth in the female.

Adiposity, as measured by skinfold thickness, normally increases in both males and females during early adolescence. Thereafter, males sharply lose fatness during middle and late adolescence, whereas females continue to increase in fatness. By early adulthood, the average male is about 8 per cent fat and the female is over 20 per cent fat. Losing one's "baby fat" during adolescence, therefore, may more naturally occur in a chubby boy than in an overweight girl. The teenager must integrate these striking bodily changes into his or her emerging body image and self concept, while negotiating the other developmental tasks of establishing independence from the family, feeling at ease with one's sexuality, and taking initial steps toward a chosen vocation.

The obese adolescent is at greater risk of experiencing special difficulties with these critical maturational issues.

TREATMENT

As no definite etiologic classification of obesity exists, there are no rigid guidelines for its treatment. The therapeutic approach must be individualized and in most instances will require considerable long-term commitment and motivation on the part of both the teenager and the physician. The younger adolescent brought for care by distraught parents and who has not yet experienced his or her growth spurt presents different management considerations than the older, fully developed teenager seeking help on his or her own initiative.

There are essentially five treatment modalities currently available: pharmacotherapy, surgery, dietary management, exercise, and behavior modification techniques; the last three, in our opinion, are the most appropriate for teenage patients. However, the first general goal of treatment is to establish and maintain a trusting relationship with the adolescent. This will best be achieved if the patient is seen no less frequently than one time per month, and more often if possible. For the younger teenager, in whom dieting and weight loss are not present goals and parental prodding is a source of conflict, the physician may become the friendly authority, thereby relieving the parents of the responsibility they feel to get their youngster to lose weight. For the older adolescent living in a home with pasta and pastry-loving parents and siblings, the physician can be a provider of support as well as guidance toward independent buying and preparing of most of his or her meals. Ideally, total family motivation to lose weight lightens the burden of any teenager living at home.

The cheerful, bright adolescent with close friends, several outside interests and some prior successes in school or sports, may respond enthusiastically to dietary advice. The sullen, inactive and isolated youngster, often with a history of prior academic or interpersonal failures, will require closer social and psychiatric evaluation and possibly intervention prior to institution of specific treatment for obesity. The latter will frequently be viewed as alien and may only increase his frustration and list of failures.

Pharmacotherapy. Anorectic drug therapy has been shown to have little lasting effect on weight loss and is rarely indicated in teenagers. Some clinicians have suggested limited amphetamine therapy in selected older adolescents as an initial morale-building step which is part of a long-term dietary program. We find no role for such agents as thyroid extract and digitalis.

Surgery. Jejunoileal bypass surgery has recently been employed in a few massively obese adolescents with some early success reported. Such surgery carries considerable initial morbidity and long-term uncertainty and ought to be reserved for the teenager with serious medical complications who is at least twice ideal weight, and in whom all other measures have failed.

Dietary Management. When planning a teenager's diet, one must consider the individual caloric requirements of the patient. These are quite variable but are in the range of about 2900 calories per day for males and 2400 for females. With the younger pre- or intra-growth-spurt obese teenager, it is advisable to plan a diet that limits intake to approximately his caloric requirement, thereby allowing maintenance or very slow loss of weight. He will, of course, begin to be perceptibly thinner as he rapidly grows taller. The older, generally more highly motivated teenager, may tolerate greater caloric restrictions of 1000 to 1800 calories per day, aiming at a steady one to two pounds per week loss of weight. A teenager whose intake equals his caloric requirement should consume at least 10 per cent of his calories as protein. A teenager on a restricted calorie diet should receive 15 to 20 per cent of his actual intake in the form of protein. Viewed alternatively, any adolescent should consume at least 10 per cent of his calories expended in the form of protein.

The teenager can be taught to plan a few days' menus for meals and snacks within the chosen caloric range. He should learn to include foods from each of the basic groups to assure adequate nutrition, and to exchange calorically equivalent choices as he pleases. We often suggest the patient obtain a small paperback pocket book listing various foods and their caloric value. In this way, no favorite food need be entirely omitted, and eventually reasonable habits will develop which, hopefully, will become lifelong. The teenager must realize there is no cure for his obesity, but merely ways of controlling it!

Exercise. Obese teenagers may be inactive for several reasons. Their largeness clearly slows them down and competitive sports are therefore difficult for them to compete in, both physically and psychologically. Additionally, obese teenagers are often loners and the opportunities for even non-competitive physical activity with peers may be markedly few. Fortunately, however, there are numerous activities they may comfortably participate in alone which will help them expend additional calories. Examples of caloric expenditure per 30 minutes include: walking, bowling, gardening and golf at about 150 calories; cycling, tennis and dancing at about 200 calories; running and swimming at over 300 calories. One must stress continued and moderate involvement in physical conditioning and exercise, and not binges of furious activity interspersed between long periods of sedentary tasks.

Behavior Modification. Behavior modification attempts to change deviant eating patterns which result in excessive caloric intake by reinforcing change with various rewards. As a first step, the patient is asked to keep a record for several days of all the types of food he eats and the amount, the times during the day that he eats, the places where the food is eaten, and to record any associated stimuli to eat, such as boredom, loneliness, or anger. Such records serve, first, to remind the patient of his specific intake and habits, and second, to allow the physician to suggest various behavior modification techniques to the patient. With the patient's eating record in mind, many possible suggestions can be made which might include the following: eat only in the kitchen to avoid snacking while watching television or reading; eat on a small luncheon plate and not a dinner plate, use teaspoons and cake forks rather than soup spoons and dinner forks; swallow all food before putting more on the fork to avoid eating too fast; remove all snack foods from the house to avoid unplanned automatic eating; leave a small amount of food on the plate at the end of a meal; remove all serving dishes from the table to avoid automatic second servings; have other activities nearby in the event of boredom or loneliness, such as sewing, painting or woodworking, to occupy both mind and hands. In addition, patients may be advised to change their bus or walking routes to avoid tempting food stores and to allow for additional exercise.

Rewards may include money, certain privileges, gifts from parents, as well as sibling, peer and teacher approval, or alternatively, avoiding disapproval. The latter operates quite successfully in weight reducing groups, which are certainly appropriate for many teenagers.

CONCLUSION

The treatment of an obese teenager must be individualized to his particular stage of physical development and caloric needs, his pattern of physical activity and personal eating habits, and his family situation and psychosocial adjustment. Although many adolescents will initially lose some weight after a physician contact, clinical experience demonstrates few will maintain this weight loss for any significant period of time. Therefore an equally important goal must be to achieve greater socialization and normalization in their lives through physical activities, group meetings, modified eating behavior, and in a few selected patients, referral for psychotherapy. If improved socialization and weight loss become the goals, treating obese adolescents need not represent a frustrating task, but rather may have rewards for patient and physician alike.

Menstrual Disorders

ALFRED M. BONGIOVANNI, M.D.

There has recently been a growing concern about a possible relationship between certain malignancies (endometrial carcinoma) and the administration of hormones, estrogens in particular. Nevertheless this section will offer recommendations for the treatment of some conditions of childhood with such agents because the psychological handicaps of therapeutic nihilism are of great consequence and outweigh the possible risks. The treatment should be based on legitimate indications and prolonged irrational therapy must be avoided.

Primary Amenorrhea. This may be due to delayed pubescence, in which case no treatment is indicated other than reassurance. Primary ovarian failure (as in gonadal dysgenesis) or hypothalamic-hypophyseal disorders (e.g., hypogonadotropic states) require replacement therapy with ovarian hormones.

Ethinyl estradiol U.S.P., 0.02 mg. daily by mouth, from the first to the 21st day of each month is usually adequate to bring about secondary sexual development and regular menstruation. It is generally not necessary to administer progestins to achieve these results; however, if menstruation is characterized by prolonged sporadic bleeding at the end of each course, norethindrone, 5.0 mg. daily by mouth during the last sevn days, together with the estrogen may be prescribed. Some authorities would prefer to employ both agents in all instances because of some evidence that unopposed estrogen action (without intermittent progestins) may be related to uterine malignancy in later life. If the development of secondary sexual characteristics is inadequate and menstrual flow scanty, a larger daily dose of ethinyl estradiol may be used, not to exceed 0.05 mg. daily. The introduction of this course

of treatment requires precise diagnosis and should conform to the usual age of puberty within a community. In gonadal dysgenesis associated with short stature, treatment is sometimes deferred in order to permit further growth prior to epiphyseal fusion. Such a decision must be related to the attitudes of the patient. It is our rule to begin treatment intermittently, 3 months on and 3 months off, from about the age of 13½ years, and permanent continuous treatment between 15½ and 16 years. This procedure brings about partial development of secondary sexual characteristics and occasional menstruation, which usually suffices in bringing about a sense of well-being and assurance.

Other causes of primary amenorrhea such as hypothyroidism or chronic disease of other etiology should not be treated in this way. Specific treatment for the basic disorder is employed.

Secondary Amenorrhea. This is usually of psychologic origin and requires identification of recent stressful experiences and reassurance. Pregnancy and recently acquired nonendocrine diseases must be ruled out. In a few instances when the amenorrhea is especially prolonged but clearly due to psychogenic factors, three or four months of cyclic treatment as described above will usually restore normal cycles.

Functional Uterine Bleeding. This is not unusual in the early stages of the menarche when it is thought to be the result of anovulation. If the monthly or less regular menstrual flow is especially troublesome and prolonged, progestins may be given for six months. Norethindrone, 5 mg. by mouth daily, or medroxyprogesterone acetate, 10 mg. by mouth daily, may be administered during the last 5 to 7 days of each cycle. Rarely an episode of bleeding may be truly excessive and relentless. Such a single episode is usually arrested by a single intravenous administration of 25.0 mg. conjugated estrogens U.S.P. and this may be repeated once after 4 hours. This unusual occurrence, once controlled by intravenous estrogens, is best followed by three months of complete replacement treatment with both estrogens and progestins as described under primary amenorrhea. Following such a course of action, were severe bleeding to recur, it would again be controlled with intravenous estrogens if necessary, but the patient would then be referred to a gynecologist for curettage and further study.

Primary Dysmenorrhea. In the majority of cases this requires detailed discussion of the natural phenomena of menstruation and further education in such matters. Appropriate exercise and rest are to be emphasized. Congenital anomalies and pathologic conditions of the pelvic viscera are to be ruled out in the severe cases. If medication is indicated, mild analgesics such as acetaminophen, 0.3 to 0.6 gm. every 4 to 6 hours, should be tried first. The employment of narcotic drugs is to be avoided.

If the pain is severe and incapacitating, several hormonal approaches have been employed. The most simple regimen which may be successful is the use of progestins alone during the last several days of the menstrual cycle as detailed under functional uterine bleeding. This program can be continued for 6 to 8 months. If this fails, complete inhibition of ovulation for four months is usually successful. In our experience many young women who require this treatment prefer to employ agents which are not clearly identifiable as contraceptive agents. We generally avoid their use. Norethindrone, 2.5 to 10.0 mg. by mouth daily from day 5 to day 24 of the cycle, is usually effective. One may employ a combination of estrogens and progestins exactly as outlined under primary amenorrhea. When ovulation inhibition is employed for this purpose it should be used for periods of 3 to 4 months with equal intervals without any hormonal treatment. The goal is to arrive at a reasonably symptom-free interval following which no further hormones are to be employed for this purpose.

Premenstrual Tension and Edema. Reassurance and counseling with regard to the encouragement of physical activity and formal exercise with appropriate rest are employed. Salt restriction in the postovulatory phase of the cycle is recommended. Diuretics are frequently employed during this same phase. The mildest, but unfortunately often unsuccessful, drug is ammonium chloride, 1.0 gm. three times daily, during the latter half of the cycle. Hydrochlorothiazide, 12.5 mg. three times daily, can be used in the latter part of the cycle. This should be individualized and begun on the days of the cycle when the particular patient experiences the onset of the symptoms. This drug should *not* be used continuously, and adequate dietary potassium supplementation is to be recommended. If all of these measures fail and the severity of the symptoms warrant, suppression of ovulation may be used as described under primary dysmenorrhea, but should not be continued indefinitely (see above).

Venereal Disease
IRIS F. LITT, M.D.

The greatest increase in the prevalence of venereal disease in the past decade has been in individuals under the age of 19 years. Whether this represents an actual increase or reflects improved culture techniques, heightened case finding efforts by physicians caring for young people, or changes in legislation allowing for more teenagers to be examined and treated for venereal disease without parental consent, is less important than the fact that venereal diseases are common among sexually active adolescents. Accordingly, screening in this group must include cultures for the gonococcus and serologic tests for syphilis in asymptomatic males and females, as well as Papanicolaou smears in females.

Evaluation of the symptomatic patient with a discharge, genital lesion or inguinal lymphadenopathy must be even more intensive, for the treatment of each of these is different.

It should also be stressed that the management of the adolescent patient with venereal disease, even more than the adult, goes beyond diagnosis and antibiotic therapy. It includes education to prevent recurrence, encouragement to involve sexual partners in therapy, reassurance that the patient will not become sterile as a result of the disease, as well as a search for coexistent venereal diseases. Because, so often, it is the occurrence of a venereal disease that alerts the physician to the teenager's sexual activity, it may provide an opportunity to initiate discussion of other related topics such as contraception, the pelvic examination, Papanicolaou smears, pregnancy testing, as well as the patient's sexuality in general. Moreover, the occurrence of a venereal disease in a prepubertal patient should always prompt investigation into the possibility of sexual abuse of the child.

SYPHILIS

The spirochete is still exquisitely sensitive to penicillin, which remains the drug of choice for this disease.

Treatment of the pregnant patient with syphilis must be rigorous at all stages of pregnancy. Disappearance of lesions of primary or secondary syphilis can occur without therapy, and seroconversion of tests such as the VDRL to negative may take from 6 months to 2 years to be complete, so neither of these can be relied upon as indicators of successful treatment in pregnancy.

We elect to treat pregnant adolescents with syphilis with 10 million units of aqueous penicillin intravenously daily for three days if hospitalization is possible or, alternatively, with 2.4 million units of benzathine penicillin G in addition to an equal dose of aqueous penicillin intramuscularly.

The pregnant adolescent who is allergic to penicillin poses special problems for therapy. Tetracycline stains tooth buds after the fourth month of gestation. Moreover, its adverse effect on skeletal growth at any stage of pregnancy should constitute a contraindication to its use. In the second and third trimesters, treatment with cephaloridine in a dose of 0.5 gm. daily for 10 days is recommended because of its ability to pass the placenta more effectively than alternatives such as erythromycin.*

Acquired Syphilis. The patient with stigmata of primary or secondary syphilis, or a positive confirmatory serologic test, may be treated with 4.8 million units of benzathine penicillin G administered intramuscularly in two doses one week apart. The penicillin-allergic individual may be treated with tetracycline administered orally in a dose of 3 gm. a day for a 15 day period, but this is clearly inferior to penicillin.

The VDRL titer will begin to fall within a month of therapy but may not become negative until 6 months to 2 years later. Ideally, the patient should undergo a spinal tap one year after therapy to determine if retreatment is necessary on the basis of findings suggestive of neurosyphilis such as elevated spinal fluid protein cells or positive VDRL.

Incubating Syphilis. The adolescent known to have been exposed to a partner infected with syphilis, or who is at risk because of having been raped, may be treated with 4.8 million units of intramuscular procaine penicillin plus 1 gm. of oral probenecid. This is also effective therapy for presumed simultaneous exposure to gonorrhea.

GONORRHEA

During 1976 a flurry of reports of gonococcal strains resistant to penicillin, apparently due to production of B-lactamase, highlighted the importance of repeating cultures one week after therapy as a test for cure. When such resistant strains are documented, treatment should be with spectinomycin.† In all other

cases, penicillin remains the drug of choice for the treatment of gonorrhea.

The asymptomatic carrier of the gonococcus or the patient with symptomatic gonorrhea of the urethra, cervix, anus or pharynx may be successfully treated with procaine penicillin G in a dose of 2.4 million units in each buttock, administered at one time in addition to probenecid. If the patient is allergic to penicillin, treatment consists of spectinomycin, administered intramuscularly in a dose of 2 gm. for males and 4 gm. for females. Follow-up care includes repeat culture for the gonococcus as well as serial VDRL determinations in the spectinomycin-treated group because of the lack of effectiveness of this drug on incubating syphilis.

Gonococcal ophthalmitis in the neonate is treated with aqueous crystalline penicillin G intravenously in a total daily dose of 150,000 units/kg.

Complicated gonorrhea in the male is characterized by the presence of prostatitis or epididymitis and may be treated with 4.8 million units of procaine penicillin G and probenecid as above. Complicated gonorrheal infection in the female consists of salpingitis, with or without peritoneal involvement, or perihepatitis. Because of the potential for tubal dysfunction resulting from inadequate therapy, teenagers with salpingitis should be hospitalized and treated with intravenous aqueous penicillin in a dose of 10 million units daily for 10 days. The patient with acute salpingitis exhibits marked relief of pain and defervescence within 24 hours of the onset of therapy, and perihepatitis typically resolves in the same time interval. With subacute or chronic salpingitis, improvement will be less rapid, and laparoscopy with tubal cultures may be necessary if there is lack of complete resolution after 10 days of penicillin therapy.

Salpingitis in the patient allergic to penicillin is difficult to treat. Cephaloridine in a dose of 1 gm. daily for five days may be effective, but a small percentage of penicillin-allergic patients cross-react with this drug. Intravenous tetracycline is often utilized, but may be complicated by hepatotoxicity.

Disseminated gonorrhea, as commonly manifested by arthritis or dermatitis, is treated with aqueous penicillin G intravenously in a dose of 10 million units daily for three days, followed by oral ampicillin, 2 gm. daily for 10 days. The patient allergic to penicillin should be treated with tetracycline by mouth in a dose of 1.5 gm. initially, followed by 2 gm. daily for five days.

---

*Manufacturer's note: Safety of cephaloridine for use during pregnancy has not been established.

†Manufacturer's note: Safety of spectinomycin during pregnancy or in infants and children has not been established.

OTHER DISEASES

Lymphogranuloma Venereum. This disease, manifested by a perineal lesion in conjunction with marked inguinal lymphadenopathy, rectal stricture or, more rarely, perineal or bowel fistulas, may be diagnosed by an intradermal Frei test or complement fixation test. Therapy with oral tetracycline, 2 gm. each day divided equally in four doses for a total of 10 days, is usually curative.

Herpes Progenitalis (Type II). These painful ulcerations, unless viewed in their earliest stages when they are vesicular, may be difficult to distinguish from the lesions of chancroid. Symptomatic relief can be achieved in both conditions with local compresses of aluminum acetate (Burow's solution). Specific therapy for herpes is not yet available, although topical application of photosensitive dyes followed by light exposure causes some improvement and appears to decrease recurrences in adults. The safety of this mode of therapy has not been established, and treatment of young patients is not recommended. Routine Papanicolaou smears to detect carcinoma-in-situ of the cervix should be performed regularly in a teenager following herpes infection because of the premalignant nature of this infection.

Chancroid. Treatment consists of tetracycline, 2 gm. orally divided in four equal doses daily for 10 days.

Granuloma Inguinale. This is less common in adolescents than the other venereal diseases and is treated with tetracycline, 2 gm. orally divided in four equal doses daily for 10 days.

Pediculosis Pubis and Trichomonas. Although not strictly venereal diseases, these are discussed here because they may be transmitted by close contact and are frequently found in the adolescent with venereal disease. Treatment of pediculosis pubis consists of the topical application of a lotion containing benzyl benzoate or gamma benzene hexachloride. Recent reports of neurotoxicity from the absorption of these agents should serve to alert us to the importance of giving explicit instructions and limiting the dosage to one application.

Trichomonas which is symptomatic may be effectively treated with a single oral dose of 1.5 gm. of metronidazole for the patient and the same for her sexual partner.*

---

*This dosage of metronidazole is higher than that recommended by the manufacturer. Metronidazole is also contraindicated during the first trimester of pregnancy.

Condyloma Acuminata. Transmission other than by sexual contact is possible with these condylomas, but venereal spread is also known to occur commonly. Once these lesions have been distinguished from condyloma lata by inspection and VDRL testing, treatment consists of a single careful topical application to the lesion of podophyllin 20 per cent in benzoin, avoiding contact with unaffected skin and instructing the patient to wash off the caustic solution with soap and water six hours after application, or earlier if burning occurs. The patient should be reevaluated after 7 to 10 days to determine if retreatment is necessary. If the condyloma is in juxtaposition with the urethra, surgical removal may be necessary because of the danger of the podophyllin causing strictures.

Premarital Counseling for the Adolescent

PRASANNA NAIR, M.B.B.S.

Premarital counseling of the adolescent should begin long before the teenager contemplates marriage or before such exigent circumstances as the occurrence of an unplanned pregnancy. Early counseling of sexually active teenagers should be directed toward preparing them for the responsibilities of marriage, family formation, and parenting, and also for developing a general sense of social well-being. Since adolescence is a period of emotional development, varying degrees of supportive counseling are necessary to help the individual teenager develop a mature and meaningful identity within his or her own social environment.

Over the past few decades, adolescents have become sexually active at younger ages, as evidenced by increasing rates of pregnancy and venereal diseases in those aged 16 and younger. The number of births below 16 has doubled within the past 12 years and the abortion rate in 1975 was higher in this age group than in all other ages except for women over 44 (Task Force on Adolescent Pregnancy, AAP, 1976).

Growth and development has always been the pediatrician's primary concern, and the evolving sexuality of teenage patients is part of the expected developmental pattern. This evolving sexuality is to be anticipated in the routine health care plan. It is the pediatrician's responsibility to use anticipatory approaches to prevent problems faced by the sexually active teenager. Many pediatricians are now seeing children into their late teens and so they are in an ideal position to incorporate sex education and premarital counseling into the total care of their patients. This usually begins at puberty, when expected physical changes and the marked individual variations in the onset of these changes should be discussed. "Sexuality" is present at all ages, but adolescence is a period when emerging sexual drives have to be dealt with by the adolescent. Individual guidance should be provided in handling these emerging sexual feelings in ways acceptable to the adolescents, their families and society.

Pediatricians have always set up specific child health supervision schedules for the care of their preschool and school-age children. It is important to set up a similar program for the preadolescent and adolescent patient. The health care plan for the teenager begins with regularly scheduled visits to the pediatrician. A self-history questionnaire may be of help as it can be developed for the population seen by that particular pediatrician or clinic. It offers a starting point in the interview with an adolescent, which can often be difficult especially for a busy clinician. It may also touch on sensitive areas without being as embarrassing as direct questions. It is important to ensure that all answers which denote concern or problems be discussed at the interview with the patient. Aspects of health, nutrition, growth and physical development could be profitably explored at this time. The history of inheritable disorders should be followed up by appropriate genetic counseling and educational programs.

Physical examination of the adolescent includes measurements (height, weight, blood pressure), urinalysis, hemoglobin and hematocrit at scheduled intervals. Routine screening for gonorrhea and syphilis should be mandatory for sexually active individuals. Papanicolaou smear, wet preparation and rubella titers are obtained in girls, the latter if there is no record of rubella vaccination. Breasts should be examined, and girls should be taught the proper manner of self-examination. If pelvic examination is to be performed, the procedure should be discussed in detail, preferably with the aid of a demonstration model and instruments to be used. The use of a model of the reproductive system can be useful in reassuring an apprehensive adolescent.

Continuity of care is important to all patients and especially to adolescents. Involvement of staff with empathy and understanding is crucial to a successful program. Group sessions using audiovisual aids on adolescent sexuality, birth control, parenting, venereal disease and vaginitis are helpful; excellent programs are available from various groups such as Planned Parenthood and the National Clearing House for Family Planning Information. These sessions should be followed by discussion with a member of the clinic team.

The teenage girl has been the one to obtain care much more frequently than the teenage boy, so that initial contact for problems associated with sexual activity are often made by the girl. Very often the approach is oblique and the teenager who presents with headaches and abdominal pain should be asked if she is worried about being or becoming pregnant. When an adolescent presents for family planning without any complaints, has a normal menstrual history and on general physical examination appears to be developing normally for her age, the pediatrician should perform a routine gynecological examination and counsel the adolescent regarding birth control measures. More and more pediatricians now feel competent in doing gynecological examinations in adolescents. A short refresher course from a gynecologist can be of help if one has not done an examination for years. The availability of a gynecologist for consultation is important if the pediatrician takes the responsibility for family planning for the adolescent. The different methods and their effectiveness, ease, problems and relative risks should be discussed (as noted earlier, good audiovisual aids are available and the local planned parenthood center could be of help). Attempts should always be made to involve the male partner in these discussions, as many teenagers are in the process of developing mature relationships and participation of the male in family planning emphasizes the role of the male in the partnership and in the decision-making process toward family formation.

When a teenager first begins to use a family planning method, monthly visits for the first three months may be required to reinforce the importance of following through with recommendations, to allay anxiety, and to answer pertinent questions. Subsequent intervals can be lengthened depending upon the maturity and motivation of the teenager. Oral contraception can be used successfully even in young teenagers, but the need for adherence to rigid regimen makes it necessary to maintain close supervision, especially of the more immature adolescent. If menstrual periods are regular, low-estrogen pills are recommended. In teenagers 15 and younger, breakthrough bleeding may be greater on low-estrogen pills so that the pediatrician will have to adjust the dosage prescribed by individual patient response. Intrauterine devices are an effective method of contraception, although cramps, menorrhagia and endometritis may occur more frequently in the adolescent. In those adolescents in whom oral contraceptives are contraindicated, the diaphragm should be recommended, for example, adolescents with hypertension, family history of atherosclerosis or cardiovascular disease, genetically determined hyperlipidemia, significant obesity. The diaphragm requires careful education of the adolescent, who must be motivated and mature enough to use this method consistently. The condom and spermatocidal foam should be discussed when the adolescent does not want to use any of the above. The condom's positive effect in decreasing the incidence of venereal disease while at the same time preventing pregnancy should be emphasized to both boys and girls.

If a teenager is pregnant, the physician has to discuss what alternatives are available to her. Her decision regarding her pregnancy will depend on numerous factors such as her relationship with her boyfriend, her parents, her own aspirations, her maturity and the duration of her pregnancy. The choices available must be discussed with her in a nonjudgmental manner, with emphasis that a decision need not be made immediately, though there may be some urgency if a therapeutic abortion is considered. Support and counseling become important when the physician or nurse may have to help the teenager break the news to the parents and cope with the parents' despair and anger. The role here would be that of an advocate for the teenager in this crisis. Comprehensive prenatal care should be arranged if the decision is to continue with the pregnancy. If a therapeutic abortion or adoption is planned, then counseling to cope with this decision becomes essential. If the couple contemplates marriage, the physician should help them look at their future objectively since the divorce rate in teenage marriages is extremely high. The pediatrician must take an active role in counseling the adolescent couple and their family in the decision-making process. For a marriage to be successful, maturity and the capacity to love and to share in responsibilities are essential. Parenting, added to the responsibilities of marriage in a young immature couple, makes adjustment to marriage doubly difficult.

In this age of changing sexual mores and its growing recognition by the general population, physicians and other medical professionals in primary care are frequently called upon to counsel couples and to discuss sexuality, family planning and marriage in schools and with parent groups. The pediatrician should take this opportunity to emphasize that knowledge of child development and parenting is a necessary and important part of the education of our children as a preparation for family formation.

Pregnancy

LOIS B. JOHNSON, M.D.

Successful pregnancy in our society requires commitment and self-compromise, as does parenthood. Pregnancy in the adolescent, particularly the single adolescent, requires life changes which may be at variance with and disruptive to the adolescent's own needs. Planned pregnancy represents a minority of the deliveries which occur to adolescent females yearly, and elective termination now exceeds deliveries in number. The combination of unplanned pregnancy and adolescence accounts for the complex problems which pregnancy may initiate, and with which professionals attending these patients must assist.

Early diagnosis is a crucial factor and determines the extent and type of services which may be offered. Primary physicians treating adolescents must maintain a relationship which allows disclosure of possible impregnation. Once this possibility has been raised, diagnosis must be made as quickly as possible. This is well within the capacity of pediatricians if the technique of pelvic examination is re-learned. Office pregnancy testing material is available and accurate if properly applied. Diagnosis of pregnancy can be confirmed in most patients by the sixth gestational week. If diagnosis is delegated to another physician, it must be with communication of probable gestational length. Follow-up must be done to be certain that the patient was seen and what diagnosis was made.

Relationship with the patient should be maintained after diagnosis in order for crisis counseling to be initiated. The primary physician may be the most appropriate crisis counselor or, but must have time to give to the process, often very time-consuming, and have updated knowledge about community services available. Referral is often more practical, but must be made with the patient's consent and with any bias of the counselor or counseling agency to whom the patient is referred known *before* referral. Medical information pertinent to the patient for reviewing pregnancy alternatives must be given to the counselor in advance (high obstetric risk, previous pregnancies, abortions and miscarriages, emotional disorder, parenting potentiality, significant mental retardation).

Crisis counseling in adolescent pregnancy has many goals, but among the most significant are the following:

1. *Acceptance of pregnancy by the patient.* Disbelief, denial or overwhelming anxiety delays diagnosis of pregnancy and may block planning and care. A trained counselor can bring the adolescent to accept the diagnosis.

2. *Presenting the diagnosis to pertinent persons in the adolescent's life.* The counselor must often assume a role of supporting adult to adolescents announcing pregnancy to parents whose reactions they realistically or unrealistically fear. Also, in most of the United States, adolescents cannot legally be given prenatal care or follow any alternatives to pregnancy until their parents' permission is obtained. It is necessary to help parents work through their own feelings about the pregnancy in order for them to take on a supportive role for the patient. They need help to consider the role of the putative father, who is often ignored.

Others whose roles are pertinent to the families (religious advisor, relatives) may be included in consultation as long as divisiveness does not occur. Too many advisors may exaggerate the usual ambivalence of the pregnant patient and block further progress.

3. *Pregnancy alternative planning.* The counselor must be ready with facts about medical risks of continuing pregnancy, need for limitation of number of pregnancies, costs of delivery and child rearing, feasibility of child rearing in the individual's personal situation and other needs of the adolescent and future child. Medical, emotional, social, educational, vocational, religious and other life issues have implications for pregnancy and parenthood and must be considered for each of the pregnancy alternatives: continuation of pregnancy and acceptance of parenthood, completing pregnancy and relinquishing parenthood, or elective termination of pregnancy. Final decision must be acceptable to the pregnant adolescent if adjustment to the long-range plan is expected.

4. *Implementation of the plans decided upon.* The adolescent who continues pregnancy needs competent prenatal care, started as early as possible. Adolescents at particularly high risk for maternal and neonatal problems include patients underweight at impregnation, those who are obese, those with chronic illness, and patients who have become pregnant within a year of the onset of menses or in the postpartum period, as well as those with clinical problems of obstetric import, such as contracted pelvis. Where prenatal care is obtained and who directs this care are important only as long as the people involved are competent professionals perceived as caring and supportive of the patient. The same must be true of the delivery and postpartum staff. The basic prenatal work-up is similar to that for adult pregnant women.

Nutritional counseling should be given individually and prenatal vitamins prescribed, along with an iron supplement (300 mg. ferrous sulfate two or three times day) and fluoride in deficient areas. Prenatal visits should be made every 4 weeks until 30 weeks and then with increasing frequency until 36 weeks, when the patient should be seen weekly. Missed visits in adolescents may signal depression or self-destructive wishes and should be followed up by phone, preferably by a familiar member of the staff.

It is important that the pregnant adolescent have help in planning and carrying out self-determining life functions. This includes the following: *school planning* (pregnancy school, local school or school transfer or substitute); *health education,* particularly covering approaching labor, delivery, sexual activity and contraception; *parenting,* including physical and emotional needs of herself and her infant; *child care,* possible nurseries; *job planning* and necessary job finding; *counseling* with someone who can follow the progress of the adolescent and pregnancy and facilitate the maturing process which pregnancy often initiates. Counseling should continue after delivery through the early parenting years when it is still needed.

Gynecologic Procedures

LOIS B. JOHNSON, M.D.

Examination. Pelvic examinations in adolescents should be carried out in a calm gentle manner. Though the examination is not physically painful it often produces intense anxiety. The first examination should be an educational process about why and how future examinations will be done. An assistant is helpful to reassure the patient. External examination is done, then vaginal speculum insertion and visual inspection of the walls of the vagina, fornix, and the cervix. One technique employed to minimize pain is to use an adult length narrow blade speculum (Huffman). The pediatric Graves speculum is inappropriate (too short to see the fornix or cervix) unless congenital anomalies or infantile vagina are present. Lubrication of instruments is done with warm water or saline so that commercial lubricants do not obscure the Papanicolaou smears. Gonococcal cultures should be taken, and other cultures as appropriate for problems encountered (see vaginitis below). Papanicolaou smears should be taken yearly after 18 years of age or after initiation of sexual activity, whichever comes first. There is no indication for routine pelvic examination in an asymptomatic, normally menstruating, non-sexually active patient under 18 years of age. Bimanual examination is done in standard manner. A competent gynecologist able to establish rapport with adolescents is needed as a consultant for pathology.

In preadolescents it is unusual to be able to complete a full pelvic examination as described. If good cooperation is obtained, the vagina may be inspected by insertion of an open-ended glass tube or a pediatric nasal speculum. Usually, however, a finger tip vaginal or bimanual rectal examination must suffice to rule out space-occupying lesions. If visualization is imperative, pelvic examination under anesthesia is indicated.

Vaginitis. *Trichomonas vaginalis* is frequently the organism responsible for vaginitis in sexually active adolescents. Its presence should be confirmed by wet smear. Systemic treatment is usually necessary for eradication of symptoms. Females receive 250 mg. of metronidazole (Flagyl) orally three times daily for 7 days. Topical therapy is not suggested in association with systemic therapy, though an acidifying douche every third or fourth treatment day may reduce symptoms. Male sexual partners are given a similar course of therapy if the vaginitis is recurrent. Metronidazole is contraindicated in pregnancy, at which time topical treatment is used. AVC, Triple Sulfa (Sultrin) or Nylmerat vaginal creams are used intravaginally once or twice daily for 10 to 14 days. It must be remembered that trichomonas is transmitted by sexual contact, and consideration should be given to contraception as part of the therapy.

Mycotic vaginitis, usually *Candida albicans,* is common, but particularly is associated with pregnancy, diabetes, and systemic antibiotic and oral contraceptive therapy. Its thick cheesy exudate can be confirmed by wet smear or growth on Nickerson's media for 48 hours (an office incubation procedure). Treatment is local, though associated medical problems should be considered and controlled. Local treatments are 2 per cent micronazole (Monistat) vaginal cream once daily intravaginally at bed time for 14 days, or nystatin (Mycostatin) vaginal tablets, 100,000 units/tablet intravaginally once or twice daily for 14 days. Pubic skin infection of sexual partners may occur. Treatment is composed of local skin hygiene and topical application of nystatin cream until clear.

Bacterial vaginitis is appropriately identified and treatment chosen by laboratory culture. Foreign bodies and parasites should be ruled out in preadolescents, particularly in resistant or recurrent vaginal infections. Fecal contamination of the vagina is not infrequent in preadolescents. Those enteric organisms responsible usually respond to Sultrin Triple Sulfa vaginal cream inserted nightly for 10 to 14 days. Topical treatment for the specific organism involved is usually appropriate unless the organism is known to require systemic treatment (i.e., gonococcus, streptococcus, etc.) or an underlying illness necessitates unusual treatment.

Viral vaginitis is not infrequent. No specific treatment is usually employed, except bland soothing topical ointment (AVC vaginal cream). In persistent or recurrent infections and in pregnancy, the patient should be seen and followed by a gynecologist, and long-term cytologic follow-up is carried out.

Other symptoms of vaginitis occur in many situations in which infection is not present. Examples include physiologic discharge, symptoms secondary to anxiety about intercourse or pregnancy, vaginitis associated with overvigorous hygienic procedures, or side effects from vaginally inserted drugs. Treatment is dependent upon diagnosis. Reinstruction for patients overvigorous in vaginal treatments should be given. There is no indication for nontherapeutic vaginal douches unless an acidified water solution (1 quart water with 1 tablespoon white vinegar) is used once or twice weekly during heavy discharge. Vaginal hygiene sprays and perfumes are not recommended.

Contraception. The physician seeing adolescents must be aware of the possibility of sexual activity by any of his patients. After the patient is fertile, if sexual activity is occurring without desire for parenthood, contraception must be considered. If an educational counseling process regarding sexuality and sexual behavior results in goal planning and self-determination, it may be the only contraceptive therapy needed. Time limitations prevent most physicians from participating in such a process with all patients. Local areas may have such services. Nationally, the agency providing such services is Planned Parenthood, whose education division conducts teen "rap" groups. Adolescents of both sexes may be referred.

In the turmoil, experimentation and impulsivity of the adolescent developmental process, long-term adherence to goal planning is frequently unrealistic. Compliance is crucial to the success of all nonsurgical methods of contraception. The choice of contraceptive method should be based on medical suitability as well as the patient's ability to understand and follow directions and to appropriately use medical personnel.

The condom, properly applied and used in combination with foam or diaphragms, can be effective for situations of infrequent intercourse. It has the added advantage of protection against venereally transmitted illnesses.

The diaphragm may be the method of choice for contraception in patients with chronic illnesses (i.e., hematologic problems involving anemias and clotting factor abnormality, collagen diseases) when both oral contraceptives and intrauterine devices are contraindicated.

Oral contraceptives remain the method of choice for most adolescents in the United States. The sequential progestational tablets have been withdrawn from the market. Only the combined estrogen-progesterone tablets are in use. Estrogenic activity has been reduced as low as possible to prevent estrogen-associated complications. In adolescents this may result in lack of cyclic withdrawal bleeding because of inadequate endometrial stimulation, and suspicion of pregnancy may occur because of lack of menses while taking tablets. A suggested routine is to begin with a low dose oral contraceptive (e.g., Ortho-Novum 1/50-28 and Demulen 28) on the fifth day after onset of menses. If menses does not occur by the completion of the second 28 day cycle, a higher dose tablet should be chosen (e.g., Ortho-Novum 1/80-28 and Norlestrin 1/50-28). A regimen of one pill daily—the 28 day packages—gives the least chance of error in instructions and affords opportunity to check on the patient's ability to follow directions. Patients are checked every three months for weight, blood pressure, side effects and compliance.

A pelvic and cytological examination are carried out before initiation of therapy and yearly thereafter. Though it is not so stated in package literature, the first year of menses is a contraindication to oral contraceptives, since they may mask or suppress pituitary-ovarian function.

Intrauterine devices are often effective contraceptive methods for adolescents because they do not have the side effects of the oral contraceptives, and their use minimizes manipulation, mistakes and noncompliance. The device is inserted during menstruation on an outpatient basis, and anesthesia is not required. The procedure is relatively painless for a prepared patient. Contraindications are similar for those in adults. Insertion of an intrauterine device is a surgical procedure in which perforation of the uterus can occur, and parental consent for minors is obtained. Changes continue to occur in configurations of the devices suitable for use in the adolescent uterus. At present those most effective (Copper 7 or Copper T) have a life-span of only two to three years and then must be changed, a drawback for use in transient populations.

Use of any contraceptives should be individualized, and follow-up by a counselor is suggested.

Therapeutic Abortion.   Elective termination of pregnancy is a choice frequently made by adolescent females and is estimated to have represented the disposition chosen in half of all unplanned adolescent pregnancies in 1975. The procedure has obvious moral and religious implications and should be the patient's choice, not one imposed by others. Professionals involved must be able to explain the procedures involved, handle anxiety regarding pain and disfigurement, as well as be supportive during decision-making. Medical risks should be represented accurately. Parents' permission must be obtained for unmarried adolescents under 18 years.

The choice of termination procedure is dependent largely upon gestational age. Prior to the 13th week of gestation, vacuum curettage or dilation and curettage (D & C) are employed. Vacuum curettage is used most widely and carries the lowest complication rate of any termination procedure, indeed a lower complication rate than pregnancy. It does not require hospitalization or anesthesia. The cost varies but is generally $200.00 or less. Because the procedure is available legally in most metropolitan areas, travel and hospitalization are eliminated, thus making this choice financially practical for most women. Its feasibility for adolescents often is lost because of delay in diagnosis, delay in decision for termination after diagnosis, or inability to schedule and carry out the procedure before 13 weeks of gestation after the decision to terminate has been made.

Significant increase in risk to the patient exists in termination during the second trimester. Intra-amniotic instillation of hypertonic saline is usually used to induce fetal death, labor and delivery. It is not done until the uterine cavity is large enough to receive the hypertonic solution with minimal risk of injection into vessels within the uterine wall. This method may require a gestational age of at least 16 weeks. Since many physicians consider live birth and infant survival to be possible at 20 or more weeks of gestation, 20 weeks of gestation (clinically, an audible heart beat or the presence of fetal movement) may be considered the absolute upper limit for termination of pregnancy. All procedures carried out during the second trimester require hospitalization, usually for three or four days if uncomplicated. This procedure is done in perhaps only one or two cities in each state; therefore travel and living expenses must be considered in cost. The total cost is usually more than $500.00, and thus the procedure is not practicable for many adolescents and their families.

Follow-up medical care, contraception and preventive mental health care are given as indicated. Adolescents may need to repress or deny infant loss as an emotional defense at the time of the procedure. Emotional crises concerning infant loss may be precipitated later, particularly at the expected date of delivery or with relationships which are perceived or expected to lead to another pregnancy. Mental health therapy may be needed during these crises.

24

Miscellaneous

Sudden Infant Death Syndrome

ABRAHAM B. BERGMAN, M.D.

Sudden infant death syndrome (SIDS), commonly known as crib death, claims about 8000 babies a year in the United States. It is responsible for approximately 3 deaths of every 1000 live births. After the first week of life, SIDS is the most important single cause of death of infants under one year of age; it ranks second only to accidents as the greatest cause of death in children less than 15 years of age.

While SIDS has been with us since biblical times (I Kings 3:19-20), masquerading under a variety of names, it did not become generally recognized as a distinct disease entity until the early 1970's. Although we can now describe SIDS and have limited knowledge about the mechanisms that produce the end result, our state of knowledge is still limited. As with leukemia or lupus, the diagnosis can be made but the cause and means of prevention remain unknown.

Epidemiology. The incidence of SIDS, 2 or 3 cases per thousand live births, is remarkably constant throughout the world, wherever the disease has been studied. It is more likely to occur in males, low birth weight babies, low socioeconomic class families, and during seasons of upper respiratory illness. It is uncommon before two weeks and after six months of age, with the peak incidence occurring between two and four months of age. Thus a low birth weight child from a poor family who is two months old and is put to sleep with a cold is more likely to succumb to SIDS than other infants. Such events make a child more "eligible" for SIDS, yet these are *statistical* findings, more of interest to the scientist conducting research

than to the physician dealing with an individual case.

Clinical Aspects. Babies who die of SIDS seem typical of the entire population of babies in that age group. SIDS can kill fat babies as well as thin; children of rich families as well as poor—but not as frequently. Approximately half of the infants have symptoms of a cold in the week prior to death. There are two clinical features of the disease that remain constant. First, death seems to occur during an apparent period of sleep. In our Seattle series of over 600 cases, each of the very few babies who were observed to die demonstrated some lethal lesion at autopsy; they were *not* deaths from SIDS. Approximately 15 per cent of infants dying suddenly and unexpectedly demonstrate some lethal lesion at autopsy such as intracranial hemorrhage, septicemia or myocarditis. *All* of our infants diagnosed as being victims of SIDS died during *sleep*. Reputable pathologists have reported deaths from SIDS occurring during observation, so it is possible, but most uncommon. A second feature is the apparent *silent* nature of death. Even if the baby is sleeping in the same room, the parents report no cry or other sounds of distress.

Pathological Aspects. The death scene is often one of disarray. The infant is sometimes found squeezed into one corner of the bed with a blanket covering the head, causing many parents to wrongly think that the child suffocated. Blood-tinged froth emanates from the nose in about half of cases, staining the sheets and giving some parents the erroneous belief that their baby suffered an internal hemorrhage. There is usually evidence of a brief burst of spasmodic motor activity; bladder and bowels are empty; sometimes blanket fibers are found under the fingernails.

On internal examination, the lungs are filled with hemorrhagic edema fluid, and minor microscopic evidence of respiratory inflammation is often found. Intrathoracic petechiae dot the surfaces of lungs, pericardium, and thymus in about 90 per cent of infants whose deaths were the result of SIDS; the fact that these petechiae are limited to the thoracic cavity is impressive.

Viral agents have been found in about a third of victims of SIDS, the same viruses that are found in babies with ordinary colds. Viral studies are not indicated unless one is involved in a research project; their presence or absence is not helpful in determining whether or not a death was the result of SIDS.

EMOTIONAL REACTION OF PARENTS

Parents may be more affected than parents of children who die of a better known disease or whose death is expected, for two reasons: the sudden and unexpected nature of the event and the aura of mystery surrounding SIDS. Characteristic grief patterns have been described for adjusting to the loss of a loved one. With most diseases, the family has the opportunity to prepare and to begin the grieving process before death. In SIDS, of course, there is no anticipation and the entire grieving process must take place after death.

Because of the significant relationship between SIDS and socioeconomic class, a large number of families lack any personal physician and thereby are unlikely to gain sympathetic support at a time of most need. Their lack of education and low standard of living compound their feelings of guilt. They tend neither to seek help nor to participate in parent self-help groups.

Physicians can play a significant part in alleviating prolonged grief and guilt reactions among survivors. Although at present there is no proven way to prevent SIDS, it is possible to deal effectively with the family that has lost an infant to this tragedy. To optimally assist the grieving family, the following elements of a SIDS program should be present in each community:

1. Autopsies should be available for all children who die suddenly and unexpectedly and should be performed by qualified pathologists.

2. The term "sudden infant death syndrome" should be utilized as a cause of death on death certificates, when appropriate.

3. Families should be notified either by telephone or letter of the autopsy results within 24 hours.

4. Follow-up counseling and information about SIDS and the characteristic grief reactions should be provided by a knowledgeable health professional.

Autopsies are important and should be available for all infants, not only those whose families can afford them. SIDS can be certified virtually beyond a doubt with clinical and pathological findings upon a gross autopsy; it is not necessary to keep families waiting in the agony of suspense until all microscopic and laboratory studies are completed. If later findings contradict the provisional diagnosis, a decision must be made whether the new findings are truly significant to the family (such as genetic disease), or useful only in altering vital statistics.

In dealing with individual families, the physician should be familiar with the basic facts about SIDS and with the characteristic grief reactions. The two most important points to convey are: (1) your baby died of a definite disease entity (SIDS) and (2) currently, SIDS can be neither predicted nor prevented; you are in no way responsible for the infant's death.

Children are especially vulnerable to guilt feelings about the death of a sibling; their reactions are often veiled. Painful as it is, open discussion of the death among family members should be encouraged. A good indication of parental coping mechanisms with grief is determined in what they tell their children about the infant's death.

Referral or contact with voluntary agencies working with SIDS can be most supportive. Many families gain comfort from contact with other families who have lost children to SIDS. Referral to such groups is an individual consideration and should be done at the request of the family. Printed information about SIDS, which is most helpful to the family in answering the invariable questions of relatives and neighbors, can be obtained from the National SIDS Foundation.

The tragedy of SIDS, unfortunately, does not end with the death of the baby. Pervasive and long-lasting guilt reactions occur among family members; the psychiatric morbidity is enormous. The cause of SIDS itself is not yet known. The cause of the guilt *is* known—ignorance; and prevention *is* possible through informed and compassionate counseling.

The following organizations are available to provide further information about SIDS.

The National Sudden Infant Death Syndrome Foundation
310 S. Michigan Avenue
Chicago, Illinois 60604
312-663-0650

The Guild for Infant Survival
6822 Brompton Road
Baltimore, Maryland 21207
301-944-8118

The Canadian Foundation for the Study of Infant
Death
4 Lawton Boulevard
Toronto, Ontario M4B 1Z4

The Foundation for the Study of Infant Death
23 St Peter's Square
London W6 9NW

The Cot Death Society
Flat No. 4
205 St. John's Road,
Remuera,
Auckland.

Child Abuse and Neglect

HOWARD M. KLEIN, M.D.,
RICHARD M. SARLES, M.D., *and*
STANFORD B. FRIEDMAN, M.D.

Child abuse and neglect represent major
etiological factors in the morbidity and mortality of children. Three conditions are generally
necessary for child abuse to occur: a child at
high risk; a parent at high risk for abuse; and a
crisis or chronic stress situation.

Children at risk for abuse may include
those with a history of prematurity or other
neonatal problems, the mentally retarded, the
handicapped, or the child who is seen for any
reason as different or difficult to manage by
the parent. Because of early separation from
their parents for their physical or mental problems, normal parent-child attachment may not
take place and these children are seen as "special" or different.

Although the potential for child abuse
exists in every parent, there appears to be a
defect in the character structure of the abusing
parent, which during stress allows aggressive
impulses to be expressed too readily and too
severely. Many abusing parents are socially isolated and have the inability to use people constructively, leaving them without support in
times of stress. In addition, some are intellectually limited, emotionally immature, or self-centered and are therefore unable to meet
their children's needs. Finally, it is clear that in
most cases of child abuse the abusing parents
have usually been abused themselves as children.

Both crisis or chronic stress situations appear to facilitate child abuse. Problems of family disruption, such as marital strife and separation, may constitute such a stress. Children
born out of wedlock, born in close succession,
or into large families represent other problems
which may induce stress into families.

The physician should be particularly sensitive to potential child abuse when the presenting history is not compatible with the physical
findings. For example, injuries and lesions
such as cigarette burns, hot water scalds, whip
marks, bites, scratches, and bruises—especially
when incompatible with the stated clinical
history—should lend high suspicion toward
possible child abuse. Occasionally, cases of ingestion may represent manifestations of gross
child abuse or neglect. A thorough medical
and psychosocial evaluation is essential in cases
of suspected child abuse. When the diagnosis
of child abuse is in doubt, the evaluation
should include a radiological skeletal survey to
detect recent fractures and evidences of old
fractures in various stages of healing.

In cases of severe injury or when there is
question of the parents' ability to cope with the
child at home, temporary removal through
hospitalization is warranted. Evaluation of the
child-parent interaction at this time can be useful in evaluating child-rearing practices, and
formulating recommendations for treatment
and management. When possible, a home visit
by the public health nurse can also provide important data as to the safety of the home.
When indicated, the evaluation may be extended to include the child's siblings, if their
welfare is in doubt. This evaluation should be
carried out through a multidisciplinary team
effort which includes medical, nursing, and social service personnel, and the local child protective agency.

Follow-up and case management need to
be coordinated by the child protective agency
with ongoing medical support. In every case it
is important for the physician to inform the
parents of the medical staff's concern for the
possibility of child abuse as a causative factor in
their child's injury and the requirement to report the suspicion to the child protective
agency. In some cases this confrontation may
lead to anger on the parent's part and a temporary disruption of the doctor-patient relationship. Generally, however, the genuine concern of the medical team and the relief felt by
the parents in obtaining help for their impulsive abusive behavior restore and may cement
a healthy, cooperative therapeutic relationship.

Treatment of child abuse is geared toward
helping the parents compensate for the
deficiencies they may bring to the child-rearing
situation and toward creating a positive shift to
personal and family functioning. Comprehensive emergency services such as a 24-hour protective services intake, a 24-hour hotline,
emergency shelter care for children and
families, and emergency crisis nursery or day
care facilities are important treatment facilities.
In combating the social isolation, the public

health nurse can serve as an important resource because of her familiarity with community resources and the guidance and support she can provide during home visits. Parent aides, such as specially trained homemakers or "foster grandparents," can provide daily home visits to help with child care in such practical matters as babysitting and housekeeping and act as proper parent role models. Parents Anonymous is a nonprofessional self-help group organized by abusing parents themselves in order to provide each other with support and a forum for discussion of mutual problems.

Counseling abusing parents is often helpful since many of these parents often place unrealistic expectations upon the child. Counseling, therefore, should include a formal explanation of normal child development and behavior to inform the parents which behaviors to expect from their child in order to formulate realistic guidelines for discipline. In addition, counseling should be directed toward making the parent aware of society's expectations of acceptable child-rearing practices and should serve as an external "super-ego" or social conscience to strengthen the parents' weak impulse control. A further goal of counseling is to help the parents effectively utilize other adults and resources in times of stress and crises. Practical suggestions for alternatives to punishment such as a "cooling off" chair or sending the child to his room should be utilized. If corporal punishment must be used, it is important to emphasize that shaking the child should be avoided and spanking should be limited to slaps on the wrist or buttocks.

Although psychosis or severe personality disorders are present in only a small percentage of abusing parents, representing a distinct and separate subgroup apart from other child abusing parents, significant parental psychopathology may indicate the need for referral for individual or group therapy. The goal of therapeutic intervention is to increase the patient's self-esteem, trust, and interpersonal contacts to the point where the parents can relinquish their abuse-neglect pattern and replace it with one more rewarding for themselves and their children. In situations where the parent is found to be psychotic, sadistic, or otherwise severely disturbed, removal of the child from the home may be required.

When the primary care physician senses the child has pent-up fears, displays marked ambivalent feelings toward the abusing parent, or expresses the concern that he himself may have precipitated the abuse, referral to a child psychiatrist or psychologist may be indicated.

Individual and group psychotherapeutic techniques have been used with varying success and focus on the child's expression of his concerns and fears while learning to trust and interact normally with another human being.

Previous follow-up studies of abused children have shown a high morbidity without intervention aimed at strengthening the maternal-child relationship. Moreover, one recent study (Pediatrics, *59*:273, 1977) comparing abused children with those who had been in accidents and controlled for socioeconomic status concluded that lower class membership may be as potent a negative force in child development as abuse. Therefore, comprehensive pediatric care sensitive to early detection of families at high risk for child abuse would seem to be as important as actual identification of abuse cases. Using a primary prevention model, this would include early promotion of parental-child bonding and helping each family develop their own coping strategies thus fostering strength in the family unit rather than belatedly trying to patch up weaknesses.

Parenteral Fluid and Electrolyte Therapy

LAURENCE FINBERG, M.D.

GENERAL PRINCIPLES

The administration of water and electrolytes to sick children has become the principal modality for maintenance and repair of physiologic homeostasis. All who aspire to give care to infants and children must become experts if the care is to be optimal.

Water and salts may be ingested orally as in ordinary feeding and in special feedings, or fluids may be administered parenterally through veins into the circulation. Most of this discussion will deal with the parenteral route, though the use of oral fluids *when the patient's condition permits* is understood to be preferable because of the potential additional regulating function of the intestinal mucosa. A few specific circumstances for oral therapy will be described. The only parenteral route considered will be the intravenous one. At least in the United States, there is little or no need to consider hypodermoclysis, intraperitoneal fluid or other parenteral modalities.

A few important principles of electrolyte physiology and water metabolism underlie all the therapeutic advice and regimens to be suggested. A brief review of these principles will place the recommendations in a usable context and permit rational application. One should have a reasonable grasp of the composition of the body with respect to water and the important solutes. Water constitutes about 70 per cent of the lean body mass (LBM), perhaps slightly higher in the newborn infant. There is little water associated with adipose tissue, so that an estimated correction is in order for obese subjects. Infants are rarely obese, so that weight and lean body mass for them are approximately the same.

About 45 per cent of the lean body mass of infants is contained within cells, mostly muscle cells. Intracellular water contains most of its solute in ionic form. The cations in highest concentration are potassium (K^+) and magnesium (Mg^{++}). The Mg^{++} is largely bound to cell protein and changes slowly, so that few clinical conditions reflect disturbances with it. The anionic composition consists of phosphates, sulfates, bicarbonate, and organic molecules, large (such as protein) and small (such as Krebs cycle intermediates). In the muscle cell there is virtually no chloride ion (Cl^-) and although calcium (Ca^{++}) is of major importance, it appears in a concentration an order below that of concern to this subject. Cl^- does appear in red cells and other tissues, but their combined mass is less than the cell mass of muscle tissue in all but the severely undernourished. Sodium (Na^+) is found in low concentration in cell water. The exclusion of Cl^- and virtual exclusion of Na^+ has fundamental importance to both homeostasis and to planning fluid therapy, since this biologic phenomenon causes NaCl content to be the determiner of the partition of body fluids.

Extracellular fluid (ECF) consists of two subcompartments. The first is interstitial fluid, which bathes the cells and accounts for about 19 per cent of the LBM. This is slightly higher in the newborn but reaches the infant proportion within the first week. Plasma, the intravascular portion of ECF, accounts for about 6 per cent of LBM. The electrolyte content of plasma and interstitial fluid is the same with instantaneous equilibrium for most of the compartment except for the presence of 6 to 7 gm. of protein per 100 ml. (10 mEq./liter or 1.7 mOsm./kg.) in the plasma, which in turn exerts a minor Donnan effect on the concentration of the other ions. These last variations are not clinically important.

Na^+ is the principal cation, Cl^- (100 mEq./liter in plasma) and bicarbonate, HCO_3^- (22 to 25 mEq./liter) the anions. Small amounts of K^+, Ca^{++}, Mg^{++}, and $HPO_4^=$ are also present. The boundary between intracellular fluid (ICF) and ECF is maintained by transport mechanisms which extrude sodium and exclude chloride. The two fluids maintain quite constant composition while in close proximity across thin cell membranes, retaining the probable ancestral arrangement of early living cells with the primeval sea.

The plasma retains its volume despite hydrostatic pressure from the heart and permeable capillaries because of the relatively impermeable protein, the albumin being smaller than the globulins exerting more osmotic (oncotic) influence. Discussion of therapy will stress maintaining the proportionate volumes of these compartments or "spaces." Note that all of these spaces represent a nearly constant fraction of the lean mass and therefore their reconstitution when they are deficient is appropriately expressed as a fraction of the patient's weight.

Water turnover, the daily obligatory expenditure of water, relates not to mass but to heat (caloric) loss. This in turn is a function of body surface, so that either calories expended or surface area may be used as a reference denominator for daily water requirements. Table 1 shows the important conversion values for infants. We prefer to use ml./100 calories* metabolized for teaching purposes because of the more obviously fundamental association. Also, newborns, edematous subjects and a few others do not quite conform to surface area calculations for water loss.

Since neither heat loss nor surface area will be measured in actual practice, Table 1 may be used to express the water requirement in terms of weight which will change with age. A quick glance at the table shows that only about four points need be remembered to make interpolation easy. In this way ongoing water requirement may be related to its appropriate reference point, energy, which is distinct

TABLE 1. Basal Caloric Expenditure for Infants and Children*

AGE	WEIGHT (KG.)	SURFACE AREA (M^2)	CAL./KG.
Newborn	2.5–4	0.2 –0.23	50
1 week to 6 mo.	3–8	0.2 –0.35	65–70
6 to 12 mo.	8–12	0.35–0.45	50–60
12 to 24 mo.	10–15	0.45–0.55	45–50
2 to 5 years	15–20	0.6 –0.7	45
6 to 10 years	20–35	0.7 –1.1	40–45
11 to 15 years	35–60	1.5 –1.7	25–40
Adult	70	1.75	15–20

*Water expenditure equals 1 ml./cal.

*The calorie used here is the nutritionist's calorie or kilocalorie, which is 1000 of the physicist's calories. In a few years the terminology will probably shift to the joule.

from deficit (composition), which in turn relates directly to weight at all ages. There is no single common denominator which may be used for both at all ages and sizes. These considerations also emphasize the especial hazard of dehydration to the small infant whose daily water turnover is about 10 per cent of its weight while the adult turns over 2 per cent. Note that the table refers to basal conditions. In this state the water is expended approximately as follows in ml./100 calories metabolized:

Insensible water	skin, 30 ml.	
	lung, 15 ml.	
Total		45 ml.
Urine (at 300 mOsm./kg.)		50 ml.
Stool		5 ml.
Total		100 ml./100 calories or 1 ml./cal.

The assumption of 300 mOsm./kg. used for urine is a clinically useful one since the actual capacity to dilute or concentrate may reduce the obligatory urine loss by a factor of 2 in infants or 4 in older children and act as a safety factor. Many sick patients temporarily lose this capacity. Patients may be at a basal state on rare occasions. More often elevation of body temperature, movement, and increased ventilation bring the fasting bed patient to about 1.5 × basal, a usual figure for calculation. Any one of high fever, extreme movement or marked tachypnea occurring would warrant an estimate of 2 × basal, and all these together, an unlikely coincidence, might at the extreme warrant 3 × basal as a calculated expenditure. These estimates have been found useful and appropriate in clinical experience.

Partially offsetting ongoing water requirement is the production of water from metabolism. This amounts to 12 ml./100 cal. metabolized or about 12 per cent of the requirement. For short term situations in which recovery follows quickly this amount may be neglected in calculations; for problems of longer duration this water becomes potentially important and will be considered later.

Homeostasis of hydrogen ion (H^+) is closely guarded in body fluids by buffers, by the control of the Pco_2 by the lung, and by renal excretion of H^+ and base. The details of these important relationships are beyond the scope of this presentation, but awareness of the major disturbances remains important. Primary changes in Pco_2 are termed respiratory and primary changes in H^+ are termed metabolic. Acidemia and alkalemia refer to actual changes in H^+ concentration, the pH system being conventionally used and pH 7.35 to 7.45 being the normal range. Acidosis and alkalosis represent a primary change in one or the other directions with compensation holding the pH in the normal range.

The availability of accurate measurements of pH and Pco_2 in the last few years has made the practical application of quantitative acid-base physiology easier—unfortunately, also easier to abuse. Two very important cautions are warranted. First, when ventilatory and renal systems are intact and functioning, H^+ homeostasis is assured except under the most extreme circumstances. This will be further elaborated a few paragraphs below. Secondly, dissolved CO_2 (which hydrated forms an acid, H_2CO_3) traverses cell membranes and the CSF-plasma boundary much faster than HCO_3^-, the base form of the buffer system. Therefore, since:

$$HCO_3^- + H^+ \rightleftharpoons H_2CO_3 \rightleftharpoons H_2O + CO_2,$$

the administration of HCO_3^- rapidly into the ECF causes CO_2 to enter ICF and CSF disproportionately to the HCO_3^- and drives pH down (H^+ ion up). Therefore rapid change in pH in ECF may produce a "paradoxical" opposite change in cells and CSF, to the patient's disadvantage. Thus, except under very unusual circumstances, a slow rate of HCO_3^- infusion is preferred even for marked distortion of acid base-balance.

A final general principle of therapy states that a systematic approach will be far superior to a haphazard one. A system should include points of analysis, preferably the same ones used in diagnosing the physiologic disturbance. We recommend five points of analysis with periodic return to them to assess therapy. They are as follows, in order of importance, together with the most useful measurement for each:

1. Volume. There are three considerations: (a) deviation from normal—usually a deficit, rarely an excess, quantitatively a fraction of weight; (b) ongoing obligatory water requirements or maintenance, a function of energy expended over time; (c) continuing abnormal losses from pathologic states.

The best measure for clinical purposes for this most important consideration is an *accurate weight of the patient*, repeated as often as condition warrants but never less than daily. Changes in weight over 24 hours or less may be taken to represent water changes. Be careful not to use such arithmetic cumulatively.

2. Body Water Space Proportions. This is dependent on considerations of osmolar physiology. The critical determinant for the

ECF-ICF portion is the NaCl content of the body, for which the Na^+ concentration in serum serves as a guide. Too low usually means relatively increased ICF and too high means proportionately increased ECF. Albumin levels in serum similarly guide understanding of the relative plasma volume.

3. Hydrogen Ion Metabolism. The principles were touched on earlier. Emphasis should be given to the fact that if volume and space partitions are essentially restored and if lung and kidney are functioning, the homeostatic mechanisms need only minimal help, perhaps more accurately an absence of aggravation, to correct the deviation. Measurements include arterial pH, $Paco_2$, and either derived or independently measured HCO_3^-. An additional useful consideration is the "base deficit," a number indicating the metabolic H^+ disturbance after mathematically adjusting the Pco_2 to 40 mm. Hg. The contribution of this derived number of Astrup and Siggard-Anderson has given clinicians a means of quantitating the metabolic component of complex disturbances in H^+ and CO_2. Their recommended calculation for correction assumes a distribution of $0.3 \times$ body weight for a rapid correction, and 0.6 or $0.7 \times$ body weight for total correction. These numbers provide useful approximations but should be used cautiously in treatment because of problems already referred to, because complete buffering is undoubtedly more complex than the assumptions imply, and finally because over time a number of physiologic adjustments are occurring.

4. ICF Ion Deficiencies. The concern here is primarily K^+ loss, which is often considerable and on which there are empiric data for a number of disorders. Mg^{++} and $PO_4^=$ losses appear usually to have less clinical relevance. The best measure is the K^+ level in the serum, but this concentration represents the result of a complex steady state and therefore it may be normal or high in the face of considerable deficit. The HCO_3^- concentration after hydration may offer a clue here, indicating deficit of K^+ when an otherwise unexplained alkalosis is present. ECG sometimes helps.

5. Skeletal-ECF Steady States. Ionized calcium levels are sometimes altered during hydration aberrations. Total calcium gives a clue; ionized $[Ca^{++}]$ gives direct information. ECG sometimes helps here also.

MAINTENANCE FLUID THERAPY

One use for fluid therapy is to maintain hydration in a patient who cannot use the oral route either because of alimentary tract disease or as a perisurgical necessity. If the patient is at bed rest and afebrile, which is usual, the volume of the water should be of the order of 1.5 × basal requirements. The requirement for sodium is very small, perhaps as little as 0.1 mEq./100 cal. metabolized, and the tolerance in the healthy child very great, up to 10 mEq./100 cal. An allowance of 2 to 3 mEq./100 cal. metabolized therefore falls midway in the range and provides a concentration of electrolyte (together with coupled anions) to prevent osmotic forces from rupturing red cells or damaging vessels. Glucose, usually 5 per cent, also serves this protective purpose and also supplies enough calories to combat ketosis.

Potassium conservation is not so good as for sodium, so that 1.5 to 2 mEq./100 cal. metabolized is needed for balance. These calculations will result in fluids with Na^+ concentrations from 30 to 50 mEq./liter and K^+ of 15 to 25 mEq./liter. The anions should be Cl^- and any of several bases, HCO_3^-, acetate or lactate. The proportion of Cl^- to base should be optimally similar to that in ECF, about 4:1. Such solutions may be made up easily by adding electrolytes to 5 per cent glucose solutions or by purchasing ready-made maintenance solutions. The first approach offers more flexibility and pedagogic advantages to large institutions with many varied problems and a teaching program; the second offers convenience and, where the service is small, safety as well. The intravenous route may be used indefinitely, but it is not advisable to leave a needle or catheter in the same vein for more than 48 hours. Otherwise thrombophlebitis or septicemia may result.

When oral electrolyte and fluid ingestion is appropriate as in the recovery period following infantile diarrheal disease, we have successfully used the following home-made, pharmacy prepared, "ion mixture" for more than 20 years. The ingredients are prepared for mixture with a liter (quart) of water and dispensed (for home use) one day at a time as a package of dry powder.

INGREDIENTS	CONCENTRATIONS WHEN DILUTED 58 GM./LITER
KCl, 1 gm.	Na, 49 mEq./liter
NaH_2PO_4, 1.42 gm.	K, 20 mEq./liter
NaCl, 0.6 gm.	Cl, 30 mEq./liter
Na citrate, 2.93 gm.	Citrate, 29 mEq./liter
Glucose, 51.5 gm.	H_2PO_4, 10 mEq./liter
	Glucose, 5 per cent or 50 gm./liter

Similar solutions may also be purchased, though the commercial ones tend to have lower sodium concentrations, because of the public's tendency to overuse the product. A wise precaution in utilizing "ion mixture" is to instruct the mother that if thirst persists after the recommended day's allotment is complete, to give plain water ad lib.

Should anuria, severe oliguria or other special problems be present, either plain glucose water or modified mixtures either to offer or to restrict Na^+ or K^+, may be concocted. Similarly appropriate anion modification may be achieved.

When fever, increased muscular activity, or hyperventilation is present, the volume of administered fluid should be increased in accordance with the previous schedule. If an anuric or oliguric patient is to be managed, then the water allowance for urine is eliminated and all K^+ removed from the solution. Sodium salts are usually also removed unless deficits or other avenues of loss coexist. The water allocation should be reduced by another 12 ml./100 cal. representing water of oxidation. To this new low allowance may be added the previous 8 hours' urine volume if oliguria rather than anuria should be present.

MANAGEMENT OF DEHYDRATION

In managing a dehydrated patient, first analyze the disturbance in the five ways discussed earlier: *volume,* including deficit, maintenance, and abnormal continuing losses; body space proportion or *osmolal status; H^+ ion status; ICF losses;* and *ECF-skeletal steady states.* The most common pediatric problems with dehydration result from the symptoms of diarrhea and vomiting which in turn produce loss of water and salts plus denial of intake. Most commonly water and salt are lost in physiologic proportion, so that there is symmetrical (proportionate) construction of body fluid spaces. This has been called isotonic, isonatremic, or classical dehydration or when unqualified, just dehydration. When advanced in degree, circulatory deficit dominates the clinical picture. Accompanying the water and salt loss is a varying degree of metabolic acidosis (or acidemia), because intestinal losses contain relatively more base than body fluids, starvation leads to ketosis, circulatory insufficiency leads to lactic acid production, and most importantly a failing circulation interferes with the renal ability to excrete nonvolatile acids.

Before implementing therapy, consider how much fluid will be given and what the solute content should be. Volume factors have been covered and usually where a deficit is involved will come to 150 to 200 ml./kg./day when dealing with infants and less for older patients in accordance with the principles already outlined. The electrolyte content of the deficit should be taken to be that of normal ECF when dealing with isotonic dehydration: Na, 150 mEq./liter; Cl^-, 120 mEq./liter; base, 30 mEq./liter.

In fact, NaCl losses are probably about two thirds of this because some ICF is also lost. The exaggeration permits one the convenience of neglecting maintenance electrolyte entirely in the face of a significant deficit fraction. Similarly the dehydrated weight may be used for calculation and the offsetting value of water of oxidation also ignored in practical situations. If little deficit is estimated, then proceed as under consideration for maintenance. Potassium replacement must be accomplished for empirical data, and a regimen is indicated in the following paragraphs. The aim is usually about 3 mEq./kg./day in diarrheal diseases and most of the other common disorders.

The plan for 24-hour management may be best divided into three phases: emergency, repletion and early recovery. Each phase, overlapping on the other two, has a particular emphasis. The first or emergency phase is to restore as rapidly as possible the vascular volume. It should last from 30 minutes to an hour and consist of very rapid pushing of fluid intravenously in amount from 20 to 40 ml./kg., depending on choice of solution and severity of illness. This fluid may be an albumin-containing solution such as single donor plasma, whole blood, 5 per cent human albumin or one of the modified plasma preparations. If so, 20 ml./kg. given rapidly is sufficient and ends the emergency phase. In very small (<3 kg.) infants, or severely undernourished babies, the albumin solutions are advisable. Alternatively a 10 per cent glucose in water stock solution to which Na^+, 75 mEq./liter, Cl^-, 50 to 60 mEq./liter, and base (HCO_3^- or lactate), 15 to 25 mEq./liter, have been added may be given at 40 ml./kg. over 40 to 60 minutes.

There are also suitable commercial solutions of this sort. Some authors recommend Ringer's lactate for this phase. We prefer the glucose-based solution because in our hands urine formation is observed earlier, but published results show little if any differences. The emergency "push" phase should always be employed in infants with any detectable or presumed deficit to ensure circulation, even if the infant is not yet seriously ill.

The second phase lasts for the next 6 to 7 hours with its primary aim being repletion of the ECF. A 5 per cent glucose base solution is recommended and the Na concentration is reduced to about 40 mEq./liter (range 35 to 55).

K^+ should be added *as soon as urine formation is assured* at a level of 20 mEq./liter, the anions to be distributed proportioned as before unless a special problem coexists. The amount given in this period should total, together with the emergency phase, one-half of the projected fluid volume for the first 24 hours. If, as is so commonly the case, the projection had been for 200 ml./kg. in the first 24 hours, the first and second periods should have delivered 100 ml./kg. in 6 to 8 hours.

The third phase, or early recovery period, continues the second phase at a slower rate, completing the projected volume plus additions for ongoing pathologic losses in 24 hours. K^+ is an important part of this phase of therapy unless severe oliguria persists and the aim is intracellular repletion. Oral therapy may be substituted here with "ion mixture" or other suitable fluid. Table 2 summarizes the preceding paragraphs and is constructed on the assumption of a 10 per cent weight loss isotonic dehydration projected to receive 200 ml./kg. in the first 24 hours. This approach should be used as a guideline and therapy individualized in accordance with more precise diagnosis of the physiologic disturbances.

When hypernatremic dehydration is diagnosed or reasonably suspected, some modifications of the therapy are in order. First, if shock is concomitant, even early circulatory failure, the emergency phase should be only an albumin solution. After this initial infusion, proceed as next described. Second, if no shock is present, no emergency phase exists and the deficit should be replaced gradually over a 48 hour period. The rate of administration of the total volume per hour should be the same over the full 48 hours, combining the deficit and 2 days' worth of allocation. Third, the stock solution should be either 2.5 per cent or at most 5 per cent glucose. Fourth, the Na^+ concentra-

tion should be 20 to 30 mEq./liter, and *as soon as urine production is manifest,* the K^+ concentration should be maximal (40 mEq./liter). Fifth, one ampule of 10 per cent calcium gluconate should be added to every 500 ml. of administered fluid. Anions distribute as in isotonic dehydration. This regimen has been remarkably successful in minimizing all complications over the past 5 years.

When hyponatremia accompanies diarrheal disease (10 per cent or less of the time) simply increase the Na^+ concentration in phases 2 and 3 of the isotonic regimen to 100 or 120 mEq./liter. Rarely will hypertonic salt be necessary.

SPECIAL HYDRATION PROBLEMS

Hyponatremic States with Circulatory Symptoms. These conditions invariably result when salt is being lost with water, but only water is being replaced. Fistula drainage, nasogastric drainage, dialytic errors and Addison's disease constitute some of the etiologic circumstances. The patients have azotemia, dilute or absent urine, and circulatory insufficiency, though they may have a normal or even supernormal water content. Such situations are best corrected by infusion of hypertonic solutions of sodium salts. Sometimes this is the only way to save life and promptness is essential. The deficit of sodium salts must be understood as a deficit of osmotically active solute, because maldistribution of body water is the most pressing problem. The distribution for calculating the deficit then becomes the *total body water* or 70 per cent of the lean body mass.

For example: A 10 kg. baby following surgery which created an ileal fistula has been maintained in water balance, but his sodium concentration in serum is only 100 mEq./liter and his SUN is 110 mg./100 ml. A mild acidosis has occurred.

TABLE 2.   **Scheme for First 24 Hours of Rehydration in Isotonic Dehydration; Deficit = 10 Per Cent of Weight**

	PERIOD 1	PERIOD 2	PERIOD 3
Phase	Emergency	Repletion	Early recovery
Duration	½ to 1 hour	6 to 7 hours	16 to 18 hours
Emphasis for restoration	Plasma volume	ECF	ICF
Fluid composition	a. Plasma or 5 per cent albumin b. 10 per cent glucose with Na+75, Cl−55, HCO₃−20 mEq./liter	5 per cent glucose with Na+40, K+20, Cl− 40, and base− 20 mEq./liter	5 per cent glucose with Na+40, K+20, Cl− 40 to 45, and base− 15 to 20 mEq./liter
Amount in ml./kg. of body weight	a. 20 ml./kg. b. 40 ml./kg.	60 to 80 ml./kg.	100 ml./kg. plus ongoing abnormal losses

Water volume $= 0.7 \times 10 = 7$ liters
Deficit per liter $= 140 - 100 = 40$ mEq.
$7 \times 40 = 280$ mEq. Na
Presume a balanced anion proportion of 200 Cl^- and 80 HCO_3^-.

The replacement should be either with molar or 0.5 M solution. 200 ml. of molar NaCl mixed with 80 ml. of molar $NaHCO_3$ will replace the deficit of electrolyte. Customarily one-half is given over a short interval and the patient rechecked. If improvement is noted and no untoward effects have occurred the other half may be run in slowly, the whole process taking 4 to 6 hours.

Salt Poisoning. Severe salt poisoning is the reverse of the previous situation and is best treated by peritoneal dialysis using 7.5 or 8 per cent glucose as the dialyzing solution with removal every 90 minutes for two or three infusions.

Diabetic Ketoacidosis. The fluid disturbance of diabetic ketoacidosis is similar to that encountered in enteric disease plus hyperglycemia. This last often makes the disturbance similar to hypernatremia. With the addition of gradual (no hurry!) administration of insulin, the principles of therapy are similar to those for hypernatremic dehydration. In particular the correction of the acidemia should be gradual. Rapid infusion of hypertonic $NaHCO_3$ is doubly dangerous, once for the sodium and a second time for the bicarbonate. Rapid reduction of hyperglycemia predisposes to cerebral edema, also best avoided.

Ventilatory Insufficiency. In conditions of ventilatory failure, whether RDS or severe status asthmaticus, the Siggard-Anderson type of analysis is helpful to approximate the metabolic component of acidemia which is secondary to hypoxia. The respiratory component will not yield successfully to administration of base; in fact, the overall disturbance will be worsened.

Surgical Conditions. Several disorders in which joint care with surgeons is indicated present special problems. Pyloric stenosis, a rather common disorder, is one of the few which may commonly give rise to a metabolic alkalosis. This is because there is high obstruction, so that gastric but not intestinal juices are lost in vomitus. Potassium losses are marked in part because too high a blood pH encourages urinary loss of $KHCO_3$ until the K^+ loss brings about paradoxical aciduria. The management of the volume and proportionate space problems is the same as in other hydration problems. The alkalosis should never be worsened by administration of any base, and the K^+ as

KCl should be replaced as rapidly as is safe both pre- and postoperatively but not intraoperatively because of possible scant urine formation. These are rare occasions for administration of NH_4Cl or even intravenous dilute HCl, but these situations are perhaps best left for experts.

In Hirschsprung's disease, the only special consideration is to remember that the large volume of fluid trapped in the colon is physiologically outside of the patient but included in his weight by the scale. The volume may easily be 5 per cent of the patient weight.

Patients burned extensively similarly develop an "edema space" which is additive to the weight by as much as 10 per cent when 50 per cent or more of body surface is involved. This fluid is unavailable to support plasma or interstitium for a period of 5 to 8 days. Allowance should be made for addition initially and delivery of the edema a week or so later.

PARENTERAL NUTRITION

Patients who have lost most of the small intestine secondary to disease or from surgery to relieve an anomaly or a disease process, as well as patients with bowel disease and severe malabsorption, where removal of enteral feeding may lead to healing of inflammatory lesions, have experienced successful intravenous alimentation, sometimes after extended periods of up to a year. This is done by placing a catheter into a large vein permitting infusion of concentrated solute loads not tolerable for peripheral veins over a day or two. The technique, however, is inherently hazardous because of the ease of contamination and of thrombus formation within the vein. In addition a variety of toxic-metabolic complications have occurred, varying with solution selected. These include hyperammonemia, other evidences of liver damage, deficiency disease and others. One aid to avoidance of deficiency of linolenic acid and trace elements has been a small weekly infusion of plasma from a donor who donates an hour after eating a high fat meal. Prematurely born infants have also been treated with these hypertonic feedings, but the results have been less clear-cut. To date the procedure remains experimental and should only be employed by groups who will treat significant numbers of patients and who will maintain a commitment to monitor each patient very closely while supervising an experienced bedside and laboratory team.

Very recently parenteral preparations containing fat have become commercially available. While the rate of adverse reactions to intravenous fat is sufficiently high to advise restriction of these preparations to large centers, it would appear that this modality will be a useful way to supply calories and avoid some of the hazards of central venous catheters.

Anesthesia: Aspects of Significance to the Pediatrician

RAYMOND B. LARAVUSO, M.D.

Preoperative Evaluation. Close cooperation and communication between pediatrician, anesthesiologist and surgeon is necessary for optimal care of the child who is to undergo anesthesia and surgery.

Any aspect of the present and past medical history can be of importance to anesthetic management. Since all anesthetic agents have profound effects on the respiratory and cardiovascular systems, particular attention must be paid to these areas. Among the most important conditions are: congenital cardiac lesions, heart failure, dehydration, anemia, asthma, upper airway obstruction or infection and pulmonary infection. Of particular interest in the history are current and past drug therapies, drug allergies and previous anesthetic and surgical experience. Patients maintained on cardiotonic or antihypertensive drugs should be maintained on these drugs until the time of surgery.

A family history of adverse anesthetic experience is important. Two conditions which have a familial incidence are prolonged paralysis following usual doses of succinylcholine and malignant hyperthermia triggered by exposure to various drugs used during anesthesia.

The physical examination of the respiratory and cardiovascular systems is of particular importance to the anesthesiologist and any abnormalities must be carefully noted. The status of the upper airway must be evaluated in order to assure the ability of the anesthesiologist to maintain its patency during anesthesia and to intubate the patient if necessary.

A preoperative complete blood count and urinalysis are the minimum laboratory work necessary prior to surgery. Need for further studies will be determined by the patient's condition and contemplated surgery. For example, any child with a cardiac problem who is taking a diuretic should have serum electrolytes determined, and children with serious respiratory disease should have arterial blood gases measured.

PREOPERATIVE PREPARATION.   The goal of preanesthetic preparation is to bring the child to the operating room in the best psychological and physical condition. The child should be prepared psychologically for anesthesia and surgery. The type of preparation involved varies with the age of the patient and the anticipated anesthetic technique. Children up to age five fear most the separation from parents. This may be handled by providing the child with heavy premedication which will result in his being asleep prior to leaving the ward. Alternatively, the anesthesiologist may choose to bring the child to the operating room awake. Permitting parents to stay with the child as long as possible (including the trip to the operating room and the stay in the preoperative holding area) can be useful in these cases.

A sympathetic operating room nurse may also be of help in calming and eliciting the cooperation of a young child. If the child is to undergo a mask induction, the procedure may be facilitated by creating a game involving a space flight, astronaut mask, the smell of engine exhaust and the feeling of floating. Preparation for such a game should be begun the night prior to surgery.

Children 5 to 10 years of age fear separation but also have fear of mutilation and physical injury. Complete explanation of what is to be done for him and maximum reassurance that he will not be harmed are required. Children 8 to 14 years of age have a fear of loss of control during anesthesia, and regional anesthesia with its resulting loss of control of parts of the body may be unsuitable in this age group. This fear of loss of control can be best handled by providing the patient with a full explanation of what is going to be done and by allowing him to participate as fully as possible in his own care. This may even be carried to the point of allowing the child to hold the anesthetic mask himself as he undergoes an inhalation induction.

Physical conditions which place a patient at particular risk include upper airway obstruction, pulmonary insufficiency, cardiac failure, hypovolemia, high fever and electrolyte imbalance. Treatment of these conditions should be undertaken prior to surgery if possible. A balance must be struck between the urgency of the surgical condition and the relative risk of undergoing surgery and anesthesia without such preparation. Several examples will illustrate this concept. (1) An asthmatic who is to undergo elective surgery would be given maximal therapy prior to surgery. (2) The dehydration which often accompanies pyloric stenosis can often be treated by intravenous therapy prior to surgery. (3) A multiple trauma victim will often need to be taken immediately to the operating room where surgery and resuscitation will be conducted simultaneously.

In order to avoid pulmonary aspiration of stomach contents, patients undergoing elective surgery should have an empty stomach prior to induction of anesthesia. The period of withholding oral intake, however, must be the minimum needed to achieve this goal. Longer periods of fluid restriction will result in decreases in intravascular volume and possibly hypotension during anesthesia. A suggested regimen is a period of four hours without oral intake for infants up to the age of six months, six hours for children six to 36 months, and eight hours for those over 36 months of age. Children should not be given milk, solids, or formula for 12 hours prior to surgery, only clear liquids being permitted. Just prior to being placed NPO, all children should be awakened and given clear liquids. If this is not done, many will have a much longer period during which they have no fluid intake. Any child who must have oral intake withheld longer than recommended above, or who cannot tolerate these minimal periods, should receive intravenous fluid therapy.

Premedication must be tailored to suit the psychological and physical condition of the child, the planned anesthetic technique, and the surgical procedure to be undertaken. Some children require no premedication. For example, a healthy outpatient with whom the anesthesiologist can establish rapport may undergo inhalation induction pleasantly without any sedation. For those who do require premedication, the following is a popular regimen in healthy chidren: 0 to 6 months of age—atropine, 0.02 mg./kg. (minimum dose, 0.15 mg.); 6 to 12 months of age—atropine, 0.02 mg./kg. (minimum dose, 0.15 mg.), pentobarbital (Nembutal), 3 to 4 mg./kg.; greater than 12 months of age—atropine, 0.02 mg./kg. (minimum dose, 0.15 mg.; maximum, 0.6 mg.), morphine sulfate, 0.1 mg./kg. (maximum dose, 10 mg.), pentobarbital 3 to 4 mg./kg. (maximum dose, 120 mg.).

The above regimen for children over 12 months of age represents a "heavy" premedication and is used only for healthy children. These children will usually arrive in the operating room asleep. If a child is ill (especially those with respiratory or cardiac insufficiency or a decrease in intravascular volume), the dosage of premedication must be reduced or premedication omitted entirely.

Anesthetic Management. Children should be afforded the full range of monitoring that is appropiate to their condition and to the surgical procedure being undertaken.

Temperature control is of particular importance in children. Infants are particularly prone to heat loss due to large body surface to volume ratios as well as high minute ventilation relative to their body mass. In addition, infants less than three months of age do not shiver. Air-conditioned operating rooms, open body cavities, intravenous fluids at room temperature, the administration of cold blood and the use of unheated inspired gases will all contribute to the development of hypothermia. For these reasons, temperature must be monitored continuously to detect hypothermia and also for the early detection of the syndrome of malignant hyperthermia.

The most important measure in preventing heat loss is to warm the operating room; ambient temperatures as high as 80° F. may be required for this purpose. A heating blanket placed under a child is useful only in children weighing less than 10 kg. In using such a blanket it is important to remember that a child's head represents a large portion of the body surface area and his head must lie on the blanket. Other aids in preventing heat loss include use of warmed skin preparation solutions, warmed and humidified inspiratory gases, warmed intravenous fluids and heating lamps.

Anesthetic Agents. Halothane is the most commonly used anesthetic vapor in pediatric practice. It permits rapid and pleasant induction as well as rapid emergence at the conclusion of anesthesia. It also allows the use of high concentrations of oxygen if necessary. Halothane is a respiratory and cardiovascular depressant. Assisted ventilation is usually required if the child is allowed to breathe spontaneously during halothane anesthesia. Newborns are sensitive to the depressant action of halothane, and hypotension and bradycardia may develop rapidly in these infants.

Enflurane (Ethrane) is a recently introduced inhalation anesthetic agent. Induction and emergence are slightly quicker than with halothane and the drug produces more muscle relaxation than halothane. It has no other real advantages. Its cardiac and respiratory effects are similar to those of halothane. The drug has an excitatory effect on the central nervous system and seizures have been reported during its use, particularly during deep levels of anesthesia or during hyperventilation.

Methoxyflurane is an inhalation anesthetic which has the advantage of being a potent analgesic; however, its metabolites are toxic to the kidney. This drug is not used frequently in pediatric practice.

Nitrous oxide is an inhalation agent commonly used in combination with intravenous drugs or other inhalational agents for the maintenance of anesthesia. It is not potent enough to produce surgical planes of anesthesia in healthy children without the addition of other drugs. Nitrous oxide is more soluble in blood than is nitrogen. For this reason, it will diffuse into and expand any air-containing space in the body. It should be avoided in cases in which a child has a pneumothorax, large amounts of gas in the bowel or air in the ventricles following a pneumoencephalogram.

Intravenous barbiturates are induction agents and can be used to supplement other agents for the maintenance of anesthesia. There is some question as to the safety of using intravenous barbiturates in younger children. They are safe in healthy children over the age of six or seven. Large doses over long periods of time should be avoided, as they will result in delayed awakening at the conclusion of anesthesia. Narcotics can be used in children to supplement nitrous oxide, barbiturates and muscle relaxants in so-called "balanced" anesthetic techniques. However, the use of large doses may require continued ventilatory support at the conclusion of surgery.

Ketamine is a recently introduced anesthetic agent which can be administered intramuscularly or intravenously. Following its administration, there is a rise in blood pressure and heart rate due to sympathetic stimulation. This property may be of advantage in anesthetizing the severely debilitated or traumatized patient. Conversely, the drug should be avoided in patients who are hypertensive. Ketamine increases intracranial pressure and this effect must be taken into consideration when anesthetizing patients for neurosurgical procedures. A major disadvantage of ketamine is its production of hallucinations and bad dreams. This seems to be less of a problem in younger children, but the incidence increases with increasing age. Ketamine has little respiratory depressant effect, and upper airway reflexes are usually stimulated by the drug. In some cases, apnea may develop following its administration and it does not protect from aspiration of stomach contents.

The ease of administration of ketamine as well as its support of the cardiovascular and respiratory systems should not lead to careless use. It should be administered by experienced personnel, and the usual anesthetic equipment, monitoring devices and drugs used during the administration of any other general anesthetic should be available.

Muscle relaxants are frequently used as part of anesthetic technique. Succinylcholine is a depolarizing muscle relaxant which is fre-quently used for brief relaxation to facilitate endotracheal intubation. Its duration of action is three to five minutes. However, in some patients who have a deficiency in the pseudocholinesterase enzyme system, muscle relaxation may be prolonged. This condition has a familial incidence and should be sought in the family history. In addition, some patients may react to a single dose of succinylcholine with a sustained contraction of skeletal muscles and malignant hyperthermia.

D-tubocurarine is a nondepolarizing muscle relaxant frequently used during anesthesia. Its most important side effect is hypotension, which may be profound in a patient who is hypovolemic. All nondepolarizing muscle relaxants should be reversed at the conclusion of anesthesia if the patient is not going to be maintained on ventilatory support. If it is felt that the neuromuscular blocking effects do not require reversal at the conclusion of anesthesia, objective criteria must be documented to support this decision. This would include a vital capacity measurement of greater than 15 ml./kg. and the use of a nerve stimulator to demonstrate sustained tetanus in a peripheral muscle. Any patient in whom neuromuscular blockade has not been reversed should be watched carefully for respiratory insufficiency in the postoperative recovery room.

Pancuronium is a nondepolarizing muscle relaxant. Unlike d-tubocurarine, it does not cause hypotension. However, there is an incidence of tachycardia with its use. Like d-tubocurarine, its effects should be reversed at the conclusion of anesthesia.

Endotracheal Intubation. Uncuffed endotracheal tubes are used in children below the age of puberty in order to avoid the pressure that a cuff would exert on immature tracheal cartilages. The correct size tube is one that passes easily into the trachea and has a slight leak at the peak of positive pressure inspiration. Under no circumstances should a tube be forced into the trachea. It is important to remember that the most narrow portion of a child's airway is at the level of the cricoid cartilage. A tube which fits tightly at the level of the vocal cords will be excessively tight at the level of the cricoid.

Neonates. Transportation to and from the operating room is a critical event for a neonate. Particular attention must be paid to maintaining body temperature, and the use of portable heated incubators is essential. All blood products and all fluids which are rapidly administered to a neonate should be warmed to body temperature. Anesthesia equipment which allows the heating and humidification of inspired gases is necessary and, in addition, the anesthesiologist must have the capability of administering oxygen in concentrations of 21 to 100 per cent without the use of nitrous oxide. This can be accomplished by providing an anesthesia machine which has the capability of administering air and oxygen in any proportion. Heart rate and blood pressure must be monitored continuously and careful attention paid to the amount of fluid and blood which is lost during surgery as well as the amount administered.

Postoperatively, great care must be taken to ensure that the neonate has adequate ventilation. If there is any doubt about the child's ability to maintain adequate ventilation on his own, mechanical ventilation must be provided.

The exact fluid requirement for a sick neonate can be determined only in consultation with the pediatrician caring for the child. Some will require much more than "routine maintenance." Some neonates require much higher concentrations of dextrose than 5 per cent, whereas others are intolerant of even 5 per cent dextrose. Hypocalcemia is another problem in neonates and knowledge of the child's status with regard to this electrolyte is imperative. Studies have shown an increase in intracranial hemorrhages when neonates receive large amounts of hypertonic solution, particularly sodium bicarbonate.

Radiation Exposure in Diagnostic Roentgenology

MELVIN TEFFT, M.D.

The value of x-ray to diagnose abnormalities of childhood which may be corrected by medical and/or surgical management must be balanced by consideration of adverse effects on normal tissues. Harmful effects of radiation may be described most simply as somatic and genetic. Somatic damage may result in direct abnormality of the person who receives radiation, such as patients who develop a malignancy. Genetic effects, which may be produced in the person who receives radiation, will not be observed until the next or succeeding generations.

Estimation of an induction rate of malignancy due to radiation has included observations in atomic bomb survivors in Japan, atomic bomb fallout from testing in the Marshall Islands in the 1950's, and therapeutic radiation for benign conditions, such as the enlarged thymus, and for malignant neoplasms. Estimated doses of radiation which these children received have exceeded radiation exposure to the whole body and critical organs which will be delivered from most diagnostic roentgenographic examinations. Such estimated doses exceeded 50 R and averaged 100 to 300 R. This is to be compared with a skin exposure dose of 0.01 R for a single posteroanterior chest film or 0.43 R for a lateral view of the lumbar spine in a three year old child. Obviously, multiple diagnostic film examinations will increase the overall exposure of these children as will other radiographic techniques, such as certain methods of fluoroscopy. For instance, with the use of older fluoroscopic units for cardiac catheterization examinations, the dose of radiation to the posterior skin surface may reach 60 R.

Malignancies related to atomic exposure or therapeutic doses have included leukemia and thyroid carcinoma. Younger children may be more sensitive to developing these lesions, although a threshold age is not clearly defined. It has been estimated that 20 additional cases of acute or chronic myeloid leukemia may be induced over a 10 to 20 year period (1 to 2 cases annually) if 10^6 persons receive 1 rad per year of whole body radiation. The spontaneous rate of leukemia is raised by a factor of 1.4 to 1.025 per rad of whole body exposure.

However, at least in two groups of children, those that received radiation for benign thymic enlargement and those who were treated for a malignancy and developed a later second "unrelated" neoplasm, other factors must be considered. Could the etiologic factors of developing an enlarged thymus relate to later malignancy if radiation was not utilized? The incidence of malignancy in such a group of untreated children has not been reported. Does a child treated for a malignant lesion have a propensity to develop second unrelated malignancies? This has been observed in large series of cancer patients as unrelated to the mode of original treatment.

Radiation as a causative agent in developing neoplasia cannot be excluded when one reviews the various available reports including our own experience. Therefore, it is necessary to limit radiation exposure in young children to all but necessary examinations. Although the exact limits of exposure are not established, cumulative doses may raise the risk of neoplastic induction.

Genetic effects of radiation are difficult to ascertain. Individuals may experience a spontaneous rate of mutation of 0.2 mutations per generation. Doses of radiation which range from 3 to 150 R (average 80 R) may double this rate. Damage is cumulative and proportional to total dose, irrespective of the time over which the dose is delivered.

It has been estimated that if a whole generation of parents receive 1 rad to the gonad before they conceive, 15 radiation-induced autosomal dominant mutations might occur in first generation decendents. This would represent an increase of 0.2 percent over the spontaneous rate for such mutations. Less than an increase of 2 per cent sex-linked mutations would occur. An increase of 0.1 per cent of "genetic deaths" might occur in 10^6 zygotes, whereas 1 rad to the gonads per parent generation of 10^6 people might result in 1.9×10^3 "genetic losses" in the 10 ensuing generations. This is to be compared with a spontaneous rate of 2.4×10^6.

The mutations produced are permanent and will affect succeeding generations. However, the process of "natural selection" may eliminate many such mutations. Since the reproductive cycle is lengthy, harmful genes may be eliminated very slowly over several succeeding generations. For example, mutations which lead to a chronic and debilitating illness may affect secondarily the ability to reproduce and thus end the transfer of mutated genes to suceeding generations. Mutations may affect certain organ systems and cause early death before reproduction of successive generations can occur.

The decision for using diagnostic radiographic procedures should rest with the referring physician who must evaluate the information to be gained with the ability to treat a condition which, if untreated, would lead to the adverse medical well-being of his patient. However, this decision can only be reached in consultation with the diagnostic radiologist who is able to evaluate the types of procedures which may be necessary and the means by which these procedures can be refined to limit radiation exposure to the patient.

With present day modern x-ray equipment, much can be done to limit radiation exposure. These refinements include using image intensification and video adapters rather than the older fluoroscopic units, adjustment of tube voltage and filtration for single films, limiting the number of films per examination, restricting the field of exposure with cones and collimators, using external shielding where applicable to protect certain critical organs, such as the gonads, and adequate patient immobilization to ensure that only the area under examination is in the beam of radiation.

For instance, lower x-ray voltage and diminished filtration of the x-ray tube, the use of grid cassettes and Bucky trays, and nonscreen film all tend to increase radiation exposure to the patient. Newer x-ray tubes allow for lower exposures by allowing increased voltage and filtration. Grids are not useful to examine small anatomic volumes and should not be used routinely. Although nonscreen film gives finer detail, regular film and cassettes should be used whenever possible to achieve lower radiation doses. High-speed screens permit reduction in exposure, even at higher voltages. The size of the x-ray beam should be limited by collimators or cones since reducing the aperture reduces the size of the primary beam and secondarily diminishes the contribution of scattered radiation. Since the distance from any anatomic site to the gonads is less for small children, indirect scattered radiation to the gonads could be higher than in older children even when such a distant site as the skull is being examined. External lead shielding cannot protect from such secondary contributions of exposure. This factor should be considered in ordering examinations of very young children and in the refinement of technique and number of films obtained. Patient immobilization is vital. Fluoroscopy should be used as little as possible since even with an image intensifier, the dose received is higher than when single films are obtained under refined techniques.

The gonadal dose to a boy of three years from a single posteroanterior chest film may be 0.7 R due to scattered radiation, whereas an older boy of 10 years will receive only 0.2 R because the center of his thorax is at a relatively greater distance from his gonads. Scattered doses to the ovaries from a single anteroposterior film of the skull may be 0.40, 0.18 and 0.08 MR at ages 6 months, 4 years, and 12 years, respectively. The dose to the gonads decreases by a factor of 100 when the thorax is examined as compared with pelvic examinations. It is reduced by 1000 in the examination of the head and neck. A single film of the pelvis in a 6 month old infant may deliver 27 MR. In general, radiography of the upper torso delivers two to three times the dose to the ovaries than to the testes; examination of the pelvis delivers direct dose to ovaries but only scattered dose to the scrotum, and results in a difference of an order of magnitude.

Older boys receive higher doses of radiation to the testes when the pelvis is examined, since increasing voltage due to thicker tissues increases the scatter contribution. Conversely, younger children may receive higher gonadal dose when the thorax is examined if the collimater of the x-ray unit is not well defined. When the collimator limits the direct beam to the thoracic cavity, the gonadal dose in boys is less than 0.1 MR per film at any age. However, if the direct beam encompasses the whole body, as may happen in very young children during a chest examination, the dose to the gonads at any age may be 50 to 200 times greater. Similarly, the gonad dose may be increased even when skull examination is undertaken if the beam is not well collimated to include only the area of the skull.

Examination of the urinary tract can yield gonadal doses of up to 4.8 rads per examination if care to limit the dose is not used. Similarly, examination of hips in infants, as for dysplasia, may yield high gonadal doses. Reduction of gonadal doses can be achieved in several ways during these examinations. For instance, small tube voltages result in superfluous patient exposure. Raising the voltage as high as a minimal required film contrast permits may diminish the image contrast but decreases exposure of the patient.

In the range of 70 to 80 kvp, with a 8 to 12 cm. depth as in the pelvis of small children, a 2 mm. external lead shield over the gonads reduces the female gonad dose by 70 to 80 per cent, provided the shield is accurately placed. Using a lead capsule around the male gonads, the incident radiation dose is too small to measure and is probably less than 10 microrads for a single exposure. This compares to a dose of 0.3 to 0.7 millirad measured just outside the lead capsule. However, placement of the lead shield for female gonadal shielding is accurate in only 60 per cent of patients. In 30 per cent of patients, one ovary may remain unshielded and neither ovary may be shielded in another 5 per cent of patients due to the variability of ovarian position in the pelvis in young children. In general, if external lead shielding is used to diminish the doses to the ovaries, the average exposure per film will be approximately equal to the natural radiation exposure for a period of eight days.

External lead shielding can be utilized in boys during examinations of the urinary tract and large bowel and can be used in both sexes during examination of the hips. However, examination of the large bowel (barium enema) and of the urinary tract in girls does not allow for routine ovarian shielding during the entire examination if one is to evaluate areas of the bladder and of the bowels. Shielding of ovaries may be utilized at least for some films during many of these examinations depending upon the nature of the information desired. Reducing the number of films to the minimum necessary to obtain the information will reduce overall patient exposure.

For evaluation of the urinary tract, the intravenous pyelogram generally includes a "scout" film followed by 1 to 2 post injection films. One of these post injection films may use a lead shield placed over the ovaries, whereas the second film will probably necessitate evaluation of the bladder and thus direct the radiation to the ovaries. However, when there is an obstructive lesion, one or more delayed films may be obtained over a period of several hours. The value of such films should be balanced by the information obtained versus the dose to be received.

In essence, the average intravenous pyelogram delivers to the female gonads a dose between 40 to 60 millirad (standard deviation 20 to 100 millirads). One intravenous pyelogram could expose the female patient to an average gonad dose which corresponds to approximately 50 to 120 per cent of that caused by the average annual radiation from natural sources.

On the other hand, the primary beam of radiation should not strike the male gonads. Such "shielding" can be undertaken by careful collimation and the use of external lead capsules. Using careful collimation, doses to the scrotum should not exceed 25 to 40 millirads. With an external lead shield, the dose will be immeasurable and therefore less than 10 millirads.

Patients who exhibit vesicoureteric reflux as a cause of "obstruction" and chronic or recurrent urinary tract infection may undergo cystourethrograms. In such procedures, the male gonads may "fall" into the primary beam since lateral and oblique projections will be necessary to evaluate the urethra. The desired information will require a dynamic examination and thus fluoroscopic evaluation is necessary. However, fluoroscopy with image intensification and television monitoring will reduce the overall dose as compared with other methods. An average dose of 200 to 300 millirads per cystourethrogram (standard deviation of 120 to 380 millirads) may be observed, which is a doubling or tripling the annual natural dose to the gonads in a girl. Total doses of 30 to 40 millirads may be delivered to the gonads of boys (standard deviation 10 to 60 millirads), but this can be diminished to immeasurable levels with the use of a firmly fitted lead capsule about the gonads.

The rapidity of the act of micturition may make cinemaphotography necessary to evaluate the dynamic changes. The film dose of 35 microR per frame may result for a total examination dose of 840 microrads per second. However, a videotape recorder may reduce these doses to 5 microR per second with a maximum of 20 microR per second necessary for a good recording.

Seventy mm. image intensification allows for considerable reduction in gonadal dose. With standard screens, the film dose is approximately 500 microR. With image intensification and the 70 mm. camera, the dose can be reduced to 1/10 (50 microR). Four conventional spot films on older fluoroscopic units are equivalent to 40 exposures with the 70 mm. camera.

Therefore evaluation of the urinary tract may require a female gonadal exposure of 50 millirads, with a male gonadal exposure of 10 millirads despite careful shielding. In addition, a female gonadal dose of 250 millirads may be obtained by cystourethrograms and a male gonadal dose of 40 millirads with the same procedure.

It has been estimated that a program of urinary tract evaluation in children using two intravenous pyelograms in 30 years may increase the risk of leukemia by 0.016 to 0.02 per cent of the spontaneous risk. The risk to children with chronic nonobstructive polynephritis may be increased by 0.096 to 0.12 per cent if 12 intravenous pyelograms are obtained over a period of 30 years. Urinary tract obstruction might raise the risk by 0.24 to 0.3 per cent, depending upon the numbers of examinations which might be obtained for that diagnosis.

Obviously, these figures are based upon the numbers of examinations obtained in the lifetime of a patient with the diagnosis of urinary tract abnormality, the types of examinations which are obtained, and the refinements which may be undertaken.

It would be helpful for the referring physician to instruct the patient and/or his parents to maintain a "log" of examinations which have been obtained so that a cumulative radiation exposure record, when available, can be a source of reminder as to how the exposures add up and may be a factor in the decision to obtain radiographic examinations in the individual patient.

High Fever

JOHN F. RYAN, M.D.

The rational therapy for correcting hyperthermia is to treat successfully the causative disease state. Most commonly, fever is due to a shift of the central thermostat of the anterior hypothalamus to a higher level. This is followed by increased metabolism to bring the temperature of the blood perfusing this area to the appropriate warmth. The shift frequently is caused by pyrogenic activity, and symptomatic therapy can be administered (such as aspirin and acetaminophen) that lowers the thermostatic setting of the hypothalamus, which decreases metabolic response and thereby lowers body temperature. Administered by rectum, the dosage of aspirin is variable, but may be as follows: infants under 1 year, 150 mg. (2.5 grains); children 1 to 5 years, 300 mg. (5 grains); and children 5 to 10 years, 600 mg. (10 grains). These doses may be repeated three or four times at four hour intervals, but prolonged use may involve danger of salicylism.

Acetaminophen (Tylenol) has become more popular in recent years due to decreased incidence of poisoning in children. The suggested oral dosage is as follows (every 4 hours): infants under 1 year, 60 mg.; children 1 to 3 years 120 mg.; children 3 to 6 years, 180 mg; and over 6 years, 240 mg. For maximum effect, both aspirin and acetaminophen can be used together. For this method, the dose of aspirin should be halved.

A second reason for high fever may be a hypermetabolic state in which the central thermoregulatory mechanisms are bypassed and cells of the body uncontrollably produce heat. This type of fever is exemplified by malignant hyperthermia, a syndrome more frequently recognized in the past decade characterized by tachycardia, tachypnea, metabolic and marked respiratory acidosis, hyperkalemia, myoglobinemia, and sudden extremely high fever. It usually presents during an uncomplicated anesthesia and surgery. The mortality at present is approximately 60 per cent. Treatment consists of stopping the anesthesia, hyperventilation, administering 100 per cent oxygen, administration of sodium bicarbonate according to blood gas determinations, administration of iced fluids intravenously for cooling, lavage of body cavities for cooling, injection of mannitol and furosemide to promote diuresis and prevent myoglobin cast formation, administration of procainamide, 15 mg./kg. over approximately a 10 minute period intravenously with EKG control, and maintenance of at least a 2 ml./kg./hr. urinary output.

At what point should any fever be treated? Obviously, this varies with the disease state. The stress of upper respiratory infection causing a 103°F. fever in an otherwise healthy child does not present the metabolic threat that the same temperature does when recorded in a gravely ill child following open heart surgery. Until recently, it was felt that temperatures greater than 105-106°F. could be associated with protein breakdown and a possible fatal outcome.

At our hospital in the past 3½ years, nine patients have had temperatures greater than 108°F. None of these patients died or suffered neurological sequelae as a result of hyperthermia. One patient did succumb 24 hours later from hyperkalemia, but he had been lucid in the interval following the temperature spike. Also, recent cancer therapy using marked hyperthermia has been utilized without pathophysiologic consequences. The most important factors in preventing cerebral damage from hyperthermia seem to be sustaining good cerebral perfusion by maintaining normovolemia, supporting cardiovascular status, monitoring and correcting blood gas (PO_2, Pco_2, pH) and electrolyte abnormalities.

To prevent febrile convulsions and to protect infants and children from possible stress if their fevers persist and their conditions deteriorate, it seems reasonable to counteract any temperature rise greater than 103° F. actively.

Classically, alcohol rubs and ice packs placed in the groin have been utilized. An efficient method we use is intravenous refrigerated saline. Cold saline not only cools the blood without directly stimulating skin cold receptors which stimulate increased oxygen consumption, but also the fluid and electrolyte deficit is corrected simultaneously. Cold intravenous fluids for fever are less uncomfortable than ice packs and, unless large volumes are given rapidly via a central line, there is not the danger of adverse myocardial response. Room temperature should be reduced to approximately 65° F. Fans and cooling blankets can also be employed.

It is important to monitor the patient's temperature during the febrile period. The simplest method is by a continuous recording thermistor placed rectally. Often the calibration of these probes is faulty, and use of a mercury thermometer once to act as a check is reasonable. Axillary placement is also useful if the rectum is unavailable. The arm opposite the one in which the intravenous has been placed is preferable so that the cold solutions coursing through the axillary veins will not give a false low reading.

Tympanic temperature monitoring will yield core temperature (as will probes placed in the lower one-third of the esophagus or the nasopharynx), but these methods are usually only useful in the unconscious patient.

Most methods of external cooling may cause shivering, which tends to increase muscular activity, increase oxygen demand and maintain or even increase the temperature.

Chlorpromazine (Thorazine) or one of the related phenothiazines is effective in lowering body temperature in the control of shivering, and may be used as an adjunct to active external cooling. All of these drugs have definite side effects which must be recognized. Chlorpromazine may cause hypotension, but if the blood pressure is carefully observed, the drug can be used more effectively than most of the newer and less familiar drugs. Chlorpromazine should be given by intermittent intramuscular administration in small doses (approximately 0.2 mg./kg.).

Once the patient's temperature reaches 101° F., vigorous cooling should cease lest hypothermia occur.

Colic

EDWARD B. SHAW, M.D.

"Colic" usually refers to the pain caused by obstruction of a hollow abdominal viscus. Infantile colic probably is related to spasmodic intestinal obstruction which may result from immature neurologic control of motility. The baby appears to be in great distress, draws up the legs, clenches fists, expels large amounts of flatus, and cries loudly and interminably.

Attacks usually recur daily, especially in late afternoon and early evening. The baby acts as though he is hungry and sucks greedily at a bottle or pacifier but with only momentary relief (young infants seem to interpret any pain as hunger). These attacks usually abate spontaneously at about 3 months of age, and are known as the "three month colic."

The pain is much too common to be related to disorders such as enzyme deficiencies, and the type of feeding makes little difference. In some instances the pain may be caused by hunger because of inadequate supply of breast milk or formula. A change of feeding has insignificant value, although the grandmothers of a generation ago insisted on changing to a very dilute sweetened condensed milk formula which seemed to be somewhat effective; in spite of its obvious nutritional deficiencies, the babies continued to thrive surprisingly well.

Prevention. Because the symptoms seem to result from trapping of large amounts of air in the intestine, every effort should be made to avoid the swallowing of air. The baby should be fed in a more or less upright position, never lying flat in the crib, or with a propped bottle. After feeding, the baby should be "burped" to expel the gas bubble which may be passed along to increase intestinal distress.

Treatment.   Changes in the type or frequency of feeding are generally ineffective. Certain drugs which incorporate atropine or atropine-like substances have been advocated but results are poor and if entrusted to the mother incur the danger of overdosage. Approximately 8 mg. of phenobarbital is sometimes effective and can be given several times a day as necessary. An old remedy can hardly be suggested seriously, except that it is sometimes more effective than anything else, i.e., a teaspoonful of gin or whiskey in a small amount of sweetened water.

Gentle dilatation of the rectal sphincter with a well lubricated little finger often causes an evacuation of flatus which seems to relieve the infant's distress. Mechanical appliances have been recommended but they are not usually worthwhile in this situation.

At the age of 2 to 3 months, the infant is not especially susceptible to psychological input. However, the mother who is so distraught by the constant interruption of her sleep and her concern about the baby's welfare may reflect this concern to her baby. The result is an infant who is equally tense and unhappy, and therefore a victim of emotions which exaggerate his symptoms of distress. Infantile colic cannot be entirely a matter of the psychological relationship between the mother and infant; however the pediatrician must reassure the mother that the condition is not grave and will terminate before long. The use of the phrase "three month colic" is a great comfort to parents who are so delighted to have produced an offspring, but find that they have a diminutive monster who makes life unbearable for them. They should be assured that the colic will not persist indefinitely and that it does not come from any serious defect in the baby.

Genetic Disease

Diagnosis, Counseling and Prevention

HAROLD M. NITOWSKY, M.D.

Recent dramatic advances in knowledge of human genetics and genetic diseases and in the techniques for diagnosis or detection of genetic abnormalities have resulted in a comparable increase of interest in genetic counseling. Genetic counseling has been defined as "a communication process which deals with the human problems associated with the occurrence, or the risk of occurrence, of a genetic disorder in a family. This process involves an attempt by one or more appropriately trained persons to help the individual or family (1) comprehend the medical facts, including the diagnosis, the probable course of the disorder, and the available management; (2) appreciate the way heredity contributes to the disorder, and the risk of recurrence in specified relatives; (3) understand the options for dealing with the risk of recurrence; (4) choose the course of action which seems appropriate to them in view of their risks and their family goals and act in accordance with that decision; and (5) make the best possible adjustment to the disorder in an affected family member and/or to the risk of recurrence of that disorder."

Traditionally, prognosis in medicine refers to the forecast of the course and outcome of a disorder in a patient with a particular disease. In contrast genetic prognosis, which is an important component of the counseling process, deals with predictions or estimates of the probability of recurrence of a genetic abnormality in the progeny or relatives of an individual with the disorder.

The term genetic prognosis implies an interest in prevention; indeed, for those genetic disorders with high recurrence risks, one of the major purposes of genetic counseling is to provide couples with sufficient information to arrive at a rational decision with respect to family planning or limitation of family size. Unlike prevention in other areas of medicine, the individual with a genetic disorder or parents who are carriers of a genetic abnormality are themselves the major effective agents for the prevention of genetic disease. They may be informed about possible risks, but the choice of having children is theirs. Some potential parents, knowing there is a serious risk of transmission of a genetic disorder, will refrain from parenthood or, if already parents, from having additional children, and thus to some extent lessen the burden of genetic disease for society. In a free society, it is not possible to impose such a decision, and genetic counseling has retained as its primary focus the provision of genetic information as a service to individuals. Whatever contribution is made thereby to the well-being of the community as a whole is only incidental.

Advances in medical genetics have added new dimensions and new complexities to the responsibilities of the genetic counselor. The increasing utilization of amniocentesis, and new developments for genetic diagnosis permit detection of a variety of genetic abnormalities during fetal life. Thus many risks can be defined directly and need not be inferred from statistical probabilities. The liberalization of social attitudes and elimination of legal restrictions in regard to therapeutic abortion have increased the possibility of prevention of the birth of infants with serious, incapacitating or life-threatening genetic abnormalities. Thus the scope as well as the potential of genetic counseling has been greatly expanded. These developments have raised ethical, moral and social issues about the prevention of genetic disease.

In considering human disease as part of a broad spectrum, at one extreme are the conditions that are entirely genetic in causation and at the other extreme the nutritional deficiencies and infectious diseases that are almost entirely due to environmental factors. Between the two extremes are many relatively common conditions, such as diabetes mellitus and certain congenital malformations, in which both genetic and environmental factors are involved. Disorders that are entirely genetic in etiology either are chromosomal abnormalities or are due to single gene mutations (unifactorial). The latter are individually rare, the mode of inheritance is simple (dominant, recessive, or X-linked), and the chances of recurrence are high (greater than 1 in 10). Conditions that etiologically are partly genetic are generally due to interaction between many genes and the environment (multifactorial). These disorders are common, the mode of inheritance is complex, and the chances of recurrence are usually low (less than 1 in 10).

Before providing genetic advice it is essential to investigate the family pedigree; at the minimum this should include information about the health of all first-degree relatives, i.e., parents, siblings and children of the person seeking such advice. If the disorder is not severe it may be possible to trace it back through several generations. On the other hand, if the condition is severe, affected individuals may not have survived to have children and to transmit the disease to subsequent generations. In many cases the affected individual is the only person in the family with the defect, which is usually the result of a new mutation.

SINGLE GENE MUTATIONS

Autosomal dominant traits affect both males and females and often show great variation in expressivity. For example, in a patient with osteogenesis imperfecta the only manifestation of the disease may be blue sclerae, whereas other individuals, even in the same family, can be very severely affected with multiple fractures. Sometimes the gene may not express itself at all, in which case it is said to be nonpenetrant. This phenomenon may explain apparent skipped generations in certain pedigrees. On the other hand, careful examination often shows that the skipped individual has definite although mild manifestations, representing a forme fruste of the disorder. Careful clinical examination of both apparently healthy parents of a child with an autosomal dominant disorder is therefore essential before the possibility of a new mutation can be considered.

If an individual with an autosomal dominant anomaly marries a normal person, the chance that any child will be affected is 50 per cent. Some autosomal genes are expressed more frequently in one sex than in the other. This is referred to as sex-influenced inheritance. For example, hemochromatosis is much more common in males than in females, who often do not develop symptoms until after menopause.

Autosomal recessive traits also affect both sexes, and since only homozygotes manifest the disorder, the heterozygous parents are unaffected. The chance for two heterozygotes to have an affected child is 25 per cent with each pregnancy. Unlike the situation with an autosomal dominant trait, it is generally impossible to trace the disease through several generations. All the affected individuals in a family are usually in one sibship. The parents of a child with a rare recessive disorder are often related, since relatives are more likely to have inherited the same gene from a common ancestor. The rarer a disorder the higher the incidence of consanguinity. However, the fact that in a particular family the parents are not related does not preclude the condition from being recessively inherited.

An X-linked recessive trait is one that is due to a mutant gene on the X chromosome. Hemizygous males (with the mutant gene on their single X chromosome) are affected, but heterozygous females (carriers) are usually normal. Diseases inherited in this manner are transmitted by healthy female carriers and by affected males if the disorder is not severe or is treatable. All the daughters of an affected male will be carriers, and all his sons will be normal. In severe X-linked disorders, such as Duchenne muscular dystrophy, affected males do not survive to have children, and the disorder is transmitted by female carriers. In the case of a woman who is a carrier of Duchenne muscular dystrophy, on the average half her sons will be affected and half her daughters will be carriers.

Quite often in serious X-linked conditions there is only one affected male in a family.

Such a sporadic case may be the result of a new mutation in the X chromosome that is inherited from the mother. However, there is also the possibility that the mother might be a carrier, the mutant gene by chance not having been transmitted to any of her male relatives but inherited only through the female line, perhaps for several generations.

MULTIFACTORIAL INHERITANCE

There are many fairly common conditions in which there is a definite familial tendency, the proportion of affected relatives being greater than in the general population. However, the proportion of affected relatives is often of the order of 5 per cent and therefore much less than would be expected for single gene mutations. Although the low familial incidence in some of these conditions has been ascribed to genes being incompletely penetrant, this explanation is unsatisfactory. It is much more likely that such conditions are caused by many genes and the effects of environment, or the so-called multifactorial inheritance.

In multifactorial inheritance it may be assumed that there is some hypothetic underlying attribute that is related to the causation of the disease. This is referred to as the individual's liability, which includes not only his genetic predisposition but also the environmental circumstances that render him more or less likely to develop the disease in question. Further, it may be assumed that the curve of liability has a normal distribution in both the general population and in relatives, but the curve for the latter is shifted to the right. In the general population the proportion of individuals above the threshold for manifestation of the disorder constitutes the population incidence. Among relatives the proportion above the threshold is the familial incidence. This model has been applied to measurable characteristics (such as stature and intelligence) and has also been used to explain the familial incidence of such conditions as diabetes mellitus, congenital pyloric stenosis, cleft lip with and without cleft palate, anencephaly and spina bifida, clubfoot, and congenital dislocation of the hip.

In conditions in which the inheritance is believed to be multifactorial, there are several consequences of the model depicted. The incidence will be greatest among the relatives of more severely affected individuals, because they presumably are more extreme deviants along the curve of liability. By similar reasoning it would also be expected that the incidence among siblings born subsequent to the index case would be greater the more affected relatives there were in the family. In spina bifida, for example, after the birth of a single affected child the incidence among subsequent siblings is approximately 4 per cent, but it is 10 per cent after the birth of two affected children, and evidence suggests the risk is higher still if another close relative is also affected.

RECURRENCE RISK

Estimation of the risk of recurrence in the individual case depends on a precise diagnosis and an established etiology. Before giving genetic counseling, a careful clinical examination and investigation of the affected individual are essential. In order to arrive at the correct diagnosis it may be necessary to refer to death certificates and autopsy and biopsy reports. It may also be necessary to examine the parents or other relatives in certain situations. Without such information it may not be possible to give reliable genetic advice.

In establishing the etiology the pedigree should include information on the health of at least all first-degree relatives, consanguinity, abortions, maternal exposure to radiation, drugs and infections during pregnancy, and details of any birth trauma. Finally, the possibility of genetic heterogeneity must always be considered. The literature should be searched for information on this point and on the relative frequencies of the various modes of inheritance. When the precise diagnosis is known and the mode of inheritance is clearly established, genetic counseling is usually straightforward and is based on expected mendelian ratios. However, in the case of autosomal recessive conditions, an individual (whether homozygous or heterozygous) is unlikely to have affected children unless the spouse also carries the same mutant gene, which is unlikely if the condition is rare.

In fairly common conditions in which genetic factors appear to play a part but where there is no simple mode of inheritance, the risks of recurrence are based on the observed frequencies of the conditions among relatives of affected individuals, so-called empiric risks. Many of these conditions are probably heterogeneous; they include disorders of various causation. Empiric risk figures are therefore unsatisfactory, as they merely represent an average figure for any one condition. A list of empiric risk figures for some common disorders is shown in Table 1. If a genetic etiology for a particular condition has not been established, and yet the family history clearly suggests a particular mode of inheritance, then genetic counseling should be based on the family history, since this condition may represent a unique situation.

In general, trisomy 21 (Down syndrome),

TABLE 1. Empiric Risks for Some Common Disorders

DISORDER	INCIDENCE (%)	SEX RATIO M:F	NORMAL PARENTS HAVING A SECOND AFFECTED CHILD (%)	AFFECTED PARENT HAVING AN AFFECTED CHILD (%)	AFFECTED PARENT HAVING A SECOND AFFECTED CHILD (%)
Anencephaly	0.20	1:2	2	—	—
Cleft palate only	0.04	2:3	2	7	15
Cleft lip +/− cleft palate	0.10	3:2	4	4	12
Club foot	0.10	2:1	3	3	10
Congenital heart disease (all types)	0.60	—	1 to 4	1 to 4	—
Pyloric stenosis	0.30	5:1			
Male index			2	4	13
Female index			10	17	38
Spina bifida	0.30	2:3	4	—	—

trisomy 13, trisomy 18, and other chromosomal abnormalities are usually the result of errors in meiosis during gametogenesis, and the chances of recurrence are small. However, if one of the parents happens to be a mosaic or carries a balanced translocation, the situation is different. If one of the parents is a mosaic, it may be difficult to give reliable genetic advice, because it is impossible to estimate what proportion of the parental gonadal tissue is normal. If one of the parents carries a translocation, genetic counseling depends on the cytogenetic findings and the sex of the carrier parent.

A common problem arises when healthy parents have a child with a particular disorder or abnormality and there is no history on either side of the family of anyone similarly affected. There are several possible explanations for such a situation. First, the disorder may be a phenocopy, perhaps due to maternal exposure during pregnancy. Second, it may be due to a chromosomal abnormality, but apart from Down syndrome most disorders associated with specific chromosome abnormalities are rare, and the chances of recurrence are small. A third possibility is that of a new autosomal dominant mutation, in which case there is little chance of recurrence in subsequent children. This is a distinct possibility if the condition is known to be inherited as an autosomal dominant, if it is always fully penetrant, and if on examination both parents are found to be unaffected. Fourth, it might be an autosomal recessive disorder. Evidence in favor of this etiology would be parental consanguinity or the demonstration that both parents are heterozygotes by an appropriate biochemical or other type of test. Finally, it could represent an X-linked recessive disorder. It is important to recognize this possibility, be-

cause an unaffected sister might then be a carrier. Clinical evidence might suggest this mode of inheritance. It might also be possible to demonstrate a biochemical or other abnormality in the mother but not in the father, which would suggest that the disorder was X-linked.

PRENATAL DIAGNOSIS

Amniocentesis for prenatal diagnosis of fetal abnormalities has added a new dimension to the prediction of risks for inheritance of genetic disorders. Heretofore the genetic counselor has estimated the risks for occurrence of a genetic abnormality in future progeny from an analysis of the family history, information about the mode of genetic transmission of the disorder, and other data. Now, however, amniocentesis permits evaluation of the status of each fetus, independently and with relative certainty for a broad spectrum of genetic abnormalities. As a result of the liberalization of abortion laws and the development of safe and accurate techniques for prenatal diagnosis, selective termination of pregnancy if the fetus is affected can be offered as a means to prevent the birth of an infant with a condition that is lethal or that may result in irremediable mental or physical handicaps. However, since many types of fetal abnormalities cannot be diagnosed by currently available methods, amniocentesis offers no guarantee that the infant will be free of all possible abnormalities.

Various techniques have been developed for detecting abnormalities in the human fetus in utero. These may conveniently be divided into those that study the fetus directly and those that study the fetus indirectly from changes in the mother's urine or blood. Some techniques for studying the fetus directly include radiography for skeletal abnormalities, amniography and fetography for soft tissue abnormalities, sonography, and fetal electrocardiography. However, these techniques may be of limited value in early pregnancy. Biopsy of membranes, placenta and fetus is still at the experimental stage, as is direct visualization of the fetus (fetoscopy), which may prove particularly valuable in the antenatal diagnosis of conditions requiring samples of fetal blood.

The usual approach to antenatal diagnosis of genetic disease is the study of amniotic fluid and its contained cells. Amniotic fluid cells are of fetal origin, being largely derived from the surface layers of the fetal skin but with contributions from other sources such as the buccal mucosa and amnion. The origin of the amniotic fluid itself is more complex and depends on the stage of gestation. Specimens of amniotic fluid are generally obtained by aspiration through the abdominal wall (transabdominal amniocentesis). This technique is carried out after the 14th week of gestation when the uterus rises above the symphysis pubis and the volume of amniotic fluid is large enough to sample safely. Experience indicates that the transabdominal approach is a relatively safe technique that entails little risk to the mother (such as hemorrhage or infection) or to the fetus (precipitation of abortion, trauma). The findings of a collaborative study sponsored by the National Institute of Child Health and Human Development indicate that the overall risk of amniocentesis is less than 0.5 per cent.

Uncultured amniotic fluid cells have been used for biochemical and histologic studies but these methods are probably too unreliable for diagnosing most biochemical disorders in utero or are too nonspecific to be of value. The main use of uncultured cells is for sex prediction based on sex chromatin and fluorescence studies. From the former the number of X chromosomes can be determined, and from the latter the number of Y chromosomes. However, there are limitations to these techniques, so that it is important to confirm the findings by chromosome studies on cultured cells.

The main indications for chromosome studies on cultured amniotic fluid cells are in families in which one of the parents is a mosaic or carries a translocation that in the unbalanced state may cause severe physical or mental abnormality, or increased maternal age, since the latter is associated with an increased fetal risk for various chromosomal abnormalities. The main application of chromosome studies of amniotic cell cultures has been in the antenatal diagnosis of Down syndrome. Because of the increased risk of trisomy 21 with maternal age (as high as 1 in 60 over age 40), it

has been recommended that amniocentesis be offered to all pregnant women over 35 years of age.

There are several pitfalls and limitations of antenatal chromosome studies. One of the most serious problems is the possible misinterpretation of a karyotype that morphologically appears normal, but contains a chromosome rearrangement that may be associated with severe physical or mental abnormality. In general, if both products of a reciprocal translocation cannot be recognized in one of the parents, then antenatal chromosome studies are probably not justified in a pregnancy at risk. However, these difficulties are less likely with the newly introduced banding techniques that permit precise identification not only of individual chromosomes but also of structural rearrangements of the chromosomes.

An important development in recent years has been the use of cultured amniotic fluid cells for the antenatal diagnosis of inherited biochemical disorders. This usually involves the demonstration of reduced activity of a particular enzyme in cell extracts. Many enzyme activities have been demonstrated in cultured amniotic fluid cells, and therefore genetic disorders associated with deficiency of these enzymes have been diagnosed or are potentially diagnosable in utero (Table 2). On a worldwide basis sickle cell anemia is probably the most common serious genetic disorder affecting man. Until recently it was believed that hemoglobin β-chain synthesis was not switched on until around the time of birth, and therefore there seemed little prospect of being able to diagnose sickle cell anemia in utero. However, recent studies have shown that β-chain synthesis begins in early fetal life, and provided the technical difficulties of obtaining specimens of fetal blood can be overcome, it may soon be possible to diagnose sickle cell anemia in utero. It is likely that during the next few years there will be a substantial increase in the number of inherited metabolic disorders that can be diagnosed antenatally.

An important prerequisite of using amniotic cell cultures for biochemical diagnosis is the establishment of reliable control values for enzymes in normal amniotic fluid cells. Recent observations suggest that cultures of amniotic fluid cells consist of cells with different biochemical properties and morphologic characteristics. The implication of these studies is that it is essential to establish normal biochemical properties for each cell type if an accurate antenatal diagnosis of a disorder is to be made. Further, the activities of a number of enzymes have been shown to vary during the

TABLE 2.   Some Hereditary Biochemical Disorders That Have Been or Are Diagnosable In Utero

ENZYME	DISORDER
Hexosaminidase A	Tay-Sachs disease
α-1, 4-glucosidase	Pompe's disease
Acid phosphatase	Acid phosphatase deficiency
α-galactosidase	Fabry's syndrome
Sphingomyelinase	Niemann-Pick disease
Hypoxanthine guanine phosphoribosyl trans-ferase	Lesch-Nyhan syndrome
Arylsulfatase A	Metachromatic leukodystrophy
β-galactosidase	Generalized gangliosidosis
Branched-chain keto acid decarboxylase	Maple syrup urine disease
Gal-1-phosphate uridyl transferase	Galactosemia
Cystathionine synthetase	Homocystinuria
L-Iduronidase	Hurler syndrome
Cystine accumulation	Cystinosis
Glucocerebrosidase	Gaucher's disease
Amylo-1,6-glucosidase	Type III glycogen storage disease
Amylo-(1,4,1,6)-trans-glucosidase	Type IV glycogen storage disease
Argininosuccinase	Argininosuccinic-aciduria
Histidase	Histidinemia
G-6-PD	G-6-PD deficiency
Endonuclease	Xeroderma pigmentosum
Valine transaminase	Hypervalinemia
Cystathioninase	Cystathioninuria
Phytanic acid oxidase	Refsum's disease
Ornithine carbamyl-transferase	Hyperammonemia
Arginase	Argininemia
Fucosidase	Fucosidosis
α-mannosidase	Mannosidosis

cycle of cell growth in culture. Accordingly, control material ideally should be amniotic fluid cells from normal fetuses of comparable gestational age that have been grown in culture for approximately the same length of time, in the same medium, and under identical conditions, and then harvested at the same stage in the growth cycle as amniotic fluid cells from a fetus at risk.

Biochemical analysis of supernatant amniotic fluid as a means of diagnosing genetic disease in utero would have considerable advantage over the methods that depend on study of cultured amniotic fluid cells, which is technically difficult and requires several weeks before results can be obtained. However, the former approach is likely to be of value only in those metabolic disorders that are associated with changes in urinary composition (since amniotic fluid is largely derived from fetal urine after the first trimester) and that are not diet-dependent.

Genetic abnormalities not associated with any specific biochemical or chromosomal abnormality present a problem in antenatal diagnosis. However, in certain congenital abnormalities, and particularly in malformations of the central nervous system such as spina bifida and anencephaly, changes occur in the biochemical composition of amniotic fluid that are of value in antenatal diagnosis. Thus there is a significant increase in the level of alpha fetoprotein in amniotic fluid in more than 90 per cent of fetuses with anencephaly or open neural tube defects.

For some fetal genetic disorders not associated with any biochemical or chromosomal abnormality, genetic linkage may be helpful for prenatal diagnosis. The underlying principle is that the loci for a marker trait and the particular disorder in question should be closely linked on the same chromosome and therefore should be likely to segregate together in a particular family, and the marker trait should be detectable in amniotic fluid or its contained cells. Two such linkages have been described: the loci for G-6-PD and hemophilia A and the loci for ABH-secretor status and myotonic dystrophy. Since the loci for G-6-PD and hemophilia A are closely linked on the X chromosome and since the G-6-PD phenotype can be determined in amniotic fluid cells, this may be valuable in the antenatal diagnosis of hemophilia in populations in which G-6-PD variants are common. Second, the loci for secretor status and myotonic dystrophy are within measurable distance of each other, and the secretor status of the fetus can be determined from amniotic fluid in early pregnancy.

Not all clinics or hospitals are equipped to carry out diagnostic amniocentesis and the culture of amniotic fluid cells in situations in which there is a high or clear-cut risk for a fetal disorder. Since cultures of amniotic cells can be grown several days after the procedure if properly handled, it may be preferable to develop selected centers for these studies. Future application of amniocentesis in pregnancies at risk for chromosomal or biochemical abnormalities may require the mobilization of laboratory resources on a regional or national basis to permit the most efficient delivery of optimal services at the lowest possible cost.

GENETIC ADVICE

Factors that influence the parents' decisions as to whether they will accept the risk of having an affected child include the severity of the abnormality, whether there is an effective treatment, statistical risk, and their religious attitudes, socioeconomic status, and education. The genetic counselor usually does not try to influence the parents' decision, although when the risks involved are high, advice in regard to family limitation may be indicated.

Contraception is not the only course of action open to parents faced with this problem. Other alternatives include sterilization or artificial insemination (if the father is affected). Following the liberalization of abortion laws, termination of pregnancy is another possibility if the mother becomes pregnant with substantial risk of serious abnormality. Selective abortion has also become a possibility whereby a pregnancy may be terminated when it is known that the fetus is abnormal.

There is ample evidence to suggest that a significant number of persons in the population are at high risk of having a child with a serious hereditary disorder and are unaware of the fact. In the past the finding of such individuals has often been a matter of chance, depending largely on the awareness of their physician. Therefore, there may be justification for setting up genetic registers in which families at high risk are recorded, so that individuals in these families can be followed up and given appropriate counseling when they reach childbearing age.

An important recent advance has been the development of methods for the identification of heterozygous carriers for mutant genes. Although such individuals are usually asymptomatic, the ability to detect a qualitative or quantitative alteration in a specific gene product or to measure an abnormality in a metabolic function as a result of the presence of a mutant allele may permit identification of the heterozygote. Although this development tends to blur the distinction between dominance and recessiveness insofar as a measurable departure from the "normal" phenotype can be discerned, retention of the distinction is of practical value.

Obviously, there are important applications of heterozygote detection for genetic counseling. While there seems to be little justification or need for the widespread application of the techniques for carrier detection in the general population, this may be of value in high-risk population groups. For example, Tay-Sachs disease occurs in about 1 out of every 3000 births among Ashkenazic (European) Jews in the United States. The frequency of the mutant gene is 0.015, and the prevalence of carriers in this population is about 1 in 30 individuals. Since the carrier for the Tay-Sachs mutant allele can be easily detected by a decrease in serum hexosaminidase-A activity, it is important to screen Jewish couples prior to marriage or childbearing despite a negative history for the disease on both sides of the family. A similar argument could be made for testing the partners of all consanguineous matings, especially when they are related as first cousins and when there has been a history in the family of one of the inborn metabolic abnormalities in which the carrier state can be identified.

Air Travel

GORDON BORKAT, M.D.,
and JEROME LIEBMAN, M.D.

Air travel has developed into the most expeditious means of transportation, whether for pleasure or medical reasons. The primary concern in choosing air travel must be the welfare of the individual and, if there are known medical problems, the unique potential hazards of flight should be taken into consideration.

SYSTEMS TO BE CONSIDERED FOR AIR TRAVEL

Eyes.   Certain types of surgery involve injection of air into the anterior chamber. This must be completely resorbed before flying to avoid the problem of expanding gases. Contact lens wearers may have pain and decreased vision from loss of corneal epithelium after a long flight. This might be due to rapid drying of tears from low humidity and air vents, or decreased oxygen available at the cellular level from low atmospheric PO_2. Such persons should be advised to wear glasses for the flight, or liberally use artificial tears.

Ears.   The closed volume of the middle ear is affected by rapid changes in pressure, particularly on descent, by the development of a barotitis media. Change in shape of the tympanic membrane causes pain. Any maneuver which opens the nasopharyngeal end of the eustachian tube should change the volume of the middle ear and equalize pressure on both sides of the tympanic membrane. Older children should swallow or yawn. Infants, who have shorter and wider eustachian tubes, usually have fewer symptoms, but can cry or suck if they have difficulty. If there is a recently healed perforation of the tympanic membrane, it may reopen because of the rapidly changing pressures. However, an open perforation is not a contraindication to flying, as pressures on both sides will always be equal.

Mouth.   Trauma to the mouth involving fractures with wiring of the jaws shut may be a contraindication to air travel. In the event of motion sickness with vomiting, aspiration could be a serious problem.

Respiratory System.   Persons with upper respiratory infections should be permitted to fly. Because of swelling of the tissues near the eustachian tube, however, barotitis media may be more serious. Such patients should be treated with decongestants.

Patients with acute and chronic sinusitis may experience renewed severe pain from changing gas volume and should be treated with decongestants.

Chronic upper airway obstructive disease is not a problem if it is mild. However, in more severe states, especially during sleep, the oxygen gradient from atmosphere to alveolus increases. There is further hypoxia as well as carbon dioxide retention. In addition to the potentially dangerous low tissue oxygen, the low PO_2 and pH can lead to pulmonary arteriolar vasoconstriction with acute pulmonary artery hypertension.

Chronic asthma under good control is not a contraindication to flying if gas exchange is good. Acute asthmatic attacks should be treated before flight, whereas the chronic asthmatic patient should be given prophylactic medication.

Patients who have chronic obstructive pulmonary disease such as cystic fibrosis are at risk from three factors. First, they have a marked alveolar-arterial oxygen gradient. If they have an arterial PO_2 greater than 50 mm. Hg at ground level, the reduced atmospheric PO_2 will probably still supply adequate tissue oxygen levels. Otherwise, increased environmental oxygen (25 to 30 per cent) should be supplied during flight. Careful control of oxygen must be observed so that the hypoxic respiratory drive is not inhibited. Second, enclosed pulmonary cysts are subject to gas expansion with occasional pneumothorax. This also causes a large alveolar-arterial oxygen gradient. Depending on the degree of involvement, patients have been reported to die from pneumothorax. Finally, decreased humidity causes thickening of secretions and makes pulmonary toilet more difficult. Therefore, administered oxygen should be humidified.

Primary pulmonary artery hypertension with systemic arterial undersaturation should preclude air travel without supplemental oxygen. There is loss of effective perfusion to a significant segment of lung with a large alveolar-arterial gradient. Additionally, there is usually a decreased cardiac output with delivery of less oxygenated blood to the tissues.

A patient with parenchymal pulmonary disease with residual cystic changes, such as the the Mikity-Wilson syndrome, resolved staphylococcal pneumonia, and tuberculosis with cavitation may undergo pneumothorax. These patients should use air travel only with great caution.

Cardiovascular System. As a general rule, patients with moderately cyanotic congenital heart disease may be permitted to fly. Even though atmospheric PO_2 decreases, there should be adequate oxygen delivery to the tissues, owing to increased oxygen extraction, increased 2,3-DPG, and good cardiac output. Patients who have moderate congestive heart failure with pulmonary edema have increased alveolar-arterial oxygen gradients and should be treated medically before flying, or receive increased oxygen during the flight.

Older children who have obstructive problems of the left side of the heart, such as aortic stenosis, may be allowed to fly, but they should be discouraged from performing isometric exercise such as carrying luggage or heavy packages. The markedly increased blood pressure during these activities imposes a large workload on the myocardium. The combination of the decreased oxygen supply associated with high altitude and the increased myocardial oxygen demands associated with isometric exercise provide a potential for sudden death. The latter is extremely rare, however.

Hematology. Inadequate hemoglobin causes low oxygen carrying capacity and supplies insufficient oxgyen for tissue needs. If the anemia is severe, with hemoglobin less than 8 gm. per 100 ml., it should be improved by transfusion before flying. Patients with sickle cell anemia or sickle cell trait who might have symptoms due to hypoxia should be carefully managed during flight. At the first sign of sickle crisis with pain, rest and increased atmospheric oxygen by mask may resolve symptomatology. Methemoglobinemia can be a contraindication to air travel.

Gastrointestinal System. Under normal circumstances a small amount of increased gas volume is not significant. However, if there is intestinal obstruction, gas expansion can cause severe pain. Active peptic ulcers, rare in children, have been known to perforate, and flying should be recommended with caution.

Following abdominal surgery, it is advisable to wait two weeks before flying to prevent wound dehiscence. Gas expansion can cause abdominal distention and subsequent opening of the incision.

Endocrine System. Patients with endocrinological disorders of any kind may fly. However, patients with diabetes mellitus must carefully follow their usual times of medications and meals so as not be become hypoglycemic.

Central Nervous System. Children with seizure disorders may have exacerbations during flight either because of hypoxia or the alkalosis associated with hyperventilation. Appropriate anticonvulsant controls should be instituted before flying, or increased oxygen should be administered.

After ventriculography or encephalography, air travel should not take place for one week. Expansion of injected gases may cause severe neurologic symptoms.

Children with emotional disorders may fly. However, they should be controlled by medication or restraint, if necessary, so that there is not danger to themselves or other passengers.

OTHER CONSIDERATIONS

Pregnancy. There is no contraindication to air travel at any time during pregnancy. During the last week of pregnancy it is advisable for a physician to approve flying if it does not seem that labor is imminent. Lap belts must be used and worn low, at the brim of the pelvis. In the event of accident, the uterus and fetus are therefore protected. Caution in moving about the airplane should be observed, as there is a shift of the center of gravity and instability when walking.

Infectious Diseases. Regardless of the disease, children who are not in imminent danger may fly, unless they have an internationally quarantineable disease. The major consideration is the safety of other passengers. In general, children are relatively isolated during flight, and are not significantly contagious. Recommendations for immunization should be determined by currently acceptable pediatric practice and the destination of the traveler. Information may be obtained from the Public Health Service.

Motion Sickness. Children prone to motion sickness may be given dimenhydrinate or meclizine hydrochloride* approximately one hour before flight.

EMERGENCY MEDICAL TRANSPORTATION

In spite of the previously mentioned risks involved with commercial air transportation in relatively well infants and children, many critically ill patients undergo flight.

The most common emergency situations involve multiple trauma, cyanotic congenital heart disease, prematurity, and congenital anomalies requiring immediate surgery in the newborn period. If appropriate personnel and

---

*Manufacturer's precaution: Usage of meclizine hydrochloride in the pediatric age group is not recommended because clinical studies establishing safety and efficacy have not been done.

equipment are available, *no* patient is too ill to fly.

In conjunction with many major pediatric centers, arrangements can be made to fly critically ill patients either by helicopter or fixed-wing aircraft. This is often done with the aid of the Air Force, the Air National Guard, or private air ambulance services.

Informed Consent

NORMAN FOST, M.D., M.P.H.

THE PURPOSE OF CONSENT

Consent ("to feel together. . . to agree") in the medical setting serves ethical as well as legal purposes. The primary ethical duty is to respect the autonomy of patients, meaning their right to accept or reject proposed medical care. In the words of Cardozo: "Every human being . . . has a right to determine what shall be done with his own body." This includes the right to make a wrong decision, so a physician cannot paternalistically treat a patient, or manipulate information to extract consent, without incurring liability.

While much attention has been centered on the ethical dimension in the experimentation setting, legal issues have generated more interest in the context of ordinary medical care. This article focuses on consent in the therapeutic nonexperimental setting. For a discussion of consent to experimentation involving children, the reader is referred elsewhere (Curr. Prob. Pediat., 6:1-31, 1976).

THE ELEMENTS OF CONSENT

When the Sterling Library—an enormous gothic building housing the Yale University Library—was completed, the librarian asked that the following inscription be carved over the entrance: "This is not the library; the library is inside." Similarly, physicians may confuse the *consent form* with informed consent. The written, signed statement is only one piece of evidence that informed consent has occurred. The practitioner is well advised, on ethical and legal grounds, to pay closer attention to the process than the form, although both are important.

Given the infinite variety of clinical interactions, it is impossible to design one form which will fit all circumstances, but the following items should ideally be included in the consent process:

1. A description of the proposed treatment in language which can be understood by the patient (or his guardian).

2. Alternatives to the proposed treatment.

3. Risks of death or serious bodily injury in the proposed treatment.

4. Problems of discomfort and recuperation that are anticipated.

5. Any additional information which other physicians would usually disclose in similar circumstances.

Since there are practical limitations to attaining this ideal goal in every patient contact, the essential question is how much to disclose. While many jurisdictions only require the physician to disclose what other members of his profession would disclose in similar circumstances, there is a recent trend toward allowing courts, rather than doctors, to decide what constitutes reasonable disclosure. This legal standard requires disclosure of risks which are *material* to a decision, meaning risks which would lead a reasonable person, in the patient's circumstances, to decline the treatment. For example, likely risks of common knowledge and trivial consequences, such as the discomfort of drawing blood, need not be disclosed, but even risks as rare as one in one million must be stated if they would lead a reasonable person to decline treatment.

An example of the latter is the famous case of *Wyeth v. Davis*, in which an adult, whose risk for contracting natural polio was less than the 1:1,000,000 chance of contracting it from vaccine, successfully sued for nondisclosure during a mass immunization campaign. The question is whether the particular patient, given that information, would have decided differently. Since a patient might deceitfully make such a claim after the fact, some have preferred the more "objective" standard of whether a reasonable person, in the patient's circumstances, would have decided differently with full disclosure. A reasonable person would be influenced by the severity and probability of risk, and therefore, as each rises, the informing should be more explicit.

Although it may be true in many cases that more information results in less comprehension, the physician concerned with protecting himself legally should err on the side of overinforming. The central point is that it is the patient who has the right to accept the risks and go ahead with treatment. When the likely benefits are clear and the risks trivial (as in routine immunization of infants or antibiotic treatment of documented streptococcal pharyngitis), most would consent and formalities are less important. It is when the need for treatment is less clear (as in elective surgery), the risks are high, and alternatives exist, that the process should be as explicit as is reasonably possible.

The physician is obviously not required to disclose risks which are unknown, but he can be expected to know as much as others in his field. He cannot, however, reliably use the defense of only disclosing as much as his colleagues do, since the law may take the view, depending on the jurisdiction, that his colleagues are not serving the patient's interest in making autonomous decisions.

An increasing number of states are enacting statutes which define the requirements for disclosure more precisely. They are usually more permissive, from the physician's view, than the court cases summarized above, in that they equate the patient's signature with the process of informing. A sample form from the Ohio statute is reproduced on page 834. While this form only refers to some of the details of the informing process, a more cautious approach would be to include in the form all the relevant facts which were presented, or to have someone witness the discussion.

WHEN IS CONSENT NOT REQUIRED?

Four justifications might be given for bypassing the requirements for consent:

1. *Presumed consent,* as in an emergency, when the patient cannot consent, or when there is insufficient time to contact a guardian. The assumption is that a reasonable person would consent to life-saving or health-preserving emergency treatment.

2. *Implied consent,* as in situations when the patient (or guardian) does not object to procedures which are simple, and whose risks are either common knowledge or extremely remote and commonly appreciated as remote (such as a physical examination or a fingerstick).

3. *Waived consent,* meaning the patient expressly asks not to be informed.

4. *Therapeutic privilege,* meaning that in the physician's judgment it is not in the patient's best interest to know. This privilege to withhold information should be confined to circumstances where there is evidence that the patient will be harmed by the information itself, usually because it is emotionally upsetting. One should be cautious about paternalistic withholding of information for the purpose of channeling a decision in the direction which the physician prefers.

Finally, consent from the patient is not required when he is not competent to consent, but an appropriate guardian must then provide permission. This will be discussed further below.

CONSENT FOR MEDICAL PROCEDURE AND ACKNOWLEDGMENT OF RECEIPT OF RISK INFORMATION

State law requires us to obtain your consent to your contemplated surgery or other medical procedure. What you are being asked to sign is simply a confirmation that we have discussed your contemplated operation or medical procedure and that we have given you sufficient information upon which to make a decision whether to have the operation or medical procedure and any choice as to the type of operation or medical procedure of your own free will. We have already discussed with you the common problems or undesired results that sometimes occur. We wish to inform you, not to alarm you. If you wish, however, we can go into more elaborate details or more unlikely problems. If you do not, that is also your privilege. Please read the form carefully and check the appropriate boxes. Ask about anything that you do not understand. We will be pleased to explain it. I hereby authorize and direct_____, with associate or assistants of his choice to perform the following surgical, diagnostic, or medical procedure on_____, my_____, as we have agreed upon.   relationship

I further authorize the doctors to perform any other procedure that in their judgment is advisable for my well being. Details of this operation have been explained to me. Alternative methods of treatment, if any, have also been explained to me as have the advantages and disadvantages of each. I am advised that though good results are expected, the possibility and nature of complications cannot be accurately anticipated and that therefore there can be no guarantee as expressed or implied either as to the result of surgery or as to cure.

Degree and kind of risks known to be associated with this procedure, including anesthesia; each marked box indicates some risks that are associated with this procedure:

	Comments
Death	_____
Brain Damage	_____
Quadriplegia (paralysis of all arms and legs)	_____
Paraplegia (paralysis of both legs)	_____
Loss of organ	_____
Loss of an arm or leg	_____
Loss of function of organ	_____
Loss of function of an arm or leg	_____
Disfiguring scars	_____

The doctor has explained to me the most likely complications or undesired results that might occur in this operation or medical procedure and I understand them. The doctor has offered to detail the less likely complications of [sic] undesired results which, even if rare, could occur.

_____I do_____I do not wish to have a full description of all the possible complications given to me.

I hereby authorize and direct the above named physician with associates or assistants to provide such additional services as they might deem reasonable and necessary including, but not limited to, the administration of any anesthetic agent, or the services of the X-ray department or laboratories, and I hereby consent thereto.

I hereby state that I have read and understand this consent and that all blanks were filled in prior to my signature.

Date:_____Time_____a.m. p.m.

Signature of Patient _____
Signature of Relative (where required) _____
Witness _____

I certify that I have personally completed all blanks in this form and explained them to the patient or his representative before requesting the patient or his representative to sign it.

_____(signature of named physician)

Model consent form from Ohio. Ohio is the only state which sets forth a model consent form in its statute, providing that if this form is properly used, consent shall be presumed to be valid. (Ohio Statutes, Sect. 2317.54 (D).)

THE LIMITS OF CONSENT

It is widely appreciated that the consent process is, in many instances, an "elaborate ritual." While information may be provided by the physician, messages sent often do not correspond to messages received, and truly informed consent is not easily obtained. These difficulties are not an excuse for not trying, and liability generally results from failure to make a sincere attempt rather than for trying and failing. Both legislatures and courts have emphasized *disclosure*, not *understanding*.

There are several reasons for maintaining high standards of disclosure, even if they result in imperfect comprehension. First, disclosure is a necessary, though insufficient, condition for understanding. Second, many patients will benefit from the process and exercise their autonomy. Third, reemphasis of the importance of disclosure serves to remind the physician of the patient's right to refuse treatment according to his values rather than the physician's.

It is also widely recognized that the informing process may meet all requirements in a technical sense, but still be biased and even determine the patient's response because of the manner of presentation. Whether the physician *should* introduce his value preferences into his practice is a much larger subject, beyond the scope of this article.

Finally, it should be realized that consent, even when fully informed, does not justify all actions. Consent is not an excuse for negligence.

SPECIAL PROBLEMS IN PEDIATRICS

The obvious incompetence of most children requires that someone speak for them in consenting to medical care. This authority has generally been assigned to parents, but there are two circumstances in which this might be questioned.

At the boundary between adolescence and adulthood there is increasing recognition of the right of children to consent to medical care without parental involvement. This has been most explicit in matters involving sexuality, where barriers to communication between parent and child may lead the child to abstain from seeking medical assistance if parental consent were required. Such withdrawal has contributed to massive public health problems of venereal disease, unwanted pregnancy, and unsafe illegal abortions for hundreds of thousands of adolescents.

Every state now allows minors (of varying ages) to obtain treatment for venereal disease without parental consent, and many have statutes regarding contraceptive services and abortion. Even in the absence of a specific statute, the United States Supreme Court has recently prohibited states from withholding abortion and contraceptive services from minors. Moreover, the law in practice is different from the law as written, and few, if any, physicians have ever been sued for providing medical care without parental consent to a child over the age of 15 years.

In addition to these specific sexual problems, minors may be considered as adult in their ability to consent if they are emancipated or otherwise fall under the mature minor doctrine. An *emancipated minor* is one who is apparently no longer under parental control, evidenced by such facts as living away from home, managing his own financial affairs, or making the majority of decisions relating to the conduct of his life. According to Hofmann and Pilpel, the *mature minor* doctrine permits consent to medical care by unemancipated minors who are of "sufficient intelligence to understand the nature and consequences of the treatment they are consenting to."

The other circumstance in which parental consent may not be legitimate is when the parent appears not to be acting in the best interest of the child. Gross abuse and neglect are obvious examples. More controversial problems arise in newborns with major birth defects, where the parent's authority to refuse life-saving treatment is acknowledged in practice but may be in violation of several statutes. This dilemma exemplifies the special complexity of consent for the pediatrician, who must balance his obligation to let the patient's guardian decide, with an attitude of questioning whether the guardian is serving the child's best interest.

Index

837

We invite your help to keep

CURRENT PEDIATRIC THERAPY

in tune with your needs

Use this postcard to tell us whether there is a subject you sought and failed to find, or a discussion you considered not sufficiently helpful or perhaps even out of date. We will do our best to improve the next edition.

SYDNEY S. GELLIS, M.D.

BENJAMIN M. KAGAN, M.D.

Albert E. Meier
Associate Medical Editor

_____

_____

_____

_____

_____

_____

Name_____

Address_____

City_____State_____ZIP_____